# Anterior Knee Pain and Patellar Instability

Vicente Sanchis-Alfonso
(Editor)

# Anterior Knee Pain and Patellar Instability

Second Edition

Springer

*Editor*
Vicente Sanchis-Alfonso, M.D., Ph.D.
International Patellofemoral Study Group
International ACL Study Group
Hospital 9 de Octubre
Hospital Arnau de Vilanova
School of Medicine
Catholic University of Valencia
Valencia
Spain

ISBN 978-1-4471-6826-3 ISBN 978-0-85729-507-1 (eBook)
DOI 10.1007/978-0-85729-507-1
Springer London Dordrecht Heidelberg New York

British Library Cataloguing in Publication Data
A catalogue record for this book is available from the British Library



*Cover design:* eStudioCalamar, Figueres/Berlin

Printed on acid-free paper

Springer is part of Springer Science+Business Media (www.springer.com)

*To my mother with all my love.*

*To my sister, Mari Carmen, who has shown great courage in her battle against breast cancer.*

*To the oncologist, Ana Lluch-Hernández, for her compassion in the treatment of her patients. The peace and serenity she conveys is invaluable.*

*The royalties from this book will go to the "Fundación Investigación Clínico de Valencia (INCLIVA) – Department of Hematology and Oncology – Breast Cancer Unit."*

# Foreword to the Second Edition

I am particularly pleased to write the introduction to this fine compendium of ideas, as Dr. Sanchis Alfonso has been a leader in the understanding of patellofemoral pain origins. This topic has fascinated me my entire career in orthopedic surgery, and has been a focus of most of my research and teaching. In 1985, I published our findings of nerve injury in the peripatellar retinaculum of patients with patellar imbalance and anterior knee pain, helping to establish the link between pain and patellofemoral malalignment. Dr. Sanchis Alfonso has not only added substance and scientific evidence to the link between musculoskeletal stress and neural changes causing pain, he has now brought together many good thinkers and scientists to present interesting and sometimes divergent points of view in this current volume. The great philosopher Hegel stated: "it is through the tension of opposites that we come to a higher truth."

Through computer simulated knee mechanical function noted in this book, Elias and Cosgarea demonstrate how articular loads can be tracked accurately and that even small aberrations of mechanical function can cause considerable alterations of stress transmitted through articular surfaces. Similarly, retinacular restraints around the patellofemoral joint will experience profound changes of loading when alignment is off, overuse is extreme, surgical balancing is not precise, and at extremes of laxity or tightness. Such is the nature of patellar and peripatellar stress and the relative anoxia caused by abnormal loading of peripatellar structure leading to cytokine elaboration and resulting pain. Thank you Dr. Sanchis Alfonso.

I believe this book is a wonderful compendium of current patellofemoral thought, not designed as a cookbook with easy answers, because there are many complex problems around the anterior knee and few easy answers. Rather, Dr. Sanchis-Alfonso's text contains many independent thinkers and scientists with a variety of approaches and concepts, some validated, some not, but all important in our search of the patellofemoral "holy grail." I encourage the reader to think, along with the authors of this textbook, synthesizing ideas and considering carefully how each concept presented here applies to the individual patient, always emphasizing nonoperative and simple measures whenever possible, but recognizing the importance of appropriate surgery when necessary for the relief of pain and suffering in the challenging patients with recalcitrant patellofemoral pain and instability.

In closing, I want to summarize my 32 years of experience with patellofemoral patients by saying that I believe a critical underlying concept for treating many patients with patellofemoral dysfunction is to recognize that the structural imbalance we see in patients with patellofemoral malalignment is at the root of much patellofemoral pain and instability. Therefore, our challenge is to restore balance and reduce excessive patellofemoral stress in these patients, using nonoperative measures including rest when possible, but designing necessary surgery to absolutely minimize both articular and periarticular damage while restoring patellofemoral balance as precisely as possible.

John P. Fulkerson, M.D.
Clinical Professor of Orthopaedic Surgery
University of Connecticut School of Medicine
Farmington, CT, USA

# Foreword to the First Edition

Anterior knee pain is one of the really big problems in my specialty, sports orthopaedic surgery, but also in all other types of orthopaedic surgery. Many years ago Sakkari Orava in Finland showed that among some 1,311 Finnish runners, anterior knee pain was the second most common complaint. In young school girls around 15 years of age, anterior knee pain is a common complaint. In ballet classes of the same age as much as 60–70% of the students complain of anterior knee pain. It is therefore an excellent idea of Dr. Sanchis-Alfonso to publish a book about anterior knee pain and patello-femoral instability in the active young.

He has been able to gather a group of extremely talented experts to help him write this book. I am particularly happy that he has devoted so much space to the non-operative treatment of anterior knee pain. During my active years as a knee surgeon, one of my worst problems was young girls referred to me for surgery of anterior knee pain. Girls that already had had 8–12 surgeries for their knee problem – surgeries that had rendered them more and more incapacitated after each operation. They now came to me for another operation. In all these cases, I referred them to our pain clinic for careful analysis, pain treatment followed by physical therapy. All recovered but had been the victims of lots of unnecessary knee surgery before they came to me.

I am also happy that Suzanne Werner in her chapter refers to our study on the personality of these anterior knee pain patients. She found that the patients differ from a normal control group of the same age. I think this is very important to keep in mind when you treat young patients with anterior knee pain.

In my mind physical therapy should always be the first choice of treatment. Not until this treatment has completely failed and a pain clinic recommends surgery, do I think surgery should be considered.

In patello-femoral instability the situation is different. When young patients suffer from frank dislocations of the patella, surgery should be considered. From my many years of treating this type of patients, I recommend that the patients undergo an arthroscopy before any attempts to treat the instability begins. The reason is that I have seen so many cases with normal X-rays that have 10–15 loose bodies in their knees. If these pieces consist of just cartilage, they cannot be seen on X-ray. When a dislocated patella jumps back, it often hits the lateral femoral condyle with considerable force. Small cartilage pieces are blasted away as well from femur as from the patella. If they are overlooked they will eventually lead to blockings of the knee in the future.

The role of the medial patello-femoral ligament can also not be overstressed. When I was taught to operate on these cases, this ligament was not even known.

I also feel that when patellar instability is going to be operated on, it is extremely important that the surgeon carefully controls in what direction the instability takes place. All instability is not in lateral direction. Some patellae have medial instability. If someone performs a routine lateral release in a case of medial instability, he will end up having to repair the lateral retinaculum in order to treat the medial dislocation that eventually occurs. Hughston and also Teitge have warned against this in the past.

It is a pleasure for me to recommend this excellent textbook by Dr. Vicente Sanchis-Alfonso.

Ejnar Eriksson, M.D., Ph.D.
Professor emeritus of Sports Medicine
Karolinska Institute, Stockholm, Sweden

## BOOK REVIEWS TO THE FIRST EDITION

### J. Bone Joint Surg. (Am) 88: 1908, 2006

*"The book has a refreshingly new and somewhat eclectic perspective on patellofemoral disorders that departs from the conventional teaching on this subject, which, in this writer's opinion, has come to somewhat of standstill over the past twenty years"*

*"This book should be read and owned by orthopaedic trauma surgeons, physical therapists, athletic trainers, general orthopaedic surgeons, orthopaedic sports-medicine physicians, and any other clinician who treats injuries and conditions of the knee. I walked away from this book with more questions than answers, and, when it comes to anterior knee pain, I think that is the nature of the beast. Perhaps that is the sign of being taught by an authentic sage"*

Louisville, Kentucky — Craig S. Roberts, M.D.

### Eur. J. Orthop. Surg. Traumatol. 19: 515–522 519, 2009

*"This excellent work is very complete, accessible to the non-specialist. It is a model which should be a work of specialized orthopaedists, essential to any surgeon being interested in pathology of the knee"*

Nancy, France — Patrice Diebold, M.D.

# Preface

This monograph reflects my deep interest in the pathology of the knee, particularly that of the extensor mechanism, and to emphasize the great importance I give to the concept of subspecialization, this being the only way to confront the deterioration and mediocrity of our specialty, Orthopaedic Surgery; and to provide our patients with better care. In line with the concept of subspecialization, this book necessarily required the participation of various authors. Although the authors are from different nationalities and different schools of thought I hope it is a homogenous product for the reader. In fact, I do not think there is a lack of cohesion between the chapters. Now, there are certain variations in form, but not in the basic content, regarding some topics dealt with by different authors. Thus it is evident that a few aspects remain unclear and the controversy continues.

With this book, we draw upon the most common pathology of the knee, even though it is the most neglected, the least known, the most problematic and controversial topic (The Bane of the Knee Surgeon, The Black Hole of Orthopaedics, Low Back Pain of the Knee). To begin with, the terminology is confusing (The Tower of Babel). Our knowledge of its etiopathogeny is also limited, therefore its treatment is one of the most complex among the different pathologies of the knee. On the other hand, we also face the problem of frequent and serious diagnostic errors that may lead to unnecessary operations. The following data reflect this problem: 11% of patients in my series underwent an unnecessary arthroscopy, and 10% were referred to a psychiatrist by physicians who had previously been consulted.

This book is organized into parts which have been reformatted from the first edition. Unlike other publications, this work gives great importance to the etiopathogeny; the latest theories are presented regarding the pathogeny of anterior knee pain and patellar instability, although in an eminently clinical and practical manner (Part I). In agreement with John Hunter, I think that to know the effects of an illness is to know very little; to know the cause of the effects is what is important. However, we do not forget the diagnostic methods or the therapeutic alternatives, surgical and nonsurgical, emphasizing minimal procedures and nonsurgical methods. Similarly, much importance is given to anterior knee pain following ACL reconstruction. Further, the participation of diverse specialists (orthopaedic surgeons, physiotherapists, rehabilitation specialists MDs, radiologists, biologists, pathologists, physiologists, psychologists, bioengineers, and plastic surgeons), that is, their multidisciplinary approach, affords us a wider vision of this pathology. In this second edition a new section has been added (Part II) where new technologies for the evaluation of the extensor mechanism are discussed (upright weight bearing MRI, real-time MRI, PET-CT imaging, physiologic imaging of cartilage, computational modeling, kinetic analysis, and kinematic analysis). The third part of this monograph is given over to the discussion of complex clinical cases (Part III). I believe we learn far more from our own mistakes, and those of other specialists, than from our successes ("*To Err is Human…*", Alexander Pope). We deal with oft-operated patients with sequelae due to operations, well indicated and performed or not, but where there were complications ("*Learn from the mistakes of others – you can never live long enough to make them all yourself*" John Luther). The diagnoses reached and how the cases were resolved are explained in detail ("*Good results come from experience, experience from bad results*," Professor Erwin Morscher). In Part IV (Surgical Techniques – "How I do it") the surgical techniques that are in use today for the patellofemoral joint are described in detail. They are described by the surgeons who have designed the technique, who are recognized by their colleagues as "masters" in their specialty. Moreover, they come with a descriptive DVD. In this second edition, I have also added a section with the personal thoughts about anterior knee pain and patellar instability (Part V) of two highly recognized and respected orthopaedic surgeons, Alan C Merchant and Scott F Dye, who give us their personal and authorized view about this controversial problem.

Deliberately the same subject is analyzed by different authors, of different nationalities, all with international prestige. The goal is to see how each one of them approaches a controversial condition/treatment (for example, proximal femoral osteotomy vs distal femoral osteotomy in the surgical treatment of a patient with femoral anteversion, isokinetics yes vs isokinetics no, etc.). Oddly enough, depending on the country of origin, indications may vary. I believe that with this approach (different opinions with their own reasoning) the reader is the one who will benefit.

The first objective I have laid out in this book is to highlight the soaring incidence of this pathology, and the impact on young people, athletes, workers, and the economy. The second goal is to improve prevention and diagnosis in order to reduce the economic and social costs of this condition. The final objective is to improve health care in these patients. This, rather than being an objective, should point to the way forward.

"Anterior Knee Pain and Patellar Instability" is addressed to orthopaedic surgeons (both general and those specialized in knee surgery), specialists in sports medicine, rehabilitation specialists, MDs, and physiotherapists.

Thus, we feel that with this approach, this monograph will fill an important gap in the literature about the pathology of the extensor mechanism of the knee. However, we do not intend to substitute any studies on patellofemoral pathology, but rather to complement them ("*All in all, you're just another brick in the wall*," Pink Floyd, The Wall). Although the information contained herein will evidently require future revision, it serves as an authoritative reference on one of the most problematic entities currently in the pathology of the knee. We hope this book will be a reference in the future from our youngest to our oldest colleagues. We trust that the reader will find this work useful, and consequently, be indirectly valuable for patients.

Valencia, Spain Vicente Sanchis-Alfonso, M.D., Ph.D.

# Acknowledgments 1

I wish to express my sincere gratitude to my friend and colleague, Dr. Donald Fithian, who I met in 1992 during my stay in San Diego, California for all I learned, together with his invaluable help, for which I will be forever grateful. My gratitude also goes out to all members of the International Patellofemoral Study Group for their constant encouragement and inspiration.

Further, I have had the privilege and honor to count on the participation of outstanding specialists who have lent prestige to this monograph. I thank all of them for their time, effort, dedication, kindness, as well as for the excellent quality of their contributing chapters. All have demonstrated generosity in sharing their great clinical experience in a clear and concise form. I am in debt to you all. Personally, and on behalf of those patients who will undoubtedly benefit from this work, thank you.

Last but not least, I am extremely grateful to both Springer-Verlag in London for the confidence shown in this project, and to Mr. Sreejith Viswanathan and his production team from SPi Global (Chennai, India) for completing this project with excellence from the time the cover is opened until the final chapter is presented.

Valencia, Spain — Vicente Sanchis-Alfonso, M.D., Ph.D.

# Acknowledgments 2

With all my appreciation to the
International Patellofemoral Study Group
And very especially to
Professor John P. Fulkerson and to Professor Alan C. Merchant

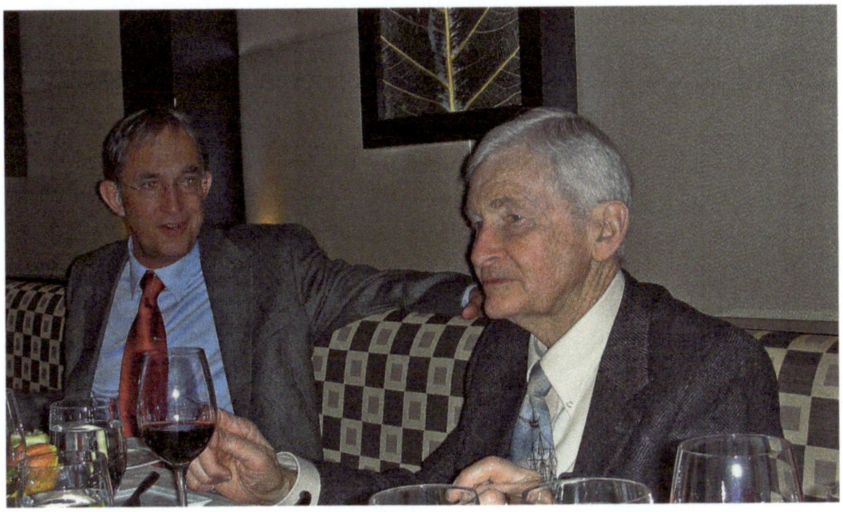

John Fulkerson (left) and Al Merchant (right), Dinner of the International Patellofemoral Study Group Meeting, Boston, 2006

*If we have been able to see further it is because we stood on the Shoulders of Giants*

*Sir Isaac Newton*

# Contents

# Video Contents

# Contributors

**Håkan Alfredson M.D., Ph.D.** Professor, Sports Medicine Unit, Department of Surgical and Perioperative Sciences, Umeå University, Umeå, Sweden

**Jack T. Andrish M.D.** Department of Orthopaedic Surgery, Center of Sports Health, Cleveland Clinic, Cleveland, OH, USA

**Francisco Aparisi M.D., Ph.D.** Department of Radiology, Hospital Universitario La Fe, Valencia, Spain

**Carlos M. Atienza Mech. Eng., Ph.D** Instituto de Biomecánica de Valencia (IBV), Universidad Politécnica de Valencia, Grupo de Tecnología Sanitaria (GTS-IBV), CIBER-BBN, Valencia, Spain

**Carolina Ávila-Carrasco Mech. Eng.** Instituto de Biomecánica de Valencia (IBV), Universidad Politécnica de Valencia, Grupo de Tecnología Sanitaria (GTS-IBV), CIBER-BBN, Valencia, Spain

**Sarvottam Bajaj B.E.** Division of Sports Medicine, Rush University Medical Center, Chicago, IL, USA

**Eszter Baló M.D.** Orthopaedic & Trauma Department, Uzsoki Hospital, Budapest, Hungary

**Lachlan Batty M.B.B.S., B.Med.Sc.** The Alfred Hospital, Melbourne VIC, Australia

**José María Baydal-Bertomeu Mech. Eng.** Instituto de Biomecánica de Valencia (IBV), Universidad Politécnica de Valencia, Valencia, Spain

**Gary Beaupré Ph.D.** Research Career Scientist, VA Rehabilitation Research and Development Center, Palo Alto, CA, USA

**Vicente Belloch-Ugarte M.D.** MR Unit – Clínica ERESA, Hospital Universitario La Fe, Valencia, Spain

**Kim Bennell Ph.D.** Professor and Director, Centre for Health, Exercise and Sports Medicine, Physiotherapy, School of Health Sciences, The University of Melbourne, Melbourne, VIC, Australia

**Thor F. Besier Ph.D.** Auckland Bioengineering Institute, The University of Auckland, Auckland, New Zealand

**Roland M. Biedert M.D.** Associate Professor, Sportclinic Villa Linde, Swiss Olympic Medical Center Magglingen-Biel, University of Basel, Biel, Switzerland

**Mario Bizzini M.S., P.T.** Research Associate, Orthopedics, F-MARC, Schulthess Klinik Zurich, Zurich, Switzerland

**José Ignacio Blanes-Mompó M.D., Ph.D.** Department of Vascular Surgery, Hospital de Manises, Valencia, Spain

**Lars Blønd M.D.** Department of Orthopaedic Surgery, Gildhøj Private Hospital, Copenhagen, Denmark

**Tommaso Bonanzinga M.D.** Biomechanics Laboratory, Istituto Ortopedico Rizzoli, Bologna, Italy

**Danilo Bruni M.D.** Biomechanics Laboratory, Istituto Ortopedico Rizzoli, Bologna, Italy

**José Antonio Calvo M.D., Ph.D.** Department of Orthopaedic Surgery, Hospital General Universitario Gregorio Marañón, Madrid, Spain

**Andrea Castelli Biomed. Eng.** Instituto de Biomecánica de Valencia (IBV), Universidad Politécnica de Valencia, Valencia, Spain

**Brian J. Cole M.D., M.B.A.** Professor, Departments of Orthopaedics & Anatomy and Cell Biology, Division of Sports Medicine, Section Head, Cartilage Restoration Center at Rush, Rush University Medical Center, Chicago, IL, USA

**Marco Collarile M.D.** Orthopaedic Department and Knee Surgery Center, Sacro Cuore Don Calabria Hospital, Negrar, Verona, Italy

**Jill L. Cook Ph.D.** School of Primary Health Care, Monash University, Melbourne, Australia

**Alex Cortés M.D., Ph.D.** Instituto de Biomecánica de Valencia (IBV), Universidad Politécnica de Valencia, Valencia, Spain

**Andrew J. Cosgarea M.D.** Professor, Department of Orthopaedic Surgery, Johns Hopkins University, Baltimore, MD, USA

**Enrique Cuñat P.T.** Physiotherapy, Clínica Enrique Cuñat Pomares, Alfara del Patriarca, Valencia, Spain

**Patrik Danielson M.D., Ph.D.** Associate Professor, Department of Integrative Medical Biology, Section for Anatomy, Faculty of Medicine, Umeå University, Umeå, Sweden

**David Dejour M.D.** Lyon Ortho Clinic, Lyon, France

**Scott Delp Ph.D.** Professor Department of Bioengineering, Stanford University, Stanford, CA, USA

**Julio Doménech M.D., Ph.D.** Department of Orthopaedic Surgery, School of Medicine, Catholic University of Valencia, Valencia, Spain

**Christine Draper Ph.D.** Department of Bioengineering, Stanford University, Stanford, CA, USA

**Scott F. Dye M.D.** Associate Clinical Professor of Orthopaedic Surgery, University of California, San Francisco, CA, USA

**Eric W. Edmonds M.D.** Assistant Clinical Professor, Sports Medicine Program Consultant, Department of Orthopaedic Surgery, University of California, San Diego CA, USA
Pediatric Orthopaedic and Scoliosis Center, Rady Children's Hospital, San Diego, CA, USA

**John J. Elias Ph.D.** Senior Research Scientist, Calhoun Research Lab, Akron General Medical Center, Akron, OH, USA

**Lars Ejerhed M.D., Ph.D.** Associate Professor, Orthopaedic Department, University of Gothenburg, NU-Hospital Organization, Trollhättan/Uddevalla, Sweden

**Pieter J. Erasmus M.D.** Honorary Consultant, University of Stellenbosch, Mediclinic, Die Boord, Stellenbosch, South Africa

**Ejnar Eriksson M.D., Ph.D.** Professor emeritus of Sports Medicine Karolinska Institute, Stockholm, Sweden

**Eveline Erni P.T., M.A., C.C.T.T.** Clinical Director, Pivotal Physical Therapy PLLC, Network Member, Hospital for Special Surgery, New York, NY, USA

**Begoña Espejo Ph.D.** Associate Professor, Department of Methodology of the Behavioural Sciences, University of Valencia, Valencia, Spain

**Jack Farr M.D.** Professor, Director, Voluntary Clinical, Orthopaedic Surgery, IU School of Medicine, OrthoIndy Knee Care Institute, Cartilage Restoration Center of Indiana, Indianapolis, IN, USA

**Donald C. Fithian M.D.** Southern California Permanente Medical Group, El Cajon CA, USA

**Sture Forsgren M.D., Ph.D.** Professor, Department of Integrative Medical Biology, Anatomy, Umeå University, Umeå, Sweden

**Michael Fredericson M.D.** Associate Professor, Department of Orthopaedics, Stanford University, Stanford, CA, USA

**Heather Freeman P.T., D.H.S.** Research Coordinator/Medical Writer, Shelbourne Knee Center, Methodist Hospital, Indianapolis, IN, USA

**John P. Fulkerson M.D.** Clinical Professor of Orthopaedic Surgery, University of Connecticut School of Medicine, Farmington, CT, USA

**José David Garrido-Jaén Mech. Eng.** Instituto de Biomecánica de Valencia (IBV), Universidad Politécnica de Valencia, Valencia, Spain

**Pablo Gelber M.D., Ph.D.** Department of Orthopaedic Surgery and Traumatology, Hospital de la Santa Creu i Sant Pau, Universitat Autònoma de Barcelona, Barcelona, Spain

**Giovanni Giordano M.D.** Biomechanics Laboratory, Istituto Ortopedico Rizzoli, Bologna, Italy

**Pau Golanó M.D.** Laboratory of Arthroscopic and Surgical Anatomy, Department of Pathology and Experimental Therapeutics, Human Anatomy Unit, Faculty of Medicine, University of Barcelona, Barcelona, Spain

**Garry Gold M.S., M.D.** Associate Professor, Department of Radiology, Stanford University, Stanford, CA, USA

**Jason Gould M.D.** Resident in Orthopedic Surgery, Mount Sinai Medical Center, New York, NY, USA

**Ronald P. Grelsamer M.D.** Chief Patellofemoral Reconstruction, Mount Sinai Medical Center, New York, NY, USA

**László Hangody M.D., Ph.D., D.Sc.** Professor, Head of Department, Department of Orthopaedics, Uzsoki Hospital, Budapest, Hungary

**Francesco Iacono M.D.** Biomechanics Laboratory, Istituto Ortopedico Rizzoli, Bologna, Italy

**Andreas B. Imhoff M.D.** Professor, of Orthopaedic Surgery and Traumatology, Director Department of Orthopaedic Sports Medicine, Klinikum Rechts der Isar, University of Munich, Munich, Germany

**Jüri Kartus M.D., Ph.D.** Professor, Orthopaedic Department, University of Gothenburg, NU-Hospital Organization, Trollhättan/Uddevalla, Sweden

**James Kercher M.D.** Division of Sports Medicine, Rush University Medical Center, Chicago IL, USA

**Karim Khan M.D., Ph.D.** Professor, Centre for Hip Health and Mobility (CHHM), University of British Columbia, Vancouver, Canada

**Najeeb Khan M.D.** Southern California Permanente Medical Group, San Marcos CA, USA

**Elizaveta Kon M.D.** Biomechanics Laboratory, Istituto Ortopedico Rizzoli, Bologna, Italy

**Emily E. Krodel M.D.** Indiana University School of Medicine, Indianapolis, IN, USA

**Maurilio Marcacci M.D.** Professor, Istituto Ortopedico Rizzoli, Bologna University, Bologna, Italy

**Giulio Maria Marcheggiani Muccioli M.D.** Biomechanics Laboratory, Istituto Ortopedico Rizzoli, Bologna, Italy

**Susana Marín-Roca Mech. Eng.** Instituto de Biomecánica de Valencia (IBV), Universidad Politécnica de Valencia, Valencia, Spain

**Vicente Martinez-Sanjuan M.D., Ph.D.** Profesor of Radiology, MR and CT Unit, ERESA-Hospital General Universitario, Valencia, Spain

**Francisco Martínez-Soriano M.D., Ph.D.** Professor, Department of Human Anatomy and Embriology, University of Valencia, Valencia, Spain

**Jenny McConnell B.App.Sci. (Phty), Grad. Dip. Man. Ther., M. Biomed. Eng.** Private Practitioner McConnell & Clements Physiotherapy, Sydney, Australia

**Fiona McManus** Centre for Health, Exercise and Sports Medicine, Physiotherapy, School of Health Sciences, The University of Melbourne, VIC, Australia

**Alan C. Merchant M.D.** Clinical Professor, Emeritus Medical Staff, Department of Orthopedic Surgery, Stanford University School of Medicine, Stanford, CA, USA Department of Orthopedic Surgery, El Camino Hospital, Mountain View, CA, USA

**Joan C. Monllau M.D., Ph.D.** Department of Orthopaedic Surgery and Traumatology, Hospital de la Santa Creu i Sant Pau, Universitat Autònoma de Barcelona, Barcelona, Spain
Arthroscopy Unit, ICATME, Institut Universitari Dexeus, Universitat Autònoma de Barcelona, Barcelona, Spain

**Carmen Monserrat M.D.** Department of Radiology, Hospital Arnau de Vilanova, Valencia, Spain

**Erik Montesinos-Berry M.D.** Department of Ortopaedic Surgery, Hospital de Manises, Valencia, Spain

**Tomas Movin M.D., Ph.D.** Associate Professor, Director of Emergency Department, Karolinska Institutet, Karolinska University Hospital, Stockholm, Sweden

**Maurice Y. Nahabedian M.D., FACS** Associate Professor of Plastic Surgery, Department of Plastic Surgery, Georgetown University, Washington, DC, USA

**Jan Näslund Ph.D.** Department of Physiology and Pharmacology, Karolinska Institutet, Stockholm, Sweden

**Maria Pia Neri M.D.** 3th Orthopaedic and Traumatologic Clinic, Istituto Ortopedico Rizzoli, Bologna, Italy

**Eiki Nomura M.D.** Department Director, Orthopaedic Surgery, International Goodwill Hospital, Yokohama, Japan

**Fermín Ordoño M.D., Ph.D.** Department of Neurophysiology, Hospital Arnau de Vilanova, Valencia, Spain

**Lars Öhberg M.D., Ph.D.** Department of Radiation Sciences, Diagnostic Radiology, Umeå, Sweden

**Saikat Pal Ph.D.** Department of Bioengineering, Stanford University, Stanford CA, USA

**Xavier Pelfort M.D.** Department of Orthopaedic Surgery and Traumatology, Hospitals IMAS. Universitat Autònoma de Barcelona, Barcelona, Spain
Arthroscopy Unit, ICATME, Institut Universitari Dexeus, Universitat Autònoma de Barcelona, Barcelona, Spain

**María Francisca Peydro-De Moya M.D., Ph.D.** Instituto de Biomecánica de Valencia (IBV), Universidad Politécnica de Valencia, Valencia, Spain

**Jaime M. Prat-Pastor M.D., Ph.D.** Instituto de Biomecánica de Valencia (IBV), Universidad Politécnica de Valencia, Grupo de Tecnología Sanitaria (GTS-IBV), CIBER-BBN, Valencia, Spain

**Fernando Revert-Ros** Biomedicina, Centro de Investigación Príncipe Felipe, Valencia, Spain

**Esther Roselló-Sastre M.D., Ph.D.** Department of Pathology, Hospital Universitario Dr. Peset, Valencia, Spain

**Paulo Renato Saggin M.D.** Instituto de Ortopedia e Traumatologia (I.O.T.), Passo Fundo, RS, Brazil

**Michael J. Salata M.D.** Division of Sports Medicine, Rush University Medical Center, Chicago, IL, USA

**Vicente Sanchis-Alfonso M.D., Ph.D.** Orthopaedic Surgeon, Professor of Orthopaedic Surgery, International Patellofemoral Study Group, International ACL Study Group, Hospital 9 de Octubre, Hospital Arnau de Vilanova, School of Medicine, Valencia Catholic University, Valencia, Spain

**Martin Sauerschnig M.D.** Department of Orthopaedic Sports Medicine, Klinikum Rechts der Isar, University of Munich, Munich, Germany

**Juan Saus-Mas** Biomedicina, Centro de Investigación Príncipe Felipe, Valencia, Spain

**Philip B. Schtötle M.D.** Orthopädie am Zürichberg, Zurich, Switzerland

**Alexander Scott B.Sc. (PT), Ph.D.** Assistant Professor, Department of Physical Therapy, Faculty of Medicine, University of British Columbia, Vancouver, BC, Canada

**Agustín Serrano M.D.** Department of Orthopaedic Surgery, Hospital de Manises, Valencia, Spain

**K. Donald Shelbourne M.D.** Associate Clinical Professor, Shelbourne Knee Center at Methodist Hospital, Indiana University School of Medicine, Indianapolis, IN, USA

**Alfredo Subías-López M.D.** Department of Orthopaedic Surgery, Hospital Universitario Dr. Peset, Valencia, Spain

**Robert A. Teitge M.D.** Professor, Program Director and Co-director Orthopaedic Research, Department of Orthopaedics, Wayne State University School of Medicine, Detroit, MI, USA

**Marc Tey M.D.** Arthroscopy Unit, ICATME, Institut Universitari Dexeus, Universitat Autònoma de Barcelona, Barcelona, Spain

**Mathieu Thaunat M.D.** Department of Orthopedic Surgery, Hopital André Mignot, Le Chesnay, France

**Roger Torga-Spak M.D.** Faculty of Orthopaedics and Traumatology, Department of Surgery, Instituto Universitario CEMIC, Buenos Aires, Argentina

**Philippe M. Tscholl M.D.** Sportclinic Villa Linde, Swiss Olympic Medical Center Magglingen-Biel, Biel, Switzerland

**Scott E. Urch M.D.** Associate Clinical Professor Shelbourne Knee Center at Methodist Hospital, Indiana University School of Medicine, Indianapolis, IN, USA

**Alfonso Valverde-Navarro M.D.** Department of Human Anatomy and Embriology, University of Valencia, Valencia, Spain

**Damien Van Tiggelen P.T.** Department of Rehabilitation Sciences and Physical Therapy, Faculty of Medicine, Ghent University, Ghent, Belgium, Department of Traumatology and Rehabilitation, Military Hospital Queen Astrid, Brussels, Belgium

**Javier Vaquero M.D., Ph.D.** Professor, Chairman, Department of Orthopaedic Surgery, Universidad Complutense de Madrid, Hospital General Universitario Gregorio Marañon, Madrid, Spain

**Jordi Vega M.D.** Department of Orthopedic and Trauma Surgery, Hospital Asepeyo Sant Cugat, Sant Cugat del Vallés, Barcelona, Spain

**Suzanne Werner Ph.D.** Professor, Chairman, Research Coordinator, Stockholm Sports Trauma Research Center, Karolinska institutet, Stockholm, Sweden Capio Artro Clinic, Stockholm, Sweden

**Lotta Willberg M.D.** Capio Artro Clinic, Karolinska Institute, Stockholm, Sweden

**Tine Willems** Department of Rehabilitation Sciences and Physical Therapy, Faculty of Medicine, Ghent University, Ghent, Belgium

**Erik Witvrouw Ph.D.** Department of Rehabilitation Sciences and Physical Therapy, Faculty of Medicine, Ghent University, Ghent, Belgium

**Stefano Zaffagnini M.D.** Biomechanics Laboratory, Istituto Ortopedico Rizzoli, Bologna, Italy

# Part I

# Etiopathogenic Bases and Therapeutic Implications

# Background: Patellofemoral Malalignment Versus Tissue Homeostasis

1

## Myths and Truths About Patellofemoral Disease

Vicente Sanchis-Alfonso

## 1.1 Introduction

Anterior knee pain* is the most common knee complaint seen in adolescents and young adults, in both the athletic and nonathletic population, although in the former, its incidence is higher. The rate is around 9% in young active adults.[69] Its incidence is 5.4% of the total injuries and as high as a quarter of all knee problems treated at a sports injury clinic.[15] Nonetheless, I am convinced that not all cases are diagnosed and hence the figure is bound to be even higher. Furthermore, it is to be expected that the number of patients with this complaint will increase because of the increasing popularity of sport practice. On the other hand, a better understanding of this pathology by orthopedic surgeons and general practitioners should lead to this condition being diagnosed more and more frequently. Females are particularly predisposed to it.[13] Anatomic factors such as increased pelvic width and resulting excessive lateral thrust on the patella, and postural and sociological factors such as wearing high heels and sitting with legs adducted can influence the incidence and severity of this condition in women.[25] Moreover, it is a nemesis to both the patient and the treating physician, creating chronic disability, limitation from participation in sports, sick leave, and generally diminished quality of life.

Special mention should be made of the term "patellar tendinitis," closely related to anterior knee pain. In 1998, Arthroscopy published an article by Nicola Maffulli and colleagues[50] that bore the title "Overuse tendon conditions: Time to change a confusing terminology." Very aptly, these authors concluded that the clinical syndrome characterized by pain (diffuse or localized), tumefaction, and a lower sports performance should be called "tendinopathy." The terms tendinitis, paratendinitis, and tendinosis should be used solely when in possession of the results of an excision biopsy. Therefore, the pervasive clinical diagnosis of patellar tendinitis, which has become the paradigm of overuse tendon injuries, would be incorrect. Furthermore, biopsies in these types of pathologies do not prove the existence of chronic or acute inflammatory infiltrates, which clearly indicate the presence of tendinitis. Patellar tendinopathy is a frequent cause for anterior knee pain, which can turn out to be frustrating for physicians as well as for athletes, for whom this lesion can well mean the end of their sports career. This means that in this monograph, we cannot leave out a discussion of this clinical entity, which is dealt with, in depth, in Chaps. 15, 16, and 27.

Finally, anterior knee pain is also a well-documented complication and the most common complaint after anterior cruciate ligament (ACL) reconstruction. Because of the upsurge of all kinds of sports, ACL injuries have become increasingly common and therefore their surgical treatment is currently commonplace.† The incidence of anterior knee pain after ACL

V. Sanchis-Alfonso
International Patellofemoral Study Group,
International ACL Study Group, Hospital 9 de Octubre,
Hospital Arnau de Vilanova, School of Medicine,
Catholic University of Valencia, Valencia, Spain
e-mail: vicente.sanchis.alfonso@gmail.com

*Term that describes pain in which the source is either within the patellofemoral joint or in the support structures around it.

†In the general population, an estimated 1 in 3000 individuals sustains an ACL injury per year in the United States,[36] corresponding to an overall injury rate of approximately 80,000[31] to 100,000[36] injuries annually. The highest incidence is in individuals 15–25 years old who participate in pivoting sports.[31]

V. Sanchis-Alfonso (ed.), *Anterior Knee Pain and Patellar Instability*,
DOI: 10.1007/978-0-85729-507-1_1, © Springer-Verlag London Limited 2011

reconstruction with bone-patellar tendon-bone (B-PT-B) autografts is from 4% to 40%.[23] Moreover, anterior knee pain is also a common complaint, from 6% to 12.5% after 2 years, with the use of hamstring grafts.[4,10,46,63] For the reasons mentioned above, we believe it is interesting to carry out a detailed analysis in this book of the appearance of anterior knee pain secondary to ACL reconstructive surgery, underscoring the importance of treatment, and especially, prevention. In order to not to fall into the trap of dogmatism, the problem is analyzed by different authors from different perspectives (see Chaps. 18 and 19).

## 1.2 The Problem

In spite of its high incidence, anterior knee pain syndrome is the most neglected, the least known, and the most problematic pathological knee condition. This is why the expression "Black Hole of Orthopaedics" that Stanley James used to refer to this condition is extremely apt to describe the current situation. On the other hand, our knowledge of the causative mechanisms of anterior knee pain is limited, with the consequence that its treatment is one of the most complex among the different pathologies of the knee. As occurs with any pathological condition, and this is not an exception, for the correct application of conservative as well as operative therapy, it is essential to have a thorough understanding of the pathogenesis of the same (see Chaps. 2–6, 9, and 14–19). This is the only way to prevent the all-too-frequent stories of multiple failed surgeries and demoralized patients, fact that is relatively common for the clinical entity under scrutiny in this book as compared with other pathological processes affecting the knee (see Chaps. 24 and 26).

Finally, diagnostic errors, which can lead to unnecessary interventions, are relatively frequent in this pathologic condition. As early as 1922, in the German literature, Georg Axhausen[5] stated that "chondromalacia" can simulate a meniscal lesion resulting in the removal of normal menisci. In this connection, Tapper and Hoover,[65] in 1969, suspected that over 20% of women who did badly after an open meniscectomy had a patellofemoral pathology. Likewise, John Insall,[38] in 1984, stated that patellofemoral pathology was the most common cause of meniscectomy failure in young patients, especially women. Obviously, this failure was a result of an erred diagnosis and, consequently, of a mistakenly indicated surgery. At present, the problem of diagnostic confusion is still the order of the day. The following data reflect this problem. In my surgical series, 11% of patients underwent unnecessary arthroscopic meniscal surgery, which, far from eradicating the symptoms, had worsened them. An improvement was obtained, however, after realignment surgery of the extensor mechanism. Finally, 10% of patients in my surgical series were referred to a psychiatrist by physicians who had previously been consulted.

The question we ask ourselves is: Why is there less knowledge about this kind of pathology than about other knee conditions? According to the International Patellofemoral Study Group (IPSG),[41] there are several explanations: (1) the biomechanics of the patellofemoral joint is more complex than that of other structures in the knee; (2) the pathology of the patella arouses less clinical interest than that of the menisci or the cruciate ligaments; (3) there are various causes for anterior knee pain; (4) there is often no correlation between symptoms, physical findings, and radiological findings; (5) there are discrepancies regarding what is regarded as "normal"; and (6) there is widespread terminological confusion ("The Tower of Babel"). As regards what is considered "normal" or "abnormal," it is interesting to mention the work by Johnson and colleagues,[68] who makes a gender-dependent analysis of the clinical assessment of asymptomatic knees. We discuss some of the conclusions of this interesting study below.

In 1995, the prevailing confusion led to the foundation by John Fulkerson of the United States and Jean-Yves Dupont of France of the IPSG in order to advance in the knowledge of the patellofemoral joint disorders by intercultural exchange of information and ideas. The condition is of such high complexity that even within this group there are antagonistic approaches and theories often holding dogmatic positions. Moreover, to stimulate research efforts and education regarding patellofemoral problems, John Fulkerson created in 2003 the Patellofemoral Foundation. The Patellofemoral Foundation sponsors the "Patellofemoral Research Excellence Award" to encourage outstanding research leading to improved understanding, prevention, and treatment of patellofemoral pain or instability. I want to emphasize the importance to improve prevention and diagnosis in order to reduce the economic and social costs of this pathology (see Chaps. 8, 10, 11, and 18).

Moreover, this foundation sponsors the "Patellofemoral Traveling Fellowship" to promote better understanding and communication regarding patellofemoral pain, permitting visits to several centers, worldwide, that offer opportunities to learn about the complexities of patellofemoral pain.

This chapter provides an overview of the most important aspects of etiopathogenesis of anterior knee pain and analyzes some myths and truths about patellofemoral disease.

## 1.3 Historical Background. Internal Derangement of the Knee and Chondromalacia Patellae. Actual Meaning of Patellar Chondral Injury

Anterior knee pain in young patients has historically been associated to the terms "internal derangement of the knee" and "chondromalacia patellae." In 1986, Schutzer and colleagues[61] published a paper in the Orthopedic Clinics of North America about the CT-assisted classification of patellofemoral pain. The authors of that paper highlight the lack of knowledge that besets this clinical entity when they associate the initials of internal derangement of the knee (IDK) with those of the phrase "**I** **D**on't **K**now," and those of chondromalacia patellae (CMP) with those of "**C**ould be – **M**ay be – **P**ossibly be." Although we think that nowadays this is certainly an exaggeration, it is true that the analogy helps us underscore the controversies around this clinical entity, or at least draw people's attention to it.

The expression "internal derangement of the knee" was coined in 1784 by British surgeon Leeds William Hey.[48] This term was later discredited by the German school surgeon Konrad Büdinger, Dr. Billroth's assistant in Vienna, who in 1906, described fissuring and degeneration of the patellar articular cartilage of spontaneous origin,[7] and in 1908 in another paper described similar lesions of traumatic origin.[8] Although Büdinger was the first to describe chondromalacia, this term was not used by Büdinger himself. Apparently, it was Koenig who in 1924 used the term "chondromalacia patellae" for the first time, although according to Karlson this term had already been used in Aleman's clinic since 1917.[1,26] What does seem clear is that it was Koenig who popularized the term. Büdinger considered that the expression "internal derangement of the knee" was a "wastebasket" term. And he was right, since the expression lacks any etiological, therapeutic, or prognostic implication.

Until the end of the 1960s, anterior knee pain was attributed to chondromalacia patellae. Stemming from the Greek *chondros* and *malakia*, this term translates literally as "softened patellar articular cartilage." However, in spite of the fact that the term "chondromalacia patellae" has historically been associated with anterior knee pain, many authors have failed to find a connection between both.[11,47,57] In 1978, Leslie and Bentley reported that only 51% of patients with a clinical diagnosis of "chondromalacia" had changes on the patellar surface when were examined by arthroscopy.[47] In 1991, Royle and colleagues[57] published in Arthroscopy a study in which they analyzed 500 arthroscopies performed in a 2-year period, with special reference made to the patellofemoral joint. In those patients with pain thought to be arising from this joint, 63% had "chondromalacia patellae" compared with a 45% incidence in those with meniscal pathological findings at arthroscopy. They concluded that patients with anterior knee pain do not always have patellar articular changes, and patellar pathology is often asymptomatic (Fig. 1.1). In agreement with this, Dye[18] did not feel any pain during arthroscopic palpation of his extensive lesion of the patellar cartilage without intraarticular anesthesia. In this regard, it would be remembered that the articular cartilage is devoid of nerve fibers and, therefore, cannot hurt.

Surgeons often refer to patellar cartilage changes as chondromalacia, using poor defined grades. According to the IPSG,[41] we should use the term chondral or cartilage lesion, and rather than resorting to grades in a classification, providing a clear description of the injury (e.g., appearance, depth, size, location, acute vs. chronic clinical status). Although hyaline cartilage cannot be the source of pain in itself, damage of articular cartilage can lead to excessive loading of the subchondral bone, which, due to its rich innervation, could be a potential source of pain. Therefore, a possible indication for very selected cases could be a resurfacing procedure such as autologous single-stage patellofemoral cartilage repair, autologous two-stage chondrocyte patellofemoral cartilage repair, patellofemoral allografts, and patellofemoral arthroplasty (see Chaps. 42–46).

According to the IPSG,[41] the term chondromalacia should not be used to describe a clinical condition; it is

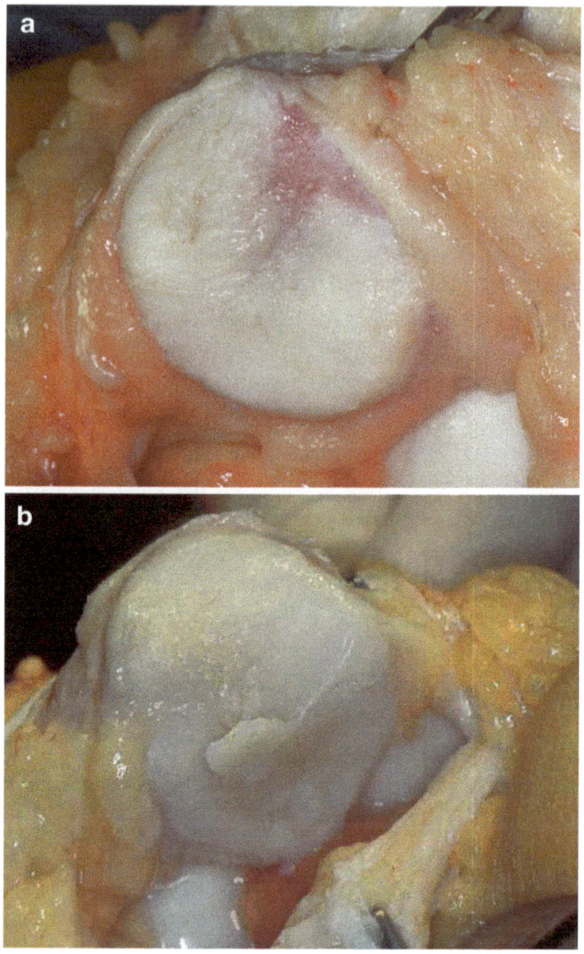

**Fig. 1.1** The intensity of preoperative pain is not related to the seriousness or the extension of the chondromalacia patellae found during surgery. The most serious cases of chondromalacia arise in patients with a recurrent patellar dislocation, who feel little or no pain between their dislocation episodes (**a**). Chondral lesion of the patella with fragmentation and fissuring of the cartilage in a patient with PFM that consulted for anterior knee pain (**b**)

merely a descriptive term for morphologic softening of the patellar articular cartilage. In conclusion, this is a diagnosis that can be made only with visual inspection and palpation by open or arthroscopic means and it is irrelevant. In short, chondromalacia patellae is not synonymous with patellofemoral pain. Thus, the term chondromalacia is also, using Büdinger's own words, a "wastebasket" term as it is lacking in practical utility. In this way, the following ominous 1908 comment from Büdinger about "internal derangement of the knee" could be applied to chondromalacia[21]: "[It] will simply not disappear from the surgical literature. It is the symbol of our helplessness in regards to a diagnosis and our ignorance of the pathology."

Although I am aware of the fact that traditions die hard, the term "chondromalacia patellae" should be excluded from the clinical terminology of current orthopedics for the reasons I have expressed. More than one century has elapsed and this term is still used today, at least in Spain, by clinicians, by the staff in charge of codifying the different pathologies for our hospitals' databases, as well as by private health insurers' lists of covered services.

The term chondromalacia is a twentieth century mistake. Unfortunately, we always make the same mistakes. Currently, the expression patellofemoral pain syndrome has replaced the term chondromalacia patellae. That is, one nonsense term as chondromalacia has been replaced by another nonsense term as patellofemoral pain syndrome. According to Dr. Teitge (IPSG member), it is not a diagnosis but an admission of ignorance.

## 1.4 Patellofemoral Malalignment

In the 1970s, anterior knee pain was related to the presence of patellofemoral malalignment (PFM).[‡] In 1968, Jack C. Hughston (Fig. 1.2) published an article on subluxation of the patella, which represented a major turning point in the recognition and treatment of patellofemoral disorders.[34] In 1974, Al Merchant, in an attempt to better understand patellofemoral biomechanics, introduced the axial radiograph of the patellofemoral joint.[54] The same author suggested, also in 1974, the lateral retinacular release as a way of treating recurrent patellar subluxation.[53] In 1975, Paul Ficat, from France, popularized the concept of patellar tilt, always associated with increased tightness of the lateral retinaculum, which caused excessive pressure on the lateral facet of the patella, leading to the "lateral patellar compression syndrome" ("Syndrome d'Hyperpression Externe de la Rotule").[20] According to Ficat, lateral patellar compression syndrome would cause hyperpressure in the lateral patellofemoral compartment and hypopressure in the medial patellofemoral compartment. Hypopressure and

[‡] We define PFM as an abnormality of patellar tracking that involves lateral displacement or lateral tilt of the patella, or both, in extension, that reduces in flexion.

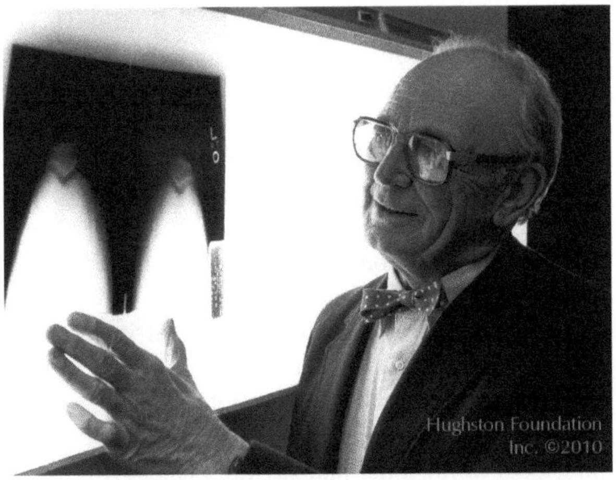


**Fig. 1.2** Jack C. Hughston, MD (1917–2004). One of the founding fathers of Sports Medicine (© The Hughston Foundation, Inc)

the disuse of the medial patellar facet would cause malnutrition and early degenerative changes in the articular cartilage because of the lack of normal pressure and function. This may explain why early chondromalacia patellae is generally found in the medial patellar facet. Hyperpression also would favor cartilage degeneration, which might explain the injury of the lateral facet. Two years later, in 1977, Ficat and Hungerford[21] published "Disorders of the Patellofemoral Joint," a classic of knee extensor mechanism surgery and the first book in English devoted exclusively to the extensor mechanism of the knee. In the preface of the book, these authors refer to the patellofemoral joint as "the forgotten compartment of the knee." This shows what the state of affairs was in those days. In fact, before the 1970s, only two diagnoses were used relating to anterior knee pain or patellar instability: chondromalacia patellae and recurrent dislocation of the patella. What is more, the initial designs for knee arthroplasties ignored the patellofemoral joint. In 1979, John Insall published a paper on "patellar malalignment syndrome"[37] and his technique for proximal patellar realignment, used to treat this syndrome.[40] According to Insall, lateral loading of the patella is increased in malalignment syndrome. In some cases, this causes chondromalacia patellae, but it does not necessarily mean that chondromalacia is the cause of pain.[38] In this way, in 1983, Insall and colleagues reported that anterior knee pain correlates better to malalignment rather than with the severity of chondromalacia found during surgery.[39] Fulkerson and colleagues have also emphasized the importance of PFM and excessively tight lateral retinaculum as a source of anterior knee pain.[24,28,61] Finally, in 2000, Ronald Grelsamer,[29] from the IPSG, stated that malalignment appears to be a necessary but not sufficient condition for the onset of anterior knee pain.[§] According to Grelsamer,[29] pain seems to be set off by a trigger (i.e., traumatism). In this sense, Grelsamer[30] tells his patients that "people with malaligned knees are akin to someone riding a bicycle on the edge of a cliff. All is well until a strong wind blows them off the cliff, which may or may not ever happen." Although it is more common to use the term malalignment as a malposition of the patella on the femur, some authors, as Robert A Teitge, from the IPSG, use the term malalignment as a malposition of the knee joint between the body and the foot with the subsequent effect on the patellofemoral mechanics (see Chap. 14).

In a previous paper,[59] we postulated that PFM, in some patients with patellofemoral pain, produces a "favorable environment" for the onset of symptoms, and neural damage would be the main "provoking factor" or "triggering factor." Overload or overuse may be another "triggering factor." In this sense, in our surgical experience, we have found that in patients with symptoms in both knees, when the more symptomatic knee is operated on, the symptoms in the contralateral less symptomatic malaligned knee, disappear or decrease in many cases, perhaps because we have reduced the load in this knee; that is, it allows us to restore joint homeostasis. In this connection, Thomee and colleagues suggested that chronic overloading and temporary overuse of the patellofemoral joint, rather than malalignment, contribute to patellofemoral pain.[67]

For many years, PFM has been widely accepted as an explanation for the genesis of anterior knee pain and patellar instability in the young patient. Moreover, this theory had a great influence on orthopedic surgeons, who developed several surgical procedures to "correct the malalignment." Unfortunately, when PFM was diagnosed, it was treated too often by means of surgery. A large amount of surgical treatments has been described, yielding extremely variable results. Currently, however, the PFM concept is questioned by

[§] However, many patients with patellofemoral pain have no evidence of malalignment, whatsoever.[67] Therefore, if PFM is a necessary condition for the presence of patellofemoral pain, how could patellofemoral pain be occurring in patients without malalignment?

many, and is not universally accepted to account for the presence of anterior knee pain and/or patellar instability. In fact, the number of realignment surgeries has dropped dramatically in recent years, due to a reassessment of the paradigm of PFM. Moreover, we know that such procedures are, in many cases, unpredictable and even dangerous; they may lead to reflex sympathetic dystrophy, medial patellar dislocations, and iatrogenous osteoarthrosis (see Chaps. 24 and 26). We should recall here a phrase by Doctor Jack Hughston, who said: "There is no problem that cannot be made worse by surgery" (see Chaps. 24–26 and 46). Among problems with the knee, this statement has never been more relevant than when approaching the extensor mechanism. Therefore, we must emphasize the importance of a correct diagnosis (see Chap. 8) and nonoperative treatment (see Chaps. 12 and 13).

However, there are patients in whom PFM is the primary cause of their pain, due to cyclical soft tissue and/or bone overload, but they represent in my clinical practice a small percentage of all patients with anterior knee pain. Moreover, in my experience, most of these patients were iatrogenically malaligned, that is, patients with multiple structurally/biomechanical-oriented surgeries.

### 1.4.1 Criticism

The great problem of the PFM concept is that not all malalignments, even of significant proportions, are symptomatic. Even more, one knee may be symptomatic and the other not, even though the underlying malalignment is entirely symmetrical (Fig. 1.3). On the other hand, patients with normal patellofemoral alignment on computed tomography (CT) can also suffer from anterior knee pain (Fig. 1.4). Therefore, PFM cannot explain all the cases of anterior knee pain, so other pathophysiological processes must exist. Moreover, PFM theory cannot adequately explain the variability of symptoms experienced by patients with anterior knee pain syndrome.

Finally, we must also remember that it has been demonstrated that there are significant differences between subchondral bone morphology and geometry of the articular cartilage surface of the patellofemoral joint, both in the axial and sagittal planes[6] (Fig. 1.5). Therefore, a radiographical PFM may not be real and it could induce us to indicate a realignment surgery than could provoke involuntarily an iatrogenic PFM leading to a worsening of preoperative symptoms. This would be another point against the universal acceptance of the PFM theory. Moreover, this could explain also the lack of predictability of operative results of realignment surgery.

### 1.4.2 Critical Analysis of Long-Term Follow-Up of Insall's Proximal Realignment for PFM. What Have We Learned? Clinical Relevance

In agreement with W.S. Halsted, I think that the operating room is "a laboratory of the highest order." As occurs with many surgical techniques, and realignment

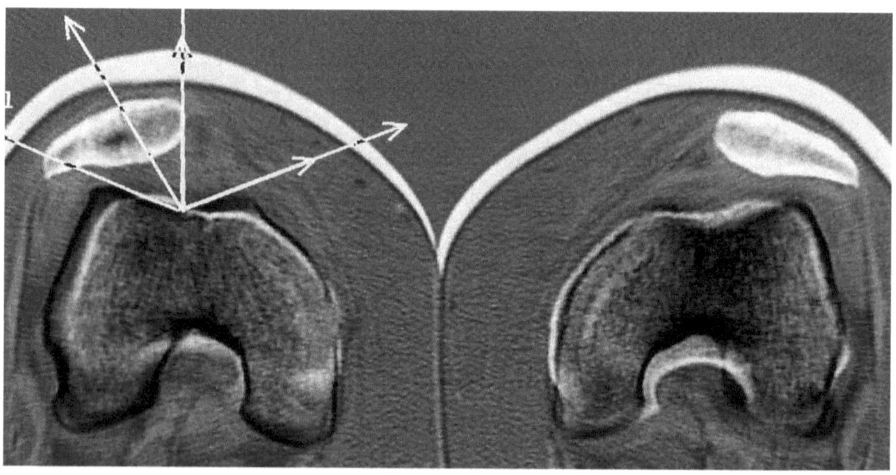

**Fig. 1.3** CT at 0° from a patient with anterior knee pain and functional patellofemoral instability in the right knee, however the left knee is completely asymptomatic. In both knees, the PFM is symmetric

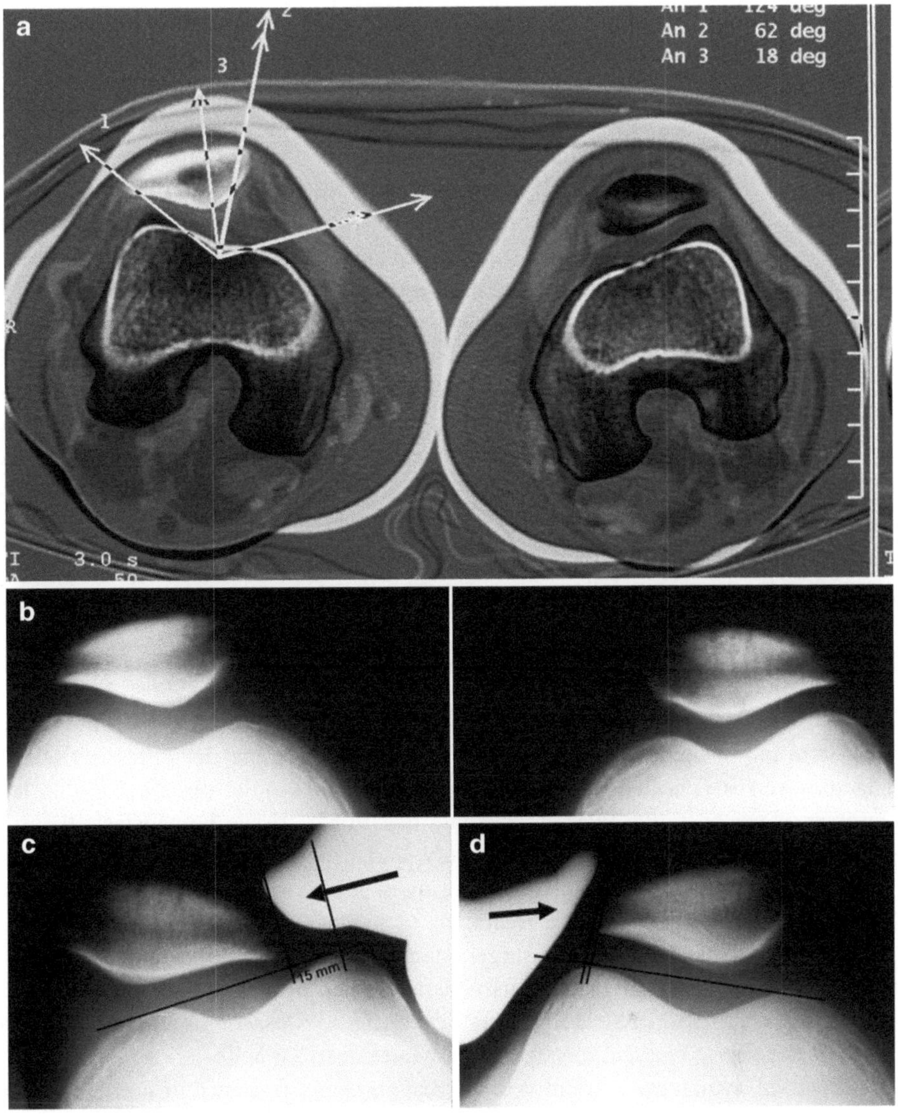


**Fig. 1.4** CT at 0° from a patient with severe anterior knee pain and patellofemoral instability in the left knee (**a**). This knee, which was operated on 2 years ago, performing an Insall's proximal realignment, was very symptomatic in spite of the correct patellofemoral congruence. Fulkerson test for medial subluxation was positive. Nevertheless, the right knee was asymptomatic despite the PFM. Conventional radiographs were normal and the patella was seen well centered in the axial view of Merchant (**b**). Axial stress radiograph of the left knee (**c**) allowed us to detect an iatrogenic medial subluxation of the patella (medial displacement of 15 mm). Note axial stress radiograph of the right knee (**d**). The symptomatology disappeared after surgical correction of medial subluxation of the patella using iliotibial tract and patellar tendon for repairing the lateral stabilizers of the patella

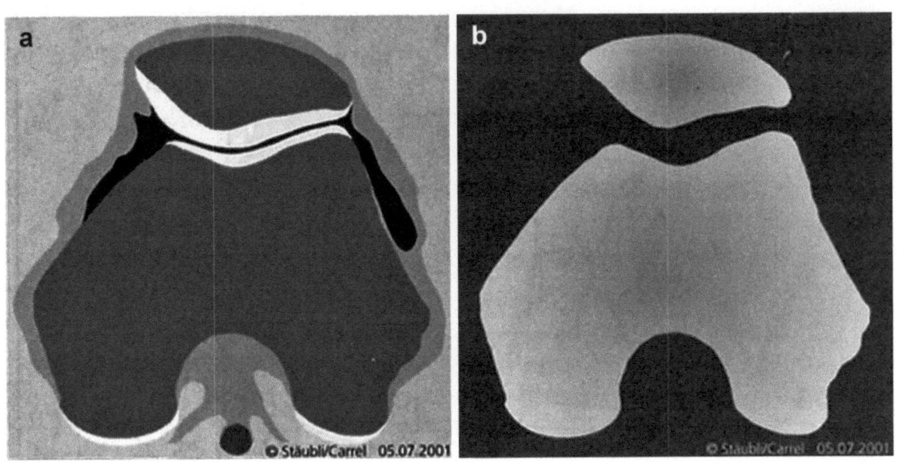


**Fig. 1.5** Scheme of gadolinium-enhanced MR arthrotomogram of the left knee in the axial plane. Note perfect patellofemoral congruence (**a**). Note patellofemoral incongruence of the osseous contours (**b**) (Reprinted from Staeubli[64], with permission from Elsevier)

surgery is not an exception, after wide usage, surgeons may question the basic tenets and may devise clinical research to test the underlying hypothesis; in our case the PFM concept.

In this way, we have evaluated retrospectively 40 Insall's proximal realignments (IPR) performed on 29 patients with isolated symptomatic PFM.[¶] The average follow up after surgery was 8 years (range 5–13 years). The whole study is presented in detail in Chap. 4.

One of the objectives of this study was to analyze whether there is a relationship between the presence of PFM and the presence of anterior knee pain or patellar instability.

In my experience, IPR provides a satisfactory centralization of the patella into the femoral trochlea in the short-term follow-up.[58] However, this satisfactory centralization of the patella is lost in the CT scans performed in the long-term follow-up in almost 57% of the cases. That is, IPR does not provide a permanent correction in all the cases. Nonetheless, this loss of centralization does not correlate with a worsening of clinical results. Furthermore, I have not found, in the long-term follow-up, a relation between the result, satisfactory versus nonsatisfactory, and the presence or absence of postoperative PFM. I speculate that PFM could influence the homeostasis negatively, and that realignment surgery could allow the restoring of joint homeostasis when nonoperative treatment of symptomatic PFM fails. Realignment surgery temporarily would unload inflamed peripatellar tissues, rather than permanently modify PFM. Moreover, according to Dye, postoperative rest and physical therapy are most important in symptoms resolution than realignment itself. Once we have achieved joint homeostasis, these PFM knees can exist happily within the envelope of function without symptoms. Moreover, in my series, 12 patients presented with unilateral symptoms. In nine of them, the contralateral asymptomatic knee presented a PFM and only in three cases was there a satisfactory centralization of the patella into the femoral trochlea.

We can conclude that not all patellofemoral maligned knees show symptoms, which is not surprising, as there are numerous examples of asymptomatic anatomic variations. Therefore, PFM is not a sufficient condition for the onset of symptoms, at least in postoperative patients. Thus, no imaging study should give us an indication for surgery. History and physical exam must point toward surgery and imaging only to allow us to confirm clinical impression (see Chap. 8).

To think of anterior knee pain or patellar instability as somehow being necessarily tied to PFM is an oversimplification that has positively stultified progress toward better diagnosis and treatment. The great danger in using PFM as a diagnosis is that the unsophisticated or unwary orthopedic surgeon may think that he or she has a license or "green light" to correct it with misguided surgical procedures that very often make the patients' pain worse (see Chaps. 24, 26 and 46).

## 1.5 Tissue Homeostasis Theory

In the 1990s, Scott F. Dye, of the University of California, San Francisco, and his research group, came up with the tissue homeostasis theory.[16,17] The initial observation that led to the development of the tissue homeostasis theory of patellofemoral pain was made by Dye, when a patient with complaints of anterior knee pain without evidence of chondromalacia or malalignment, underwent a technetium 99 m methylene diphosphonate bone scan evaluation of the knees in an attempt to assess the possible presence of covert osseous pathology. The bone scan of that individual manifested an intense diffuse patellar uptake in the presence of normal radiographic images. This finding revealed the presence of a covert osseous metabolic process of the patella in a symptomatic patient with anterior knee pain and normal radiographic findings.

The tissue homeostasis theory is in agreement with the ideas expressed by John Hilton (1807–1876) in his famous book *Rest and Pain.*[48] "The surgeon will be compelled to admit that he has no power to repair directly any injury … it is the prerogative of Nature alone to repair … his chief duty consists of ascertaining and removing those impediments which thwart the effort of Nature." Moreover, this is in agreement with the ideas exposed by Thomas Sydenham (1624–1689), "the father of English Medicine," and a cardinal figure in orthopedics in Britain and the world, who looked back to Hippocrates who taught that Nature was the physician of our diseases. According to Sydenham,

[¶] We define the term "isolated symptomatic PFM" as anterior knee pain or patellar instability, or both, with abnormalities of patellar tracking during physical examination verified with CT scans at 0° of knee flexion, but with no associated intraarticular abnormality demonstrated arthroscopically the doctor's task was to supplement, not to supplant Nature.[48]

The tissue homeostasis theory states that joints are more than mechanical structures – they are living, metabolically active systems. This theory attributes pain to a physiopathological mosaic of causes such as, increase of osseous remodeling, increase of intraosseous pressure, or peripatellar synovitis that lead to a decrease of what he called "Envelope of Function" (or "Envelope of Load Acceptance").

According to Dye,[16] the "Envelope of Function" describes a range of loading/energy absorption that is compatible with tissue homeostasis of an entire joint system; that is, with the mechanisms of healing and maintenance of normal tissues. Obviously, the Envelope of Function for a young athlete will be greater than that of sedentary elderly individual. Within the Envelope of Function is the region termed Zone of Homeostasis (Fig. 1.6a). Loads that exceed the Envelope of Function but are insufficient to cause a macrostructural failure

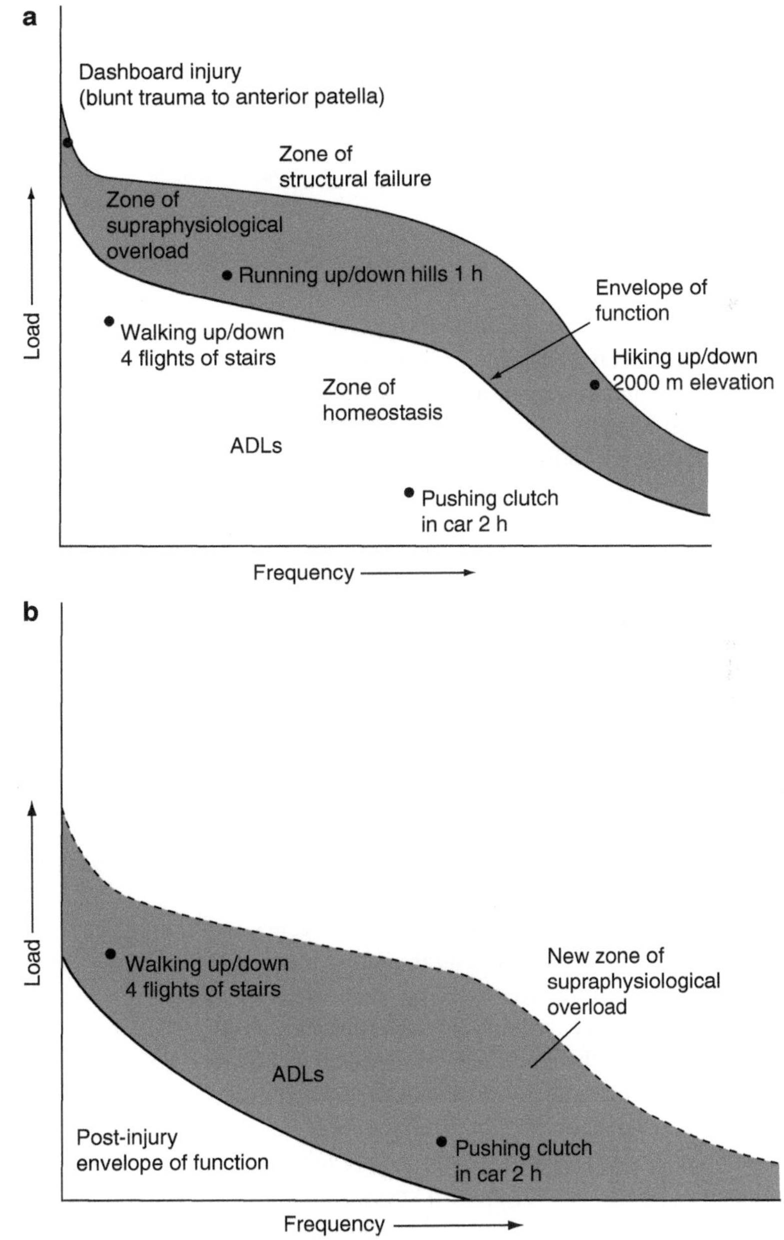


**Fig. 1.6** The Dye envelope of function theory. (**a**) Zone of Homeostasis, Envelope of Function and Zone of Structural Failure. (**b**) Post-injury envelope of function. (**c**) Decreasing loading to within the new envelope of function allows normal healing processes

**Fig. 1.6** (continued)

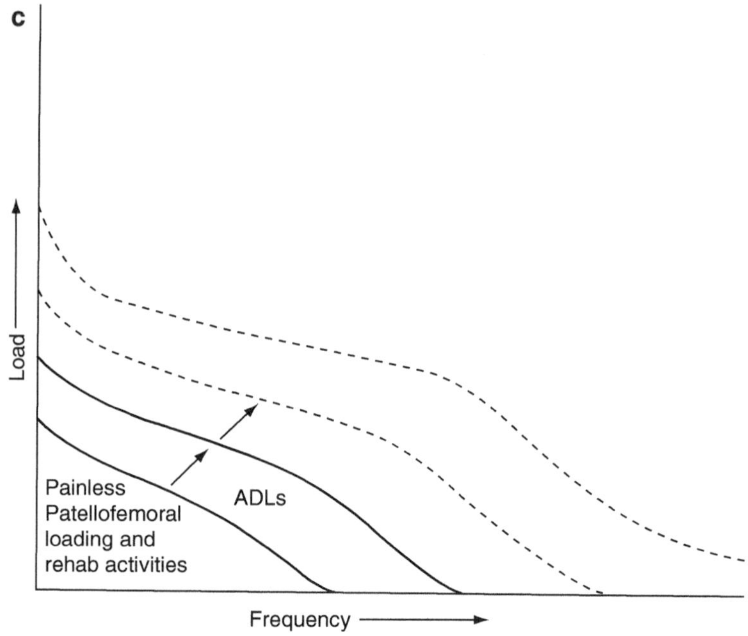


are termed the Zone of Supraphysiologic Overload (Fig. 1.6a). If sufficiently high forces are placed across the patellofemoral system, macrostructural failure can occur (Fig. 1.6a).

For Dye,[16] the following four factors determine the Envelope of Function or Zone of Homeostasis: (1) anatomic factors (morphology, structural integrity, and biomechanical characteristics of tissue); (2) kinematic factors (dynamic control of the joint involving proprioceptive sensory output, cerebral and cerebellar sequencing of motor units, spinal reflex mechanisms, and muscle strength and motor control); (3) physiological factors (the genetically determined mechanisms of molecular and cellular homeostasis that determine the quality and rate of repair of damaged tissues); and (4) treatment factors (type of rehabilitation or surgery received).

According to Dye, the loss of both osseous and soft tissue homeostasis is more important in the genesis of anterior knee pain than structural characteristics. To him, it matters little what specific structural factors may be present (i.e., chondromalacia patellae, PFM, etc.) as long as the joint is being loaded within its Envelope of Function, and is therefore asymptomatic. He suggests that patients with patellofemoral pain syndrome are often symptomatic due to supraphysiological loading of anatomically normal knees components.[16] In fact, patients with anterior knee pain often lack an easily identifiable structural abnormality to account for the symptoms. The Envelope of Function frequently diminishes after an episode of injury to the level where many activities of daily living, previously well tolerated (e.g., stair climbing, sitting down in and arising out of chairs, pushing the clutch of a car), become sufficiently high (supraphysiological loads for that patient) to lead to subversion of tissue healing and continued symptoms (Fig. 1.6b). Decreasing loading to within the newly diminished Envelope of Function allows normal tissue healing processes (Fig. 1.6c).

Finally, according to Dye, many instances of giving way, in patients with patellofemoral pain, could represent reflex inhibition of the quadriceps, which results from transient impingement of swollen, innervated peripatellar soft tissues, such as inflamed synovium in patients with normal alignment.

### 1.5.1 Clinical Relevance

Patients with an initial presentation of anterior knee pain frequently will respond positively to load restriction within their Envelope of Function and pain-free rehabilitation program. Moreover, Dye believes that enforced rest after realignment surgery could also be important in symptom resolution. Even if patients, parents, and trainers are apt to stubbornly reject any suggestion to introduce changes into the patient's activities and training routine demanding an urgent surgical procedure, orthopedic surgeons should under no circumstances alter their opinions and recommendations, however strong the pressure exerted upon them may be. Trainers, physical therapists, and physicians all have a high degree of responsibility and need to behave in an ethical way.

## 1.6 Patellofemoral Malalignment Theory Versus Tissue Homeostasis Theory

From a biomechanical point of view, there are two factors that can contribute to pain: (1) PFM and (2) joint loading, that depends on intensity and duration of activity. Thus, the presence of PFM would reduce the person's envelope of loading potential; that is, a person with PFM and minimal-to-moderate joint loading can have the same overloading of the subchondral bone, which is richly innervated, as someone without PFM and high loading. Presumably, this is because PFM reduces patellofemoral contact area, which in turn would result in elevated stress across the joint.

In essence, the proponents of tissue homeostasis theory look at PFM as representing internal load shifting within the patellofemoral joint that may lower the threshold (i.e., decrease of the Envelope of Function) for the initiation and persistence of loss of tissue homeostasis leading to the perception of patellofemoral pain. Pain always denotes loss of tissue homeostasis. From this perspective, there is no inherent conflict between both theories. However, these are not two coequal theories. Tissue homeostasis theory easily incorporates and properly assesses the clinical importance of possible factors of PFM, whereas the opposite is not true.

In conclusion, I truly believe that both theories are not exclusive, but complementary. In my experience, a knee with PFM can exist happily within its envelope of function, but once it is out, for example by overuse, training error, patterns of faulty sports movements, or traumatism, it can be harder to get back within it, and realignment surgery could be necessary in very selected cases when nonoperative measures fail. The objective of surgery is to restore balance in a way that normalizes loading of both retinacular and osseous structures.

## 1.7 Myths and Truths About Patellofemoral Disease

*Myth*: *Anterior knee pain and patellar instability are always self-limited and therefore active treatment is unnecessary. The natural history of this pathological entity is always benign*

Traditionally, anterior knee pain syndrome is considered to be a self-limited condition without long-term sequelae. This is true for many cases but cannot be regarded as a "golden rule." A large percentage of patients experience spontaneous recoveries; indeed, many patients remain asymptomatic even without specific treatment. In the case of some of our patients, 10 years elapsed from the onset of symptoms until the time of surgery; their symptoms not only failed to improve but they worsened in spite of the passage of time and of the patient's restricting or even abandoning sports practice. These same patients obtained excellent or good results after correction of their symptomatic PFM, which persisted in the long-term follow-up (see Chap. 4). Milgrom and colleagues[55] performed a prospective study to determine the natural history of anterior knee pain caused by overactivity. At 6 years follow-up, half of the knees originally with anterior knee pain were still symptomatic, but in only 8% of the originally symptomatic knees was the pain severe, hindering physical activity. Clinical experience shows that a prolonged and controlled active conservative treatment generally solves the problem. On the other hand, trying to negligently ignore the problem causes disability in some patients. Unfortunately, the patient's own ambition, as well as that of their parents and coaches prevails over their doctor's judgment, which is necessarily based on avoiding for at least 3–6 months any sports movement which could cause pain. That is, the fact that this process is on occasion self-limited should not make us forget the need to indicate active treatment in all cases. This means that the process we are studying is reversible at least until a certain point has been reached. The question we ask ourselves is: where is the point of no return?

Primary patellar dislocation is not a trivial condition either. It is true that with the passage of time the frequency of recurrent dislocations tends to diminish, but each episode is a potential source for a chondral injury.[29] A long-term assessment of patients (mean follow-up of 13 years) reveals that conservative treatment of patellar dislocation results in 44% of redislocations and 19% of late patellofemoral pain.[49]

Also, there are studies that establish a connection between PFM and patellofemoral and tibiofemoral osteoarthrosis.[26,42] Now, osteoarthrosis is a long-term hazard, both with or without a surgical procedure.[29] Davies and Newman[12] carried out a comparative study to evaluate the incidence of previous adolescent anterior knee pain syndrome in patients who underwent patellofemoral replacement for isolated patellofemoral osteoarthrosis in comparison with a matched group of patients who underwent unicompartmental replacement for isolated medial compartment osteoarthrosis. They found that the incidence of adolescent anterior knee pain syndrome and patellar instability was higher ($p<0.001$) in the patients who underwent patellofemoral replacement for isolated patellofemoral osteoarthrosis (22% and 14%, respectively) than in those who underwent unicompartmental replacement for isolated medial compartment osteoarthrosis (6% and 1%, respectively). They conclude that anterior knee pain syndrome is not always a self-limiting condition given that it may lead to patellofemoral osteoarthrosis. On the other hand, Arnbjörnsson and colleagues[3] found a high incidence of patellofemoral degenerative changes (29%) after nonoperative treatment of recurrent dislocation of the patella (average follow-up time 14 years with a minimum follow-up time of 11 years and a maximum follow-up time of 19 years). Bearing in mind that the mean age of the patients at follow-up was 39 years, they conclude that recurrent dislocation of the patella seems to cause patellofemoral osteoarthrosis. In conclusion, PFM's natural history is not always benign.

Quite often, symptomatic PFM is associated with a patellar tendinopathy.[2] The latter has also been called a self-limited pathology. It has been shown that it is not a benign condition that subsides with time, that is, it is not a self-limited process in athletes.[51] Normally, the injury progresses and when it gets to Blazina's stage III, it generally becomes irreversible and leads to the failure of conservative treatment.[51]

*Myth*: *Anterior knee pain is related to growth, and therefore once the patient has fully grown symptoms will disappear*

Anterior knee pain has also been related to growing pains. It is true that in young athletes during their maximum growth phase ("growth spurt"), there can be an increase in the tension of the extensor mechanism as a consequence of some "shortcoming" or "delay" in its development vis-à-vis bone growth. There may exist also a delay in the development of the VMO with regard to other muscles in the knee and therefore a transient muscle imbalance may ensue. But, it is also true that quite often parents tell us that the doctor their child saw told them that when the child stopped growing, the symptoms would go away and that, nevertheless, these persist once the child has fully grown.

*Myth*: *Anterior knee pain in adolescents is an expression of psychological problems*

Many physicians believe that anterior knee pain is a sign of psychological problems. Consequently, this condition has been associated with a moderate elevation of hysteria and, to a lesser degree, hypochondria with the problem in the knee being considered an unconscious strategy to confront an emotional conflict.[43] Likewise, it has been shown that, on some occasions, in adolescent women, anterior knee pain with no evident somatic cause can represent a way to control solicitous or complacent parents.[43] What cannot be questioned is that anybody at whatever age can somatize or try to attract other people's attention through some disease. In spite of this, one should be very cautious when it comes to suggesting to parents that their child's problem is wholly psychological. Nonetheless, it has to be recognized that these types of patients present with a very particular psychological profile (see Chap. 9). Furthermore, there are patients with objective somatic problems who disproportionately exaggerate their pain because of some associated psychological component or secondary emotional or financial gains.

Unfortunately, in my personal current surgical series (84 patients, 102 knees), there are 8 patients (7 females and 1 male) who had been referred to a mental health unit. Strangely enough, these patients' problem was satisfactorily addressed by surgery, which shows that the problem was not psychological. In addition, both the histological and the immunohistochemical and immunochemical techniques-based studies of the lateral patellar retinacula of these patients showed objective alterations that made it possible for us to detect that the pain had a neuroanatomic base. In short, the orthopedic surgeon has the duty to rule out mechanical problems as well as other pathologies that may cause anterior knee pain before blaming the pain on "emotional problems" or "feigning."

*Myth: Patellofemoral crepitation is in itself an indication of dysfunction*

A very common symptom that worries patients very much is patellofemoral crepitation. Crepitation is indicative of an articular cartilage lesion in the patella or in the femoral trochlea. Nonetheless, some patients who present with crepitation have a macroscopically intact cartilage at the moment of performing the arthroscopy.[30] The crepitation could be caused by alterations in the synovial or in other soft tissues.

The International Knee Documentation Committee (IKDC)[32] stated: "The knee is normal when crepitation is absent." However, this statement cannot be upheld after Johnson and colleagues[68] published their 1998 paper in *Arthroscopy* on the assessment of asymptomatic knees. Indeed, patellofemoral crepitation has a great incidence in asymptomatic women (94% in females versus 45% in males).[68] Patellofemoral crepitation has been associated with the lateral subluxation of the patella, but Johnson and colleagues[68] have observed that lateral subluxation of the patella in asymptomatic persons is more common in males than in females (35% versus 19%). Crepitation is not always present in patients with significant pain. Furthermore, when it is present, it does not necessarily cause anterior knee pain. In short, since crepitation is frequent in asymptomatic knees, its presence is more significant when it is absent from the contralateral knee or when there is some kind of asymmetry. The concept of knee asymmetry in the genesis of unilateral anterior knee pain is discussed by KD Shelbourne in Chap. 5.

*Myth: VMO is responsible for patellar stability*

It has been stated that the vastus medialis obliquus (VMO) is responsible for patellar stability, but we have not found convincing evidence in the literature for this belief; and, as ligaments are the joint stabilizers, this premise would appear to be faulty. In theory, the VMO resists lateral patellar motion, either by active contraction or by passive muscle resistance. In this way, in Farahmand's study,[19] lateral patellar force-displacement behavior was not affected by simulated muscle forces at any flexion angle from 15° to 75°. On the other hand, the orientation of the VMO varies greatly during knee flexion. The VMO's line of pull most efficiently resists lateral patellar motion when the knee is in deep flexion, at which time trochlear containment of the patella is independent of soft tissues influences (see Chap. 7).

It seems likely that operations that advance the VMO include tightening of the underlying medial patellofemoral ligament (MPFL), and it would be responsible for the success of the surgical technique (see Chap. 4). In this sense, we must note that the VMO tendon becomes confluent with the MPFL in the region of patellar attachment. Therefore, it would be more logical to protect the VMO and address the ligament deficiency surgically as needed (see Chap. 7).

*Controversy: Should the Q angle be measured? If so, how should it be measured? Is this of any use?*[29,56]

Another aspect that normally receives great importance in the physical examination of these patients in their Q angle, to the extent that some authors regard it as one of the criteria to be used for indicating a realignment surgery. Nonetheless, values considered to be normal vary greatly across the different studies carried out. In addition, there are no scientific criteria that correlate the incidence of patellofemoral pathology with the Q angle measure. Nowadays, some believe that the Q angle, as it is calculated, is not a very accurate way of measuring the patella's alignment since the measurement is made in extension and a laterally subluxating patella would lead to a falsely low measurement. In sum, even if Q angle measurement has traditionally been used in the clinical assessment of patients with patellofemoral pathology, currently the usefulness of this measurement is uncertain in spite of the multiple studies performed to date. A realignment surgery must never be justified on the basis of a high Q angle. The real controversy at present is how to measure the Q angle.

*Myth: Lateral release is a minor risk-free surgical procedure*

Over the years, lateral retinacular release has been recommended for a number of specific patellofemoral conditions[22]: recurrent lateral patellar dislocations or subluxations, chronic lateral subluxation – fixed lateral position, excessive lateral pressure syndrome, lateral retinacular tightness, and retinacular neuroma. A possible explanation for this wide range of surgical indications could be that some orthopedic surgeons consider the lateral release as a minor risk-free surgical procedure. However, I believe in agreement with Ronald Grelsamer that "There is no such thing as minor surgery – only minor surgeons." Surprisingly, in a survey of the IPSG,[22] on isolated lateral retinacular release, published in 2004 in *Arthroscopy*, most respondents (89%) indicated that this surgical procedure is a legitimate treatment, but only on rare occasions (1–2% of surgeries performed, less than five lateral releases a year). Furthermore, strong consensus (78%) existed that objective evidence should show lateral retinacular tension if a lateral release is to be performed.

Although lateral retinacular release is a simple procedure, it can lead to significant complications (see Chaps. 24, 26 and 46). In biomechanical studies, lateral release has been shown: (1) to reduce lateral tilt of the patella in cases in which tight lateral retinaculum is seen on CT scans,[27] (2) to increase passive medial displacement of the patella,[62,66] and (3) to increase passive lateral displacement of the patella.[14] Finally, in cadaver knees without preexisting lateral retinacular tightness, lateral release had no effect on articular pressures when the quadriceps were loaded.[33]

In conclusion, indiscriminate use of lateral release is of little benefit and can often cause increased symptoms. That is the reason why lengthening of the lateral retinaculum is the therapy chosen by authors such as Roland Biedert.

*Reality*: *Patellofemoral pathology leads to diagnostic error and, therefore, to inappropriate treatments and to patients being subjected to multiple procedures and to a great deal of frustration*

All myths and controversies analyzed throughout the present chapter could lead the reader to attribute importance to things that in actual fact are unimportant (i.e., crepitation) or, on the contrary, to underrate or cast aside complaints like anterior knee pain or functional patellar instability, considering them to be either a psychological problem or a condition bound to subside with time. Sometimes we do not go far enough, which may lead us to overlook other pathologies (diagnostic errors leading to therapeutic errors). In other cases, we overdo it and treat cases of malalignment that are not symptomatic. So, we have seen patients with symptoms of instability, who were treated for malalignment when what they really had was instability caused by a tear in their ACL.

We have also seen patients treated for a meniscal injury who really had isolated symptomatic PFM. In this connection, it is important to point out that McMurray's test, traditionally associated with meniscal pathology, can lead to a medial–lateral displacement of the patella and also cause pain in patients with PFM. Finally, it is worrying to see how many patients are referred to outpatient orthopedic surgery practices in our hospitals with an MRI-based diagnosis of a tear in the posterior horn of the medial meniscus, who during clinical examination present with anterior knee pain and no meniscal symptoms. It is a proven fact that given the overcrowding of outpatient units' orthopedic services and because of social pressure, as time passes, doctors tend to conduct more superficial physical examinations and to order more MRIs. In this way, we must remember the statement by Dr. Casscells[9]: *Technology: a good servant, but a bad master.* According to Augusto Sarmiento, former Chairman of the American Academy of Orthopedic Surgeons (AAOS), MRIs are unfortunately replacing the physical examination when it comes to assessing a painful joint.[60] MRI is not a panacea and, what's more, it gives rise to false positives. Patients' great faith in technology and their skepticism regarding their doctors and an increasingly dehumanized medical practice has resulted in the failure of partial arthroscopic meniscectomies owing to a bad indication, in frustrated patients, and in the squandering of resources. In 1940, Karlson[44] wrote the following about chondromalacia patellae: "The diagnosis is difficult to make and the differential diagnosis of injury to the meniscus. – causes special difficulties, as in both these ailments [meniscal and patellar pathology] there is a pressure tenderness over the medial joint space." Hughston endorsed these words when he stated, first in 1960 and then in 1984[35]: "The orthopaedic surgeon who has not mistaken a recurrent subluxation of the patella for a torn meniscus has undoubtedly had a very limited and fortunate experience with knees and meniscectomies." Just think of the sheer amount of arthroscopies performed unnecessarily on the basis of a complaint of anterior knee pain!

Nowadays, this problem has been magnified because of the relative ease with which meniscectomies are indicated and performed thanks to the benefits of arthroscopy. In a lecture delivered at the Conference of the Nordic Orthopaedic Federation held in Finland in 2000, Augusto Sarmiento stated that the number of unnecessary surgeries (including arthroscopies) carried out in our field in the United States is extremely high.[60] It is therefore essential to underscore the importance of physically examining the patient (see Chap. 8).

Finally, another source of frustration for the patient is the lack of communication with his or her doctor (dehumanized medicine), which may lead to unrealistic expectations. It is essential for the patient to understand the difficulties inherent in treating patellofemoral problems. This is the only way in which patients can be satisfied after surgery even if their symptoms do not disappear completely.

*Reality*: *Treatment should be customized*

It is very important to identify the pathological alteration responsible for the clinical aspect of this clinical entity to select the most effective treatment options based on clinical findings (made-to-measure treatment). This will yield the most satisfactory results. At present, minimal intervention (e.g., specific soft tissue excision of painful tissue[45]), and nonsurgical methods are emphasized (see Chaps. 12 and 13). Obviously, if the etiology of patellofemoral pain and patellar instability is multifactorial, then the evaluation must be multifactorial, and the treatment should be multifactorial also.[52] This should lead to a simplified treatment plan. We must find out what is wrong and fix it; that is, we must address specific identifiable pathology (e.g., peripatellar synovitis, serious rotational alterations, etc.). In the few patients who require surgery, a minimalist surgical approach is the best in most cases.[17,45] We agree with the statement of Philip Wiles in 1952: "However important surgery may be now, it should be the aim of all doctors, including surgeons, to limit and ultimately abolish it."[48]

## 1.8 Conclusions

The pathology we discuss in the present monograph presents itself with a multifactorial etiology and a great pathogenic, diagnostic, and therapeutic complexity.

The consideration of anterior knee pain to be a self-limited condition in patients with an underlying neurotic personality should be banished from the orthopedic literature.

Our knowledge about anterior knee pain has evolved throughout the twentieth century. While until the end of the 1960s this pain was attributed to chondromalacia patellae, a concept born at the beginning of the century, after that period, it came to be connected with abnormal patellofemoral alignment. More recently, the pain was put down to a wide range of physiopathological processes such as peripatellar synovitis, the increment in intraosseous pressure, and increased bone remodeling. We are now at a turning point. New information is produced at breakneck speed. Nowadays, medicine in its entirety is being reassessed at subcellular level, and this is precisely the line of thought we are following in the approach to anterior knee pain syndrome. Still to be seen are the implications that this change of mentality will have in the treatment of anterior knee pain syndrome in the future, but I am sure that these new currents of thought will open the doors for us to new and exciting perspectives that could potentially revolutionize the management of this troublesome condition in the new millennium we have just entered. Clearly, we are only at the beginning of the road that will lead to understanding where anterior knee pain comes from.

## References


1. Aleman O. Chondromalacia post-traumatica patellae. *Acta Chir Scand.* 1928;63:194.
2. Allen GM, Tauro PG, Ostlere SJ. Proximal patellar tendinosis and abnormalities of patellar tracking. *Skeletal Radiol.* 1999;28:220-223.
3. Arnbjörnsson A, Egund N, Rydling O. The natural history of recurrent dislocation of the patella. Long-term results of conservative and operative treatment.. 1992;74():140-142.
4. Aune AK, Holm I, Risberg MA, et al. Four-strand hamstring tendon autograft compared with patellar tendon-bone autograft for anterior cruciate ligament reconstruction. A randomized study with two-year follow-up. *Am J Sports Med.* 2001;29:722-728.
5. Axhausen G. Zur pathogenese der arthritis deformans. *Arch Orthop Unfallchir.* 1922;20:1.
6. Bosshard C, Staubli HU, Rauschning W. Konturinkongruenz von gelenkknorpeloberflachen und subchondralem knochen des femoropatellargelenkas in der sagittalen ebene. *Arthroskopie.* 1997;10:72-76.
7. Budinger K. Üeber ablösung von gelenkteilen und verwandte prozesse. *Dtsch Z Chir.* 1906;84:311-365.
8. Budinger K. Üeber traumatische knorpelrisse im kniegelenk. *Dtsch Z Chir.* 1908;92:510.
9. Casscells SW. Technology: a good servant, but a bad master. *Arthroscopy.* 1990;6:1-2.
10. Corry IS, Webb JM, Clingeleffer AJ, et al. Arthroscopic reconstruction of the anterior cruciate ligament. A comparison of patellar tendon autograft and four-strand hamstring tendon autograft. *Am J Sports Med.* 1999;27:444-454.
11. Dandy DJ, Poirier H. Chondromalacia and the unstable patella. *Acta Orthop Scand.* 1975;46:695-699.

12. Davies G, Newman JH Does adolescent anterior knee pain lead to patello femoral arthritis?. *10th Congress European Society of Sports Traumatology, Knee Surgery and Arthroscopy*. Rome, *Book of Abstracts*, 2002:353
13. DeHaven KE, Lintner DM. Athletic injuries: comparison by age, sport, and gender. *Am J Sports Med*. 1986;14:218-224.
14. Desio SM, Burks RT, Bachus KN. Soft tissue restraints to lateral patellar translation in the human knee. *Am J Sports Med*. 1998;26:59-65.
15. Devereaux MD, Lachmann SM. Patello-femoral arthralgia in athletes attending a sports injury clinic. *Br J Sports Med*. 1984;18:18-21.
16. Dye SF. The knee as a biologic transmission with an envelope of function: a theory. *Clin Orthop*. 1996;325:10-18.
17. Dye SF, Staubli HU, Biedert RM, et al. The mosaic of pathophysiology causing patellofemoral pain: therapeutic implications. *Oper Tech Sports Med*. 1999;7:46-54.
18. Dye SF, Vaupel GL, Dye CC. Conscious neurosensory mapping of the internal structures of the human knee without intra-articular anesthesia. *Am J Sports Med*. 1998;26: 773-777.
19. Farahmand F, Tahmasbi MN, Amis AA. Lateral force-displacement behaviour of the human patella and its variation with knee flexion – a biomechanical study in vitro. *J Biomech*. 1998;31:1147-1152.
20. Ficat P, Ficat C, Bailleux A. Syndrome d'hyperpression externe de la rotule (S.H.P.E). *Rev Chir Orthop*. 1975;61: 39-59.
21. Ficat P, Hungerford DS. *Disorders of the Patello-Femoral Joint*. Baltimore: Williams & Wilkins; 1977.
22. Fithian DC, Paxton EW, Post WR, et al. Lateral retinacular release: a survey of the International Patellofemoral Study Group. *Arthroscopy*. 2004;20:463-468.
23. Fu FH, Bennett CH, Ma CB, et al. Current trends in anterior cruciate ligament reconstruction. Part 2: operative procedures and clinical correlations. *Am J Sports Med*. 2000;28: 124-130.
24. Fulkerson JP. The etiology of patellofemoral pain in young, active patients: a prospective study. *Clin Orthop*. 1983;179:129-133.
25. Fulkerson JP, Arendt EA. Anterior knee pain in females. *Clin Orthop*. 2000;372:69-73.
26. Fulkerson JP, Hungerford DS. *Disorders of the Patellofemoral Joint*. Baltimore: Williams & Wilkins; 1990.
27. Fulkerson JP, Schutzer SF, Ramsby GR, et al. Computerized tomopraphy of the patellofemoral joint before and after release and malalignment. *Arthroscopy*. 1987;3:19-24.
28. Fulkerson JP, Tennant R, Jaivin JS. Histologic evidence of retinacular nerve injury associated with patellofemoral malalignment. *Clin Orthop*. 1985;197:196-205.
29. Grelsamer RP. Patellar malalignment. *J Bone Joint Surg*. 2000;82-A:1639-1650.
30. Grelsamer RP, McConnell J. *The Patella. A Team Approach*. Gaithersburg: An Aspen Publication; 1998.
31. Griffin LY, Agel J, Albohm MJ, et al. Noncontact anterior cruciate ligament injuries: risk factors and prevention strategies. *J Am Acad Orthop Surg*. 2000;8:141-150.
32. Hefti F, Muller W, Jakob RP, et al. Evaluation of knee ligament injuries with the IKDC form. *Knee Surg Sports Traumatol Arthrosc*. 1993;1:226-234.
33. Huberti HH, Hayes WC. Contact pressures in chondromalacia patellae and the effects of capsular reconstructive procedures. *J Orthop Res*. 1988;6:499-508.
34. Hughston JC. Subluxation of the patella. *J Bone Joint Surg*. (1968;50(A):1003-1026.
35. Hughston JC, Walsh WM, Puddu G. *Patellar Subluxation and Dislocation. Saunders Monographs in Clinical Orthopaedics*, vol. 5. Philadelphia: WB Saunders; 1984.
36. Huston LJ, Greenfield ML, Wojtys EM. Anterior cruciate ligament injuries in the female athlete. Potential risk factors. *Clin Orthop*. 2000;372:50-63.
37. Insall J. "Chondromalacia Patellae": patellar malalignment syndrome. *Orthop Clin North Am*. 1979;10:117-127.
38. Insall J. *Surgery of the Knee*. New York: Churchill Livingstone; 1984 & 1993.
39. Insall JN, Aglietti P, Tria AJ Jr. Patellar pain and incongruence II: clinical application. *Clin Orthop*. 1983;176: 225-232.
40. Insall J, Bullough PG, Burnstein AH. Proximal "tube" realignment of the patella for chondromalacia patellae. *Clin Orthop*. 1979;144:63-69.
41. International Patellofemoral Study Group. Patellofemoral semantics. The Tower of Babel. *Am J Knee Surg*. 1997;10: 92-95.
42. Iwano T, Kurosawa H, Tokuyama H, et al. Roentgenographic and clinical findings of patellofemoral osteoarthritis. *Clin Orthop*. 1990;252:190-197.
43. Johnson LL. *Arthroscopic Surgery. Principles & Practice*. St. Louis: The C.V. Mosby Company; 1986.
44. Karlson S. Chondromalacia patellae. *Acta Chir Sacand*. 1940;83:347-381.
45. Kasim N, Fulkerson JP. Resection of clinically localized segments of painful retinaculum in the treatment of selected patients with anterior knee pain. *Am J Sports Med*. 2000;28: 811-814.
46. Larson RV. Complications and pitfalls in anterior cruciate ligament reconstruction with hamstring tendons. In: Malek MM, ed. *Knee Surgery. Complications, Pitfalls and Salvage*. New York: Springer; (2001:77-88.
47. Leslie IJ, Bentley G. Arthroscopy in the diagnosis of chondromalacia patellae. *Ann Rheum Dis*. 1978;37:540-547.
48. Levay D. *The History of Orthopaedics*. Park Ridge: The Parthenon Publishing Group; 1990.
49. Mäenpää H, Lehto MUK. Patellar dislocation. The long-term results of nonoperative management in 100 patients. *Am J Sports Med*. 1997;25:213-217.
50. Maffulli N, Khan KM, Puddu G. Overuse tendon conditions: time to change a confusing terminology. *Arthroscopy*. 1998;14:840-843.
51. Martens M, Wouters P, Burssens A, et al. Patellar tendinitis: pathology and results of treatment. *Acta Orthop Scand*. 1982;53:445-450.
52. Merchant AC 33 years in the PF joint. What have I learned?. VIII International Patellofemoral Study Group Meeting; 2003;Naples.
53. Merchant AC, Mercer RL. Lateral release of the patella: a preliminary report. *Clin Orthop*. 1974;103:40.
54. Merchant AC, Mercer RL, Jacobsen RH, et al. Roentgenographic analysis of patellofemoral congruence. *J Bone Joint Surg*. 1974;56(A):1391-1396.

55. Milgrom C, Finestone A, Shlamkovitch N, et al. Anterior knee pain caused by overactivity: a long term prospective followup. *Clin Orthop*. 1996;331:256-260.
56. Post WR. Clinical evaluation of patients with patellofemoral disorders. *Arthroscopy*. 1999;15:841-851.
57. Royle SG, Noble J, Davies DR, et al. The significance of chondromalacic changes on the patella. *Arthroscopy*. 1991;7: 158-160.
58. Sanchis-Alfonso V, Gastaldi-Orquín E, Martinez-SanJuan V. Usefulness of computed tomography in evaluating the patellofemoral joint before and after Insall's realignment. Correlation with short-term clinical results. *Am J Knee Surg*. 1994;7:65-72.
59. Sanchis-Alfonso V, Roselló-Sastre E. Anterior knee pain in the young patient – what causes the pain? "Neural model". *Acta Orthop Scand*. 2003;74:697-703.
60. Sarmiento A. The future of our specialty. *Acta Orthop Scand*. 2000;71:574-579.
61. Schutzer SF, Ramsby GR, Fulkerson JP. Computed tomographic classification of patellofemoral pain patients. *Orthop Clin North Am*. 1986;17:235-248.
62. Skalley TC, Terry GC, Teitge RA. The quantitative measurement of normal passive medial and lateral patellar motion limits. *Am J Sports Med*. 1993;21:728-732.
63. Spicer DD, Blagg SE, Unwin AJ, et al. Anterior knee symptoms after four-strand hamstring tendon anterior cruciate ligament reconstruction. *Knee Surg Sports Traumatol Arthrosc*. 2000;8:286-289.
64. Staeubli HU, Bosshard C, Porcellini P, et al. Magnetic resonance imaging for articular cartilage: cartilage-bone mismatch. *Clin Sports Med*. 2002;21:417-433.
65. Tapper EM, Hoover NW. Late results after meniscectomy. *J Bone Joint Surg*. 1969;51(A):517-526.
66. Teitge RA, Faerber WW, Des Madryl P, et al. Stress radiographs of the patellofemoral joint. *J Bone Joint Surg*. 1996; 78(A):193-203.
67. Thomee R, Restrom P, Karlsson J, et al. Patellofemoral pain syndrome in young women. I. A clinical analysis of alignment, pain parameters, common symptoms and functional activity level. *Scand J Med Sci Sports*. 1995;5: 237-244.
68. van Johnson LL, Dyk E, Green JR, et al. Clinical assessment of asymptomatic knees: comparison of men and women. *Arthroscopy*. 1998;14:347-359.
69. Witvrouw E, Lysens R, Bellemans J, et al. Intrinsic risk factors for the development of anterior knee pain in an athletic population: a two-year prospective study. *Am J Sports Med*. 2000;28:480-489.

# 2 In Search of the Etiology of Anterior Knee Pain

Jan Näslund

## 2.1 Introduction

Because pain is often the only manifest symptom in patients suffering from anterior knee pain (AKP), an in-depth analysis of this subjective emotion may yield valuable information about this elusive knee condition. This book chapter focuses on pain perception and its mechanisms, physiology, and evolutionary context. In the last 10 years, new insights have contributed to our understanding of pain. Those that focus on pain and the role of homeostatic tissue regulation and are related to AKP will be discussed.

## 2.2 The Knee Region: A Common Location of Pain

The knee region is a common anatomic location of pain. Pain in this region occurs in persons of all ages. Epidemiological studies found that young persons report regular perception of knee pain when asked,[4,31] and 11% of young children report incidence of everyday knee pain.[23] In adults, knee osteoarthrosis is one of the major causes of chronic pain.[18]

Pain in the knee region also occurs in disparate diagnoses. Bilateral trigger points in this region are mandatory for a diagnosis of fibromyalgia.[42] Pain in the knee region is also the pain that is first and most often reported in decompression sickness.[52]

J. Näslund
Department of Physiology and Pharmacology, Karolinska Institute, Stockholm, Sweden
e-mail: jan.e.naslund@ki.se

One reason for the knee's susceptibility to pain may be evolutionary in nature. Millions of years ago, our ancestors who used four limbs for locomotion rose to walk on two legs. To accommodate this change, anatomical and biomechanical adaptation of the knee joint was key; perhaps this was possible only through compromise?

## 2.3 Pain Classifications

Pain was traditionally classified according to clinical relevance, physiology, or mechanism.[43] The International Association for the Study of Pain (IASP) recently suggested a new system that classifies pain in four main groups[69]:

- *Nociception* (acute pain)
- *Inflammatory pain* (pain during reestablishment of homeostasis)
- *Functional pain* (pain caused by a pathological reorganization of the nervous system)
- *Neuropathic pain* (pain caused by known nerve injury or a disease that is known to cause nerve damage)

This system would classify the pain experienced by patients suffering from AKP into one of two groups: inflammatory pain or functional pain. AKP would normally not be classed as acute pain (nociception) because most studies report a pain duration of 3–6 months for this condition. But Brushoj and colleagues have questioned this consensus and proposed that acute AKP be regarded a subgroup of patellofemoral pain syndrome (PFPS).[11] Also, AKP has seldom been classed as neuropathic pain, and there is little current evidence to do so now. Inclusion criteria for neuropathic pain were recently changed.[41]

V. Sanchis-Alfonso (ed.), *Anterior Knee Pain and Patellar Instability*,
DOI: 10.1007/978-0-85729-507-1_2, © Springer-Verlag London Limited 2011

Long-standing chronic pain was traditionally described in terms such as "burning" or "shooting" and often regarded as neuropathic. Involvement of damaged nerve tissue is now a mandatory criterion. Despite this, Jensen et al. hypothesized that a subgroup of AKP patients do suffer from neuropathic pain.[35] Using quantified sensory testing (QST), bedside neurological tests, and case histories, the authors found considerable heterogeneity and overlap in degree and type of nervous system aberration – but no APK patient subgroup was identified as having neuropathic pain.

## 2.4 Inflammation and Immune Reactions

Distinguishing between inflammatory pain and functional pain is not always easy. The dominant problem is a clear and unambiguous definition of inflammation.

*Inflammation* is an old term, commonly used and well-known in medical circles, however ill defined.[56] Its main use is for describing sharp and intense reactions to tissue damage – *acute inflammation.* The cardinal signs of inflammation – rubor, tumor, calor, dolor, and function laesa (loss of function) – define what we today recognize as a classic acute inflammatory response; for example, sequelae to traumatic cell injury. These physiological processes give rise to the cardinal signs:

- Increased vascular permeability
- Vasodilation
- Increased granulation tissue
- Initiation of pain
- Reflex muscle inhibition
- Disruption of tissue structure
- Fibro- and metaplasia

But various time-dependent reactions indicate that some inflammatory processes are not of an acute nature. And inflammatory reactions can vary due to the type of stimulus. Three main types occur:

- Exogenous stimuli – for example, microbes
- Endogenous stimuli
- Activation of the adaptive immune system

The most effective initiation of inflammation occurs when microbes (bacteria, viruses, or fungi) gain unwanted access to various areas of our bodies. Cells and molecules of the innate immune system immediately react to these invaders.[1] Activation of cells, molecules, and mediators follows a fairly typical course – *inflammation.* Granulocytes (polymorphonuclear leukocytes) and edema are typical signs of acute inflammation.

Injuries to somatic cells or tissues will also initiate an inflammation. In this second type of inflammation, stimuli are endogenous, as opposed to exogenous stimuli involved in the first type. When cells in our body are damaged, substances and structures that are normally stored inside the cells are released and initiate an inflammatory reaction. The inflammatory cascade of cells, molecules, and mediators resembles – but is not exactly like – the one that occurs in response to an exogenous stimulus. Endogenous stimuli evoke different kinds of mediators, cells, and reactions.

The third type of inflammatory reaction is an activation of the adaptive immune system. The adaptive immune system uses inflammation to kill microbes because it lacks an inherent ability to do so. This interaction between inflammation and immune reaction is typical for the human body.

Once they begin, inflammatory processes follow a predetermined course and cease first when the initial causes are eradicated – healing then ensues. These processes are time dependent. When the stimulus cannot be eliminated, inflammation continues, changing in nature.

*Subacute* or *chronic inflammation* are terms that have been applied to ongoing inflammation, but likewise, they are ill defined. Tissue that contains increased amounts of monomorphonuclear leukocytes (lymphocytes, monocytes, macrophages, and plasma cells) and fibrosis is undergoing what is commonly known as chronic inflammation. Unfortunately, *chronic* often implies a nonhealing or irreversible condition. Alternatively, *degeneration* has been used to denote the status of tissue with fibrosis and no indications of acute inflammation (mediators, cells, and molecules). Obviously, a new approach for understanding and defining inflammatory reactions is needed.[24,56]

To recap, inflammation is the body's response to injury and homeostatic disturbances. Together with the immune system, inflammation not only senses and reacts to threat and damage but also initiates tissue healing – all critical aspects in maintaining the health of an organism. A growing body of evidence shows that inflammatory processes are a key factor in homeostatic maintenance, and thus, in what previously were considered to be unavoidable aging processes. Inflammation is nearly always present – recognition of its role in the disease process, in response to and in the initiation of, is growing.[63] Some aspects of inflammatory processes are constantly involved in homeostasis – the adjustments that an organism makes to its physiological processes to maintain internal equilibrium. But some aspects of inflammation also interact with other physiological systems, so a simple model is elusive. Inflammatory processes are involved in nearly all acute and chronic diseases – such as, cancer, AIDS, transplant rejection, obesity, diabetes, musculoskeletal disorders (atherosclerosis, tendon pain, myopathy), Alzheimer's disease, and aging.[24] Future treatment of these diseases will require a deeper understanding of inflammation, and its role in homeostasis of the body. Maybe inflammation should not be understood as being the cause of a disease but as the way the body handles gentle as well as serious hazards to homeostasis?

Inflammation is an umbrella term encompassing reactions at various levels: clinical, physiological, molecular, cellular, and intracellular. During particular tissue damage, some or all of the reactions may occur, and a time-dependent cascade of complex interactions could occur at all levels (Fig. 2.1). After removal of pathogens and dead cells, inflammatory processes act to foster healing of damaged tissue. In other words, phagocytosis and remodeling of new tissues are two ways inflammatory processes help maintain somatic homeostasis.

As mentioned above, activation of the immune system is a pathway that commonly initiates normal inflammatory responses. Many cells express receptors of the innate immune system; examples include macrophages and mast cells, both known to be present during inflammation. When these effector cells are

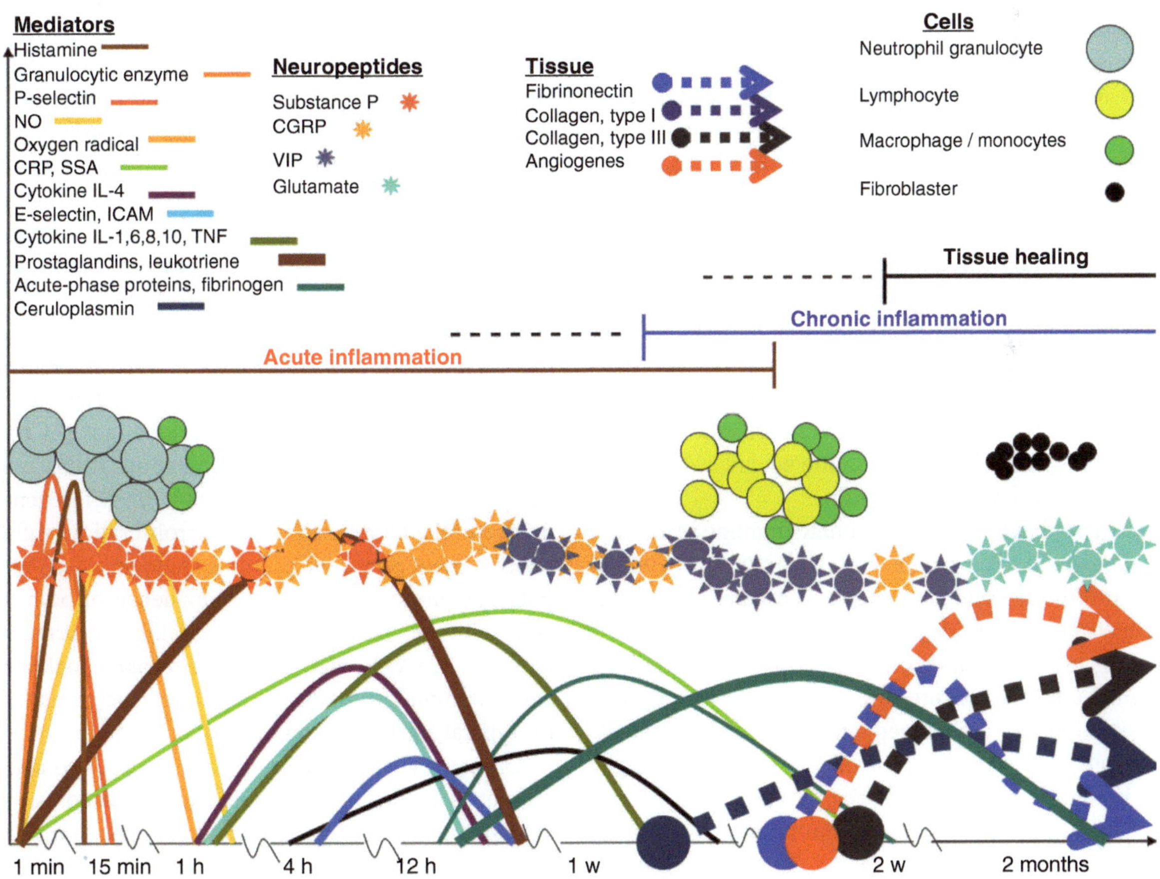


**Fig. 2.1** Cells, neuropeptides, and mediators involved in inflammatory processes

activated, they initiate a rapid response marked by release of inflammatory mediators and cytokines (Fig. 2.1). Cytokines (e.g., interleukin-1 [IL-1] and tumor necrosis factor [TNF]) stimulate inflammation.

Inflammation cannot continue unabated without serious hazard to the host. Hence, complex processes have evolved to suppress these responses, repair local damage, and reestablish homeostasis. Immune responses are designed to be self-limited, so processes that initiate resolution are also triggered. For instance, a subset of T-cells promotes resolution of inflammation and tissue repair. As part of the repair process, fibroblasts and other mesenchymal cells produce collagen and other components of the extracellular matrix. These counter-regulatory systems ultimately reestablish homeostasis.

After minor disturbances of homeostasis that only create mild reactions (e.g., syntheses of proteins, increases in metabolism, mild hypoxia, and oxidative stress), some inflammatory reactions will appear but will be scarcely detectable. Previously, despite similarities to inflammation, these mild reactions were seldom recognized as part of inflammation. *Homeostasis* and *immune reactions* describe these physiological processes. So to sum, inflammation is one of the immune system's first responses to injury, infection, or irritation to reestablish homeostasis.

An inflammatory background has been proposed for some chronic diseases, such as cardiovascular disease, diabetes, irritable bowel syndrome (IBS), and cancer. Patients with these diseases present elevated levels of cytokines. Innate immune cells preferentially produce proinflammatory cytokines, which indicates that the immune system has an elevated activation status. Low-grade immune activation occurs during intermittent or chronic inflammation.

Macrophages coordinate innate immune responses; they respond to environmental input signals by initiating resolution of inflammation. These cells play vital homeostatic roles, display remarkable plasticity, and can change their physiology in response to environmental cues. Accordingly, a spectrum of macrophage populations are recognized, among others: classically activated macrophages, wound-healing macrophages, and regulatory macrophages.[44] Macrophages can respond to (1) endogenous stimuli that are generated following injury or infection and (2) signals produced by immune cells. These are examples of the close relationship between various types of inflammation and the immune system.

Per the above, discussing inflammation solely from an acute perspective could lead to false conclusions since inflammation should be viewed as a process that ultimately reestablishes homeostasis.[20] But inflammation can have several etiologies, and this fact is poorly recognized, as evinced in the current discussion on whether tendinopathy should be called *tendinitis* or *tendinosis*.

The healing process that begins with an acute inflammation – that is, peripheral sensitization together with release of substances such as histamine, substance P, prostaglandins, calcitonin gene-related peptide (CGRP), nerve growth factor (NGF), and C-reactive proteins (CRP) – in the presence of neutrophil granulocytes and macrophages alters its nature in a matter of hours, days, or weeks. In this later stage, most cells are lymphocytes and monocytes, with vasoactive intestinal polypeptide (VIP) and glutamate being the dominant neuropeptides (Fig. 2.1).[56] Chronic inflammation might also occur without an initial period of acute inflammation.

The initial stimulus determines the ensuing inflammatory cascade. In the last stage, production of collagen and angiogenesis complete the healing process – and the inflammation dissipates. After several months, patients with long-standing Achilles tendon pain, not surprisingly, present increased levels of glutamate and angiogenesis.[3] Problems in comparing results of various studies seem to arise from the *definition of inflammation* used.

The neuronal cholinergic pathway plays a major role in immune reactions. Lately, also nonneuronal cholinergic pathways have been described, an indication of the importance of acetylcholine (ACh) in immune responses and in inflammation. It has previously been reported that stimulation of ACh receptors induce collagen deposition, cell proliferation, inflammatory remodeling, and promote angiogenesis.[25] When Forsgren and colleagues report evidence of both Ach and Ach receptors in chronically painful tendons, this indicates the existence of a nonneuronal cholinergic anti-inflammatory pathway that might be responsible for typical signs of chronic inflammation.

Organs that sustain chronic inflammation sometime present a multifaceted, multilayered response that involves epithelial to mesenchymal transition, fibroblast activation, recruitment of inflammatory cells, and cellular regeneration at sites of damage.[33] This results in a maladaptive accumulation of extracellular matrix, a condition known as fibrosis.

As mentioned before, some of these inflammatory processes may arise despite lack of observable cell death. Also, the nervous system itself is able to initiate inflammatory reactions (neurogenic inflammation). The major role played by peripheral nerves in initiating and terminating inflammatory reactions must not be forgotten.[1]

Tissue remodeling occurs during the regulation of homeostasis. Excluding visible initial acute inflammation, some of the processes described in chronic inflammation are similar to those in homeostasis. Hypoxia and apoptosis are among the most relevant stimuli in muscle and bone tissue remodeling. But no acute inflammatory processes occur in muscle cell regeneration (protein synthesis) or bone remodeling. Apoptosis occurs as a normal component in most tissues and this kind of cell death does not necessarily signify a physiological problem. The apoptotic process gives rise to a large number of signal molecules that affect the behavior of cells. Apoptosis occurs with minimal or no inflammatory response and even stimulates production of anti-inflammatory molecules.[48] By contrast, necrosis initiates a typical inflammatory response. For the sake of clarity, it must be mentioned that apoptosis of osteocytes, which is involved in the modeling and remodeling of bone tissue, induces TNF-alpha activity, a pro-inflammatory cytokine.[39] Again, defining *inflammation* is troublesome.

Pain perception is part of the inflammatory process. It occurs in acute inflammation, in immune reactions, and in chronic inflammation. But the pain mechanisms that underlie inflammation, immune reactions, and homeostasis may differ substantially.[17] Because the role of some inflammatory mediators – prostaglandin E (PGE), bradykinin, substance P, adenosine triphosphate (ATP), IL-6, TNF – includes triggering pain signals, pain could be considered a homeostatic emotion that facilitates regulation of homeostasis.[17]

Apart from pain stimulation, substance P induces primarily vasodilation and increased levels are correlated to inflammatory reactions. Increased levels of substance P containing nerves have been found in the lateral retinaculum in AKP patients.[54] This suggests an inflammatory process in the knee. Since increased levels of substance P are found in chronic inflammatory diseases like rheumatoid arthritis and Mb Crohn, type of inflammation in AKP is a matter of debate.

## 2.5 Pain Mechanisms: Peripheral and Central Sensitization, Allodynia, and Hyperalgesia

The classical Cartesian view of pain is that of a homogeneous sensory entity, mediated by a specialized high threshold sensory system that extends from the periphery through the spinal cord, brain stem, and thalamus to the cerebral cortex. But multiple mechanisms that were detected in the nervous system responsible for pain of different etiologies challenge this view. Pain is a subjective experience, it is highly complex, and it is related to nociceptive input in a nonlinear fashion – but despite this, significant pro-and anti-nociceptive modulations affect the perception of this phenomenon.[8]

When pain transforms from an acute (an alarm signal) to a chronic state (a sustained challenge), sections of the nervous system (peripheral nociceptors and neurons in the dorsal horn and various areas of the brain) reorganize. Furthermore, this reorganization continues in the chronic state and has an impact on which signals reach the cortex and are recognized as pain.[5] Apart from pain's influence on cortical functions, continuous reorganization of the supraspinal brain areas responsible for descending modulations of pain occurs. Although unrecognized, descending modulation of afferent signals within the nociceptive pathways is continuous since ongoing afferent action potentials are essential to homeostatic regulation. Normally, descending modulation of afferent impulses in nociceptive pathways prevents all perception of pain – afferent impulses are transmitted from the periphery to higher levels but stop short of the cortical areas of the brain. The exception is when pain is needed to regulate homeostasis.[17]

Perception of acute pain (*nociception*) caused by a noxious stimulus is mediated by a specialized high-threshold sensory system – the nociceptive system. To prevent tissue damage, learned behavior associates certain categories of stimuli with danger that must be avoided. Noxious stimuli are linked with an intense, unpleasant sensation. Accordingly, pain is multidimensional, with sensory, cognitive, and emotional aspects. The sensation generated by acute pain must be so strong that immediate attention is required.

If tissue damage occurs despite the nociceptive defensive system, the body's imperative shifts from protecting against noxious, potentially damaging stimuli to promoting healing of the injured tissue (homeostasis). Pain during inflammatory processes – *inflammatory pain* per

Woolf's definition – is designed to accomplish this goal.[69] In this state, sensitivity (peripheral and central sensitization) increases so that stimulation of the affected area, which would normally not cause pain, now does. As a result, contact with or movement of the injured part is avoided until repair is complete, minimizing further damage. Inflammatory pain typically decreases as damage and inflammatory responses resolve.[69]

In the absence of acute tissue injury, evoked pain may arise from a low-intensity, normally innocuous stimulus, such as a light touch to the skin (mechanical receptors), or it may be an exaggerated and prolonged response to a noxious stimulus. The first condition is *allodynia* and the latter *hyperalgesia.* Allodynia is suggested to be the pain mechanism behind delayed onset muscle soreness (DOMS),[65] and perhaps represents a lower degree of alertness since this pain is not a true alarm signal. The heightened sensitivity of the nervous system that develops during prolonged inflammation can lead to pain onset in the absence of peripheral noxious stimuli (i.e., mechanical allodynia). Two major challenges in pain management are to:

- Identify the mechanisms – peripheral or central plasticity – responsible for producing allodynia and hyperalgesia.
- Find a means of normalizing sensitivity and preventing the changes from becoming established.

## 2.6 Hypoxia and Allodynia

Sometimes, mechanical allodynia is the best way for the human body to signal pain or discomfort. It is important to understand why this is so. For instance, what homeostatic problem does *the emotion of pain* signal in AKP? Perhaps bone tissue hypoxia.[47,53] And in a sprained ankle, what homeostatic problem does *the perception of pain* signal? Most likely acute tissue damage and acute inflammation.

Mechanical allodynia implies that although homeostasis is suboptimal, no acute threatening event is present, while in acute inflammation, the tissue must not be used or loaded, and high threshold nociceptors are sensitized to transmit this information.

Normally, long-standing, continuous C-fiber activity causes allodynia.[5] This continuous C-fiber activity could be a result of:

- Afferent activity starting as action potentials in nociceptors that eventually become sensitized (peripheral sensitization)
- Chemical stimuli, as in a hypoxic state[60]
- Free polymodal nerve endings that react to several stimuli

Some somatic cells – such as neurons and heart muscle cells – depend exclusively on aerobic metabolism. A short period without oxygen could be disastrous. Other cells – such as leucocytes and erythrocytes – depend exclusively on anaerobic energy production. Muscle cells are capable of anaerobic metabolism for some time. For a few minutes, type II cells can produce ATP in the absence of oxygen.

Bone cells also depend exclusively on aerobic energy production, but they are able to sustain hypoxia for hours during surgery. What impact this might have in the long term is still unknown. Hypoxia in bone tissue has been reported to cause stress fracture,[50] osteoarthrosis,[16] osteoporosis,[51] and AKP.[46,53] It is possible that these diagnoses share the same pain mechanism – mechanical allodynia caused by long-standing afferent signals transmitted in response to chemical stimuli during hypoxia.

On the other hand, intermittent hypoxia is considered one of the most important stimuli in bone remodeling. The Gross and colleagues studies have shown that disuse induces osteocyte hypoxia and that bone hyperemia is locally mediated and precedes onset of disuse-induced intracortical resorption.[29,30] Thus, the same stimulus – hypoxia – initiates bone-cell remodeling *and* causes bone-cell death. The parameters (intensity, duration) for the different reactions are still unknown.

As global regulators of oxygen homeostasis, hypoxia-inducible factors (HIFs) facilitate oxygen delivery *and* adaptations to oxygen deprivation by regulating angiogenesis, erythropoiesis, anaerobic glycolysis, and cellular proliferation (collagen I) and apoptosis.[66] And although HIF signaling appears to play a pivotal role in inflammation,[33] the functional role of HIF in chronic disease conditions is not well understood.

## 2.7 Bone Tissue, Blood Flow, and Hypoxia

Cardiovascular disease and osteoporosis are major public health problems that frequently coexist and account for significant morbidity and mortality in the aging population. Bone and vascular tissue share similar pathological features, and accumulating evidence indicates a pathophysiological link between osteoporosis and cardiovascular disease. An age-independent association between progressive atherosclerotic calcification and bone loss has been observed, as has an association between low bone mineral density and mortality due to stroke and cardiovascular disease.[67]

Atherosclerotic calcification is a regulated process with many cellular mechanisms similar to bone formation and resorption. In osteoporosis – as in atherosclerosis – excess lipids accumulate beneath the vascular intima and perivascular area in bones. In the biology of atherosclerosis, inflammation and oxidative stress play a key role – markers of inflammation are increased and correlate with the severity of the atherosclerotic process.[40] The vascular inflammatory response is a complex process that leads to thrombosis, hypoxia, angiogenesis, neointimal thickening, and atherosclerosis. Changes in bone metabolism in patients with AKP suggest an association between hypoxia, bone metabolism, and pain.[12,46,53]

Basic knowledge of how blood flow – and oxygen delivery – is regulated in bone tissue is limited. Because the role of central and peripheral mechanisms in the regulation of blood flow is unknown, the cause of reduced blood flow in bone is also unknown. Shim and Peterson observed that the most potent regulator of bone blood flow in rabbits is the metabolic control mechanism.[59] Blood flow appears to be closely related to oxygen and carbon dioxide tension, pH, and acid metabolites in blood. But in some human bones, a specific mechanism was found to regulate blood flow. For instance, in adults, most of the blood supply to the head of the femur is derived from retinacular vessels on the posterolateral surface of the femoral neck and arise from the medial femoral circumflex artery.[6] This circumstance explains why blood flow to the caput femoris is sensitive to rotation of the femur.

Brookes and Revell suggested that since aging is accompanied by marrow ischemia, periosteal vessels are increasingly responsible for blood supply to the cortex.[10] So the direction of blood flow in long bones could change during senescence. In the elderly, overall vascular patterns in irregular and flat bones vary substantially from the vascular organization of long bones in young persons – young long bones lack the high degree of periosteal blood supply found in older bones.

The patellar bone is situated anterior to the femur in the knee region. Superficially, it comprises a thin layer of cortical bone that surrounds a center composed of trabecular bone. The patella has no bone marrow cavity. Intraosseous vessels in the patellar bone are encased in rigid, unyielding bony cylinders. Five to six main arteries enter the patellar rete and form an arterial circle. These arteries also supply the distal end of the femur and the proximal region of the tibia. Anatomically, they are entirely responsible for arterial blood supply throughout the knee joint.[38] The pain in AKP may be diffuse in character and located in the anterior portion of the knee. Since arterial supply is the same for all bony parts of the knee joint, a peripatellar pain location does not contradict a hypoxic etiology.

## 2.8 Muscle Activity and Reactive Blood Flow in Bone

An important function of muscles is their role as blood pumps.[62] Wang and colleagues[64] showed that impaired venous circulation reduced interstitial blood flow in bone. Since muscle contractions pump venous blood, it is reasonable to suppose that a long-term reduction or cessation of muscle contractions could cause venous congestion in bones.

Physical exercise appears to increase blood flow to bones, but study results are so far uneven and stem mostly from animal research.[2] Kalliokoski and colleagues reported that *muscle exercise hyperemia* is more widespread if extended periods of muscle work occur at a level where aerobic metabolism is the primary source of energy.[36] The Gross and colleagues[28] study on dogs running on a treadmill found vascular constriction in bone and vasodilation in adjacent muscles.

Marked variations in measured rates of bone blood flow possibly reflect differing metabolic demands of various bone regions. Colleran and colleagues[15] suggested that the inability to precisely regulate blood flow makes bone tissue more susceptible to fluid shifts, which might play a functional role as a stimulus for skeletal remodeling. In muscle tissue, local hypoxia is known to be vital for peripheral blood flow, even though most details of this process are still unknown. Hypoxia is also a possible regulator of microcirculation in bone tissue, but this has not yet been studied in humans.

We have recently found (unpublished) that patellar bone blood flow is influenced by the type of muscle contractions that occur in the surrounding muscle compartments (m. Vastus lateralis). Bone reactive hyperemia was greater after anaerobic muscle work than after aerobic work. This finding supports the Utah Paradigm, which proposes that muscle contractions are key stimuli for bone health.[26]

## 2.9 Functional Pain

Woolf proposed a new mechanism-based pain classification.[69] As mentioned, AKP is probably best classified as inflammatory pain or functional pain. Although inflammatory and functional pains have different etiologies, they share some characteristics: (1) the pain may arise spontaneously in the apparent absence of any peripheral stimulus and (2) it may be evoked by stimuli. Evoked pain may arise from a low-intensity, normally innocuous stimulus, such as a light touch to the skin or normal non-recognized afferent homeostatic action potentials.

Functional pain is an evolving concept. No neurologic deficit or peripheral abnormality has been detected in this type of pain – it arises due to abnormal responsiveness or abnormal functioning of the nervous system in which heightened gain or sensitivity of the sensory apparatus amplifies symptoms. Several common diagnoses have features that suggest functional pain[69]:

- Fibromyalgia
- Irritable bowel syndrome (IBS)
- Some forms of noncardiac chest pain
- Tension-type headache
- Low back pain (LBP)
- Temporomandibular dysfunction (TMD)

AKP shares many of the characteristics reported in these chronic pain conditions.

It is not known why the central nervous system in patients with functional pain displays abnormal sensitivity or hyperresponsiveness. Still, functional pain is the result of abnormal central processing of normal input. Several lines of evidence support the concept of an altered pain modulatory system (either a dysfunctional descending inhibition or enhanced descending facilitation) in chronic pain states. Recent studies provide evidence that active afferent inhibition of nociceptive input is one way in which cognition modulates pain perception.[8]

In functional pain diagnoses, pain-related psychiatric comorbidity – such as depression, anxiety, and sleeping disorders – are of interest since cognitive and emotional aspects of pain experience are important. Psychological variables, such as catastrophizing, anxiety, and depression, have been implicated in AKP,[14,34,61,68] raising the suspicion that AKP may have nonorganic causes.

Patients with functional pain undergo a different spectrum of treatment modalities – cognitive behavior therapy (CBT) and anti-depressant medication – than patients with inflammatory pain. This leads to the fundamental issue of whether (1) the descending modulatory system in chronic pain patients is faulty or (2) psychological factors like hypervigilance, catastrophizing, and anxiety hinder these patients from an adequate engagement of pain modulation systems. So, it should not be surprising that patients who have had chronic pain for many years develop depression and a passive attitude.

## 2.10 Anterior Knee Pain in Children and Adolescents

Nonspecific AKP probably has varying etiologies and thus varying pain mechanisms. In children and adolescents, bone growth in relation to the apophysis can trigger an inflammatory reaction when excess stress is put on a musculotendinous junction adjacent to the apophysis. In the knee region, this reaction can occur at apex patellae (Mb Sinding-Larsen, Johansson) and at tuberositas tibiae (Mb Osgaard-Schlatter).

An acute inflammation may occur in response to too much strain. But even in non-acute periods, apophyses are known to produce feelings of pain or discomfort during stress. Since bone growth is warranted and programmed in this situation, peripheral sensitization is probably not the optimal pain mechanism for regulating homeostasis – allodynia is most likely a better regulator of physical activity. A slightly disturbed homeostasis should not induce alarm signals.

Pain from the patellar tendon after intensive use of m. quadriceps is commonly called jumper's knee – or patellar tendinopathy. This diagnosis refers to an overuse problem that causes an inflammatory reaction. Although distinguishing clinically between jumper's knee and Mb Sinding-Larsen, Johansson is nearly impossible in adolescents, it is important for choice of treatment regime. Regions of the skeleton that are undergoing growth are by nature weak and vulnerable. In children and adolescents, the apophysis will be weaker than the attached tendons while in adults, bone tissue is better able to withstand impact. Different pain mechanisms in the two conditions are probable.

AKP-related research has studied populations of varying ages. Clinical reports of remission or healing of AKP following conservative treatment are common. But as Kannus and colleagues observed, about 30% of AKP patients still have pain years later.[37] These conflicting opinions might arise because bone growth-related pain diminishes with time and ceases when mature bone is established. If AKP has a different etiology, healing may be time independent.

Dye and colleagues reported that, in the knee region, the anterior synovium, the fat pad, and the joint capsule are most sensitive to nociceptive stimuli.[22] Direct trauma and indirect impacts can cause inflammatory reactions in these structures. In the case of direct trauma, the duration of acute inflammation will be brief. But if hypoxia is the source of the inflammatory reaction, and if the hypoxic state continues, a radically different situation occurs.

Because long-standing hypoxia induces central sensitization, the most obvious symptom would be mechanical allodynia. Clinically, typical findings in AKP are activity-induced pain (climbing stairs) and movie sign pain (sitting with flexed knees for prolonged periods). Mechanical allodynia explains these symptoms well.

Exploring the cause of a hypoxic state is critical for treatment success. Sanchis-Alfonso hypothesized that short, periodic episodes of ischemia in the lateral retinaculum is a probable etiology of AKP.[53] The ischemia could trigger neural proliferation of nociceptive axons (substance P-positive nerves), mainly in a perivascular location. The Näslund and colleagues study on pulsatile blood flow in the patellar bone found that flexing the knee 90° significantly reduced blood flow in AKP patients but not in controls.[47] This decrease in blood flow might explain not only the suggested ischemia but also the increased bone metabolism that several studies report, since short episodes of ischemia trigger bone remodeling.[12,21,46]

Sensitivity to cold surroundings is a common clinical feature in AKP. Ben-Eliyahu reported disturbances in knee skin temperature regulation and Selfe and colleagues suggested a cold test for diagnostic purposes.[7,57,58] This is all compatible with the current theory of tissue homeostasis used to explain the genesis of AKP.[20]

But several factors could have an impact on homeostasis. In adolescence, bone growth is vital and is the most prominent factor regulating homeostasis. In school, youth sit daily for hours with flexed knees. Many adults also spend their working days in a sitting position. Combined with impaired arterial supply to knee bones, these circumstances might prevent time-dependent healing and initiate chronic inflammation.

## 2.11 Treatment Modalities and Pain-Relieving Mechanisms in Anterior Knee Pain

Conservative treatment is the first choice for dealing with unspecified AKP. But there are many modalities, and no consensus has been reached. A probable pain mechanism – if one could be found – would help determine the best treatment modality.[69] But in lieu of a pain mechanism, the next best course is to retrospectively analyze effects of various treatment regimes to explore possible etiologies and pain mechanisms. The current treatment modalities that are most interesting are discussed below in relation to pain mechanism.

### *2.11.1 Muscle Exercises*

Any treatment regime comprising muscle exercises – straight leg raises (isometric muscle activity), open or closed chain exercises (dynamic muscle activity), hip muscle exercises, or functional exercises for the lower extremities – will increase blood flow to the knee region and help decrease any hypoxia. Pain relief after muscle activity could indicate that hypoxia is the main pain mechanism, especially if movie sign pain is a symptom (see the mechanical allodynia section).

Physical activity is also being increasingly advocated in chronic pain treatment. But explanations of the exact mechanisms behind treatment effects are sparse. One proposal is the release of endogenous opioids. But production of endogenous opioids increases only when physiological stress is apparent and recognized, and the low amount and intensity of exercises commonly used in AKP regimes make it unlikely that endogenous opioids explain the pain relief experienced after lower extremity exercises.

Increased muscle strength after successful rehabilitation has sometimes been suggested as an explanation of pain relief. But if this were so, pain would also arise due to hypotrophy induced by muscular inactivity, and this has not yet been shown. More likely, muscular defects in AKP patients should be viewed as a *consequence* of pain and muscular inactivity – not a cause.

### 2.11.2 Sympathetic Blockades

Butler-Manuel successfully used sympathetic blockades to treat AKP patients who presented increased bone metabolism on scintigraphy.[12] With sympathetic-mediated pain, blockades of sympathetic tone not only have pain-relieving effects, but will also increase blood flow and eventually decrease hypoxia.

### 2.11.3 Nonsteroid Anti-inflammatory Drugs (NSAIDs)

The anti-inflammatory effect of NSAIDs arises from inhibition of prostaglandin synthesis, largely by inhibiting the cyclooxygenase (COX) enzymes, which catalyze the conversion of arachidonic acid to prostaglandins. This synthesis usually occurs in the acute phase of an inflammation when arachidonic acid is freed from a phospholipid molecule. Accordingly, NSAIDs decrease pain mostly in the acute phase of inflammation. The Heintjes and colleagues study on unspecified AKP and NSAIDs found such treatment to have questionable effects, which suggests that the pain in AKP is not prostaglandin mediated or caused by acute inflammatory reactions.[32]

### 2.11.4 Taping

The pain-relieving effect of taping regimes has not yet been satisfactorily explained. Although various taping techniques have been presented, exactly how and where the tape is attached to the patellar bone appears to be less important.[13] It might be that allodynia is inhibited when other afferent stimuli are imposed. The proprioceptive role of the tape touching the skin is one example of increased afferent signals able to inhibit allodynia. Taping might also stimulate tactile C fibers responsible for the sense of well-being.[49]

### 2.11.5 Knee Braces

Apart from inducing afferent signals through skin stimulation, knee braces may also raise skin temperature in the knee region. Most knee braces for patients with AKP are made of neoprene – a material known to increase skin temperature. Afferent signals transmitting a sense of higher temperature could cause pain reduction via the well-known gate-control theory.

### 2.11.6 Acupuncture

A systematic review on the quality of randomized controlled trials of nonoperative AKP treatment found acupuncture to have the highest methodology score.[9] Because classic deep acupuncture *and* superficial needling produce the same pain relief, important clues for explaining pain mechanisms should be sought in the CNS.[45] Sandberg and colleagues[55] found that both deep and superficial acupuncture may increase peripheral blood flow, so it is possible that acupuncture normalizes hypoxia and allodynia.

### 2.11.7 Surgery

Biomechanically, the knee joint is considered to be one of the most complicated joints in our body. Fulkerson proposed that biomechanical abnormalities are responsible for malfunctions of the patellofemoral contact, which then produce irritation and inflammation.[27]

Although surgery has been advocated for correcting malalignment and has been performed when conservative treatment fails, it is now rarely recommended in patients with AKP – especially not in children and adolescents.[19]

After surgery, an immediate pain-relieving effect is often experienced. Several explanations for this pain relief have been proposed. One is that denervation occurring in surgery could be responsible. But surgery nearly always means that physical activity decreases for some time and pain causing activities are avoided. The reactive hyperemia following any surgery in the knee region might also help normalize hypoxia and thus be beneficial.

## 2.12 Conclusions

In any long-term pain condition, a causal explanation is important to seek. One is that a mild disturbance of homeostasis, so mild that it is clinically undetectable, could signal pain. Pain mechanisms differ depending on onset stimulus, immune reactions, and type of inflammation, so distinguishing possible pain mechanisms is valuable. Analyzing inflammatory mediators and immune cells may reveal meaningful information in the search for a diffuse AKP etiology. Retrospective analyses of prior treatment modalities may also yield important clues. This chapter has argued that hypoxia suits well as an etiological factor in AKP.

## References


1. Abbas AK, Lichtman AH. *Basic Immunology: Functions and Disorders of the Immune System*. Philadelphia: Saunders Elsevier; 2007.
2. Albertazzi P, Steel SA, Botazzi M. Effect of intermittent compression therapy on bone mineral density in women with low bone mass. *Bone*. 2005;37:662-668.
3. Alfredson H. The chronic painful Achilles and patellar tendon: research on basic biology and treatment. *Scand J Med Sci Sports*. 2005;15:252-259.
4. Andersson HI, Ejlertsson G, Leden I, et al. Chronic pain in a geographically defined general population: studies of different age, gender, social class, and pain location. *Clin J Pain*. 1993;9:174-182.
5. Apkarian AV, Baliki MN, Geha PY. Towards a theory of chronic pain. *Prog Neurobiol*. 2009;87:81-97.
6. Beaulé PE, Campbell P, Lu Z, et al. Vascularity of the arthritic femoral head and hip resurfacing. *J Bone Joint Surg*. 2006;88-A(Suppl 4):85-96.
7. Ben-Eliyahu D. Infrared thermographic imaging in the detection of sympathetic dysfunction in patients with patellofemoral pain syndrome. *J Manipulative Physiol Ther*. 1992;3:164-170.
8. Bingel U, Tracey I. Imaging CNS modulation of pain in humans. *Physiology*. 2008;23:371-380.
9. Bizzini M, Childs JD, Piva SR, et al. Systematic review of the quality of randomized controlled trials for patellofemoral pain syndrome. *J Orthop Sports Phys Ther*. 2003;33:4-20.
10. Brookes M, Revell WJ. *Blood Supply of Bone*. London: Springer; 1998.
11. Brushøj C, Henriksen BM, Albrecht-Beste E, et al. Acute patellofemoral pain: aggravating activities, clinical examination, MRI and ultrasound findings. *Br J Sports Med*. 2008; 42:64-67.
12. Butler-Manuel PA. Sympathetically mediated anterior knee pain. *Acta Orthop Scand*. 1992;63:90-93.
13. Callaghan MJ, Selfe J, McHenry A, et al. Effects of patellar taping on knee joint proprioception in patients with patellofemoral pain syndrome. *Man Ther*. 2008;13:192-199.
14. Carlsson AM, Werner S, Mattlar CE, et al. Personality in patients with long-term patellofemoral pain syndrome. *Knee Surg Sports Traumatol Arthrosc*. 1993;1:178-183.
15. Colleran NP, Wilkerson MK, Bloomfield SA, et al. Alterations in skeletal perfusion with simulated microgravity: a possible mechanism for bone remodeling. *J Appl Physiol*. 2000;89:1046-1054.
16. Conaghan PG, Vanharanta H, Dieppe PA. Is progressive osteoarthritis an atheromatous vascular disease? *Ann Rheum Dis*. 2005;64:1539-1541.
17. Craig AD. A new view of pain as a homeostatic emotion. *Trends Neurosci*. 2003;26:303-307.
18. Dieppe PA, Lohmander S. Pathogenesis and management of pain in osteoarthritis. *Lancet*. 2005;365:965-973.
19. Dixit S, DiFiori JP, Burton M, et al. Management of patellofemoral pain syndrome. *Am Fam Physician*. 2007;75:194-202.
20. Dye SF. The pathophysiology of patellofemoral pain. *Clin Orthop Relat Res*. 2005;436:100-110.
21. Dye SF, Chew MH. The use of scintigraphy to detect increased osseous metabolic activity about the knee. *J Bone Joint Surg*. 1993;75:1388-1406.
22. Dye SF, Vaupel GL, Dye CC. Conscious neurosensory mapping of the internal structures of the human knee without intraarticular anesthesia. *Am J Sports Med*. 1998;26:773-777.
23. Fearon I, McGrath PJ, Achat H. 'Booboos': the study of everyday pain among children. *Pain*. 1996;68:55-62.
24. Firestein GS, Corr M. Common mechanisms in immune-mediated inflammatory disease. *J Rheumatol*. 2005;32(Suppl 73): 8-13.
25. Forsgren S, Grimsholm O, Jönsson M, et al. New insight into the non-neuronal cholinergic system via studies on chronically painful tendons and inflammatory situations. *Life Sci*. 2009;84:865-870.
26. Frost HM. A 2003 update of bone physiology and Wolff"s law for clinicians. *Angle Orthod*. 2004;74:3-15.
27. Fulkerson JP et al. *Disorders of the Patellofemoral Joint*. 4th ed. Philadelphia: Lippincott Williams & Wilkins; 2004.

28. Gross PM, Marcus ML, Heistad DD. Measurements of blood flow to bone and marrow in experimental animals by means of the microsphere technique. *J Bone Joint Surg*. 1981;6: 1028-1031.
29. Gross TS, Damji AA, Judex S, et al. Bone hyperemia precedes disuse-induced intracortical bone resorption. *J Appl Physiol*. 1999;86:230-235.
30. Gross TS, Poliachik SL, Ausk BJ, et al. Why rest stimulates bone formation: a hypothesis based on complex adaptive phenomenon. *Exerc Sport Sci Rev*. 2004;32:9-13.
31. Hasselström J, Liu-Palmgren J, Rasjö-Wrååk G. Prevalence of pain in general practice. *Eur J Pain*. 2002;6:375-385.
32. Heintjes E, Berger MY, Bierma-Zeinstra SM, et al (2004) Pharmacotherapy for patellofemoral pain syndrome. *Cochrane Database Syst Rev*. 3: CD003470.
33. Higgins DF, Kimura K, Iwano M, et al. Hypoxia-inducible factor signaling in the development of tissue fibrosis. *Cell Cycle*. 2008;7:1128-1132.
34. Jensen R, Hystad T, Barheim A. Knee function and pain related to psychological variables in patients with long-term patellofemoral pain syndrome. *J Orthop Sports Phys Ther*. 2005;35:594-600.
35. Jensen R, Kvale A, Baerheim A. Is patellofemoral pain neuropathic? *Clin J Pain*. 2008;24:384-394.
36. Kalliokoski KK, Kemppainen J, Larmola K, et al. Muscle blood flow and flow heterogeneity during exercise studied with positron emission tomography in humans. *Eur J Appl Physiol*. 2000;83:395-401.
37. Kannus P, Natri A, Paakkala T, et al. An outcome study of chronic patellofemoral pain syndrome. Seven-year follow-up of patients in a randomized, controlled trial. *J Bone Joint Surg*. 1999;81-A:355-363.
38. Kirschner MH, Menck J, Nerlich A, et al. The arterial blood supply of the human patella. Its clinical importance for the operating technique in vascularized knee joint transplantations. *Surg Radiol Anat*. 1997;19:345-351.
39. Kogianni G, Mann V, Noble BS. Apoptotic bodies convey activity capable of initiating osteoclastogenesis and localized bone destruction. *J Bone Miner Res*. 2008;6:915-927.
40. Libby P. Inflammation in atherosclerosis. *Nature*. 2002; 420:868-874.
41. Loeser JD, Treede RD. The Kyoto protocol of IASP basic pain terminology. *Pain*. 2008;137:473-477.
42. Mease P. Fibromyalgia syndrome: review of clinical presentation, pathogenesis, outcome measures, and treatment. *J Rheumatol*. 2005;32(Suppl 75):6-21.
43. MelzackP Wall P. *Textbook of Pain*. 4th ed. London: Harcourt Publishers Limited; 2000.
44. Mosser DM, Edwards JP. Exploring the full spectrum of macrophage activation. *Nat Rev Immunol*. 2008;8:958-969.
45. Näslund J, Näslund UB, Odenbring S, et al. Sensory stimulation (acupuncture) for the treatment of idiopathic anterior knee pain. *J Rehabil Med*. 2002;34:231-238.
46. Näslund J, Odenbring S, Näslund UB, et al. Diffusely increased bone scintigraphic uptake in patellofemoral pain syndrome. *Br J Sports Med*. 2005;39:162-165.
47. Näslund J, Waldén M, Lindberg LG. Decreased pulsatile blood flow in the patella in patellofemoral pain. *Am J Sports Med*. 2007;35:1668-1673.
48. Noble B. Microdamage and apoptosis. *Eur J Morphol*. 2005;42:91-98.
49. Olausson HW, Cole J, Vallbo A, et al. Unmyelinated tactile afferents have opposite effects on insular and somatosensory cortical processing. *Neurosci Lett*. 2008;436:128-132.
50. Otter MW, Qin YX, Rbin CT, et al. Does bone perfusion/reperfusion initiate bone remodeling and the stress fracture syndrome? *Med Hypotheses*. 1999;53:363-368.
51. Pennisi P, Signorelli SS, Riccoben S, et al. Low bone density and abnormal bone turnover in patients with atherosclerosis of peripheral vessels. *Osteoporos Int*. 2004;15:389-395.
52. Ryles MT, Pilmanis AA. The initial signs and symptoms of altitude decompression sickness. *Aviat Space Environ Med*. 1996;10:983-989.
53. Sanchis-Alfonso V. Patellofemorale schmerzen. *Orthopade*. 2008;37:835-840.
54. Sanchis-Alfonso V, Roselló-Sastre E, Subías-Lopez A. Neuroanatomic basis for pain in patellar tendinosis ("jumper's knee"): a neuroimmunohistochemical study. *Am J Knee Surg*. 2001;14:174-177.
55. Sandberg M, Zhang Q, Styf J, et al. Non-invasive monitoring of muscle blood perfusion by photoplethysmography: evaluation of a new application. *Acta Physiol Scand*. 2005;183: 335-343.
56. Scott A, Khan KM, Roberts R, et al. What do we mean by the term "inflammation"? A contemporary basic science update for sports medicine. *Br J Sports Med*. 2004;38:372-380.
57. Selfe J, Harper L, Pedersen I, et al. Cold legs: a potential indicator of negative outcome in the rehabilitation of patients with patellofemoral pain syndrome. *Knee*. 2003;10:139-143.
58. Selfe J, Karki A, Stevens D. A review of the role of circulatory deficit in the genesis of patellofemoral pain. *Phys Ther Rev*. 2002;7:169-172.
59. Shim SS, Patterson FP. A direct method of qualitative study of bone blood circulation. *Surg Gynecol Obstet*. 1967;125: 261-268.
60. Soe HS, Kim HW, Roh DH, et al. A new rat model for thrombus-induced ischemic pain (TIIP); development of bilateral mechanical allodynia. *Pain*. 2008;139:520-532.
61. Thomee P, Thomee R, Karlsoon J. Patellofemoral pain syndrome: pain, coping strategies and degree of well-being. *Scand J Med Sci Sports*. 2002;12:276-281.
62. Trueta J. The role of the vessels in osteogenesis. *J Bone Joint Surg*. 1963;45-B:402-418.
63. Vodovotz Y, Constantine G, Rubin J, et al. Mechanistic stimulation of inflammation: current state and future prospects. *Math Biosci*. 2009;217:1-10.
64. Wang L, Fritton SP, Weinbaum S, et al. On bone adaption due to venous stasis. *J Biomech*. 2003;36:1439-1451.
65. Weerakkody NS, Percival P, Hickey MW, et al. Effects of local pressure and vibration on muscle pain from eccentric exercise and hypertonic saline. *Pain*. 2003;105:425-435.
66. Wenger RH, Stiehl DP, Camenisch G. Integration of oxygen signaling at the consensus HRE. *Sci STKE*. 2005;2005(306): re12.
67. Whitney C, Warburton D, Frohlich J, et al. Are cardiovascular disease and osteoporosis directly linked? *Sports Med*. 2004;34:779-807.
68. Witonski D. Anterior knee pain syndrome. *Int Orthop*. 1999;23:341-344.
69. Woolf CJ. Pain: moving from symptom control toward mechanism-specific pharmacologic management. *Ann Intern Med*. 2004;140:441-451.

# 3 Biological Causes of Anterior Knee Pain

Vicente Sanchis-Alfonso, Esther Roselló-Sastre, Juan Saus-Mas, and Fernando Revert-Ros

## 3.1 Introduction

Despite an abundance of clinical and basic science research, anterior knee pain syndrome or patellofemoral pain syndrome (PFPS) remains, according to John Insall, an orthopedic "enigma" ("Black hole of Orthopedics"). The numerous treatment regimes that exist for PFPS highlight the lack of knowledge regarding the etiology of the pain. At present, no theory provides a comprehensive explanation of the true nature of this pathologic condition or how to hasten its resolution in a safe and reliable way. This chapter reviews the literature and synthesizes our research on anterior knee pain pathophysiology. This topic is clinically relevant because patient management will be greatly simplified when we understand what the causes are for anterior knee pain in the young patient.

We are fully aware that anterior knee pain cannot be blamed on one single factor, but rather a multiplicity of factors is involved. Peripheral neurologic signals resulting in perceived pain can only come from innervated structures. Articular cartilage has no nerve endings. However, the infrapatellar fat pad, subchondral bone, the synovium, the medial and lateral retinaculum all have a rich nerve supply, and each of these structures, individually or in combination, could be a potential source of nociceptive output resulting in the perception of pain at any given moment. Moreover, we must also consider some influencing factors such as: gender, overuse, instability, psychological factors, and patellofemoral malalignment* (PFM) with the subsequent retinacular and subchondral overload. Therefore, it is very likely that different subgroups of PFPS exist. One way to shed some light on the etiology of pain would be the histological study of the above-mentioned anatomical structures.

## 3.2 "Neural Model" in the Genesis of Anterior Knee Pain. Neuroanatomic Bases for Anterior Knee Pain in the Young Patient

Based on our histological studies,[61,62,65-69] we have developed what we call "Neural Model"[63] as an explanation for the genesis of anterior knee pain in the young patient.

Most of our studies on anterior knee pain pathophysiology[61,62,65-67] have been focused on the lateral retinaculum (67 specimens analyzed) retrieved during patellofemoral realignment surgery. There is clinical support to believe that this anatomical structure plays a key role in the genesis of anterior knee pain in the young patient.[10,20,23,34,40,61,62,64-67,83]

Patients with patellar symptoms can be divided into two groups: those with anterior knee pain as the main

V. Sanchis-Alfonso (✉)
International Patellofemoral Study Group, International ACL Study Group, Hospital 9 de Octubre,
Hospital Arnau de Vilanova, School of Medicine,
Catholic University of Valencia, Valencia, Spain
e-mail: vicente.sanchis.alfonso@gmail.com

*We define patellofemoral malalignment (PFM) as an abnormality of the patellar tracking in the sense of lateral displacement of the patella or lateral tilt of the patella or both in extension that is reduced in flexion

V. Sanchis-Alfonso (ed.), *Anterior Knee Pain and Patellar Instability*,
DOI: 10.1007/978-0-85729-507-1_3, © Springer-Verlag London Limited 2011

complaint and those with patellar instability as the predominant symptom. To obtain a homogeneous population, we have included only those patients in our study group[61,62,65-67] who had: (1) tenderness over the lateral retinaculum and excessive lateral tightness in the cases in which the main symptom was pain; and patients who had instability in the lateral direction in the cases in which the predominant symptom was instability, (2) PFM demonstrated with CT, (3) no previous knee surgery, (4) no peripatellar tendinosis and bursitis, and (5) no associated intraarticular pathology (synovitis, meniscal tears, ACL/PCL tears, osteoarthritis) confirmed arthroscopically. Given that our objective was to study "pain," the patellar instability group was used as control group.

According to Fulkerson,[18] in patients with PFM, there is an adaptative shortening of the lateral retinaculum as a consequence of the lateral displacement of the patella. With knee flexion, the patella migrates medially into the femoral trochlea,[60] which produces a recurrent stretching on the shortened lateral retinaculum that may cause nerve changes such as neuromas and neural myxoid degeneration.[18,20]

### 3.2.1 Morphologic Neural Changes into the Lateral Retinaculum

Some studies have suggested neural damage into the lateral retinaculum as a possible source of pain in the young patient. In 1985, Fulkerson and colleagues[20] described for the first time nerve damage (demyelination and fibrosis) in the lateral retinaculum of patients with intractable patellofemoral pain requiring lateral retinacular release or realignment of the patellofemoral joint. The changes observed by these authors in the retinacular nerves resembled the histopathologic picture of Morton's interdigital neuroma. Later, in 1991, Mori and colleagues[50] published a paper in which they analyzed histologically the lateral retinaculum of 35 knees of 22 patients suffering from anterior knee pain. They found severe degenerative neuropathy in 9 knees, moderate changes in 9, and slight in 11; the remaining 6 knees were normal. Like these authors, we have also observed in many cases, in the lateral retinaculum, chronic degenerative nonspecific changes in nerve fibers, with myxoid degeneration of the endoneurium, retraction of the axonal component, and perineural fibrosis (Fig. 3.1).[65,67] Likewise, a smaller group of specimens presented nerve fibers mimicking amputation neuromas seen in other parts of the body[65,67] (Fig. 3.1). However, we have found no inflammatory component associated with vascular or nerve structures that could explain the presence of pain in these patients, except for a population of mast cells immersed in the fibrous bands surrounding vessels (Fig. 3.2). Regarding neuromas, we have seen a clear relationship between their presence and anterior knee pain.[62,65,67] In contrast, we have found no relationship between neural myxoid degeneration and anterior knee pain.[62,65]

Nerve damage occurs diffusely in the affected retinaculum, and therefore one must consider the possibility of multiple neurologic sequelae in the peripatellar region. A possible consequence of this nerve damage could be an altered proprioceptive innervation.[20] Baker and colleagues observed abnormal knee joint position sense (proprioception) in subjects with PFPS.[32] This is in agreement with the clinical study of Jerosch and Prymka in 1996,[33] which revealed a highly significant reduction in knee proprioception after patella dislocation, explained by the damage of neuroproprioceptive fibers.[33,81]

Current research shows the importance of proprioceptive information from joint mechanoreceptors for proper knee function. Connective tissues, in addition to their mechanical function, play an important role in transmitting specific somatosensory afferent signals to the spinal and cerebral regulatory systems. Thus, the giving-way in patients with PFPS can be explained, at least in part, because of the alteration or loss of joint afferent information concerning proprioception due to the nerve damage of the ascendent proprioception pathway or a decrease of healthy nerve fibers capable of transmitting proprioceptory stimuli.[65] In conclusion, it seems likely that, to a certain degree, the instability in patients with PFPS depends not only on mechanical factors (such as patella alta, soft tissue dysplasia, and patellar and trochlear dysplasia) but also on neural factors (proprioceptive deficit both in the sense of position, and in slowing or decrease of stabilizing and protective reflexes).[19,24,33,81] Jensen and colleagues[32] demonstrated an abnormal sensory function in the painful and non-painful knee in some subjects with long-lasting unilateral PFPS. A dysfunction of the peripheral and/or the central nervous system may cause neuropathic pain in some individuals with PFPS.

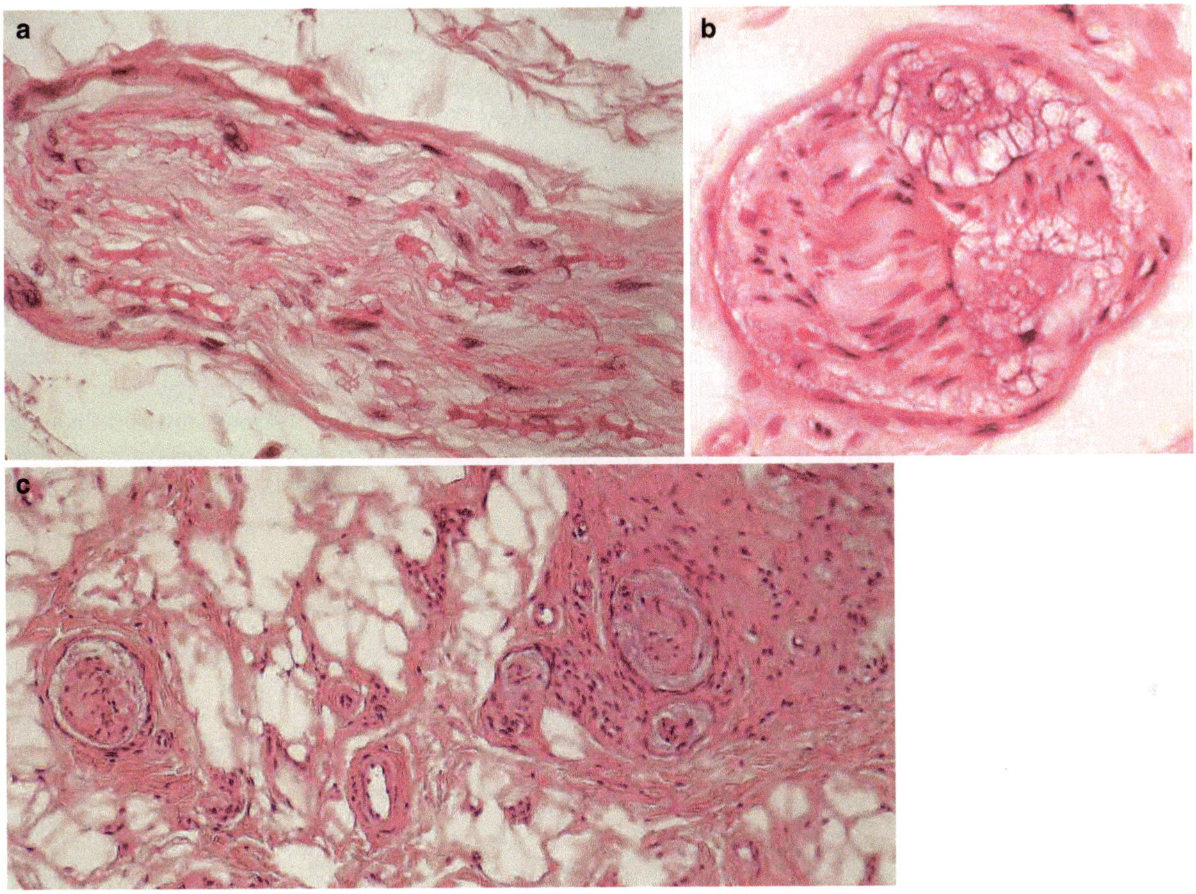


**Fig. 3.1** Histologic features of a normal nerve (**a**), a nerve with neural myxoid degeneration (**b**), and a tissular neuroma (**c**) in the lateral retinaculum. (Hematoxylin-Eosin stain) (**b** – Reproduced from Sanchis-Alfonso et al.[65] Reprinted by permission from Thieme, **c** – Reproduced from Sanchis-Alfonso et al.[65], copyright © 1998, Reprinted by permission of SAGE Publications)

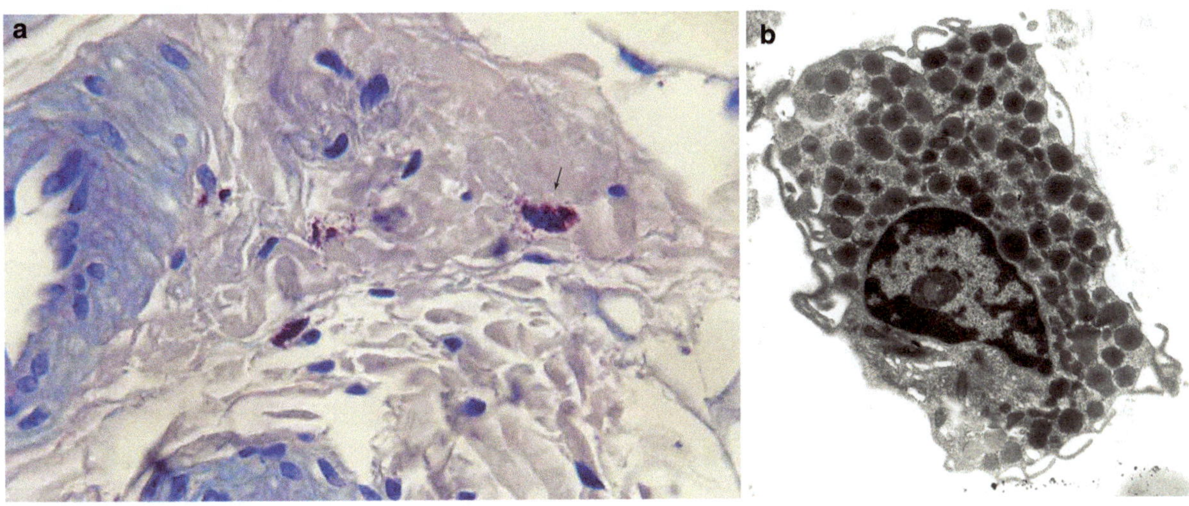


**Fig. 3.2** Mast cells are abundant in the stroma (*arrow*), mainly in a perivascular disposition. Some of them show a degranulation process (activated mast cells) (**a**) (Giemsa stain). Ultrastructural image of a mast cell of the lateral retinaculum with its cytoplasm full of chemotactic granules, (TEM) (**b**) (**a** – Reproduced from Sanchis-Alfonso et al.[62] copyright © 2000, Reprinted by permission of SAGE Publications)

### 3.2.2 Relationship Between Hyperinnervation into the Lateral Retinaculum and Anterior Knee Pain. Immunohistochemical Analysis for Neural Markers

Our studies have suggested hyperinnervation into the lateral retinaculum as a possible source of anterior knee pain in the young patient.[65,67] Thus, we found an increase in the number of nerves in the lateral retinaculum of patients with painful PFM, with higher values in those with severe pain compared with those with moderate or light pain.[67] Moreover, we have seen that the lateral retinaculum of the patients with pain as the predominant symptom showed a higher innervation pattern than the medial retinaculum or the lateral retinaculum of patients with patellar instability as the main symptom.[62] This nerve ingrowth, consisted of myelinated (specifically immunoreactive to S-100 protein) and unmyelinated nerve fibers (specifically immunoreactive to neurofilament protein [NF]) (Fig. 3.3) with a predominant nociceptive component.[62]

The nociceptive properties of at least some of these nerves are evidenced by their substance P (SP) immunoreactivity. SP, which is found in primary sensory neurons and C fibers (slow-chronic pain pathway), is involved in the neurotransmission pathways of nociceptive signals.[3,5-7,13,17,26,36-38,56,82,83] SP was detected in the axons of big nerve fibers, in free nerve endings, and in

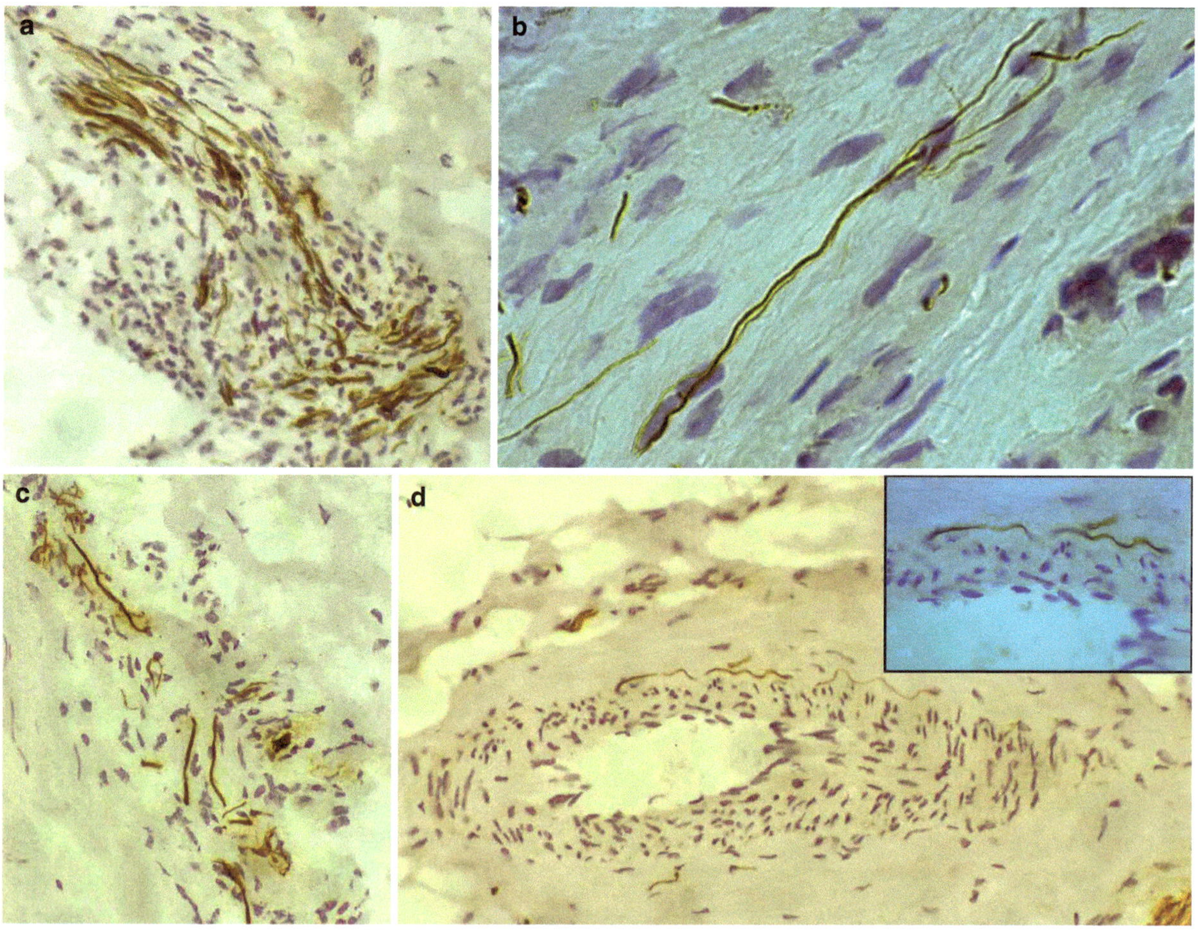


**Fig. 3.3** An increased innervation is evident in the connective tissue, showing microneuromas (**a**) and free nerve endings immersed in the stroma (**b**), or next to small vessels (**c**). Vascular innervation is also increased with tiny axons arranged like a necklace in the adventitia (**d**) (**a–c** – Reproduced from Sanchis-Alfonso et al.[62] copyright © 2000, Reprinted by permission of SAGE Publications)

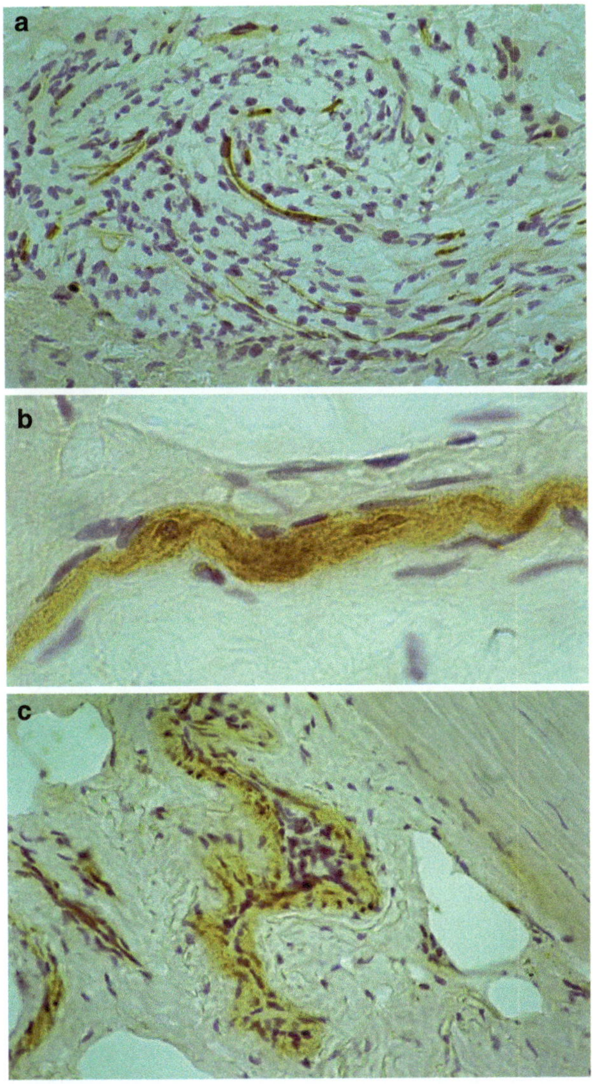


**Fig. 3.4** Neuromas are rich in nociceptive axons, as can be demonstrated studying substance P (**a**). Substance P is present in the axons of the nerves and in the free nerve endings with a granular pattern (**b**), and can be observed in the vessel walls in some patients with painful symptoms (**c**). (Immunohistochemistry for Substance P. Frozen sections) (**a**, **b** – Reproduced from Sanchis-Alfonso et al.[62] copyright © 2000, Reprinted by permission of SAGE Publications)

the vessel walls in some patients with pain as predominant symptom[62] (Fig. 3.4). Nociceptive fibers, that is, neural fibers with intra-axonal SP, were lower in number than NF fibers, indicating that not all the tiny perivascular or interstitial nerves were nociceptive.[62] Interestingly, our finding that SP fibers were more abundant in the lateral retinaculum than in its medial counterpart (13 specimens of medial retinaculum analyzed) reinforce the role of the lateral retinaculum as a main source of pain in these patients.[62] Moreover, we have observed that the number of these nociceptive fibers was higher in PFM patients suffering from pain as the main symptom than in those with instability as the predominant symptom (with little or no pain between instability episodes).[62]

Nerve ingrowth is mostly located within and around vessels[62,65,67] (Fig. 3.5). Thus, we have seen, in the lateral retinaculum of patients with painful PFM, S-100 positive fibers in the adventitial and within the muscular layer of medium and small arteries, resembling a necklace. S-100 protein is a good marker when studying nerves, because of its ability to identify Schwann cells that accompany the axons in their myelinated part. It is well known that myelinated fibers lose their myelin sheath before entering into the muscular arterial wall, but this was not the case in our patients. Since we were studying by S-100 immunostaining only the myelinated fibers, and the myelin sheath is supposed to be lost before the nerve enters the muscular arterial wall, we were surprised by the identification of S-100-positive fibers within the muscular layer of medium and small arteries. Therefore, our findings may be considered as an increase in vascular innervation. We have demonstrated that vascular innervation was more prominent (94%) in patients with severe pain, whereas this type of hyperinnervation was found in only 30% of the patients with light or moderate pain.[67] Our findings are in agreement with the statement of Byers that postulated in 1968, that pain in the osteoid osteoma could be generated and transmitted by vascular pressure-sensitive autonomic nerves.[11]

In reviewing the literature, we have seen that hyperinnervation is also a factor implicated in the pathophysiology of pain in other orthopedic abnormalities such as chronic back pain, and jumper's knee.[13,17,68] On the other hand, pain has also been related with vascular innervation in some pathologies as is the case of an osteoid osteoma,[28] where the authors found an increase in perivascular innervation in all their cases, postulating that pain was more related with this innervation than with the release of prostaglandin $E_2$. Grönblad and colleagues[25] have also found similar findings in the lumbar pain of the facet syndrome. Finally, Alfredson and colleagues[4] related pain in Achilles tendinosis with vasculo-neural ingrowth.

We have demonstrated that hyperinnervation is associated with the release of neural growth factor (NGF),

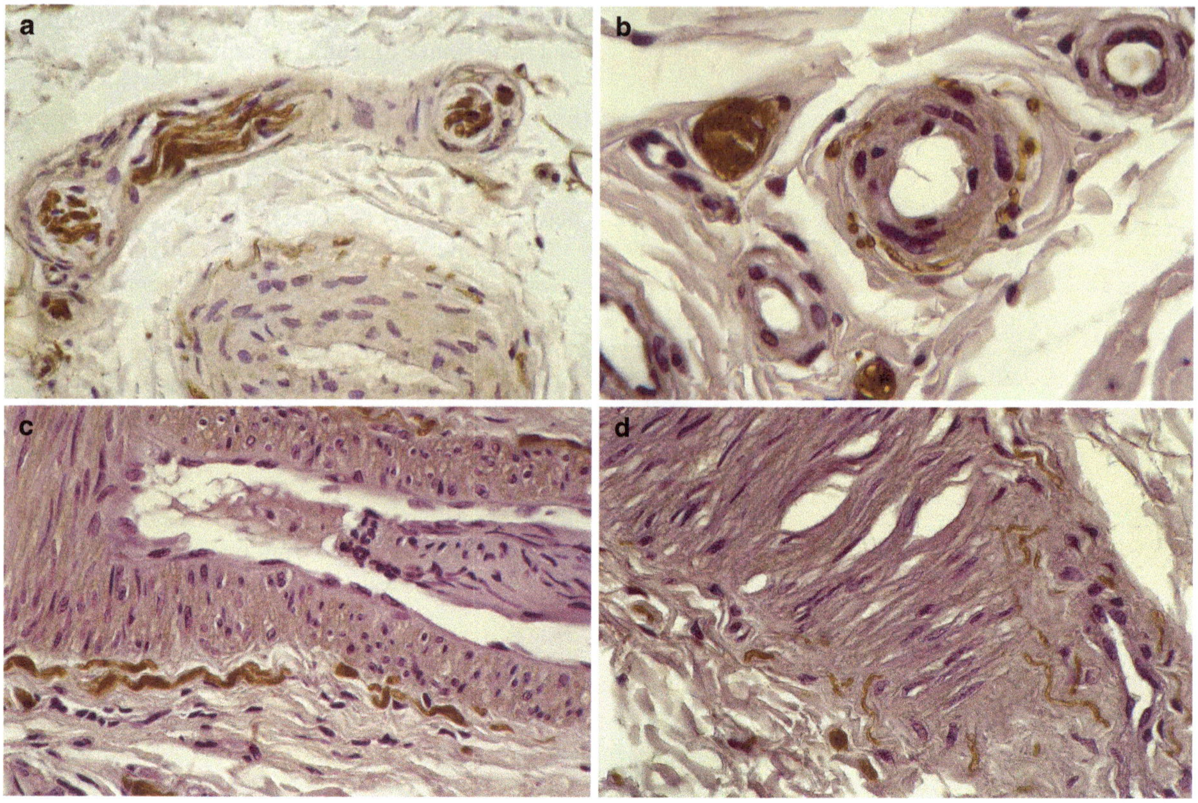


**Fig. 3.5** An increase in periadventitial innervation is detectable in our patients expressed as a rich vascular network made up of tiny myelinated fibers that, from the arterial adventitia, enter into the outer muscular layer, conforming a necklace (**a**, **b**). Transversal section (**c**) and tangential section (**d**). (Immunohistochemistry for protein S-100) (Reproduced from Sanchis-Alfonso et al.[65] copyright © 1998, Reprinted by permission of SAGE Publications)

a polypeptide that stimulates axonogenesis.[66] NGF adopted a granular pattern in the cytoplasm of Schwann cells of the thick nerve fibers and in the muscular wall of the arterial vessels and the amount of staining for this neurotrophin was related with increased perivascular innervation[62] (Fig. 3.6). NGF has two biologically active precursors: a long form of approximately 34 kDa of molecular weight, and a short form of 27 kDa.[14] We have found, in the lateral retinaculum of patients with painful PFM, the 34 kDa precursor. The fact that some of the nerve fibers of the lateral retinaculum express NGF means that these nerve fibers must still be in a proliferative phase.[66] As expected, we found that NGF is higher in patients with pain that in those with instability as the main symptom[66] (Fig. 3.7). Gigante and colleagues[23] have also found NGF and TrkA expression into the lateral retinaculum of patients with PFM, but not in patients with jumper's knee or meniscal tears. TrkA (the NGF receptor) plays a crucial role in pain sensation.

However, NGF is related not only to neural proliferation in vessels and perivascular tissue but also to the release of neuroceptive transmitters, such as substance P.[44] We postulate that both mechanisms are involved in the pathogenesis of anterior knee pain in patients with PFM. Thus, we suggest that two pathobiological mechanisms may lead to symptomatic PFM: (1) pain as the main symptom, with detectable levels of NGF that cause hyperinnervation and stimulus of SP release; and (2) instability as the predominant symptom, with lower levels of local NGF release, less neural proliferation, and less nociceptive stimulus.[66] This means that there must be other factors acting on a PFM to cause pain versus instability as the main symptom. Maybe, PFM may not have anything to do with the appearance of pain (PFM = "non-participating guest"). In other words, symptoms appear to be related to multiple factors with variable clinical expressions, and our imperfect understanding of these factors may explain the

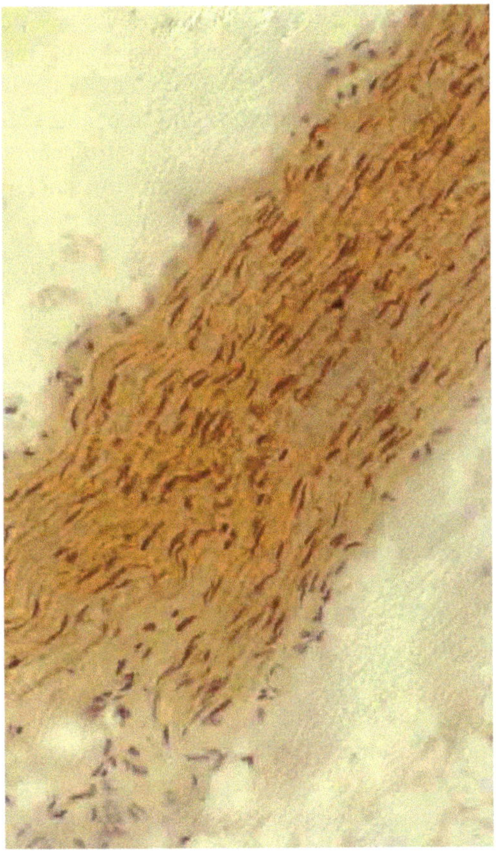

Fig. 3.6 NGF is present in thick nerves in the axons in a granular distribution and in the cytoplasm of the Schwann cells

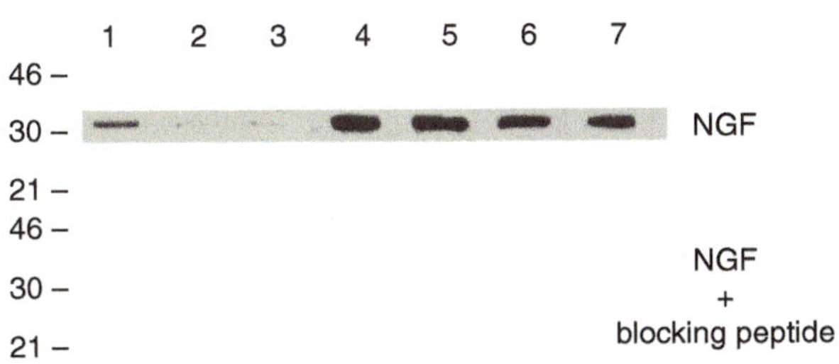


**Fig. 3.7** Immunoblotting detection of NGF, showing a thick band located at the level of NGF precursor in patients with pain (cases 4,5,6,7) and absence or a very thin band in the patients with instability as the main symptom (cases 1,2,3). The numbers at the *left* indicate molecular mass in kDa

all-too-frequent failure to achieve adequate symptom relief with the use of realignment procedures.

The question is: which are the mechanisms that stimulate NGF release in these patients? We hypothesize that periodic short episodes of ischemia could be the primary mechanism of NGF release, hyperinnervation, and therefore could be implicated in pain, at least in a subgroup of patients with PFPS.[61]

## 3.3 Which Is the Basic Cause of the Disease? Role of Ischemia in the Genesis of Anterior Knee Pain. "Loss of Vascular Homeostasis"

Despite the numerous publications concerning PFPS, the basic cause of the disease, that is the pain-provoking mechanism, is controversial. Rethinking the pathogenesis of PFPS and exploring new pain mechanisms could lead to changes in the assessment and management of this syndrome. The findings in our studies are in agreement with the biologically orientated perspective of the genesis of pain proposed by Scott Dye.[15] Our results indicate that vascular problems also affect the tissue homeostasis. We propose the loss of vascular homeostasis as an intrinsic mechanism of pain, at least, in a subgroup of anterior knee pain patients.

### *3.3.1 Definition of Tissue Homeostasis, Ischemia, and Hypoxia*

The term homeostasis is defined by Guyton and Hall[27] as the maintenance of constant conditions in the internal environment. The concept of tissue homeostasis involves all the molecular and biochemical processes that result in the normal maintenance of living structures and which is restored in an automatic biologic process homeostasis (healing) following a distressing event or series of events (overuse). At present, osseous homeostasis can be sensitively and geographically manifested by the use of PET (Positron Emission Tomography) scans with the use of flourine.[18] However, no method exists to sensitively and geographically manifest soft tissue homeostasis. Clinically, the presence of musculoskeletal soft tissue homeostasis is manifested by the absence of pain, tenderness, warmth, or swelling, while the loss of musculoskeletal soft tissue homeostasis is most often indicated by the presence of pain, tenderness, warmth, and swelling, that is, the classical signs of inflammation.

Hypoxia is a pathological condition in which the body as a whole (generalized hypoxia) or in part (tissue hypoxia) is deprived of an adequate supply of oxygen. It could be the result of a reduced supply of arterial blood or venous stasis (ischemic hypoxia), insufficient oxygen saturation (hypoxic hypoxia), or low hemoglobin (anemic hypoxia). Ischemia is an absolute or relative shortage of blood supply caused by vasoconstriction or blockage of the blood vessels supplying or draining the tissue.

### 3.3.2 Basic Science

According to some authors, NGF synthesis can be induced by ischemia.[1,42,85] Moreover, it has been shown that NGF stimulates neural sprouting and hastens neural proliferation in vessels walls,[30,35] and this is precisely the pattern of hyperinnervation that is seen in the lateral retinaculum of patients with painful PFM.[62,65,67] Similar changes have been studied in animal models and are present in the coronary innervation of patients with myocardial infarcts and brain ischemia.[1,35,42] Thus, we hypothesize that short episodes of tissular ischemia, due to a mechanism of vascular torsion or vascular bending, may be the main problem in painful PFM.[61,62,66,67] Vascular bending could be induced mechanically by medial traction over the retracted lateral retinaculum, due to PFM, with knee flexion.

We have demonstrated histologic retinacular changes associated with hypoxia in painful PFM.[67] In this way, we find lesions that can lead to tissular anoxia such as arterial vessels with obliterated lumina and thick muscular walls, which are reminiscent of hypertensive vascular changes frequently seen in other sites (as the kidney) but not expected in young healthy patients.[61,67] In addition, we find other lesions that are a consequence of ischemia such as infarcted foci of the connective tissue, myxoid stromal degeneration, and ultrastructural findings related with anoxia (degenerated fibroblasts with autophagic intracytoplasmic vacuoles, endothelial cells with reduplication of the basal lamina, young vessels with endothelial cells containing active nuclei and conspicuous nucleoli and neural sprouting)[39,59,61,67,75] (Fig. 3.8). In Fig. 3.8f and g, we can see the phenomenon of neural sprouting: after axonal damage has been established due to ischemia, the distal end of the axon degenerates and subsequent regeneration occurs in the swollen end of the proximal axon. The neuronal body is able to produce new microtubules and microfilaments that arrive to the swollen end of the proximal axon and induce neural sprouting. Schwann cells try to surround and to engulf the new axons giving a typical image of neural regeneration. We ought to bear in mind that, at experimental level, it has been found that neural sprouting finishes when NGF infusion ends.[30]

Another phenomenon related with ischemia is angiogenesis, given that chronic ischemia leads to VEGF-release, inducing hypervascularization in order to satisfy the needs of the tissue.[74] We have performed a quantitative analysis of vascularization into the lateral retinaculum excised at the time of surgical patellofemoral realignments using a pan-vascular marker, anti-Factor VIII-related antigen.[67] Factor VIII is one of the three functional components of the antihemophilic factor and is synthesized by endothelial cells of blood vessels; hence, it is considered as a specific marker for endothelial cells.[51] Thus, we found an increase in the number of vessels in the lateral retinaculum of patients with painful PFM, with higher values in the severe pain group compared with those of moderate or light pain.[67] Moreover, as expected, we found a positive linear correlation between number of vessels and number of nerves.[67]

Tissular ischemia induces vascular endothelial growth factor (VEGF) release by fibroblasts, synovial cells, mast cells, or even endothelial cells.[43,48,52,86] Following these principles, we performed a study of VEGF expression into the lateral retinaculum of patients with PFM by immunohistochemistry and immunoblot.[67] VEGF is a potent hypoxia-inducible angiogenic factor that causes hypervascularization.[9,29,31,43,46,48,58,74,78] VEGF release begins 8 h after hypoxia and the peptide disappears in 24 h, if the ischemic crisis is over.[29] Therefore, VEGF positivity reflects that, at this moment, we face an ischemic process, or better said, we are between 8 and 24 h from the onset of the transitory ischemic episode. However, given the fact that the average life of VEGF is very short, its negativity has no significance regarding the presence or not of a transitory ischemic process.

Although this process has been well documented in joints affected by rheumatoid arthritis and osteoarthritis,[9,31,52,57,86] it has never been documented in PFM until our study.[67] In our series, VEGF production was seen in stromal fibroblasts, vessel walls, certain endothelial cells, and even nerve fibers, as much in axons as in

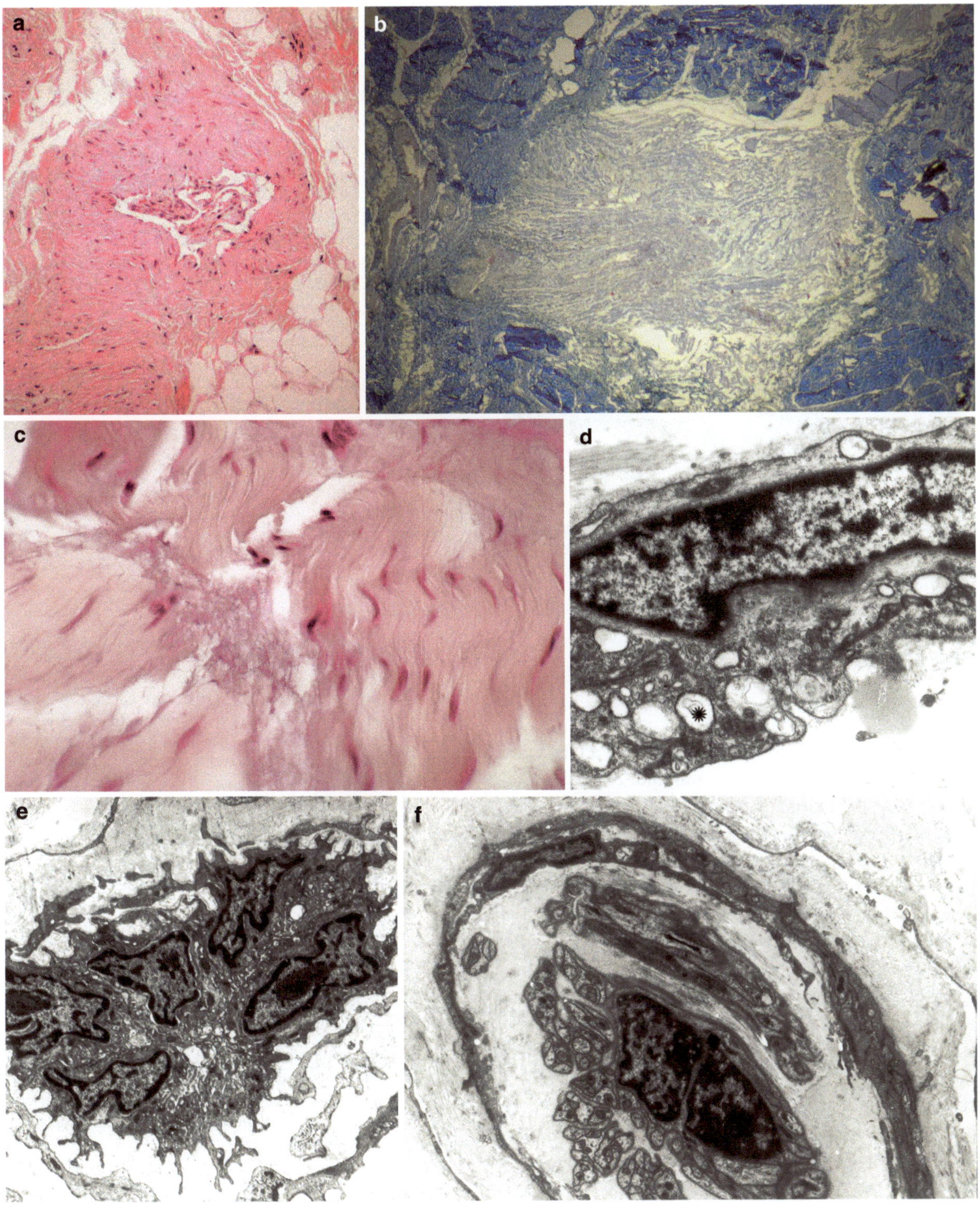


**Fig. 3.8** (**a**) Arterial vessel in the retinacular tissue can show a prominent and irregular endothelium and thick muscular walls or even an irregular reduction of the vascular lumen. (Hematoxylin-Eosin stain). (**b**) Infarcted foci in the connective tissue showing a degenerative pattern of the collagen fibers, with loss of the fibrillar component and accumulation of myxoid material in the interstitium, (Masson's Trichrome stain). (**c**) Myxoid stromal degeneration in the middle of the fibrous retinacular tissue (Hematoxylin-Eosin stain). (**d**) Degenerative changes in fibroblasts (increased autophagic vacuoles – *asterisk* –) secondary to hypoxia (TEM). (**e**) Young vessels with endothelial cells containing active nuclei and conspicuous nucleoli. (**f**) Neural sprouting is detected ultrastructurally as a bunch of tiny axons immersed in the Schwann cell cytoplasm. (**g**) Neural sprouting detail (**b** – Reproduced with permission from Sanchis-Alfonso et al.[61])

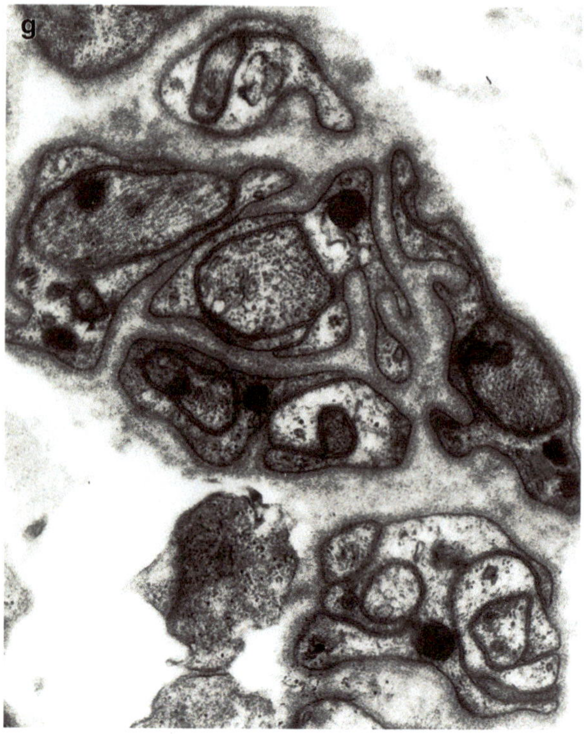


**Fig. 3.8** (continued)

perineurum[67] (Fig. 3.9). We complemented immunohistochemistry to identify and locate VEGF with immunoblotting to detect even minimal expression of VEGF. Our immunohistochemical findings were confirmed by immunoblot analysis. VEGF levels were higher in patients with severe pain than in those with light–moderate pain, whereas the protein was barely detectable in two cases with light pain[67] (Fig. 3.10).

VEGF expression is absent in normal joints[31] although inflammatory processes can stimulate its release.[9,31,57] In such cases, synovial hypoxia secondary to articular inflammation is supposed to trigger VEGF production.[31] However, we have not observed inflammatory changes in the lateral retinaculum in our cases.[65,67] Furthermore, it has been reported that peripheral nervous system hypoxia can simultaneously trigger VEGF and NGF synthesis via neurons[12] inflammatory or stromal cells.[1,42,85] VEGF induces hypervascularization and NGF induces hyperinnervation. Both facts have been observed in our cases.[65,67] We have concluded that ischemia could be the main trigger for the pain in PFPS, at least in a subgroup of patients with PFPS.

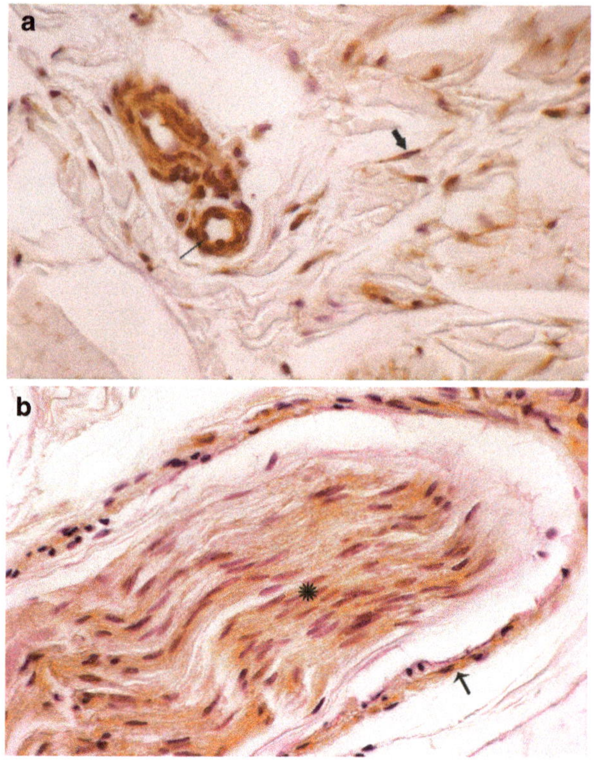


**Fig. 3.9** VEGF is present in small vessels (wall and endothelium) (*thin arrow*) and in perivascular fibroblasts (*thick arrow*) in patients with moderate to severe pain (**a**). Some cases have VEGF expression even in the perineural sheath (*thin arrow*) and inside the axons (*asterisk*) (**b**). (Immunohistochemistry for VEGF)

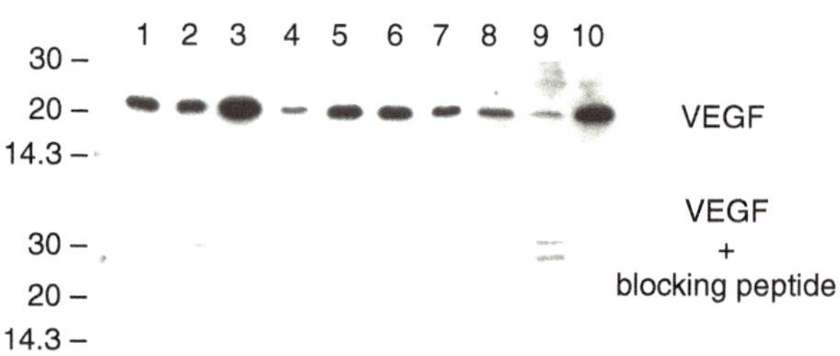


**Fig. 3.10** Immunoblotting detection of VEGF, showing a thicker band in cases with severe pain, whereas it is hardly expressed in two patients in whom instability and not pain was the main problem. (Severe pain: cases 2,3,10; moderate pain: cases 1,5,8; and light pain: cases 4,6,7,9)

### 3.3.3 Clinical Studies

We believe that PFPS may be caused by vascular disturbance. However, the role of vascular insufficiency in PFPS has not been studied extensively from a clinical point of view. In fact, up to now, only a few clinical papers allude to the possibility of hypoxia as a factor in the pathogenesis of anterior knee pain.

Sandow and Goodfellow[70] investigated the natural history of anterior knee pain in adolescents. They observed in a study sample of 54 adolescent girls that 9 out of 54 (16.7%) had pain that was aggravated by cold weather. According to Selfe and colleagues,[72] the proximal part of the rete patellae is very superficial, and therefore it is vulnerable to thermal environmental stress, resulting in greater hypoxia during cold weather. More recently, Selfe and colleagues[71] studied the clinical outcome in a sample of patients categorized as hypoxic, that is to say, PFPS patients with "cold knees" (his or her legs felt cold even in warm surroundings). Fourteen out of 77 (18%) of the patients were classified as "cold sufferers" (a percentage very similar to that of Sandow and Goodfellow). They studied local hypothermia by means of infrared thermography. The authors concluded that the patients categorized as hypoxic reported greater pain levels and responded worse to an exercise-based treatment than non-hypoxic patients. Gelfer and colleagues,[21] using single-photon emission computed tomography (SPECT), also found a relationship between transient patellar ischemia following total knee replacement and clinical symptoms of anterior knee pain. In the same sense, Jan Naslund[53] also observed, using photoplethysmography, which is a reliable technique for estimating blood flow in bone tissue, that an ischemic mechanism (decreased blood flow in the patellar bone) is involved in the pathogenesis of pain in PFPS. Moreover, Naslund[53] also observed in half of PFPS patients an accelerated bone remodeling in any of the bony compartments of the knee joint that may be due to a dysfunctioning sympathetic nervous system and cause intermittent ischemia and pain. Selfe and colleagues[72] classified anterior knee pain syndrome patients into three groups: hypoxic, inflammatory, and mechanical. However, ischemia may be the pain-provoking factor in all three groups given that inflammatory changes can develop not only after ischemia but also after mechanical damage to the vascular system.[53,84] Ischemia could also be caused by higher intraosseous pressure, redundant axial loading, or decreased arterial blood flow.[53]

## 3.4 Histological Findings in Chronic Tendinopathy. In Defense of Our Results

Our histological results are in agreement with those of Messner and colleagues[47] in experimentally induced Achilles tendinosis. Their histologic evaluation of tendinosis showed: hyperinnervation, hypervascularization, and increased immunoreactivity for substance P. In addition, Alfredson and colleagues[4] found vasculoneural ingrowth in the structurally changed part of the chronic painful Achilles tendinosis tendons, which possibly can explain the pain suffered by these patients. Thus, in our experience we[68] found neovascularization and hyperinnervation with nerve fibers ingrowth showing a histological pattern of neural sprouting, with vascular hyperinnervation and stromal neuromatous changes in chronic patellar tendinosis. We must remember that Achilles tendinosis and patellar tendinosis are a consequence of repetitive overloading of the Achilles/patellar tendon, that is to say, microtraumas, and is related to activity duration and intensity, a mechanism similar to symptomatic PFM. Therefore, the results of these studies lend credibility to the validity of our histological results.

## 3.5 Author's Proposed Anterior Knee Pain Pathophysiology

We hypothesize that short and repetitive episodes of tissular ischemia, due maybe to a mechanism of vascular torsion or vascular bending, which could be induced by a medial traction over a retracted lateral retinaculum, could trigger the release of NGF and VEGF on PFM. Once NGF is present in the tissues, it induces hyperinnervation, attraction of mastocytes, and substance P release by free nerve endings.[44] In addition, VEGF induces hypervascularization and plays also a role, increasing neural proliferation.

Free nerve endings, slowly adapting receptors that mediate nociception, are activated in response to the deformation of tissues resulting from abnormal tensile and compressive forces generated during flexoextension of the knee, or in response to the stimulus of chemical agents such as histamine, bradykinin, prostaglandins, and leukotrienes.[36,76,77] Therefore, SP is released from peripheral endings of nociceptive afferents as a result of noxious chemical or mechanical stimulation. The nociceptive information relayed by these free nerve endings is responsible, at least in part, for the pain.

Once SP is liberated on the connective tissue, the neuropeptide induces as well the release of prostaglandin E2, one of the biochemical agents known to stimulate nociceptors.[3] The activation of nociceptive pathways by prostaglandins could be one of the many mechanisms involved in the transmission of pain from knees with PFM. Moreover, SP stimulates mast cells, facilitating a degranulation process, which may release in the media another nonneurogenic pain mediator, histamine.[26] Numerous mast cells have been identified into the lateral retinaculum of our patients.[62] Mast cells have been also related with the release of NGF,[54,62] contributing to the hyperinnervation and indirectly causing more pain. Furthermore, SP has been shown to induce the release of collagenase, interleukin-1, and tumor necrosis factor-alpha (TNF) from synoviocytes, fibroblasts, and macrophages, which could participate in the genesis of patellar instability by degradation of soft tissues.[3,6] SP has recently been implicated as well in bone resorption both in vitro and in vivo, which can explain at least in part the osteoporosis associated in many cases of anterior knee pain (Fig. 3.11).[73] Finally, SP and VEGF stimulate endothelial cell proliferation and migration,[7] which are essential in the development of a new vascular network that may promote tissue repair, but indirectly maintain the vicious circle.

Woolf[84] described from a clinical point of view four types of pain: (1) Nociceptive pain – transient pain in response to noxious stimulus. (2) Homeostatic pain – pain that promotes the healing of injured tissue, that is the cascade of events that participate in the reestablishment of homeostasis. (3) Neuropathic pain – spontaneous pain and hypersensitivity to stimulus in association with damage of the nervous system. (4) Functional pain – pain resulting from abnormal central processing of normal input. Homeostatic pain may include specific symptoms such as allodynia (pain due to stimulus that does not normally provoke pain) and hyperalgesia (a heightened response to a stimulus that is normally painful). The phenomenon of rest pain in PFPS ("movie sign") might be an example of allodynia, that is, pain arising from non-nociceptive afferent activity due to central sensitization and can be induced by ischemia.[49] In theory, all these mechanisms could be involved in the pathophysiology of pain in PFPS.

## 3.6 Other Anatomical Structures Responsible for Anterior Knee Pain: Synovium, Infrapatellar Fat Pad, and Subchondral Bone

The conscious neurosensory characteristics of the internal components of the human knee have been documented by instrumented arthroscopic palpation without intraarticular anesthesia by Scott Dye.[16] Subjectively, he graded the sensation from no sensation (0) to severe pain (4), with a modifier of either accurate spatial localization (A) or poor spatial localization (B). The nature of the intraarticular sensation was variable, ranging from 0 on the patellar articular

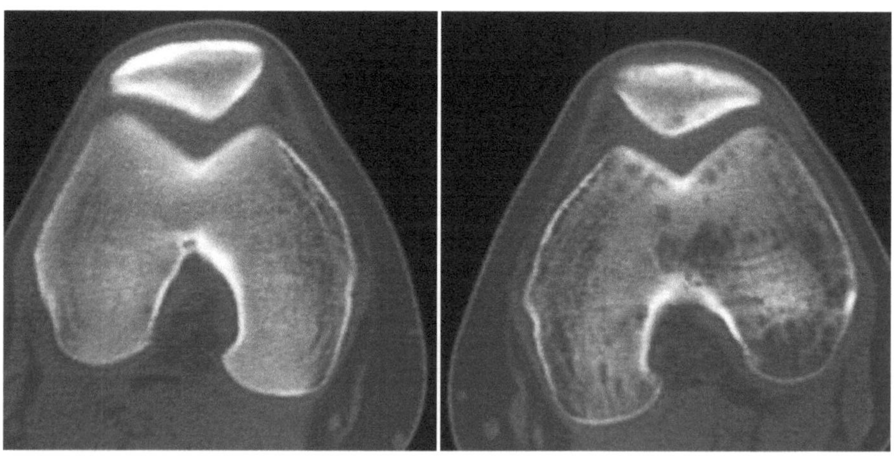

**Fig. 3.11** Osteoporosis associated to anterior knee pain syndrome (left knee)

cartilage to 4A on the anterior synovium, fat pad, and joint capsule. The sensation arising from the cruciate ligaments ranged from 1 to 2B in the midportion, and from 3 to 4B at the insertion sites. The sensation from the meniscal cartilages ranged from 1B on the inner rim to 3B near the capsular margin. Dye[16] stated that innervation of most intraarticular components of the knee is probably crucial for tissue homeostasis.

The synovium has a rich nerve supply of type IVa free nerve endings and fibers containing SP.[10] Peripatellar synovitis is described by Dye as one of the most common causes of anterior knee pain due to a mechanism of impingement.[15] Likewise, repetitive impingement of a medio- or suprapatellar plica between the patella and the femur can also be a cause of anterior knee pain.

The Hoffa fat pad is also a richly innervated structure containing SP – immunoreactive nerve fibers and type IVa free nerve endings that transmit pain.[10] Therefore, the Hoffa fat pad could be another source of pain. Impingement of the fat pad, which could stimulate free nerve endings, is possible during eccentric load in jumping or running and during straight leg rising.[10] Moreover, a tight lateral retinaculum may cause fat pad irritation and therefore pain.[10] Chronic irritation of the synovium with joint effusion leads to swelling of the fat pad, and the risk of impingement behind the patellar tendon increases. In patients with Hoffa's disease, the irritation of free nerve endings due to a mechanism of impingement of the infrapatellar fat pad produces pain as the knee approaches terminal extension.[41] The improvement in pain and function after arthroscopic resection of the Hoffa fat pad[41] could be explained for the denervation effect of the operation.

Moreover, we have seen in the infrapatellar fat pad adjacent to the inferior pole of the patella, in patients with jumper's knee or chronic patellar tendinopathy, a rich vascular net consisting mainly in newly formed capillaries with endothelial hyperplasia and irregular lumen or even solid tubes.[68] We have found hyperinnervation, predominantly of free nerve endings next to the bone–tendon junction that could be implicated in the mechanism of pain.[68] Moreover, we have seen pathologic neural changes such as free myelinated nerve fibers showing an histological pattern of "nerve sprouting" (similar to that observed in the regeneration after sectioning a nerve) (Fig. 3.12), increased vascular innervation with nerve fibers entering the adventitia and the muscular layer, giving the artery a brown necklace appearance, and finally neuroma-like formations that could also be implicated in the genesis of pain.[68,69] Denervation could also explain the good results of arthroscopic shaving of the fat pad adjacent to the inferior pole of the patella in the treatment of chronic patellar tendinopathy.[55,80]

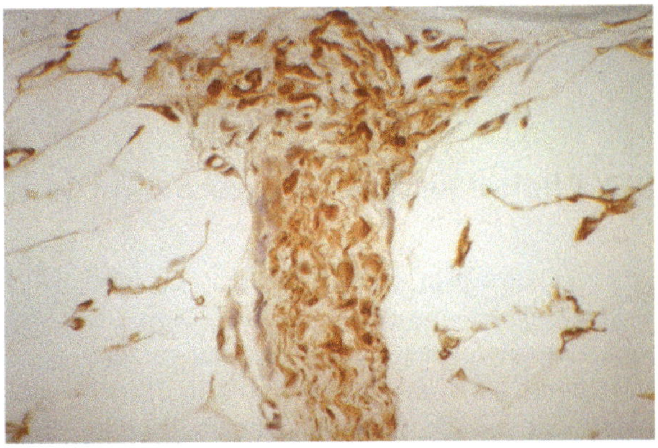

**Fig. 3.12** Medium-size nerves near the osteotendinous insertion suffer a "nerve sprouting" process, losing their perineurium sheath and liberating their tiny nerve branches (anti-S 100 protein)

Finally, subchondral patellar bone could be another source of pain due to its rich nerve supply. Maralcan and colleagues[45] analyzed the topographic anatomy of the innervation of the patella. Unlike other papers that emphasize in the medial innervation, these authors found that two nerves reached the patella, one from the vastus medialis and the other one from the vastus lateralis. After selective local anesthetic injections in the entry points of these nerves in patients with PFPS, they found a decrease of anterior knee pain. However, they were unable to find any other neural structures around the patella. The precise description of the entry points of these nerves into the patella could be useful for performing selective denervation. Barton and colleagues[8] have demonstrated that the density of intraosseous nerves was greatest in the medial and central portions of the patella, with a significant paucity in the lateral portion. These authors documented intraosseous nerves in association with intraosseous arterial capillaries and, less frequently, not associated with vessels. These intraosseous nerves could relay nociceptive information as a result of mechanical stimulation. This mechanical stimulation could be due to the increment of intraosseous pressure (intraosseous edema) or the increment of the subchondral bone pressure (due to failure of energy absorption of the articular cartilage secondary to the decrease of the contact area – PFM – or secondary to chondral damage).

## 3.7 Clinical Relevance. Future Directions

Anterior knee pain depends not only on mechanical factors, but also on neural factors. Our findings provide support for the clinical observation that lateral retinaculae plays an important role in anterior knee pain syndrome. The resolution of pain by realignment surgery, as we have seen in our series,[60] does not necessarily mean that PFM caused these symptoms. We agree with Abraham and colleagues,[2] who suggested that pain relief after realignment surgery may be attributed, in part, to denervation. In the same sense, Vega and colleagues,[79] in 2006, described electrosurgical arthroscopic patellar denervation for the treatment of patients with intractable anterior knee pain and no or minimal malalignment.

Moreover, realignment surgery would not only achieve the effect of denervation mentioned above, but it would also eliminate the tensile and compressive forces that are produced in the lateral retinaculum with knee flexion–extension, that stimulate free nerve endings (a type of nociceptor),[36] and would break the ischemia – hyperinnervation – pain circle.

If the "neural model" of anterior knee pain proves to have certain validity, it would lead, in many cases, to therapeutic recommendations to alleviate pain more effectively and safer than the attempts to correct "malalignment." Thus, specific unloading, a selective pharmaceutical approach, that is to say, medications that affect neural pain transmission (e.g., drug inhibitors of synthesis and release of SP, or SP receptor antagonists), or pharmaceutical options for the treatment of neuropathic pain such as pregabalin[22] could be of interest in the treatment of pain in these patients. Finally, if we demonstrate that regional anoxia plays a key role in the genesis of pain, topical periferic vasorelaxant drugs could also be of special interest in the treatment of pain in these patients, as well as protecting the knees from a decrease in blood flow by means of limitations in time spent with knee in flexion as well as protecting the knees from a cold environment. Moreover, ice application in these patients may cause an increase of symptoms due to a significant decrease of blood flow.

We suggest proprioceptive neuromuscular training as a beneficial aspect of rehabilitation programs following realignment knee surgery to improve function and knee proprioception and therefore decrease the risk of reinjury. Moreover, the fact that the instability is due, in part, to proprioceptive deficit may explain that McConnell taping or bracing can improve considerably the stability, in spite of their doubtful biomechanical efficacy, by increasing proprioceptive feedback.

We are now at a turning point. Nowadays, medicine in its entirety is being reassessed at a subcellular level, and this is precisely the line of thought we are following in the approach to PFPS. Still to be seen are the implications that this change of mentality will have in the treatment of PFPS in the future, but we are sure that these new trends of thought will open the doors to new and exciting perspectives that could potentially revolutionize the management of this troublesome pathologic condition in the new millennium we have just entered. Clearly, we are only at the beginning of the road that will lead to understanding where anterior knee pain comes from.

## 3.8 Summary

We review the pathophysiology of anterior knee pain in the young patient. Emphasis is placed on newer findings. We have developed what we call the "Neural Model" as an explanation for the genesis of anterior knee pain. We have demonstrated a neuroanatomical basis for PFPS in the young patient and the clinical observation that the lateral retinaculum may have a key role in the origin of this pain. According to our studies, we hypothesize that periodic short episodes of ischemia in the lateral retinaculum could be implicated in the pathogenesis of anterior knee pain, at least in a subgroup of anterior knee pain patients, by triggering neural proliferation of nociceptive axons (substance P positive nerves), mainly in a perivascular location. Our findings are compatible with the tissue homeostasis theory widely accepted currently to explain the genesis of anterior knee pain. If the "neural model" of anterior knee pain proves to have a certain validity, it would lead in many cases to therapeutic recommendations to alleviate pain more effectively and safer than the attempts to correct "malalignment." Moreover, we believe that instability in patients with PFPS can be explained, at least in part, because of the damage of nerves of the lateral retinaculum, which can be related with proprioception. Our findings, however, do not preclude the possibility of pain arising in other anatomical structures such as infrapatellar fat pad, synovium, and subchondral bone.

## References


1. Abe T, Morgan DA, Gutterman DD. Protective role of nerve growth factor against postischemic dysfunction of sympathetic coronary innervation. *Circulation.* 1997;95:213-220.
2. Abraham E, Washington E, Huang TL. Insall proximal realignment for disorders of the patella. *Clin Orthop Relat Res.* 1989;248:61-65.
3. Ahmed M, Bergstrom J, Lundblad H, et al. Sensory nerves in the interface membrane of aseptic loose hip prostheses. *J Bone Joint Surg.* 1998;80-B:151-155.
4. Alfredson H, Ohberg L, Forsgren S. Is vasculo-neural ingrowth the cause of pain in chronic Achilles tendinosis? An investigation using ultrasonography and colour Doppler, immunohistochemistry, and diagnostic injections. *Knee Surg Sports Traumatol Arthrosc.* 2003;11:334-338.
5. Ashton IK, Ashton BA, Gibson SJ, et al. Morphological basis for back pain: the demonstration of nerve fibers and neuropeptides in the lumbar facet joint capsule but not in ligamentum flavum. *J Orthop Res.* 1992;10:72-78.
6. Ashton IK, Roberts S, Jaffray DC. Neuropeptides in the human intervertebral disc. *J Orthop Res.* 1994;12:186-192.
7. Ashton IK, Walsh DA, Polak JM, et al. Substance P in intervertebral discs binding sites vascular endothelium human annulus fibrosus. *Acta Orthop Scand.* 1994;65:635-639.
8. Barton RS, Ostrowski ML, Anderson TD, et al. Intraosseous innervation of the human patella: a histologic study. *Am J Sports Med.* 2007;35:307-311.
9. Berse B, Hunt JA, Diegel RJ, et al. Hypoxia augments cytokine-induced vascular endothelial growth factor secretion by human synovial fibroblasts. *Clin Exp Immunol.* 1999;115:176-182.
10. Biedert RM, Sanchis-Alfonso V. Sources of anterior knee pain. *Clin Sports Med.* 2002;21:335-347.
11. Byers PD. Solitary benign osteoblastic lesions of bone osteoid osteoma benign osteoblastoma. *Cancer.* 1968;22: 43-57.
12. Calzà L, Giardino L, Giuliani A, et al. Nerve growth factor control of neuronal expression of angiogenetic and vasoactive factors. *Proc Natl Acad Sci USA.* 2001;98:4160-4165.
13. Coppes MH, Marani E, Thomeer RT, et al. Innervation of "painful" lumbar discs. *Spine.* 1997;22:2342-2349.
14. Dicou E, Pflug B, Magazin M, et al. Two peptides derived from the nerve growth factor precursor are biologically active. *J Cell Biol.* 1997;136:389-398.
15. Dye SF, Staubli HU, Biedert RM, et al. The mosaic of pathophysiology causing patellofemoral pain: therapeutic implications. *Oper Tech Sports Med.* 1999;7:46-54.
16. Dye SF, Vaupel GL, Dye CC. Conscious neurosensory mapping of the internal structures of the human knee without intra-articular anesthesia. *Am J Sports Med.* 1998;26: 773-777.
17. Freemont AJ, Peacock TE, Goupille P, et al. Nerve ingrowth into diseased intervertebral disc in chronic back pain. *Lancet.* 1997;350:178-181.
18. Fulkerson JP. The etiology of patellofemoral pain in young active patients: a prospective study. *Clin Orthop Relat Res.* 1983;179:129-133.
19. Fulkerson JP, Hungerford DS. *Disorders of the Patellofemoral Joint.* Baltimore: Williams & Wilkins; 1990.
20. Fulkerson JP, Tennant R, Jaivin JS, et al. Histologic evidence of retinacular nerve injury associated with patellofemoral malalignment. *Clin Orthop Relat Res.* 1985;197:196-205.
21. Gelfer Y, Pinkas L, Horne T, et al. Symptomatic transient patellar ischemia following total knee replacement as detected by scintigraphy. A prospective, randomized, double-blind study comparing the mid-vastus to the medial para-patellar approach. *Knee.* 2003;10:341-345.
22. Gidal B, Billington R. New and emerging treatment options for neuropathic pain. *Am J Manag Care.* 2006;12:S269-S278.
23. Gigante A, Bevilacqua C, Ricevuto A, et al. Biological aspects in patello-femoral malalignment. In: *Book of Abstracts, 11th Congress European Society of Sports Traumatology, Knee Surgery and Arthroscopy.* Athens: Springer; 2004:218.
24. Grelsamer RP, McConnell J. *The Patella. A Team Approach.* Gaithersburg: An Aspen Publication; 1998.
25. Grönblad M, Korkala O, Konttinen YT, et al. Silver impregnation and immunohistochemical study of nerves in lumbar facet joint plical tissue. *Spine.* 1991;16:34-38.
26. Grönblad M, Weinstein JN, Santavirta S. Immunohistochemical observations on spinal tissue innervation. A review of hipothetical mechanisms of back pain. *Acta Orthop Scand.* 1991;62:614-622.
27. Guyton AC, Hall JE. *Textbook of Medical Physiology.* Philadelphia: WB Saunders Co; 1996.
28. Hasegawa T, Hirose T, Sakamoto R, et al. Mechanism of pain in osteoid osteomas: an immunohistochemical study. *Histopathology.* 1993;22:487-491.
29. Hayashi T, Sakurai M, Abe K, et al. Expression of angiogenic factors in rabbit spinal cord after transient ischaemia. *Neuropathol Appl Neurobiol.* 1999;25:63-71.
30. Isaacson LG, Crutcher KA. The duration of sprouted cerebrovascular axons following intracranial infusion of nerve growth factor. *Exp Neurol.* 1995;13:174-179.
31. Jackson JR, Minton JAL, Ho ML, et al. Expression of vascular endothelial growth factor in synovial fibroblasts is induced by hipoxia and interleukin 1ß. *J Rheumatol.* 1997; 24:1253-1259.
32. Jensen R, Hystad T, Kvale A, et al. Quantitative sensory testing of patients with long lasting patellofemoral pain síndrome. *Eur J Pain.* 2007;11:665-676.
33. Jerosch J, Prymka M. Knee joint propioception in patients with posttraumatic recurrent patella dislocation. *Knee Surg Sports Traumatol Arthrosc.* 1996;4:14-18.
34. Kasim N, Fulkerson JP. Resection of clinically localized segments of painful retinaculum in the treatment of selected patients with anterior knee pain. *Am J Sports Med.* 2000; 28:811-814.

35. Kawaja MD. Sympathetic and sensory innervation of the extracerebral vasculature: roles for p75NTR neuronal expression and nerve growth factor. *J Neurosci Res*. 1998;52: 295-306.
36. Kocher MS, Fu FH, Harner ChD. Neuropathophysiology. In: Fu FH, Harner ChD, Vince KG, eds. *Knee Surgery*. Baltimore: Williams and Wilkins; 1994:231-249.
37. Konttinen YT, Grönblad M, Antti-Poika I, et al. Neuro-immunohistochemical analysis of peridiscal nociceptive neural elements. *Spine*. 1990;15:383-386.
38. Korkala O, Grönblad M, Liesi P, et al. Immunohistochemical demonstration of nociceptors in the ligamentous structures of the lumbar spine. *Spine*. 1985;10:156-157.
39. Kraushaar BS, Nirschl RP. Tendinosis of the elbow (tennis elbow). *J Bone Joint Surg*. 1999;81-A:259-278.
40. Krompinger WJ, Fulkerson JP. Lateral retinacular release for intractable lateral retinacular pain. *Clin Orthop Relat Res*. 1983;179:191-193.
41. Kumar D, Alvand A, Beacon JP. Impingement of infrapatellar fat pad (Hoffa's disease): results of high-portal arthroscopic resection. *Arthroscopy*. 2007;23:1180-1186.
42. Lee TH, Kato H, Kogure K, et al. Temporal profile of nerve growth factor-like immunoreactivity after transient focal cerebral ischemia in rats. *Brain Res*. 1996;713:199-210.
43. Liu Y, Cox SR, Morita T, et al. Hypoxia regulates vascular endothelial growth factor gene expression in endothelial cells. Identification of a 5′ enhancer. *Circ Res*. 1995;77:638-643.
44. Malcangio M, Garrett NE, Cruwys S, et al. Nerve growth factor- and neurotrophin-3-induced changes in nociceptive threshold and the release of substance P from the rat isolated spinal cord. *J Neurosci*. 1997;17:8459-8467.
45. Maralcan G, Kuru I, Issi S, et al. The innervation of patella: anatomical and clinical study. *Surg Radiol Anat*. 2005;27: 331-335.
46. Marti HJ, Bernaudin M, Bellail A, et al. Hypoxia-induced vascular endothelial growth factor expression precedes neovascularization after cerebral ischemia. *Am J Pathol*. 2000; 156:965-976.
47. Messner K, Wei Y, Andersson B, et al. Rat model of Achilles tendon disorder. A pilot study. *Cells Tissues Organs*. 1999;165:30-39.
48. Minchenko A, Bauer T, Salceda S, et al. Hypoxic stimulation of vascular endothelial growth factor expression in vitro and in vivo. *Lab Invest*. 1994;71:374-379.
49. Mitchell AC, Fallon MT. A single infusi6n of intravenous ketamine improves pain relief in patients with critical limb ischemia: results of a double blind randomised controlled trial. *Pain*. 2002;97:275-281.
50. Mori Y, Fujimoto A, Okumo H, et al. Lateral retinaculum release in adolescent patellofemoral disorders: its relationship to peripheral nerve injury in the lateral retinaculum. *Bull Hosp Jt Dis Orthop Inst*. 1991;51:218-229.
51. Mukai K, Rosai J, Burgdorf WH. Localization of factor VIII-related antigen in vascular endothelial cells using an immunoperoxidase method. *Am J Surg Pathol*. 1980;4:273-276.
52. Nagashima M, Yoshino S, Ishiwata T, et al. Role of vascular endothelial growth factor in angiogenesis of rheumatoid arthritis. *J Rheumatol*. 1995;22:1624-1630.
53. Naslund J. *Patellofemoral pain syndrome. Clinical and pathophysiological considerations*. Thesis. Karolinska Institutet, Stockholm; 2006.
54. Nilsson G, Forsberg-Nilsson K, Xiang Z, et al. Human mast cells express functional TrkA and are a source of nerve growth factor. *Eur J Immunol*. 1997;27:2295-2301.
55. Ogon P, Maier D, Jaeger A, et al. Arthroscopic patellar release for the treatment of chronic patellar tendinopathy. *Arthroscopy*. 2006;22:462.e1-462.e5.
56. Palmgren T, Grönblad M, Virri J, et al. Immunohistochemical demonstration of sensory and autonomic nerve terminals in herniated lumbar disc tissue. *Spine*. 1996;21:1301-1306.
57. Pufe T, Petersen W, Tillmann B, et al. The splice variants VEGF121 and VEGF189 of the angiogenic peptide vascular endothelial growth factor are expressed in osteoarthritic cartilage. *Arthritis Rheum*. 2001;44:1082-1088.
58. Richard DE, Berra E, Pouyssegur J. Angiogenesis: how a tumor adapts to hypoxia. *Biochem Biophys Res Commun*. 1999;266:718-722.
59. Richardson EP, DeGirolami U. *Pathology of the Peripheral Nerve*. Philadelphia: W.B. Saunders Company; 1995.
60. Sanchis-Alfonso V, Gastaldi-Orquín E, Martinez-SanJuan V. Usefulness of computed tomography in evaluating the patellofemoral joint before and after Insall's realignment. Correlation with short-term clinical results. *Am J Knee Surg*. 1994;7:65-72.
61. Sanchis-Alfonso V, Roselló-Sastre E. Proliferaci6n neural e isquemia. *Rev Patol Rodilla*. 1998;3:60-63.
62. Sanchis-Alfonso V, Roselló-Sastre E. Immunohistochemical analysis for neural markers of the lateral retinaculum in patients with isolated symptomatic patellofemoral malalignment. A neuroanatomic basis for anterior knee pain in the active young patient. *Am J Sports Med*. 2000;28:725-731.
63. Sanchis-Alfonso V, Roselló-Sastre E. Anterior knee pain in the young patient – what causes the pain? "Neural model". *Acta Orthop Scand*. 2003;74:697-703.
64. Sanchis-Alfonso V, Roselló-Sastre E, Martinez-SanJuan V. Pathogenesis of anterior knee pain syndrome and functional patellofemoral instability in the active young. A review. *Am J Knee Surg*. 1999;12:29-40.
65. Sanchis-Alfonso V, Roselló-Sastre E, Monteagudo-Castro C, et al. Quantitative analysis of nerve changes in the lateral retinaculum in patients with isolated symptomatic patellofemoral malalignment. A preliminary study. *Am J Sports Med*. 1998;26:703-709.
66. Sanchis-Alfonso V, Roselló-Sastre E, Revert F. Neural growth factor expression in the lateral retinaculum in painful patellofemoral malalignment. *Acta Orthop Scand*. 2001; 72:146-149.
67. Sanchis-Alfonso V, Roselló-Sastre E, Revert F, et al. Histologic retinacular changes associated with ischemia in painful patellofemoral malalignment. *Orthopedics*. 2005;28: 593-599.
68. Sanchis-Alfonso V, Roselló-Sastre E, Subías-López A. Mechanisms of pain in jumper's knee. A histological and immunohistochemical study. *J Bone Joint Surg*. 1999; 81-B((Supp I)):82.
69. Sanchis-Alfonso V, Roselló-Sastre E, Subías-López A. Neuroanatomic basis for pain in patellar tendinosis ("jumper's knee"): a neuroimmunohistochemical study. *Am J Knee Surg*. 2001;14:174-177.
70. Sandow MJ, Goodfellow JW. The natural history of anterior knee pain in adolescents. *J Bone Joint Surg*. 1985;67-B: 36-38.

71. Selfe J, Harper L, Pedersen I, et al. Cold legs: a potential indicator of negative outcome in the rehabilitation of patients with patellofemoral pain syndrome. *Knee*. 2003;10: 139-143.
72. Selfe J, Karki A, Stevens D. A review of the role of circulatory deficit in the genesis of patellofemoral pain. *Phys Ther Rev*. 2002;7:169-172.
73. Sherman BE, Chole RA. A mechanism for sympathectomy-induced bone resorption in the middle ear. *Otolaryngol Head Neck Surg*. 1995;113:569-581.
74. Shweiki D, Itin A, Soffer D, et al. Vascular endothelial growth factor induced by hypoxia may mediate hypoxia-initiated angiogenesis. *Nature*. 1992;359:843-845.
75. Society for Ultrastructural Pathology. *Handbook of Diagnostic Electron Microscopy for Pathologists-in-Training*. New York, Tokyo: Igaku-Shoin Medical Publishers Committee; 1995.
76. Soifer TB, Levy HJ, Soifer FM, et al. Neurohistology of the subacromial space. *Arthroscopy*. 1996;12:182-186.
77. Solomonow M, Ambrosia RD. Neural reflex arcs and muscle control of knee stability and motion. In: Scott WN, ed. *Ligament and Extensor Mechanism Injuries of the Knee: Diagnosis and Treatment*. St. Louis: Mosby-Year Book; 1991:389-400.
78. Steinbrech DS, Mehrara BJ, Saadeh PB, et al. Hypoxia regulates VEGF expression and cellular proliferation by osteoblasts in vitro. *Plast Reconstr Surg*. 1999;104:738-747.
79. Vega J, Golano P, Perez-Carro L. Electrosurgical arthroscopic patellar denervation. *Arthroscopy*. 2006;22:1028. el-3.
80. Willberg L, Sunding K, Forssblad M, et al. Ultrasound- and Doppler-guided arthroscopic saving to treat jumper's knee: a technical note. *Knee Surg Sports Traumatol Arthrosc*. 2007;15:1400-1403.
81. Wilson AS, Lee HB. Hypothesis relevant to defective position sense in a damaged knee. *J Neurol Neurosurg Psychiatry*. 1986;49:1462-1463.
82. Witonski D, Wagrowska-Danielewicz M. Distribution of substance-P nerve fibers in the knee joint in patients with anterior knee pain syndrome. *Knee Surg Sports Traumatol Arthrosc*. 1999;7:177-183.
83. Wojtys EM, Beaman DN, Glover RA, et al. Innervation of the human knee joint by substance-P fibers. *Arthroscopy*. 1990;6:254-263.
84. Woolf CJ. Pain: moving from symptom control toward mechanism-specific pharmacologic management. *Ann Intern Med*. 2004;140:441-451.
85. Woolf CJ, Allchorne A, Safieh-Garabedian B, et al. Cytokines, nerve growth factor and inflammatory hyperalgesia: the contribution of tumour necrosis factor alpha. *Br J Pharmacol*. 1997;121:417-424.
86. Yamada T, Sawatsubashi M, Yakushiji H, et al. Localization of vascular endothelial growth factor in synovial membrane mast cells: examination with "multi-labelling subtraction immunostaining". *Virchows Arch*. 1998;433:567-570.

# Pathogenesis of Anterior Knee Pain in the Active Young: Is There a Relation Between the Presence of Patellofemoral Malalignment and Pain?

4

## What Have We Learned from Realignment Surgery?

Vicente Sanchis-Alfonso, Fermín Ordoño, Alfredo Subías-López, and Carmen Monserrat

## 4.1 Introduction

For many years, patellofemoral malalignment (PFM), an abnormality of patellar tracking that involves lateral displacement or lateral tilt of the patella (or both) in extension that is reduced in flexion, was widely accepted as an explanation for the genesis of anterior knee pain and patellar instability, the most common knee complaints in clinical practice in young patients.[11,16,18,19,23,24,28] Moreover, this concept had a great influence on orthopaedic surgeons, who developed several surgical procedures to "correct the malalignment," such as Insall's proximal realignment (IPR).[20] Currently, however, this concept is questioned by many, and is not universally accepted to account for the presence of anterior knee pain and/or patellar instability. In fact, the number of realignment surgeries has dropped dramatically in recent years, due to a reassessment of the paradigm of PFM. Despite a large body of literature on patellofemoral realignment procedures, little information is available on the in-depth long-term results of these surgical procedures.[1,2,8] It has been the common practice in our institution to evaluate patients carefully with regular follow-ups, scrutinizing their results so that we may learn from them and continually improve our techniques and outcomes.

The current retrospective clinical study was conducted to critically evaluate the long-term results of the operative treatment of "isolated symptomatic PFM," recalcitrant to conservative treatment, by IPR, in order to clarify the following points: (1) whether there is a relationship between the presence of PFM and the presence of anterior knee pain; (2) long-term response of vastus medialis obliquus (VMO) muscle fibers to increased resting length; and (3) incidence of patellofemoral osteoarthritis after IPR surgery.

## 4.2 Patients and Methods

### 4.2.1 Subjects

From 1991 through 1999, 59 IPRs were performed on 45 patients by the first author (V.S-A). To obtain a homogeneous population, we included in the study group only those cases with the following criteria: (1) PFM demonstrated with CT at 0º of knee flexion; (2) no previous knee surgery; (3) no associated intra-articular pathology (such as synovial plica, meniscal tears, ACL/PCL tears or osteoarthrosis) confirmed arthroscopically or by X-rays; and (4) IPR as an isolated surgical procedure. Moreover, we excluded patients involved in workman's compensation or other pending litigation

V. Sanchis-Alfonso (✉)
International Patellofemoral Study Group,
International ACL Study Group,
Hospital 9 de Octubre, Hospital Arnau de Vilanova,
School of Medicine, Catholic University of Valencia,
Valencia, Spain
e-mail: vicente.sanchis.alfonso@gmail.com

V. Sanchis-Alfonso (ed.), *Anterior Knee Pain and Patellar Instability*,
DOI: 10.1007/978-0-85729-507-1_4, © Springer-Verlag London Limited 2011

claims and patients who had recurrent dislocation of the patella associated with Down syndrome. Sixteen of 45 surgical patients were excluded because they did not meet the aforementioned criteria or they were not available for follow-up.

Thus, only 40 IPRs (20 right and 20 left) performed on 29 patients composed the study group. There were 26 females and 3 males. The average age at the onset of symptoms was 16 (range 10–23 years). Onset of symptoms was secondary to a twisting injury while participating in sports in 16 cases (40%), and secondary to a fall on the flexed knee in one case (2.5%). In 23 cases (57.5%), the onset of symptoms occurred spontaneously without injury. Surgery was performed after a mean of 24 months following onset of symptoms (range 2 months – 11 years). The main motive that led the patient to surgery was disabling patellofemoral pain in 21 cases (52.5%) and patellar instability in 19 cases (47.5%). Therefore, two populations were analyzed in this study: "patellar pain patients with PFM" (group I) and "patellar instability patients with PFM" (group II). For the purposes of this paper, the term patellar instability is used to describe giving way as a result of the patella partially slipping out of the trochlea, and dislocation (complete displacement of the patella out of the trochlea). The average age of the patients at the time of surgery was 19 (range 11–26 years). Eleven patients (38%) were operated on both knees. The average follow-up after surgery was 8 years (range 5–13 years). This series had been evaluated clinically at medium-term (average follow-up after surgery: 3 years) (unpublished data). The average age of patients at the time of follow-up was 27 (range 21–36 years).

### 4.2.2 Diagnostic Criteria for Isolated Symptomatic PFM

We define patients with "isolated symptomatic PFM" as those with anterior knee pain, or patellar instability, with abnormalities of patellar tracking during the physical examination, verified with computed tomography (CT) at 0° and 30° of knee flexion, and no associated intra-articular pathology shown during arthroscopy.[26]

### 4.2.3 Patient Selection for IPR

The operation was indicated in young patients (even with open physis) with severe and persistent peripatellar pain and/or patellar instability (with or without recurrent dislocation of the patella), with Q angle <20°, in which CT demonstrated PFM type 1 (subluxation without tilt) or 2 (subluxation with tilt), according to the classification of Schutzer and colleagues,[32] that produced significant disability for daily living activities (ADL), and that did not improve generally after a minimum of 6 months following standard nonoperative treatment.[25] Only in three of our cases, the patient was operated on before 6 months after onset of symptoms because of severe instability with various episodes of falling to the ground. Nonoperative treatment includes physical therapy, medication, counseling, modification of activities, stopping certain activities, and most important, time. Generally, surgery should be considered as a last recourse after all conservative options have been exhausted.

### 4.2.4 Surgical Technique

A proximal realignment, as described by Insall,[19] was performed on all patients. A lateral retinacular release extending along the most distal fibers of the vastus lateralis (vastus lateralis obliquus), the lateral patellar edge, and the lateral edge of the patellar tendon was always performed before the medial imbrication. Medial capsular tightening was achieved by overlapping the medial flap on the patella; the medial flap extends from the upper edge of the VMO into the quadriceps tendon over the patella and above the patellar tendon. Realignment was effected by advancing the vastus medialis laterally and distally, which was held with several preliminary sutures. After realignment, the knee was moved through the range of motion, and the tracking of the patella in the femoral sulcus was assessed. The patella was determined to be centralized if it tracked entirely within the intercondylar sulcus, with no medial or lateral tilt and/or subluxation.

### 4.2.5 Follow-Up Evaluation

We conducted comprehensive follow-up evaluation. All studies were performed by the same examiners, who were blinded to the clinical results.

The clinical results were rated according to the Cincinnati symptom rating scale,[5] Lysholm score,[21] Tegner activity level,[34] and Cincinnati patient perception scale of the overall condition of the knee.[5]

We used the visual analog scale to report the severity of pain, which allows us to quantify numerically (numerical scale) the pain through a 10 cm bar with 1 cm gradations. Pain is rated from 0 to 10, with 0 representing the absence of pain and 10 indicating excruciating pain. Moreover, this permits us to quantify verbally the pain (verbal scale): light (0–3.3), moderate (3.3–6.6), and severe pain (6.6–10).[33]

Roentgenographic staging of patellofemoral osteoarthritis was made in all the patients, except in two due to pregnancy, (37 knees) at the follow-up examination with the axial view X-rays at 45° flexion of the knee, using the method of Merchant.[22] Moreover, preoperative radiographs were reviewed in all the patients. Signs of retropatellar osteoarthritis were rated according to the Sperner classification: Stage 1: subchondral sclerosis, no osteophyte formation; Stage 2: osteophyte formation on the patella; Stage 3: patellofemoral joint space narrowing, marked osteophytes on the patella and femoral condyles; and Stage 4: gross narrowing or complete obliteration of joint space.[36] Osteoarthrosis in Stage 1 was excluded from this study, because it may vary among investigators due to its slight changes. Moreover, CT examinations at 0° of knee flexion at the long-term follow-up examination were made in all patients, except in two due to pregnancy, (37 knees) following a previously well-described technique, given that it is an acceptable way to detect subtle PFM.[25]

Finally, surface electromyographic (SEMG) analysis of amplitude and voluntary activity pattern of VMO and vastus lateralis muscle (VL) of both knees was made in all the patients operated on one knee, the contralateral knee being asymptomatic (12 patients, 24 knees). The contralateral asymptomatic knee was used as a control. Amplitude analyses were conducted to evaluate the magnitude and timing of muscle activity. Voluntary activity pattern was rated in four grades according to the classification of Buchthal.[6] Voluntary activity pattern measures in an indirect way the number of motor units, very useful when there is suspicion of muscle atrophy or hypertrophy. Electromyography data were collected with the Esaote Reporter® (Florence, Italy) electromyography system of four channels, with a program specifically designed for this study, with two channels fitted out, 5 s of sweep screen, filters of 100 Hz and 1 kHz, and 10 mV of amplitude. After skin preparation, which included shaving and cleaning with isopropyl alcohol, surface electrodes were placed on the muscle belly and tendinous attachment of both VMO and VL. A ground electrode was placed on the contralateral aspect of the thigh. We confirm optimal electrode placement by observation and palpation of the patient's quadriceps during isometric contraction with the knee extended. We evaluated the VMO and VL during five maximum voluntary isometric contractions with knee extension, of at least 2 s, following a previously well-described technique.[16] The amplitude was obtained by calculating the average of the amplitudes of each of the five contractions. Between each pair of contractions enough time was left for the muscle to rest. All the patients were able to complete the test without problems or pain. In both knees, we calculated SEMG ratios for VMO:VL function to assess muscle balance.

### 4.2.6 Statistical Analyses of Data

Statistical analysis was performed using the software SPSS version 10.0 (SPSS Inc., Chicago, Illinois) for Windows. Data are presented as mean ± SD. Descriptive statistics, Student's *t*-test, Chi-square test, Fisher's test, and Pearson's correlation coefficient were used for the analysis. A $P$ value $<0.05$ was accepted as reflecting statistical significance. Finally, to determine if we had enough knees in this study to show a clinically significant difference, we performed a power analyses.

## 4.3 Results

### 4.3.1 Clinical Results

At long-term follow-up, all the patients demonstrated improvement based on pain, instability, knee function, activity level, and subjective perception of the condition of her or his knee.

### 4.3.2 Group I (Patellar Pain Patients with PFM; 21 Knees)

Referring to pain, according to the Cincinnati symptom rating scale, preoperatively, 52.4% of the patients had severe pain, constant and not relieved, with ADL; 28.6% had moderate pain, frequent and limiting, with ADL; 9.5% had pain only with severe work/sports activities; 4.8% were able to do ADL without pain, but they had pain with light work/sports activities; and 4.8% had pain only with moderate work/sports activities. Postoperatively, at long-term follow-up, 42.9% of the patients had no pain; 23.8% had pain only with strenuous work/sports, but they were able to do moderate works/sports without pain; 23.8% had pain only with moderate work/sports; 5% had moderate pain with ADL; and 9.5% had pain with light work/sports. Concerning instability, according to the Cincinnati symptom rating scale, preoperatively, 94.4% of the patients, suffered partial giving-way (partial knee collapse but no fall to the ground) and 5.6% total giving-way (knee collapse with actual falling to the ground). Postoperatively, at long-term follow-up, 90.5% had no instability and 9.5% suffered giving-way.

According to Lysholm's score, preoperatively 71% of the knees were catalogued as poor and 29% as fair. Postoperatively, at long-term follow-up, the results were excellent in 8 cases (38%), good in 10 (47.6%), fair in 1 (4.7%), and poor in 2 (9.5%). The preoperative Lysholm score averaged 49.76 (SD, 19.94; range 12–76). The postoperative Lysholm score averaged 95.15 (SD, 4.76; range 88–100) at the medium-term follow-up. At long-term follow-up, it averaged 89 (SD, 13.19; range 53–100). There was no statistically significant worsening when comparing the results at medium– and long-term follow-ups ($p=0.178$; $1-\beta=55.2\%$). Tegner activity score improved from $0.73 \pm 1.01$ to $3.44 \pm 1.01$ at long-term follow-up.

Subjectively, according to the Cincinnati patient perception scale, preoperatively, 60% of the knees were catalogued as fair (moderate limitations that affected ADL, no sports possible) and 40% as poor (significant limitations that affected ADL). Postoperatively, at long-term follow-up, 19% of the knees were catalogued as normal (the patient is able to do whatever he or she wishes with no problems), 57% as good (some limitations with sports, but the patient can participate), and 24% as fair. In six patients with bilateral symptoms operated on the most symptomatic knee, the contralateral nonoperated knee was pain-free in the follow-up.

### 4.3.3 Group II (Patellar Instability Patients with PFM; 19 Knees)

Referring to pain, according to the Cincinnati symptom rating scale, preoperatively, 61.1% of the patients had moderate pain, frequent and limiting, with ADL; 11.1% had severe pain constant and not relieved, with ADL; 5.6% had pain only with severe work/sports activities; 5.6% were able to do ADL without pain, but they had pain with light work/sports activities; and 5.6% had pain only with moderate work/sports activities. Postoperatively, at long-term follow-up, 68.4% of the patients had no pain; 15.8% had pain only with strenuous work/sports, but they were able to do moderate work/sports without pain; 10.5% had moderate pain with ADL; and 5.3% had pain only with moderate work/sports. Concerning instability, according to the Cincinnati symptom rating scale, preoperatively, 83.3% of the patients suffered total giving-way and 16.7% partial giving-way. Postoperatively, at long-term follow-up, 94.7% had no instability and 5.3% suffered giving-way.

According to Lysholm's score, preoperatively, 78% of the knees were catalogued as poor and 22% as fair. Postoperatively, at long-term follow-up, the results were excellent in 13 cases (68%), good in 4 (21%), fair in 1 (5%), and poor in 1 (5%). The preoperative Lysholm score averaged 47.56 (SD, 16.31; range 17–76). The postoperative Lysholm score averaged 96.63 (SD, 3.20; range 90–100) at the medium-term follow-up. At long-term follow-up, it averaged 92.89 (SD, 11.05; range 54–100). There was no statistically significant worsening when comparing the results at medium- and long-term follow-ups ($p=0.256$; $1-\beta=88.6\%$). Tegner activity score improved from $1.08 \pm 1.19$ to $4.36 \pm 0.5$ at long-term follow-up.

Subjectively, according to the Cincinnati patient perception scale, preoperatively, 66.7% of the knees were catalogued as poor and 33.3% as fair. Postoperatively, at long-term follow-up, 42.1% of the knees were catalogued as normal (excellent), 47.4% as good, 5.3% as fair, and 5.3% as poor.

In only one knee (5.2%) a redislocation of the patella occurred spontaneously without traumatism 7 years after surgery; until then, this knee had an excellent result (Lysholm score 95 points). Since then, the result was catalogued as poor (Lysholm score 54 points). We had 2 cases (10.5%) of knee motion limitation, which required manipulation under general anesthesia with an excellent result at 6 and 8 years of follow-up (Lysholm scores 95 and 96 points).

There were no statistically significant differences at long-term follow-up of Lysholm scores in both groups

($p=0.321$; $1-\beta=70.4\%$) with equal variances assumed ($F$ [18, 20]=0.565, $p=0.457$).

### 4.3.4 Image Analyses

Postoperative CT at 0° of knee flexion, at long-term follow-up, demonstrated PFM type 1 or 2 according to the classification of Schutzer and colleagues[32] in 21 cases (56.75%). In the other 16 cases (43.24%), there was a satisfactory centralization of the patella in the femoral trochlea. Eighteen out of 21 cases (85.7%) that presented PFM had a satisfactory result (excellent or good), while the other 3 cases (14.3%) presented a poor result. Fourteen out of 16 cases (87.5%) that presented a satisfactory centralization of the patella had a satisfactory result, while the other 2 cases (12.5%) presented a fair result. There is no relation between the result (satisfactory vs unsatisfactory) and the presence or no presence of PFM ($\chi^2=0.025$, $p=0.875$) (Figs. 4.1 and 4.2). In 12 patients, in whom the contralateral non-operated knee was completely asymptomatic, we found objective PFM in 9 cases, and in 3 cases we found a satisfactory centralization.

Preoperatively, we found no radiographic degenerative changes in any case. Roentgenographic assessment, at long-term follow-up, revealed no detectable signs of retropatellar osteoarthritis in 34 (92%) out of 37 operated knees evaluated by x-rays. One patient had a narrowing of the patellofemoral joint gap (6 years of follow-up, Lysholm score 94 points); one patient had marked osteophytes on the patella and femoral condyles with a narrow joint gap (12 years of follow-up, Lysholm score 91 points) (Fig. 4.3); and one patient had marked osteophytes on the patella and femoral condyles without a narrow joint gap (6 years of

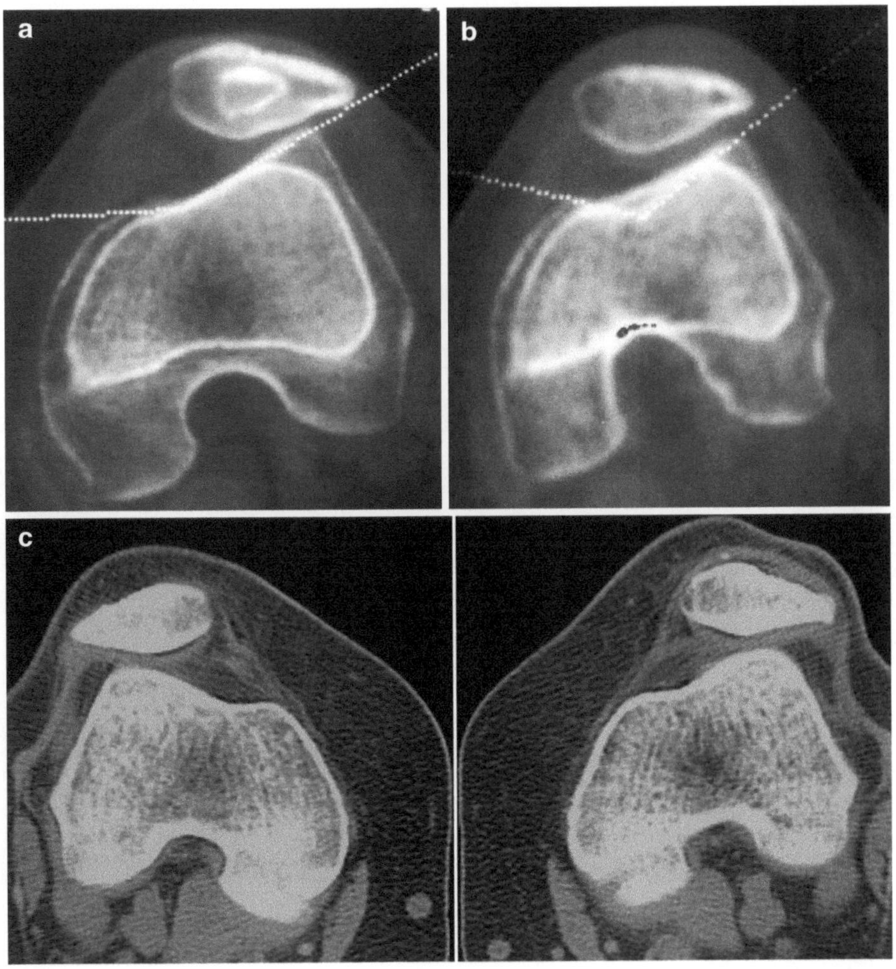


**Fig. 4.1** CT at 0° of knee flexion. (**a**) Preoperative CT: PFM. (**b**) At short-term follow-up after IPR, there is a correct patellofemoral congruence. (**c**) At long-term follow-up (13 years after IPR), we can observe a bilateral asymptomatic PFM (**a** – Reproduced from Sanchis-Alfonso et al.[28], Reprinted by permission from Thieme)

follow-up, Lysholm score 96 points). In the last patient, we found a severe patellar chondropathy during surgery. In the three cases, the contralateral asymptomatic knee had not osteoarthritic changes.

### 4.3.5 SEMG Analysis

We found in all the cases a normal voluntary activity pattern (grade IV according to the classification of Buchthal[6]), in both VMO and VL (Fig. 4.4). VMO amplitude of the operated knee averaged 1.30 ± 0.54. VMO amplitude of the nonoperated knee averaged 1.23 ± 0.53. We found no statistically significant differences between the amplitude of VMO of the operated knee, in comparison with the VMO of the contralateral asymptomatic knee ($p = 0.506$). VL amplitude of the operated knee averaged 1.27 ± 0.39. VL amplitude of the nonoperated knee averaged 1.41 ± 0.53. Neither have we found statistically significant differences between the amplitude of VL of the operated knee, in comparison with the VL of the contralateral asymptomatic knee ($p = 0.189$). The average VMO:VL ratio in the operated knee was 1.06 (range 0.51–1.96). The average VMO:VL ratio in the nonoperated knee was 0.9 (range 0.42–1.82). We found no statistically significant differences between the VMO:VL ratio of the operated knee, in comparison with the VMO:VL ratio of the contralateral asymptomatic knee ($F^{1,24} = 1.768$; $p = 0{,}1972$) (Fig. 4.5), although in the operated knee, the muscle balance was better (Fig. 4.6). We have found a linear correlation between the VMO and VL in the operated knee (Pearson's correlation coefficient = 0.592, $p = 0.043$). In contrast, we have not found a linear correlation between the VMO and VL in the nonoperated knee (Pearson's correlation coefficient = 0.550, $p = 0.064$).

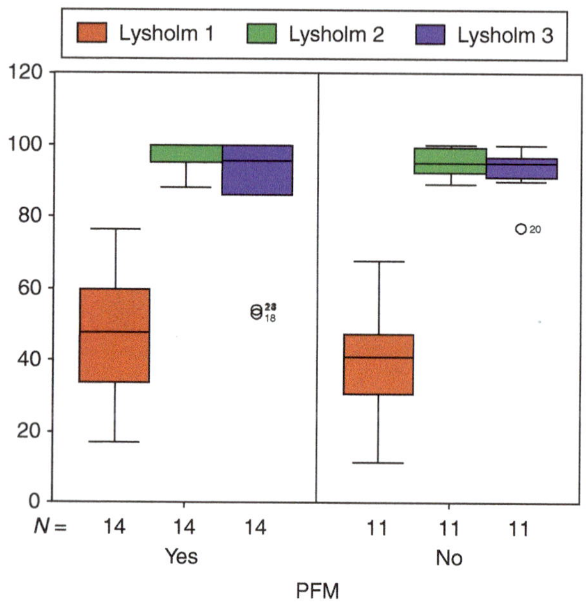


**Fig. 4.2** Lysholm scores of the patients with and without PFM. Lysholm 1 = Preoperative Lysholm score; Lysholm 2 = Lysholm score at medium-term follow-up; Lysholm 3 = Lysholm score at long-term follow-up

## 4.4 Discussion

Patients with patellar symptoms can be divided into two groups: those with patellar instability and those with anterior knee pain. Instability has a clear

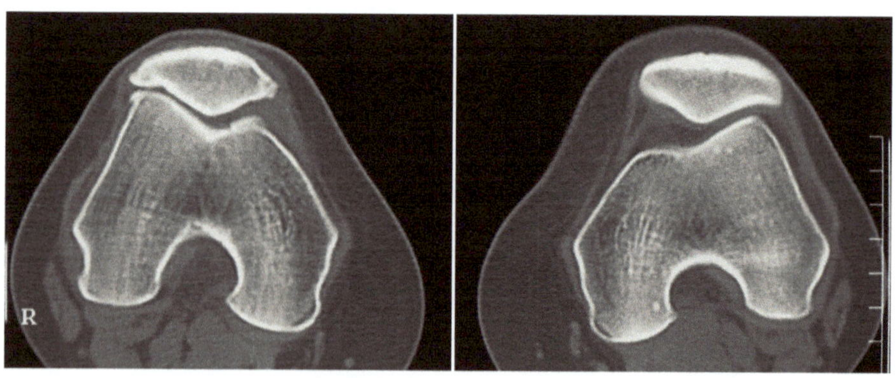


**Fig. 4.3** CT images at 0° of knee flexion from a female 36 years old operated on 12 years ago of the right knee with an Insall's proximal realignment. We can see osteophytes on the patella and femoral condyles with a visible narrowing of the patellofemoral joint gap (right knee). However, clinical result at 12 years follow-up was good. The left knee is asymptomatic despite the PFM

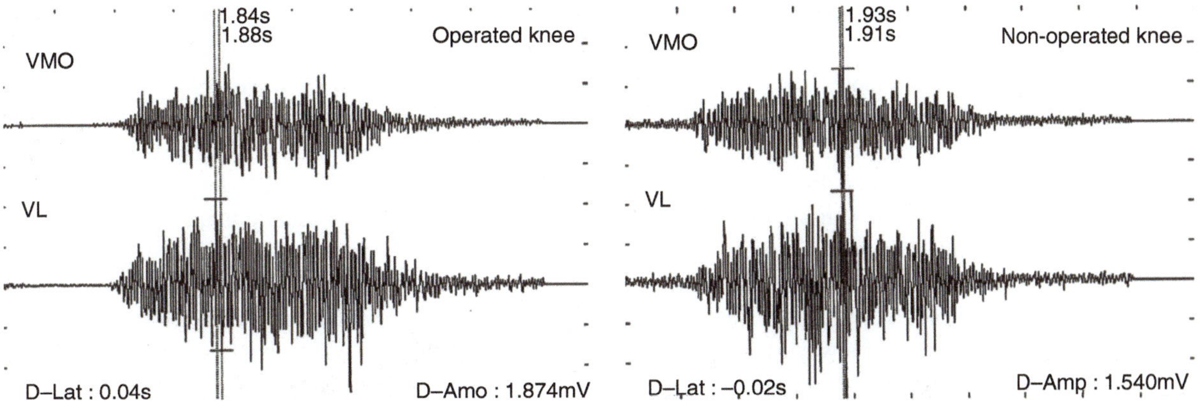


**Fig. 4.4** SEMG activity of the VMO of the operated knee and VMO of the contralateral asymptomatic nonoperated knee. SEMG activity of the VL of the operated knee and VL of the contralateral asymptomatic nonoperated knee

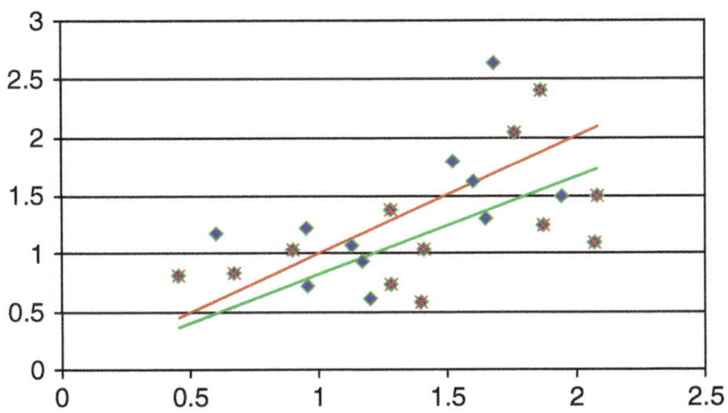


**Fig. 4.5** VMO:VL ratio of the operated knee (*green line*) vs. nonoperated knee (*red line*). *Asterisk* = nonoperated knee. *Rhombus* = operated knee

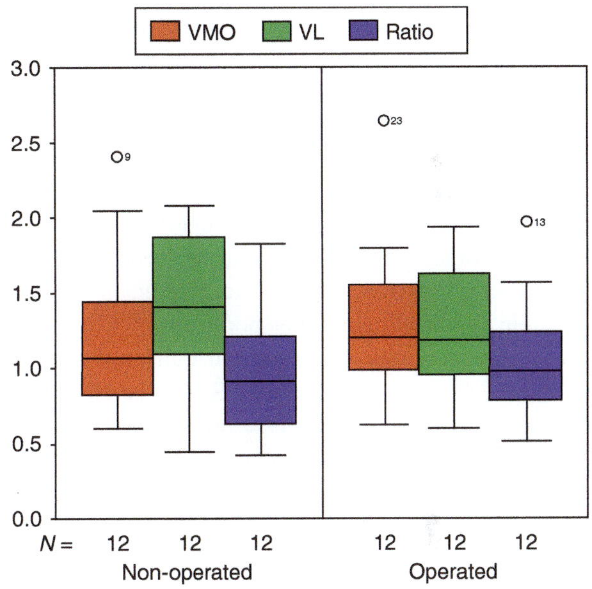


**Fig. 4.6** Amplitude of the VMO and VL of the operated knee and the contralateral asymptomatic nonoperated knee. VMO:VL ratio of the operated knee vs. nonoperated knee

biomechanical basis. In fact, in the 1990s, attention began to be focused on the medial patellofemoral ligament (MPFL) as a restraint of lateral patellar translation, and the traditional approach of *"realign"* the quadriceps has been replaced by the reconstruction of the MPFL.[13] On the contrary, the causative mechanisms of patellar pain remain less well understood, in spite of its high prevalence. In the 1970s, the PFM concept was widely accepted as an explanation for the genesis of anterior knee pain and patellar instability,[11,16,18,19,23,24,28] and influenced the way orthopedic surgeons evaluated and treated such patients. More recently, in the 1990s, Scott Dye came up with the tissue homeostasis theory.[9] For this author, the loss of both osseous and soft tissue homeostasis is more important in the genesis of anterior knee pain than structural characteristics. In fact, patients with anterior knee pain often lack an easily identifiable structural abnormality to account for the symptoms.[9] Likewise, we have patients with no PFM who have recurrent patellar dislocations. Thus, the main objective of this paper is to reassess critically a concept from the 1970s, the PFM, based on our personal experience in IPR surgery.

The first goal of our study was to identify whether there is a relationship between the presence of PFM and the presence of anterior knee pain. A fact that could reflect the relationship between PFM and symptoms would be the diminishment or disappearance of symptoms with realignment surgery, as we have seen in a previous paper.[25] Moreover, IPR, in our experience, provides a satisfactory centralization of the patella in the femoral trochlea, which is detected in postoperative CT scans performed between 3 and 6 months after surgical treatment.[25] Therefore, our satisfactory clinical results could be attributed to restoration of patellofemoral congruence. This fact is said to support the malalignment theory. In this sense, Insall and colleagues[20] reported that nonsatisfactory results (by either persistent pain or instability) were related to the existence of postoperative residual malalignment, whereas if patellofemoral congruence was reestablished, the results were almost always good or excellent. In contrast, as shown by Wojtys and colleagues, there are authors who have failed to show objective improvements of malalignment after isolated lateral release, despite the fact that this procedure frequently lessens pain.[35]

Therefore, the resolution of pain or instability by realignment surgery, as we have seen in our series, does not necessarily mean that PFM caused these symptoms. The success of realignment surgery may be due to factors independent of patellofemoral alignment such as denervation of the patella, postoperative extensive rest (unload), and postoperative physical therapy. Some studies have implicated neural damage and hyperinnervation, into the lateral retinaculum as a possible source of pain in this population.[15,29,30] In this way, we agree with Abraham and colleagues,[1] who suggested that pain relief after IPR may be attributed in part to denervation. Because the sensory innervation of the patella comes in large part from its superomedial aspect via branches of the saphenous nerve, some authors have postulated that operations on the medial side of the patella, such as IPR, work simply by further denervation of the patella.[16] Moreover, IPR would also eliminate the tensile forces that are produced in the retracted lateral retinaculum of patients with chronic lateral patellar subluxation during knee flexion–extension, which would stimulate free nerve endings; finally it would break the ischemia–hyperinnervation–pain circle.[14,27,30,31]

Interestingly, in the present study, we have found that the satisfactory centralization of the patella in the femoral trochlea, obtained at short-term follow-up,[25] is lost in the CT scans performed at long-term follow-up in almost 57% of the cases. So, proximal realignment does not provide a permanent correction of patellofemoral congruence in all the cases. Nonetheless, this loss of centralization does not correlate with a worsening of clinical results. Furthermore, we have not found, in the long-term follow-up, a relation between the results, satisfactory vs. nonsatisfactory, and the presence or absence of postoperative PFM. So, if the presence of PFM is crucial in the genesis of anterior knee pain: Why have we not found differences at long-term follow-up between the results and the presence or absence of PFM? We speculate that PFM could influence the tissue homeostasis negatively, and that realignment surgery could allow the restoring of joint homeostasis when nonoperative treatment of symptomatic PFM fails. Realignment surgery temporarily would unload peripatellar tissues, rather than permanently modify PFM. Once we have achieved joint homeostasis, these PFM knees can exist happily within the envelope of function without symptoms.

On the other hand, in our series, 12 patients presented with unilateral symptoms. In nine of them, the contralateral asymptomatic knee presented a PFM and only in three cases was there a satisfactory centralization of the patella into the femoral trochlea. That is, there is a poor relationship between malalignment and symptoms. In other words, not all PFM are symptomatic. So, if the presence of PFM is crucial in the genesis of anterior knee pain: How can we account for unilateral symptoms in patients with similar morphologic characteristics of their patellofemoral joints? With regards to unilateral pain in the presence of bilateral PFM, it is said that all of us load one limb more than the other, usually the dominant limb. This loading difference could be enough to cause unilateral pain. Moreover, when one knee starts to hurt, overall activity tends to decrease. Perhaps in this situation, the loading on the other side could be insufficient to reach the pain threshold. However, we have not seen loading differences between limbs even during high demanding activities as occurs in sports, for example jumping with pivoting. According with this, we have not found a relation between the lateral limb dominance and the affected side in the cases with unilateral pain.

Finally, in six patients with bilateral symptoms operated on the most symptomatic knee, the contralateral nonoperated knee was pain-free in the follow-up. Moreover, in my experience, 91% of patients with anterior knee pain improve with conservative treatment (unpublished data). So, if the presence of PFM is crucial in the genesis of anterior knee pain: Why do symptoms disappear without any change in the patellofemoral alignment? We speculate that loss of both tissue and bone homeostasis is more important than structural characteristics in the genesis of anterior knee pain.

In conclusion, we have observed that not all PFM knees show symptoms. Therefore, PFM is not a sufficient condition for the onset of symptoms. Moreover, it is not crucial for the genesis of pain given that there are many patients with anterior knee pain without PFM. As a consequence of our findings, it is mandatory to reassess the concept of PFM in the genesis of anterior knee pain. We believe that the pain generator is not the malalignment.

It has been stated that the VMO is responsible for patellar stability, but we have not found convincing evidence in the literature for this belief; and, as ligaments are the joint stabilizers, this premise would appear to be faulty. In theory, the VMO resists lateral patellar motion, either by active contraction, or by passive muscle resistance. In this way, in Farahmand's study,[10] lateral patellar force-displacement behavior was not affected by simulated muscle forces at any flexion angle from 15 to 75°. Regarding resisting lateral patellar displacement, the orientation of the VMO varies greatly during knee flexion. The VMO's line of pull most efficiently resists lateral patellar motion when the knee is in deep flexion, at which time trochlear containment of the patella is independent of soft tissues influences.[3,10,17] The question is: How can we explain our satisfactory results with IPR regarding instability? It seems likely that operations that advance the VMO, such as IPR, include tightening of the underlying MPFL, and it would be responsible for the success of the surgical technique. In this sense, we must note that the VMO tendon becomes confluent with the MPFL in the region of patellar attachment.[12] Therefore, it would be more logical to protect the VMO and address the ligament deficiency surgically as needed.

Advancement of the VMO to increase passive stiffness would have unpredictable effects, because the long-term response of VMO muscle fibers to increased resting length is unknown. We have used SEMG to record muscle action potentials with skin surface electrodes. This is, to our knowledge, the first report specifically addressing long-term response of VMO muscle fibers to increased resting length. We have not found differences between the amplitude of VMO of the operated knee, in comparison with the VMO of the contralateral asymptomatic knee. Neither have we found differences between the amplitude of VL of the operated knee, in comparison with the VL of the contralateral asymptomatic knee. Moreover, we have found VMO:VL ratios within the limits of normality.[7] EMG relationship for each muscle could be problematic if the relationships demonstrate nonlinearity, but this was not the case in our patients. In this sense, we have found a linear correlation between VMO and VL in the operated knee. Therefore, IPR does not provoke an imbalance in the patellofemoral joint. However, we must remember that SEMG VMO:VL activity of each knee of unilaterally symptomatic patients was similar to each other but different from that in knees of healthy subjects.[16] Finally, we found no deficit of the voluntary activity pattern of VMO. Therefore, we can conclude that advancement of VMO has no deleterious effects on VMO from the SEMG point of view.

Muscle activity results in compressive patellofemoral joint forces. It is possible that the generation of high joint reaction forces may be partially responsible for the osteoarthritis that can occur after realignment surgery.[4,8] Crosby and Insall have not found late osteoarthritis after soft tissue corrections without movement of the tibial tubercle.[8] However, Zeichen and colleagues[36] have found patellofemoral osteoarthritis in 36.8% of the patients at medium-term follow-up after IPR. We have found retropatellar osteoarthritis in only 3 knees (8%). Furthermore, clinical results are not comparable with degenerative changes presented at long-term follow-up.

## 4.5 Summary

This study is not intended to advocate for a particular surgical technique, but it does provide insight into improving our understanding of the pathophysiology of anterior knee pain syndrome. Our objectives were: to identify a relationship, or lack of one, between the presence of PFM and the presence of anterior knee pain; to analyze the long-term response of VMO muscle fibers to increased resting length; and to determine the incidence of patellofemoral osteoarthritis after IPR surgery. Our findings indicate (1) that not all PFM knees show symptoms, that is, PFM is not a sufficient condition for the onset of symptoms, at least in postoperative patients; (2) that the advancement of VMO has no deleterious effects on VMO; and (3) that IPR does not predispose to retropatellar osteoarthritis.

**Acknowledgments** The authors gratefully acknowledge the invaluable assistance of Professor Jesús Basulto from the University of Sevilla, Spain, with the statistical analysis, and Paco Ferriz for his technical assistance in CT studies.

## References


1. Abraham E, Washington E, Huang TL. Insall proximal realignment for disorders of the patella. *Clin Orthop Relat Res*. 1989;248:61-65.
2. Aglietti P, Buzzi R, De Biase P, et al. Surgical treatment of recurrent dislocation of the patella. *Clin Orthop Relat Res*. 1994;308:8-17.
3. Ahmed AM, Duncan NA. Correlation of patellar tracking pattern with trochlear and retropatellar surface topographies. *J Biomech Eng*. 2000;122:652-660.
4. Arnbjornsson A, Egund N, Rydling O. The natural history of recurrent dislocation of the patella. Long-term results of conservative and operative treatment. *J Bone Joint Surg*. 1992;74-B:140-142.
5. Barber-Westin SD, Noyes FR, McCloskey JW. Rigorous statistical reliability, validity and responsiveness testing of the Cincinnati knee rating system in 350 subjects with uninjured, injured, or anterior cruciate ligament-reconstructed knees. *Am J Sports Med*. 1999;27:402-416.
6. Buchthal F. *An Introduction to Electromyography*. Glydendal: Scandinavian University Books; 1957.
7. Cerny K. Vastus medialis oblique/vastus lateralis muscle activity ratios for selected exercises in persons with and without patellofemoral pain syndrome. *Phys Ther*. 1995;75:672-683.
8. Crosby EB, Insall J. Recurrent dislocation of the patella. Relation of treatment to osteoarthritis. *J Bone Joint Surg*. 1976;58-A:9-13.
9. Dye SF, Staubli HU, Biedert RM, et al. The mosaic of pathophysiology causing patellofemoral pain: therapeutic implications. *Operat Tech Sports Med*. 1999;7:46-54.
10. Farahmand F, Tahmasbi MN, Amis AA. Lateral force-displacement behaviour of the human patella and its variation with knee flexion – a biomechanical study in vitro. *J Biomech*. 1998;31:1147-1152.
11. Ficat P, Ficat C, Bailleux A. Syndrome d'hyperpression externe de la rotule (S.H.P.E). *Rev Chir Orthop*. 1975;61:39.
12. Fithian DC, Nomura E, Arendt E. Anatomy of patellar dislocation. *Operat Tech Sports Med*. 2001;9:102-111.
13. Fithian DC, Paxton EW, Cohen AB. Indications in the treatment of patellar instability. *J Knee Surg*. 2004;17:47-56.
14. Fulkerson JP. The etiology of patellofemoral pain in young active patients: a prospective study. *Clin Orthop Relat Res*. 1983;179:129-133.
15. Fulkerson JP, Tennant R, Jaivin JS. Histologic evidence of retinacular nerve injury associated with patellofemoral malalignment. *Clin Orthop Relat Res*. 1985;197:196-205.
16. Grelsamer RP, McConnell J. *The Patella. A Team Approach*. Gaithersburg: An Aspen Publication; 1998.
17. Heegaard J, Leyvraz PF, Van Kampen A. Influence of soft structures on patellar three-dimensional tracking. *Clin Orthop Relat Res*. 1994;299:235-243.
18. Hughston JC. Subluxation of the patella. *J Bone Joint Surg*. 1968;50-A:1003-1026.
19. Insall JN. "Chondromalacia Patellae": patellar malalignment syndrome. *Orthop Clin North Am*. 1979;10:117-127.
20. Insall J, Bullough PG, Burnstein AH. Proximal "tube" realignment of the patella for chondromalacia patellae. *Clin Orthop Relat Res*. 1979;144:63-69.
21. Lysholm J, Gillquist J. Evaluation of knee ligament surgery results with special emphasis on use of a scoring scale. *Am J Sports Med*. 1982;10:150-154.
22. Merchant AC. Radiography of the patellofemoral joint. *Operat Tech Sports Med*. 1999;7:59-64.
23. Merchant AC, Mercer RL. Lateral release of the patella: a preliminary report. *Clin Orthop Relat Res*. 1974;103:40.
24. Merchant AC, Mercer RL, Jacobsen RH. Roentgenographic analysis of patellofemoral congruence. *J Bone Joint Surg*. 1974;56-A:1391-1396.
25. Sanchis-Alfonso V, Gastaldi-Orquín E, Martinez-SanJuan V. Usefulness of computed tomography in evaluating the patellofemoral joint before and after Insall's realignment. Correlation with short-term clinical results. *Am J Knee Surg*. 1994;7:65-72.
26. Sanchis-Alfonso V, Roselló-Sastre E. Immunohistochemical analysis for neural markers of the lateral retinaculum in patients with isolated symptomatic patellofemoral malalignment. A neuroanatomic basis for anterior knee pain in the active young patient. *Am J Sports Med*. 2000;28:725-731.
27. Sanchis-Alfonso V, Roselló-Sastre E. Anterior knee pain in the young patient – what causes the pain? "Neural model". *Acta Orthop Scand*. 2003;74:697-703.
28. Sanchis-Alfonso V, Roselló-Sastre E, Martinez-SanJuan V. Pathogenesis of anterior knee pain syndrome and functional patellofemoral instability in the active young. A review. *Am J Knee Surg*. 1999;12:29-40.
29. Sanchis-Alfonso V, Roselló-Sastre E, Monteagudo-Castro C, et al. Quantitative analysis of nerve changes in the lateral retinaculum in patients with isolated symptomatic patellofemoral malalignment. A preliminary study. *Am J Sports Med*. 1998;26:703-709.
30. Sanchis-Alfonso V, Roselló-Sastre E, Revert F. Neural growth factor expression in the lateral retinaculum in painful patellofemoral malalignment. *Acta Orthop Scand*. 2001;72:146-149.
31. Sanchis-Alfonso V, Roselló-Sastre E, Revert F, et al. Histologic retinacular changes associated with ischemia in painful patellofemoral malalignment. *Orthopedics*. 2005;28:593-599.
32. Schutzer SF, Ramsby GR, Fulkerson JP. The evaluation of patellofemoral pain using computerized tomography. A preliminary study. *Clin Orthop Relat Res*. 1986;204:286-293.
33. Scott J, Huskisson EC. Graphic representation of pain. *Pain*. 1976;2:175-184.
34. Tegner Y, Lysholm J. Rating systems in the evaluation of knee ligament injuries. *Clin Orthop Relat Res*. 1985;198:43-49.
35. Wojtys EM, Beaman DN, Glover RA, et al. Innervation of the human knee joint by substance-P fibers. *Arthroscopy*. 1990;6:254-263.
36. Zeichen J, Lobenhoffer P, Gerich T, et al. Medium-term results of the operative treatment of recurrent patellar dislocation by Insall proximal realignment. *Knee Surg Sports Traumatol Arthrosc*. 1999;7:173-176.

# Unilateral Anterior Knee Pain as a Sign of Knee Asymmetry

5

K. Donald Shelbourne and Emily E. Krodel

## 5.1 Introduction

Anterior knee pain is a common complaint and reason for people to seek orthopedic medical care, in either a general or sports medicine practice. It affects a wide range of patients, from highly competitive athletes to the aging population. Despite its prevalence, however, anterior knee pain remains a poorly understood entity that has not been well studied in the literature. "Anterior knee pain" is a nonspecific term that can result from a host of etiologies, including malalignment, muscular imbalance, overuse, trauma, and biochemical substance changes. Although these are all reasonable causes of pain, we have found that unilateral anterior knee pain can oftentimes simply be attributed to asymmetry between the knees. This pain can be improved in a nonoperative manner in most cases, and rehabilitative techniques should be initiated prior to pursuing a surgical treatment. This chapter will offer a description of symmetric knees, a mechanism for the development of unilateral anterior knee pain, and specific evaluation and rehabilitation strategies.

## 5.2 Knee Symmetry

People without knee soreness or pain have symmetric knees. Symmetry between the knees is necessary for people to perform everyday activities comfortably and for athletes to function at a high level. As simple of a concept as this may be, it often seems to go unrealized by both patients and physicians. When comparing an asymptomatic person's right leg and left leg, they should not only look the same, but also have equal knee range of motion, leg strength, and knee stability. When viewed radiographically, femoral size, femoral notches, patella tendon length, and patella size are equal.

Many physicians fail to understand or appreciate these underlying similarities between knees. This can result in an insufficient clinical evaluation for knee pain. In an orthopedic practice devoted to the treatment of knee problems, we have evaluated many patients who have seen other physicians for the same knee problem. We have observed that many physicians failed to look at the patient's non-problematic knee as part of their examination. Examining the patient's "normal" knee first is essential to get a baseline for what the involved knee should resemble in terms of anatomy and functionality. Since "normal" varies from person to person, it is absolutely necessary to get an idea of what the baseline is for each individual. Similarly, this also includes obtaining x-rays of both knees, not just the involved side.

## 5.3 Mechanism for Asymmetry

The author's present philosophy on the development and management of unilateral anterior knee pain is a result of over 20 years of listening to and carefully observing patients. As we have analyzed the results of thousands of patients, it has become apparent that this nonspecific knee pain can largely be attributed to asymmetry between knees. This asymmetry can result

K.D. Shelbourne (✉)
Shelbourne Knee Center at Methodist Hospital,
Indiana University School of Medicine, Indianapolis, IN, USA
e-mail: acldoc@aclmd.com

V. Sanchis-Alfonso (ed.), *Anterior Knee Pain and Patellar Instability*,
DOI: 10.1007/978-0-85729-507-1_5, © Springer-Verlag London Limited 2011

from both reversible and irreversible knee problems and can manifest itself in a variety of ways. What follows is a description of a deconditioned knee and a proposed mechanism for the development of unilateral anterior knee pain.

Patients tend to seek treatment when they have an injury or condition causing asymmetry between their knees. They become concerned when one knee does not feel like the other one. Patients have difficulty localizing the pain and will tend to place a hand over the painful knee, complaining that it "hurts all over." The underlying problem could be reversible, such as an overuse injury or minor trauma. The problem could also be something irreversible such as osteoarthritis or post-meniscectomy. It is possible to have both reversible abnormalities and irreversible ones. At other times, patients may not recall an injury at all. For whatever reason, the patient began to favor one leg, which resulted in a discrepancy between the knees.

A "deconditioned" knee is one that has lost range of motion and/or strength, each of which alters the normal function of the knee.[7] A typical scenario for developing this lost function usually begins with a patient who has done something abnormal to one knee, whether it was realized at the time or not. There does not need to be anything anatomically wrong with the joint; the knee might just bother the patient to a small extent. Regardless of the specific etiology, the patient proceeds to favor that knee by standing solely on the normal knee rather than using both legs equally as a way to avoid worsening the pain. Patients who favor one knee subconsciously stop using the involved leg and will develop a flexion contracture of the knee by avoiding weight bearing on the leg and by keeping the knee bent. A flexion contracture causes a loss of leg strength. As the leg becomes weaker, the patient favors it even more, which further exacerbates the problem.

In most patients who lack knee symmetry in some respect, activities like running and walking, which require equal use of each leg, tend to cause discomfort in the deconditioned knee. This discomfort is commonly described as anterior knee pain. After favoring the knee for so long, the involved knee lacks strength and range of motion. When the patient attempts to return to certain activities, the weak leg struggles to keep up with the normal one and the knee becomes tired and painful by the end of the day.

The natural course of action for most individuals is to rest the knee to see if the pain improves. Patients feel like they are helping themselves along in the recovery process by staying off of it. It is also common for a patient to schedule an appointment with an orthopedic surgeon at this point. Unfortunately, many orthopedists will offer similar advice by recommending cessation of activities that precipitate the knee pain. Not surprisingly, the pain usually persists and may even become worse. An MRI scan is frequently ordered to evaluate for pathology. More often than not, in patients older than 40, abnormalities such as a degenerative medial meniscus tear or articular cartilage damage will be present. The joint pathology present may not be related to the symptoms in the knee, and the same pathology may also be present in the noninvolved knee. Not only does a surgical procedure in this scenario fail to correct the underlying problem of knee asymmetry, it oftentimes exacerbates the knee pain. In our experience, the cycle of knee pain, rest, and disuse causes limitation of normal knee range of motion. Subtle, but significant, loss of normal knee range of motion causes anterior knee pain. Without proper rehabilitation to regain full range of motion, a surgery to treat the joint pathology will not be effective. When rehabilitation is the initial treatment provided, with a goal of encouraging normal use of the extremity and correcting for a loss of motion, surgery can be avoided. However, the recognition of this type of knee asymmetry needs to be recognized.

## 5.4 Evaluation Methods

To perform a proper evaluation of unilateral anterior knee pain, it is absolutely essential to keep the principles of knee symmetry in mind. The assessment of knee pain can be divided into several elements, each of which involves evaluating both knees. The clinician can initially begin to formulate an idea of the cause of knee pain by obtaining a thorough history and carefully observing the patient's habits. Next, the anatomy of the knees needs to be examined, both by physical exam and radiographic means. Afterward, each knee should be evaluated objectively in regards to motion and strength. Again, it is extremely important to use the opposite knee as a guide as to what normal should be, especially if the patient considers the other knee to be normal.[11]

An observation we have made in recent years of evaluating many patients for a second opinion is how surprised some patients are when we have them wear shorts to view the knees and then actually touch both knees for the physical examination. All too often, patients have had MRI scans performed on their knee without any physical examination being done. Given that many people have abnormalities in the joint, it is disturbing to us that physicians make treatment decisions based on radiographic findings without correlating the findings to both the detailed history and physical examination of an involved knee to a noninvolved knee.

### 5.4.1 Clinical Examination

An appropriate knee examination can begin once the patient is dressed in loose-fitting athletic shorts. The patient should initially be observed in a standing position, with attention to quadriceps muscle atrophy, limb alignment,[6] and size of the lower extremity. When a patient has been walking more on his or her toes due to a stiff knee, the gastrocnemius muscles may be hypertrophied in that leg. It is also possible that the patient walks with a flat foot gait with the foot turned out and the calf size may be decreased. The involved lower extremity may also become edematous due to weakness of the leg muscles and subsequent impaired venous return.

If rising from a seated position, it should be noted if the patient seems to use both legs equally to stand. If not, he or she will primarily use the stronger leg to rise from the chair. It is then important to note weight-bearing ability and on which leg the patient appears to stand. Ideally, a patient should be able to stand on both legs equally, with each knee locked in full extension. When the knee is fully extended, the patient can stand with the knee locked and the quadriceps muscles can relax. This is why people can stand for long periods of time without muscle fatigue.

Patients with an acute injury or a flexion contracture will stand with their weight shifted to the uninvolved extremity, with the involved knee slightly bent (Fig. 5.1). If a significant flexion contracture is present, this will be an obvious finding. However, if the patient is lacking only a couple of degrees of full extension compared to the normal knee, the difference will be subtle. It is similar to a door that appears to be shut but is not completely shut to where you hear the click of the door closing. Even a few degrees of extension

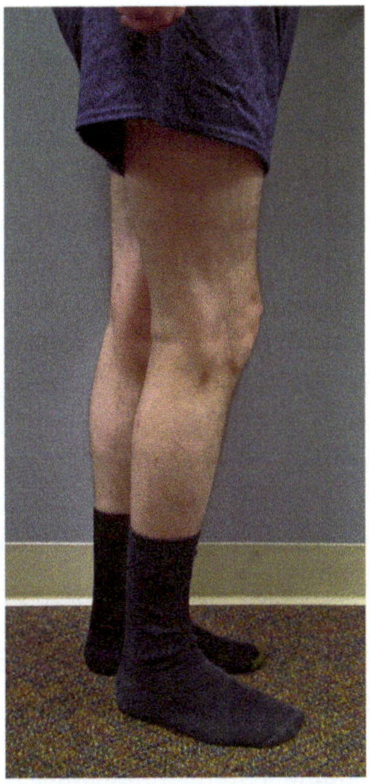

**Fig. 5.1** Patients with knee pain typically favor one leg by standing on the normal knee and leaving the painful knee bent

loss can keep a patient from being able to stand comfortably and equally on both legs. While this may temporarily make the knee feel better to the patient, if the patient continues to keep the knee slightly bent, it may lead to a deconditioned knee causing anterior knee pain. The patient may not be aware of the slight loss of extension because it feels better with rest, but the extension loss causes problems with every day activities such as walking and stairs such that it alters the normal gait pattern and subsequently causes a loss of strength.

It is also important to observe the patient during ambulation. Patients with anterior knee pain may have only minor gait deficits.[8] The patient is then asked to squat down as far as possible, without bending at the waist, in an attempt to sit on his heels. Sometimes, the patient will lean toward the unaffected extremity while squatting. This is a more telling test of knee flexion than passive stretching because the joint is overloaded while squatting.

The uninvolved extremity should always be tested first in order to establish a baseline to which the bothersome knee can be compared. Examining the normal knee can also reduce patient apprehension.[8] The next step in evaluation is to have the patient hop on one foot, if able, testing the normal extremity first. If the patient refuses to jump on the involved side due to anxiety, the test is obviously positive. A patient who agrees to hop on the involved foot, but with difficulty will usually attempt to maintain balance with more pronounced arm movements. Also, patients are more able to hop on their toes on the normal side, whereas they will want to land and roll back toward their heels on the affected side and will usually hesitate before the next hop.

Next, we examine the patient while sitting on the side of the examination table with legs bent. We ask the patient to straighten each knee actively while we check for crepitus and a lag in knee extension. Pain and crepitus with increasing knee flexion implies a more proximal location of an articular lesion on the patella.[6] Patellar tracking is also observed during knee extension to determine if and when the patella moves out of the trochlea laterally, yielding a positive J-sign.[11] The patellofemoral joint and surrounding soft tissues are palpated for tenderness. The distal quadriceps muscles and tendon, patella, prepatellar bursa, retinaculi, facets, plica, patellar tendon, tibial tubercle, and joint lines should all be examined.[6]

The patient is then asked to swing his or her legs onto the table and lie supine. In the process of doing this, the examiner should continue to observe the patient's habits. Sometimes, a patient with a weak lower extremity will pick up the involved limb with his hands to move it onto the table. This is yet another sign that the patient has been favoring that leg. The patient needs to have both heels on the table to be able to check for a flexion contracture and external rotation of the hip, in which the foot of the affected extremity will be angled laterally (Fig. 5.2). While both legs are extended side-by-side on the table with toes pointed toward the ceiling, the examiner should note the height of each patella from the table. If one knee is more bent, that patella will be further off of the table (Fig. 5.3). Another way to check for a flexion contracture is for the examiner to slide his hand under each knee, palm up, and ask the patient to contract the quadriceps in an attempt to press down on the hand (Fig. 5.4). There will be a notable difference in the case of a flexion contracture. Also, a discrepancy in the depth of quadriceps muscle contractions between legs may be visualized as an additional sign of asymmetry.

One of the most important components of the physical examination when evaluating anterior knee pain is an assessment of knee hyperextension for each leg. The physician can do this by placing a hand just above the knee to stabilize the femur and lifting the patient's heel off the table with the other hand (Fig. 5.5). Most individuals exhibit some degree of hyperextension. Based on data obtained from a group of uninjured

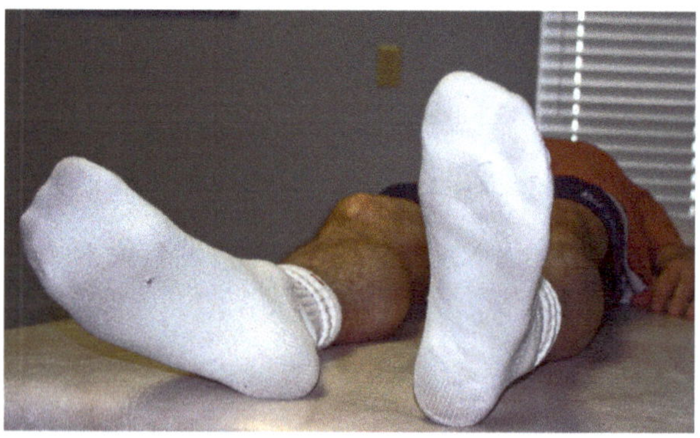

**Fig. 5.2** As part of the physical examination, we have the patient lie supine on the examination table and observe the position of the legs. Patients who favor a knee by keeping it bent can be identified easily because they will have one leg and foot rotated externally

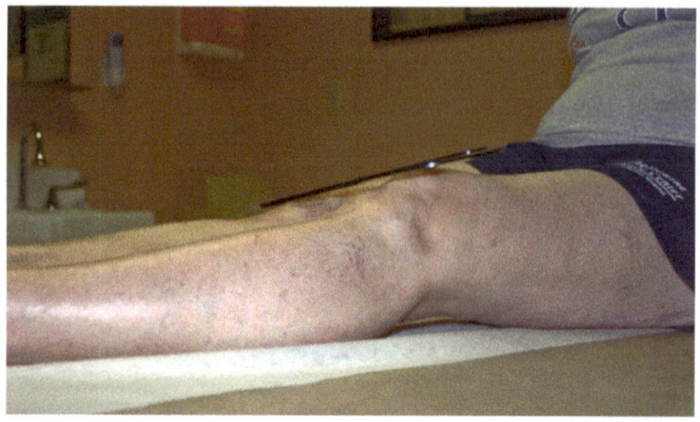

**Fig. 5.3** Lack of normal knee extension can be observed by placing an object over the top of the knees. The bent knee will be the higher side

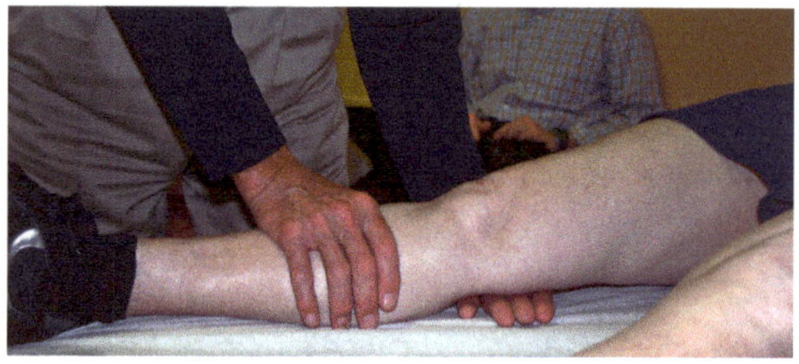

**Fig. 5.4** To critically evaluate small degrees of extension loss, the examiner can place his or her palm behind the patient's knee and evaluate whether the patient can actively extend the knee so that the back of the knee touches the palm

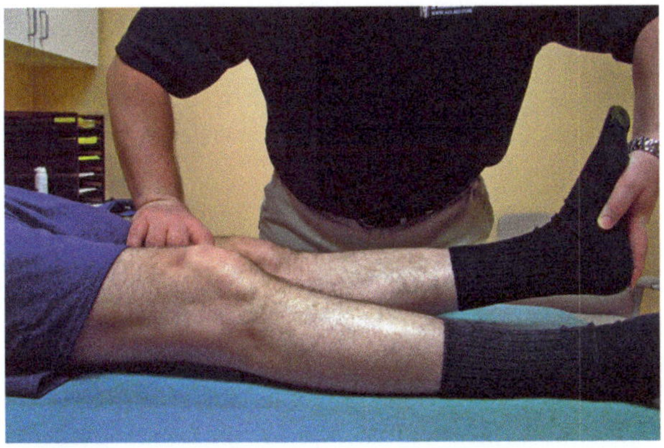

**Fig. 5.5** To evaluate for knee hyperextension, the examiner places one hand above the knee to hold down the thigh and places the other hand on the foot to raise the foot passively to bring the knee into hyperextension. Not only can you evaluate the degree of hyperextension but also how easily the knee moves into hyperextension

athletes, DeCarlo and Sell[2] found that males average 5° of hyperextension compared to 6° of hyperextension in females, with 96% of all people having some degree of hyperextension in their knees.

To complete a thorough knee examination, the physician should also assess passive flexion by gently allowing the foot to drop with the hip flexed. Hamstring flexibility is evaluated by flexing the hip to 90° and extending the knee. During this maneuver, the examiner can feel for patellofemoral crepitus. Quadriceps muscle flexibility can be evaluated with the patient lying prone and having the patient bend both knees to be able to compare heel heights. Other ways to evaluate knee symmetry include performing McMurray's, Lachman's, patella tilt, posterior drawer, pivot shift, and varus and valgus laxity tests and checking for joint line tenderness.

### 5.4.2 Radiographic Evaluation

Multiple radiographic images are obtained to compliment the physical examination. Most patients complain of anterior knee pain unilaterally, so it is important to obtain radiographs of both knees so joint abnormalities can be compared between knees. The most helpful view is a bilateral 45° flexed weight-bearing posteroanterior radiograph, which was described by Rosenberg and colleagues.[5] It can show development variations, osteochondritis dissecans, fractures, and other knee joint pathology that may cause anterior knee pain.[6] This view is most useful because its orientation allows the best visualization of joint space narrowing to evaluate for asymmetric osteoarthritis. If joint space narrowing is present, particularly in the medial compartment, a posterior horn radial medial meniscus tear is usually present because the meniscus gets extruded with narrowing.

An interesting observation that we have made is that although asymmetric joint space narrowing is abnormal, it does not always correlate with the knee having pain. If a patient has significant osteoarthritis but consistently performs exercises that encourage knee symmetry, such as cycling, he or she can be relatively asymptomatic. When this observation is compared to a person with normal radiographs but also a flexion contracture, the need for symmetric knees becomes apparent. The person with a knee flexion contracture will likely be the one complaining of knee pain.

Lateral view radiographs are taken with each knee flexed to 60° to be sure the patellar tendon is under tension. The method described by Blackburne and Peel[1] is used to determine patella baja or patella alta. To specifically assess the patellofemoral joint, the Merchant view radiograph[3] is also obtained. It, too, is a bilateral view of the knees bent at 45°, but is taken axially and is not weight-bearing. It is useful to evaluate the location of each patella in its respective trochlear groove.[11] It is also important to compare the density between each patella. If a patient has favored one leg for a significant amount of time, the patella of the affected leg can be markedly osteopenic.

In general, MRI evaluation is not needed to determine treatment. MRI scans for people over the age of 30 will most likely show some abnormalities, but these abnormalities may not be the cause of symptoms. Viewing MRI scans can lead to over-treatment of articular cartilage defects and small meniscus tears.

### 5.4.3 Objective Testing

It is also extremely important to evaluate a patient's strength and range of motion in an objective fashion. This needs to be performed at the time of initial evaluation and at subsequent visits in order to monitor the patient's progress. Without objective data, it is difficult to define an endpoint of treatment.

Knee range of motion measurements are taken using a goniometer, as described by Norkin and White,[4] and recorded in a-b-c format, with "a" representing the degree of knee hyperextension, "b" representing the degree short of 0° extension, and "c" representing the degree of flexion. Isokinetic quadriceps muscle strength is tested using a Cybex dynamometer or a leg-press test. If the patient's knee is too painful to perform the test at the initial visit, however, this can be delayed until the first therapy visit.

### 5.4.4 Subjective Testing

International Knee Documentation Committee (IKDC) subjective questionnaires are also used to assess symptoms, function, and sports activity in patients with a variety of knee disorders. It is a reliable, responsive, and validated instrument of evaluation.

## 5.5 Rehabilitation

The treatment of nonspecific anterior knee pain can be a very frustrating problem for the patient, orthopedic surgeon, and physical therapist. Many orthopedists are at a loss when surgical interventions fail to improve a patient's symptoms, or in some cases, worsen them. We have adapted our approach to treatment strategies in order to improve final outcomes. In our experience, a majority of anterior knee pain can be treated successfully with proper physical therapy, specifically rehabilitation to improve symmetry. This should be attempted before seeking an operative solution in most cases.

In our clinic, we have worked diligently to follow up regularly with our patients to monitor their progress. This has allowed us to formulate specific rehabilitation protocols in terms of types and frequencies of exercises. It has also permitted us to sort the beneficial modalities from the ones that fail to address the underlying problem. Some treatment options such as weight loss, medication, braces, and arthroscopy do not improve knee extension, and therefore will not yield symmetric knees.

As a general guideline, the patient should be seen frequently in the clinic throughout the rehabilitation period by both the physician and therapist. This is done in order to assess the degree of improvement and continue the subsequent management plan. The patient needs to be cooperative, motivated, and exhibit patience while being treated for this problem.[10]

The main thing to remember during the rehabilitative period is that patients desire a pair of normal knees. Because the definition of normal can vary between individuals, the aim is essentially to achieve symmetry between knees. This needs to address both knee range of motion and leg strength. Sometimes, physical therapists fail to recognize or treat loss of normal knee range of motion and concentrate only on leg strength. The initial goal is to restore full knee extension, including hyperextension, as compared to the non-problematic knee. Once extension has been equalized, the next objective is to regain flexion if a discrepancy existed between knees. Only after full range of motion has been obtained can the patient begin to work aggressively to improve strength. It is difficult to increase strength when patients lack full terminal extension. In our experience, when strengthening and range of motion exercises are combined, little progress is made for either goal. Patients spend only 30 min to 1 h a day performing rehabilitation exercises. When a patient has a flexion contracture, he or she will not be able to use the leg normally throughout the day with standing, walking, stairs, etc. If a patient can achieve full knee extension and be taught to use the leg normally with these daily activities, leg strength will naturally increase as well.

Achieving full extension is of primary importance. Loss of extension is usually more symptomatic compared with flexion loss, and is reported to be associated with patellofemoral pain, quadriceps muscle weakness, and overall poor knee function.[10] Again, it is important to remember that most people can hyperextend their knees past 0°. A physical therapy program should emphasize obtaining normal extension before flexion, because improving both extension and flexion loss is difficult to address simultaneously. Normal flexion can usually be regained better once full extension is achieved. Once full knee range of motion is achieved, specific strengthening of the quadriceps muscle can be introduced.

Full extension can be maintained through a combination of rehabilitation exercises such as prone hangs, heel props (Fig. 5.6), and towel extension exercises

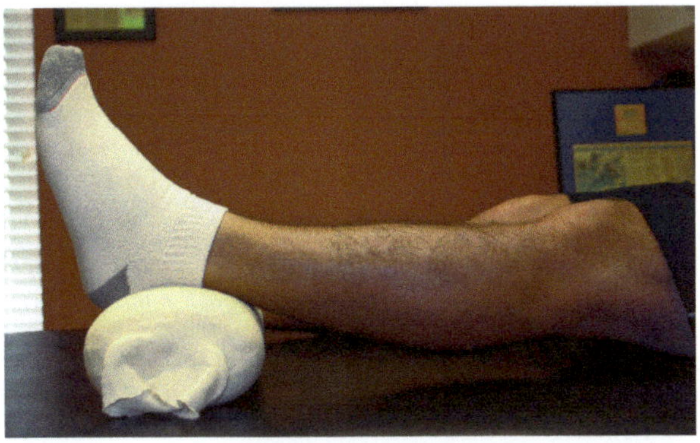

**Fig. 5.6** Heel prop exercise is used to increase knee extension. This exercise is also used to measure for knee hyperextension

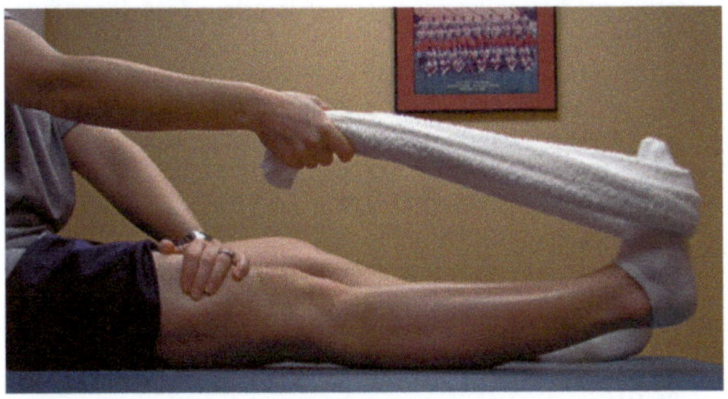

**Fig. 5.7** Towel extension exercise is used to increase knee extension. The patient holds onto the ends of a towel and loops the middle of the towel around the foot. While holding down the thigh, the patient can pull on the ends of the towel to bring the knee into hyperextension

(Fig. 5.7), and gait and posture training. The most effective method to obtain full knee extension is to instruct patients how to improve their daily habits with activities of daily living to help maintain the knee extension that is gained by exercises. They need to be aware of their stance and make a conscious effort to stand on the involved extremity with the knee locked out in full extension via an active quadriceps muscle contraction.[7] A knee extension device such as an Elite Seat (Kneebourne Therapeutics, Noblesville, Indiana) can also be helpful when dealing with flexion contractures, as it can be very difficult to improve range of motion, particularly extension, through exercises only.

Upon normalization of knee extension, the rehabilitation program can progress to include flexion exercises if a deficit is present. Active and passive flexion exercises include wall slides while lying supine, heel slides while sitting, and stationary bicycle riding with progressive lowering of the seat.[10]

Once range of motion is restored, patients may begin low-impact aerobic exercise on a stationary bike, elliptical, or stair-stepping machine. Light strengthening exercises should also be initiated at this point. These can include single leg press, single leg extension, quarter squats, and step-down exercises.

Swelling in the knee joint is another cause of asymmetry, so an attempt to minimize this should be made. At any point during the rehabilitative period, patients can be encouraged to ice their knee for swelling and soreness as needed. If cryotherapy is not sufficient, over-the-counter anti-inflammatory medications may be a reasonable suggestion. In some cases, a cortisone injection might also be appropriate in order to control pain to the extent that the patient is comfortable enough to commence physical therapy.

Despite our best efforts with therapy and nonoperative rehabilitation, conservative treatment does not always sufficiently improve anterior knee pain. At this time, surgery might be a suitable next step in certain situations. However, a trial of therapy is still pertinent to the overall treatment plan. As a result of studying our patients over the years, we have noticed the importance of preoperative rehabilitation programs. If full knee range of motion and leg strength are regained before an operation, the postoperative rehabilitation is much easier. If a patient is unable to fully flex and extend the knee before a surgical procedure, they will not be able to do so immediately afterward.[9]

## 5.6 Summary

Anterior knee pain is a common complaint in the orthopedic community. It is nonspecific in nature and can be frustrating to treat. Symmetry between the knees is necessary for people to perform everyday activities comfortably and for athletes to function at a high level. Through observation and research on thousands of patients, we have found that unilateral anterior knee pain can largely be attributed to asymmetry between knees, in particular the loss of full knee extension. Loss of full knee extension can be caused by many factors. Regardless of the specific etiology, patients favor one knee by standing solely on the normal knee rather than using both legs equally. Patients subconsciously stop using the involved leg and a flexion contracture can develop when they avoid weight bearing on the leg and they keep the knee bent. As the leg becomes weaker, the patient favors it even more and the knee can become "deconditioned." Even small degrees of extension loss can cause anterior knee pain. Our experience has shown that the most important objective to keep in mind when dealing with anterior knee pain is the restoration and maintenance of symmetry between knees. This is primarily accomplished by treating any deficits in knee range of motion first followed by improving leg strength with appropriate rehabilitative exercises and instructions for correct symmetrical use of the legs with daily activities.

## References


1. Blackburn JS, Peel TE. A new method of measuring patellar height. *J Bone Joint Surg Br.* 1977;59-B:241-242.
2. DeCarlo MS, Sell KE. Normative data for range of motion and single-leg hop in high school athletes. *J Sports Rehabil.* 1997;6:246-255.
3. Merchant A. Patellofemoral malalignment and instabilities. In: Ewing JW, ed. *Articular Cartilage and Knee Joint Function: Basic Science and Arthroscopy.* Raven Press: New York; 1990:79-91.
4. Norkin CC, White DJ. *Measurement of Joint Motion: A Guide to Goniometry.* 3rd ed. Philadelphia: FA Davis Co; 2003.
5. Rosenberg TD, Paulos LE, Parker RD, Coward DB, Scott SM. The forty-five degree posteroanterior flexion weight-bearing radiograph of the knee. *J Bone Joint Surg Am.* 1988;70:1479-1483.
6. Shelbourne KD, Adsit WS. Conservative care of patellofemoral pain. In: *The Patella.* New York: Springer; 1994: 1-15.
7. Shelbourne KD, Biggs A, Gray T. Deconditioned knee: the effectiveness of a rehabilitation program that restores normal knee motion to improve symptoms and function. *North Am J Sports Phys Ther.* 2007;2:81-89.
8. Shelbourne KD, Freeman HE. Nonoperative management of acute medial collateral ligament injuries. *Tech Knee Surg.* 2007;6(2):93-98.
9. Shelbourne KD, Klotz C. What I have learned about the ACL: utilizing a progressive rehabilitation scheme to achieve total knee symmetry after anterior cruciate ligament reconstruction. *J Orthop Sci.* 2007;11:318-325.
10. Shelbourne KD, Patel DV, Martini DJ. Classification and management of arthrofibrosis of the knee after anterior cruciate ligament reconstruction. *Am J Sports Med.* 1996;24: 857-862.
11. Urch SE, Shelbourne KD. Treatment algorithm for patellar dislocation or malalignment. *Indiana Orthop J.* 2008;2: 86-91.

# Biomechanical Bases for Anterior Knee Pain and Patellar Instability

# 6

Vicente Sanchis-Alfonso, Carolina Ávila-Carrasco, Jaime M. Prat-Pastor, Carlos M. Atienza, and Enrique Cuñat

## 6.1 Introduction

The mechanical theory has received more attention than the neural hypothesis to explain the genesis of anterior knee pain (AKP) and patellar instability.[2,16-24,27,31,33-35,42,51,57-59,69,70] Patellofemoral malalignment (PFM) and the excessive patellofemoral joint reaction (PFJR) forces have been identified as the two main causes of subchondral bone overload and consequently, of AKP. Mechanical factors like malalignment between the joint surfaces, unbalanced muscle pull, excessive knee valgus (increased Q angle), and quadriceps contractures, contribute to the production of excessive forces on the patellofemoral joint (PFJ) surface. For this reason, understanding the biomechanics of the patellofemoral mechanism and identifying the resulting forces involved in dynamic and static knee positions is a basic prerequisite for the successful treatment of patients with patellofemoral pathology.[3]

Subchondral bone overload, with the consequent increment of the subchondral intraosseous pressure, is a direct result of PFM. However, subchondral bone overload can also be increased when the knee, with or without malalignment, is subject to an overuse or to a direct or indirect traumatism, frequently observed in the practice of sports. Indeed, 49% of the patients in our surgical series suffered an indirect traumatism during sport activities before the onset of symptoms, and 5% of them suffered a direct hit.[59] Furthermore, certain attitudes that are necessary to adopt in some sports (inherently) can contribute, on one hand, to the increase of the subchondral bone overload due to the increment of the PFJR force, and on the other hand to the increment of the Q angle.

Sport is an important agent in the pathogenesis of AKP and in the functional patellar instability as seen by the fact that 73% of our operated patients (unpublished data) used to play energetic sports (volleyball, basketball, handball, football, rhythmic gymnastics, or hockey) of level I (4–7 days a week of practice) or level II (1–3 days a week of practice) before the symptoms started. In addition to this, the degree of pain was related to the patient's level of activity. It is worth remembering the undoubted relation between sport activities and the articular overuse concept. Overuse is defined in general terms as a repetitive microtrauma of a sufficient degree to overcome the regeneration capacity of the tissues.[52] In all types of tissues, the microtraumatism, caused by the application of repetitive tensions, produces microlesions in the collagen fibers, in addition to direct or indirect effects on the vascular supply. Using the wrong technique, or training inadequately (including overtraining), and not employing the right equipment, are additional factors for the onset of the overuse syndromes.

## 6.2 Reaction Forces Generated by the Impacts Produced While Running and Jumping

Running, jumping, turning, and swiveling are an important part of many energetic sports as mentioned before. Of these, jumping is the main culprit in the

V. Sanchis-Alfonso (✉)
International Patellofemoral Study Group,
International ACL Study Group,
Hospital 9 de Octubre,
Hospital Arnau de Vilanova, School of Medicine,
Catholic University of Valencia, Valencia, Spain
e-mail: vicente.sanchis.alfonso@gmail.com

V. Sanchis-Alfonso (ed.), *Anterior Knee Pain and Patellar Instability*,
DOI: 10.1007/978-0-85729-507-1_6, © Springer-Verlag London Limited 2011

origin of chronic lesions of the knee. Furthermore, jumping is one of the main causes of patellar tendinopathy ("jumper's knee"), which is a typical example of an overuse knee lesion, and in 49% of our cases, it was linked to a symptomatic PFM (unpublished data). The reaction forces generated between the foot and the ground when landing after a jump from the standing position and then transmitted through the musculoskeletal system from feet to head, can be up to five times the weight of the player (i.e., for volleyball players during landing after a blocking maneuver)[3,49] and up to nine times when the jump follows a previous run.[46] If to this we add that jumping is a repetitive gesture, it is understandable how damaging it can become for the player's knee. For instance, a player of the NBA is thought to jump at least 70 times per match.[47] The heavy weight and great height of the basketball players are additionally negative factors. On the other hand, during running, the impact forces against the ground reach two to three times the body weight.[12] Moreover, other different maneuvers executed during a match, as v-cuts or defensive shuffles, can produce ground reaction forces between 2 and 3.5 times the body weight.[15]

These repetitive and high loads on the knee have a cumulative effect during the training and competition periods, without forgetting the sport practice by adolescents in physical education classes, which on its own or associated to other predisposing factors, can cause the onset of the symptoms. These sport movements are inevitable and are part of the sport itself, but they can be mitigated.

## 6.3 Importance of Footwear, Ground Surface, and Personal Technique in the Origin and Prevention of Lesions

The human body has some natural systems of shock absorption to protect itself from the effect derived from jumping and running: soft heel tissue, pronation of the hindfoot, ankle dorsiflexion, knee flexion, menisci, articular cartilage, and hip flexion.[11,40] As pointed out by Gross and Nelson,[25] the series of articular movements on landing from a vertical jump starts with the distal joints to end in the proximal ones (metatarsophalangeal, midtarsal, subtalar, ankle, knee, and hip joints). The knee and the hip play a primary role in the process of shock absorption after a jump, whereas the foot pronation (subtalar joint) is the main shock absorber when running.[40] However, this knee flexion with a positive effect as a shock absorber also shows a negative effect as it increases the PFJR force, as will be seen in the next section. On the other hand, the total strength of the impact suffered by the organism depends not only on the applied force, but also on the time that force is being applied. It is considered a good technique of dissipation or absorption of the impact when the force is distributed along a certain period of time. Shock absorption can be incremented by using these natural mechanisms (i.e., good sport technique, speed of the fall) or by using external materials (i.e., appropriate footwear and adequate playing surface). In this way, prevention of lesions related to overuse or reduction of the negative impact of certain inevitable stresses on the knee like running and jumping is probably possible.

Footwear can contribute to reducing the reaction force after impact in three ways: (1) increasing the natural shock-absorbing mechanisms (appropriate heel insole to increase heel fat shock-absorbing role and a strong heel stiffener to prevent hyperpronation), (2) supplementing the aforesaid mechanisms (good-quality sole materials, air chambers, and insoles), and (3) avoiding limiting the natural shock-absorbing mechanisms like heel dorsiflexion (boot-type footwear increases the charges transmitted to the muscular skeletal system by limiting ankle mobility, as opposed to the shoe-type footwear). Overlooking these rules in sport, footwear will increase the impact stresses when jumping and running and therefore, it will produce an overload of the knee and will favor the development of chronic overload lesions. Having a well-supported ankle (boot-type footwear) reduces the shock-absorbing efficiency when running and swiveling, very frequent gestures in handball, therefore this type of footwear is not recommended for this sport.[55] Finally, having the sole empty at midfoot level would allow a certain independence of movement between the forefoot and the hindfoot, reducing shoe rigidity. This would favor the mobility of the midtarsal joint (natural shock-absorbing system).

Excessive adherence of shoe to the playing surface is another lesion-producing factor. On the other hand, lack of this adherence can, as well, be the cause of lesions. In handball, for instance, it is necessary to have a good adherence between shoe and court as there are frequent changes in direction and breaking movements in this sport.[55] When practiced in a pavilion, sports shoes with "caramel soles," called thus because of their aspect, are used. These soles have a great parquet adherence; this increases the performance, but they are not advisable because this adherence can cause a knee lesion. It has been said that a pattern under the head of the first metatarsal should be added to the specific sole pattern to facilitate turning over this area, reducing the overload on the knee joint, and thus counteracting the adherence of the sole to the playing surface. An excessive adherence can cause lesions. For instance, rhythmic gymnastics on a mat should be practiced barefoot or with slippers, as normal sports shoes could cause a severe knee lesion due to the excessive adherence of the shoe to the mat (avoidable technical error).

Finally, worn-out sport shoes are a negative factor, as the adherence and shock-absorbing mechanisms have lost their efficiency (avoidable factor).[11,12] The fact that these types of shoes are worn for too long is related to their high price, and for this reason some athletes opt for funny and dangerous solutions, for example, soaking the soles of their shoes in Coca-Cola, Reflex, honey, lacquer, or something that the handball players call "stick," a resin that they put on their hands to prevent the ball from slipping. The final aim is to increase the adherence of the shoe to the court.

Regarding the playing surface, a high percentage of amateur sportsmen and sportswomen in our environment play and train on hard surfaces, such as cement or asphalt. These hard surfaces favor the development of overload lesions due to the fact that the reaction forces after the impacts caused by jumping and running are very high. Ideally, they should train and play over parquet or synthetic materials with a high shock-absorbing capacity. The problem is the lack of properly fitted sports pavilions.

## 6.4 Patellofemoral Joint Reaction Force. Patellofemoral Contact Areas

Different pathologies can modify the physiological patellofemoral contact surface, but generally speaking, a reduction of the reaction force in the PFJ is associated with pain reduction. It is therefore necessary to determine the value that such a reaction force can reach in each sport movement and for each rehabilitation exercise, or at least to determine what knee positions are associated with maximum values of these reaction forces.

Isolating the knee joint, in a schematic way, as can be seen in Fig. 6.1a, shows that the forces acting on the PFJ during knee extension are the quadriceps muscular force ($F_Q$), the force transmitted to the patellar tendon ($F_{PT}$), and the reaction force generated on the PFJ ($F_{PFJR}$). In a simple way, if the force transmitted to the patellar tendon and the one exerted by the quadriceps are equal (this hypothesis is more inaccurate for higher degrees of flexion), the PFJR force can be determined graphically, as we can see in Fig. 6.1b.

Using the graphic method, it is easy to observe that for a certain quadriceps muscle force, the PFJR force increases with the angle of knee flexion, therefore it is minimal at complete extension[2,19,23,34,51,70,74] (Fig. 6.2a). For example, for a quadriceps force of 1,000 N (approximately 100 kg) and a flexion of 5°, the PFJR force is around 60 kg, whereas if flexion reaches 90° the reaction force increases to values around 130 kg (Fig. 6.2a). This would increase for higher flexion values. The patellar articular cartilage is one of the thickest in the body, which is very useful to withstand these great compressive loads. In numerous sports, the

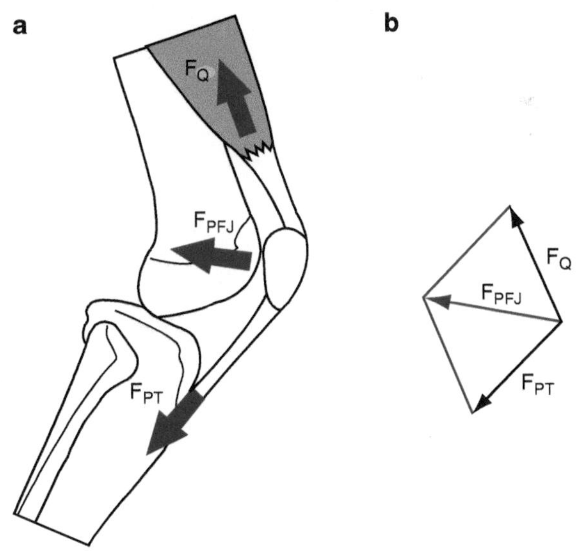


**Fig. 6.1** (**a**) Simplified scheme of the forces acting on the patellofemoral joint. (**b**) Graphic calculation of the patellofemoral reaction force. $F_Q$ force upon quadriceps, $F_{PT}$ force transmitted to the patellar tendon, $F_{PFJ}$ reaction force upon the patellofemoral joint

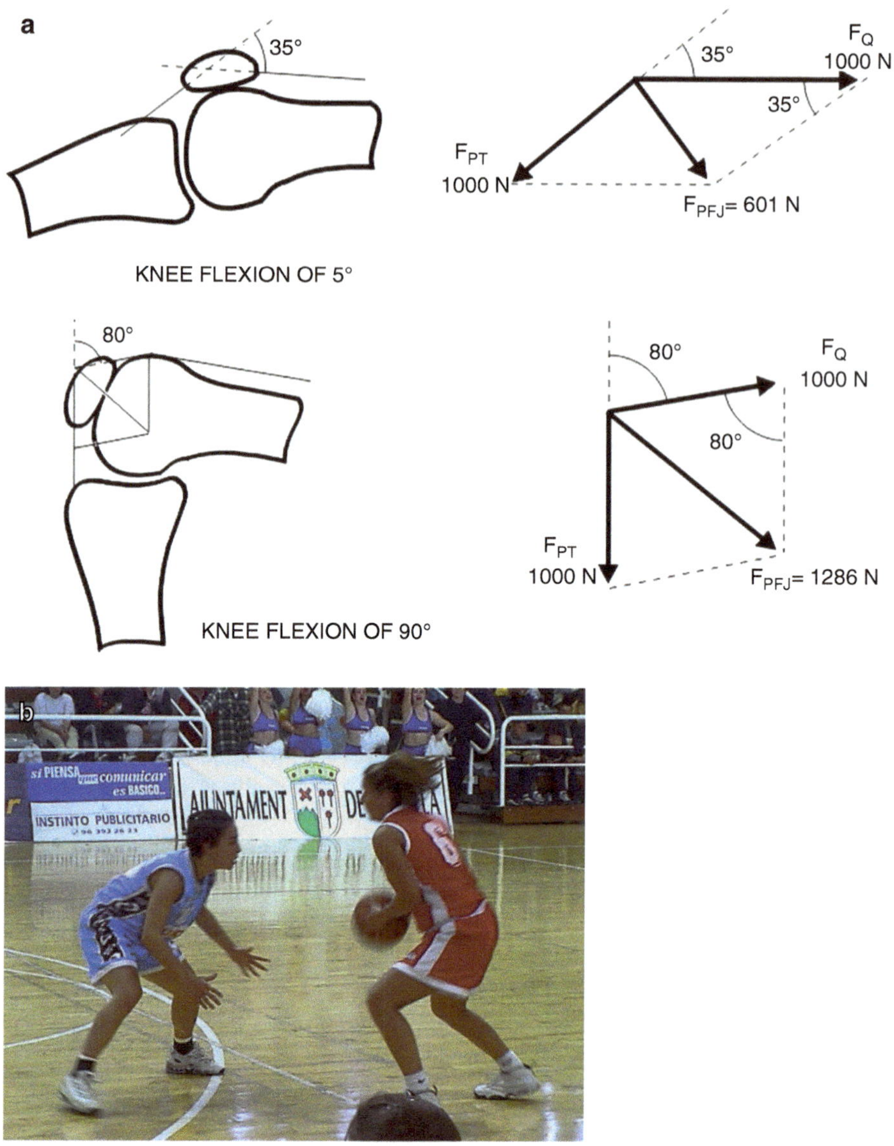


**Fig. 6.2** (**a**) Patellofemoral reaction force determined for a knee flexion of 5° and 90° with a quadriceps muscle force of 1,000 N. (**b**) The reaction force increases as the knee flexion increases. Positions of maintained knee flexion are frequent in sports (Fig. b is reproduced with permission of Promo Sport)

repetitive and maintained knee flexion positions are frequent, producing increases in the PFJR forces and subjecting the patellar cartilage to a maximal risk despite its thickness (Fig. 6.2b).

It is necessary to apply the concept of moment (product of a force and the distance from its line of action to a point) to estimate the quadriceps extension force that has to be applied in certain positions (Fig. 6.3). The flexion moment due to external forces (in the figure 60 kg of body weight) has to be balanced by an extensor moment, which, in a simplified way, can be due to the quadriceps only. The flexion moment is calculated multiplying the force that bends the joint (body weight) by the distance of its line of action (the line which passes through the center of gravity) to the center of rotational movement (which coincides with the point of joint contact between the femur and the tibia). Also, the extensor moment will be equal to the quadriceps force multiplied by the distance of its line of action (roughly the medial line of the patella) to the center of rotation. For a position like the one depicted in Fig. 6.3a with a flexion of 45°, the distance from the body weight action line to the center of the joint is approximately 5 cm and coincides with the distance between the line of action of the extensor force to the same center. Therefore, the

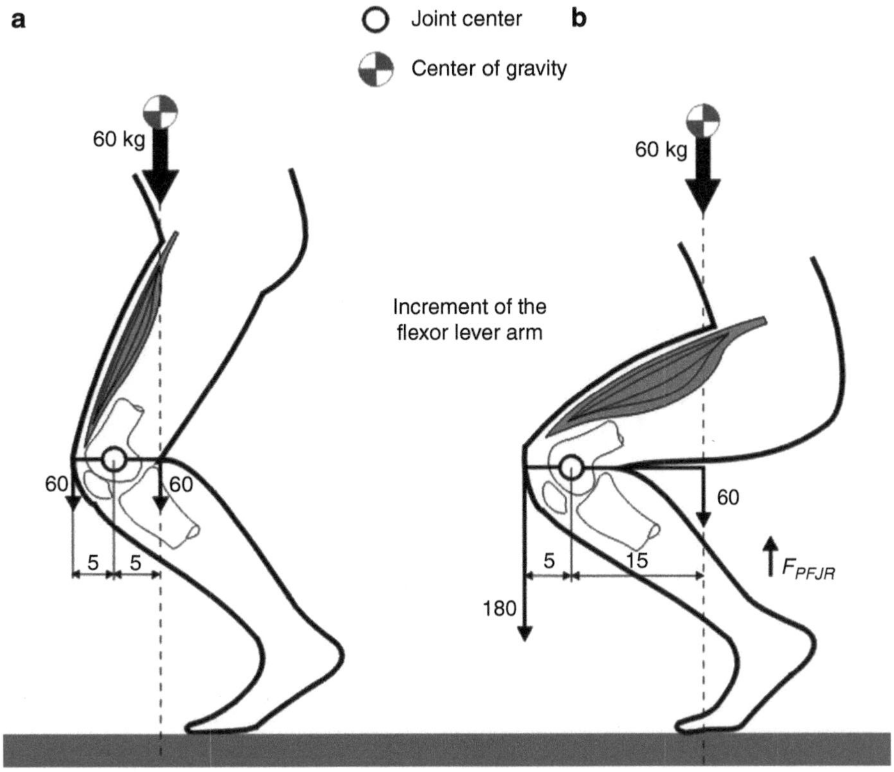


**Fig. 6.3** (**a**, **b**) Body weight line of action and quadriceps extension force applied to different positions of knee flexion. Effect of the increment of the flexor lever arm upon the reaction force in the patellofemoral joint ($F_{PFJR}$) (Units of force kg, and distance cm)

extensor force should also coincide with the body weight force. If knee flexion increases to 115° (Fig. 6.3b), the distance of the body weight action line to the joint center increases threefold (15 cm), and for the same body weight, the extensor force has to increase in the same proportion, reaching a value of 180 kg. For a given quadriceps force, the increase in reaction force is a little more than one and a half times the former when passing from 45° to 115° of flexion; therefore, while quadriceps force increases threefold, reaction force does so more than four and a half times.

From these simple mechanical considerations, the great importance of knee flexion becomes very clear, during extensor exercises, upon the PFJR force, which is directly related to the joint pain.

The reaction force at the PFJ during walking is 0.5 times the body weight[54]; climbing up and down stairs increases the loads 3.5 times the body weight and for squatting movements, the value can reach around 3 times the body weight.[44]

Certain activities of daily life are responsible for the increase in the reaction force of the PFJ. This would be the reason why climbing up and down stairs, crouching, bicycle riding, and sitting for some time with the knees bent, like in the cinema or in a car, cause pain in the group of patients we are studying. However, it is important to underlie that for some of these movements, like squats, the human subject can lean forward to move the center of mass, tilt the hip reducing the knee joint moment, and therefore, lower the PFJR force significantly (Fig. 6.4).[6] That is, one way of reducing the PFJ reaction force would be to associate a hip flexion, as this approximates the line of action of the body weight to the knee.

In summary, the PFJR force not only increases with knee flexion due to the resultant force increment, but also because of the flexor lever arm, which requires a quadriceps response and increases in length. As a general rule, it is not advisable to bend the knees excessively when they are under strain (e.g., supplementary weight (Fig. 6.5), speed, short breaking distance, etc.). It becomes clear that, with a good personal technique and a good training technique, it is possible to partially lessen the bad effect of the PFJR force. Additionally, we can understand how loss of weight, obviously when the patient is overweight, is an important part in the treatment of this type of patients. Obesity is one of the

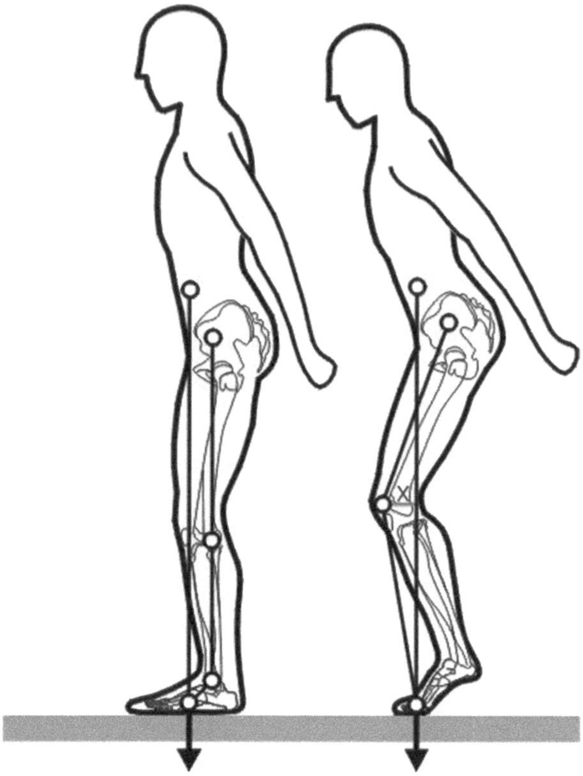

**Fig. 6.4** Effect of the hip flexion on the reaction force in the patellofemoral joint

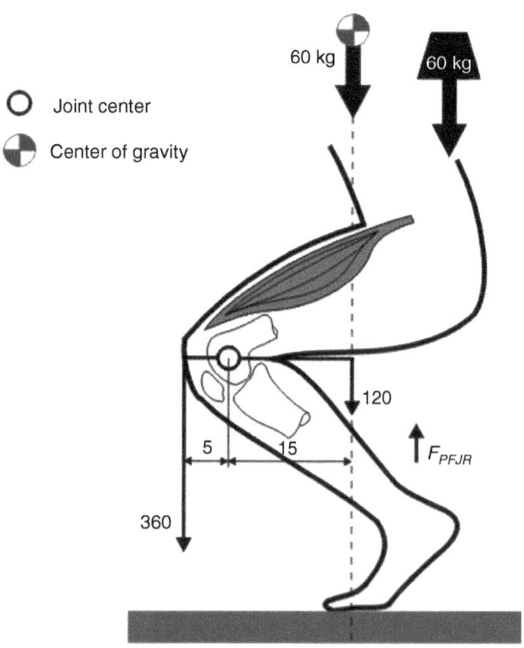


**Fig. 6.5** Effect of the complementary weights (60 kg) upon the patellofemoral joint reaction force ($F_{PFJR}$) (Units of force kg, and distance cm)

main factors in the overloading of the PFJ and cannot be overlooked in the treatment.

Another important factor to study is PFJ stress (pressure) (reaction force/contact surface). Eisenhart-Rothe and colleagues[18] have analyzed the three-dimensional kinematics and contact area of the PFJ of healthy volunteers by 3D image postprocessing. During knee flexion (30–90°), patellofemoral contact areas increased significantly in size (134 mm$^2$ vs. 205 mm$^2$). Besier and colleagues[6] also studied the PFJ contact areas and showed the existence of differences between gender and physiologic loading conditions as well. So, under weight-bearing conditions, they found that contact areas increase by an average of 24%.

Therefore, for healthy persons during knee flexion, an increase of the reaction force is related to a bigger contact surface and a moderate increase in PFJ pressures. On the contrary, contact stress (pressure) at the PFJ increases in PFM during knee flexion in the same or higher proportion as a consequence of a patellofemoral contact area decrease. Brechter and Powers[9] have studied the patellofemoral stress during walking in persons with and without patellofemoral pain (PFP). On average, PFJ stress was significantly greater in subjects with PFP compared with control subjects during level walking. The observed increase in PFJ stress in the PFP group was attributed to a significant reduction in PFJ contact area, as the PFJR forces were similar between these two groups.

However, Heino and Powers[28] found that during stair ascending and descending, subjects with PFP did not exhibit excessive PFJ stress. The reduction in the knee extensor moments and PFJR forces appeared to be a compensatory strategy aimed at keeping joint stress within acceptable limits. This was accomplished by reducing the walking speed.

Hamstring and triceps surae contractures can have an indirect effect in the patellofemoral dynamics as they increase the reaction force at the PFJ, as these contractures produce a maintained flexion of the knee. Lastly, a quadriceps contracture directly increases the contact pressure between patella and femur.

In a similar way, anterior knee pain after intra-articular reconstruction of the anterior cruciate ligament (ACL) with a bone-patellar tendon-bone autograft is related more to a maintained flexion contracture of the knee, and therefore, to an increment of

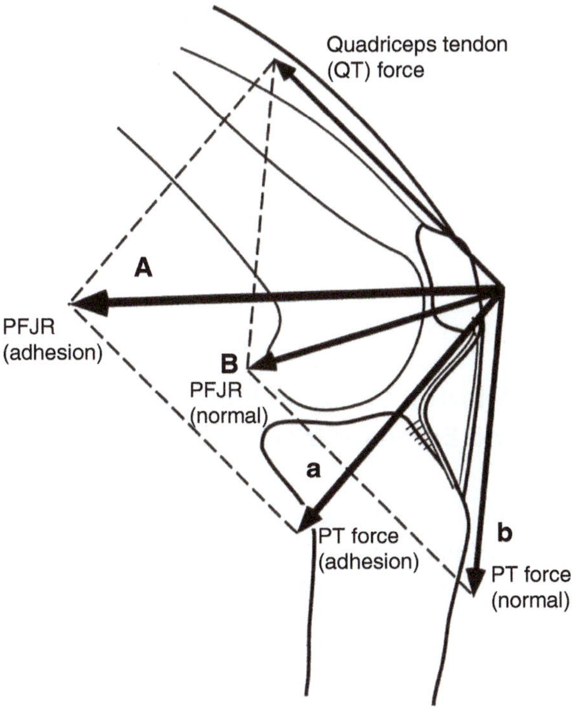


**Fig. 6.6** Patellofemoral joint reaction force ($F_{PFJR}$) in a knee with patellar tendon adhesions to the proximal tibial surface (Reproduced from Ahmad[1]. Reprinted by permission of SAGE Publications)

the reaction force of the PFJ, than to the actual graft harvesting.[37,60,62] Because of this, regaining full hyperextension of the knee early after ACL surgery is advisable, as it is clear that it does not affect, negatively, knee stability in the long term.[62] An unstable knee is better tolerated by the patient than a stable one with a permanent flexion deformity. The latter is one of the causes of AKP. Anterior knee pain after ACL surgery has also been related to the patellar tendon pretibial adhesions that produce an increase in the PFJR force (Fig. 6.6).[1]

## 6.5 Q Angle and Valgus Vector

The Q angle implies the existence of a vector pointing laterally with contraction of the quadriceps, called the valgus vector (Fig. 6.7a), which favors not only the lateral subluxation of the patella, counteracted by the medial patellofemoral ligament, but also an increase of the traction tensions at the insertion of the patellar tendon in the lower patellar pole. This Q angle increases when there is hip anteversion, external tibial torsion, genu valgum, tightness of the fascia lata and of the

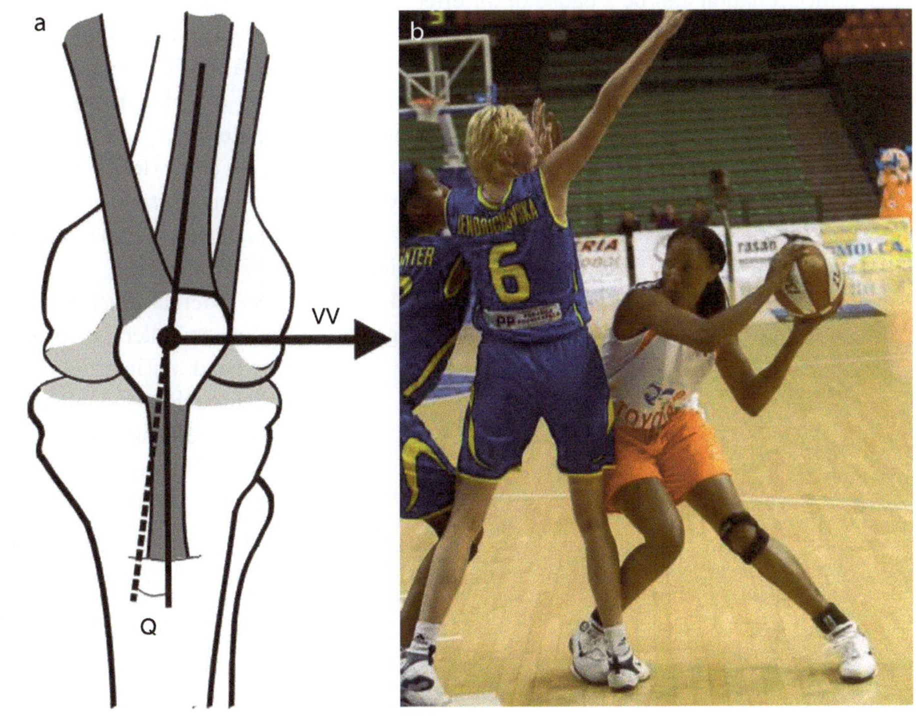


**Fig. 6.7** (**a**) Q angle and valgus vector (VV). The Q angle imposes a valgus vector in the last degrees of extension. (**b**) In many sport positions, knee valgus is strained, which increases the Q angle and the valgus vector (Fig. b is reproduced with permission from ROS CASARES/JACOBO PAYA)

iliotibial band, gluteus medius weakness, and pronated feet. Women have a wider pelvis (gynecoid pelvis), which favors greater knee valgus with the consequent pronation of the feet and a bigger Q angle. This angle is also increased in certain attitudes practiced in sports (Fig. 6.7b). As the knee starts to flex, the tibia derotates, diminishing the Q angle and the valgus vector. From 20° or 30° of flexion, resistance to lateral subluxation is mainly provided by the lateral femoral condyle.

Out of all these factors, a pronated foot is one of the most important in the etiology of patellofemoral pain[69] (Table 6.1). A pronated foot should not be mistaken with flat foot, as it is not necessary for the foot to be flat to suffer an excessive pronation. Pronation is not a position, it is a function. An excessive pronation leads to[53,69]: (1) an increase in the Q angle; (2) an anterior displacement of the proximal tibia, with the consequent flexion of the knee and because of this an increase in the PFJR force; (3) an increase of the impact forces which reach the knee joint, due to the calcaneal eversion, which is, therefore, unable to increase its eversion, (we must remember that calcaneal eversion constitutes an important shock-absorbing mechanism, to lessen the impact forces when jumping or running); and (4) an internal tibial rotation that affects the PFJ dynamics.

There is a high correlation between asymmetrical pronators and leg length discrepancy.[43] Unilateral subtalar joint pronation can be a cause or an effect in leg length discrepancy. This unilateral pronation can increase the Q angle and result in anterior knee pain.[14] Nevertheless, up to now, there are no studies relating the anterior knee pain to leg length discrepancy.[53] These problems associated to pronated foot justify the occasional use of orthopedic insoles in the treatment of anterior knee pain.

These factors could explain the frequent association between jumper's knee and symptomatic PFM that we have found in our series. Therefore, in this group of patients, it is necessary to carry on a complete physical examination, not only of the knee but of the whole limb, with special attention dedicated to the foot structures. The association between hip anteversion, in-facing patellae, external tibial torsion, pronated feet (positive Helbing sign [medial arching of the Achilles tendon]), and bayonet sign is known in the orthopedic bibliography as the "miserable malalignment syndrome"[70] (Fig.6.8).

**Table 6.1** Etiology of pronation

| |
|---|
| *Intrinsic causes* |
| Forefoot varus |
| Hindfoot varus |
| Tibial varus |
| *Extrinsic causes* |
| Flexibility deficit (triceps surae, hip flexors, iliotibial tract, hip rotators, and hamstrings) |
| Resistance deficit (ankle inversion, hip rotators, gluteus medius, and/or lumbar quadratus) |
| Leg length discrepancy |

From Wallace and Sullivan[69]

## 6.6 Relation Between Morphotype and Extensor Mechanism Pathology

Lower limb possibilities of malalignment in the different spatial planes are: (1) frontal plane (*genu valgum and genu varum*); (2) sagittal plane (*genu recurvatum and genu flexum*); and (3) transversal plane (femoral and tibial torsion).

Valgus knees (*genu valgum*) show the tibial tuberosity further lateral than normal and following this an increase in the Q angle that will be even bigger when there is external tibial torsion.[68] In *genu varum*, the tibial tuberosity is placed more medial than in normal knees and it provokes not only an important overload in the medial compartment of the knee, but also a moderate overload in the medial region of the patellofemoral joint.[68]

*Genu recurvatum* is frequently associated with patella alta. This type of knee, more frequent in women, shows a higher incidence of recurrent dislocation of the patella, especially when it is associated with *genu valgum* and external tibial torsion.[68] In addition to this, *genu recurvatum* is frequently associated to AKP.[68] *Genu flexum* is also associated with AKP as it increases the PFJR force.

An external tibial torsion produces lateral tilt, lateral rotation, and lateral displacement of the patella.[67] On the other hand, an internal tibial torsion causes medial tilt, medial rotation, and medial displacement of the patella.[67]

Such deformities as increased femoral anteversion or internal femoral torsion are closely related to patellofemoral pathology.[38] Both produce an increase of the quadricipital angle, which causes excessive lateral displacement of the patella when the muscle contracts. This leads to an excess of tension on the medial patellofemoral ligament (MPFL) as well as of the stresses on the lateral side of the patella and the trochlea. Initially, this induces pain and later it causes instability, chondromalacia, and patellofemoral osteoarthritis.[38]

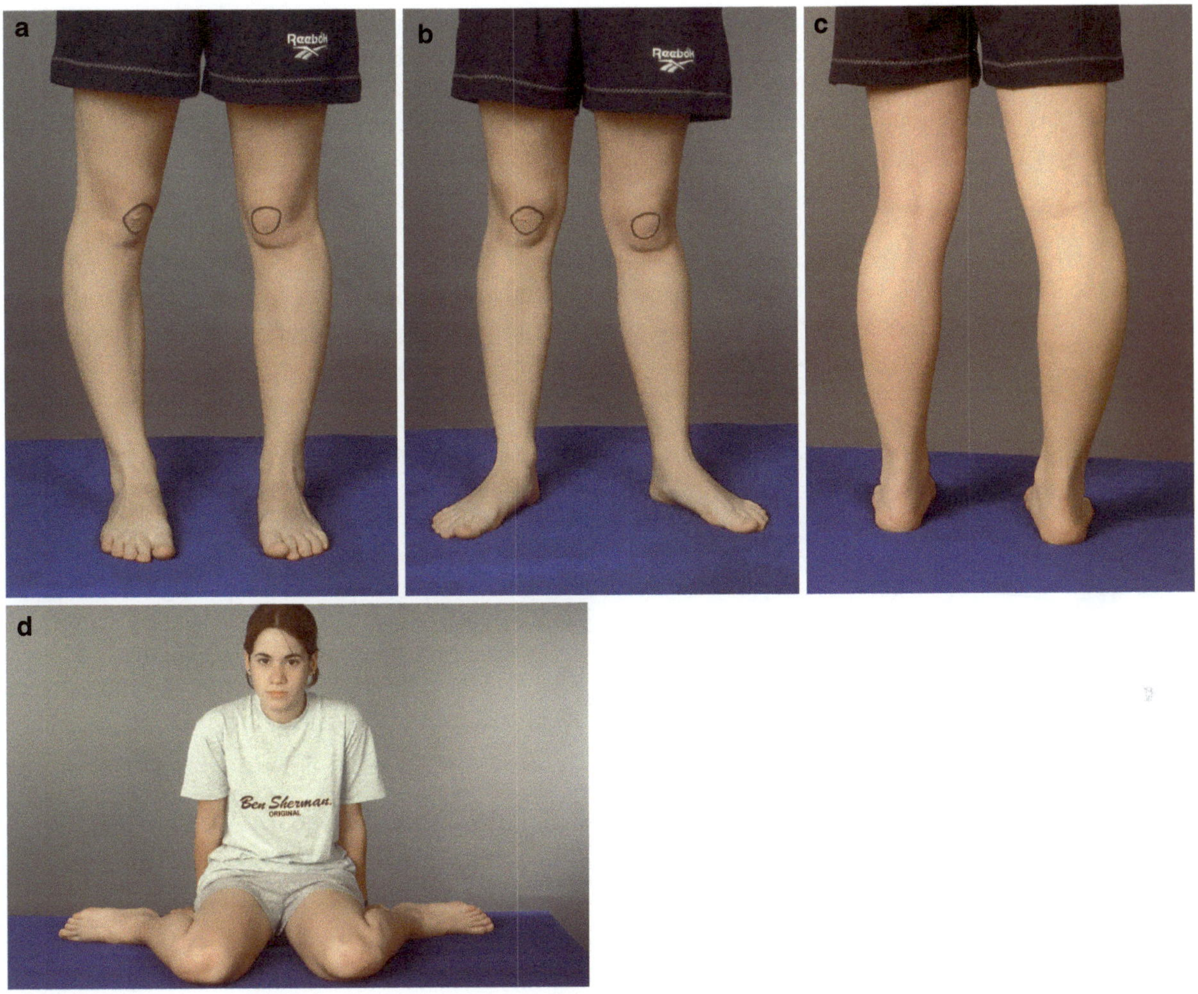


**Fig. 6.8** "Miserable malalignment syndrome" is characterized by inward-looking patellae (**a**), external tibial torsion (**b**), pronated right foot with positive Helbing´s sign (medial bowing of the Achilles tendon) (**c**), and femoral neck anteversion (**d**) (Reproduced from Sanchis-Alfonso[59]. Reprinted by permission from Thieme)

Pain causes inhibition atrophy of the quadriceps, which aggravates the symptoms. Quadriceps exercises occasionally cause an overload of the knee joint that increases the pain and the inhibition of the muscle, paradoxically causing greater atrophy.

Kijowski and colleagues[38] observed statistically significant changes in the contact area and in the contact pressure of the PFJ with femur rotation. Internal rotation of the femur (e.g., secondary to an excessive femoral anteversion) induces an increase in the contact area and pressure on the lateral side of the PFJ and a decrease of both on the medial side of the same joint. Obviously, external rotation produces the opposite effects. In addition to this, these authors proved that internal rotation of the femur up to 30° produces a statistically significant increase of the MPFL tension when the knee is at 30° of flexion. These alterations could be partially responsible for the frequency of patellofemoral pathology in people with an abnormal rotational femoral alignment.

## 6.7 Swimming as an Example of Pain by Overuse

To highlight the importance of excessive valgus and PFJR force in the pathology we are dealing with, we will look at swimming.[56] Knee pain in this sport is a paradigm of pain by overuse, as in this competitive sport, there is no weight-bearing or contact. In freestyle, backstroke, and butterfly, there is a knee flexion associated with every "kick," with a repetitive contraction of the quadriceps that can lead to an AKP caused by a patellofemoral cumulative overload (Fig. 6.9). In addition to this, when pushing against the wall, when starting and turning, a strong contraction of quadriceps with the knee in high flexion takes place, with an increment of the PFJR force. Another cause for this pain could be an increase in the valgus alignment and external tibial torsion, which are both normal components of the breaststroke kick (Fig. 6.10).

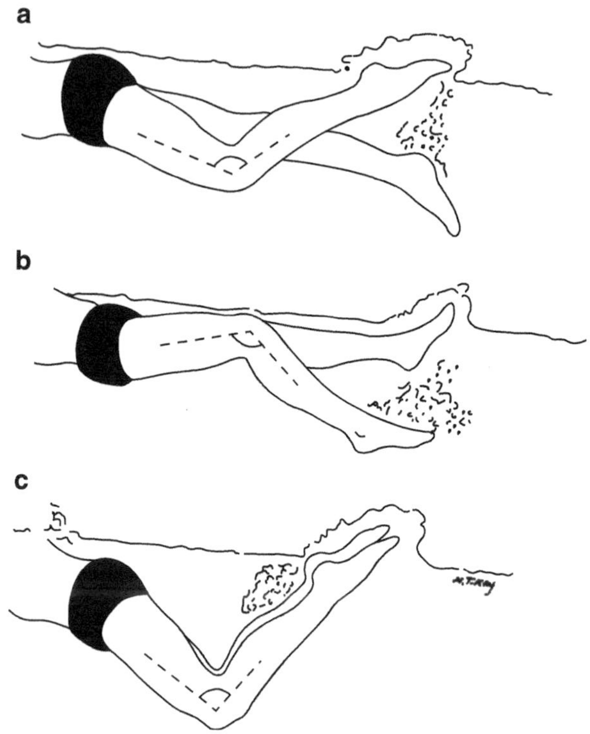


**Fig. 6.9** Flexion of the knee in freestyle (**a**), backstroke (**b**), and butterfly (**c**). Degree of flexion associated with each impulse (Reprinted from Rodeo[56], with permission from Elsevier)

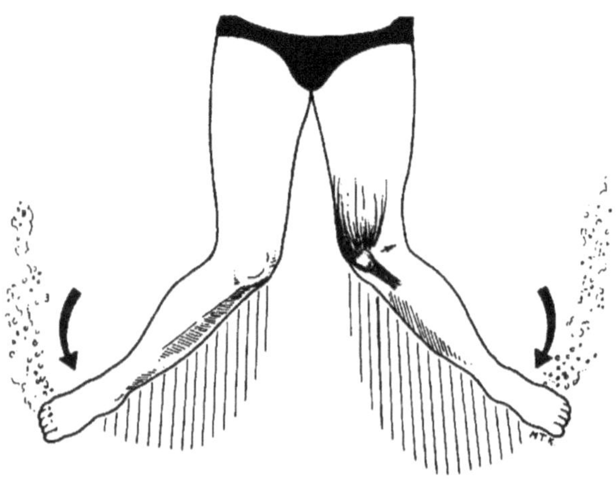

**Fig. 6.10** Position of the lower limbs in breast stroke (Reprinted Rodeo[56], with permission from Elsevier)

## 6.8 Impingement Mechanism Between the Inferior Pole of the Patella and the Posterior Surface of the Proximal Third of the Patellar Tendon

Maintained and repetitive hyperflexion knee positions are often present in sports (Fig. 6.11). These positions would favor the impingement of the inferior pole of the patella against the posterior surface of the patellar tendon proximal third. This is the pathogenic theory of the patellar tendinopathy ("jumper's knee") proposed by some authors.[36] In fact, the maneuver that is demonstrative of the jumper's knee is in fact a reproduction of the impingement mechanism (Fig. 6.11d).

## 6.9 Anatomical Factors Associated with Patellar Pain and Instability. Anatomical Predisposing Anomalies. "Imbalance" as an Alternative to "Malalignment"

The aforementioned factors as well as other predisposing anatomical factors, such as insufficiency of the vastus medialis obliquus (VMO) muscle, a lax medial retinaculum, patellar dysplasia, trochlear dysplasia, patella alta, and generalized ligamentous laxity (Fig. 6.12) contribute to start or aggravate the patellar pain and instability.[13,16-20,23,24,30,34,42,51,58,63,70,72] These factors contribute to create what could be called a "knee at risk" or a "favorable environment" for the development of the AKP syndrome and patellar functional instability. One isolated factor might be insignificant, but when there are many associated factors, these are cumulative. The association of these factors varies among patients, and causing a great variety of symptoms. That is why there are many types of clinical presentations.

Among all these anatomical factors, possibly the main one is the VMO insufficiency, since this muscle plays an essential role in the dynamic stabilization of

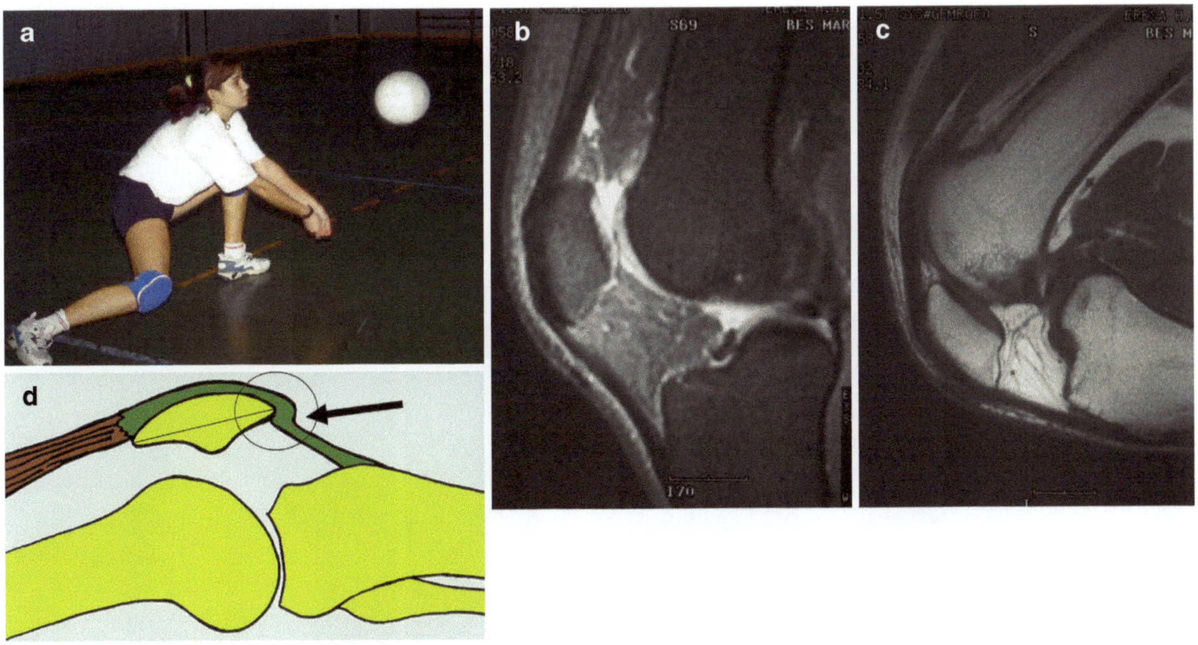

**Fig. 6.11** (**a**) Volleyball player with her left knee in a maintained hyperflexion position (increase of the patellofemoral joint reaction force). The right knee is forced into excessive valgus and, eventually, will sustain an indirect or direct traumatism. (**b, c**) Functional study of the knee by magnetic resonance in a patient with right jumper's knee and a highly positive Puddu's maneuver. With flexion of the knee, the inferior patellar pole impinges on the patellar tendon posterior aspect in its proximal end. The patient referred severe pain in the knee after any position with maintained hyperflexion. He had problems with everyday activities like driving a car. (**d**) Scheme to show Puddu's maneuver producing impingement of the patellar inferior pole upon the patellar tendon

the patella, opposing its lateral displacement during the first degrees of flexion. The VMO fibers exert a force that actively displaces the patella medially during the first degrees of knee flexion. The electrical activity of the VMO fibers is twice as much as the rest of the quadriceps.[39] An imbalance of this 2:1 proportion can lead to a lateral patellar displacement at knee extension caused by traction of the vastus lateralis. In this sense, patellar tilt and a high patellofemoral congruence angle could be considered a measurable expression of the quadricipital dysplasia. This VMO insufficiency could be secondary to a high insertion (congenitally) or to a disuse atrophy (acquired). Floyd and colleagues[21] suggest that many cases of recurrent dislocation of the patella are caused by a primary muscular defect (abundance of abnormal muscular fibers type 2C). On the other hand, Robert Teitge, distinguished member of the International Patellofemoral study Group (IPSG), does not believe that the VMO is responsible for patellar stability.[65] In his opinion, patellar stability depends on the geometry of bone and ligaments, the MPFL being the main one, whereas the medial meniscopatellar ligament has only a secondary role.[65] This way of thinking coincides with that of many other authors (see Chap. 7).

The medial retinacular laxity can be secondary to its tear after a dislocation or to an elongation secondary to a tense lateral retinaculum, chronic effusion, or recurrent external subluxation of the patella.

Dejour and colleagues[16] believe that the trochlear dysplasia is the distinctive finding in the objective patellar instability, and the high frequency of bilateral cases (92.5%) makes them think that it is a constitutional anomaly.

Insall and colleagues[30] and Blackburn and Peel[8] have highlighted the role that patella alta plays in patellar instability, which is logical thinking considering that this patella has a longer stretch outside the femoral trochlea with knee flexion and extension and therefore, is less stable than a normal patella. Moreover, knees with patella alta show an increase in the PFJR force.[2] Patellar tilt and patella alta are present in both knees in more than 90% of the cases with objective patellar instability, even when one of them is asymptomatic.[16] This finding highlights the fact that patellar tilt and patella alta are not a consequence of the dislocation,

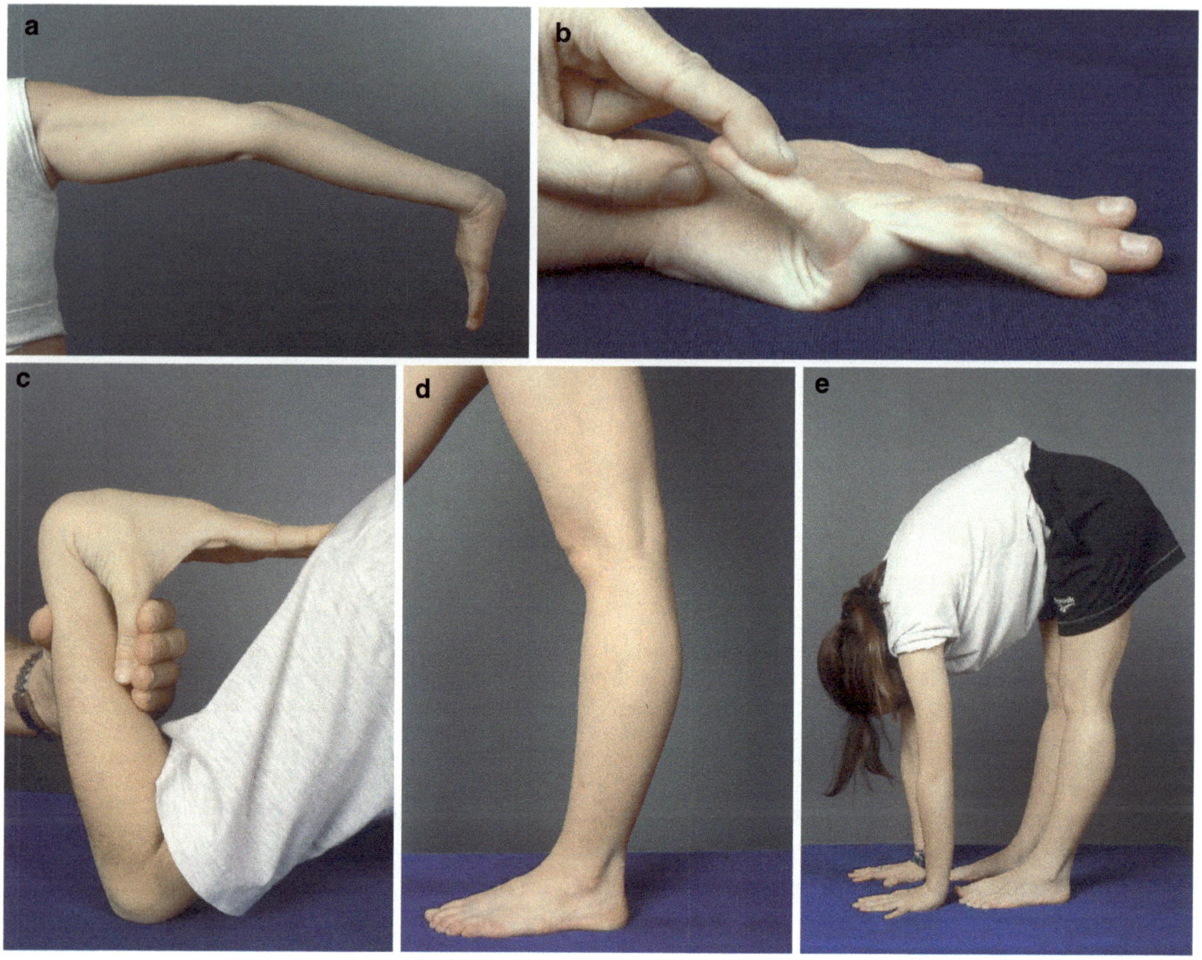


**Fig. 6.12** Generalized ligamentous laxity criteria: elbow hyperextension >10° (**a**), fifth finger passive hyperextension >90° (**b**), passive thumb to forearm contact (**c**), knee hyperextension >10° (**d**), palms in contact with the ground with knees extended (**e**). Ligamentous laxity exists when the patient can do three or more of these tests

but of a constitutional anomaly: the quadricipital dysplasia. Ward and Powers[71] have studied the influence of patella alta on PFJ stress during normal and fast walking. People with patella alta demonstrated a greater calculated patellofemoral stress during fast walking. This was the result of reductions in the contact area as joint reaction forces were similar between groups. Luyckx and colleagues[41] demonstrated that the maximal patellofemoral contact force and contact pressure increase significantly with increasing patellar height.

Finally, generalized ligamentous laxity[13,63] has to be taken into account, especially because of its clinical consequences related to the association between acute patellar dislocation and chondral lesion. Stanitski[63] studied the relationship between joint hypermobility and chondral lesion after an acute patellar dislocation and found that the chondral lesion was 2.5 times more frequent in the patients without joint hypermobility than in the ones that showed generalized ligamentous laxity.

## 6.10 Mechanism of Pain Production According to the Mechanical Theory

The patellar articular cartilage lesion is the result of the application of tangential forces on the PFJ or of compression forces that do not disperse in an adequate way on the patellar articular surface. As we have mentioned before, the increase of the compression force is produced during activities that require an increase of knee flexion, or as a consequence of a direct trauma, situations that happen frequently in sport practice or everyday life (falls, traffic accidents), given the protective function of the patella.

As a consequence of the direct or indirect traumatisms that the patella sustains without malalignment, but more so with it, the articular cartilage lesion is caused by the release of arachidonic acid, which could initiate a series of biochemical changes leading to the release of cathepsin with the consequent progressive degradation of the articular cartilage, probably mediated by prostaglandins.[23] Furthermore, prostaglandin E causes bone resorption, which induces an internal bone remodeling (intense bone metabolism) that can cause a painful patella. The intra-articular presence of degradation products of the cartilage produces a chemical synovitis ("gunk synovitis"[54]) that could explain the popliteal pain that sometimes accompanies the AKP syndrome. The hypothesis of the chemical synovitis is favored by the clinical finding that a simple arthroscopic lavage could improve the pain in these patients. On the other hand, the abnormal pressure transmitted to the subchondral bone due to the softening of the patellar articular cartilage stimulates the subchondral nerves and the remodeling of the subchondral bone. These phenomena could constitute another mechanism of pain production. Therefore, the patella itself could be the main source of pain in some patients.

It is then clear to see the overlapping of the mechanical and neural theories. Furthermore the intraosseous hypertension secondary to the microscopic stress fractures caused by the alteration of the load transmission to the subchondral bone, which follows the articular cartilage failure, could also be another cause of anterior knee pain.[26] Brill[10] observed, nevertheless, that gammagraphies are not often positive in young sports players who suffer from AKP. This could be due to the fact that the cause of their anterior knee pain lies fundamentally in the peripatellar tissues and in the patellar tendon. This coincides with our clinical observations. A positive gammagraphic result would then be an objective clue for the indication of a decompression surgery (e.g., anteromedial transfer of the tibial tubercle by Fulkerson).

Finally, the pain threshold in the subchondral bone could be surpassed, even with an intact cartilage, under an excessive stress or under a strong force (sport or direct trauma), or else under a normal stress applied on a knee with PFM.

## 6.11 Clinical Relevance

Because of the complexity and variability in the pathogenesis of the clinical entity we are now studying, it is easy to understand how difficult it is to establish the most appropriate treatment for each individual case. More than 100 surgical treatments have been described with different percentages of success, which reflects a problematic situation from the point of view of the pathogenesis, diagnostics, and treatment.[4,16,19,23,32,34,35,50,51,57,58,61,66,70,73] Therefore, it is essential to identify the pathological factor responsible for the clinical manifestations of each patient in order to select the most effective treatment based on clinical findings ("made to measure" treatment). This policy will give us the most satisfactory results.

Given the aspects treated in this chapter and in Chap. 3, the importance of the following elements in the treatment of the clinical picture is easily understandable: (1) when the symptoms appear, we must stop the sport activity; (2) treatment for pain and for tissue normalization (galvanic or continuous current, iontophoresis, diadynamic currents, Travert currents, transcutaneous electric stimulation (TENS), pulsating ultrasound, phonophoresis, cryotherapy, technique of deep transverse friction or technique by Cyriax); (3) stretching exercises (hamstrings, quadriceps, iliotibial tract, gastrocnemius, and lateral retinaculum); (4) strengthening of the quadriceps (with special attention to the VMO), gluteous medius, and posterior tibial muscle; (5) proprioception exercises; and (6) knee braces, functional bandages, and foot insoles.

Some of the aspects that, if overlooked or unknown, may lead to erroneous treatments and iatrogenic problems will be analyzed next.

### *6.11.1 How Should the Quadriceps Muscle Be Strengthened? Closed Versus Open Kinetic Chain Exercises. Eccentric Versus Concentric Phase Exercises*

Historically, treatment of patellofemoral pain has focused on strengthening the VMO to improve dynamic patellar stability. However, there is no conclusive

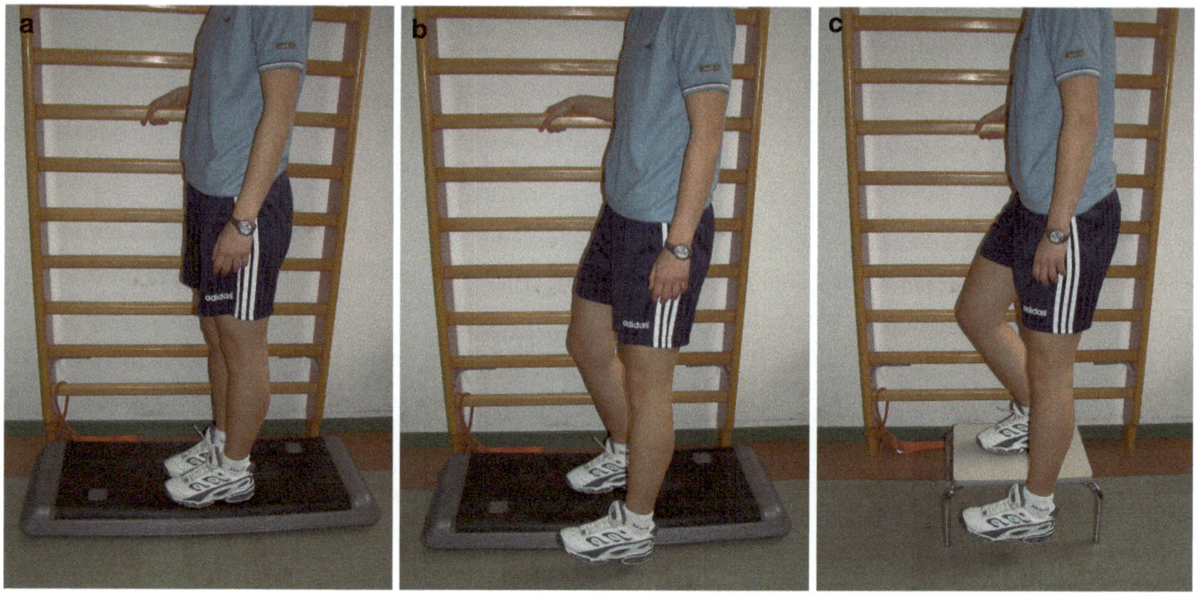

**Fig. 6.13** Exercises for quadriceps (*of the right leg*) in closed kinetic chain (lateral step) with eccentric work. (**a**) Starting position. (**b**) Strengthening position. (**c**) Strengthening position with a higher step

evidence that specific exercises can be performed to selectively recruit the VMO. It may be that successful treatment of patellofemoral pain can be achieved by general quadriceps strengthening exercises.[48]

At present, the best exercises to strengthen the quadriceps in patients with patellofemoral dysfunction in the intermediate and advanced phases of the treatment, are the techniques of closed kinetic chain (mini-squatting, lateral step (Fig. 6.13), bicycling with a high saddle, etc.) in the last degrees of extension (from 0° to 30°), as the joint is subject to the minimal pressures (stresses).[57] Furthermore, the strengthening of the VMO is favored if the mini-squatting is associated to an adduction of the hips, which can be achieved with the use of a balloon. The clinical experience shows that patients with PFJ problems seem to tolerate best the exercises of leg press (closed kinetic chain) through the functional mobility range (less contact pressure [force times area] upon the PFJ), but they tend to present an increase of the symptoms during the leg extension exercises in open kinetic chain against resistance, in the functional mobility range (greater contact pressure [force times area] upon the PFJ).[64] Additionally, many patients without problems in the PFJ develop symptoms after this last type of exercises.[64] Our philosophy should be to regain the muscular resistance along a painless arc of flexion. In the process of rehabilitation, pain is the best guide. The expression "lack of pain, lack of progress" is not applicable to the rehabilitation of the extensor mechanism.

The eccentric isotonic exercises (Fig. 6.14) constitute a vital part in the muscular strengthening program as a weakness of the muscles in the eccentric phase could increment the reaction forces in the PFJ.[45] It has been demonstrated that patients with AKP and patellar instability develop a larger torsional moment in the quadriceps concentric contraction than in the eccentric one.[5] On the contrary, the isotonic exercises against resistance in the concentric phase should be prohibited (this would be a sentence to the "electric chair" for the knee). It is important to point out that there could be risk of lesions when performing eccentric work with maximal loads, for which we advise doing this type of exercise with less than maximal and progressively controlled loads, always following the golden rule of "absence of pain."

In summary, the indication or contraindication of the different types of exercises seems to be mainly related to the contact pressure generated in the PFJ and to the major or minor friction that can cause pain. The location of a chondral lesion can also influence exercise prescription. For example, if the patient has a painful proximal lesion on the patella, exercises between 60° and 90° of flexion should be avoided.[48]

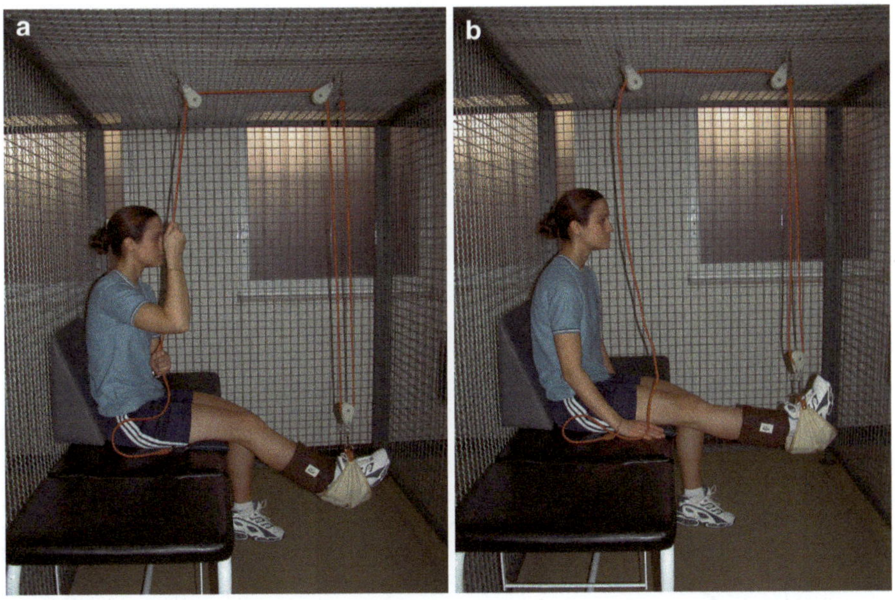


**Fig. 6.14** Strengthening of quadriceps in open kinetic chain with eccentric work. Patient sitting down (in Rocher cage). (**a**) With the help of pulleys, the patient extends the limb. (**b**) After that she flexes the knee, exercising the quadriceps in eccentric phase

Steinkamp and colleagues[64] have studied the different mechanical effects of quadriceps rehabilitation exercises in closed and open kinetic chains. As this is very important, we will deal with the subject in detail. The parameters used to show the differences between these two types of rehabilitation therapy were: (1) the articular moment in the knee; (2) the PFJR force; and (3) the pressure (stress) in the PFJ. It is worth analyzing the clinical significance of these three parameters to be able to understand the obtained results.

The articular moment of the knee flexion–extension movement is the total of all the forces that favor knee joint flexion or extension movements, which, because they act at different distances from the geometrical center of the knee, create a different moment in this joint. For instance, if we hang a 2-kg weight at the ankle joint in a sitting individual with the knee in extension, the generated moment in the knee (flexion moment, as this weight would tend to flex the knee) would be greater than the one generated by hanging the same weight at the center of the leg (shin), as in this case the force is the same (2 kg) but the flexion moment generated in the knee (force x distance to the center of the knee) is smaller. Therefore, depending on the magnitude and direction of the acting force and on the distance to the geometrical center of the knee, the flexion moments (they tend to flex the knee) or extension moments can vary according to the exercise. Since the main function of the quadriceps is to extend the knee, the greater the flexor moment generated, the greater the muscular activity that the quadriceps muscle will have to develop to oppose this flexion force.

The reaction force in the PFJ corresponds to a much simpler concept and refers to the global force in a perpendicular direction between the femoral and patellar articular surfaces in each of the angles of joint flexion, as we have mentioned before. It seems logical to suppose that more pain will be produced in this joint as the reaction forces increase with any movement of the knee. Articular pressure can make the results vary as we will see next.

The stress (pressure) in the PFJ tells us about the distribution of the global reaction force in this joint (reaction force/contact surface). Therefore, the smaller the contact surface, the greater the joint pressures will be. In spite of being completely different from a mechanical point of view, we could compare this to the explanation of the articular moment. With reference to the pressures, we have to talk about the values of the reaction force magnitude and the contact surface, and we have to realize, paradoxically, that with a small reaction force and reduced contact surfaces, higher pressures can be produced than with bigger reaction forces acting on wide contact surfaces. In a similar way to what was explained about the reaction forces, the presence of high stresses (pressures) while doing rehabilitation exercises will be associated with an increase in the articular pain.

In Fig. 6.15, the three parameters (moment, reaction force, and pressures) are analyzed in different

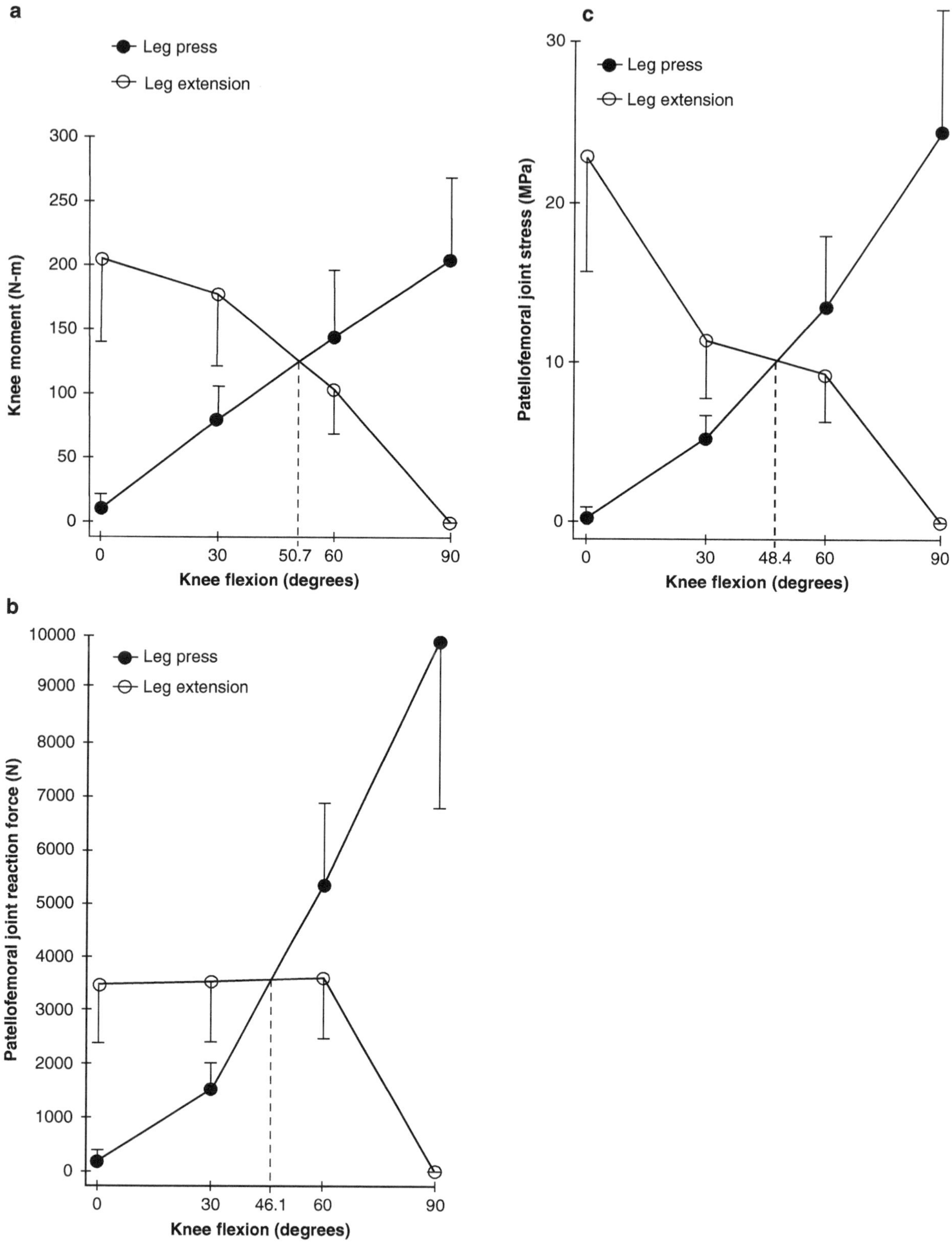


**Fig. 6.15** (**a**) Comparative values of the articular moment at 0°, 30°, 60°, and 90° in open and closed kinetic chains. (**b**) Comparative values of the reaction force at 0°, 30°, 60°, and 90° in open and closed kinetic chains. (**c**) Comparative values of the pressures at 0°, 30°, 60°, and 90° in open and closed kinetic chains (Reproduced from Steinkamp[64]. Reprinted by permission of SAGE Publications)

amounts of knee flexion and with the two rehabilitation methods proposed. It is clear that the exercises in closed kinetic chain have a minimum in complete extension and a maximum in flexion of 90°. The flexion moment arm of the knee increases as the angle of knee flexion increases and therefore, greater quadriceps and patellar tendon tension is required to counteract the increasing flexion moment arm, resulting in greater PFJR force as the knee flexes.

In a similar way, the exercises in open kinetic chain show a minimum at 90° and a maximum in extension, which coincides with the intuitive appreciation that maximal relaxation of the quadriceps happens at 90° of flexion. Analyzing Fig. 6.15, it becomes clear that the rehabilitation graphics in open and closed kinetic chains cross at one point, which corresponds with a definite flexion angle (50.7° [articular moment], 46.1° [reaction force], and 48.4° [pressure]). These intersecting values indicate that below them, the closed kinetic chain exercises cause smaller moments, lesser reaction forces, and smaller pressure in the PFJ, and due to that they are less harmful for the patient. Nevertheless, beyond these intersecting values, the open chain exercises are the ones with smaller moment, reaction forces, and pressure.

Similar results were found by Hungerford and Barry[29] who compared patellofemoral contact stresses between open kinetic chain knee extension against a 9-kg load and squatting under body weight. The contact stress was less for open kinetic chain knee extension against a 9-kg load than when squatting under body weight between 90° and 53° of knee flexion. The contact stress was less when squatting under body weight than when performing open kinetic chain knee extension against a 9-kg load between 0° and 53° of flexion.

Both of the above studies indicate that patellofemoral joint stress can be increased or decreased depending on the mode (open or closed kinetic chain) and flexion angle at which the exercise is performed. Both open and closed kinetic chain exercises can be used in the treatment of patients with patellofemoral pain if performed within a pain-free range. Closed kinetic chain exercises may be better tolerated by the patellofemoral joint in the range of 0±45° of knee flexion. In this range, suggested exercises include step-ups, mini-squats, and leg presses. Open kinetic chain exercises may be better tolerated by the patellofemoral joint in the ranges between 90±50° and 20±0° of knee flexion. In these ranges, suggested exercises include short arc isotonics, multiple angle isometrics, straight leg raises, and quadriceps sets. Open and closed chain exercises should be performed within a safe range of motion to allow quadriceps activation while minimizing patellofemoral joint reaction forces. The evidence suggests that both types of exercises should be incorporated into rehabilitation programs.[7,48]

## 6.12 Summary

The anterior knee pain syndrome and functional patellar instability in the active young person is one of the most complex knee disorders, with a multiple factor and highly variable pathogenesis, with intermingling mechanical and neurological factors. Probably, the neural factor is the cause of the well-established symptoms in patients with certain mechanical anomalies and a knee overuse.

The word "overuse" is closely linked to sport, which is one of the most popular activities nowadays. In addition to favoring personal relationship, sport is a source of physical and mental health. It is amusing, relaxing, it encourages a sense of discipline, fellowship, team spirit, and will to excel. Therefore, we ought to encourage it and support those who practice it. But sport can be the cause of lesions, and it is the orthopedic surgeon's duty not only to diagnose and heal them, but also to play an active role in the education of the patient to prevent them. This prevention implies detecting persons and risk situations and taking an active part in the education of the sports player by means of teaching healthy habits (e.g., training of the proprioception). It could be said that the sport lesions are not accidental ones, as many of them can be prevented. If the doctor, the physiotherapist, the physical trainer, and the administration do not cooperate in this prevention, the practice of sport should not be encouraged.

Taking into account that overuse, training errors, and specific patterns of mobility in each sport can be important factors in the appearance of symptoms, it is then easy to understand that reeducating the patient is necessary for the success of treatment and the prevention of relapses. To achieve this, it is necessary to analyze the gait and to video analyze how the patient practices the sport. Any treatment program overlooking reeducation (training of brain "software", altering the expectations and the lifestyle) will fail in the long run. In addition to that, the surgeon, the patient, and his family should judge whether it is convenient for the patient himself to continue practicing the same sport at the same level as before the onset of the symptoms. One has to be realistic when counseling the patient's return to sport. We have to keep in mind that not everyone is fit to practice a sport, for instance people who show important biomechanical alterations in the alignment of the lower limbs.

## References


1. Ahmad CS, Kwak SD, Ateshian GA, et al. Effects of patellar tendon adhesion to the anterior tibia on knee mechanics. *Am J Sports Med*. 1998;26:715-724.
2. Amis AA, Farahmand F. Biomechanics of the knee extensor mechanism. *Knee*. 1996;3:73-81.
3. Bellemans J. Biomechanics of anterior knee pain. *Knee*. 2003;10:123-126.
4. Bellemans J, Cauwenberghs F, Witvrouw E, et al. Anteromedial tibial tubercle transfer in patients with chronic anterior knee pain and subluxation-type patellar malalignment. *Am J Sports Med*. 1997;25:375-381.
5. Bennett JG, Stauber WT. Evaluation and treatment of anterior knee pain using eccentric exercise. *Med Sci Sports Exerc*. 1986;18:526-530.
6. Besier ThF, Draper ChE, Gold GE, et al. Patellofemoral joint contact area increases with knee flexion and weight-bearing. *J Orthop Res*. 2005;23:345-350.
7. Bizzini M, Biedert R, Maffiuletti N, et al. Biomechanical issues in patellofemoral joint rehabilitation. *Orthopade*. 2008;37(864):866-871.
8. Blackburne JS, Peel TE. A new method of measuring patellar height. *J Bone Joint Surg*. 1977;59-B:241-242.
9. Brechter JH, Powers CM. Patellofemoral stress during walking in persons with and without patellofemoral pain. *Med Sci Sports Exerc*. 2002;34:1582-1593.
10. Brill D. Sports nuclear medicine. Bone imaging lower extremity pain athletes. *Clin Nucl Med*. 1984;8:101-116.
11. Brizuela G, Ferrandis R, Llana S. Aspectos epidemiológicos del calzado para baloncesto. *Arch Med Deporte*. 1996;13: 391-396.
12. Brizuela G, Llana S, Ferrandis R. Aspectos epidemiológicos del balonmano y su relación con el calzado. *Arch Med Deporte*. 1996;13:267-274.
13. Carter C, Sweetnam R. Familial joint laxity and recurrent dislocation of the patella. *J Bone Joint Surg*. 1958;40-B: 664-667.
14. Chambers MRC. Running on leg length discrepancy. *Athletes World*. 1983;6:55-58.
15. Dayakidisa MK, Boudolos K. Ground reaction force data in functional ankle instability during two cutting movements. *Clin Biomech*. 2006;21:405-411.
16. Dejour H, Walch G, Nove-Josserand L, et al. Factors of patellar instability: an anatomic radiographic study. *Knee Surg Sports Traumatol Arthrosc*. 1994;2:19-26.
17. Eifert-Mangine M, Bilbo JT. Conservative management of patellofemoral chondrosis. In: Mangine RE, ed. *Clinics in Physical Therapy. Physical Therapy of the Knee*. 2nd ed. New York: Churchill Livingstone; 1995:113-142.
18. Eisenhart-Rothe R, Siebert M, Bringmann C, et al. A new in vivo technique for determination of 3D kinematics and contact areas of the patello-femoral and tibio-femoral joint. *J Biomech*. 2004;37:927-34.
19. Ficat P, Hungerford D. *Disorders of the Patellofemoral Joint*. Baltimore: Williams & Wilkins; 1977.
20. Fithian DC, Mishra DK, Balen PF, et al. Instrumented measurement of patellar mobility. *Am J Sports Med*. 1995; 23:607-615.
21. Floyd A, Phillips P, Khan MR, et al. Recurrent dislocation of the patella. Histochemical and electromyographic evidence of primary muscular pathology. *J Bone Joint Surg*. 1987; 69-B:790-793.
22. Fu FH, Seel MJ, Berger RA. Patellofemoral biomechanics. In: Fox JM, Del Pizzo W, eds. *The Patellofemoral Joint*. New York: McGraw-Hill Inc; 1993:49-62.
23. Fulkerson JP, Hungerford DS. *Disorders of the Patellofemoral Joint*. Baltimore: Williams & Wilkins; 1990.
24. Fulkerson JP, Shea KP. Current concepts review: disorders of patellofemoral alignment. *J Bone Joint Surg*. 1990;72-A:1424-1429.
25. Gross TS, Nelson RC. The shock attenuation role of the ankle during landing from a vertical jump. *Med Sci Sports Exerc*. 1988;20:506-514.
26. Gruber MA. The conservative treatment of chondromalacia patellae. *Orthop Clin North Am*. 1979;10:105-115.
27. Guzzanti V, Gigante A, Di Lazzaro A, et al. Patellofemoral malalignment in adolescents. Computerized tomographic assessment with or without quadriceps contraction. *Am J Sports Med*. 1994;22:55-60.
28. Heino Brechter JG, Powers ChM. Patellofemoral joint stress during stair ascent and descent: a comparison of persons with and without patellofemoral pain. *Gait Posture*. 2002;16:115-123.
29. Hungerford DS, Barry BS. Biomechanics of the patellofemoral joint. *Clin Orthop*. 1979;144:9-15.
30. Insall J. "Chondromalacia patellae": patellar malalignment syndrome. *Orthop Clin North Am*. 1979;10:117-127.
31. Insall J. *Surgery of the Knee*. New York: Churchill Livingstone; 1993.
32. Insall J, Aglietti P, Tria A. Patellar pain and incongruence. *Clin Orthop*. 1983;176:225-232.
33. Insall J, Bullough PG, Burnstein AH. Proximal "tube" realignment of the patella for chondromalacia patellae. *Clin Orthop*. 1979;144:63-69.
34. Insall J, Goldberg V, Salvati E. Recurrent dislocation and the high-riding patella. *Clin Orthop*. 1972;88:67-69.
35. Johnson LL. *Arthroscopic Surgery. Principles & Practice*. St Louis: The C.V. Mosby Company; 1986.
36. Johnson DP, Wakeley ChJ, Watt I. Magnetic resonance imaging of patellar tendonitis. *J Bone Joint Surg*. 1996;78-B:452-457.
37. Kartus J, Magnusson L, Stener S, et al. Complications following arthroscopic anterior cruciate ligament reconstruction.

A 2–5-year follow-up of 604 patients with special emphasis on anterior knee pain. *Knee Surg Sports Traumatol Arthrosc.* 1999;7:2-8.

38. Kijowski R, Plagens D, Shaeh SJ, et al. The effects of rotational deformities of the femur on contact pressure and contact area in the patellofemoral joint and on strain in the medial patellofemoral ligament. Presented at the Annual Meeting of the International Patellofemoral Study Group, Napa Valley, San Francisco, CA, September 1999.
39. Lieb FJ, Perry J. Quadriceps function: an EMG study under isometric conditions. *J Bone Joint Surg.* 1971;53-A: 749-758.
40. Llana S, Brizuela G. Estudio biomecánico de los impactos en los saltos. *Biomecánica.* 1996;5:103-107.
41. Luyckx T, Didden K, Vandenneucker H, et al. Is there a biomechanical explanation for anterior knee pain in patients with patella alta? Influence of patellar height on patellofemoral contact force, contact area and contact pressure. *J Bone Joint Surg.* 2009;91-B:344-350.
42. Mäenpää H, Lehto MUK. Patellar dislocation has predisposing factors. A roentgenographic study on lateral and tangential views in patients and healthy controls. *Knee Surg Sports Traumatol Arthrosc.* 1996;4:212-216.
43. Mannello DM. Leg length inequality. *J Manipulative Physiol Ther.* 1992;15:576-590.
44. Mason JJ, Leszko F, Johnson T, et al. Patellofemoral joint forces. *J Biomech.* 2008;41:2337-2348.
45. Maunder T. Conservative treatment of patellofemoral joint problems. *Knee.* 1996;3:104.
46. McClay Y, Robinson J, Andriacchi T, et al. A profile of ground reaction forces in professional basketball. *J Appl Biomech.* 1994;10:222-236.
47. McClay Y, Robinson J, Andriacchi T, et al. A kinematic profile of skills in professional basketball players. *J Appl Biomech.* 1994;10:205-221.
48. McGinty G, Irrgang JJ, Pezzullo D. Biomechanical considerations for rehabilitation of the knee. *Clin Biomech.* 2000;15:160-166.
49. McNair PJ, Prapavessis H. Normative data of vertical ground reaction forces during landing from a jump. *J Sci Med Sport.* 1999;2:86-88.
50. O'Neill DB. Open lateral retinacular lengthening compared with arthroscopic release. A prospective, randomized outcome study. *J Bone Joint Surg.* 1997;79-A:1759-1769.
51. Pickett JC, Radin EL. *Chondromalacia of the Patella.* Baltimore: Williams & Wilkins; 1983.
52. Pitner MA. Pathophysiology of overuse injuries in the hand and wrist. *Hand Clin.* 1990;6:355-364.
53. Post WR. Clinical evaluation of patients with patellofemoral disorders. *Arthroscopy.* 1999;15:841-851.
54. Reilly DT, Martens M. Experimental analysis of quadriceps muscle force and patellofemoral joint reaction force for various activities. *Acta Orthop Scand.* 1972;43:126.
55. Robinson JR, Frederick EC, Cooper LB. Systematic ankle stabilization and the effect on performance. *Med Sci Sports Exerc.* 1986;18:625-628.
56. Rodeo SA. Knee pain in competitive swimming. *Clin Sports Med.* 1999;18:379-387.
57. Sanchis-Alfonso V. *Cirugía de la Rodilla. Conceptos actuales y controversias.* Madrid: Médica Panamericana; 1995.
58. Sanchis-Alfonso V, Gastaldi-Orquin E, Martinez-SanJuan V. Usefulness of computed tomography in evaluating the patellofemoral joint before and after Insall's realignment. Correlation with short-term clinical results. *Am J Knee Surg.* 1994;7:65-72.
59. Sanchis-Alfonso V, Roselló-Sastre E, Martinez-SanJuan V. Pathogenesis of anterior knee pain syndrome and functional patellofemoral instability in the active young. A. *Am J Knee Surg.* 1999;12:29-40.
60. Sanchis-Alfonso V, Subías-López A, Monteagudo-Castro C, et al. Healing of patellar tendon donor defect created after patellar tendon autograft harversting. A long-term histological evaluation in the lamb model. *Knee Surg Sports Traumatol Arthrosc.* 1999;7(6):340-348.
61. Scuderi G, Cuomo F, Scott WN. Lateral release and proximal realignment for patellar subluxation and dislocation. *J Bone Joint Surg.* 1988;70-A:856-861.
62. Shelbourne KD, Trumper RV. Preventing anterior knee pain after anterior cruciate ligament reconstruction. *Am J Sports Med.* 1997;25:41-47.
63. Stanitski CL. Articular hypermobility and chondral injury in patients with acute patellar dislocation. *Am J Sports Med.* 1995;23:146-150.
64. Steinkamp LA, Dillingham MF, Markel MD, et al. Biomechanical considerations in patellofemoral joint rehabilitation. *Am J Sports Med.* 1993;21:438-444.
65. Teitge RA. Treatment of complications of patellofemoral joint surgery. *Oper Tech Sports Medicine.* 1994;2(4): 317-334.
66. Trillat A, Dejour H, Couette A. Diagnostic et traitement des subluxations récidivantes de la rotule. *Rev Chir Orthop.* 1964;50:813-824.
67. Van Kampen A, Huiskes R. The three dimensional tracking pattern of the human patella. *J Ortho Res.* 1990;8:372-382.
68. Vilarrubias JM. *Patología del Aparato Extensor de la Rodilla.* Barcelona: Editorial JIMS; 1986.
69. Wallace LA, Sullivan MF. Foot alignment and knee pathology. In: Mangine RE, ed. *Clinics in Physical Therapy. Physical Therapy of the Knee.* 2nd ed. New York: Churchill Livingstone; 1995:87-110.
70. Walsh WM. Patellofemoral joint. In: DeLee Drez, ed. *Orthopaedic Sports Medicine. Principles and Practice.* Philadelphia: W.B. Saunders Company; 1994:1163-1248.
71. Ward SR, Powers CM. The influence of patella alta on patellofemoral joint stress during normal and fast walking. *Clin Biomech.* 2004;19:1040-1047.
72. Waryasz GR, McDermott AY. Patellofemoral pain syndrome (PFPS): a systematic review of anatomy and potential risk factors. *Dyn Med.* 2008;7:9.
73. Weiker GT, Black KP. The anterior femoral osteotomy for patellofemoral instability. *Am J Knee Surg.* 1997;10:221-227.
74. Wirhed R. *Habilidad atlética y Anatomía del Movimiento.* Barcelona: Edika-Med; 1989.

# Anatomy of Patellar Dislocation

# 7

Najeeb Khan, Donald C. Fithian, and Eiki Nomura

## 7.1 Introduction

Patellar dislocation can lead to disabling sequelae such as pain and recurrent instability, particularly in young athletes.[9,29,33,59,80,87,102] In recognition of its importance, more than 100 different procedures have been described for the treatment or prevention of recurrent patellar instability after the initial dislocation.[63,83] Surgical treatment has not been uniformly successful.[8,12,27,32,38,57,69,75,86,104,136] The wide array of surgical approaches suggests general uncertainty among authors about the most appropriate treatment. Widespread reports of mixed results[19,24,27,31,32,38,48,77,83,97,132] or outright failure[8,104] of surgical treatment suggest that such uncertainty is justified.

Despite the enormous volume of literature on patellofemoral instability and anterior knee pain, there was until recently little attention given to the structures that are injured during patellar dislocation, and the contributions these injured structures make in controlling patellar motion in the intact knee. Since the early 1990s, some investigators have focused on the individual components of the knee extensor mechanism that limit lateral patellar motion.[2,21,30,42,44,45,58,60] In vivo studies of the surgical pathology[1,10,52,72,105,116,126,134] and magnetic resonance (MR) imaging studies[72,91,105,116,126] have reported the pathoanatomy of the primary dislocation with specific attention to injuries within structures thought to play a role in controlling lateral patellar displacement. The importance of these lines of research is that they have focused attention on: (1) the pathological anatomy of the initial dislocation event, and (2) the specific components of the extensor mechanism that limit lateral patellar displacement in the normal knee. This represents a novel approach to the clinical problem of the unstable patella, which holds promise for new therapeutic approaches that may enhance our understanding and treatment of this challenging problem. The purpose of this chapter is to bring the results and implications of this body of research into perspective within the context of the prevailing literature on patellar dislocation.

## 7.2 Anatomy

The medial patellofemoral ligament (MPFL) was first described by Warren and Marshall[138] in 1979. Several authors report that the MPFL is present in all knees,[46,58,107,133] whereas Conlan et al.[30] and Aragao et al.[6] found the MPFL in 88%. The anatomy of the medial and anterior knee structures has been described in detail by Warren and Marshall,[138] Kaplan,[70] Reider,[113] Terry,[131] Davis and Fithian,[37] and Baldwin.[11]

Warren and Marshall delineated a three-layered arrangement of tissue planes. Layer 1 includes the superficial medial retinaculum (SMR), which courses from the anteromedial tibia and extends proximally to blend with fibers of the superficial medial retinaculum over the distal patella. The medial patellotibial ligament (MPTL) is an obliquely oriented band of fibers coursing from the anteromedial tibia and blending with the fibers of the retinaculum to insert on the medial border of the patella.[30,42,131] Warren and Marshall considered the

N. Khan (✉)
Southern California Permanente Medical Group,
San Marcos, CA, USA
e-mail: najeebkhan@mac.com

V. Sanchis-Alfonso (ed.), *Anterior Knee Pain and Patellar Instability*,
DOI: 10.1007/978-0-85729-507-1_7, © Springer-Verlag London Limited 2011

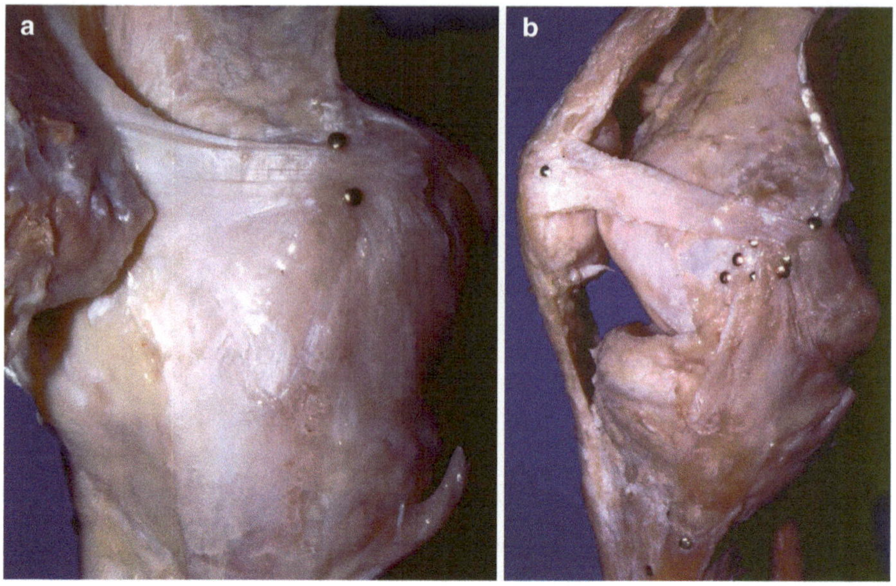


**Fig. 7.1** Macroscopic observation of the MPFL. When the VMO is reflected, the (**a**) MPFL can be seen. (**b**) With VMO resected, the full course of the MPFL is seen. Two pins are placed at the femoral attachment (From Nomura et al.[106])

MPFL, along with the superficial medial collateral ligament (MCL), to be part of layer 2.[138] On the medial knee, the adductor tubercle is superior and posterior to the medial epicondyle. The MCL originates primarily from the medial epicondyle, whereas the adductor tubercle serves as the attachment for the adductor magnus.

Anatomic studies report differing origins for the MPFL, including the medial femoral epicondyle,[10,58,70,113,138] anterior to the medial femoral epicondyle,[46] superoposterior to the medial femoral epicondyle,[106,107] and the adductor tubercle,[30,131] with a common insertion at the superomedial two-thirds of the patella. As the MPFL extends anteriorly, its fibers fuse with the undersurface of the vastus medialis tendon as shown in Fig. 7.1.[106,113] In sum, the "MPFL passes from the medial femoral epicondyle and adductor tubercle to the superomedial two-third of the patella fusing anteriorly with the inferior surface of the VMO."[138]

Baldwin[11] dissected 50 knees and reported two origins for the MPFL: (1) A 10.6 mm transverse origin in the groove between the medial epicondyle and adductor tubercle, and (2) an oblique origin from the proximal 30 mm of the leading edge of the superficial MCL. These origins combine to join the VMO and insert onto the ventral edge of the patella adjacent to the articular cartilage over a span of 28.2 ± 5.6 mm. Aragao et al.[6] reported in a similar anatomic study of 17 knees that the width of the patellar insertion of the MPFL ranged from 16 to 38.8 mm, with a mean of 27.9 mm.

The reported size and robustness of the MPFL varies considerably among anatomical cadaver studies. Reider could not even identify the MPFL in some specimens.[113] Conlan found it to be variable, representing a distinct structure in 29 of 33 fresh frozen cadaver knees.[30] In 2 of 25 knees that were tested for patellar mobility, the ligament was not grossly palpable. Both these knees demonstrated greater than average lateral mobility. In a study of nine fresh frozen cadavers, Desio et al. reported that the MPFL was identified in all specimens, though its size was variable.[42] In a second study of fresh frozen human cadaver knees reported by the same group, the MPFL again was present in all specimens.[21] Hautamaa et al.[58] reported a palpable band running along undersurface of the distal vastus medialis obliquus (VMO), attaching to both the medial femoral epicondyle and the proximal two-thirds of the patella.[58] These fibers represent the MPFL, which is distinguishable from the tendon of the VMO as it courses between the femoral epicondyle and the patella, without interposition of muscle fibers. Amis et al. report the tensile strength of the MPFL to be 208N, with a standard deviation of 90N.[98]

Nomura[106] observed in 2 of 30 knees that the MPFL inserted not directly into the medial border of the patella, but into the medial aspect of the quadriceps tendon immediately proximal to its insertion at the patella. Nomura reported the dimensions of the MPFL in detail along its length, and described the relationship of the MPFL to the VMO tendon[106] (Fig. 7.2). Figure 7.3 shows the relationship of the MPFL to the VMO as they approach their respective insertions, viewed from the femoral perspective.

Whether the MPFL is isometric or anisometric is not a settled issue. Nomura et al. found that the MPFL

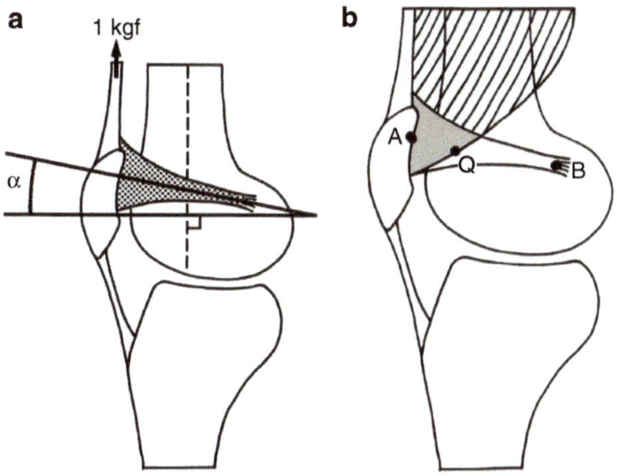


**Fig. 7.2** (**a**) The axis of the MPFL deviates proximally from a line drawn perpendicular to the femoral axis. (**b**) The VMO tendon becomes confluent with the MPFL in the region from Q to A (From Nomura et al.[106])

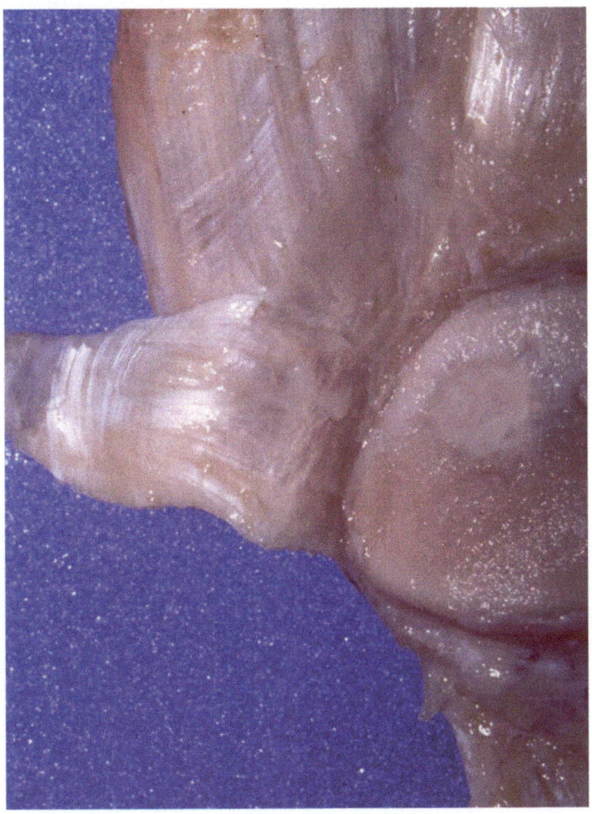

**Fig. 7.3** The MPFL and VMO as seen from the perspective of the femur (From Nomura et al.[106])

was slightly relaxed at 15–30° of knee flexion and tight at other angles, suggesting that the natural structure is not isometric.[107] In contrast, Steensen et al. showed in a cadaveric study that[129] (1) the MPFL was nearly isometric during knee flexion from 0° to 90°, demonstrating an average change in length of 1.1 mm, and (2) the most isometric portion of the MPFL is from the inferior patellar attachment to the superior femoral attachment.

Layer 3 includes the medial patellomeniscal ligament (MPML), a condensation of fibers along the medial border of the infrapatellar fat pad,[42] which inserts on the inferomedial one-third of the patella, distal to the MPFL insertion.[30,42]

The nerve supply of the patella and surrounding structures is described in numerous studies. There are three constant nerves at the medial knee.[62] The termination of the medial femoral cutaneous nerve usually travels superficially to the sartorius, but can also travel in Hunters canal to either perforate or remain deep to the sartorius. It courses 1 cm distal to the adductor tubercle, bisects the patella, and continues to the lateral aspect of the knee. The infrapatellar branch of the saphenous nerve courses approximately 3 cm posterior to the medial femoral condyle and terminates near the tibial tubercle. The terminal branch of the nerve to the vastus medialis becomes intra-articular after sending a branch to the MCL.

## 7.3 Normal Limits of Lateral Patellar Motion

The two components of the knee extensor apparatus that primarily affect the limits of passive mediolateral patellar motion, as depicted in Fig. 7.4 are: (1) bony constraint due to congruity between the patella and the femoral trochlea,[93,140] and (2) soft tissue tethers. The combination of articular buttress and soft tissue tension determines the limits of passive patellar displacement.

Studying the complex articular geometry of the patellofemoral joint between 30 and 100° of knee flexion, Ahmed[2] reported that mediolateral patellar translation was controlled by the passive restraint provided by the topographic interaction of the patellofemoral contacting surfaces. In particular, patellar medial–lateral translation was controlled by the trochlear topography, while retropatellar topography also had a significant role in the control of patellar rotations ("tilt" and "spin"). Heegard[60] observed that constraint within the femoral groove dominated over the stabilizing effect of the soft tissues through most of the range of motion in normal cadaver knees. At full extension,

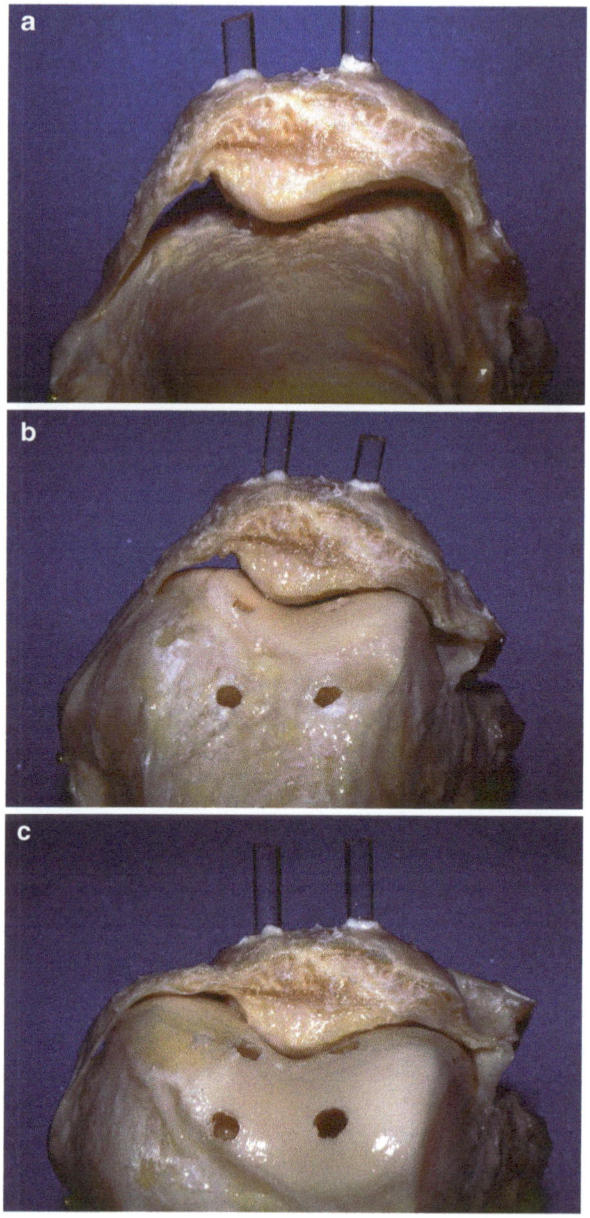


**Fig. 7.4** Axial view of the patellofemoral articulation at (**a**) 0°, (**b**) 60°, and (**c**) 120° flexion with a 1-kg load applied to the quadriceps (From Nomura et al.[107])

however, when there was little or no contact between patella and femur, the influence of the retinacula was greatest relative to that of the trochlea.[60] Fig. 7.5 shows the patellofemoral relationships at various angles of flexion. The differences between the intact and dissected knee kinematics suggested that patellar motion was controlled by the transverse soft tissue structures near extension, and by the patellofemoral joint geometry during further flexion.[60]

Farahmand et al.[44] measured the patellar lateral force-displacement behavior at a range of knee flexion angles and extensor muscle loads in normal human cadaver specimens. They reported that a 5-mm lateral patellar displacement required a constant displacing force (i.e., the patella had constant lateral stability) up to 60° knee flexion, with a significant increase in the force at 90° knee flexion. In a related study, Farahmand et al.[45] measured the trochlear depth and sulcus angle throughout the range of patellofemoral contact, and reported that the trochlear groove did not deepen with progressive knee flexion. These studies suggest that, with respect to the limits of mediolateral patellar motion in normal human knees, the trochlear shape assumes a dominant role at an early stage of knee flexion, and simulated muscle forces do not greatly enhance the constraint provided by the passive stabilizers.[44]

The contribution of specific medial retinacular structures to restraint against lateral patellar displacement has been studied in normal cadaver knees using sequential cutting methods.[30,42,58,107] Ligamentous retinacular structures that may be relevant to lateral patellar instability include: (1) the superficial medial patellar retinaculum (MPR),[113] (2) the medial patellotibial ligament (MPTL),[131] (3) the medial patellomeniscal ligament (MPML),[30,42,58] and (4) the MPFL.[21,30,42,58,107,113] These studies have consistently shown that the MPFL is the primary ligamentous restraint against lateral patellar displacement.

Nomura[107] studied the anatomy and contributions of the MPFL and superficial medial retinaculum in restraining lateral patellar displacement using ten fresh frozen human knee specimens. Lateral shift ratios were measured during the application of a 10 N laterally directed force with the knee in 20–120° of flexion. Isolated sectioning of the MPFL greatly increased lateral displacement in the range of knee flexion studied, and isolated MPFL reconstruction restored patellar displacement to within normal limits.[107]

In selective cutting studies of human cadaver medial retinacular tissues, the MPFL has consistently been shown to provide the primary restraint against lateral patellar displacement. Conlan reported the MPFL contributed 53% of the restraining force against lateral patellar displacement.[30] In Desio's study, the MPFL contributed an average of 60 ± 13% (range 41–80%) of

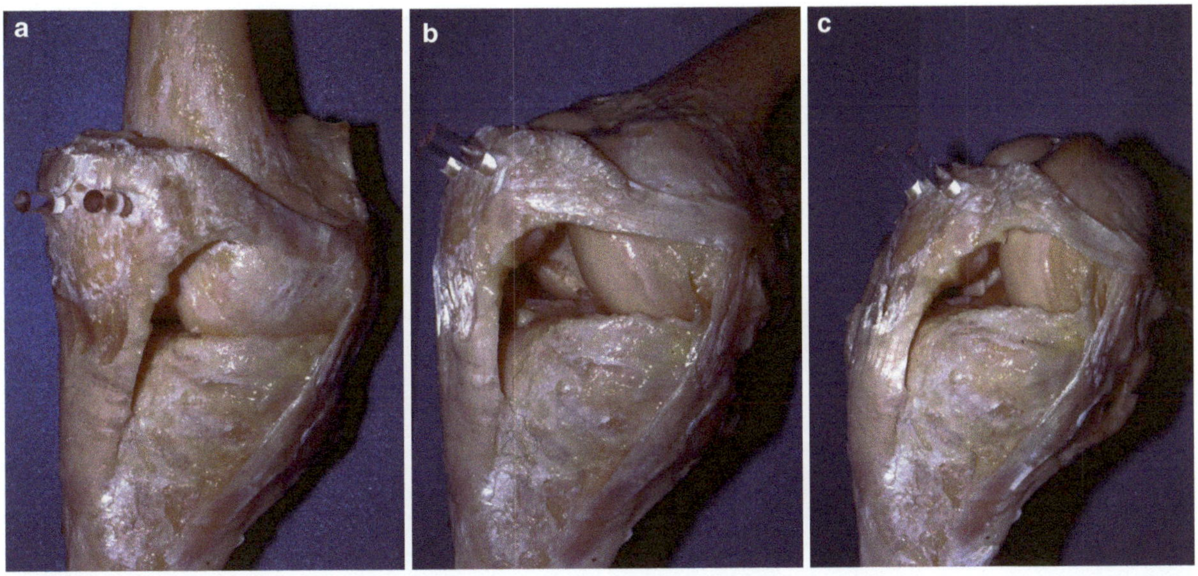


**Fig. 7.5** Anterolateral view of the patellofemoral articulation at (**a**) 0°, (**b**) 60°, and (**c**) 120° flexion with a 1-kg load applied to the quadriceps (From Nomura et al.[106])

the restraining force against lateral patellar displacement in cadaver knees.[42] Interestingly, Desio et al. reported that isolated lateral release actually reduced resistance to lateral displacement.[42] Hautamaa et al. observed that isolated section of the MPFL increased lateral patellar displacement 50% compared to intact knees.[58] Repair of the MPFL alone restored lateral mobility to within normal values.[58,107] Repair of more superficial retinacular tissues, as typically seen with "medial reefing," was neither necessary nor sufficient to restore stability.[58,107]

Although the vastus medialis obliquus (VMO)[63,81,118] is oriented to resist lateral patellar motion either by active contraction or by passive muscle resistance, the effect of muscle forces on patellar motion limits has not been defined clearly. With respect to resisting lateral patellar displacement, the orientation of the VMO varies greatly during knee flexion, as shown in Fig. 7.6. The VMO's line of pull most efficiently resists lateral patellar motion when the knee is in deep flexion, when trochlear containment of the patella is quite independent of soft tissue influences.[2,44,60] In Farahmand's study, lateral patellar force-displacement behavior was not affected by variations in simulated muscle forces at any flexion angle from 15° to 75°.[44]

In addition to the patellofemoral stability that is derived primarily from bony geometry when the knee is in a flexed position,[60] the application of as little as 5-lb load to the central slip of the quadriceps tendon with the knee at 30° flexion was shown to cause a measurable reduction in patellar displacement in response to medially or laterally directed 5-lb force.[58] As in other articulations, the magnitude and direction of joint compressive forces affect patellofemoral kinematics. This is particularly true during active muscle contraction. Powers et al.[112] have shown that appropriate anatomical modeling of muscle forces affects patellofemoral contact pressures. Muscle activity can affect patellar motion either by increasing joint reaction force or by generating net medializing or lateralizing force vectors within the patellofemoral joint. Therefore, depending upon whether the muscle forces tend to reduce or displace the patella with respect to the trochlea, muscle activity has an inconsistent effect on patellar kinematics.[88] If quadriceps activation reduces the patella, it prevents medial or lateral displacement and protects against dislocation; if quadriceps activation displaces the patella from the trochlea, it can cause dislocation if the passive medial restraints (ligaments) and lateral trochlear buttress fail to contain the patella.

Even when muscles are aligned so as to center the patella in the trochlea, they must be activated in order to do so. While it is possible that passive muscle tension in

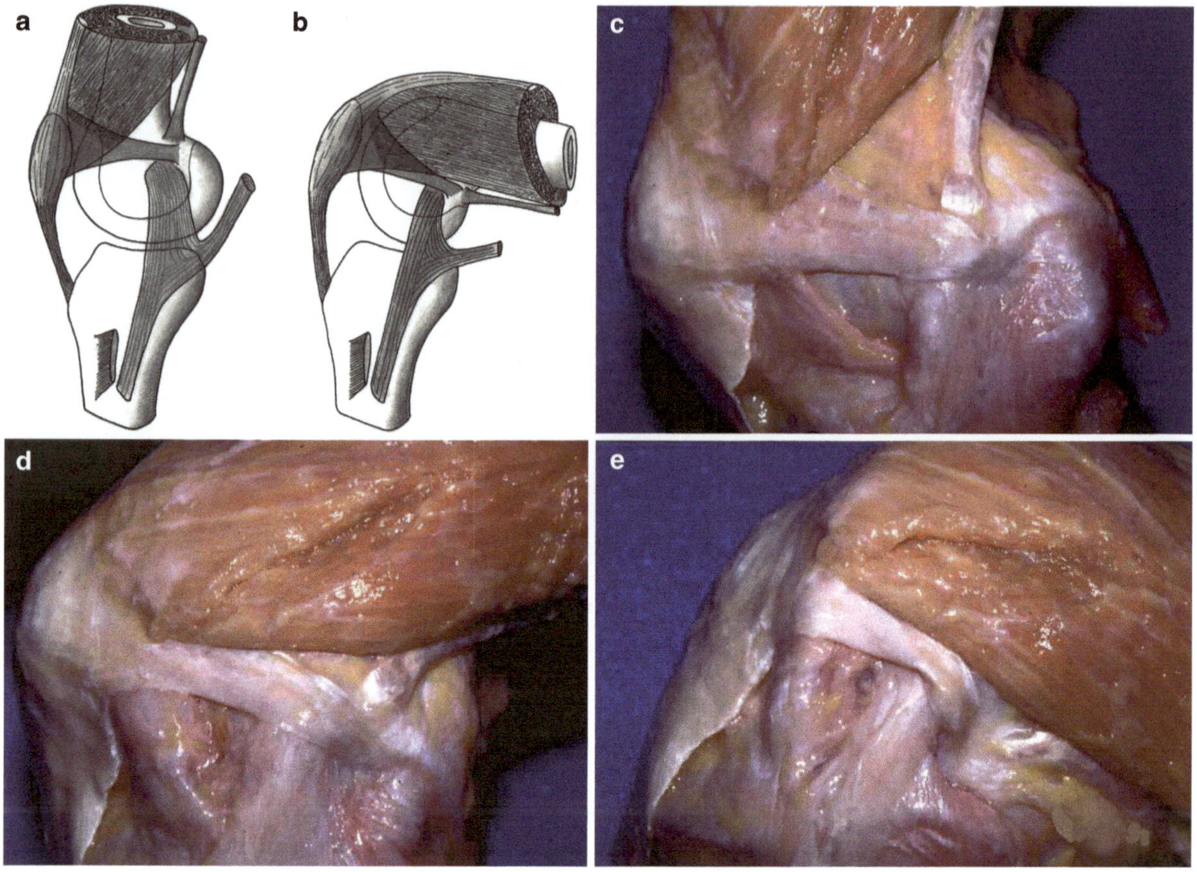


**Fig. 7.6** (**a**) Schematic drawing of the relationships between the VMO and the MPFL. (**b**) The vastus medialis overlies the distal one-third of the MPFL (From Nomura et al.[106]). Its angle of pull relative to the MPFL fibers changes dramatically as the knee is flexed. (**c**) 0°, (**d**) 60°, (**e**) 120° (From Nomura et al.[107])

the vastus medialis obliquus (VMO) resists lateral patellar displacement, this possibility has not been studied. Muscles are designed to do work associated with limb control and locomotion; for them to substitute for passive stabilizers is inefficient. Muscle activity requires effort and results in compressive joint forces in order to compensate for ligamentous laxity. It is possible that the generation of high joint reaction forces may be partially responsible for the arthrosis that can occur after realignment surgery for recurrent patellar dislocation.[8,32] Advancement of the VMO in order to increase passive stiffness would have unpredictable effects because the long-term response of VMO muscle fibers to increased resting length is unknown.

In summary, muscle contraction can have inconsistent and unpredictable effects on joint mobility; it can either cause or prevent abnormal joint motions depending on the magnitude and direction of the resultant muscle force relative to the ligament deficiency.[13,36] Since muscle forces can reduce the apparent limits of joint motion by increasing joint contact force and reducing shear compliance, care must be taken when examining a joint for instability that the muscles are relaxed.[34,35,122] Alternatively, muscle forces that displace a joint in the direction of its pathologic laxity will result in subluxation.[36] The alignment of the extensor mechanism determines whether quadriceps contraction will tend to reduce the patella in the trochlea or displace it from the trochlea. However, the normal patella cannot be dislocated because the passive restraints prevent it from being displaced from the trochlea.[49,58,130] There exists no evidence that any amount of malalignment will cause dislocation unless the passive stabilizers are damaged. On the other hand, a hypermobile patella is unstable using Noyes's definition,[110] even if the muscles are realigned to eliminate lateralizing forces. Using this definition of patellar instability, excessive passive laxity is the essential element in instability of the patellofemoral joint, and the role of extensor alignment and muscle forces is not clear.

## 7.4 Anatomical Features of Acute Patellar Dislocators: The "Patella at Risk"

It has long been appreciated that there are anatomical features that seem to be characteristic of patellar instability.[4,18,139] Several of these features can, either alone or in combination, reduce "containment" of the patella within the trochlear groove, thus predisposing the patella to dislocation. A knee with one or more of these abnormalities may therefore be characterized as possessing a "patella at risk" for dislocation. In fact, Heywood[61] noted that the mechanism in such knees was rarely traumatic. Cash[25] and others[59,84] have noted an association between what have been called "dysplastic features" and the risk of redislocation after primary patellar dislocation, although Larsen[76] reported such a preponderance of dysplastic features among their study population that they were unable to demonstrate a specific association between most abnormalities and the risk of recurrent dislocation.

The typical "morphotype"[78] of the patellar dislocator has been characterized extensively as an adolescent female[50,82] with ligamentous laxity and multiple developmental anomalies,[84,115] including patella alta,[76,115] trochlear dysplasia,[40] and rotational and angular bony malalignment.[65,100,132] Trochlear dysplasia and patella alta, which reduce the "containment" of the patella within the femoral trochlea at any given flexion angle compared to the normal knee, contribute directly to the risk of recurrent patellar dislocation by reducing the relative height of the lateral trochlear buttress.

First described by Albee in 1915,[4] and reported on axial views by Brattstrom in 1964,[18] dysplasia of the femoral sulcus is widely felt to be the most critical anatomical abnormality predisposing individuals to lateral patellar dislocation because the patella is not securely contained within the trochlea.[20,67,73,76,101,119] This situation puts the remaining patellar stabilizers at a disadvantage and increases their susceptibility to failure, which would produce a subluxation or dislocation. Trochlear dysplasia can be identified on a merchant view radiograph by measuring a sulcus angle of more than 145°.[89]

Dejour[40] defined the "crossing sign" as an intersection of the deepest part of the femoral groove with the most prominent aspect of the lateral femoral trochlear facet when viewed from a strict lateral projection on plain radiographs. This finding has high diagnostic value for the presence of patellar instability. The eminence represents the overhang of the trochlear end line in relation to the anterior cortex of the femur, which takes the shape of a beak or bump at the junction of the groove and the anterior femoral cortex.

Dejour et al.[39] compared radiographs and computed tomography (CT) scans of knees with "objective" patellar instability, contralateral asymptomatic knees, and control knees. Four "relevant" factors were identified in knees with symptomatic patellar instability: (1) trochlear dysplasia (85%), as defined by the crossing sign (96%) and quantitatively expressed by the trochlear bump, pathological above 3 mm or more (66%), and the trochlear depth, pathologic at 4 mm or less; (2) "quadriceps dysplasia" (83%), which they defined as present when the patellar tilt in extension was more than 20° on the CT scans; (3) patella alta (Caton-Deschamps) index greater than or equal to 1.2 (24%); and (4) tibial tuberosity-trochlear groove (TT-TG) distance, which they defined as pathological when greater than or equal to 20 mm (56%). The factors appeared in only 3–6.5% of the control knees. Like many other authors before and since, they concluded from these data that the etiology of patellar instability is multifactorial.

Patella alta is also strongly associated with patellar dislocation,[9,15,16,26,54,66,71,74,76,79,108,115,124,139] and is the only factor that leads to patellar dislocation without trochlear dysplasia. A high-riding patella may be seen in spastic neuromuscular disorders such as cerebral palsy,[5] but is idiopathic in most cases of patellar instability.[26] Geenen et al. reported that little trauma was required to produce a dislocation in patients with patella alta.[53] It was his opinion that patella alta was the only significant contributing factor in patellar dislocation because a high-riding patella does not engage the trochlea in time to control the rotational and lateralizing forces produced by weightbearing activities.[53] Ward et al. compared patellofemoral alignment on MRIs of normal and patella alta knees and found that subjects with patella alta had 20% more lateral patellar displacement and 39% more lateral patellar tilt at 0° of flexion. In addition, subjects with patella alta had 19% less patellofemoral contact area from 0° to 60°.[137]

Hvid[64] and Nietosvaara[101] have shown evidence that patella alta may contribute to dysplasia of the trochlea because of altered patellofemoral mechanics during skeletal development. Whatever its affect on trochlear development, a patella such as the one shown in Fig. 7.7 can be viewed as balanced upon the convexity of the femoral shaft for a good part of early knee flexion. In such a knee, the medial soft tissue restraints are virtually alone in establishing the limits of lateral patellar displacement, and surely are at risk of sudden or gradual failure.

Because the patella is a sesamoid bone, its position and rotation are widely used to indicate the condition of the surrounding soft tissues. Extensor mechanism malalignment is a poorly defined abnormality of patellar position or rotation described on static radiographs that is often reported in the setting of patellar instability. It has been studied using axial views[43,56,90,93,96,120,121,125,139] and lateral views.[88,95,100,109] While it must be acknowledged that there is more to patellofemoral mechanics than bony architecture, it is doubtful that malalignment as measured in these studies offers specific evidence or clear indications as to the pathologic anatomy involved. It has already been shown that the subchondral bone does not accurately reflect the topography of the articular surface.[101,103,128] Given the limitations of radiographs, it is quite possible that they are equally imprecise in defining the condition of the ligaments and muscles around the patella. Patellar tilt and lateral subluxation, the two most frequently observed abnormalities, are caused by imbalance in the soft tissues.[39] However, these effects can be produced by muscle imbalance,[15,39,41,63,65] medial laxity,[7] by lateral tightness,[120] by degenerative wear of the lateral patellar cartilage,[47,120] or a combination. Thus, the finding of tilt or lateral subluxation is ambiguous and offers only a vague suggestion as to the pathologic anatomy of the soft tissues.

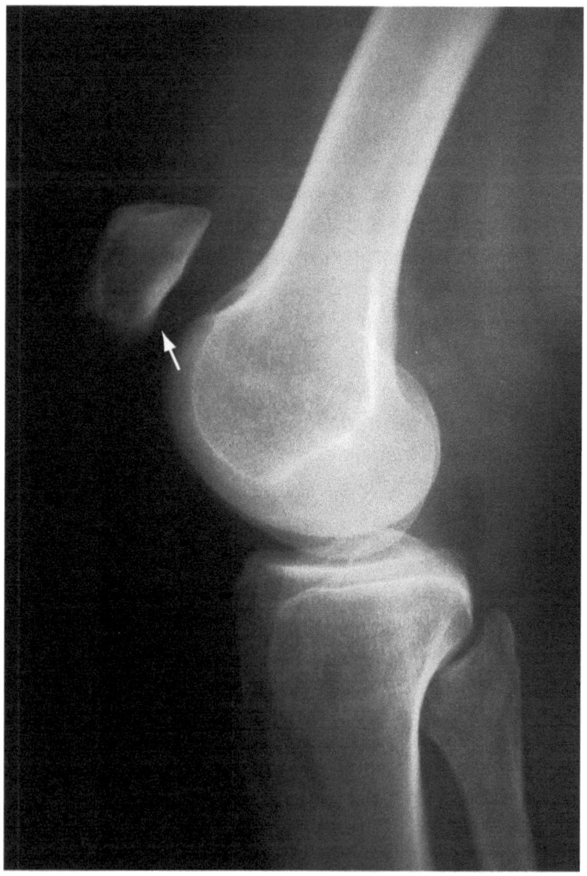

**Fig. 7.7** Lateral radiograph taken after reduction of a lateral patellar dislocation. Note that even at the moderate degree of flexion shown, the inferior pole of the patella (as marked by the *arrow*) has barely entered the trochlear groove

The Q-angle is rarely helpful, as it is imprecise and changes with patellar mobility. If a patella is subluxed laterally, the Q-angle measurement is falsely low. On the other hand, femoral and tibial torsion can play a role in patellar instability, with the largest lateral force placed on the patella when the tibia rotates externally in terminal knee extension. A distance between the tibial tuberosity and the trochlear groove (TT-TG as measured on axial imaging) that exceeds 20 mm is nearly always associated with patellar instability.[39]

Soft tissue dysplasias are seen more commonly among patellar dislocators than among normal subjects.[14,55,68,109,115,127] Ligamentous hyperlaxity, which has been described in patients with patellar instability,[3,23,61,115,127] can reduce the ability of the medial ligamentous tethers to resist lateral patellar displacement. Dysplasia of soft tissues can contribute directly to patellar dislocation if it results in hyperlaxity of the ligaments responsible for preventing lateral patellar displacement.[61,127] Muscular weakness or imbalance has been associated with patellar instability,[50,63,92] but it is unknown if this weakness is a cause or effect. Whether this weakness or imbalance is developmental[109] or the result of dislocations[13,49,51,65,91,116] is not known. That primary muscular dysplasia is directly responsible for patellar dislocation has not been conclusively shown, but muscular imbalance can produce a dislocation in a knee where the passive patellar restraints are already deficient.

Familial history of patellar dislocations has been reported to increase the risk of failed surgical stabilization.[86] Reportedly, at least some of the anatomical factors that contribute to patellar instability are heritable.[14,94,114]

## 7.5 Pathoanatomy of Patellar Dislocation

Acute lateral patellar dislocation may result in specific medial retinacular injuries,[13,17,46,116,126] and the location and extent of the injuries should be documented as a part of a thorough examination.[13] Medial retinacular tenderness and bloody effusion have been used by numerous authors to document that a patellar dislocation has occurred.[13,29,52,59,76,85,102,134] In a retrospective series of 55 patients who underwent surgery for acute primary patellar dislocation, Vanionpää et al. reported that the medial retinaculum was ruptured in 54 and stretched in one patient.[134]

MR imaging has enhanced the accuracy of noninvasive methods for documenting retinacular injury.[21,72,91,105,116,126] Comparison studies evaluating the diagnostic accuracy of MR imaging for identifying complete retinacular injuries have shown 95–100% agreement between preoperative MR films and the findings at surgical exploration.[21,72,116]

The location of MPFL injury in acute dislocation has been studied by multiple authors, with a variety of findings. O'Donoghue thought that the majority of cases involved avulsion of the medial retinaculum from the patella.[111] Sargent shared this view.[117] In contrast, Avikainen et al. reported that 14 of 14 patients who underwent surgical exploration for acute patellar dislocation had avulsion of the MPFL from its femoral attachment.[10] Sallay et al. reported a retrospective study of MR imaging and early surgical exploration and repair.[116] The study sample included 23 patients collected over a 5 year period, who had presented with acute primary (first-time) patellar dislocation. Preoperative MR revealed a tear of the MPFL at the adductor tubercle in 87% of cases. Distal (parapatellar) MPFL injury, indicated by increased MR signal, was noted as well in 43% of knees, though only one patient appeared to have a complete rupture at that location. Arthroscopic evaluation was unrevealing in the "majority" of cases, with only three knees showing subsynovial hemorrhage in the medial gutter near the adductor tubercle. Open surgical dissection revealed avulsion of the MPFL from the adductor tubercle in 94% of knees. Marangi et al. reported a prospective series of 56 patients who underwent MR imaging for primary acute lateral patellar dislocation.[91] Sixty-three percent of patients had evidence of medial retinacular injury. Approximately half of all complete retinacular ruptures (27% of injured knees) were noted near the patellar insertion of the MPFL. Nine percent had complete rupture of the MPFL at the adductor tubercle. Importantly, retinacular injury was commonly noted at more than one location along the course of the MPFL (Fig. 7.8). Because this imaging study was part of a larger natural history study of patellar dislocation, surgical exploration was not performed. This weakens the conclusions because the MR findings were not confirmed by direct anatomical inspection. The finding that the medial retinacula are commonly injured at multiple locations provides context for the finding that isolated repair of the MPFL is usually unsuccessful.[28]

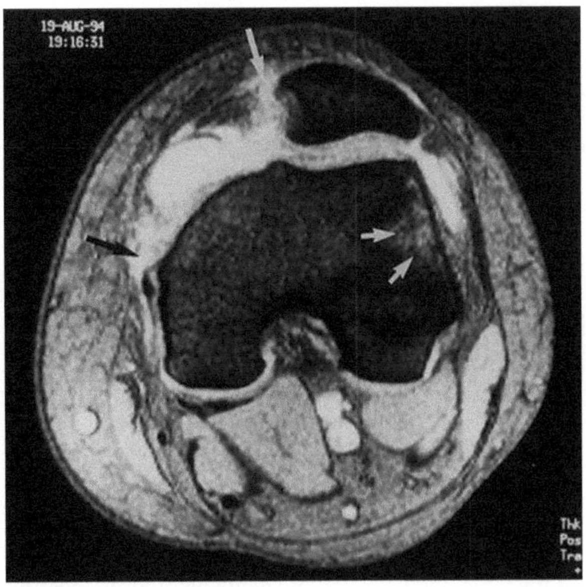


**Fig. 7.8** Axial MR image following lateral patellar dislocation. Note complete discontinuity of signal in the area of the MPFL (indicative of complete rupture) both at the medial femoral epicondyle (*black arrow*) and at the medial border of the patella (*long white arrow*). Lateral condylar marrow edema is also seen (*short white arrows*)

In a more recent study, Silanpaa et al. reported on MRI data of acute dislocators where 66% of the MPFL ruptures were femoral, 21% midsubstance, and 13% patellar.[123] After a mean follow-up of 7 years, 15 patients reported patellar instability (including painful subluxations and patellar re-dislocations). Of this group, 13 had a femoral injury, one patellar, and one midsubstance. The important conclusion of this study is that an MPFL injury at the femoral attachment in primary traumatic patellar dislocations predicts subsequent patellar instability.

Burks et al. reported a simulation of patellar dislocation using normal cadaver knees that directly compared MR and gross anatomical findings.[21] Ten fresh frozen cadaver knees underwent lateral patellar translation equal to 135% of the patellar width. They performed MR imaging, then dissected the medial structures to determine where ligamentous injuries had occurred, and correlated the surgical findings with the MR images. The MPFL was injured in 8 of 10 knees. The location of injury varied, but the most frequent site of injury was at the femoral attachment of the MPFL. The MPML also was avulsed from the inferomedial patella in 8 of 10 specimens. MR images showed MPFL injury in 6 of 10 knees: two at the femur, three at the patella, and one at both the patella and the femur. The authors felt that MR evidence of retinacular injury or avulsion fracture along the medial border of the patella represented injury to the insertion of the MPML, whereas retinacular injury near the femoral attachment of the retinaculum represented injury to the MPFL.

Nomura[105] evaluated the remnants of the MPFL of 67 knees of 64 patients, 18 with acute patellar dislocation and 49 with chronic patellar dislocation. The MPFL injuries of the acute cases could be classified into 2 groups: avulsion and in-substance tears. The chronic cases fell into 3 groups: those with loose femoral attachment (9 knees), those with scar tissue formation or abnormal scar branch formation (29 knees), and those with no evidence or continuity of the ligament (absent type) (11 knees). The authors concluded that incompetence of the MPFL was a major factor in the occurrence of recurrent patellar dislocation and/or an unstable patella following acute patellar dislocation in their study sample.[105]

Clearly, retinacular injury is evident following the primary dislocation event in most cases where the retinaculum is inspected, and the injury usually involves the MPFL. The evidence presented above suggests strongly that residual laxity of the ligament is primarily responsible for patellar instability after the initial dislocation event. Injury to the MPFL may occur at more than one location along its length during the dislocation.[21,91,116] The question arises as to whether the ligament must be repaired at the site of injury for it to function normally. It has not been determined whether a rupture of the MPFL results, after healing, merely in lengthening of the ligament, as in MCL injuries,[99] or in a completely incompetent ligament, as in ACL injuries. Because of its close proximity and anatomical similarities to the MCL, we have hypothesized that the MPFL will heal at an increased length. If acute operative repair is undertaken, failure to identify any and all locations of disruption can jeopardize the success of the repair.

Two recent randomized controlled trials compared nonoperative treatment and repair of the MPFL in acute patellar dislocation. Christiansen et al.[28] randomized 80 patients with primary patella dislocation at a mean of 50 days after injury to either bracing or surgery. The surgical technique for all patients was an anchor-based reattachment to the adductor tubercle. The re-dislocation rate was 17% and 20% in the operative and conservative groups, respectively, showing no significant difference. This study assumes that MPFL rupture occurs at the adductor tubercle and does not attempt to identify the location of MPFL rupture in its surgical group. A similar study done by Camanho et al.[22] did address the location of MPFL rupture in the acute dislocators. The authors repaired the MPFL at the site of injury, as determined by MRI, in eight acute dislocators and found no recurrences compared to a 50% recurrence rate in the nonoperative group at a mean follow-up of 40.4 months. Of the 17 patients in the operative group, 10 were found to have an MPFL injury at the patella, and 7 at the femur. These results suggest that surgical repair of a discrete lesion in the MPFL in the acute dislocator may decrease recurrence. These results have not been duplicated, and are not applicable to the recurrent dislocator.

The documentation of significant retinacular injury in a large number of first-time dislocators has implications for the risk of recurrent dislocation. Garth,[52] Ahmad,[1] Sallay,[116] Sargent,[117] and Vanionpää[135] have all reported satisfactory results after acute repair of the injured retinaculum. Christiansen et al. reported more recently[28] that isolated repair of the MPFL after primary dislocation did not decrease the risk of re-dislocation, ostensibly due to weakening of the repaired ligament to such a degree that it cannot withstand any new trauma that lateralized the patella. Nevertheless, some natural history studies have seemed to suggest that the absence of retinacular injury, a less traumatic mechanism of injury, and familial history of patellar instability predicted a higher risk of re-dislocation.[86,87] It may be that the anatomical predisposition is the most important factor in predicting recurrence after the initial dislocation event. It may also be that specific structures, when injured, also play a role in recurrent instability. The relative contributions of all factors remain to be elucidated.

## 7.6 Summary and Future Directions

Patella dislocation often occurs in knees with an identifiable anatomic predisposition. Yet the initial dislocation event itself often results in injury to the medial ligaments responsible for restraining the patella. The central question for the immediate future is: what anatomical features play major roles in determining the risk of primary dislocation and recurrent instability. Note that these are not the same thing. Though many clinical studies combine primary and recurrent dislocators, it is not clear that the two groups represent the same population. The authors believe that failure to distinguish between them is partly responsible for the confusion that remains about patellofemoral instability.

Other areas of particular interest, at this time, include the biology of MPFL healing and studies comparing the surgical pathology of primary and recurrent dislocations. It is not known how the location of MPFL injury affects its healing potential, and longitudinal studies have not been published showing tissue healing over time after dislocation.

Finally, prospective clinical trials are needed to narrow the range of surgical approaches and compare their success rates in specific clinical scenarios. The anatomical concepts presented in this paper provide principles that could be used to design such studies.

**Acknowledgments** The authors wish to thank the members of the International Patellofemoral Study Group, whose collaboration inspires and informs our work.

## References

1. Ahmad CS, Stein BE, Matuz D, et al. Immediate surgical repair of the medial patellar stabilizers for acute patellar dislocation. A review of eight cases. *Am J Sports Med.* 2000; 28:804-810.
2. Ahmed AM, Duncan NA. Correlation of patellar tracking pattern with trochlear and retropatellar surface topographies. *J Biomech Eng.* 2000;122:652-660.
3. Ahstrom JP. Osteochondral fracture in the knee joint associated with hypermobility and dislocation of the patella. Report of eighteen cases. *J Bone Joint Surg.* 1965;47-A:1491-1502.
4. Albee RH. The bone graft wedge in the treatment of habitual dislocation of the patella. *Med Rec.* 1915;88:257-259.
5. Aparicio G, Abril JC, Albinana J, et al. Patellar height ratios in children: an interobserver study of three methods. *J Pediatr Orthop.* 1999;8-B:29-32.
6. Aragão JA, Reis FP, de Vasconcelos DP, et al. Metric measurements and attachment levels of the medial patellofemoral ligament: an anatomical study in cadavers. *Clinics (Sao Paulo).* 2008;63:541-544.
7. Arendt E: Personal Communication, 1996.
8. Arnbjornsson A, Egund N, Rydling O, et al. The natural history of recurrent dislocation of the patella. Long-term results of conservative and operative treatment. *J Bone Joint Surg.* 1992;74-B:140-142.
9. Atkin DM, Fithian DC, Marangi KS, et al. Characteristics of patients with primary acute lateral patellar dislocation and their recovery within the first 6 months of injury. *Am J Sports Med.* 2000;28:472-479.
10. Avikainen VJ, Nikku RK, Seppanen-Lehmonen TK. Adductor magnus tenodesis for patellar dislocation. Technique and preliminary results. *Clin Orthop Relat Res.* 1993;297:12-16.
11. Baldwin JL. The anatomy of the medial patellofemoral ligament. *Am J Sports Med.* 2009;37:2355-2361.
12. Barbari S, Raugstad TS, Lichtenberg N, et al. The Hauser operation for patellar dislocation. 3-32-year results in 63 knees. *Acta Orthop Scand.* 1990;61:32-35.
13. Bassett FH. Acute dislocation of the patella, osteochondral fractures, and injuries to the extensor mechanism of the knee. In: *American Academy of Orthopedic Surgeons Instructional Course Lecture.* Rosemont: American Academy of Orthopaedic Surgeons; 1976:40-49.
14. Beighton PH, Horan FT. Dominant inheritance in familial generalised articular hypermobility. *J Bone Joint Surg.* 1970;52-B:145-147.
15. Bernageau J, Goutallier D, Debeyre J, et al. New exploration technic of the patellofemoral joint. Relaxed axial quadriceps and contracted quadriceps. *Rev Chir Orthop Reparatrice Appar Mot.* 1975;61(Suppl 2):286-290.
16. Blackburne JS, Peel TE. A new method of measuring patellar height. *J Bone Joint Surg.* 1977;59-B:241-242.
17. Boden BP, Pearsall AW, Garrett WE Jr, et al. Patellofemoral instability: evaluation and management. *J Am Acad Orthop Surg.* 1997;5:47-57.
18. Brattstrom H. Shape of the intercondylar groove normally and in recurrent dislocation of patella: a clinical and x-ray anatomical investigation. *Acta Orthop Scand Suppl.* 1964; 68:134-148.

19. Brown DE, Alexander AH, Lichtman DM. The Elmslie-Trillat procedure: evaluation in patellar dislocation and subluxation. *Am J Sports Med.* 1984;12:104-109.
20. Buard J, Benoit J, Lortat-Jacob A, et al. The depth of the patellar groove of the femur (author's transl). *Rev Chir Orthop Reparatrice Appar Mot.* 1981;67:721-729.
21. Burks RT, Desio SM, Bachus KN, et al. Biomechanical evaluation of lateral patellar dislocations. *Am J Knee Surg.* 1998; 11:24-31.
22. Camanho G, Viegas A, Bitar A, et al. Conservative versus surgical treatment for repair of the medial patellofemoral ligament in acute dislocations of the patella. *Arthroscopy.* 2009;25:620-625.
23. Carter C, Sweetnam R. Familial joint laxity and recurrent dislocation of the patella. *J Bone Joint Surg.* 1958;40-B: 664-667.
24. Cartier P, Cistac C, Maulaz D. Results of surgical treatment of patellar disequilibrium. Apropos of 311 cases. *Acta Orthop Belg.* 1989;55:395-409.
25. Cash JD, Hughston JC. Treatment of acute patellar dislocation. *Am J Sports Med.* 1988;16:244-249.
26. Caton J, Mironneau A, Walch G, et al. Idiopathic high patella in adolescents. Apropos of 61 surgical cases. *Rev Chir Orthop Reparatrice Appar Mot.* 1990;76:253-260.
27. Chrisman OD, Snook GA, Wilson TC. A long-term prospective study of the Hauser and Roux-Goldthwait procedures for recurrent patellar dislocation. *Clin Orthop Relat Res.* 1979;144:27-30.
28. Christiansen SE, Jakobsen BW, Lund B, et al. Isolated repair of the medial patellofemoral ligament in primary dislocation of the patella: a prospective randomized study. *Arthroscopy.* 2008;24:881-887.
29. Cofield RH, Bryan RS. Acute dislocation of the patella: results of conservative treatment. *J Trauma.* 1977;17: 526-531.
30. Conlan T, Garth WP Jr, Lemons JE. Evaluation of the medial soft-tissue restraints of the extensor mechanism of the knee. *J Bone Joint Surg.* 1993;75:682-693.
31. Cox JS. Evaluation of the Roux-Elmslie-Trillat procedure for knee extensor realignment. *Am J Sports Med.* 1982;10:303-310.
32. Crosby EB, Insall J. Recurrent dislocation of the patella. Relation of treatment to osteoarthritis. *J Bone Joint Surg.* 1976;58-A:9-13.
33. Dandy DJ. Recurrent subluxation of the patella on extension of the knee. *J Bone Joint Surg.* 1971;53-B:483-487.
34. Daniel DM. Assessing the limits of knee motion. *Am J Sports Med.* 1991;19:139-147.
35. Daniel DM. Diagnosis of a ligament injury. In: Daniel DM, Akeson WA, O'Connor JJ, eds. *Knee Ligaments: Structure, Function, Injury, and Repair.* New York: Raven Press; 1990:3-10.
36. Daniel DM, Lawler L, Malcom L, et al. The quadriceps – anterior cruciate ligament interaction. *Orthop Trans.* 1982; 6:199-200.
37. Davis DK, Fithian DC. Techniques of medial retinacular repair and reconstruction. *Clin Orthop Relat Res.* 2002; 402:38-52.
38. DeCesare WF. Late results of Hauser procedure for recurrent dislocation of the patella. *Clin Orthop Relat Res.* 1979;140:137-144.
39. Dejour H, Walch G, Nove-Josserand L, et al. Factors of patellar instability: an anatomic radiographic study. *Knee Surg Sports Traumatol Arthrosc.* 1994;2:19-26.
40. Dejour H, Walch G, Neyret P, et al. Dysplasia of the femoral trochlea. *Rev Chir Orthop Reparatrice Appar Mot.* 1990; 76:45-54.
41. Delgado-Martinez AD, Estrada C, Rodriguez-Merchan EC, et al. CT scanning of the patellofemoral joint. The quadriceps relaxed or contracted? *Int Orthop.* 1996;20:159-162.
42. Desio SM, Burks RT, Bachus KN. Soft tissue restraints to lateral patellar translation in the human knee. *Am J Sports Med.* 1998;26:59-65.
43. Dixon AM. Demonstration of lateral patellar subluxation: the 30 degrees LR projection lateral rotation. *Radiogr Today.* 1991;57:20-21.
44. Farahmand F, Tahmasbi MN, Amis AA. Lateral force-displacement behaviour of the human patella and its variation with knee flexion – a biomechanical study in vitro. *J Biomech.* 1998;31:1147-1152.
45. Farahmand F, Senavongse W, Amis AA. Quantitative study of the quadriceps muscles and trochlear groove geometry related to instability of the patellofemoral joint. *J Orthop Res.* 1998;16:136-143.
46. Feller JA, Feagin JA Jr, Garrett WE Jr. The medial patellofemoral ligament revisited: an anatomical study. *Knee Surg Sports Traumatol Arthrosc.* 1993;1:184-186.
47. Ficat RP, Philippe J, Hungerford DS. Chondromalacia patellae: a system of classification. *Clin Orthop Relat Res.* 1979;144:55-62.
48. Fielding JW, Liebler WA, Krishne Urs ND, et al. Tibial tubercle transfer: a long-range follow-up study. *Clin Orthop Relat Res.* 1979;144:43-44.
49. Fithian DC, Mishra DK, Balen PF, et al. Instrumented measurement of patellar mobility. *Am J Sports Med.* 1995;23:607-615.
50. Floyd A, Phillips P, Khan MR, et al. Recurrent dislocation of the patella. Histochemical and electromyographic evidence of primary muscle pathology. *J Bone Joint Surg.* 1987;69-B:790-793.
51. Fox TA. Dysplasia of the quadriceps mechanism. Hypoplasia of the vastus medialis muscle as related to the hypermobile patella syndrome. *Surg Clin North Am.* 1975; 55:199-226.
52. Garth WP, DiChristina DG, Holt G. Delayed proximal repair and distal realignment after patellar dislocation. *Clin Orthop Relat Res.* 2000;377:132-144.
53. Geenen E, Molenaers G, Martens M. Patella alta in patellofemoral instability. *Acta Orthop Belg.* 1989;55:387-393.
54. Glimet T. Course of recurrent dislocation of the patella, patellar syndrome without dislocation and femoropatellar osteoarthritis. *Ann Radiol (Paris).* 1993;36:215-219.
55. Gunn DR. Contracture of the quadriceps muscle: a discussion on the etiology and relationahip to recurrent dislocation of the patella. *J Bone Joint Surg.* 1964;46-B:492-497.
56. Guzzanti V, Gigante A, Di Lazzaro A, et al. Patellofemoral malalignment in adolescents computerized tomographic assessment with or without quadriceps contraction. *Am J Sports Med.* 1994;22:55-60.
57. Hampson WG, Hill P. Late results of transfer of the tibial tubercle for recurrent dislocation of the patella. *J Bone Joint Surg.* 1975;57-B:209-213.

58. Hautamaa PV, Fithian DC, Kaufman KR, et al. Medial soft tissue restraints in lateral patellar instability and repair. *Clin Orthop Relat Res.* 1998;349:174-182.
59. Hawkins RJ, Bell RH, Anisette G. Acute patellar dislocations. The natural history. *Am J Sports Med.* 1986;14:117-120.
60. Heegaard J, Leyvraz PF, Van Kampen A, et al. Influence of soft structures on patellar three-dimensional tracking. *Clin Orthop Relat Res.* 1994;299:235-243.
61. Heywood AWB, Heywood AWB. Recurrent dislocation of the patella: a study of its pathology and treatment in 106 knees. *J Bone Joint Surg.* 1961;43-B:508-517.
62. Horner G, Dellon AL. Innervation of the human knee joint and implications for surgery. *Clin Orthop Relat Res.* 1994;301:221-226.
63. Hughston JC. Subluxation of the patella. *J Bone Joint Surg.* 1968;50-A:1003-1026.
64. Hvid I, Andersen LI, Schmidt H. Patellar height and femoral trochlear development. *Acta Orthop Scand.* 1983;54:91-93.
65. Insall J, Bullough PG, Burstein AH. Proximal "tube" realignment of the patella for chondromalacia patellae. *Clin Orthop Relat Res.* 1979;144:63-69.
66. Insall J, Goldberg V, Salvati E. Recurrent dislocation and the high-riding patella. *Clin Orthop Relat Res.* 1972;88:67-69.
67. Jacobsen K, Metz P. Occult traumatic dislocation of the patella. *J Trauma.* 1976;16:829-835.
68. Jeffreys TE. Recurrent dislocation of the patella due to abnormal attachment of the ilio-tibial tract. *J Bone Joint Surg.* 1963;45-B:740-743.
69. Juliusson R, Markhede G. A modified Hauser procedure for recurrent dislocation of the patella. A long-term follow-up study with special reference to osteoarthritis. *Arch Orthop Trauma Surg.* 1984;103:42-46.
70. Kaplan EB. Factors responsible for the stability of the knee joint. *Bull Hosp Joint Dis.* 1957;18:51-59.
71. Kimberlin GE. Radiological assessment of the patellofemoral articulation and subluxation of the patella. *Radiol Technol.* 1973;45:129-137.
72. Kirsch MD, Fitzgerald SW, Friedman H, et al. Transient lateral patellar dislocation: diagnosis with MR imaging. *Am J Roentgenol.* 1993;161:109-113.
73. Kujala UM, Osterman K, Kormano M, et al. Patellofemoral relationships in recurrent patellar dislocation. *J Bone Joint Surg.* 1989;1-B:788-792.
74. Lancourt JE, Cristini JA. Patella alta and patella infera. Their etiological role in patellar dislocation, chondromalacia, and apophysitis of the tibial tubercle. *J Bone Joint Surg.* 1975;57-A:1112-1115.
75. Lanier BE. Stuck medial patella: unusual complication of a Hauser-Hughston patellar-shaving procedure. *NY State J Med.* 1977;77:1955-1957.
76. Larsen E, Lauridsen F. Conservative treatment of patellar dislocations. Influence of evident factors on the tendency to redislocation and the therapeutic result. *Clin Orthop Relat Res.* 1982;171:131-136.
77. Larsen E, Varmarken JE. Recurrent dislocation of the patella. Two principles of treatment prospectively studied. *Acta Orthop Belg.* 1988;54:434-438.
78. Lerat JL. Morphotypes of patellar instability. *Rev Chir Orthop Reparatrice Appar Mot.* 1982;68:50-52.
79. Leung YF, Wai YL, Leung YC. Patella alta in southern China. A new method of measurement. *Int Orthop.* 1996;20:305-310.
80. Levy AS, Wetzler MJ, Lewars M, et al. Knee injuries in women collegiate rugby players. *Am J Sports Med.* 1997;25:360-362.
81. Lieb FJ, Perry J. Quadriceps function. An anatomical and mechanical study using amputated limbs. *J Bone Joint Surg.* 1968;50-A:1535-1548.
82. MacNab I. Recurrent dislocation of the patella. *J Bone Joint Surg.* 1952;34-B:957.
83. Madigan R, Wissinger HA, Donaldson WF. Preliminary experience with a method of quadricepsplasty in recurrent subluxation of the patella. *J Bone Joint Surg.* 1975;57-A:600-607.
84. Maenpaa H, Lehto MU. Patellar dislocation has predisposing factors. A roentgenographic study on lateral and tangential views in patients and healthy controls. *Knee Surg Sports Traumatol Arthrosc.* 1996;4:212-216.
85. Maenpaa H, Lehto MU. Patellar dislocation. The long-term results of nonoperative management in 100 patients. *Am J Sports Med.* 1997;25:213-217.
86. Maenpaa H, Lehto MU. Surgery in acute patellar dislocation – evaluation of the effect of injury mechanism and family occurrence on the outcome of treatment. *Br J Sports Med.* 1995;29:239-241.
87. Maenpaa H, Huhtala H, Lehto MU. Recurrence after patellar dislocation. Redislocation in 37/75 patients followed for 6–24 years. *Acta Orthop Scand.* 1997;68:424-426.
88. Maldague B, Malghem J. Significance of the radiograph of the knee profile in the detection of patellar instability. Preliminary report. *Rev Chir Orthop Reparatrice Appar Mot.* 1985;71(Suppl 2):5-13.
89. Malghem J, Maldague B. Depth insufficiency of the proximal trochlear groove on lateral radiographs of the knee: relation to patellar dislocation. *Radiology.* 1989;170:507-510.
90. Malghem J, Maldague B. Patellofemoral joint: 30 degrees axial radiograph with lateral rotation of the leg. *Radiology.* 1989;170:566-567.
91. Marangi K, White LM, Brossmann J, et al. Magnetic resonance imaging of the knee following acute lateral patellar dislocation. 63rd Annual Meeting of the American Academy of Orthopaedic Surgeons, Atlanta, February 22–26, 1996.
92. Mariani PP, Caruso I. An electromyographic investigation of subluxation of the patella. *J Bone Joint Surg.* 1979;61-B:169-171.
93. Merchant AC, Mercer RL, Jacobsen RH, et al. Roentgenographic analysis of patellofemoral congruence. *J Bone Joint Surg.* 1974;56:1391-1396.
94. Miller GF. Familial recurrent dislocation of the patella. *J Bone Joint Surg.* 1978;60-B:203-204.
95. Moller BN, Krebs B, Jurik AG. Patellofemoral incongruence in chondromalacia and instability of the patella. *Acta Orthop Scand.* 1986;57:232-234.
96. Morscher E. Indications and possibilities of patella wedge osteotomy. *Orthopade.* 1985;14:261-265.
97. Morshuis WJ, Pavlov PW, de Rooy KP. Anteromedialization of the tibial tuberosity in the treatment of patellofemoral pain and malalignment. *Clin Orthop Relat Res.* 1990;255:242-250.

98. Mountney J, Senavongse W, Amis A, et al. Tensile strength of the medial patellofemoral ligament before and after repair or reconstruction. *J Bone Joint Surg*. 2005;87-B:36-40.
99. Murphy PG, Frank CB, Hart DA. The cell biology of ligaments and ligament healing. In: Jackson DW, ed. *The Anterior Cruciate Ligament: Current and Future Concepts*. New York: Raven Press; 1993:165-177.
100. Murray TF, Dupont JY, Fulkerson JP. Axial and lateral radiographs in evaluating patellofemoral malalignment. *Am J Sports Med*. 1999;27:580-584.
101. Nietosvaara Y, Aalto K. The cartilaginous femoral sulcus in children with patellar dislocation: an ultrasonographic study. *J Pediatr Orthop*. 1997;17:50-53.
102. Nietosvaara Y, Aalto K, Kallio PE. Acute patellar dislocation in children: incidence and associated osteochondral fractures. *J Pediatr Orthop*. 1994;14:513-515.
103. Nietosvaara Y. The femoral sulcus in children. An ultrasonographic study. *J Bone Joint Surg*. 1994;76-B:807-809.
104. Nikku R, Nietosvaara Y, Kallio PE, et al. Operative versus closed treatment of primary dislocation of the patella. Similar 2-year results in 125 randomized patients [see comments]. *Acta Orthop Scand*. 1997;68:419-423.
105. Nomura E. Classification of lesions of the medial patellofemoral ligament in patellar dislocation. *Int Orthop*. 1999;23:260-263.
106. Nomura E, Fujikawa T, Takeda T, et al. Anatomical study of the medial patellofemoral ligament. *Orthop Surg Suppl*. 1992;22:2-5.
107. Nomura E, Horiuchi Y, Kihara M. Medial patellofemoral ligament restraint in lateral patellar translation and reconstruction. *Knee*. 2000;7:121-127.
108. Norman O, Egund N, Ekelund L, et al. The vertical position of the patella. *Acta Orthop Scand*. 1983;54:908-913.
109. Nove-Josserand L, Dejour D. Quadriceps dysplasia and patellar tilt in objective patellar instability. *Rev Chir Orthop Reparatrice Appar Mot*. 1995;81:497-504.
110. Noyes FR, Grood ES, Torzilli PA. Current concepts review. The definitions of terms for motion and position of the knee and injuries of the ligaments. *J Bone Joint Surg*. 1989;71-A:465-472.
111. O'Donoghue DH. *Treatment of Injuries to Athletes*. 3rd ed. Philadelphia: Saunders; 1976:600-617.
112. Powers CM, Lilley JC, Lee TQ. The effects of axial and multi-plane loading of the extensor mechanism on the patellofemoral joint. *Clin Biomech (Bristol Avon)*. 1998;13:616-624.
113. Reider B, Marshall JL, Koslin B, et al. The anterior aspect of the knee joint. *J Bone Joint Surg*. 1981;63-A:351-356.
114. Rouvillain JL, Piquion N, Lepage-Lezin A, et al. A familial form of bilateral recurrent dislocation of the patella with major trochlea dysplasia. *Rev Chir Orthop Reparatrice Appar Mot*. 1998;84:285-291.
115. Runow A. The dislocating patella. Etiology and prognosis in relation to generalized joint laxity and anatomy of the patellar articulation. *Acta Orthop Scand Suppl*. 1983;201: 1-53.
116. Sallay PI, Poggi J, Speer KP, et al. Acute dislocation of the patella. A correlative pathoanatomic study. *Am J Sports Med*. 1996;24:52-60.
117. Sargent JR, Teipner WA. Medial patellar retinacular repair for acute and recurrent dislocation of the patella – a preliminary report. *J Bone Joint Surg Am*. 1971; 53-A:386.
118. Scharf W, Weinstrabl R, Firbas W. Anatomic studies of the extensor system of the knee joint and its clinical relevance. *Unfallchirurg*. 1986;89:456-462.
119. Schutzer SF, Ramsby GR, Fulkerson JP. Computed tomographic classification of patellofemoral pain patients. *Orthop Clin North Am*. 1986;17:235-248.
120. Schutzer SF, Ramsby GR, Fulkerson JP. The evaluation of patellofemoral pain using computerized tomography. A preliminary study. *Clin Orthop Relat Res*. 1986;204: 286-293.
121. Shelbourne KD, Porter DA, Rozzi W. Use of a modified Elmslie-Trillat procedure to improve abnormal patellar congruence angle. *Am J Sports Med*. 1994;22:318-323.
122. Shoemaker SC, Daniel DM. The limits of knee motion. In vitro studies. In: Daniel DM, Akeson WH, O'Connor JJ, eds. *Knee Ligaments: Structure, Function, Injury, and Repair*. New York: Raven Press; 1990:153-161.
123. Sillanpää PJ, Peltola E, Mattila V, et al. Femoral avulsion of the medial patellofemoral ligament after primary traumatic patellar dislocation predicts subsequent instability in men: a mean 7-year nonoperative follow-up study. *Am J Sports Med*. 2009;37:1513-1521.
124. Simmons E, Cameron JC. Patella alta and recurrent dislocation of the patella. *Clin Orthop Relat Res*. 1992;274: 265-269.
125. Somer T, Bokorov B. The axial image of the femoropatellar joint. *Med Pregl*. 1985;38:283-287.
126. Spritzer CE, Courneya DL, Burk DL, et al. Medial retinacular complex injury in acute patellar dislocation: MR findings and surgical implications. *Am J Roentgenol*. 1997;168:117-122.
127. Stanitski CL. Articular hypermobility and chondral injury in patients with acute patellar dislocation. *Am J Sports Med*. 1995;23:146-150.
128. Staubli HU, Durrenmatt U, Porcellini B, et al. Anatomy and surface geometry of the patellofemoral joint in the axial plane. *J Bone Joint Surg*. 1999;81-B:452-458.
129. Steensen RN, Dopirak RM, McDonald WG III. The anatomy and isometry of the medial patellofemoral ligament: implications for reconstruction. *Am J Sports Med*. 2004;32:1509-1513.
130. Teitge RA, Faerber WW, Des Madryl P, et al. Stress radiographs of the patellofemoral joint. *J Bone Joint Surg*. 1996;78-A:193-203.
131. Terry GC. The anatomy of the extensor mechanism. *Clin Sports Med*. 1989;8:163-177.
132. Trillat A, DeJour H, Couette A. Diagnostic et traitement des subluxations recidivantes de la rotule. *Rev Chir Orthop (Paris)*. 1964;50:813-824.
133. Tuxoe JI, Teir M, Winge S, et al. The medial patellofemoral ligament: a dissection study. *Knee Surg Sports Traumatol Arthrosc*. 2002;10:138-140.
134. Vainionpaa S, Laasonen E, Patiala H, et al. Acute dislocation of the patella. Clinical, radiographic and operative findings in 64 consecutive cases. *Acta Orthop Scand*. 1986;57:331-333.

135. Vainionpaa S, Laasonen E, Silvennoinen T, et al. Acute dislocation of the patella. A prospective review of operative treatment. *J Bone Joint Surg*. 1990;72-B:366-369.
136. Wall JJ. Compartment syndrome as a complication of the Hauser procedure. *J Bone Joint Surg*. 1979;61-A:185-191.
137. Ward SR, Terk MR, Powers CM. Patella alta: association with patellofemoral alignment and changes in contact area during weight-bearing. *J Bone Joint Surg*. 2007;89-A: 1749-1755.
138. Warren LF, Marshall JL. The supporting structures and layers on the medial side of the knee: an anatomical analysis. *J Bone Joint Surg*. 1979;61:56-62.
139. Wiberg G. Roentgenographic and anatomic studies on the patellofemoral joint.With special reference to chondromalacia patella. *Acta Orthop Scand*. 1941;12:319-410.
140. Willems S, Litt R, Albassir A, et al. Comparative study of a series of normal knees and a series of knees with patellar instability. *Acta Orthop Belg*. 1989;55:339-345.

# 8 Evaluation of the Patient with Anterior Knee Pain and Patellar Instability

Vicente Sanchis-Alfonso, Erik Montesinos-Berry, Agustin Serrano, and Vicente Martínez-Sanjuan

## 8.1 Introduction

When dealing with patients suffering from anterior knee pain and patellar instability, a thorough anamnesis as well as a complete and careful physical examination are the main means to reach a correct diagnosis and once this is done, to start the most appropriate treatment. Imaging studies are only a help to confirm the diagnosis or to complement the data obtained by the history and examination of the patient. This chapter provides an overview of the most important aspects of the history, physical examination, emotional and psychiatric evaluation, imaging studies, and arthroscopic evaluation. Obviously, if the etiology of patellofemoral pain and patellar instability is multifactorial, then the evaluation must also consider all the different factors.

## 8.2 History

The first diagnostic step is a thorough history. This is the main clue for an exact diagnosis. For instance, absence of a traumatic episode or presence of bilateral symptoms should lead toward patellofemoral pathology and against meniscal derangement in the young patient; on the contrary, the presence of effusion suggests intra-articular pathology (e.g., meniscal rupture, pathologic plicae, osteochondral or chondral loose bodies, synovial pathology, peripatellar synovitis) rather than a peripatellar condition. A small effusion, however, may be present with a patellofemoral syndrome. However, polyarthralgias are not a part of the pathology we are now dealing with.

Patients with patellar symptoms can be divided into two groups: those with anterior knee pain, and those with patellar instability. We must determine if the main complaint is pain or instability. It is common to have symptoms in both knees that may change from one knee to the other over time. This is a tip-off for a patellofemoral problem.

Generally, the onset of symptoms is insidious, without trauma, reflecting an overuse condition or an underlying malalignment. Overuse can be the result of a new activity or of the increase in time, frequency or intensity of a previous work or sports activity. In these cases, history should be oriented to determine which supraphysiologic loading activity or activities are of importance in the origin of anterior knee symptoms. Identification and rigorous control of the activities associated with the initiation and persistence of symptoms is crucial for the treatment success. For example, patients with left anterior knee pain should avoid driving a car with a clutch for prolonged periods of time because it aggravates the symptoms. In these cases, patient education is crucial to prevent recurrence. In other cases, symptoms can be secondary to a direct (e.g., automobile accident in which the anterior knee strikes the dashboard ["*dashboard knee*"]) or indirect (internal rotation of the femur on an externally rotated tibia in a flexed and valgus knee position) knee trauma.

Pain is often described as dull with occasional episodes of acute sharp pain. Pain rarely is constant and asymptomatic periods are frequent. It is difficult for the patient with anterior knee pain to pinpoint the area

V. Sanchis-Alfonso (✉)
International Patellofemoral Study Group,
International ACL Study Group,
Hospital 9 de Octubre, Hospital Arnau de Vilanova,
School of Medicine, Catholic University of Valencia,
Valencia, Spain
e-mail: vicente.sanchis.alfonso@gmail.com

V. Sanchis-Alfonso (ed.), *Anterior Knee Pain and Patellar Instability*,
DOI: 10.1007/978-0-85729-507-1_8, © Springer-Verlag London Limited 2011

of pain, placing his or her hand over the anterior aspect of the knee when we ask them to locate the pain. However, the pain can also be medial, lateral or popliteal. Generally, patients have multiple painful sites, with different pain intensity. Pain related to extensor mechanism is typically exacerbated by physical activity, descending stairs (which requires eccentric quadriceps contraction), or after prolonged sitting, for instance during a long trip by car or prolonged sitting in a cinema ("*movie sign*" or "*theater sign*"), and improves by extending the knee. A constant and severe pain way out of proportion to physical findings must make us think of psychological issues or reflex sympathetic dystrophy (RSD) even when the classic vasomotor findings are absent.[27] Finally, constant burning pain indicates a neuromatous origin.

One must not forget the possibility of pain secondary to a posterior cruciate ligament (PCL) deficiency when there has been a knee trauma. This is a well-known cause for anterior knee pain, given that PCL tears increase patellofemoral joint reaction force by posterior displacement of the tibial tuberosity.[27] It is also important to examine the integrity of the anterior cruciate ligament (ACL) as anterior knee pain is present in 20–27% of patients with ACL chronic insufficiency.[27]

Regarding instability, "*giving-way*" episodes due to ACL or meniscal tears are brought about by rotational activities, whereas "*giving-way*" episodes related to patellofemoral problems are associated to activities that do not imply rotational strains,[13] and are a consequence of a sudden reflex inhibition and/or atrophy of the quadriceps muscle.

Patients sometimes report locking of the knee, which usually is only a catching sensation; however they are able to actively unlock the knee, and therefore this type of locking should not be confused with the one experienced by patients with meniscal lesions. Another symptom is crepitus, which should not be mistaken with the snapping sensation more consistent with a pathologic plica.

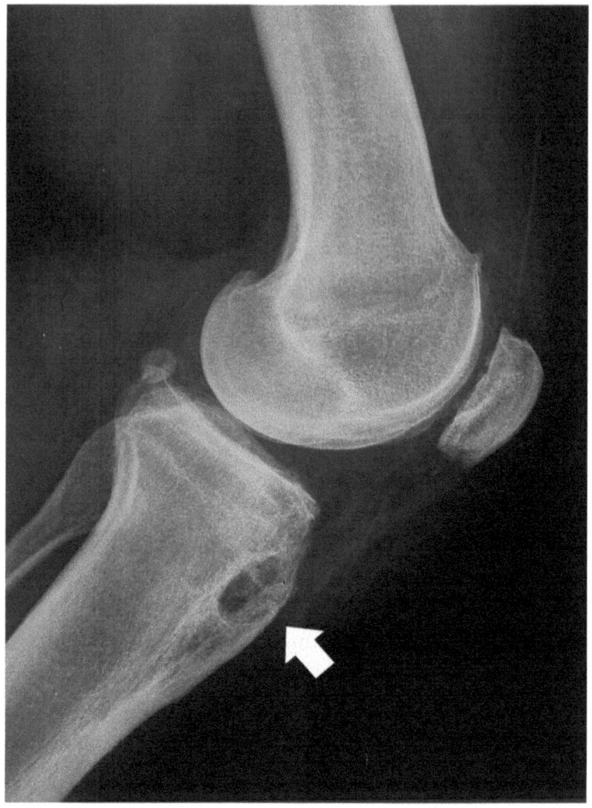

**Fig. 8.1** The most important diagnostic tool is the finger. The location of pain is extremely helpful to make the diagnosis and to plan the treatment. Lateral X-ray of a patient who underwent a Maquet procedure that shows an asymptomatic patellofemoral osteoarthritis. He suffered from highly localized pain on the lytic lesion he had of the proximal tibia (*arrow*). Curettage and bone grafting of the lesion solved his anterior knee pain

## 8.3 Physical Examination

The second diagnostic step is a complete and careful physical examination. It is essential. Its primary goal is to locate the painful zone, and to reproduce the symptoms (pain and/or instability). The location of the pain can indicate which structure is injured; this is extremely helpful to make the diagnosis and to plan the treatment. The most important diagnostic tool is the finger! (Fig. 8.1). Both legs should be examined.

In the first place, pain ought to be tested. The lateral retinaculum should be felt and assessed carefully. Tenderness somewhere over the lateral retinaculum, especially where the retinaculum inserts into the patella, is a very frequent finding (90%) in patients with anterior knee pain.[11] We perform the patellar glide test (Fig. 8.2) to evaluate lateral retinacular tightness. This test is performed with the knee flexed 30° and the quadriceps relaxed. The patella is divided into four longitudinal quadrants and is displaced medially. A medial translation of one quadrant or less is suggestive of excessive lateral tightness.[27] With this test, pain is elicited over the lateral retinaculum. The patellar tilt test can also detect a tight lateral retinaculum, and should always be done (Fig. 8.3). In a normal knee, the patella can be lifted from its lateral edge farther than the transepicondylar axis, with a fully extended knee.

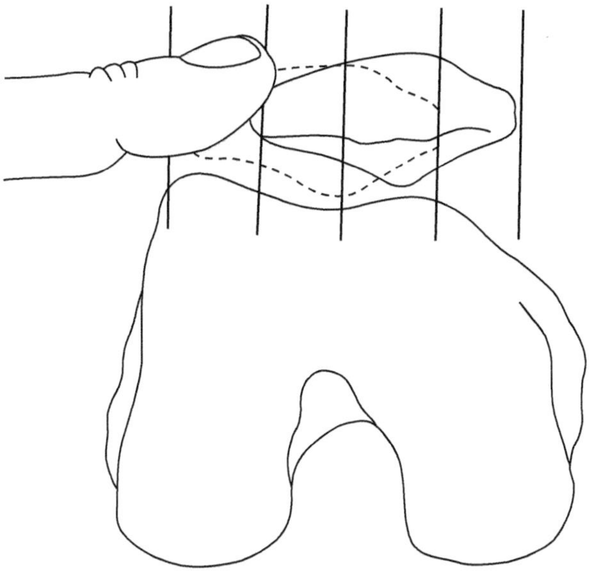

**Fig. 8.2** Patellar glide test. The patellofemoral joint is mentally divided into quadrants and patellar mobility is assessed in both directions

On the contrary, a patellar tilt of 0° or less indicates a tight lateral retinaculum. Lateral retinacular tightness is very common in patients with anterior knee pain, and it is the hallmark of the excessive lateral pressure syndrome described by Ficat et al.[10] In those cases with anterior knee pain after ACL reconstruction we passively "tilt" the inferior pole of the patella away from the anterior tibial cortex to rule out pretibial patellar tendon adhesions.

The axial compression test of the patella (or patellar grind test) should be part of the systematic examination as it elicits anterior knee pain originating in the patellofemoral articular surfaces (patellar and/or trochlear subchondral bone). We also perform the sustained knee flexion test, which when positive (appearance of pain) means that the patella is the origin of the pain, and it is caused by an increase of the intraosseous pressure.[16] To perform the axial compression test (Fig. 8.4) we compress the patella against the trochlea with the palm of the hand at various angles of knee flexion. In addition, this test enables us to determine the location of the lesion in the patellar articular cartilage. With knee flexion, the patellofemoral contact zone is displaced proximally in the patella and distally in the femur. Thus, proximal lesions will yield pain and crepitation at approximately 90° of knee flexion. On the contrary, distal lesions are tender in the early degrees of knee

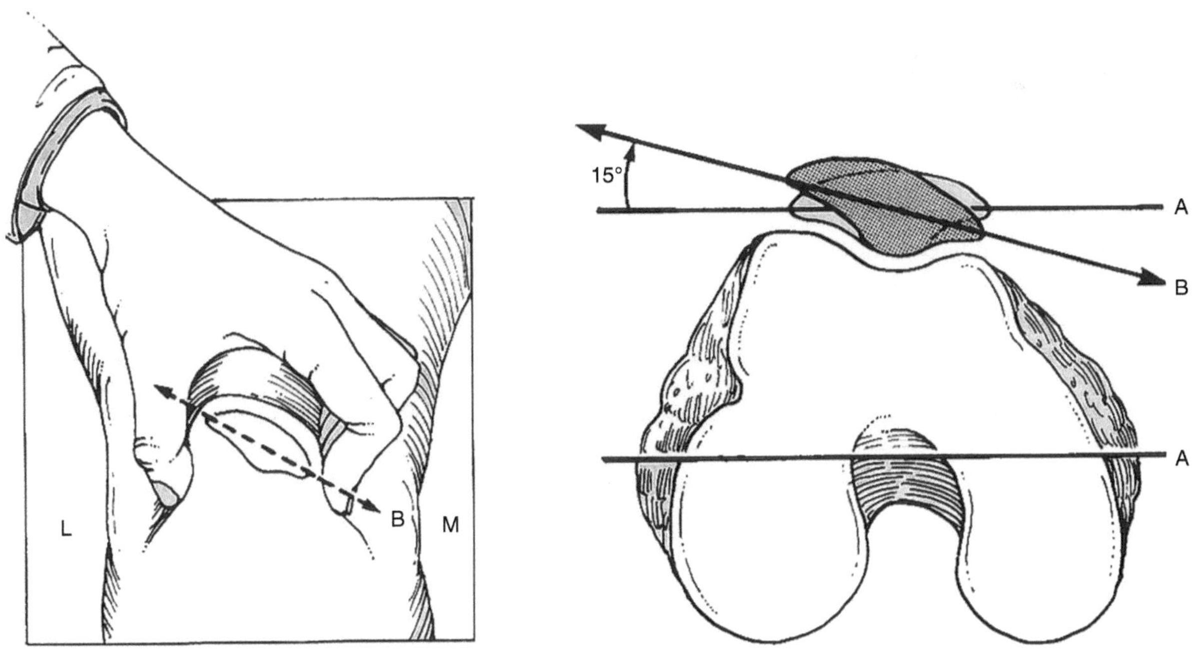


**Fig. 8.3** Patellar tilt test (Reprinted from Scuderi,[41] p. 79, with permission from Springer-Verlag)

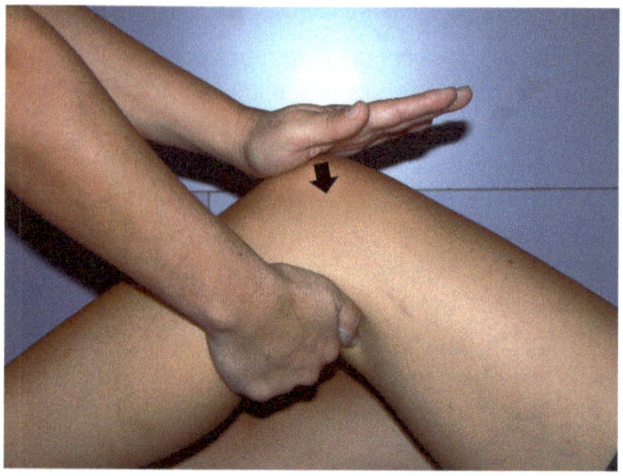

**Fig. 8.4** Axial compression patellar test. We compress the patella against the trochlea with the palm of the hand (*black arrow*)

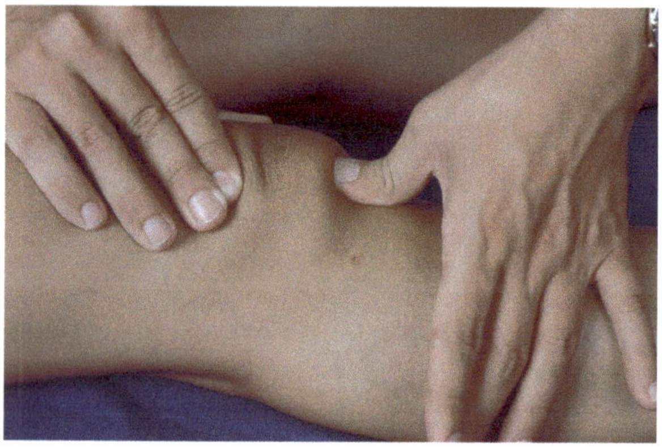

**Fig. 8.5** Palpation on the distal pole of the patella and the proximal patellar tendon

flexion. For the sustained knee flexion test, the patient lies supine on a couch with his or her knee extended and relaxed. The knee is then flexed fully and kept firmly in a sustained flexion for up to 45 s. The test is positive if the patient complains of increasing pain after a pain-free interlude of 15–30 s.

Allen and colleagues[2] have found, in patients referred with anterior knee pain, a significant association between proximal patellar tendinosis and abnormal patellar tracking. Therefore, in order to rule-out patellar tendinopathy, palpation of the inferior pole of the patella ought to be carried out in all cases (Fig. 8.5). To perform this test we press downward on the proximal patella, with which the inferior pole of the patella tilt anteriorly. This maneuver lets us palpate the proximal patellar tendon attachment. However, quite often there is mild tenderness at the attachment of the

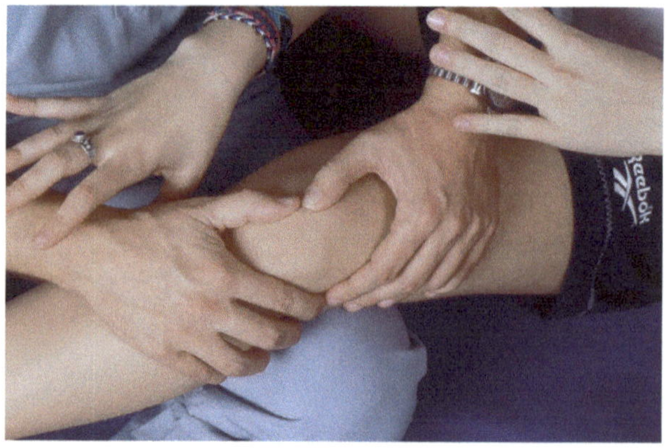

**Fig. 8.6** Patellar apprehension test

patellar tendon at the inferior pole of the patella in individuals who play sports. Thus, only moderate and severe tenderness should be valued. Moreover, Hoffa's fat pad should always be felt as it can be a source of pain as well.[14] Finally, existing scars should be palpated and Tinel's sign performed to detect neuromas. Injecting a local anesthetic will confirm this diagnosis by immediate relief of pain (see Chap. 25).

In the second place, patellar instability ought to be tested. It is extremely important that the surgeon evaluates the direction of the instability. We must note that not all instabilities are in a lateral direction; some patellas have medial instability and some patients suffer from multidirectional instability.

Generally, the most frequent direction of instability is lateral. Fairbanks patellar apprehension test (Fig. 8.6), when positive (pain and muscle defensive contraction on lateral patellar displacement with 20°–30° of knee flexion), indicates that lateral patellar instability is an important part of the patient's problem. This test may be so positive that the patient withdraws the leg rapidly when the examiner approaches the knee with his or her hand, preventing thus any contact, or he or she grabs the examiner's arm. However, Sallay and colleagues[29] found that only 39% of patients who sustained a patellar dislocation had a positive apprehension test. To help achieve greater diagnostic accuracy, Ahmad and colleagues[1] described the "moving patellar apprehension test" that can be performed in an office setting (Fig. 8.7). This test has a sensitivity of 100%, a specificity of 88.4%, a positive predictive value of 89.2%, a negative predictive value of 100%, and an accuracy of 94.1%.[1] This dynamic provocative test

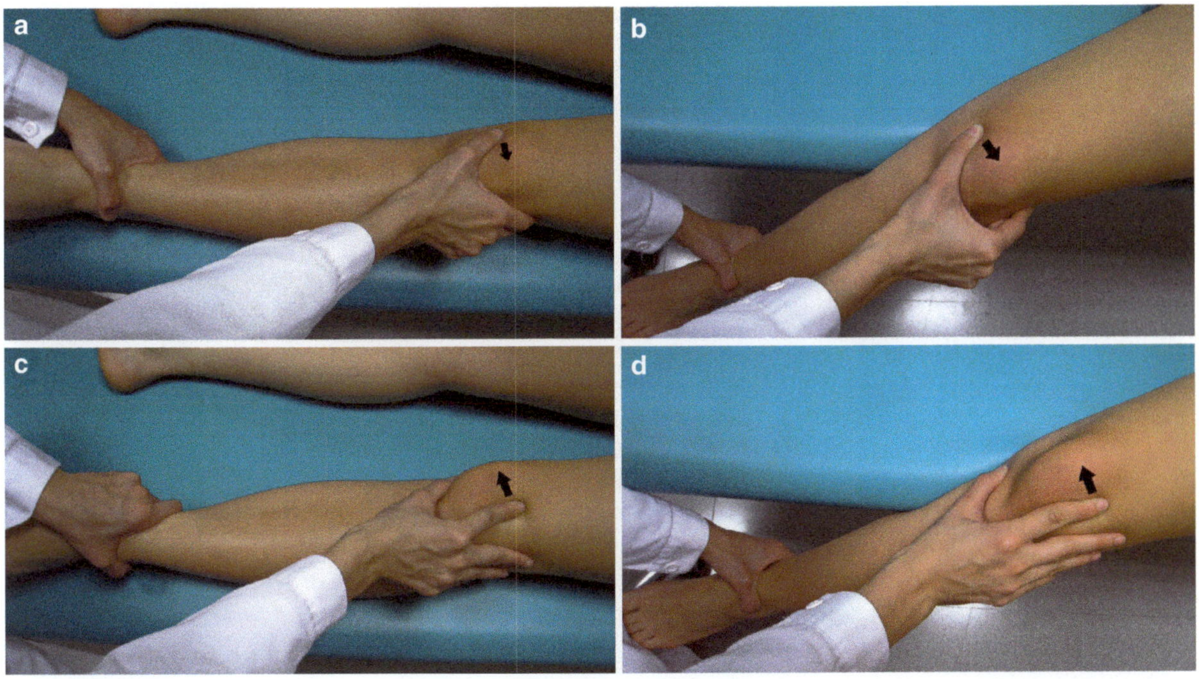


**Fig. 8.7** The moving patellar apprehension test begins with the knee held in full extension and the patella is manually translated laterally (*black arrow*) with the thumb (**a**). The knee is then flexed to 90° and then brought back to full extension while the lateral force on the patella (*black arrow*) is maintained (**b**). In the second part of the test, the knee is started in full extension (**c**), brought to 90° of flexion (**d**), and then back to full extension while the index finger is used to translate the patella medially (*black arrow*). For a positive test, in the first part, the patient expresses apprehension and may activate his or her quadriceps in response to apprehension. However, in the second part of the test, the patient experiences no apprehension and allows free flexion and extension of the knee

is similar in concept to the pivot shift test for ACL-deficient knee.

In order to evaluate instability we also perform the patellar glide test. A medial or lateral displacement of the patella greater than or equal to three quadrants, with the patellar glide test, is consistent with incompetent lateral or medial restraints[27] (Fig. 8.8).

Medial patellar instability is much less frequent than lateral patellar instability, but should be suspected, especially in patients who remain symptomatic after unnecessary or excessive realignment surgery or lateral retinacular release (see Chaps. 24, 26, 32, 33 and 46). Medial patellar instability provokes a sudden, dramatic giving-way worse than before surgery. Our primary method for diagnosis of medial patellar subluxation is the Fulkerson's relocation test[12] (Fig. 8.9). To perform this test we hold the patella slightly in a medial direction with the knee extended. Then, we flex the knee while letting go of the patella, which causes the patella to go into the femoral trochlea. In patients with medial subluxation this test reproduces the patient's symptom. If this test is positive, we should put on an appropriate brace (e.g., Trupull brace, DJ Orthopedics, Vista, California) that should diminish or eliminate the symptoms. This is another way to confirm our diagnosis before indicating a surgical treatment.

It is very important to assess the flexibility of quadriceps, hamstring and gastrocnemius muscles and that of the iliotibial band, as the pathology under scrutiny is often associated with a decreased flexibility of these structures. Tightness of these structures indicates the need for specific stretching exercises and possible training modification.

To test quadriceps flexibility the patient lies prone and the knee is passively flexed with one hand while stabilizing the pelvis with the other hand to prevent compensatory hip flexion (Fig. 8.10). We can measure the quadriceps tightness as degrees of prone knee flexion. Suggestions of quadriceps retraction are[39]: (1) asymmetry, that is to say, a different flexion of one knee compared to the other, (2) feeling of tightness in the anterior aspect of the thigh, and (3) elevation of the pelvis due to flexion of the hip. It is important to assess

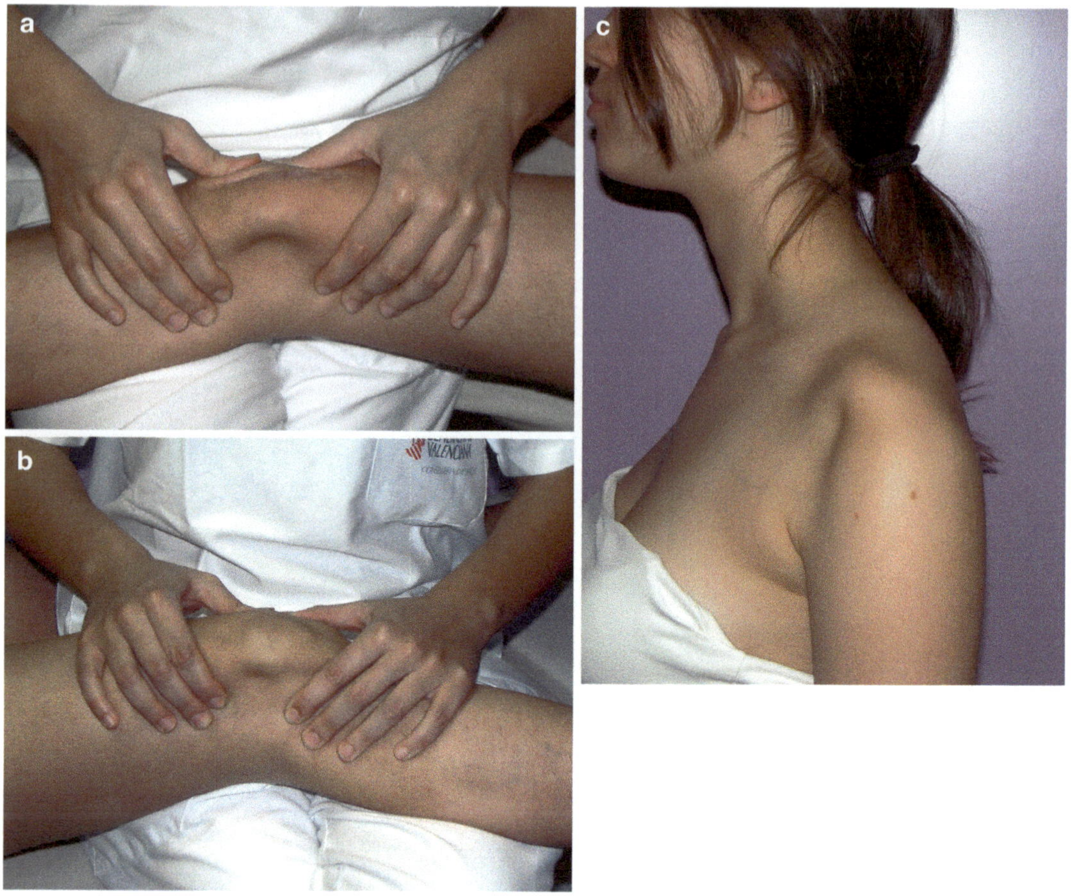

**Fig. 8.8** Patellar glide test in a patient with multidirectional instability. Pathologic lateral displacement of the patella (**a**). Contralateral asymptomatic knee (**b**). We have seen an image (**a**) similar to the sulcus sign observed in patients with multidirectional instability of the shoulder (**c**)

quadriceps contracture as this can increase in a direct way the contact pressure between patella and femur.

To test hamstring flexibility the patient lies supine with the hip at 90° of flexion. The patient is then asked to straighten his or her knee (Fig. 8.11). If complete extension is not possible, there is a hamstring contracture, and its amount is measured by the popliteal angle. Most young athletic individuals have popliteal angles between 160° and 180°.[27] Hamstring tightness implies an increase in the quadriceps force necessary to extend the knee, which augments the patellofemoral joint reaction (PFJR) force. Hamstring tightness could also be associated with spondylolisthesis.

We evaluate gastrocnemius tightness performing a passive ankle dorsiflexion with the knee extended and the foot in slight inversion (Fig. 8.12). Normally this should reach 15° from the neutral position.[39] This test also serves to rule out lumbar radiculopathy or a herniated nucleus pulposus manifesting itself as an anterior knee pain (referred pain). Tightness of the gastrocnemius, in the same way as hamstrings tightness, increases the PFJR force, producing a maintained flexed position of the knee. Moreover, limited ankle dorsiflexion results in increased subtalar joint pronation, that causes an increment of tibial internal rotation with deleterious effects on patellofemoral biomechanics.[27]

The iliotibial band (ITB) is often tight in patients who have patellofemoral pain. This causes lateral patellar displacement and tilt as well as weakness of the medial patellar retinaculum. We use Ober's test to assess ITB flexibility (Fig. 8.13). To perform this test, the patient lies on the side opposite the affected leg with the hip and knee of the bottom leg fully flexed to eliminate the lumbar lordosis. Then, the examiner flexes the affected knee and hip at 90°. After that, he passively abducts the affected hip as far as possible and extends the thigh so that it is in line with the rest of the

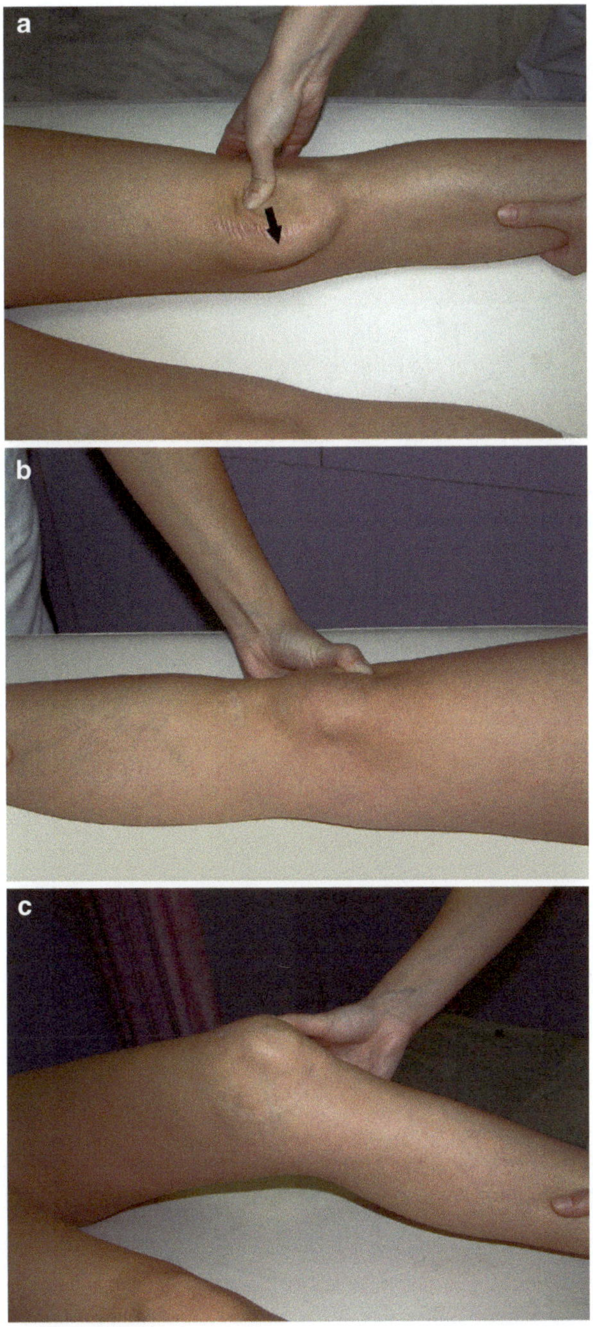

**Fig. 8.9** Fulkerson's relocation test. We hold the patella slightly in a medial direction (*black arrow*) with the knee extended (**a**). Contralateral asymptomatic knee (**b**). Then, we flex the knee while letting go the patella, which causes the patella to go into the femoral trochlea (**c**)

body (neutral position), which places the ITB on maximal stretch. Palpation of the ITB just proximal to the lateral femoral condyle during maximal stretch will cause severe pain in patients who have excessive ITB tightness. At this position, we ask the patient to relax,

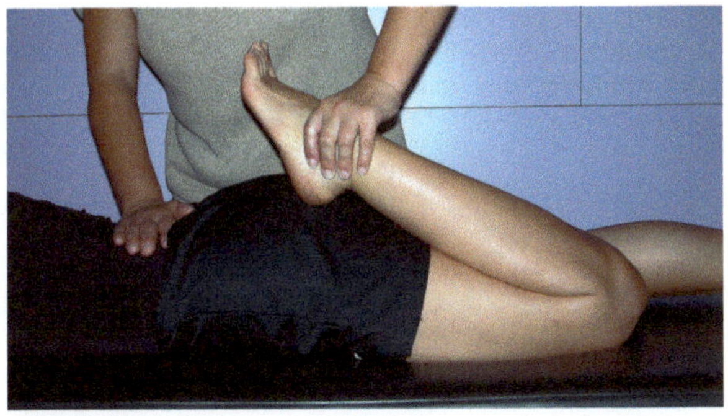

**Fig. 8.10** Evaluation of quadriceps flexibility

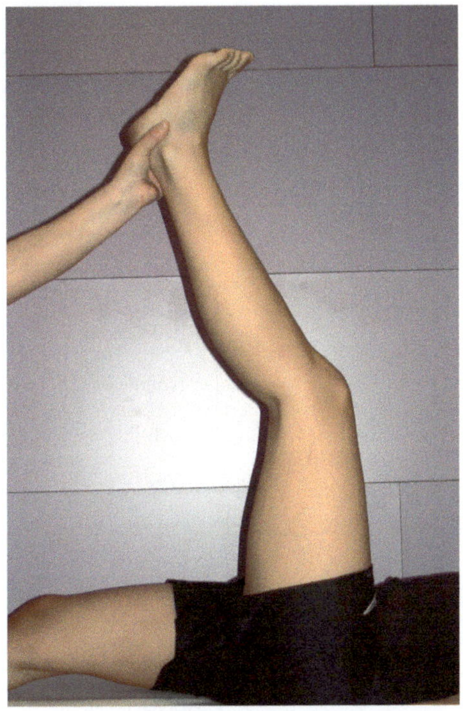

**Fig. 8.11** Evaluation of hamstrings flexibility

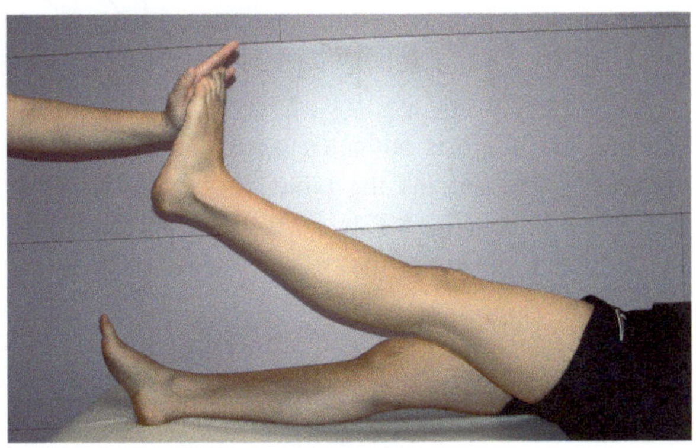

**Fig. 8.12** Evaluation of gastrocnemius flexibility

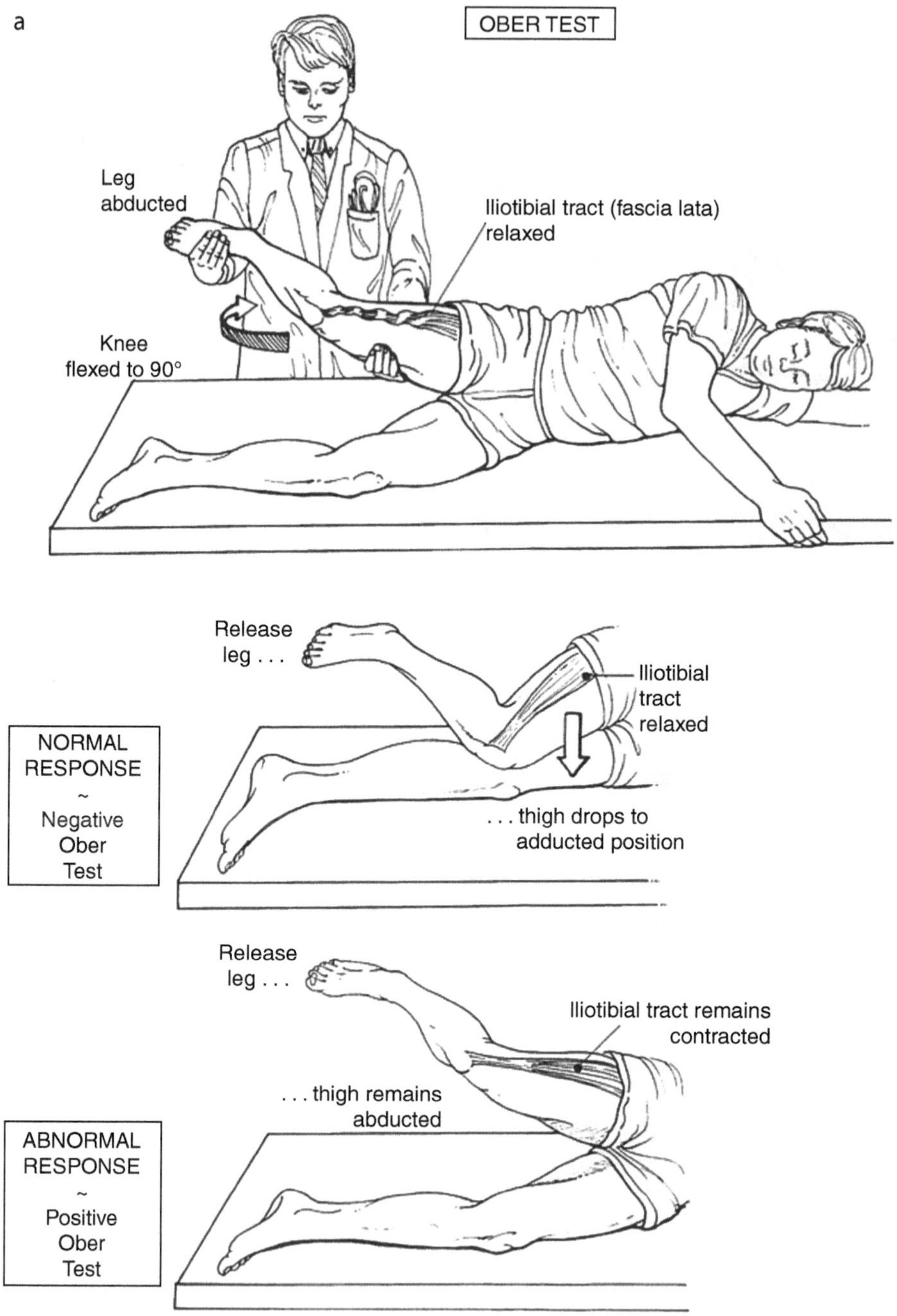


**Fig. 8.13** (**a**) Ober's test. (Reprinted from Scuderi,[41] p. 80, with permission from Springer-Verlag). (**b**, **c**) Positive test

and then the thigh is adducted passively. If the thigh remains suspended off the table, the test is positive (shortened ITB) (Fig. 8.13b, c). If the thigh drops into an adducted position, the test is negative (normal ITB).

As we have seen, patients suffering from patellofemoral problems usually show a flexibility deficit, but some may have hypermobility. It is, therefore, important to evaluate the presence of ligament laxity, as is shown in Chap. 6. Thus, patellar dislocation is six times more frequent in hypermobile patients compared to age-matched controls.[28] Furthermore, articular injuries during patellar dislocation are less frequent in hypermobile patients.[28, 36] In addition to this, these patients may show excessive skin laxity (Fig. 8.14). The presence of Ehlers–Danlos syndrome should be

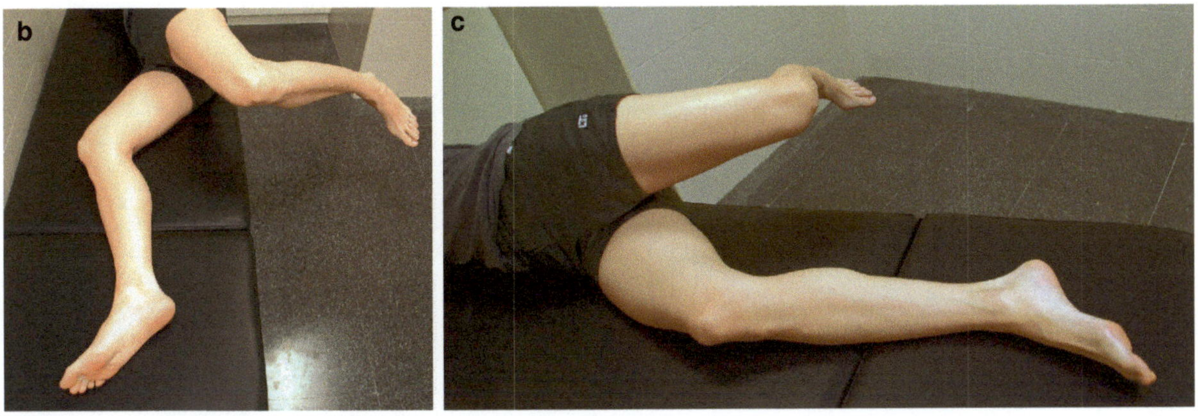


**Fig. 8.13** (continued)

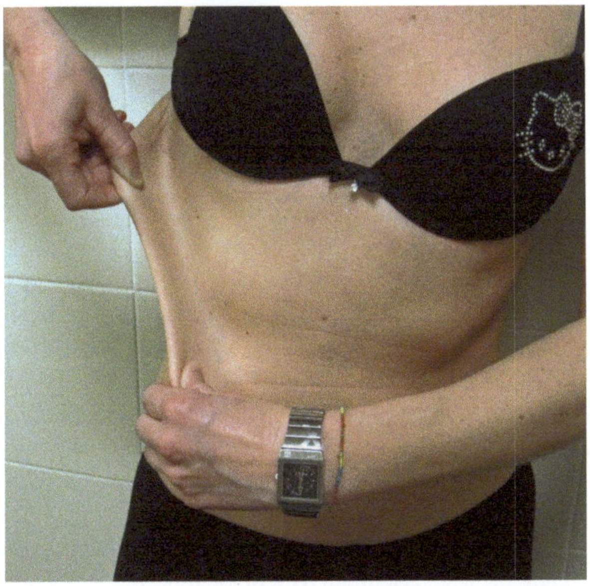

**Fig. 8.14** Skin laxity in Ehlers–Danlos syndrome

ruled out due to the serious systemic complications that may be present.

It is very important to evaluate quadriceps atrophy. When the quadriceps is weak, it fails in its role of shock absorber, and therefore patellofemoral loads increase.[27] This could explain the pain while descending stairs. Patients with an anterior knee pain syndrome usually have a visible and palpable atrophy of the vastus medialis obliquus (VMO) muscle. In 1984, Spencer and colleagues[35] published a study designed to elucidate the role of knee effusion in producing the reflex inhibition and subsequent atrophy of the quadriceps. They found that VMO inhibition is produced with approximately 20–30 mL of intra-articular fluid.[35] This may result in dynamic malalignment, which might explain the possibility of anterior knee pain after surgery for a meniscal or ligamentous injury. Thus, control of effusion is essential for adequate rehabilitation.

Patellar tracking should be examined using the "J" sign (Fig. 8.15). With the patient seated on the examination table and the legs hanging over the side with the knees flexed 90°, he or she is asked to extend the knee actively to a fully extended position. Normally, the patella follows a straight line as the knee is extended. However, as the knee is extended the patella runs proximally and laterally describing an inverted "J" when patellofemoral malalignment (PFM) is present.

As stated in Chap. 6, examination of the feet is essential, as pronated feet (Fig. 8.16) have an important role in the origin of anterior knee pain.

Moreover, leg-length measurement is also important because leg-length discrepancy may be associated with anterior knee pain in the short leg.[27]

Anomalies of the normal knee alignment (genu varum, genu valgum, genu flexum, and genu recurvatum) and rotational abnormalities of the femur and tibia have to be taken into account, as it is shown in Chaps. 6, 14, 34, 36 and 37. In this context, increased femoral anteversion (Fig. 8.17) and internal torsion are closely related to patellofemoral pathology.[22] An increased range of the internal over the external rotation by 30° or more indicates femoral anteversion.[20] Increase in femoral anteversion and internal femoral torsion cause an increase in the quadricipital angle, which produces a greater lateral displacement of the patella on quadriceps contraction. This leads to an

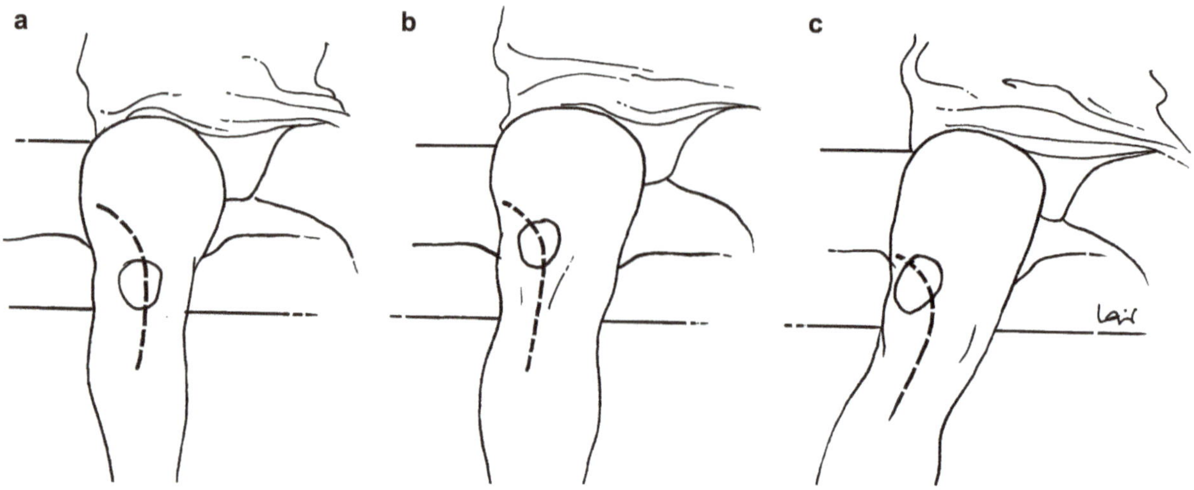


**Fig. 8.15** The "J" sign. When the knee is extended from 90° (**a**) to 0° (**c**) the patella describes an inverted J-shaped course. Intermediate position between 90° and 0° (**b**)

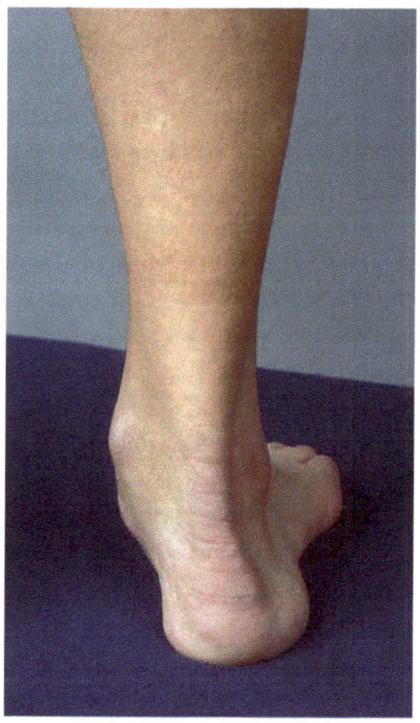

**Fig. 8.16** Pronated foot

increase in the medial patellofemoral ligament tension, as well as in the stresses upon the lateral side of the patella and the trochlea. This is initially the cause of pain and, later on, of instability, chondromalacia, and patellofemoral osteoarthrosis.[22] The pain itself causes quadriceps atrophy, which makes symptoms worse. Quadriceps exercises prescribed by the doctor often produce an overload to the damaged joint, which increases quadriceps inhibition, and paradoxically are the cause of greater atrophy. On the other hand, if the hip mobility is limited and painful, this may indicate the presence of hip pathology (e.g., Perthes disease, slipped capital femoral epiphysis, or osteoarthrosis of the hip) manifesting itself as an anterior knee pain. Therefore, it is very important to evaluate patient's hips to rule out referred pain to the knee. The physician should consider the possibility of referred pain, from the hip or lumbar spine, when no tenderness is elicited about the knee itself. Moreover, a hip flexion contracture (Fig. 8.18) must be ruled out because it results in increased knee flexion when walking, and therefore in increased PFJR force.[27]

Finally, the evaluation of the stability of the knee ligaments (i.e., Lachman test, pivot shift, and posterior drawer maneuvers) is very important to identify factors that may contribute to anterior knee pain and instability in the young patient.

## 8.4 Emotional and Psychiatric Evaluation

We must rule out an organic cause of anterior knee pain before saying the patient has psychosocial problems or he or she is malingering (see Chap. 9). Furthermore, we must not forget that patients with psychogenic pain can also have an organic cause associated.

There are patients who report false symptoms (e.g., attributable to secondary gain in a work compensation or medical-legal case). The difficulty lies in the fact

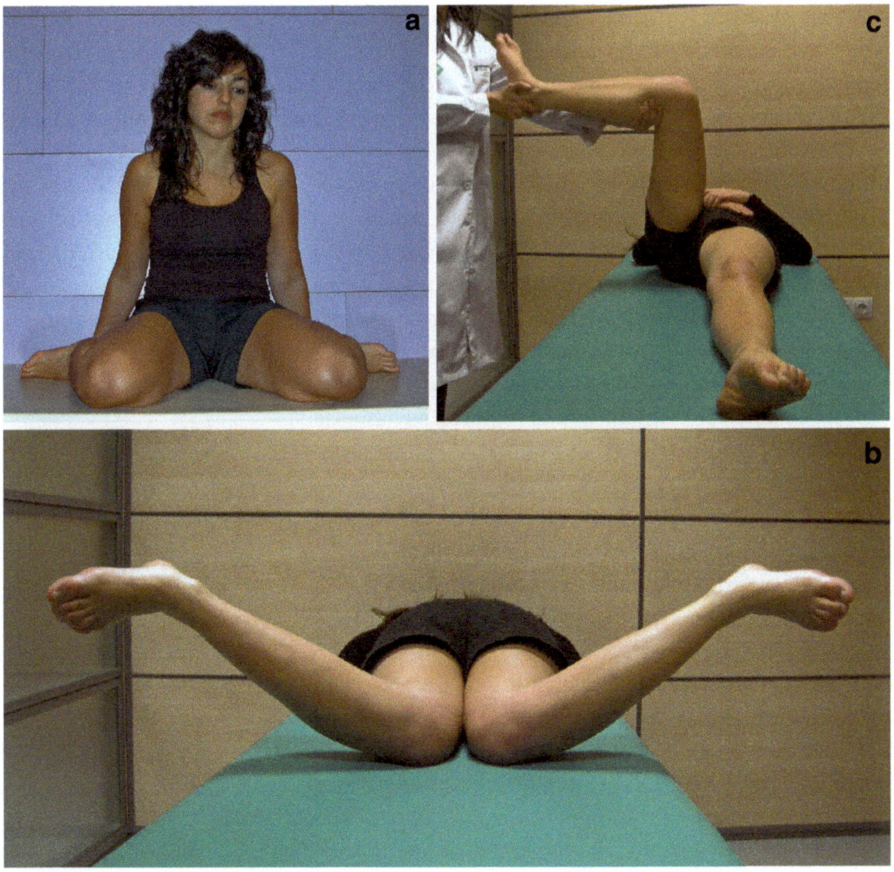


**Fig. 8.17** Increased femoral anteversion. (**a**) Patient sitting down. (**b**) Patient in supine position (**c**) Patient in prone position

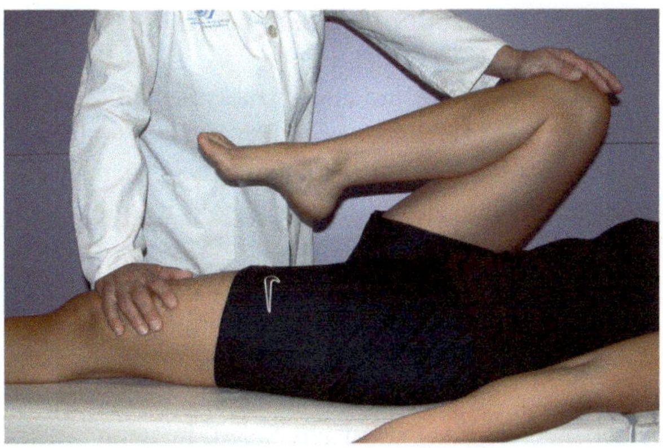

**Fig. 8.18** Evaluation of hip flexion contracture by flexing the contralateral hip completely. If the ipsilateral hip cannot lie flat on the table, hip flexion contracture is present

that whereas in patients suffering from objective structured lesions (e.g., ACL or meniscus rupture), these are easily detected, patients with patellofemoral pain syndrome very often do not show any identifiable structural abnormality. Psychological assessment is indeed very important for patients who have undergone several surgical procedures.

Thomee and colleagues[38] evaluated how patients with patellofemoral pain syndrome experienced their pain, what coping strategies they used for pain, and their degree of well-being. They concluded that the way patients with patellofemoral pain syndrome experience their pain, the coping strategies they use for their pain, and their degree of well-being were all in agreement with other patient groups who have chronic pain reported in the literature. However, the high scores reported for the catastrophizing coping strategy could indicate that these patients might have a more negative outlook on their pain and their prognosis than other groups of patients reported in orthopedic literature. In some cases, there is a moderate elevation in hysteria and hypochondriasis, an unconscious strategy to cope with emotional conflict or control over solicitous parents.[18] Carlsson and colleagues[5] found greater depression, hostility, and passive attitude in patients with long-term patellofemoral pain compared to healthy controls, matched for gender and age. Finally, Andrish has observed that anterior knee pain in some teenage females may represent a somatization of physical or sexual abuse.[7]

Therefore, it is essential to assess the emotional status of the patient. A long- lasting knee pain or an established instability with frequent falls, in the absence of a definite diagnosis by the treating doctor, can become a very stressing situation for the patient. For instance, in our series, one lady with a chronic ACL rupture and frequent falling-down episodes, who had been treated elsewhere for patellofemoral instability for 2 years, developed a hysteric blindness that required psychiatric treatment. Moreover, the patient's response to the problem and whether the associated depression is part of the orthopedic problem are also well worth assessing. We must find out whether we are dealing with a hostile, passive or a "proper" patient. It is essential to analyze the patient's behavior as well as to observe whether it is the patient or his or her mother who "*calls the shots.*"

Finally, it is worth keeping in mind the existence of the genupath.[17] The whole life and being of these persons centers around their knee symptoms, which become chronic and the cause of their failures in their private life and work commitments. With patience and persistence they can convince the orthopedic surgeon to perform a series of procedures, each one more drastic than the last. Self-mutilation can be suspected, and in most some form of litigation is used to maintain their lifestyle. Orthopedic surgeons must be on their guard, as these patients will deliberately induce them to erroneous diagnosis and inappropriate surgical procedures, when what they need is psychiatric treatment. A rule to follow is never to operate on subjective symptoms alone. To give undue attention to isolated clinical data, instead of evaluating the whole picture, can lead to important diagnostic errors.[19] This will prevent making unnecessary mistaken operative indications and their disastrous consequences.

## 8.5 Psychological Pain Versus Pain Due to Reflex Sympathetic Dystrophy: Objective Assessment

A constant and severe pain way out of proportion with physical findings makes us consider psychological issues or RSD. One way of differentiating them is by performing a differential sympathetic block.[14] This has three components: (1) injection of saline solution, (2) injection of just enough anesthetic to block the sympathetic nerves (10 cc of 0.25% procaine), and (3) injection of added anesthetic to block the sensory and motor nerves. Patients who state that with the injection of saline their pain stops or those who have pain after their entire leg has been anesthetized are malingering. Patients who respond positively to the second injection have RSD. Finally, those who respond only to the third injection have nonneurogenic pain.

## 8.6 Imaging Studies

The methods of diagnosis with imaging studies are the second diagnostic step and cannot replace the first step. Overlooking this rule can lead to diagnostic errors, followed by failed treatment and iatrogenic morbidity. A surgical indication should never be based solely on imaging techniques, since the correlation between clinical and image data is not good. The "image" only confirms the clinical impression, but the history and physical examination are the fundamental elements in the evaluation of the patient with patellofemoral pain. Nothing can replace the history and clinical examination. Another aim of the imaging studies is to quantify the pathology and to look for other pathologies.

Nowadays, there are three categories of imaging studies in patellofemoral pathology: (1) structural imaging (radiographs, computed tomography [CT], magnetic resonance imaging [MRI]), (2) metabolic imaging (technetium scintigraphy), and (3) a combination of both.

The majority of patients with patellofemoral pain will only require standard radiography (standing anteroposterior view, a true lateral view, and the low flexion angle axial view [Merchant]). Generally, until thorough nonoperative management has failed, imaging studies beyond standard radiography are not indicated. Weight-bearing anteroposterior projection allows one to evaluate varus, valgus, and joint space narrowing. The lateral view allows one to evaluate the patellar height: high-riding patella or patella alta (alta is Spanish) and low-riding patella or patella baja or infera (baja is Spanish, and infera Latin). Moreover, a true lateral X-ray (overlapping of the posterior borders of the femoral condyles

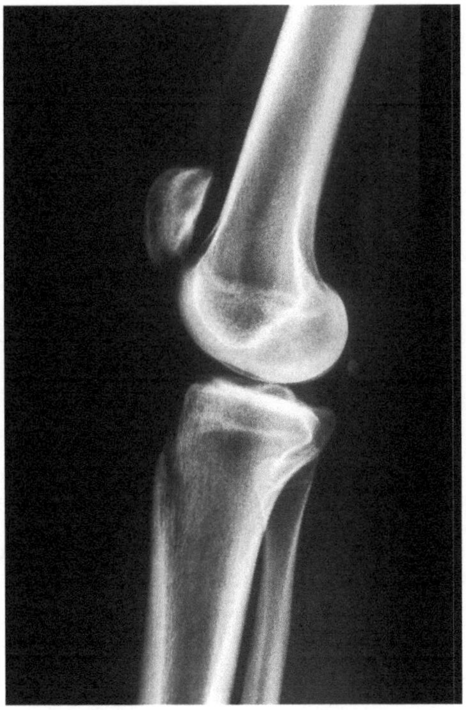

**Fig. 8.19** True lateral radiograph

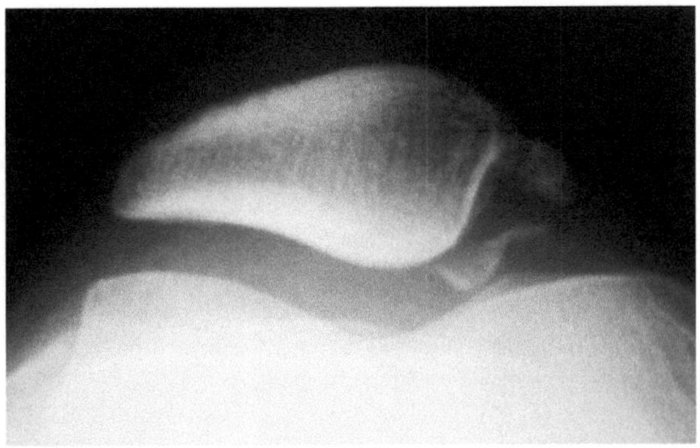

**Fig. 8.20** Merchant axial view, where two bony fragments are seen at the patellar medial border, sequelae from former dislocation episodes

[Fig. 8.19]) allows one to assess trochlear dysplasia (defined by the crossing sign and quantitatively expressed by the trochlear bump and the trochlear depth), and patellar tilt.[4, 6, 14, 24, 37] Axial views can demonstrate patellofemoral maltracking (i.e., tilt, shift, or both) when this happens beyond 30° of knee flexion, sulcus angle, loss of joint space, subchondral sclerosis, and the shape of the patella. In addition to this, an axial view can detect intra-articular bodies or secondary clues of earlier dislocation episodes; for example, medial retinacular calcification is observed sometimes on the axial views and may occur in association with recurrent subluxation (Fig. 8.20). Finally, standard X-ray allows one to rule out associated and potentially serious bony conditions such as tumors or infections.

Adequate bony geometry and competent ligamentous structures are needed to produce stability of the patellofemoral joint. The bone geometry can be seen in conventional X-ray plates, but the ligamentous tightness cannot. Unstable joints are generally congruent at rest, but stress can provoke an abnormal displacement. Axial stress X-rays[37] are useful to document hidden patellar instabilities, which could confirm clinical diagnosis. Stress X-rays can pinpoint lateral, medial, and multidirectional instabilities.

However, there are subtle cases of PFM, in fact the majority of them, which manifest themselves at the first degrees of knee flexion, in which the diagnosis is impossible by conventional radiology, since at 30° of knee flexion, the patella relocates into the femoral trochlea, because with knee flexion the patella migrates medially and distally within the trochlear groove (Fig. 8.21). CT allows us to evaluate patellar tracking from 0° to 30°, and also the tibial tuberosity–trochlear groove (TT-TG) distance. CT ought to be used after failure of conservative treatment and when realignment surgery is being considered.

By using CT scans in asymptomatic volunteers, we found that the patella is usually well-centered in the intercondylar groove in extension[30]. Schutzer and colleagues[32] identified three patterns of malalignment using CT imaging: type 1 includes patellar subluxation without tilt, type 2 is described as patellar subluxation with tilt, and type 3 is patellar tilt without subluxation. To assess patellar tilt we use the lateral patellofemoral angle (Fig. 8.21). This angle is the result of the intersection of two lines: a line that runs across the apices of the femoral condyles and another line that is drawn along the articular surface of the lateral patellar facet. This angle is normal (negative for patellar tilt) when it opens laterally, and is considered as abnormal (positive for patellar tilt) when both lines are parallel or the angle opens medially (Fig. 8.21).[9] We must note that the presence of tilt does not automatically imply that this is the source of the patient's symptoms. Regarding TT-TG distance, the mean TT-TG is 13 mm, and a distance of >20 mm with knee pain is a sign for tibial tubercle medialization surgery, particularly if the trochlea is flat.[3]

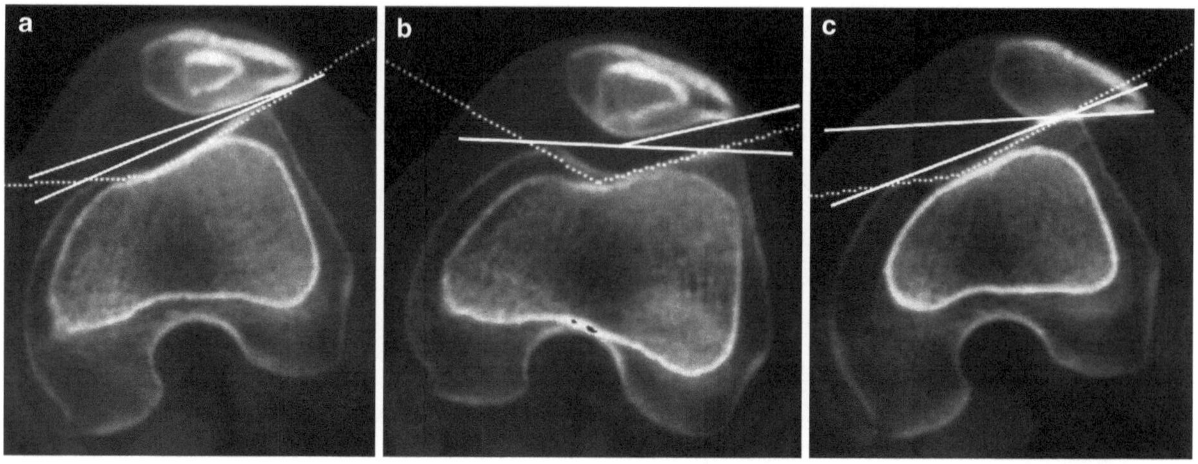


**Fig. 8.21** An 18-year-old woman, referred for anterior knee pain and patellar instability of her left knee with repeated hemarthrosis and severe giving-way with falling to the ground with activities of daily living. Conventional radiographs were normal and the patella was seen well-centered in the axial view of Merchant. CT shows PFM type 2 (**a**) with the patella relocated into the femoral trochlea at 30° (**b**). With the contraction of the quadriceps subluxation and tilt increases (**c**) (Reproduced from Sanchis-Alfonso et al.,[42] Reprinted by permission from Thieme)

Shakespeare and Fick[33] found that visual inspection of the knee is unreliable in determining the TT-TG measurement and recommended a CT before medialization of the tibial tubercle.

Furthermore, it is important to note that PFM in some cases is only a dynamic phenomenon, and in these cases CT at 0° of knee flexion with quadriceps contraction is the only way to identify PFM. A patellar subluxation with a relaxed quadriceps can remain unchanged, increase (Fig. 8.21c) or decrease (phenomenon of dynamic reposition) with quadriceps contraction.[4] On the other hand, a well-centered patella with a relaxed quadriceps can subluxate laterally or medially with quadriceps contraction.[4] The comparison of static and dynamic CT scans gives important information and helps to determine the best treatment. Stress CT in extension with a relaxed quadriceps helps document objective instability.[4] If possible, comparison of the normal with the abnormal side is more important than the absolute amount of displacement.

Finally, CT scans can detect torsional anomalies of the lower limbs (e.g., increased femoral anteversion, internal femoral torsion, tibial torsion) (see Chap. 14).

Three-dimensional computed tomography (3D-CT) does not seem to have an advantage over the conventional CT scans. 3D-CT not only shows a realistic volumetric representation of spatial relationships between the patella and femoral trochlea in the three spatial planes (sagittal, axial, and frontal) and visualization of the patellofemoral contact area in vivo,[21] but also shows with great fidelity the surface anatomy including size and location of the chondral lesions (Fig. 8.22). However, its clinical utility is seriously hindered by the inability to show undersurface detail (Fig. 8.22).

MRI is useful for evaluating moderate to severe patellar cartilage damage, although this structural damage may not necessarily be the cause of anterior knee pain. In addition, it also detects possible concomitant lesions that may worsen the symptoms or mimic patellofemoral syndrome. MRI also lets us detect patellar tracking abnormalities.[34, 40] Grelsamer and Weinstein have found an excellent correlation between clinical and MRI tilts.[15] Tilt angles less than or equal to 10° are found in patients without clinical tilt, and are considered as normal, whereas tilt angles greater than 15° are all found in subjects with clinical patellar tilt, and are considered as abnormal. In addition, MRI often shows low-grade effusions associated with symptomatic peripatellar synovitis, an under-diagnosed pathologic condition of the knee.[7] MRI plays a key role in the evaluation of acute lateral patellar dislocation[9] confirming the clinical suspicion of patellar dislocation. The most frequent MRI signs[9] of acute lateral patellar dislocation are (Fig. 8.23): contusions of the anterior portion of the lateral femoral condyle and of the medial patella, osteochondral defects, intra-articular bodies, medial retinacular injuries, and joint

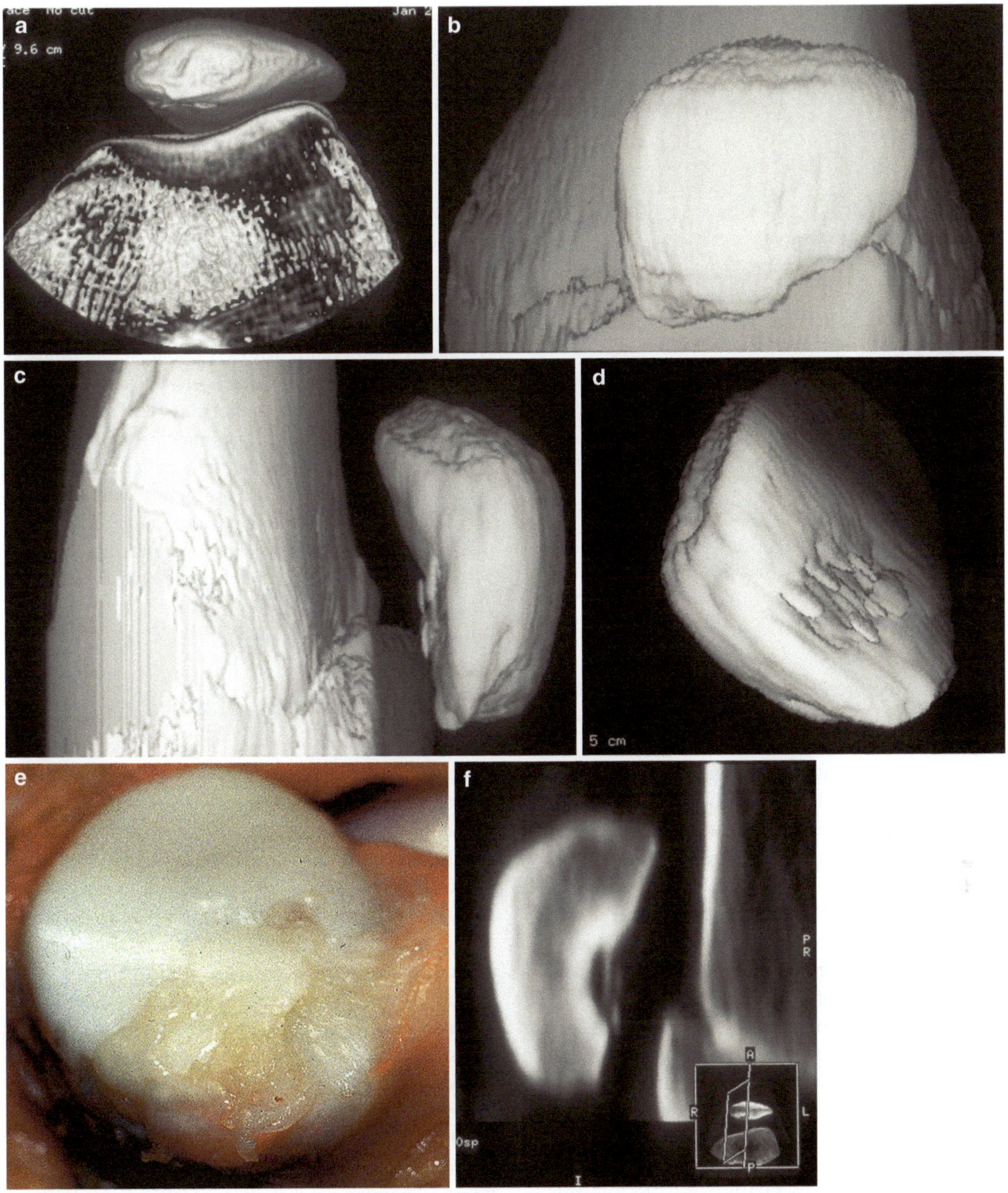


**Fig. 8.22** 3D-CT reconstruction of the patellofemoral joint. Axial plane showing degenerative changes of the articular cartilage of the medial patellar facet (**a**), frontal plane (**b**), and sagittal plane (**c**). 3D-CT shows great fidelity of the surface anatomy including size and location of the chondral lesion (**d**, **e**), although it is unable to show undersurface detail, which is clearly shown by conventional CT scans (**f**) or by MRI (**g**) [Sagittal SE T1W MR image])

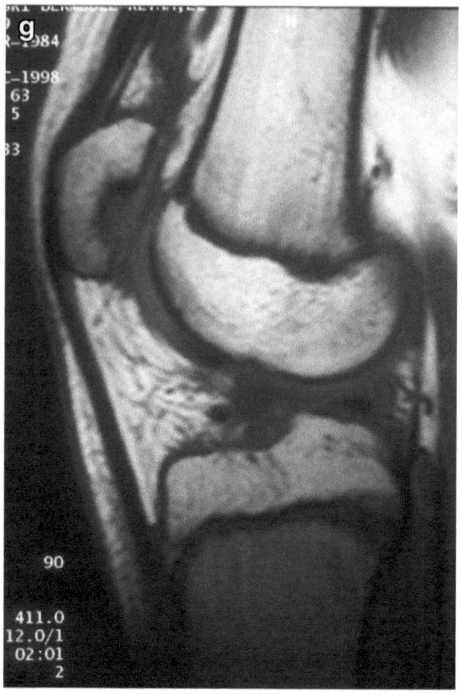


**Fig. 8.22** (continued)

effusions. Moreover, a concave impaction deformity at the inferomedial patella, similar to the Hill-Sachs lesion of the humeral head that follows anterior dislocation of the glenohumeral joint, is a specific sign of previous patellar dislocation.[9] The precise delineation of the injury pattern is crucial in the surgical planning. In addition to all this, MRI is a good method to assess patellar tendinopathy. Moreover, TT-TG can be determined reliably on MRI using either cartilage or bony landmarks. Therefore additional CT scans are not necessary.[31] Moreover, according to Schoettle and colleagues[31], the use of soft tissue landmarks (patellar tendon, deepest site of the cartilage in the trochlea) for TT-TG measurement seems more reasonable, since they represent the true points where the forces act on the patellofemoral joint during flexion–extension movement.

Finally, bone scintigraphy using 99mTc methylene diphosphonate (99mTc-MDP), may be useful in selected cases. If the patella is hot, this suggests that it is the source of pain, but does not provide a diagnosis. Dye and Boll[8] observed that about one-half of their patients with anterior knee pain presented increased patellar uptake in comparison with 4% of the control group. Biopsy demonstrated that this increased patellar uptake was secondary to the increased remodeling activity of the bone. Bone scintigraphy can detect loss of osseous homeostasis, and often correlates well with the presence of patellar pain and its resolution.[7] According to Dye and Boll[8], the bone scan commonly reverted to normal at an average time of 6.2 months (range 3–14 months), which is interpreted as restoration of osseous homeostasis. Scintigraphy may be especially useful in patients with injuries related to workers' compensation cases in which the physician wishes to establish objective findings. According to Lorberboym and colleagues[23], single-photon emission computed tomography (SPECT) bone scintigraphy is highly sensitive for the diagnosis of patellofemoral abnormalities. For these authors, SPECT significantly improves the detection of maltracking of the patella and the ensuing increased lateral patellar compression syndrome. They conclude that this information could be used to treat patellofemoral problems more effectively. SPECT bone scans may be overlaid onto an MRI or CT (fusion) to correlate bone activity with specifics of anatomy.

## 8.7 Arthroscopic Evaluation

Once surgery is indicated, and before any realignment procedure is performed, an arthroscopy should be performed. To inspect the patellofemoral joint the scope should be introduced through the superomedial portal. Arthroscopy is helpful in order to rule out any other unsuspected intra-articular pathology (e.g., synovial plicae, peripatellar synovitis, meniscus rupture) not obvious at the preoperative appraisal, that may cause symptoms that mimic patellofemoral syndrome, and to evaluate patellar articular cartilage. Arthroscopy provides valuable information about articular cartilage breakdown location, extent, and pattern, which may help with future treatment decisions. Moreover, in order to establish a prognosis it is of great interest to ascertain the site of the chondral lesion. Pidoriano and colleagues[25] pointed out that after anteromedial transfer of the tibial tubercle better results were obtained in distal or lateral lesions than in proximal or medial ones. This may be due to the surgical displacement proximally and medially of the patellofemoral tracking area.

Arthroscopy, however, produces scanty information about patellar tracking. No realignment surgical

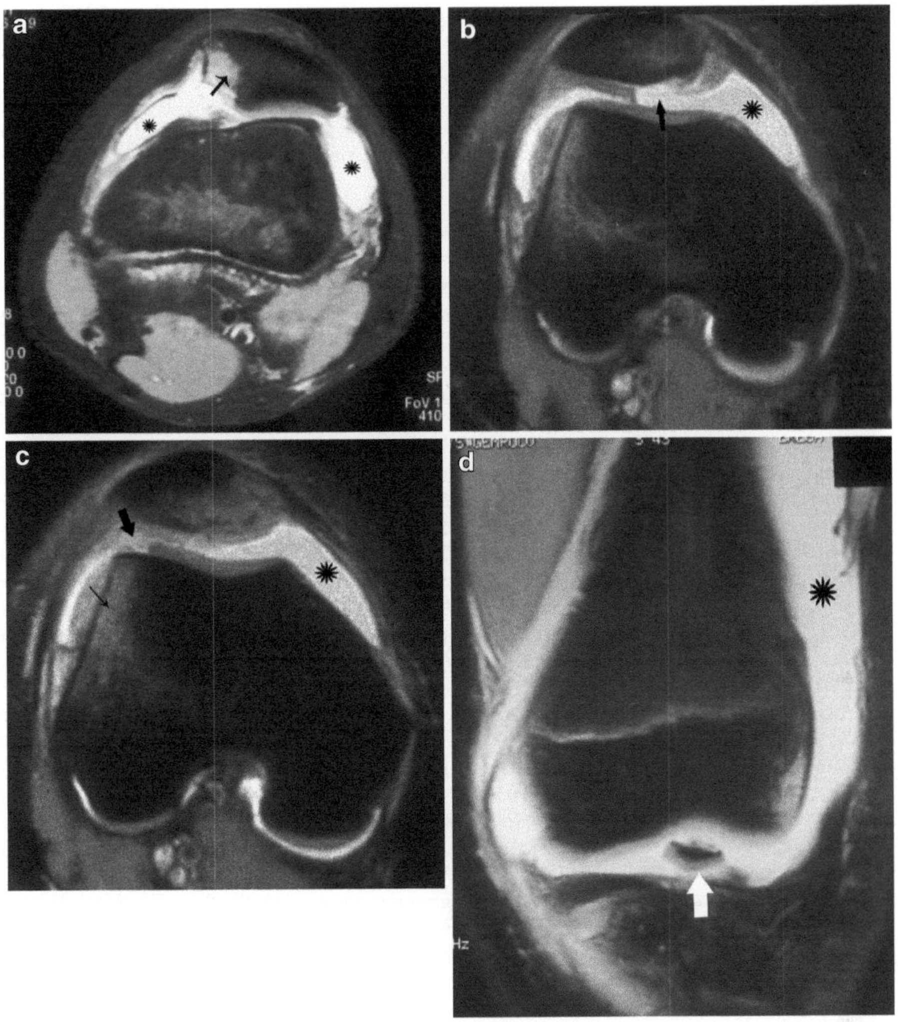


**Fig. 8.23** MRI signs of acute lateral patellar dislocation: contusions of the anterior portion of the lateral femoral condyle and of the medial patellae (*black thin arrow*), osteochondral defects (*black thick arrow*), intra-articular bodies (*white thick arrow*), and joint effusions (*asterisk*). (**a**) Axial FSE PDW Fat Sat MR image. (**b, c**) Axial FSE PDW Fat Sat MR images. (**d**) Coronal FSE PDW Fat Sat MR image

procedure ought to be based entirely upon the arthroscopic analysis of the patellofemoral congruence, as many variable factors (intra-articular pressure, portal localization, contraction versus quadriceps relaxation, tourniquet and foot position) may lead to mistaken conclusions (i.e., impression of malalignment in patients who have normal alignment).[26]

## 8.8 Summary

There is no substitute for a thorough history and a complete and careful physical examination. The history and physical examination still remain the first step for making an accurate diagnosis of anterior knee pain and patellar instability above any technique of diagnostic image. Imaging studies are a second step and can never replace the former. Surgical indications should not be based only on methods of image diagnosis as there is a poor correlation between clinical and image data. Finally, arthroscopy should be used judiciously and no realignment surgery should be based solely on the arthroscopic analysis of the patellofemoral congruence.

## References

1. Ahmad ChS, McCarthy M, Gomez JA, et al. The moving patellar apprehension test for lateral patellar instability. *Am J Sports Med.* 2009;37:791-796.
2. Allen GM, Tauro PG, Ostlere SJ. Proximal patellar tendinosis and abnormalities of patellar tracking. *Skeletal Radiol.* 1999;28:220-223.

3. Bicos J, Fulkerson JP, Amis A. The medial patellofemoral ligament. *Am J Sports Med.* 2007;35:484-492.
4. Biedert RM. *Patellofemoral Disorders. Diagnosis and Treatment.* England, UK: John Wiley & Sons Ltd; 2004.
5. Carlsson AM, Werner S, Mattlar CE, et al. Personality in patients with long-term patellofemoral pain syndrome. *Knee Surg Sports Traumatol Arthrosc.* 1993;1:178-183.
6. Dejour H, Walch G, Nove-Josserand L, et al. Factors of patellar instability: an anatomic radiographic study. *Knee Surg Sports Traumatol Arthrosc.* 1994;2:19-26.
7. Dye SF. Reflections on patellofemoral disorders. In: Biedert RM, ed. *Patellofemoral Disorders. Diagnosis and Treatment.* England, UK: John Wiley & Sons Ltd; 2004:3-17.
8. Dye SF, Boll DA. Radionuclide imaging of the patellofemoral joint in young adults with anterior knee pain. *Orthop Clin North Am.* 1986;17:249-262.
9. Elias DA, White LM, Fithian DC. Acute lateral patellar dislocation at MR imaging: injury patterns of medial patellar soft-tissue restraints and osteochondral injuries of the inferomedial patella. *Radiology.* 2002;225:736-743.
10. Ficat P, Ficat C, Bailleux A. External hypertension syndrome of the patella. Its significance in the recognition of arthrosis. *Rev Chir Orthop Reparatrice Appar Mot.* 1975;61:39-59.
11. Fulkerson JP. The etiology of patellofemoral pain in young, active patients: a prospective study. *Clin Orthop Relat Res.* 1983;179:129-133.
12. Fulkerson JP. A clinical test for medial patella tracking. *Tech Orthop.* 1997;12:165-169.
13. Gambardella RA. Technical pitfalls of patellofemoral surgery. *Clin Sports Med.* 1999;18:897-903.
14. Grelsamer RP, McConnell J. *The Patella. A Team Approach.* Gaithersburg: An Aspen Publication; 1998.
15. Grelsamer R, Weinstein C. *Patellar tilt. An MRI study. 10th Congress European Society of Sports Traumatology, Knee Surgery and Arthroscopy*, Rome, 23rd–27th April, Book of Abstracts, p. 178; 2002.
16. Hejgaard N, Arnoldi CC. Osteotomy of the patella in the patellofemoral pain syndrome. The significance of increased intraosseous pressure during sustained knee flexion. *Int Orthop.* 1987;8:189-194.
17. Jackson AM. Anterior knee pain. *J Bone Joint Surg.* 2001;83-B:937-948.
18. Johnson LL. *Arthroscopic Surgery. Principles and Practice.* St. Louis: The C.V Mosby Company; 1986.
19. Johnson LL, van Dyk E, Green JR, et al. Clinical assessment of asymptomatic knees: comparison of men and women. *Arthroscopy.* 1998;14:347-359.
20. Kantaras AT, Selby J, Johnson DL. History and physical examination of the patellofemoral joint with patellar instability. *Oper Tech Sports Med.* 2001;9:129-133.
21. Kawakubo M, Fujikawa K, Matsumoto H. Evaluation of patellofemoral joint congruence using three-dimensional computed tomography. *Knee.* 1999;6:165-170.
22. Kijowski R, Plagens D, Shaeh SJ et al. The effects of rotational deformities of the femur on contact pressure and contact area in the patellofemoral joint and on strain in the medial patellofemoral ligament. Presented at the Annual Meeting of the International Patellofemoral Study Group; 1999; Napa Valley, San Francisco, USA.
23. Lorberboym M, Ami DB, Zin D, et al. Incremental diagnostic value of 99mTc methylene diphosphonate bone SPECT in patients with patellofemoral pain disorders. *Nucl Med Commun.* 2003;24:403-410.
24. Merchant AC. Radiography of the patellofemoral joint. *Oper Tech Sports Med.* 1999;7:59-64.
25. Pidoriano AJ, Weinstein RN, Buuck DA, et al. Correlation of patellar articular lesions with results from anteromedial tibial tubercle transfer. *Am J Sports Med.* 1997;25:533-537.
26. Pidoriano AJ, Fulkerson JP. Arthroscopy of the patellofemoral joint. *Clin Sports Med.* 1997;16:17-28.
27. Post WR. History and physical examination. In: Fulkerson JP et al., eds. *Disorders of the Patellofemoral Joint.* 4th ed. Philadelphia: Lippincott Williams & Wilkins; 2004:43-75.
28. Runow A. The dislocating patella: etiology and prognosis in relation to generalized joint laxity and anatomy of the patellar articulation. *Acta Orthop Scand Suppl.* 1983;201:1-53.
29. Sallay PJ, Poggi J, Speer KP, et al. Acute dislocation of the patella. A correlative pathoanatomic study. *Am J Sports Med.* 1996;24:52-60.
30. Sanchis-Alfonso V, Gastaldi-Orquín E, Martinez-SanJuan V. Usefulness of computed tomography in evaluating the patellofemoral joint before and after Insall's realignment. Correlation with short-term clinical results. *Am J Knee Surg.* 1994;7:65-72.
31. Schoettle PhB, Zanetti M, Seifert B, et al. The tibial tuberosity – trochlear groove distance: a comparative study between CT and MRI scanning. *Knee.* 2006;13:26-31.
32. Schutzer SF, Ramsby GR, Fulkerson JP. Computed tomographic classification of patellofemoral pain patients. *Orthop Clin North Am.* 1986;17:235-248.
33. Shakespeare D, Fick D. Patellar instability – can the TT-TG distance be measured clinically? *Knee.* 2005;12:201-204.
34. Shellock FG, Mink JH, Deutsch AL, et al. Patellar tracking abnormalities: clinical experience with kinematic MR imaging in 130 patients. *Radiology.* 1989;172:799-804.
35. Spencer JD, Hayes KC, Alexander IJ. Knee joint effusion and quadriceps inhibition in man. *Arch Phys Med Rehabil.* 1984;65:171-177.
36. Stanitski CL. Articular hypermobility and chondral injury in patients with acute patellar dislocation. *Am J Sports Med.* 1995;23:146-150.
37. Teitge RA. Plain patellofemoral radiographs. *Oper Tech Sports Med.* 2001;9:134-151.
38. Thomee P, Thomee R, Karlsson J. Patellofemoral pain syndrome: pain, coping strategies and degree of well-being. *Scand J Med Sci Sports.* 2002;12:276-281.
39. Walsh WM. Patellofemoral joint. In: DeLee JC, Drez D, eds. *Orthopaedic Sports Medicine. Principles and Practice.* Philadelphia: W.B. Saunders Company; 1994:1163-1248.
40. Witonski D, Goraj B. Patellar motion analyzed by kinematic and dynamic axial magnetic resonance imaging in patients with anterior knee pain syndrome. *Arch Orthop Trauma Surg.* 1999;119:46-49.
41. Scuderi GR, ed. *The Patella.* New York: Springer; 1995.
42. Sanchis-Alfonso V, Roselló-Sastre E, Martinez-SanJuan V. Pathogenesis of anterior knee pain syndrome and functional patellofemoral instability in the active young. A review. *Am J Knee Surg.* 1999;12:29-40.

# Influence of Psychological Factors on Pain and Disability in Anterior Knee Pain Patients

9

Julio Doménech, Vicente Sanchis-Alfonso, and Begoña Espejo

## 9.1 Introduction

Pain is a constant symptom in patients with a Patellofemoral Syndrome (PFS). The definition proposed by the International Association for the Study of Pain establishes pain as "an unpleasant sensory and emotional experience associated with actual or potential tissue damage, or described in terms of such damage."[47] This definition establishes the experience of pain in a subjective manner unmatched with a measurable external stimulus. Meaning, it is a prerogative of the subject itself suffering the pain that determines if pain is present or not, regardless of any objective structural damage.

Melzack and Casey[82] proposed structuring pain in three dimensions: (1) Sensory-discriminative. It refers purely to the sensitive magnitude of pain, with which we can determine three related elements: its location, its intensity, and its quality; (2) Affective-motivational. It refers to the emotional properties that accompany the painful feeling such as fear (or anxiety), sadness (or depression), rage, or anger that facilitate or predispose for a response such as aversion, escape, avoidance, or fight; (3) Cognitive-evaluative. It refers to beliefs, thoughts, attitudes and coping strategies regarding pain, the consequences of the experience of pain, and the possible design of a conscious plan to handle the situation.

According to Melzack,[81] these categories interact with one another and influence each other, and can only be understood as a whole. In most cases, there is a high correlation between the sensory and affective dimensions, whereas when pain is more intense, it feels more uncomfortable and causes stronger avoidance and escape reactions. The effects between emotional and cognitive factors in the perception of pain are also known.[59,62,77,79] Traditionally, pain has been related to the disability that the person with a lesion suffers. This correlation is very strong in acute pain. For example, a patient with an acute patellar lesion experiences acute pain, limiting his mobility and disabling him for his ordinary activities. However, pain that becomes chronic can hardly be attributed to identifiable physiologic damage. Pain, impairment, and disability are related but are independent constructs with no connection at all.[37,127]

This correlation between chronic pain and disability is also found in chronic patients with PFS. Jensen et al.[50] studied a group of patients with PFS measuring the degree of pain with the VAS scale and the disability with the Cincinnati Knee rating system (CKRS) questionnaire, and found no significant correlation between the level of pain and the measured disability (Pearson $r = 0.33$, $p$ not significant). In another study by our research group, a significant correlation between pain and disability measured with the Lysholm questionnaire was found, but with a poor correlation index.[21] In another study of young women with PFS, no significant differences were found in the level of functional activity between patients with more knee symptoms and less symptomatic patients.[116] Therefore, we can reason that PFS causes, on one hand, pain and on the other hand, disability; being both independent dimensions with a poor correlation.

For more than a century, the treatment of musculoskeletal conditions has been based on a biomedical disease model.[65,122] This model establishes a direct and sequential relation between tissue damage and pain, between pain and functional impairment and

J. Doménech (✉)
Department of Orthopaedic Surgery, School of Medicine, Catholic University of Valencia, Valencia, Spain
e-mail: julio.domenech@ucv.es

V. Sanchis-Alfonso (ed.), *Anterior Knee Pain and Patellar Instability*,
DOI: 10.1007/978-0-85729-507-1_9, © Springer-Verlag London Limited 2011

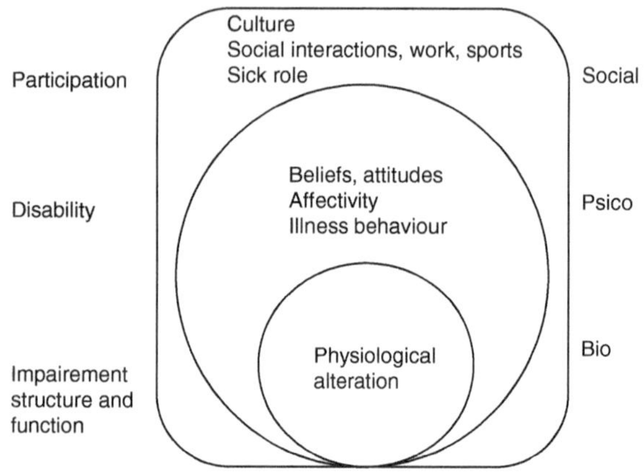


**Fig. 9.1** The Biopsychosocial model of chronic pain and disability. *ICF* International Classification of Functioning Disability and Health, *WHO* World Health Organization (Modified from Waddell[127])

disability. Therefore, the doctor's task would be to repair the damage and clear the pain, making the functional impairment and disability disappear. This model has worked well for conditions such as meniscal tears. However, for some conditions that develop with chronic pain, such as low back pain, this classical model is not enough to establish an adequate treatment.[25,36,127] In these cases, a psychosocial model that integrates patient's biological, psychological, and social elements would be more useful (Fig. 9.1).

In patients with anterior knee pain syndrome (AKPS), the biomedical model, which is very important in understanding the pathophysiology and determining adequate treatment, does not completely explain certain clinical findings. As an example, patients with AKP show different degrees of disability in their everyday life, regardless of how intense the pain is.[21,50] Furthermore, no significant correlation between structural alterations of the patellofemoral joint and disability have been observed.[45,97,116] In fact, some cases with important anatomic alterations (patellofemoral malalignment, severe patellar chondropathy) are painless.[51,74]

The biopsychosocial model would allow the development of more adequate therapeutic strategies than the biomedical model.[9,25,36] Nowadays, very few studies focus on the patient with AKP from a biologic, psychological, and social perspective, although for other conditions such as low back pain, knee osteoarthritis, fibromyalgia, or rheumatoid arthritis, many studies focus on their treatment from this perspective.[5,26,52,113]

## 9.2 Fear-Avoidance Model in Musculoskeletal Pain

In the beginning of the 1980s, several authors proposed the Fear-Avoidance Model[69,93,124,125,128] (Fig. 9.2). This model was initially developed for patients with low back pain and wanted to explain why most of the patients that suffered an episode of acute low back pain resolved spontaneously while a minority of patients developed chronic low back pain. This fear-avoidance model established the existence of many possible responses to a lesion that causes pain. Those patients who do not perceive pain as a threat and are able to cope with it satisfactorily continue their usual activities and achieve full recovery. On the other hand, patients who interpret pain in an exaggerated or catastrophic way develop fear to pain and associated behaviors in search of security, such as hypervigilance and avoidance. Although these avoidance and hypervigilance behaviors can be adaptive when coping with acute pain, they can worsen the patient's condition if the pain is chronic, because they favor disuse, depression, and increase disability. In later years, Asmudson[4] added the pain anxiety component to this model as an aggravating factor in the avoidance behavior generating circuit. The avoidance behavior would not only include limiting the movements, but also avoiding social interactions and recreational activities, which increase pain and suffering in patients.[68] Crombez[18] has even said that "the fear of pain is more disabling that pain itself."

In many crossover studies, fear and avoidance behaviors have been strongly associated with the disability present in patients with low back pain.[1,59,128,134] Also, in low back pain longitudinal studies, changes in the fear avoidance beliefs were good disability predictors.[14,33,39,43,115,135] The fear of pain and the catastrophic vision of pain also occur in pain-free people, so these beliefs can play an important role in the development of new episodes of pain. In studies performed in subjects without low back pain,[49,71,72,120] it was observed that fear of pain increased the risk of suffering episodes of low back pain, and therefore the risk of a disability was increased. Picavet[94] performed a longitudinal study in a population of 1,571 subjects without any important illness during 6 months. The results showed that for the group that indicated the initial low back pain, catastrophization

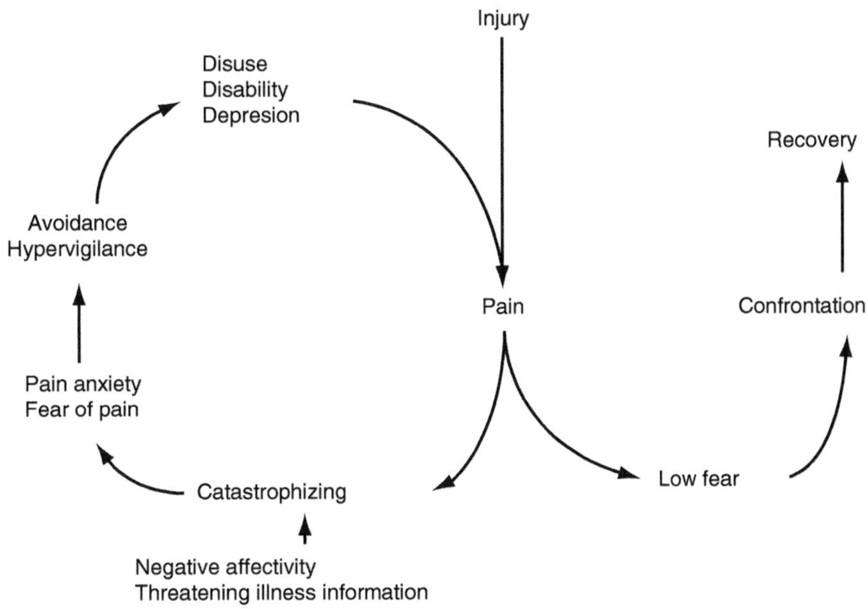


**Fig. 9.2** The fear-avoidance model of chronic pain based on the fear-avoidance model of Vlaeyen and Linton[125] and the fear-anxiety-avoidance model of Asmudson et al.[4]

and kinesiophobia were good predictors for the chronification of pain and the disability. Interestingly, in those subjects with no initial low back pain, both catastrophization and kinesiophobia, also predicted low back pain with disability during follow-up. In another study, Carragee[14] performed a 5 year follow-up in a group of 100 subjects with mild low back pain, by performing magnetic resonance imaging (MRI) and a discography, measuring their fear-avoidance beliefs with a FABQ (Fear Avoidance Beliefs Questionnaire). Surprisingly, the severe low back pain cases and disabilities had no relation with structural anomalies found in the MRI or discography, and it was the presence of fear and avoidance behaviors that turned out to be the strongest predictor in low back pain and disability.

The AKP syndrome shares with nonspecific low back pain the fact that both conditions have a low correlation between the symptoms and anomalies found in imaging studies, and both conditions tend to become chronic and cause disability. Piva[98] studied to see if changes in the fear-avoidance behaviors (measured in the FABQ modified for the knee) influenced the disability in a group of patients with AKP under conventional physical therapy treatment. They found that those patients who lowered their levels of fear and avoidance of physical activity and work, improved their level of pain and disability at the end of the treatment.

In research done by our study group,[21] 54 patients with AKP longer than a year and with severe pain were analyzed (6.3 mean in the Visual Analog Pain Scale). The ideas of fear and avoidance measured with the Tampa Kinesiophobia Scale showed a strong correlation with the patient's referred disability measured with the Lysholm score ($r=-0.59$, $p<0.001$); therefore, the greater the fear and avoidance beliefs, even greater will the disability perceived by the patient be. It is interesting to highlight that the correlation between kinesiophobia and disability was higher than the one between pain and disability. These patients also had very strong catastrophizing ideas measured through the Catastrophizing Coping Scale Questionnaire and through the catastrophic imaging subscale of the Coping Strategies Questionnaire. These beliefs also showed a statistically significant correlation with the disability ($r=-0.49$, $p<0.001$), when the perception of pain is more catastrophic, the patients perceive a higher disability.

Several studies have shown that cognitive–behavioral treatments focused on reducing these fear-avoidance behaviors and the catastrophization of pain, influencing the clinical state of patients with chronic osteoarticular pain in a positive manner.[103,109,114] This approach opens the doors for the trial of new treatment models integrating the biopsychosocial model. Therefore, psychologic therapies can work together with physical therapy and surgical therapies in AKP patients.

## 9.3 Relationship Between Cognitions and Anterior Knee Pain

### 9.3.1 Coping Strategies

In the last decades, the concept of coping with pain has become one of the most important aspects in understanding the consequences of chronic pain in the patient's health. Coping has been defined as the constantly changing cognitive and behavioral efforts that are developed to deal with specific external and/or internal demands evaluated as going beyond the individual's resources.[66] In the case of chronic pain, the patients see their pain as a source of stress for which they develop cognitive and behavioral strategies that are constantly changing to minimize the impact of pain and disability. On certain occasions, these coping strategies are positive, improving tolerance to reduce the perception of pain and disability. But on other occasions, these coping strategies are not adaptative, worsening the disease's clinical course. These differences in managing pain influence the compliance to the treatment prescribed by the doctor.

The Coping Strategies Questionnaire (CSQ)[99] has been widely used in patients with rheumatic conditions. This tool measures the frequency with which patients use different coping strategies. It is comprised of seven subscales, six cognitive (distraction, reinterpreting the painful feeling, ignoring the feeling of pain, coping self-assertion, prayer or hope, and catastrophic view), and a behavioral subscale (increase in the activity level and the behaviors that reduce the painful feeling).

Several studies have shown that patients with osteoarthritis of the knee and arthritis that have high scores in the Pain Control and Rational Thinking factors and low scores in the cognitive distortion factors (catastrophization), show low levels of disability, pain and psychological distress, as well as less behaviors associated with pain.[55,56,58,87,131] Another approach to understand the pain-coping strategies is provided by the Vanderbilt Pain Management Inventory (VPMI), which divides the strategies into passive and active.[10] The active strategies are those in which the patient is actively involved in the management of his pain, such as entertainment with other recreational activities, practicing sports, or keeping up with his daily activities. In the passive strategies, the patient leaves his pain in the hands of the doctor, talks frequently about his pain or uses medication to achieve instant relief. Passive strategies are associated with a significant increase in the risk of developing chronic pain, depression, and physical disability in several studies of patients with arthritis, osteoarthritis, and low back pain.[83,90]

Thomeé[116] studied the coping strategies in a group of 50 Swedish patients with chronic AKP using the CSQ questionnaire, and found that the scores in the different coping subscales were in accordance with the results published in other series of patients with other aetiologies of chronic pain. The most commonly used strategy was the coping self-statements and the less used was reinterpreting pain sensations. In a recent study done by our group in Spain, in a 54 patient group with chronic AKP, similar results were found regarding the frequency with which the different coping strategies are used, regardless of the cultural differences between people of the different studies. The most used strategies were the increase in behavioral activities and the coping self-statements, and the least used was reinterpreting pain sensations. The strategies that showed the highest variability among patients were the catastrophic vision and the coping self-statements.[21] In this study, we also analyzed the relationship between the pain-coping subscales and pain and disability. The catastrophic vision and prayer/hope subscales showed significant correlation with the patient's disability. Also, all of the coping strategies except the prayer/hope one had a significant relationship with the HAD. However, none of the coping strategies showed a significant relationship with the degree of pain.

The modification of the beliefs and behaviors of the patients, in order to use more adequate pain-coping strategies, can help them reduce their symptoms, increase their functional capacity, and reduce their psychological distress. Some clinical trials have shown that a cognitive–behavioral treatment combined with the usual medical treatment in patients with chronic rheumatoid pain is useful in improving their physical and psychological state.[26,31,102]

### 9.3.2 Catastrophization

The catastrophic vision of pain refers to the cognitive process by which pain is seen as an extreme threat and from which the patient suffers exaggerated negative consequences. There is growing evidence that the catastrophic vision of pain is related not only to the pain the patients mention but also to other aspects that influence the course of the illness. Some studies show that patients with musculoskeletal pain with these ideas have a higher degree of disability,[78] higher use of health resources,[100] higher use of medication,[7,48] and worse recovery after knee arthroplasty surgery.[60]

Many studies confirm a strong association between the ideas of pain catastrophization and the patient's disability in several conditions with chronic pain mainly in musculoskeletal pain.[92,101,112,118]

Besides the association with disability, the catastrophic view has been related to the degree of pain. Patients with important ideas of catastrophization mentioned higher degrees of pain, both in acute and chronic pain conditions.[11,100,101,118] Follow-up studies have also shown that the initial catastrophization ideas are related to the level of pain that a patient will point out after a surgical procedure[41,88] or after other painful conditions.[23,24,111,126]

Although the exact mechanisms by which catastrophization affects the experience of pain and disability are not well known, it has been suggested that it influences the focusing of one's attention to the painful or potentially painful process. People, who catastrophize, have difficulties in not focusing on the painful or threatening stimulus.[17,91] This intensifies fear of pain, which increases attention paid to the stimulus. Therefore, evaluating a threat, regardless of the degree of pain, is an important mediator in the perception of pain. Also, an excessively emotional evaluation of pain is associated with catastrophization, which produces a higher perception of the experience of pain.[38] In a study done with functional MRI in patients with chronic pain, it was seen that ideas of catastrophization were not only associated with a higher degree of activity in the brain's pain processing areas but also in the cortical areas related to attention, the anticipation of pain, and emotional aspects of pain.[40] In a study performed in healthy subjects in whom pain was caused by heat, higher levels of pain catastrophization were related with a higher degree of pain as well as higher duration of the heat-related pain. This suggests that catastrophization plays a facilitator role in the pain perception process.[23]

Catastrophization can be clinically measured by the catastrophization subscale of the Coping Strategies Questionnaire (CSQ).[99] There is another specific tool to measure it as well, the Pain Catastrophizing Scale (PCS).[110] This questionnaire has been widely used in clinical practice and has excellent psychometric features.

Even if the influence of the catastrophic view in chronic pain and disability has been widely studied in musculoskeletal conditions such as rheumatoid arthritis,[53,57] knee osteoarthritis[30,55,107] or low back pain,[17,84,92] we are only aware of two studies that analyze this aspect in the AKP patient. Thomeé[117] studied the pain-coping strategies in a group of AKP patients. The catastrophization subscale showed a very high score in the patients with AKP, more than double the score found in other series of rheumatoid arthritis patients. Our group studied the relationship between the catastrophization ideas (measured with the catastrophization subscale of the CSP, and also specifically with the PCS questionnaire) and the disability in a group of patients with AKP. A statistically significant correlation was found between the disability Lysholm scale score and the score obtained from the PCS questionnaire ($r=-0.49$; $p=0.001$); however, there was poorer correlation with the degree of pain ($r=0.32$; $p=0.023$).[21] In this study, we also found that catastrophization was a widely used coping strategy in chronic AKP patients.

## 9.4 Relationship Between Depression and Anterior Knee Pain

Depression is a psychopathologic condition that has been frequently associated with chronic pain. The prevalence of depression in chronic musculoskeletal pain patients is higher than in the general population. Applying strict diagnostic criteria, the prevalence of depression varies between 30% and 60% in chronic pain patients,[20,76] while in the pain-free general population, it is between 2% and 4%.[80]

The importance of this association lies in the fact that both conditions, chronic pain and depression, can interact to intensify their effects. A meta-analysis of 83 studies has shown that the severity of the depression is related not only to the presence of chronic pain, but also to its duration, the degree of pain, and the number of painful areas.[28] Regarding its influence on the disability, several studies show that depression reduces the functional capacity of patients with osteoarthritis and rheumatoid arthritis.[6,62,89] Furthermore, in patients with depression and chronic pain, if the pain is reduced, the depression symptoms improve.[28,63,130] The relationship between depression and pain is reinforced by the fact that antidepressant drugs have an analgesic effect in musculoskeletal pain patients even without depression.[108]

Even if the relationship between chronic pain and depression has been widely studied in other musculoskeletal conditions, very few studies analyze this relationship in AKP patients. Carlsson[13] used the Rorschach test in a group of patients with AKP comparing it to a control group. Patients with AKP were different than control patients in that they showed a higher depression index (DEPI > 4). Comparison with a group of psychiatric outpatients showed a higher depression rate in patients with AKP. However, Witonski[132] using the Beck Depression Inventory (BDI), found no differences between a group of 20 AKP patients with a mean age of 18 and a control group of similar age. It is possible that the difference in the results is because this last group was too young, a mean age of 18, or else because of the different type of measurement tool. Clark[15] performed a clinical trial with 81 AKP patients, assigning them randomly to four types of physical therapy treatments. Prior to this treatment, 15% of patients had borderline depression symptoms or a well-established depression measured with the Hospital Anxiety and Depression questionnaire (HAD) scale. Interestingly, the levels of depression, pain, and disability improved after 3 months and after 12 months of treatment in the four groups.

In a crossover study done by our research group, we analyzed a sample of 54 patients with chronic AKP.[21] We measured the presence of depression symptoms with the HAD questionnaire. 46.3% of our patients had a score equal or higher than 11, which is an indication of a confirmed clinical illness,[136] while the rest of the patients, except one, had a score of clinical suspicion of depression.

Therefore, in a chronic AKP patient, it is important to identify the coincidence of a depression for several reasons. The most important is that a depression increases the disability and the degree of pain and, therefore, perpetuates the condition. Another reason is that the undiagnosed and untreated depression has been related to a poor response to physical therapy or surgery. It is essential to perform a special evaluation aimed at ruling out the coexistence of a hidden depression in these patients.

## 9.5 Relationship Between Anxiety/Stress and Anterior Knee Pain

Anxiety and stress are normal emotional reactions regarding certain situations. Both anxiety and stress in a mild or moderate form are healthy and even beneficial because they motivate a person to prepare a response, either to remain vigilant or to serve as a warning when in danger. However, on occasions, it becomes dysfunctional when its level is too high or lasts too long, becoming pathological.

Anxiety expresses itself differently in patients, sometimes in emotional and cognitive manners (tension, fear, edginess, discomfort, nervousness), behavioral or motor aspects (immobility, avoidance, restlessness); however, on occasion, it is accompanied by vegetative reactions such as perspiration, palpitations, dry mouth, shaking, dizziness, or nausea.

Patients with chronic pain perceive pain as a situation that generates prolonged stress. The prevalence of anxiety in patients with chronic pain is very high.[80] The presence of anxiety influences the symptoms in these patients bidirectionally. High degrees of pain can sometimes predict anxiety symptoms[106] and conversely, anxiety increases the painful experience.[121] One of the most studied mechanisms of the effects of maladaptative anxiety in chronic pain patients is a tendency toward hypervigilance and catastrophization.[4] These tendencies amplify the perception of pain and cause behaviors that increase disability.[79]

Clark[15] found that 27% of patients with AKP who were included in a clinical trial showed anxiety symptoms measured with the HAD questionnaire, and after receiving treatment these symptoms improved. Thomeé[117] also found high levels of anxiety in a group of patients with AKP, using the STAI questionnaire (State Trait Anxiety Inventory), finding similar scores to those published for rheumatoid arthritis. Carlsson[13] measured distress/anxiety using the Rorschach test in patients with AKP and in a control group mainly of physical therapy students, finding out that patients had a high anxiety level, but with no difference from the control group. The authors will probably comment to say that this is because the students also have a high level of distress. Piva[98] studied a group of AKP patients with at least 4 weeks of pain and an average numeric scale pain of 3.6, finding a correlation with the disability and the level of anxiety measured with the Beck questionnaire, suggesting that patients with more limitations in physical function had higher anxiety levels.

In a study conducted by our working group in chronic AKP patients with important symptoms (mean VAS 6.3 and Lysholm score 50), high anxiety levels measured through the HAD questionnaire was present in 90% of patients, and above the level, considered the diagnosis of anxiety disorder in 37% of the cases. However, although no correlation between anxiety with pain or disability was found, a very significant correlation between kinesiophobia (fear of movement) and disability was found.[21]

Even if anxiety is often present in patients with chronic pain, its role in disability seems to be more related to fear. Fear and anxiety go hand in hand but are not the same thing. Anxiety is an emotional reaction to something undetermined, while in fear the threat is specific. In patients with chronic pain, fear appears as fear to pain and fear to movement, which can cause the pain and worsen the lesion.[68] Even so, anxiety itself worsens the suffering of these patients, as an entity by itself and deserves to be treated.

## 9.6 Relationship Between Personality, Mental Disorder and Anterior Knee Pain

The prevalence of mental disorders is higher in patients with chronic pain than in the general population.[20] However and despite the fact that it is a common idea in orthopedics, there seem to be no studies that support the existence of a psychopathic personality or other mental health conditions that predispose for AKP.

In a prospective study, Gatchel[37] evaluated the predictive value of a battery of mental health parameters in a large group of patients with acute low back pain to determine who would develop disability in the long term because of chronic pain. This study did not find any predictive capacity for major psychopathology in the development of disability caused by chronic pain. These findings suggest that although an association between psychopathology and chronic pain exists, we cannot state that psychopathologic conditions cause chronic pain, but they are rather a consequence of it. Other findings support this, since the incidence of psychological conditions is higher in patients with chronic musculoskeletal pain.[35,61,95] Furthermore, Dersh[20] studied the presence of psychiatric conditions in a group of 1,595 patients with chronic pain and disability caused by different musculoskekeletal conditions, finding that 64% had a psychiatric condition, compared with 15% in the general population. However, he found that this high incidence appeared only after the onset of the musculoskeletal process, suggesting that the stress associated with pain was a determining factor in the intensification of it. Some studies have found that the incidence of psychiatric conditions is lower in musculoskeletal pain patients after an effective physical therapy treatment of their condition.[86,123] In a study with 250 chronic pain patients, it was shown that personality traits and initial personality disorders were not useful to predict disability after 1 year.[70] In another study performed with patients that suffered different musculoskeletal conditions and healthy patients, it was shown that the differences in the different personality traits had a stronger correlation with psychological distress than with pain.[75]

AKP patients have been thought of as having a neurotic personality that predisposed them to suffer from chronic pain without structural damage. Some authors believe that when no structural causes are found, the condition could be explained by psychological problems (family, self-esteem, sport performance, aversion to sports).[19] Witonski[132] states that AKP could be a psychosomatic condition after finding personality disorders in these patients following the Minnesota Multiphasic Personality Inventory (MMPI) questionnaire. This questionnaire, however, has been questioned for its use with patients with rheumatic conditions, suggesting it should be used with caution in rheumatic patients.[27,54] High levels of depression, hypochondria, and hysteria measured by the MMPI reflect the level of arthritis better than the psychological status.[96] In patients who were operated on because of low back pain, high levels of psychopathology using MMPI were found; however, in an epidemiological study done in those patients on whom by chance the MMPI was used prior to the condition, the premorbid profiles were normal, which is a strong suggestion that the disease causing the chronic pain is responsible for the personality trait changes.[44,73]

Witvrow[133] studied a group of 282 asymptomatic student athletes that were followed for a 2 year period. At the beginning of the study, the student's psychological features were studied. At the end of the study, 24 patients developed AKP. Solely, the parameter "looking for social support" obtained a significant lower score in the group with pain compared with the control group, but no difference was found in neurotic and psychosomatic instability, extroversion, palliative reaction, passive reaction pattern, expression of emotions or reassuring thoughts. Studies analyzing personality traits in patients with established AKP have been performed. Fritz[32] did a prospective study in a group of 28 adolescents with AKP through the High School Personality Questionnaire (HSPQ) before evaluating the cause of their pain. The goal of the study was to verify the usefulness of this questionnaire in order to identify patients with a structural identifiable cause. After an 8 month follow-up, one third of the patients showed psychological factors associated with pain, but the personality questionnaire was not useful to differentiate between the structural cause group and the functional cause group. In another crossover study, Carlsson[13] found no alexithymic personality traits in a group of AKP patients, although patients with chronic pain did show higher levels of depression, hostility, and passive attitudes than the control group.

From the different studies to investigate the influence of personality both in chronic musculoskeletal pain and specifically in AKP patients, there is no causal relationship between personality type and a predisposition to suffer this condition.[20,64,119,127] Personality traits are very stable, while anxiety, depression, and hostility can change depending on the subject's environment even if to a certain degree they are present in every person. The most accepted belief is that the distress alterations found in patients with chronic pain seem to be a consequence of the chronic pain process itself, and not the cause of it.

## 9.7 Miscellaneous

### 9.7.1 Malingering

The DSM-IV[2] manual defines malingering as the "the intentional production of false or grossly exaggerated physical or psychological symptoms, motivated by external incentives such as avoiding military duty, avoiding work, obtaining financial compensation, evading criminal prosecution or obtaining drugs." From this definition, it is understood that a malicious behavior is associated with a secondary gain, but contrary to other mental processes, malingering is a deliberate behavior. This is what distinguishes it from other behaviors associated with pain and with which it should not be mistaken. Malingering is not really a psychological factor that modulates or is determined by the course of pain and disease. It is the own patient who is showing his intentions by misleading the clinicians through fictitious symptoms. Several methods to try to help the clinician in detecting patients who feign something have been developed, although they are not particularly reliable.[8,12,42,67,104]

The presence of this behavior in chronic pain patients is highly variable, ranging from 1.2% and 36%[3,85]; however, other authors believe it is very low.[76] Waddell[129] considers that the incidence of malingering in low back pain is low, and is frequently mistaken with behaviors associated with pain.

There are no specific studies about the prevalence of malicious pretending in the AKP patient. Extrapolating results of other chronic musculoskeletal painful processes with a similar poor correlation between physical findings and radiology, we should expect to find a similar incidence of compensation to that found in low back pain patients. Possibly, this likely relationship is lower than in other chronic pain processes because the AKP patients are normally younger than those with other chronic pain from musculoskeletal conditions. Also, malingering is associated with a situation aimed at a monetary or work compensation.[3]

### 9.7.2 Psychogenic Pain

The concept of psychogenic pain has caused controversy in different areas of medicine not only regarding its diagnosis, but mostly regarding its existence.[16] It tries to explain pain when no other alterations appear in the physical examination or complementary tests. The patient with AKP seems like the perfect situation for this type of diagnosis to come up frequently. As previously explained in this chapter, psychological factors have a big influence as modulators of AKP but there is not enough evidence to state that they are the only factors present at the onset of pain. Hendler[46] believes that psychogenic pain, if in fact does exist, has a very low prevalence (1 in 3,000 patients with chronic pain). Manchikanti,[77] after reviewing psychological aspects of chronic pain, states that psychogenic pain is an illusion. Kuch[64] performed a systematic review, concluding there was no evidence to support the theory that chronic pain is the direct result of a previous psychiatric disorder. The fact that no structural cause can be found may certainly be frustrating for the physician, but that doesn't mean there is not one. The attribution of a psychogenic origin to a great number of AKP patients can implicitly lead to not offering them the possibility of treatment. The influence of affectivity, anxiety, mood, and cognitions with chronic pain seems clear. The relationship between psychopathology, mainly depression, seems clear as well and also bidirectional. But generally, the higher prevalence of psychiatric conditions in chronic musculoskeletal pain patients appears after the onset of the musculoskeletal condition.[20,119] Kuch[64] thinks that even if the psychological condition can precede the lesion, its presence does not mean that it is the cause of the chronic pain, although it can clearly worsen the situation. To attribute pain to a psychogenic origin is as limitating as trying to understand pain from a purely structural or biologic point of view.

### *9.7.3 Somatization*

A somatization disorder is a controversial condition both in its definition and on how it's applied in the clinical practice. In the AKP patients, with no structural findings in the imaging tests, this diagnosis is frequently reached, especially if there is a history of emotional distress. However, to diagnose somatization in a patient, the criteria established in the DSM-IV[2] have to be met.

The prevalence of somatization in the AKP patient is unknown, although it is probably very low if we extrapolate the incidence published for somatization disorders in general that range from 0.2% to 1.5%.[34,105]

Those patients with a tendency toward somatization present themselves to the physician mainly with somatic symptoms more so than with psychosocial symptoms, hoping to get medical attention and symptomatic treatment.[76] This tendency begins during childhood and persists into adulthood. These patients are very heterogeneous and present themselves with a great variety of unexplained symptoms, and come frequently to the clinics. Patients with chronic pain have higher levels of hypochondria and a tendency toward somatization compared with the pain-free population.[29] It has also been stated that chronic pain patients can also confuse painful and non-painful experiences and interpret a wide variety of experiences in terms of pain, especially emotional distress and depression.[22]

## 9.8 Conclusion

AKP patients express chronic pain, but also disability. However, the correlation between pain and disability is not complete and linear. Some patients with a lot of pain show mild disability, while others with much less pain also show great disability. The disability is profoundly influenced by other emotional and cognitive factors that are associated with the perception of pain. Therefore, the clinical efforts do not have to be focused only on treating the pain as a feeling but on identifying and modifying these factors.

Can AKP have a psychological cause as it has been classically believed? We think not. There is a structural lesion that causes pain and disability, although sometimes it may not be found. The psychological factors modulate the course of the disease but are not the cause. Even so, psychological factors are of utmost importance, which is why it is essential that physicians be aware of them.

Even if the importance of emotion in pain and disability in AKP patients seems clear, disorders in negative emotions (anxiety and depression) are also sources of suffering in these patients and deserve to be treated independently from other measures taken in the course of the condition.

In many AKP patients, the classic biomedical approach has failed to provide adequate treatment despite decades of research. Given that the biopsychosocial model provides a better understanding of articular pain and has contributed to the improved treatment of other musculoskeletal conditions, it seem reasonable to think that a biopsychosocial approach would provide a useful tool for the conventional medical treatment of AKP. It is, therefore, interesting to contemplate cognitive–behavioral treatment models as another therapeutic option to help these patients.

## References


1. Al-Obaidi SM, Beattie P, Al-Zoabi B, et al. The relationship of anticipated pain and fear avoidance beliefs to outcome in patients with chronic low back pain who are not receiving workers' compensation. *Spine*. 2005;30:1051-1057.
2. American Psychiatric Association. *Diagnostic and Statistical Manual for Mental Disorders*. 4th ed. Arlington: American Psychiatric Association; 2000.
3. Aronoff GM, Mandel S, Genovese E, et al. Evaluating malingering in contested injury or illness. *Pain Pract*. 2007; 7:178-204.
4. Asmudson GJ, Norton PJ, Vlaeyen JWS. Fear avoidance models of chronic pain: an overview. In: Asmudson GJ, Vlaeyen JWS, Crombez G, eds. *Understanding and Treating Fear of Pain*. Oxford: Oxford University Press; 2004:3-24.
5. Astin J, Beckner W, Soeken K, et al. Psychological interventions for rheumatoid arthritis: a meta-analysis of randomized controlled trials. *Arthritis Rheum*. 2002;15:291-302.
6. Axford J, Heron C, Ross F, et al. Management of knee osteoarthritis in primary care: pain and depression are the major obstacles. *J Psychosom Res*. 2008;64:461-467.
7. Bedard GB, Reid GJ, McGrath PJ. Coping and self-medication in a community sample of junior high school students. *Pain Res Manag*. 1997;2:151-156.
8. Bianchini KJ, Etherton JL, Greve KW, et al. Classification accuracy of MMPI-2 validity scales in the detection of pain-related malingering: a known-groups study. *Assessment*. 2008;15:435-449.
9. Borrell-Carrió F, Suchman AL, Epstein RM. The biopsychosocial model 25 years later: principles, practice, and scientific inquiry. *Ann Fam Med*. 2004;2:576-582.
10. Brown GK, Nicassio PM. Development of a questionnaire for the assessment of active and passive coping strategies in chronic pain patients. *Pain*. 1987;31:53-64.
11. Buer N, Linton SJ. Fear-avoidance beliefs and catastrophizing: occurrence and risk factor in back pain and ADL in the general population. *Pain*. 2002;99:485-491.
12. Butcher JN, Dahlstrom WG, Graham JR, et al. MMPI-2: Inventario Multifásico de Personalidad de Minnesota-2. Manual (spanish versión A. Avila-Espada, F. Jiménez-Gómez). Madrid: TEA Ediciones; 1999.
13. Carlsson AM, Warner S, Mattlar CE, et al. Personality in patients with long term patellofemoral pain syndrome. *Knee Surg Sports Traumatol Arthrosc*. 1993;1:178-183.
14. Carragee EJ, Alamin TF, Miller JL, et al. Disographic, MRI and psychosocial determinants of low back pain disability and remission: a prospective study in subjects with benign persistent back pain. *Spine J*. 2005;5:24-35.
15. Clark DI, Downing N, Mitchell J, et al. Physiotherapy for anterior knee pain: a randomized controlled trial. *Ann Rheum Dis*. 2009;59:700-704.
16. Covington EC. Psychogenic pain. What it means, why it does not exist and how to diagnose it. *Pain Med*. 2000;1: 287-294.
17. Crombez G, Eccleston C, Baeyens F, et al. When somatic information threatens, catastrophic thinking enhances attentional interference. *Pain*. 1998;75:187-198.
18. Crombez G, Vlaeyen JW, Heuts PH, et al. Pain related fear is more disabling than pain itself: evidence on the role of pain related fear in chronic low back pain disability. *Pain*. 1999;80:329-339.
19. De Pablos J, Farrington D (2003). La rodilla dolorosa en la infancia y la adolescencia. En La rodilla infantil, Ed: J dePablos. Argon, majadahonda. pp25-36
20. Dersh J, Gatchel RJ, Polatin P, et al. Prevalence of psychiatric disorders in patients with chronic work-related musculoskeletal pain disability. *J Occup Environ Med*. 2002;44: 459-468.
21. Domenech J, Sanchis-Alfonso V, Espejo B, et al. *Factores psicológicos en el síndrome femoropatelar. Estudio analítico transversal*. Valencia: Congreso Sociedad Española Investigación en Cirugía Ortopédica (INVESCOT); 2010.
22. Dworkin SF, Wilson L, Masson DL. Somatizing as a risk factor for chronic pain. In: Grzesiak RC, Ciccone DC, eds. *Psychological Vulnerbility to Chronic Pain*. New York: Springer; 1994.
23. Edward RR, Smith MT, Stonerock G, et al. Pain-related catastrophizing in healthy women is associated with greater temporal summation of and reduced habituation to thermal pain. *Clin J Pain*. 2006;22:730-737.
24. Edwards RR, Fillingim RB, Maixner W, et al. Catastrophizing predicts changes in thermal pain responses after resolution of acute dental pain. *J Pain*. 2004;5:164-170.
25. Engel George L. The need for a new medical model. *Science*. 1977;196:129-136.
26. Evers AW, Kraaimaat FW, van Riel PL, et al. Tailored cognitive behavioral therapy in early rheumatoid arthritis for patients at risk: a randomised controlled trial. *Pain*. 2002;100:141-153.
27. Fishbain DA, Cole B, Cutler RB, et al. Chronic pain and the measurement of personality: do states influence traits? *Pain Med*. 2006;7:509-529.
28. Fishbain DA, Cutler R, Rosomoff HL, et al. Chronic pain-associated depression: antecedent or consequence of chronic pain? A review. *Clin J Pain*. 1997;13:116-137.
29. Fishbain DA, Lewis JE, Gao J, et al. Is chronic pain associated with somatization/hypochondriasis? An evidence based structured review. *Pain Pract*. 2009;9:449-467.
30. Forsythe ME, Dumbar MJ, Henningar AW, et al. Prospective relation between catastrophizing and residual pain following knee arthroplasty: two-year follow-up. *Pain Res Manag*. 2008;13:335-341.
31. Foster G, Taylor SJ, Eldridge SE, et al. Self-management education programmes by lay leaders for people with chronic conditions. *Cochrane Database Syst Rev*. 2007;CD005108.
32. Fritz GK, Bleck EE, Dahl IS. Functional versus organic knee pain in adolescents. A pilot study. *Am J Sports Med*. 1981;7:247-249.
33. Fritz JM, George S, Delitto A. The role of fear avoidance beliefs in acute low back pain: relationship with current and future disability and work status. *Pain*. 2001;94:7-15.
34. Fynk P, Hansen MS, Oxhoj ML. The prevalence of somatoform disorders among internal medical inpatients. *J Psychosom Res*. 2004;56:413-418.
35. Gatchel RJ, Garofalo JP, Ellis E, et al. Major psychological disorders in acute and chronic TMD: an initial examination. *J Am Dent Assoc*. 1996;127:1365-1374.
36. Gatchel RJ, Peng YB, Peters ML, et al. The biopsychosocial approach to chronic pain: scientific advances and future directions. *Psychol Bull*. 2007;133:581-624.

37. Gatchel RJ, Polatin PB, Mayer TG. The dominant role of psychosocial risk factors in the development of chronic low back pain disability. *Spine*. 1995;20:2702-2709.
38. Geisser ME, Robinson ME, Keefe FJ, et al. Catastrophizing, depression and the sensory, affective and evaluative aspects of chronic pain. *Pain*. 1994;59:79-83.
39. George SZ, Fritz JM, McNeil DW. Fear avoidance beliefs as measured by the fear avoidance beliefs questionnaire: change in fear avoidance beliefs questionnaire is predictive of change in self report of disability and pain intensity for patients with acute low back pain. *Clin J Pain*. 2006;22: 197-203.
40. Gracely RH, Geisser ME, Giesecke T, et al. Pain catastrophizing and neural responses to pain among persons with fibromyalgia. *Brain*. 2004;127:835-843.
41. Granot M, Ferber SG. The roles of pain catastrophizing and anxiety in the prediction of postoperative pain intensity: a prospective study. *Clin J Pain*. 2005;21:439-445.
42. Grave KW, Bianchini KJ, Etherton JL, et al. Detecting malingered pain-related disability: classification accuracy of the Portland digit recognition test. *Clin Neuropsychol*. 2009;23:850-869.
43. Grotle M, Vollestad NK, Brox JI. Clinical course and impact of fear avoidance beliefs in acute low back pain. *Spine*. 2006;31:1038-1046.
44. Hagendorn SD, Maruta T, Swanson DW, et al. Premorbid MMPI profiles of low back patients. Surgical successes versus surgical failures. *Clin J Pain*. 1985;1:177-179.
45. Haim A, Yaniv M, Dekel S, et al. Patellofemoral pain syndrome: validity of clinical and radiological features. *Clin Orthop*. 2006;451:223-228.
46. Hendler N, Bergson C, Morrison C. Overlooked physical diagnoses in chronic pain patients involved in litigation, Part 2. *Psychosomatics*. 1996;37:509-517.
47. IASP Subcomité on Taxonomy. Pain terms: a list with definitions and notes on usage. *Pain*. 1979;6:247-252.
48. Jacobson NS, Butler R. Relation of cognitive coping and catastrophizing to acute pain and analgesic use following breast cancer surgery. *J Behav Med*. 2000;19:17-29.
49. Jensen JN, Albertsen K, Borg V, et al. The predictive effect of fear-avoidance beliefs on low back pain among newly qualified health care workers with and without previous low back pain: a prospective cohort study. *BMC Musculoskelet Disord*. 2009;10:117.
50. Jensen R, Hystad T, Baerheim A. Knee function and pain related to psychological variables in patients with long-term patellofemoral pain syndrome. *J Orthop Sports Phys Ther*. 2005;35:594-600.
51. Johnson LL, van Dyk GE, Green JR, et al. Clinical assessment of asymptomatic knees: comparison of men and women. *Arthroscopy*. 1998;14:347-359.
52. Karjalainenen K, Malmivaara A, Van Tulder M, et al. Multidisciplinary biopsychosocial rehabilitation for subacute low back pain among working age adults. *Cochrane Database Syst Rev*. 2003;(2):CD002193.
53. Keefe FJ, Affleck G, Lefebvre JC, et al. Pain coping strategies and coping efficacy in rheumatoid arthritis: a daily process analysis. *Pain*. 1997;69:35-42.
54. Keefe FJ, Bonk V. Valoración psicosocial del dolor en pacientes con enfermedades reumáticas. *Rheuma Dis Clin North Am*. 1999;1:81-104.
55. Keefe FJ, Caldwell DS, Queen KT, et al. Pain coping strategies in osteoarthritis patients. *J Consult Clin Psychol*. 1987;55:208-212.
56. Keefe FJ, DS C, Queen KT, et al. Osteoarthritic knee pain: a behavioural analysis. *Pain*. 1987;28:309-321.
57. Keefe FJ, Gk B, Wallston KA, et al. Coping with rheumatoid arthritis pain: catastrophizing as a maladaptative strategy. *Pain*. 1989;37:51-56.
58. Keefe FJ, Lefebvre JC, Egert JR, et al. The relationship of gender to pain, pain behavior, and disability in osteoarthritis patients: the role of catastrophizing. *Pain*. 2000;87:325-334.
59. Keeley P, Creed F, Tomenson B, et al. Psychosocial predictors of health-related quality of life and health service utilisation in people with chronic low back pain. *Pain*. 2008;135:142-150.
60. Kendell K, Saxby B, Farrow M, et al. Psychological factors associated with short term recovery from total knee replacement. *Br J Health Psychol*. 2001;6:41-52.
61. Kinney RK, Gatchel RJ, Polatin PB, et al. Prevalence of psychopathology in acute and chronic low back pain patients. *J Occup Rehabil*. 1993;3:95-103.
62. Kojima M, Kojima T, Suzuki S, et al. Depression, inflammation, and pain in patients with rheumatoid arthritis. *Arthritis Rheum*. 2009;61:1018-1024.
63. Kroenke K, Bair MJ, Damush TM, et al. Optimized antidepressant therapy and pain self-management in primary care patients with depression and musculoskeletal pain: a randomized controlled trial. *JAMA*. 2009;301:2099-2110.
64. Kuch K. Psychological factors and the development of chronic pain. *Clin J Pain*. 2001;17:S33-S38.
65. Laín-Entralgo P. *El diagnóstico Médico. Historia y Teoría*. Barcelona: Salvat; 1982.
66. Lazarus R, Folkman S. *Stress, Appraisal and Coping*. New York: Springer; 1984.
67. Lee-Haley PR, English LT, Glenn WJ. A fake bad scale on the MMPI-2 for personal injury claimants. *Psychol Rep*. 1991;68:203-210.
68. Leeuw M, Goosens ME, Linton SJ, et al. The fear-avoidance model of musculoskeletal pain: current state of scientific evidence. *J Behav Med*. 2007;30:77-94.
69. Lethem J, Slade PD, Troup JD, et al. Outline of a fear avoidance model of exaggerated pain perception. *Behav Res Ther*. 1983;2:401-408.
70. Linder J, Poston WSC, Haddock CK, et al. Does personality or psychopathology predict disability in chronic pain patients. *Disabil Rehabil*. 2000;22:281-287.
71. Linton SJ, Boersma K, Jansson M, et al. Are fear avoidance beliefs related to the inception of an episode of back pain? A prospective study. *Psychol Health*. 1999;14:1051-1059.
72. Linton SJ, Boersma K, Jansson M, et al. The effects of cognitive behavioural and physical therapy preventive interventions on pain related sick leave. A randomized controlled trial. *Clin J Pain*. 2005;21:109-119.
73. Love PW, Peck CL. The MMPI and psychological factors in chronic low back pain. A review. *Pain*. 1987;28:1-12.
74. Macintyre NJ, Hill NA, Fellows RA, et al. Patellofemoral joint kinematics in individuals with and without patellofemoral pain síndrome. *J Bone Joint Surg*. 2006;88A:2596-2605.
75. Malmgren-Olsson EB, Bergdahl J. Temperament and character personality dimensions in patients with nonspecific musculoskeletal disorders. *Clin J Pain*. 2006;22:625-631.

76. Manchikanti L, Fellows B, Pampati, et al. Comparison of psychological status of chronic pain patients and the general population. *Pain Physician*. 2002;5:40-48.
77. Manchikanti L, Fellows B, Singh V. Understanding psychological aspects of chronic pain in interventional pain management. *Pain Physician*. 2001;5:57-82.
78. Martin M, Bradley L, Alexander R, et al. Coping strategies predict disability in patients with primary fibromyalgia. *Pain*. 1996;68:45-53.
79. McCracken LM, Faber SD, Janeck AS. Pain-related anxiety predicts non-specific physical complaints in persons with chronic pain. *Behav Res Ther*. 1998;36:621-630.
80. McWilliams LA, Cox BJ, Enns MW. Mood and anxiety disorders associated with chronic pain: an examination in a nationally representative sample. *Pain*. 2003;106:127-133.
81. Melzack R. From the gate to the neuromatrix. *Pain*. 1999;6:S121-S126.
82. Melzack R, Casey KL. *The Skin Senses*. Springfield: CC Thomas; 1968:423-443.
83. Mercado AC, Carroll LJ, Cassidy JD, et al. Passive coping as a risk factor for disabling neck and low back pain. *Pain*. 2006;117:51-57.
84. Meyer K, Tschopp A, Sprott H, et al. Association between catastrophizing and self-rated pain and disability in patients with chronic low back pain. *J Rehabil Med*. 2009;41:620-625.
85. Novy DM, Collins HS, Nelson DV, et al. Waddell signs: distributional properties and correlates. *Arch Phys Med Rehabil*. 1998;79:820-822.
86. Owen-Salters E, Gatchel RJ, Polatin PB, et al. Changes in psychopathology following functional restoration of chronic low back pain patients: a prospective study. *J Occup Rehabil*. 1996;6:215-223.
87. Parker JC, Smarr KL, Buescher KL, et al. Pain control and rational thinking: implications for rheumatoid arthritis. *Arthritis Rheum*. 1989;38:1807-1818.
88. Pavlin DJ, Sullivan MJ, Freund PR, et al. Catastrophizing: a risk factor for postsurgical pain. *Clin J Pain*. 2005;21: 83-90.
89. Peck JR, Smith TW, Ward JR, et al. Disability and depression in rheumatoid arthritis. A multi-trait, multi-method investigation. *Arthritis Rheum*. 1989;32:1100-1106.
90. Perrot S, Poiraudeau S, Kabir M, et al. Active or passive pain coping strategies in hip and knee osteoarthritis? Results of a national survey of 4,719 patients in a primary care setting. *Arthritis Rheum*. 2008;59:1555-1562.
91. Peters ML, Vlaeyen JWS, van Drunen C. Do fibromyalgia patients display hypervigiance for innocuous somatosensory stimulus? Application of a body scanning reaction time paradigm. *Pain*. 2000;86:283-292.
92. Peters ML, Vlaeyen JWS, Weber WEJ. The joint contribution of physical pathology, pain-related fear and catastrophizing to chronic back pain disability. *Pain*. 2005;113:45-50.
93. Philips HC. Avoidance behaviour and its role in sustaining chronic pain. *Behav Res Ther*. 1987;25:273-279.
94. Picavet HSJ, Vlaeyen JWS, Schouten SAG. Pain catastrophizing and kinesiophobia: predictors of chronic low back pain. *Am J Epidemiol*. 2002;156:1028-1034.
95. Pincus T, Burton AK, Vogel S, et al. A systematic review of psychological factors as predictors of chronicity/disability in prospective cohorts of low back pain. *Spine*. 2002;27: 109-120.
96. Pincus T, Callahan LF, Bradley LA, et al. Elevated MMPI scores for hypochondriasis, depression and hysteria in patients with rheumatoid arthritis reflect disease rather than psychological status. *Arthritis Rheum*. 1986;29:1456-1465.
97. Piva SR, Fitzgerald GK, Irrgang JJ, Fritz JM, et al. Associates of physical function and pain in patients with patellofemoral pain syndrome. *Arch Phys Med Rehabil*. 2009;90:285-295.
98. Piva SR, Fitzgerald GK, Wisniewski S, et al. Predictor of pain and function outcome after rehabilitation in patients with patellofemoral pain syndrome. *J Rehabil Med*. 2009; 41:604-612.
99. Rosenstiel AK, Keefe FJ. The use of coping strategies in chronic low back pain patients: relationship to patient characteristics and current adjustment. *Pain*. 1983;17:33-44.
100. Severeijns R, Vlaeyen JW, van den Hout MA, et al. Pain catastrophizing predicts pain intensity, disability, and psychological distress independent of the level of physical impairment. *Clin J Pain*. 2001;17:165-172.
101. Severeijns R, Vlaeyen JWS, Van Den Hout MA, et al. Pain catastrophizing is associated with health indices in musculoskeletal pain: a cross-sectional study in the Dutch community. *Health Psychol*. 2004;23:49-57.
102. Sharpe L, Sensky T, Timberlake N, et al. Long-term efficacy of a cognitive behavioural treatment from a randomized controlled trial for patients recently diagnosed with rheumatoid arthritis. *Rheumatology*. 2003; 42:435-441.
103. Smeets RJ, Vlaeyen JW, Kester AD, et al. Reduction of pain catastrophizing mediates the outcome of both physical and cognitive- behavioral treatment in chronic low back pain. *J Pain*. 2006;7:261-271.
104. Smith GP, Burger GK. Detection of malingering: validation of the Structured Inventory of Malingered Symptomatology (SIMS). *Am Acad Psychiatry Law*. 1997;25:183-189.
105. Smith GC, Clarke DM, Handrinos D, et al. Consultation-liaison psychiatrists'management of somatoforms disorders. *Psychosomatics*. 2000;41:481-489.
106. Soderlin MK, Hakala M, Nieminen P. Anxiety and depression in a community-based rheumatoid arthritis population. *Scand J Rheumatol*. 2000;29:177-183.
107. Sommers T, Keefe Fj, Pells J, et al. Pain catastrophizing and pain-related fear in osteoarthritis patients: relationships to pain and disability. *J Pain Symptom Manage*. 2009;37: 863-872.
108. Staiger TO, Gaster B, Sullivan MD, et al. Systematic review of antidepressants in the treatment of chronic low back pain. *Spine*. 2003;28:2540-2545.
109. Sullivan MJ, Adams H, Rhodenizer T, et al. A psychosocial risk factor- targeted intervention for the prevention of chronic pain and disability following whiplash injury. *Phys Ther*. 2006;86:8-18.
110. Sullivan HJL, Bishop SR, Pivik J. The pain catastrophizing scale: development and validation. *Psychol Assess*. 1995;7:524-532.
111. Sullivan MJ, Neish N. The effects of disclosure on pain during dental hygiene treatment: the moderating role of catastrophizing. *Pain*. 1999;79:155-163.
112. Sullivan MJ, Rodgers WM, Wilson PM, et al. An experimental investigation of the relation between catastrophizing and activity intolerance. *Pain*. 2002;100:47-53.

113. Sullivan M, Tanzer M, Stanish W, et al. Psychological determinants of problematic outcomes following total knee arthroplasty. *Pain*. 2009;143:123-129.
114. Sullivan MJ, Ward LC, Tripp D, et al. Secondary prevention of work disability: community-based psychosocial intervention for musculoskeletal disorders. *J Occup Rehabil*. 2005;15:377-392.
115. Swinkels-Meewise IEJ, Roelofs J, Shouten EGW, et al. Fear of movement/(re)injury predicting chronic disabling low back pain: a prospective inception cohort study. *Spine*. 2006;31:658-664.
116. Thomeé R, Renstrom P, Karlsson J, et al. Patellofemoral pain syndrome in young women. I. A clinical analysis of alignment, pain parameters, common symptoms and functional activity level. *Scand J Med Sci Sports*. 1995;5:237-244.
117. Thomeé P, Thomeé R, Karlsson J. Patellofemoral pain syndrome: pain, coping strategies and degree of well-being. *Scand J Med Sci Sports*. 2002;12:276-281.
118. Turner JA, Mancl L, Aaron LA. Pain-related catastrophizing: a daily process study. *Pain*. 2004;110:103-111.
119. Tyrer S. Psychosomatic pain. *Br J Psychol*. 2006;188:91-93.
120. Van Nieuwenhuyse A, Somville PR, Crombez G, et al. The role of physical workload and pain related fear in the development of low back pain in young workers: evidence from the BelCoBack study: results after one year of follow up. *Occup Environ Med*. 2006;63:247-257.
121. Varni JW, Rapoff MA, Waidron SA, et al. Effects of perceived stress on pediatric chronic pain. *J Behav Med*. 1996; 19:515-528.
122. Virchow R (1858) Die cellularpathologie in ihrer Begründung auf physiologische und pathologische Gewebenlehre. Berlin (accessed at http://books.google.es).
123. Vittengl JR, Clark LA, Owen-Salter E, et al. Diagnostic change and personality stability following functional restoration treatment in chronic low back pain patients. *Psychol Assess*. 1999;6:79-91.
124. Vlaeyen JWS, Kole Snijders AMJ, Boeren RGB, et al. Fear of movement/ (re)injury in chronic low back pain and its relation to behavioural performance. *Pain*. 1995;62:363-372.
125. Vlaeyen JWS, Linton SJ. Fear avoidance and its consequences in chronic musculoskeletal pain: a state of the art. *Pain*. 2000;85:317-332.
126. Vlaeyen JWS, Timmermans C, Rodriguez LM, et al. Catastrophic thinking about pain increases discomfort during internal atrial cardioversion. *J Psychosom Res*. 2004;56: 139-144.
127. Waddell G. *The Back Pain Revolution*. 2nd ed. London: Churchill-Livingston; 2004.
128. Waddell G, Newton M, Henderson I, et al. A fear avoidance beliefs questionnaire and the role of fear avoidance beliefs in chronic low back pain and disability. *Pain*. 1993;52: 157-168.
129. Waddell G, Pilowsky I, Bond MR. Clinical assessment and interpretation of abnormal illness behaviour in low back pain. *Pain*. 1989;39:41-53.
130. Wallis BJ, Lord SM, Bogduk M. Resolution of psychological distress of whiplash patients following treatment by radiofrequency neurotomy. A randomized double blind placebo controlled trial. *Pain*. 1997;73: 15-22.
131. Watkins KW, Shifren K, Park DC, et al. Age, pain, and coping with rheumatoid arthritis. *Pain*. 1999;82:217-228.
132. Witonski D. Anterior knee pain syndrome. *Int Orthop*. 1999;23:341-344.
133. Witvrouw E, Lysens R, Bellemans J, et al. Intrinsic risk factors for the development of anterior knee pain in an athletic population. A two-year prospective study. *Am J Sports Med*. 2000;28:480-489.
134. Woby SR, Watson PJ, Roach NK, et al. Adjustment to chronic low back pain – the relative influence of fear avoidance beliefs, catastrophizing and appraisals of control. *Behav Res Ther*. 2004;42:762-774.
135. Woby SR, Watson PJ, Roach NK, et al. Are changes in fear avoidance beliefs, catastrophizing and appraisal of control, predictive of changes in chronic low back pain and disability? *Eur J Pain*. 2004;8:201-210.
136. Zigmond AS, Snaith RP. The hospital anxiety and depression scale. *Acta Psychiatr Scand*. 1983;67:361-370.

# Uncommon Causes of Anterior Knee Pain 10

Vicente Sanchis-Alfonso, Erik Montesinos-Berry,
Francisco Aparisi-Rodriguez, and Vicente Belloch-Ugarte

## 10.1 Introduction

Anterior knee pain is a common symptom, which may have a large variety of causes. Although, patellofemoral malalignment (PFM) is a potential cause of anterior knee pain in young patients, not all malalignments are symptomatic. To think of anterior knee pain as somehow being necessarily tied to PFM is an oversimplification that has positively stultified progress toward better diagnosis and treatment of patients with anterior knee pain syndrome. PFM could be the single culprit for the pain, but it is also possible that it bears no relation whatsoever with the patient's complaint or that it is only partly to blame for the problem. PFM can exist without anterior knee pain, and anterior knee pain can exist without PFM. There are many causes of anterior knee pain, some of them related to PFM and many more not related to PFM. Likewise, we should bear in mind that there are teenage patients with anterior knee pain who lack evidence of organic pathology (i.e., their condition is of a psychosomatic nature[21]) and also patients who suffer from the "malingering syndrome." In this chapter, we analyze uncommon causes of anterior knee pain, emphasizing the fact that not all malalignments are symptomatic.

The question to be addressed is, therefore, what factor is responsible for the patient's symptoms? As with any other pathology, it is necessary to make an accurate diagnosis before embarking on a specific treatment plan. An incorrect diagnosis may lead to inappropriate or unnecessary surgical procedures, which can cause morbidity and unnecessary expenses. Moreover, an unsuitable treatment, resulting from an incorrect diagnosis, may worsen the situation. The final result could be disastrous since it may add to an already serious condition a reflex sympathetic dystrophy or an iatrogenic medial dislocation of the patella.

The goal of an orthopedic surgeon treating patients with anterior knee pain is to precisely determine the etiology of the pain since this is the only way to come up with a "tailored treatment."

## 10.2 Anterior Knee Pain Related to Patellofemoral Malalignment

There are some uncommon injuries (e.g., osteochondritis dissecans [OCD] of the patellofemoral groove, or painful bipartite patella) that result from PFM but that do not require specific treatment since healing is achieved by treating the malalignment.

OCD of the patellofemoral groove is a very rare cause of patellofemoral pain. Mori and colleagues[36] regard overuse and the excessive lateral pressure syndrome as factors involved in the development of OCD of the patellofemoral groove. These authors consider the isolated lateral retinacular release to be an effective treatment for these patients. In our own series, we have two cases of OCD of the patellofemoral groove associated with PFM that were treated with an Insall's proximal realignment, with satisfactory clinical results, leading to the healing of the osteochondral lesion, as shown by a MRI (Fig. 10.1).

Furthermore, the pain experienced by patients with a bipartite patella is, according to Mori and

V. Sanchis-Alfonso (✉)
International Patellofemoral Study Group,
International ACL Study Group,
Hospital 9 de Octubre, Hospital Arnau de Vilanova,
School of Medicine, Catholic University of Valencia,
Valencia, Spain
e-mail: vicente.sanchis.alfonso@gmail.com

V. Sanchis-Alfonso (ed.), *Anterior Knee Pain and Patellar Instability*,
DOI: 10.1007/978-0-85729-507-1_10, 

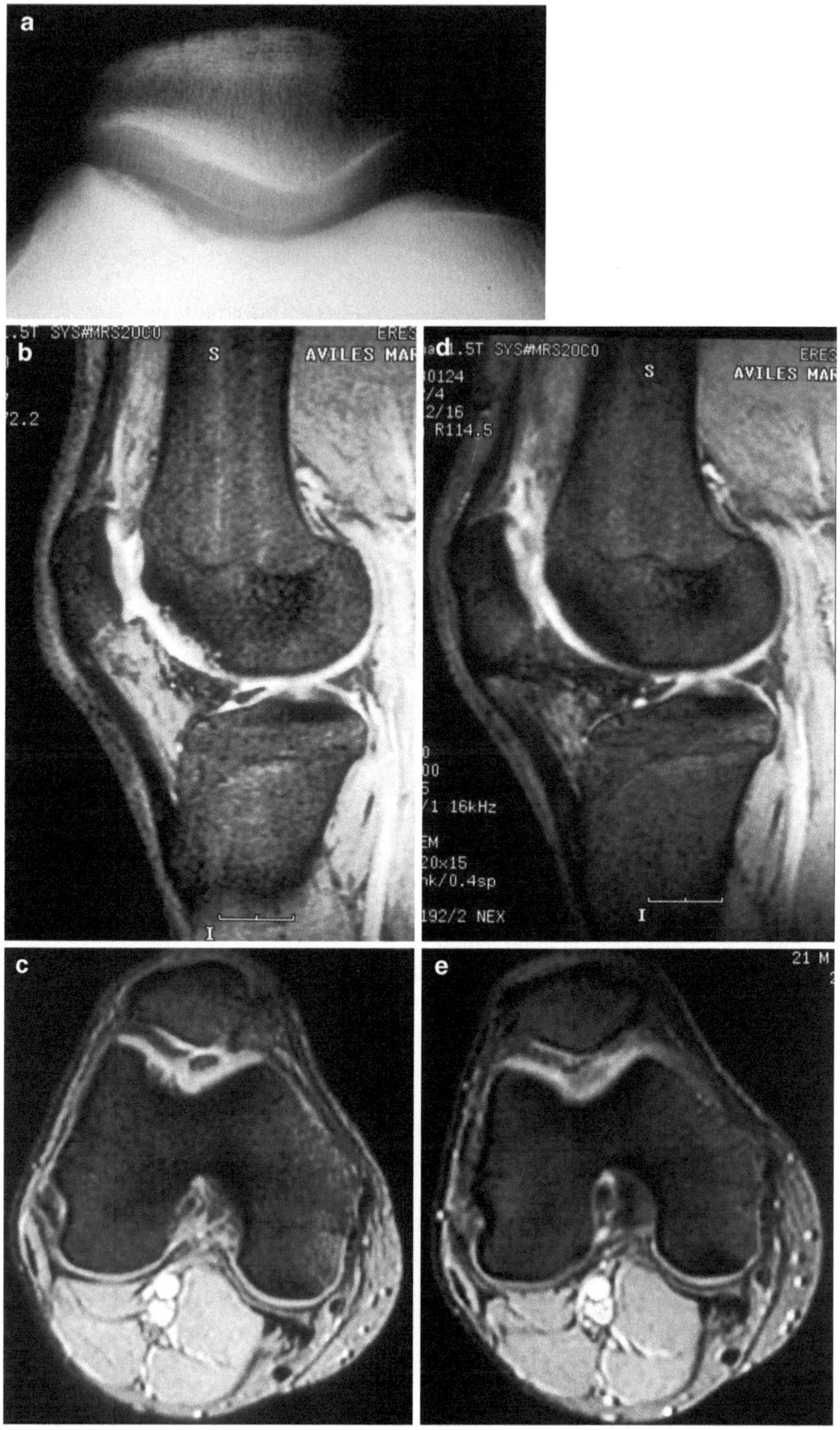


**Fig. 10.1** Osteochondritis dissecans of the patellofemoral groove in a patient with symptomatic PFM (**a**–**c**). The MRI shows the chondral lesion healed a year and a half after realignment surgery (**d**, **e**) (**b**–**e** – GrE T2* MR images)

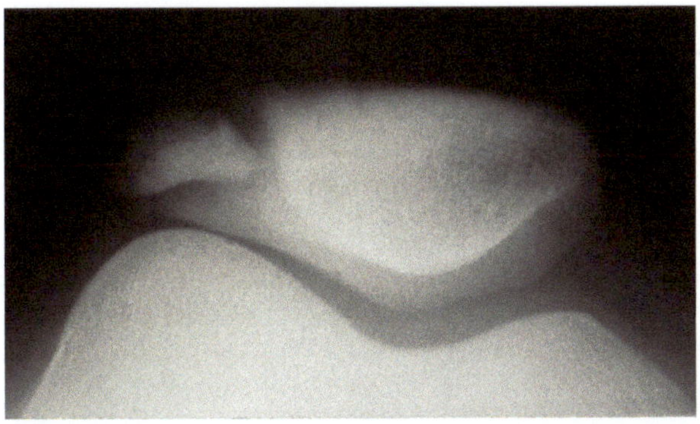

**Fig. 10.2** Bipartite patella of a volleyball player with excessive lateral pressure syndrome

colleagues,[37] a result of excessive traction by the vastus lateralis and the lateral retinaculum on the superolateral bone fragment (Fig. 10.2). These authors have observed that a modified lateral retinacular release eliminates the anterior knee pain experienced by these patients and that, in 94% of cases, induces bony union between the superolateral fragment and the rest of the patella.

## 10.3 Anterior Knee Pain Not Related to Patellofemoral Malalignment

It should be remembered that the region of the knee is home to many infrequent lesions, some of them serious, which may mimic a symptomatic PFM but which bear no relation whatsoever to it. These lesions can cause confusion and hence lead to an incorrect diagnosis, resulting in an erroneous treatment.

Within this group of infrequent lesions, it is worth mentioning the following: intramuscular hemangioma of the vastus medialis obliquus muscle[13,46] (Fig. 10.3), benign giant-cell tumor of the patellar tendon,[5] glomus tumor of Hoffa's fat pad,[18] Hoffa's fat pad disease,[11,33] localized pigmented villonodular synovitis[6,9,19,23,40,55] (Fig. 10.4), hypertrophy of the synovium in the anteromedial joint compartment following minor trauma,[7] intra-articular hemangioma,[4,41] osteoid osteoma[16] (Fig. 10.5), intra-articular ganglion[49,56] (Fig. 10.6), deep cartilage defects of the patella,[29] double patella syndrome,[8] ossification of the patellar tendon,[31] symptomatic synovial plicae,[24-26,28] iliotibial friction band syndrome[44] (Fig. 10.7), snapping pes syndrome and pes anserine bursitis and tendonitis,[3,44] semimembranous tendonitis,[44] medial collateral ligament bursitis,[44] popliteus tendonitis,[44] subluxation of the popliteus tendon,[32] proximal tibiofibular instability,[44] fabella syndrome,[44] occult localized osteonecrosis of the patella (Fig. 10.8),[47] injuries to the infrapatellar branch of the saphenous nerve such as postsurgical neuromas or trauma,[42,54] saphenous nerve entrapment,[44] stress fractures in the region of the knee[35,39,53] (Fig. 10.9), symptomatic ossicles in the anterior tuberosity of the tibia[45] (Fig. 10.10), Osgood-Schlatter apophysitis, Sinding-Larsen-Johansson apophysitis, pre-patellar bursitis ("housemaid's knee"), infrapatellar bursitis ("clergyman's knee"), infrapatellar contracture syndrome,[12]

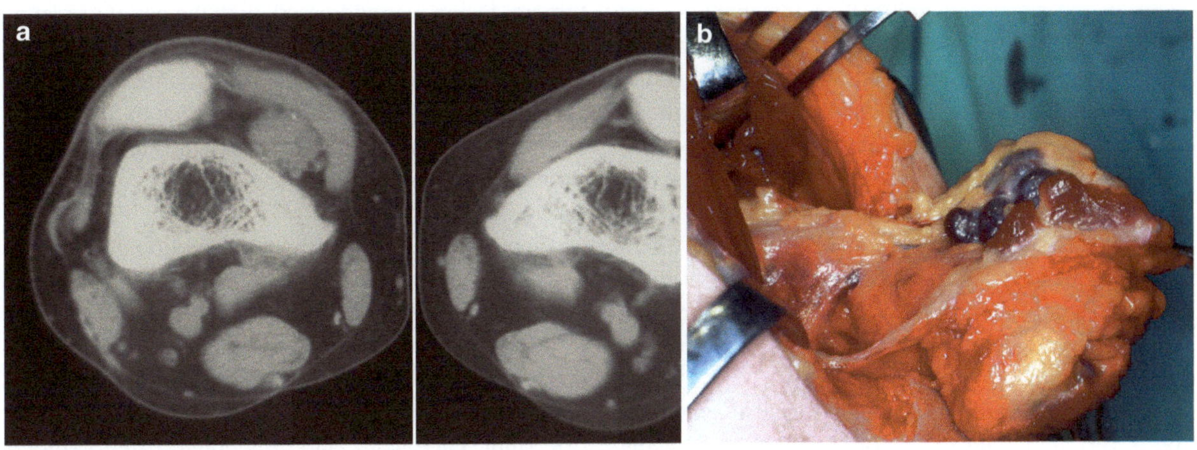


**Fig. 10.3** Intramuscular hemangioma of the vastus medialis obliquus muscle (**a**) CT image (**b**) Macroscopioc appearance (Reproduced from Sanchis-Alfonso et al.[46], with permission)

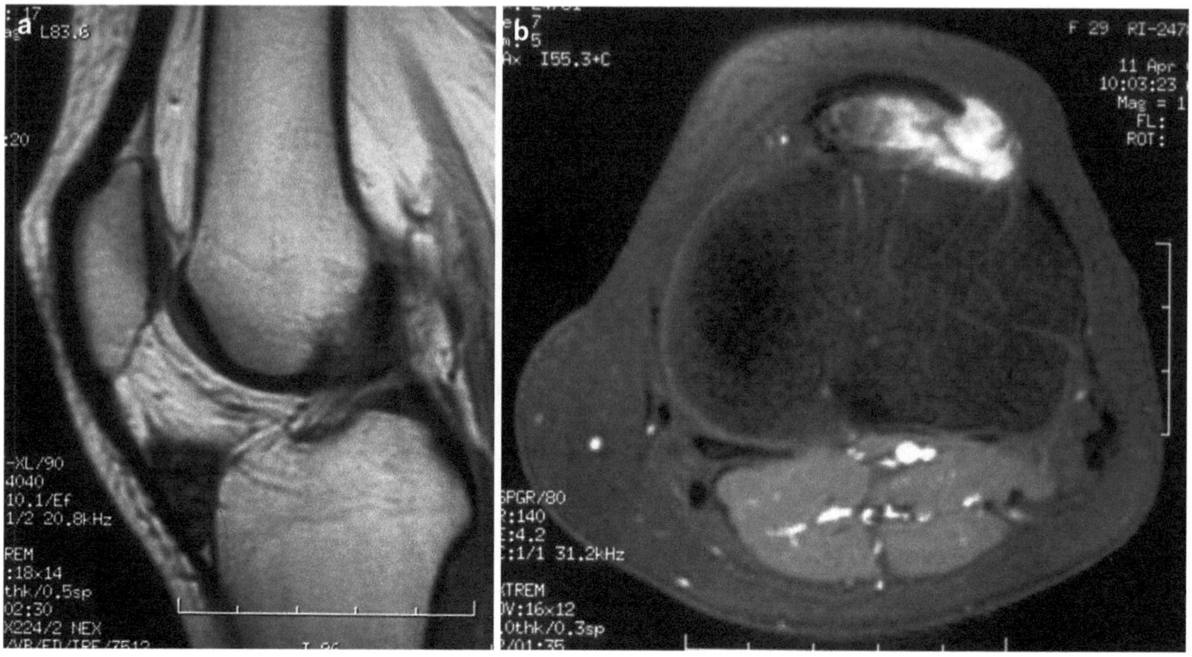


**Fig. 10.4** Localized pigmented villonodular synovitis of the Hoffa's fat pad. (**a**) Sagittal FSE T1W MR image. Hypointense lesion in the Hoffa's Fat Pad. (**b**) Axial GrE T1W + gd-DTPA. Heterogeneous enhancement lesion in the Hoffa's Fat Pad

Cyclops syndrome[45] (Fig. 10.11), osteolytic tibial cyst formation in the osseous tibial tunnel after ACL reconstruction using biodegradable interference screws (Fig. 10.12), infections,[1,10] and primary – benign as well as malignant – (Fig. 10.13) and metastatic tumors.[15,30,38]

We must remember that the clinical presentation of a musculoskeletal tumor may mimic that of an anterior knee pain syndrome. Moreover, a high proportion of primary aggressive benign or malignant bone tumors occur in the same age group than this pathological condition, and have also a predilection for the knee. According to Muscolo and colleagues,[38] poor-quality radiographs and an unquestioned original diagnosis despite persistent symptoms seems to be the most frequent causes of an erroneous diagnosis, and therefore an incorrect treatment. When a musculoskeletal tumor is initially misdiagnosed as a sports injury, its treatment may be adversely affected by the delay in diagnosis or by an inappropriate invasive procedure that can result in extension of the tumor and may close the doors on a limb-salvage surgery.[38]

Moreover, a careful thorough physical examination is very important to rule out referred pain arising from the lumbosacral spine (e.g., disc herniations, spondilolysthesis) and the hip (e.g., hip osteonecrosis, osteoid osteoma of the femoral neck, stress fractures of the femoral neck, slipped femoral epiphysis). Associated numbness or tingling suggests a lumbar problem. Referred pain from the hip usually affects the anterior aspect of the distal thigh and knee, and generally, there is decreased internal rotation and pain on hip motion. For instance, a patient in our series who was being treated elsewhere for an anterior knee pain syndrome and functional patellofemoral instability with *"associated psychological factors"* was in actual fact found to have a calcar osteoid osteoma. Once the tumoral lesion was addressed, both the patient's symptoms and large-scale quadriceps atrophy disappeared. Currently (9 years later), this patient is in a physically very demanding job, which he manages to do without any problem. In this case, the patient had knee pain resulting from a hip injury and instability was due to severe quadriceps atrophy.

Finally, we must note that in exceptional cases, the source of the anterior knee pain may be in the posterior aspect of the knee[48] (see patient 1 – case histories). For instance, in Fig. 10.14, we can see the case of a patient operated on 5 years ago with an Insall's proximal realignment of the right knee, who consulted for anterior right knee pain and functional patellofemoral instability. In the CT scan, we can see a correct patellofemoral congruence of the right knee and an osteolytic area in the lateral femoral condyle. The MRI

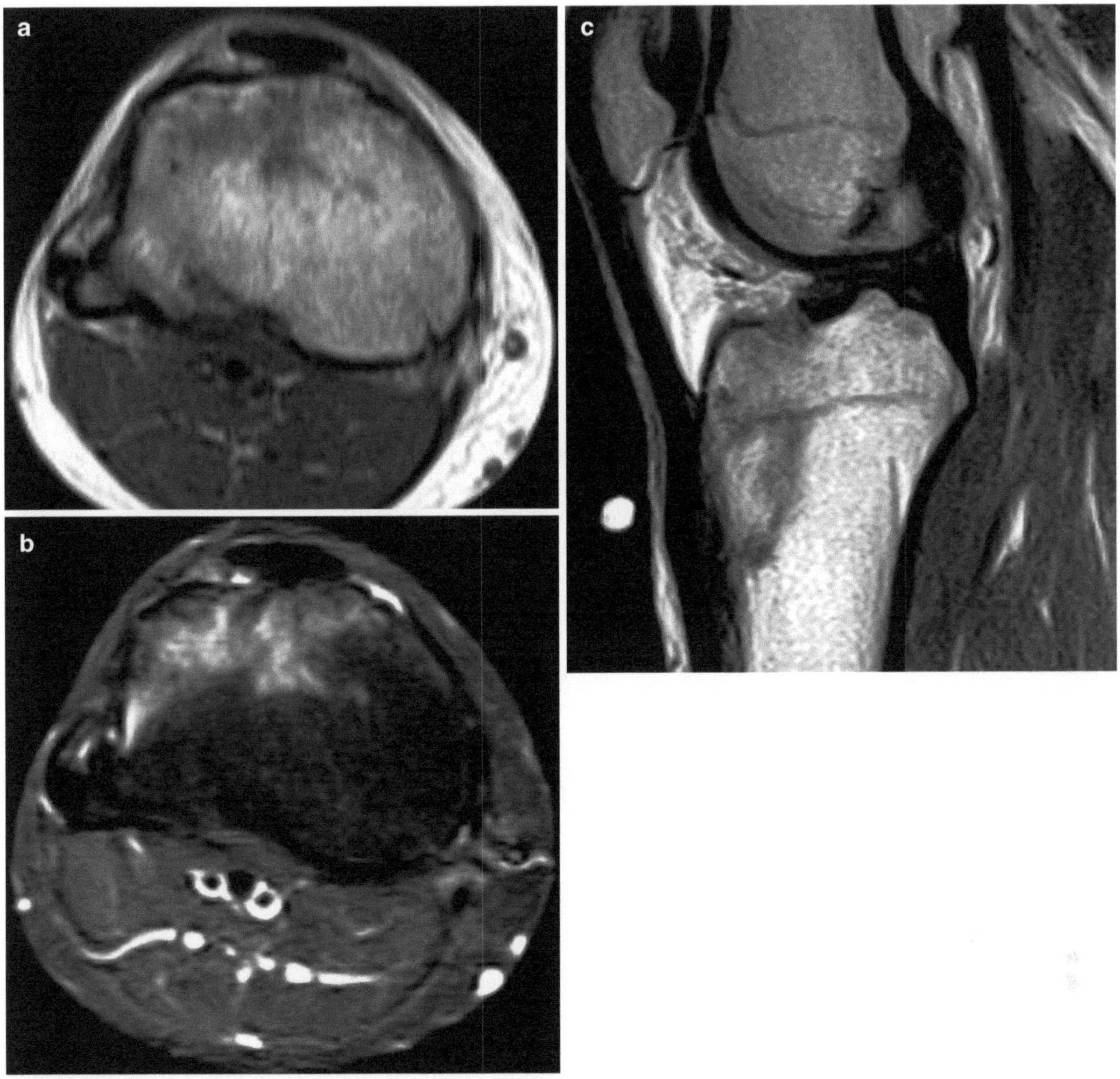


**Fig. 10.5** A subperiostial osteoid osteoma on the anterior aspect of the proximal end of the tibia is an extremely rare cause of anterior knee pain. Conventional x-rays were negative. Axial T1-weighted MR image (**a**). Axial T2-weighted MR image (with fat suppression) (**b**). Note a well-defined edematous area without significant extraosseous involvement. Sagittal T1-weighted MR image (**c**)

shows a mass in the popliteal aspect with bone involvement. Biopsy revealed a nonspecific chronic synovitis of the popliteal aspect. Symptoms of the anterior aspect of the knee disappeared after the resection of the lesion.

In conclusion, as a general rule, the more infrequent causes of anterior knee pain should be considered in the differential diagnosis of a painful knee when the treatment of the most frequent ones has proved ineffective.

## 10.4 Treat the Patient, Not the Image. Advances in Diagnostic Imaging Do Not Replace History and Physical Examination

In some cases, a distinction should be drawn between instabilities caused by an ACL tear and those caused by the patella. In our series, there is a patient who was referred to us with knee instability secondary to

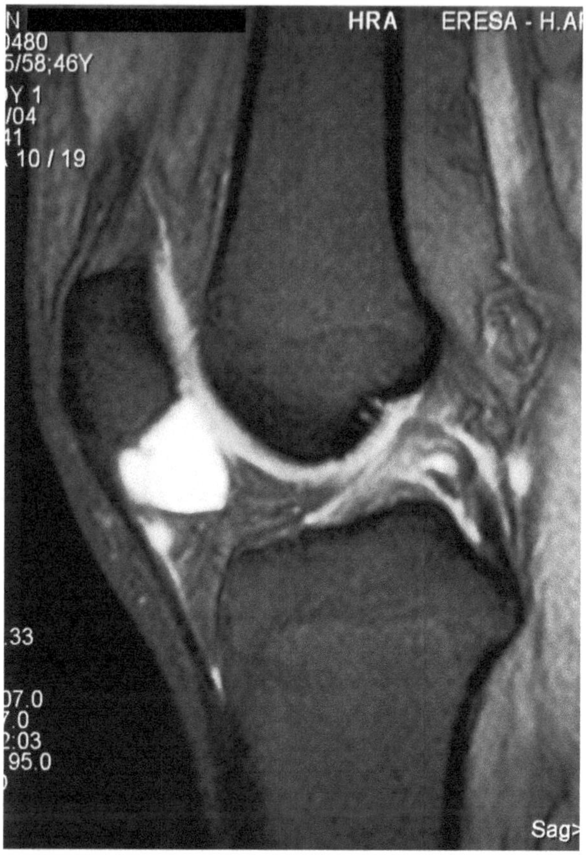


**Fig. 10.6** Sagittal FSE PDW Fat Sat MRI showing an intra-articular ganglion cyst in the Hoffa's fat pad

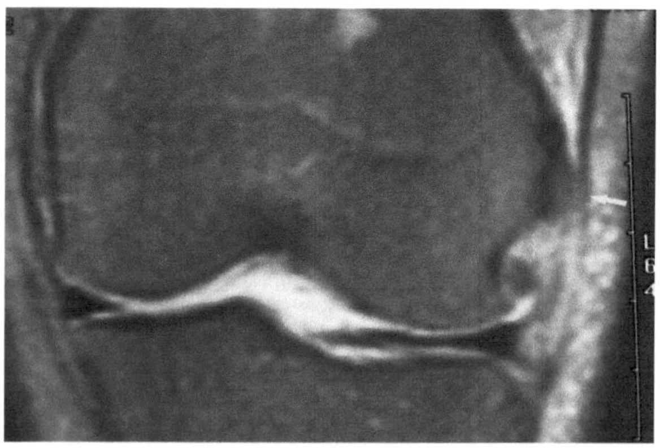

**Fig. 10.7** Coronal FSE PDW Fat Sat MRI. Illiotibial friction band syndrome in a female surfer. Note the bone exostosis of the lateral femoral condyle (*arrow*), which leads to an impingement on the iliotibial tract

indirect trauma caused by a skiing accident. The patient's MRI result was compatible with an ACL rupture (Fig. 10.15). Clinical examination revealed a normal ACL, which was confirmed arthroscopically. What this patient really had was a symptomatic PFM, which was duly treated and cured. Another patient, sent to our department with knee pain and instability, previously diagnosed by CT-scan to have PFM, actually had an ACL rupture as well as a bucket-handle tear of the medial meniscus (Fig. 10.16). We should once more stress the importance of history and physical examination vis-à-vis the use of imaging techniques.

Regarding instability, it should be emphasized that giving-way episodes due to ACL tears are normally associated with activities involving turns, whereas giving-way episodes related to patellofemoral joint disorders are associated to activities, which do not involve turns (i.e., straight movements such as walking or going downstairs). It should be remembered that quadriceps atrophy gives patients a feeling of instability, but this feeling appears without turning the knee. Obviously, clinically things tend to be more complicated, since in cases of chronic ACL tears, there is an associated quadriceps atrophy.

Moreover, we should remember that a "chondromalacia" can simulate a meniscal lesion, a fact already noted by Axhausen in 1922, resulting in the removal of normal menisci.[2] In this connection, Tapper and Hoover suspected that over 20% of women who did badly after an open meniscectomy had a patellofemoral pathology.[52] Likewise, Insall[20] stated that patellofemoral pathology was the most common cause of meniscectomy failure in young patients, especially women. These young women who have undergone a meniscectomy often end up with severe osteoarthritis (Fig. 10.17). This confusion may be due to the fact that the region where patients with patellofemoral pathology feel their pain is normally the anteromedial aspect of the knee. Another possible explanation for this diagnostic confusion might lie in the fact that the patella and the anterior horns of both menisci are connected by Kaplan's ligaments (one medial and the other lateral). Finally, unfortunately, the diagnostic error may be due to an MRI false positive. On the other hand, in a young patient (unlike an elderly one), the lack of a history of trauma makes the diagnosis of meniscal rupture unlikely. However, a history of joint effusion would tilt the scales toward a diagnosis of intra-articular pathology (e.g., meniscal rupture). To think of the sheer amount of menisci that have been needlessly sacrificed in patients with anterior knee pain syndrome! Obviously, this should nowadays be a thing of the past, given the wide array of diagnostic techniques at our disposal. Nonetheless, in spite of all the diagnostic techniques available, the key factor remains the physical examination of the patient.[22]

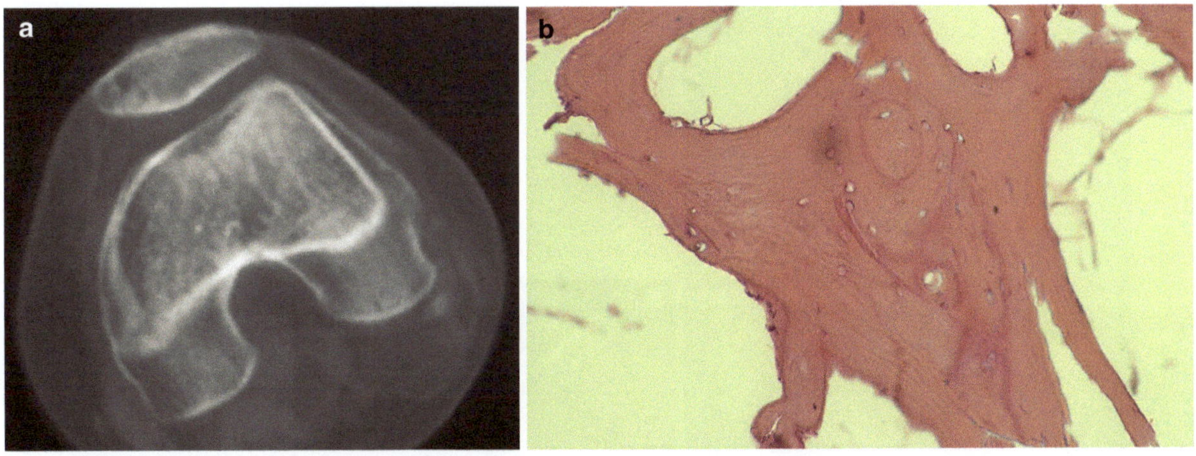

**Fig. 10.8** Localized osteonecrosis of the patella (**a**) CT image. (**b**) Microscopic appearance (Reproduced from Sanchis-Alfonso et al.[47], reprinted by permission from Thieme)

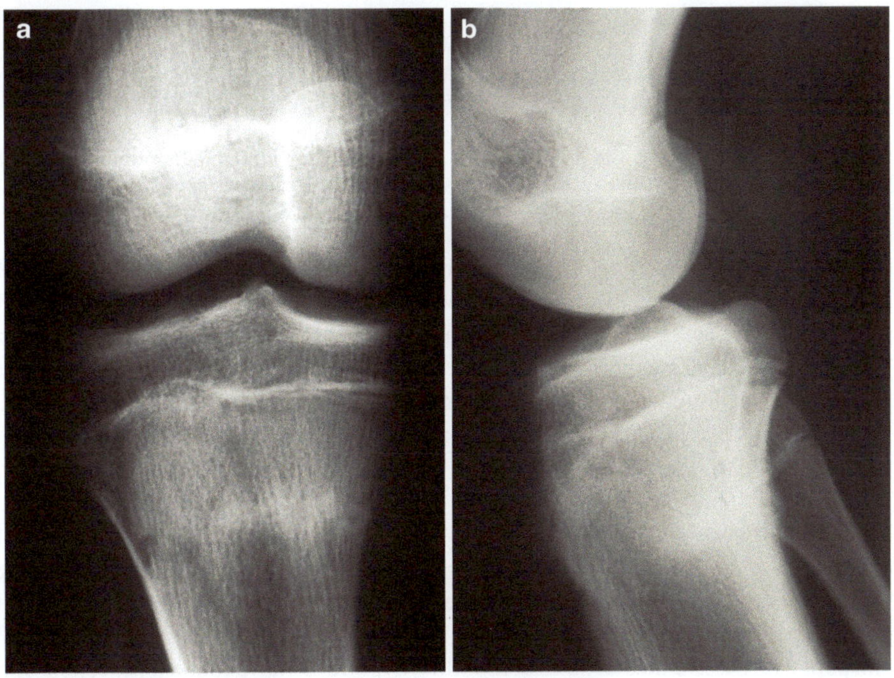

**Fig. 10.9** Stress fracture in the proximal tibia in a patient who consulted for anterior knee pain without traumatism (**a**) Anteroposterior view. (**b**) Lateral view

It should be emphasized once again that we should treat patients, not x-rays, CT scans, or MRI! Unfortunately, MRI seems to be taking the place of the clinical examination in assessing a painful joint, and this may lead to diagnostic confusion. This happens, for example, with the magic angle phenomenon, which can mislead us into diagnosing a patient without symptoms in the patellar tendon with patellar tendinopathy (Fig. 10.18). Nonetheless, MRI is obviously a very useful tool when it supplements physical examination since it can sometimes confirm a pathological condition in a patient involved in workman's compensation or other pending litigation claims (Fig. 10.19).

## 10.5 Cases Histories

### *10.5.1 Patient 1*

A 49-year-old male was referred for severe anterior right knee pain with activities of daily living and during the night for about 8 months. The pain was vague, and the patient could not specifically locate it with one finger, sweeping his fingers along both sides of the quadriceps tendon, patella, and patellar tendon. Pain did not subside with rest, medication, or physical therapy, limiting significantly his activities of daily living

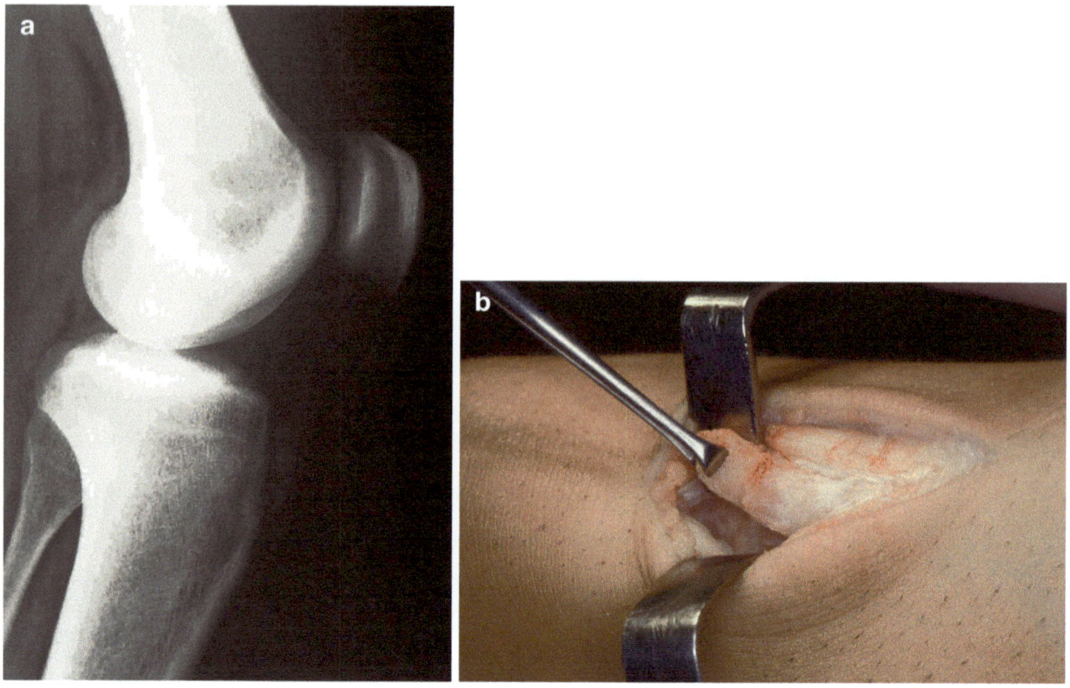


**Fig. 10.10** This is a patient who presented with swelling and pain in the anterior tibial tubercle. Lateral x-ray showing ossicles in the anterior tibial tubercle (**a**). Excision of the ossicles via a transtendinous approach (**b**)

(climbing stairs, squatting, and car driving). The patient underwent an endoscopic ACL reconstruction 1.5 years before using a four-bundled semitendinosus/gracilis graft fixed with bioabsorbable interference screws. The pain began 4 months after surgery after performing a squat of 140°, and it was progressing.

#### 10.5.1.1 Physical Examination

Physical examination revealed peripatellar and retropatellar pain with positive compression patellar test and pain with passive medial patellar mobility, hypotrophy of the quadriceps, 5° lack of full active extension, a tight gastrocnemius and calf pain that irradiated to the posterior aspect of the thigh. The remainder of the physical examination was completely normal.

#### 10.5.1.2 Which is the Source of the Anterior Knee Pain in Our Patient? Image Evaluation

This is the first question we must ask before proposing surgical treatment. To answer this question, we performed a CT at 0° of knee flexion that revealed a patellar subluxation (Fig. 10.20a). Therefore, the most obvious reply to our question would be that the source of pain was in the anterior aspect of the knee. However, if we examine in depth the CT, we can see an osteolytic area in the lateral femoral condyle and a structure that could correspond to the femoral interference screw (Fig. 10.20a). That is why, we did an MRI that clearly showed a broken divergent femoral interference screw (Fig. 10.20b), as the surgery revealed (Fig. 10.20c). MRI tilt angle according to the method described by Grelsamer and Weinstein[17] was of 10°. These authors have found an excellent correlation between clinical and MRI tilt. Tilt angles less than or equal to 10°, as in our case, are found in patients without clinical tilt, and are considered as normal, whereas tilt angles greater than 15° are all found in subjects with clinical patellar tilt, and are considered as abnormal. Therefore, the fact that in our patient the MRI tilt angle was 10° is against the source of pain being in the anterior aspect of the knee. Consequently, we postulated that anterior knee pain was secondary to a severe femoral interference screw divergence. Now, we must note that a severe femoral screw divergence is not necessarily accompanied by pain, neither in the anterior nor posterior aspects of the knee.

#### 10.5.1.3 Treatment Plan

Based on our hypothesis, we advised screw removal. Prior to surgery, we carried out an examination under general anesthesia that revealed that the knee was stable and the range of motion was complete. After that, we performed an arthroscopy that showed no abnormalities. Following arthroscopy, the patient was placed in the decubitus prone position and the femoral screw was removed through a Trickey's posterior approach. During surgery, we could see that the screw was incrusted into the lateral head of the gastrocnemius. Further, the screw was broken. The fact that the screw was broken reflects the existence

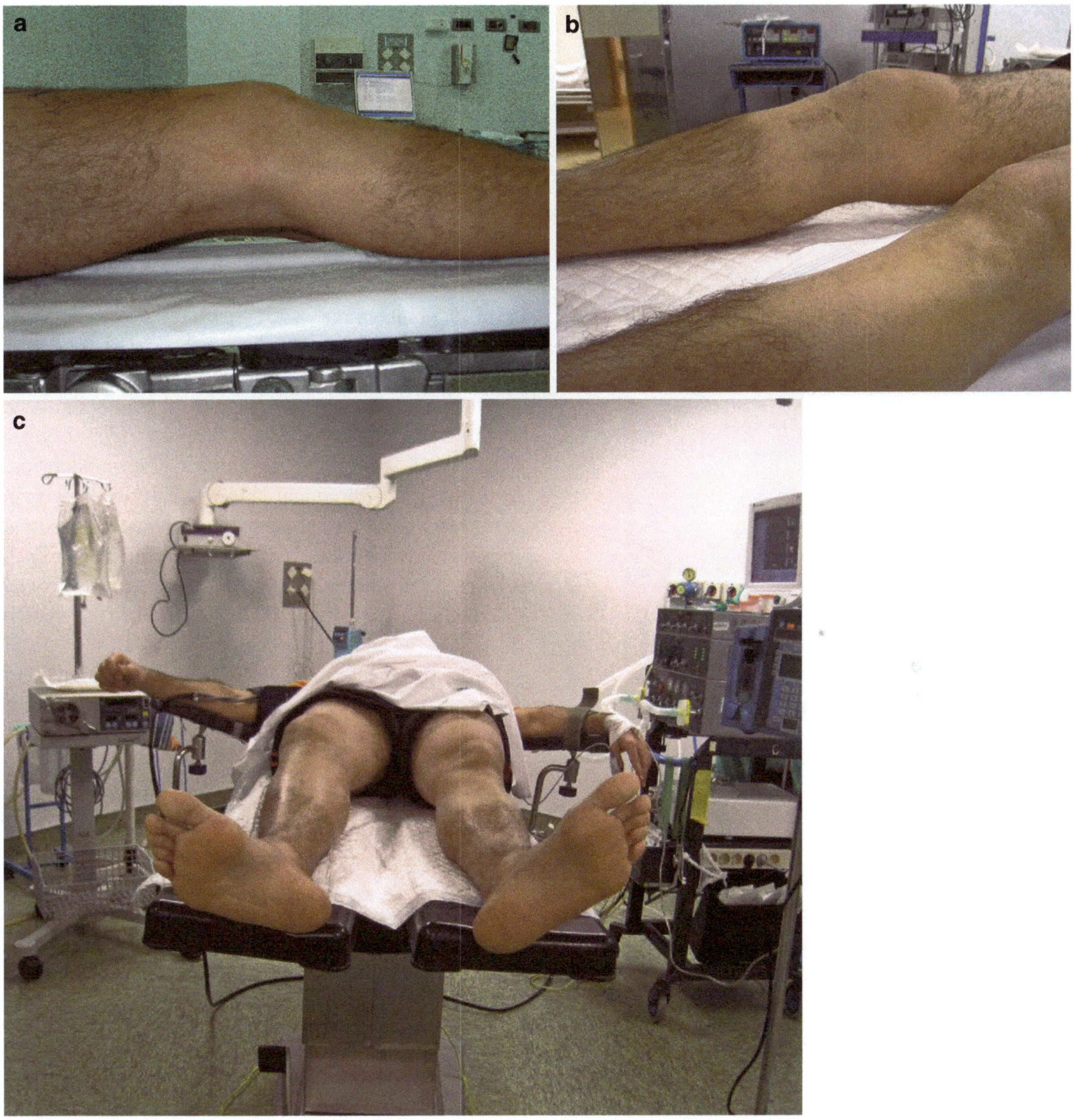

**Fig. 10.11** Anterior knee pain after ACL reconstruction with autogenous hamstrings tendons 11 months ago. (**a, b**) Lack of normal knee extension can be observed (bent knee). Patients who favor a knee by keeping it bent can be identified easily because they will have one leg and foot rotated externally (**c**). Chondral lesion of the trochlea (**d**). Cyclops syndrome (**e, f**)

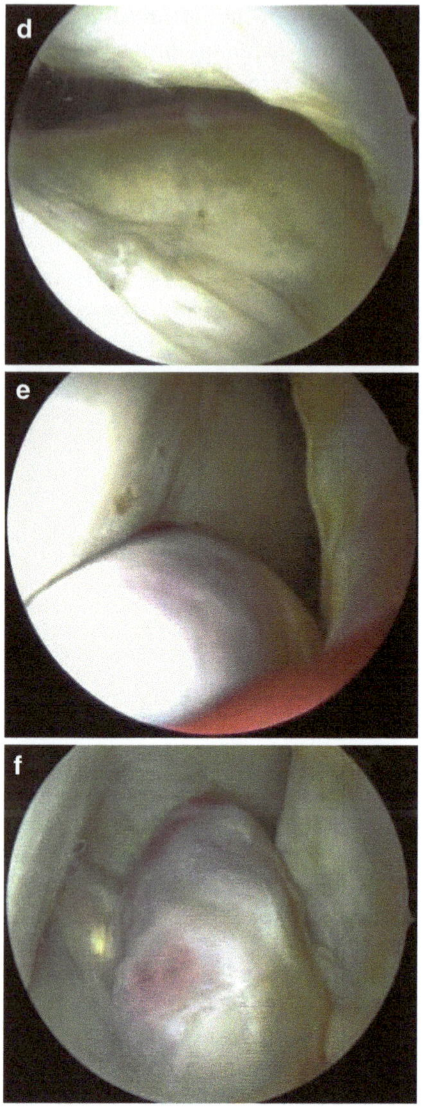


**Fig. 10.11** (continued)

of an important impingement between the screw and the surrounding soft tissues, specifically the lateral head of the gastrocnemius. We must note that the existence of impingement depends not only on the divergence in the sagittal plane, but also in the coronal plane. The fact that our patient was pain free after screw removal supports the hypothesis that the anterior knee pain source was in the posterior aspect of the knee.

#### 10.5.1.4 How Can We Explain the Anterior Knee Pain in Our Patient, Basing Ourselves on the Proposed Hypothesis?

First, because of the increment of the patellofemoral joint reaction (PFJR) force. This increment is secondary to the slight and maintained knee flexion, due to the contracture of the lateral head of the gastrocnemius provoked by irritation caused by the femoral screw. Sachs and colleagues[43] first proposed the association between anterior knee pain with flexion contracture of the knee. Later, Shelbourne and Trumper emphasized the importance of obtaining full extension to reduce the incidence of anterior knee pain after ACL reconstruction.[50] The increment of the PFJR force contributes to an increasing overload of the subchondral bone of the patella, which could explain the positive compression patellar test documented in our patient. Along the same line of thought, Strobel and colleagues[51] hypothesized that the ACL graft – PCL impingement near extension, could be a more frequent cause of anterior knee pain than we had thought after ACL reconstruction (Fig. 10.21). This impingement mechanism activates a proprioceptive reflex leading to a persistent functional extension loss while the patient is awake; this deficit disappears when the patient is anesthetized.

Second, because of the increment of the valgus vector force at the knee. This increment is secondary to the increment in foot pronation of the subtalar joint due to the contracture of the lateral head of the gastrocnemius.[14,27,34] The increment of the valgus vector could explain pain with passive medial patellar mobility.

#### 10.5.1.5 What Have We Learned from This Case?

The first lesson learned from this case is that although patellar subluxation is a potential cause of anterior knee pain, we must note that not all malalignments are

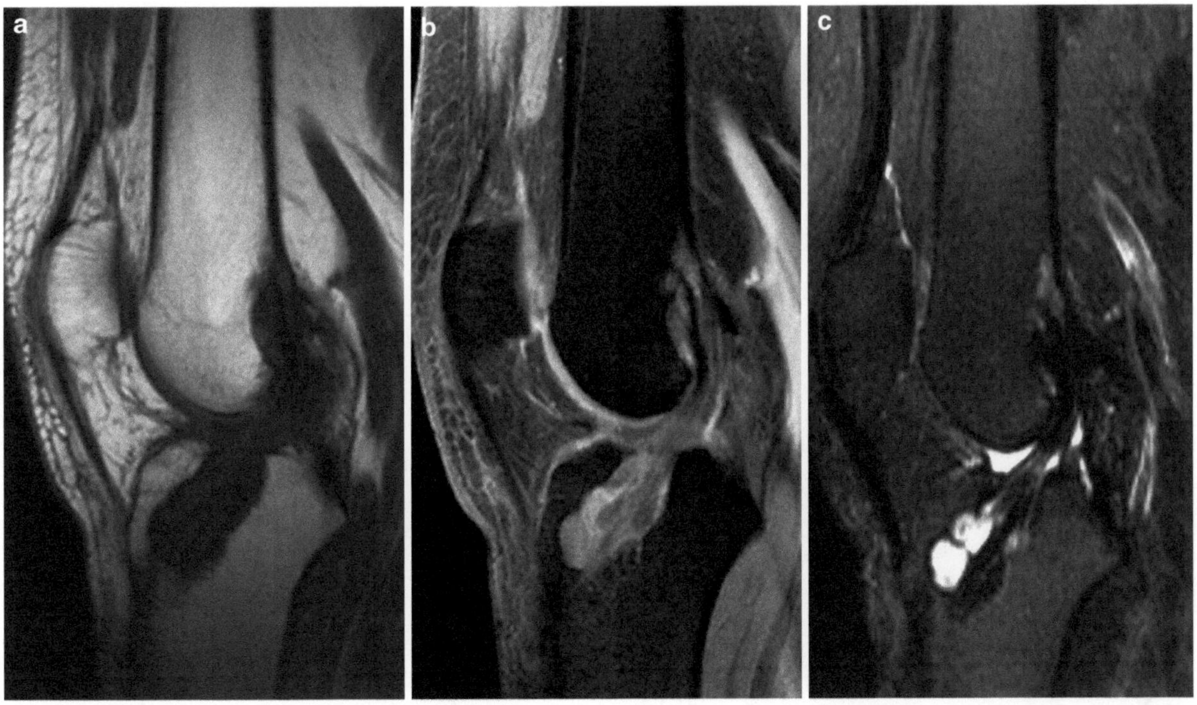


**Fig. 10.12** A 38-year-old male presented with a history of continuous chronic anterior left knee pain with daily living activities refractory to conservative treatment. The patient underwent an endoscopic ACL reconstruction 5 years before using autogenous hamstrings tendons fixed with bioabsorbable polylactic acid interference screws. An MRI showing an osteolytic tibial cyst in the tibial tunnel. (**a**) Sagittal FSE T1 weighted. A hypointense lesion is seen at the tibial tunnel. (**b**) Sagittal fat sat FSE T1 weighted following administration of paramagnetic contrast medium. There is an irregular enhancement at the wall related to the fibrous and inflammatory component of the cavity. The cyst shows no enhancement and corresponds to the central part of the cavity. (**c**) Sagittal fat sat FSE T2 weighted. The cyst is shown as a hyperintense image. The graft shows no abnormalities

symptomatic. Hence, we must always rule out other causes of anterior knee pain that can resemble the symptoms of malalignment and could lead to incorrect diagnosis and, consequently, incorrect treatment. The second lesson learned from this case is that anterior knee pain can arise in the posterior aspect of the knee.

### 10.5.2 Patient 2

An 18-year-old female presented in our outpatient clinic with a 1.5 year history of severe anterior left knee pain recalcitrant to conservative treatment. A joint effusion was aspirated twice at this interval of time, the obtained aspirate being yellowish. Moreover, the patient presented recurrent episodes of knee locking. There was no history of trauma. Pain aggravated by forced knee flexion, by ascending stairs, squatting, and prolonged sitting with a flexed knee. In the end, she had problems with activities of daily living.

#### 10.5.2.1 Physical Examination

Physical examination revealed tenderness to palpation at the anteromedial aspect of the knee. Moreover, there was a precise painful area localized at the anteromedial

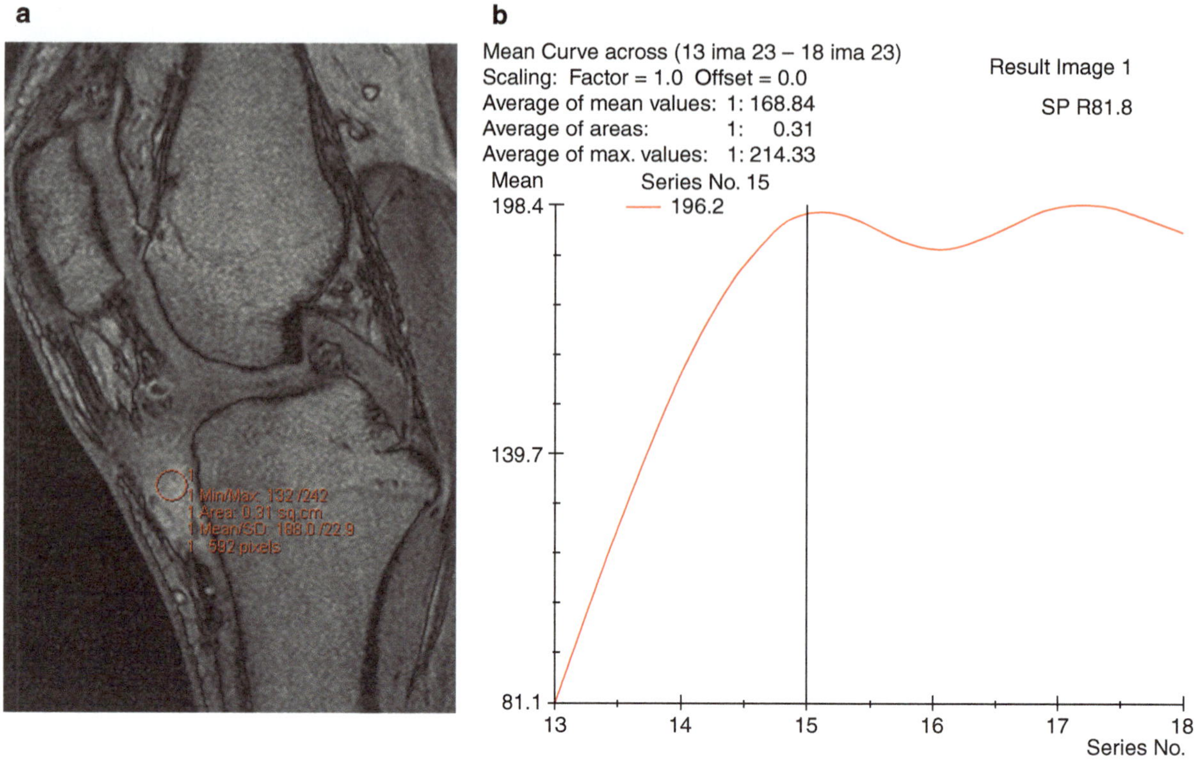


**Fig. 10.13** Extraskeletal osteosarcoma of the infrapatellar Hoffa's fat pad. (**a**) Dynamic study after in bolus paramagnetic contrast administration. 3D sagittal T1-weighted echo sequence, 6 acquisitions, 20 s duration for each one. Contrast uptaking soft tissue tumor adjacent to the anterior tibial surface. The ROI is marked (red circle) for contrast uptake curve analysis. (**b**) Graphic representation of the paramagnetic contrast uptake curve timing. The uptake intensity is represented on the vertical axis, and the series, equivalent to time units (20 s per series) is represented on the horizontal axis. The curve indicates the biological aggressive behavior of the tumor: it has a high growth slope in the initial series (13, 14, and 15), corresponding to the first minutes, reaching stable intensity values ("plateau") in the intermediate and last series (16, 17, and 18)

aspect of the knee. There were no inflammatory signs, no localized swelling, no joint effusion, no palpable mass, and the meniscal and ligamentous tests were negative. The patella was painful when mobilized. The range of motion of the knee was normal.

#### 10.5.2.2 Image Evaluation

Conventional radiography revealed no abnormalities. Because of the severity of the clinical symptoms contrasting with the paucity of the clinical examination, and the normality of routine x-rays, MRI was performed. MRI showed a well-demarcated and homogeneous solitary mass lesion within the infrapatellar Hoffa fat pad occupying the pretibial recess (Fig. 10.22). MRI tilt angle according to the method described by Grelsamer and Weinstein[17] was of 20°.

#### 10.5.2.3 Treatment Plan

Prior to resection of the lesion of the Hoffa fat pad, a routine arthroscopy was performed using standard anterolateral and anteromedial portals under general anesthesia. We found an unexpected single yellowish-brown tumor-like ovoid mass, well encapsulated, in the anteromedial aspect of the left knee, just in front of the anterior horn of the medial meniscus (Fig. 10.23a). A long pedicle attached the mass to the adjacent synovial membrane (Fig. 10.23b). According to Huang and colleagues,[19] the observation of a pedicle, as in our case, is relevant because torsion of this pedicle can produce acute knee pain. Moreover, there was a discrete involvement of the surrounding synovium with hypertrophic villous-like projections with brownish pigmentation (Fig. 10.23c). No other intra-articular abnormalities were noted. The intra-articular lesion

**Fig. 10.14** Nonspecific chronic synovitis of the popliteal aspect of the right knee. Axial CT scan at 0° of knee flexion (**a**). Sagittal GrE T2* MR images (**b**, **c**)

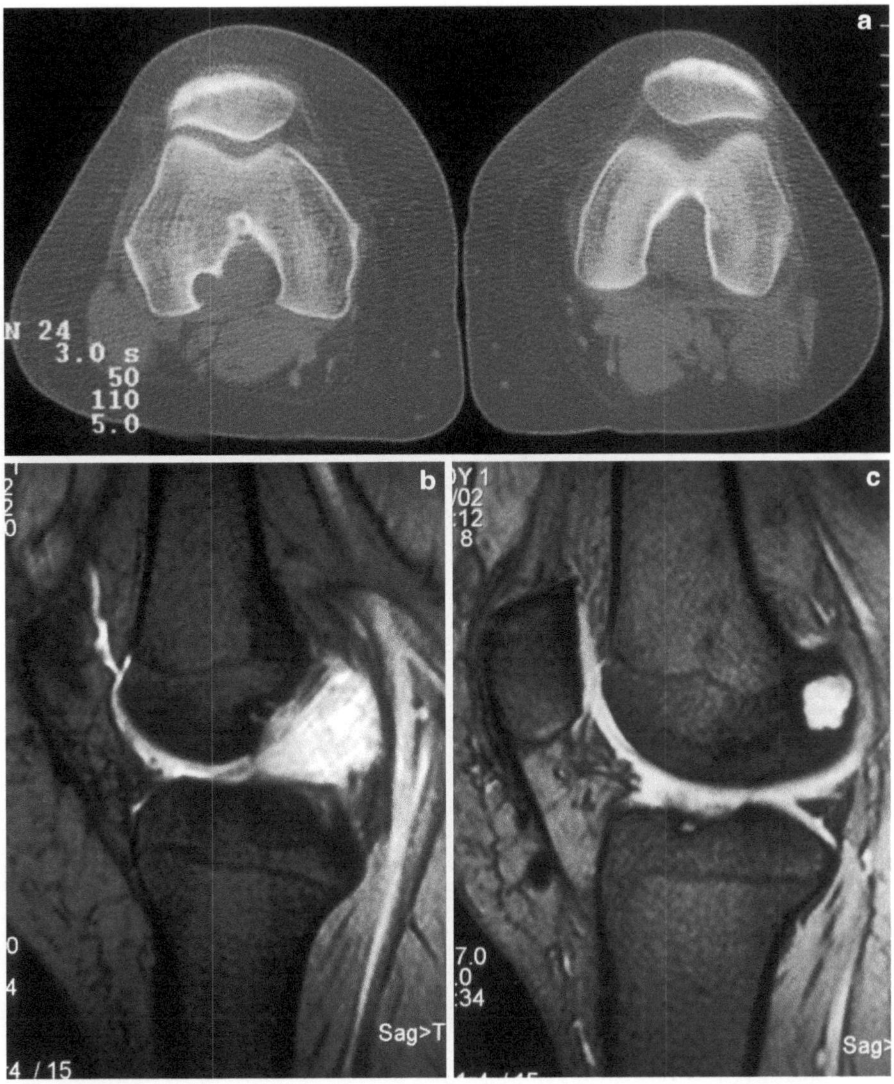


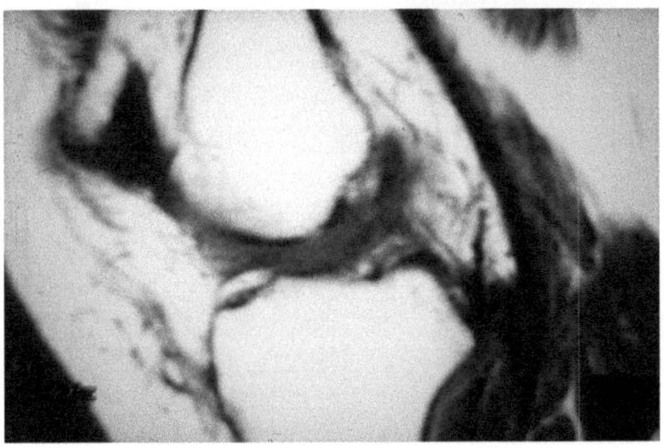

**Fig. 10.15** Sagittal SE T1W MR image. False positive detection of an ACL tear

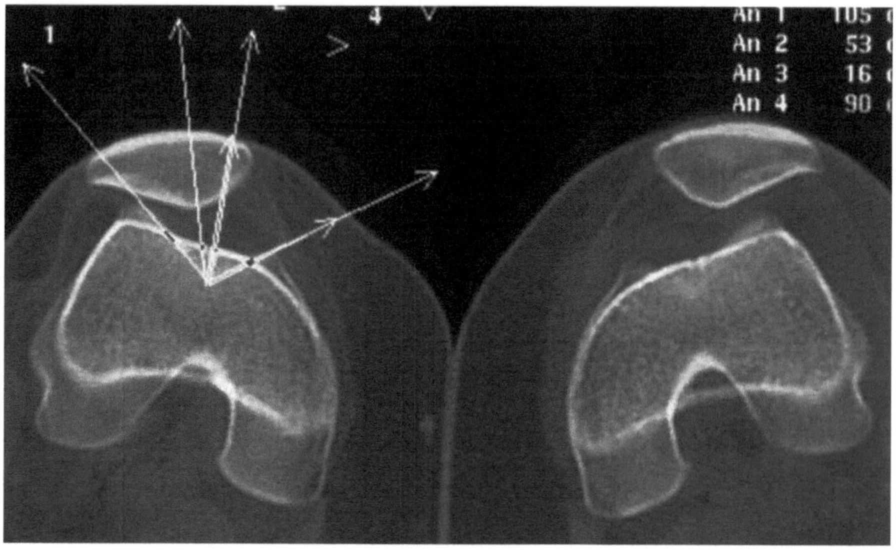


**Fig. 10.16** Asymptomatic bilateral PFM. CT scan with the knees at 0° of flexion with a relaxed quadriceps. The patient's actual problem was a chronic rupture of the ACL and a bucket-handle tear of the medial meniscus. The result of the physical examination of the extensor mechanism was negative for both knees. Two years after the CT scan was performed, the results of the physical examination of the extensor mechanism were still negative. The importance of a physical examination cannot be underestimated

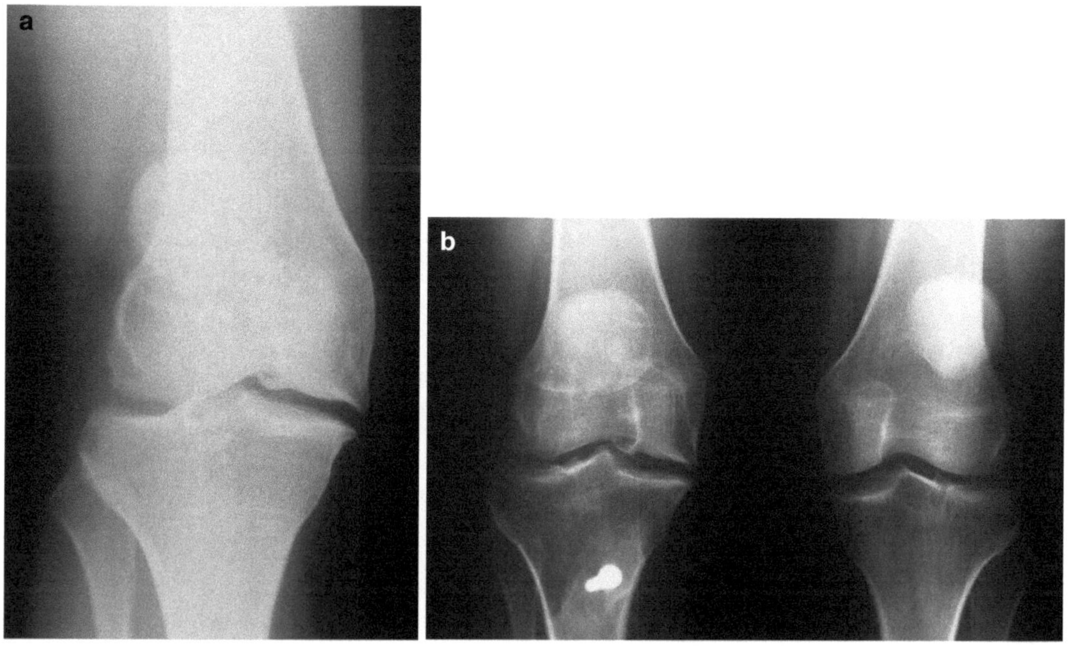


**Fig. 10.17** Post-meniscectomy osteoarthritis in a patient who had been mistakenly diagnosed with a rupture of the medial meniscus owing to a confusion between patellofemoral and meniscal pathologies (**a**). An extensor mechanism realignment surgery did away with the symptoms, which led to the first operation (**b**)

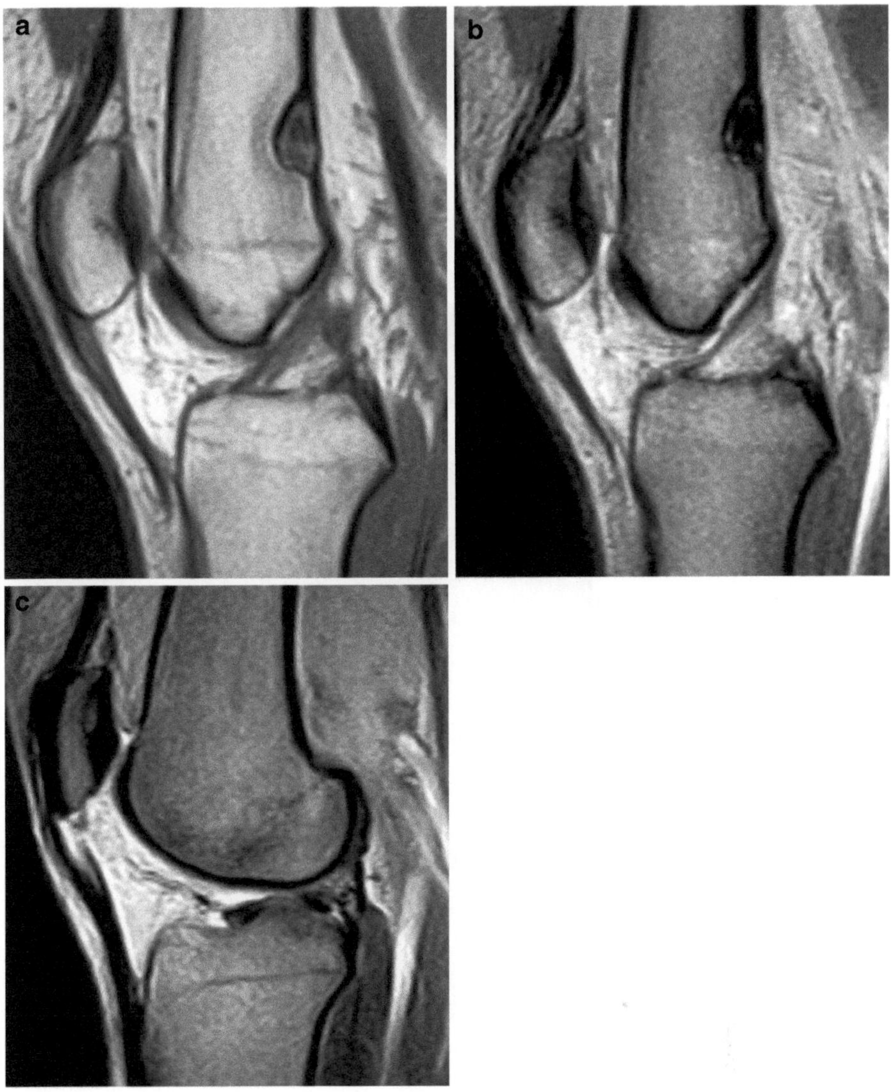


**Fig. 10.18** Magic angle phenomenon (**a**, **b**). Sagittal views, which show sequences with T1 (**a**) and T2 (GE) (**b**) – weighted images. Signal variations can be observed in the patellar tendon suggesting a structural alteration. If one looks at the image more closely, one notices that the signal variation follows the tendon's axis and that, in addition, there is no change whatsoever in its profile. This alteration corresponds to an imaging artifact arising from the magic angle phenomenon. This term covers the signal variations shown by certain structures when they are not aligned with the direction of the magnetic field (50°). This phenomenon is seen more often when the gradient echo (*GE*) technique is used. This is therefore an example of a false positive. Typical MR image of a patellar tendinopathy, T2-weighted FSE image, sagittal plane (**c**)

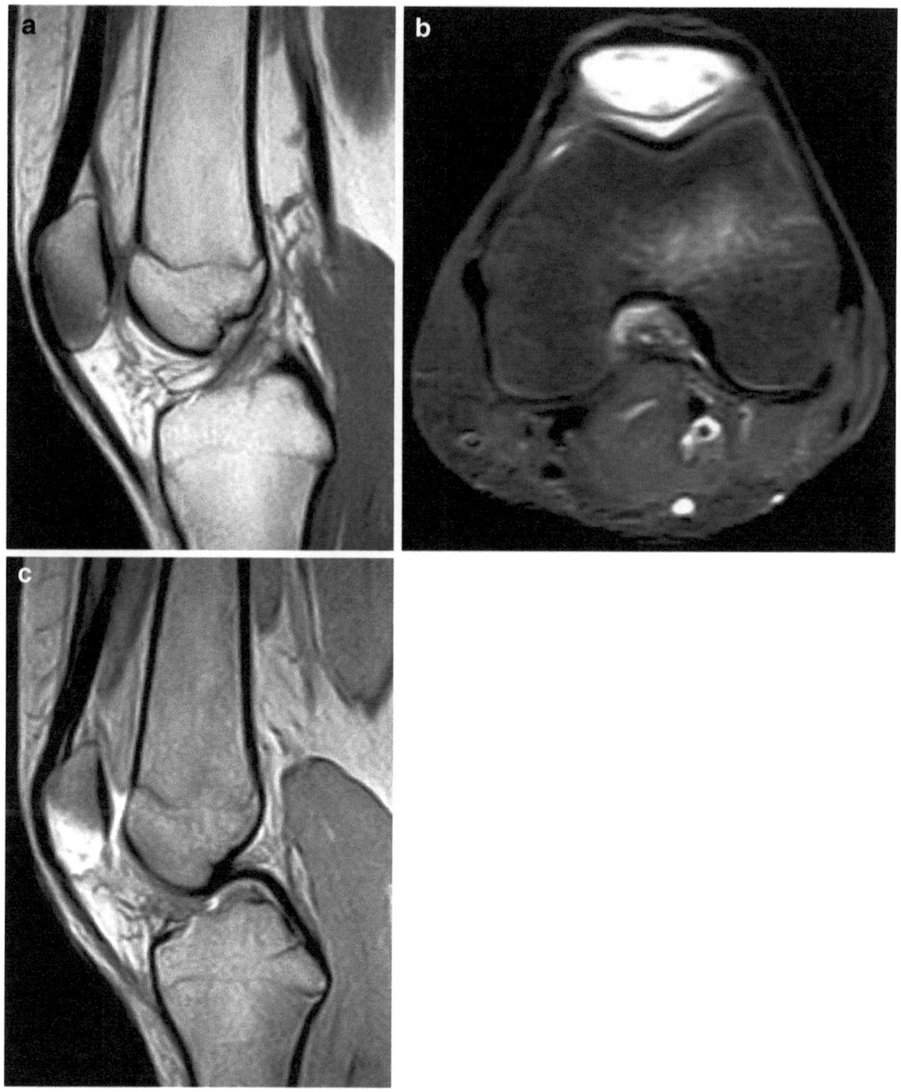


**Fig. 10.19** This patient had been suffering from anterior knee pain for several months caused by trauma due to a car accident. Conventional x-rays did not show any pathological finding. However, MRI did. (**a**) Sagittal SE T1W MR image. (**b**) Axial FSE PDW Fat Sat MR image. (**c**) Sagittal FSE T2W MR image

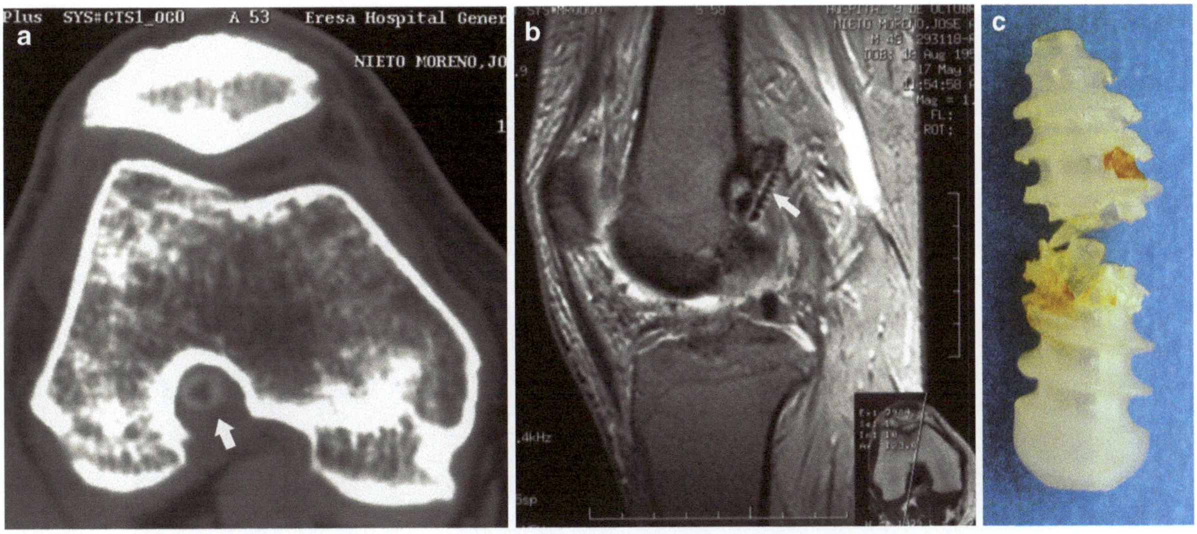


**Fig. 10.20** (**a**) Axial CT scan at 0° of knee flexion demonstrating a lateral subluxation of the patella. Femoral screw (*arrow*). (**b**) Sagittal GrE T2* MRI demonstrating a severe femoral screw/tunnel divergence. Moreover, you can note that the screw is broken (*arrow*). (**c**) Broken femoral interference screw (Reprinted from Sanchis-Alfonso and Tintó-Pedrerol[48], with permission from Elsevier)

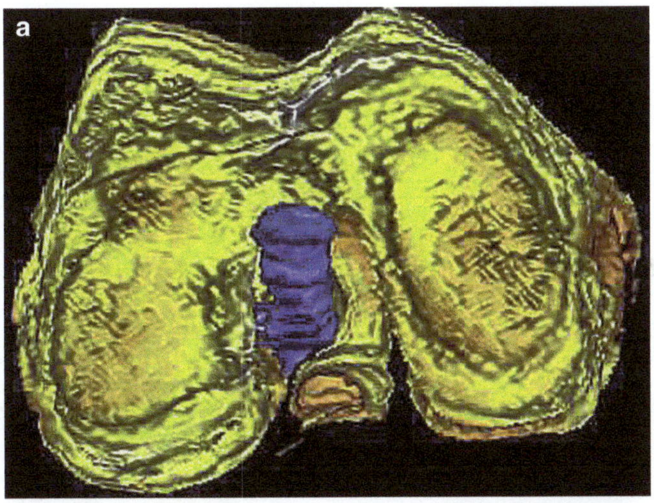


**Fig. 10.21** Anterior knee pain after ACL reconstruction in a patient with a correct patellofemoral alignment. MRI 3D reconstruction in the knee extended position demonstrated that the PCL is displaced medially and indented by a vertical ACL-graft in the coronal plane. Our patient was pain-free after an anatomical ACL-graft replacement. (**a**, **b**) T2-weighted 3D echo sequence in transverse acquisition with 3D rendering with surface algorithm with Barco Voxar 3D software. Bone structures (tibia, femur, patella) are segmented according to signal intensities. The segmentation is done by manually delineating the ACL-graft in each of the transverse planes. Bone structures are in yellow, and the ACL-graft is in blue. We can see the verticalization of the ACL-graft. (**c**) Sagittal FSE T2 2D sequence where we can see the ACL as a markedly hypointense structure

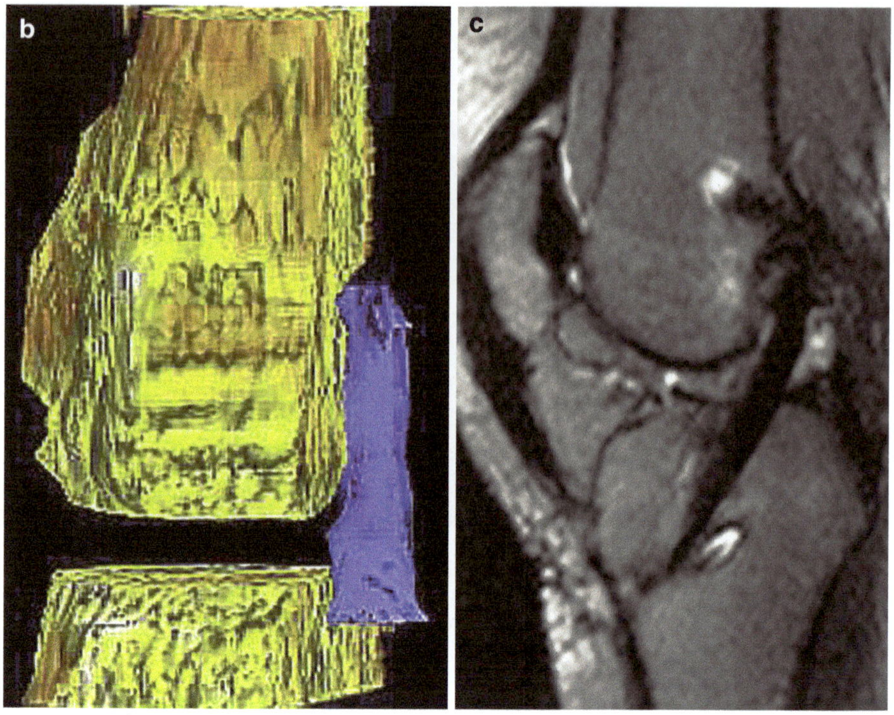


**Fig. 10.21** (continued)

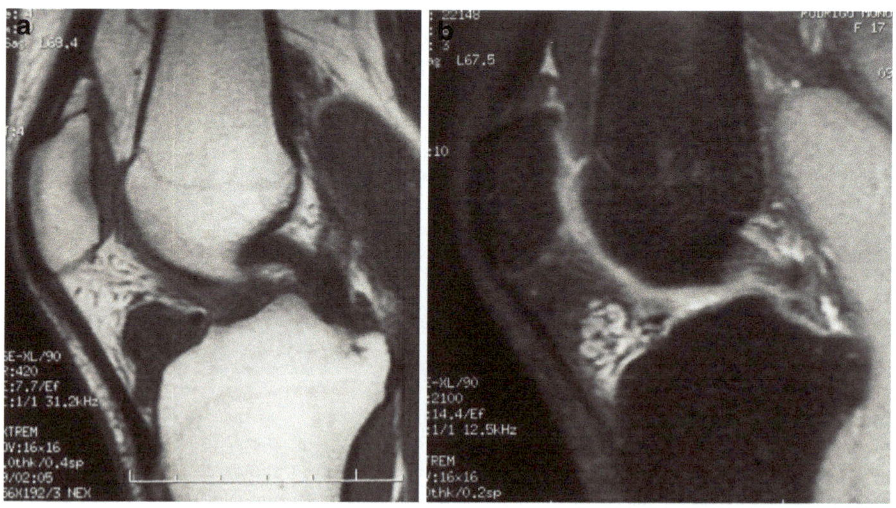


**Fig. 10.22** MRI. Sagittal plane FSE T1W, showing a rounded lesion involving the infrapatellar Hoffa's fat pad, isointense with skeletal muscle, displacing the intermeniscal ligament but without affecting either bone or the patellar tendon (**a**). Oblique sagittal plane FSE PDW with Fat Sat, showing the same lesion as in the Fig. a (**b**). The lesion appears hyperintense, of polycyclic appearance, and with hemosiderin and/or ferritin within the interior and at periphery. Likewise, no bone or tendon involvement is noted in this image

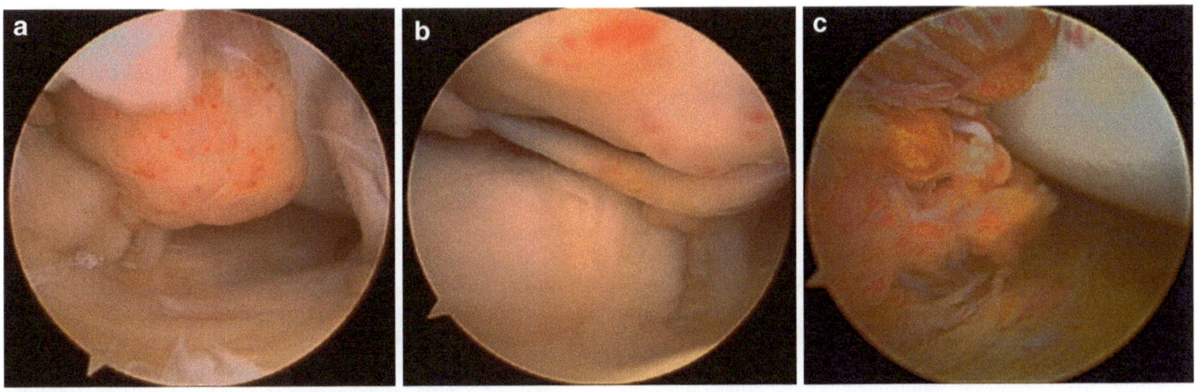

**Fig. 10.23** Arthroscopic view of the tumor. Tumor-like mass, well encapsulated, in the anteromedial aspect of the knee (**a**). Long pedicle attaching the mass to adjacent synovium (**b**). Involvement of the surrounding synovium with hypertrophic villous-like projections with brownish pigmentation (**c**)

was resected arthroscopically and easily removed through the medial portal, which had been previously enlarged with a surgical blade. The tumor was well-encapsulated and measured 1.5 cm long. After this, we performed an arthroscopic partial synovectomy of the surrounding synovitis with a motorized shaver introduced through the anteromedial portal. After arthroscopy, the solid tumor of the pretibial recess, the preoperative expected mass lesion, was removed through an anterior approach through the patellar tendon. The mass had a brownish aspect, well delimited, and 3 cm in diameter.

Both nodules, and the surrounding synovium of the intra-articular mass, were submitted for histologic study. Pathologists referred the intra-articular nodule to be a nodular form of a typical pigmented villonodular synovitis, with a proliferation of fibroblasts, giant cells, xanthomatous cells, and hemosiderin-ladened macrophages. Similar histologic features were observed in the surrounding synovium of the intra-articular mass. Nevertheless, the nodule localized in the Hoffa fat pad was considered as a nodular chronic nonspecific synovitis because, although it showed plenty of macrophages with hemosiderin deposits and xanthomatous changes, the stroma was myxoid, paucicellular, with small aggregates of lymph cells and a hyperplastic vascular pattern. The typical nodular proliferation of fibroblasts and macrophages was not present, nor were the giant cells.

The postoperative course was uneventful. The patient had a prompt and complete recovery of her symptoms and returned to her normal daily activities.

#### 10.5.2.4 What Have We Learned from This Case?

The first lesson learned from this case is that MRI not always allows us to detect synovial abnormalities, the arthroscopy being an important diagnostic and therapeutic tool. The second lesson learned from this case is that although patellar tilt is a potential cause of anterior knee pain, it is not always symptomatic. Hence, we must always rule out other causes of anterior knee pain that can resemble the symptoms of malalignment and lead to incorrect diagnosis and, consequently, incorrect treatment. Last, the presence of effusion is indicative of an intra-articular injury, a localized pigmented villonodular synovitis in our case, rather than retinacular injury.

## References


1. Alexeeff M, Macnicol MF. Subacute patellar osteomyelitis. *Knee*. 1995;1:237-239.
2. Axhausen G. Zur Pathogenese der Artritis deformans. *Arch Orthop Unfallchir*. 1922;20:1.
3. Bollen SR, Arvinte D. Snapping pes syndrome. *J Bone Joint Surg*. 2008;90-B:334-335.
4. Bruns J, Eggers-Stroeder G, von Torklus D. Synovial hemangioma – a rare benign synovial tumor. Report of four cases. *Knee Surg Sports Traumatol Arthrosc*. 1994;2:186-189.
5. Carls J, Kohn D, Maschek H. Benign giant-cell tumor of the patellar ligament. *Arthroscopy*. 1998;14:94-98.
6. Choi NH. Localized pigmented villonodular synovitis involving the fat pad of the knee. *Am J Knee Surg*. 2000; 13:117-119.
7. Chow JCY, Hantes M, Houle JB. Hypertrophy of the synovium in the anteromedial aspect of the knee joint following trauma: an unusual cause of knee pain. *Arthroscopy*. 2002;18: 735-740.
8. Cipolla M, Cerullo G, Franco V, et al. The double patella syndrome. *Knee Surg Sports Traumatol Arthrosc*. 1995;3: 21-25.
9. Delcogliano A, Galli M, Menghi A, et al. Localized pigmented villonodular synovitis of the knee: report of two cases of fat pad involvement. *Arthroscopy*. 1998;14:527-531.
10. Dhillon MS, Rajasekhar C, Nagi ON. Tuberculosis of the patella: report of a case and review of the literature. *Knee*. 1995;2:53-56.
11. Duri ZAA, Aichroth PM, Dowd G. The fat pad: clinical observations. *Am J Knee Surg*. 1996;9:55-66.
12. Ellen MI, Jackson HB, DiBiase SJ. Uncommon causes of anterior knee pain: a case report of infrapatellar contracture syndrome. *Am J Phys Med Rehabil*. 1999;78:376-380.
13. Elliot AJ, Fulkerson JP. Skeletal muscle hemangioma: a cause of unexplained pain about the knee. *Arthroscopy*. 1989;5:269-273.
14. Eng JJ, Pierrynowski MR. Evaluation of soft foot orthotics in the treatment of patellofemoral pain syndrome. *Phys Ther*. 1993;73:62-70.
15. Ferguson PC, Griffin AM, Bell RS. Primary patellar tumors. *Clin Orthop*. 1997;336:199-204.
16. Georgoulis AD, Soucacos PN, Beris AE, et al. Osteoid osteoma in the differential diagnosis of persistent joint pain. *Knee Surg Sports Traumatol Arthrosc*. 1995;3:125-128.
17. Grelsamer R, Weinstein C. Patellar tilt. An MRI study. *10th Congress European Society of Sports Traumatology, Knee Surgery and Arthroscopy, Book of Abstracts*, April 23–27, 2002, Rome:178.
18. Hardy Ph, Muller GP, Got C, et al. Glomus tumor of the fat pad. *Arthroscopy*. 1998;14:325-328.
19. Huang GS, Lee CH, Chan WP, et al. Localized nodular synovitis of the knee: MRI imaging appearance and clinical correlates in 21 patients. *Am J Radiol*. 2003;181:539-543.
20. Insall J. *Surgery of the Knee*. New York: Churchill Livingstone; 1984.
21. Johnson LL. *Arthroscopic Surgery. Principles and Practice*. St Louis: The C.V. Mosby Company; 1986.
22. Khan KM, Tress BW, Hare WSC, et al. "Treat the patient, not the x-ray": advances in diagnostic imaging do not replace the need for clinical interpretation [lead editorial]. *Clin J Sport Med*. 1998;8:1-4.
23. Kim SJ, Choi NH, Lee SC. Tenosynovial giant-cell tumor in the knee joint. *Arthroscopy*. 1995;11:213-215.
24. Kim SJ, Jeong JH, Cheon YM, et al. MPP test in the diagnosis of medial patellar plica syndrome. *Arthroscopy*. 2004;20:1101-1103.
25. Kim SJ, Kim JY, Lee JW. Pathologic infrapatellar plica: a report of two cases and literature review. *Arthroscopy*. 2002;18(5):e25.
26. Kim SJ, Shin SJ, Koo TY. Arch type pathologic suprapatellar plica. *Arthroscopy*. 2001;17:536-538.
27. Klingman RE, Liaos SM, Hardin KM. The effect of subtalar joint position on patellar glide position in subjects with excessive rearfoot pronation. *J Sports Phys Ther*. 1997;25: 185-191.
28. Kurosaka M, Yoshiya S, Yamada M, et al. Lateral synovial plica syndrome. A case report. *Am J Sports Med*. 1992;20:92-94.
29. Lorentzon R, Alfredson H, Hildingsson Ch. Treatment of deep cartilage defects of the patella with periosteal transplantation. *Knee Surg Sports Traumatol Arthrosc*. 1998;6: 202-208.
30. Lundy DW, Aboulafia AJ, Otis JB, et al. Myxoid liposarcoma of the retropatellar fat pad. *Am J Orthop*. 1997;26: 287-289.
31. Matsumoto H, Kawakabo M, Otani T, et al. Extensive posttraumatic ossification of the patellar tendon. *J Bone Joint Surg*. 1999;81-B:34-36.
32. McAllister DR, Parker RD. Bilateral subluxating popliteus tendons. A case report. *Am J Sports Med*. 1999;27:376-379.
33. McConnell J. Fat pad irritation – a mistaken patellar tendinitis. *Sport Health*. 1991;9:7-9.
34. McConnell J. Conservative management of patellofemoral problems. In: Grelsamer RP, MacConnell J, eds. *The Patella: A Team Approach*. Gaithersburg: Aspen Publishers; 1998: 119-136.
35. Meister K, Jackson AM. Longitudinal stress fracture of the patella: an autolateral release. A case report. *Am J Knee Surg*. 1994;7:49-52.
36. Mori Y, Kubo M, Shimokoube J, et al. Osteochondritis dissecans of the patellofemoral groove in athletes: unusual cases of patellofemoral pain. *Knee Surg Sports Traumatol Arthrosc*. 1994;2:242-244.
37. Mori Y, Okumo H, Iketani H, et al. Efficacy of lateral retinacular release for painful bipartite patella. *Am J Sports Med*. 1995;23:13-18.
38. Muscolo DL, Ayerza MA, Makino A, et al. Tumors about the knee misdiagnosed as athletic injuries. *J Bone Joint Surg*. 2003;85-A:1209-1214.
39. Orava S, Taimela S, Kvist M, et al. Diagnosis and treatment of stress fracture of the patella in athletes. *Knee Surg Sports Traumatol Arthrosc*. 1996;4:206-211.
40. Palumbo RC, Matthews LS, Reuben JM. Localized pigmented villonodular synovitis of the patellar fat pad: a report of two cases. *Arthroscopy*. 1994;10:400-403.
41. Pinar H, Bozkurt M, Baktiroglu L, et al. Intra-articular hemangioma of the knee with meniscal and bony attachment. *Arthroscopy*. 1997;13:507-510.
42. Pinar H, Özkan M, Akseki D, et al. Traumatic prepatellar neuroma: an unusual cause of anterior knee pain. *Knee Surg Sports Traumatol Arthrosc*. 1996;4:154-156.

43. Sachs RA, Daniel DM, Stone ML, et al. Patellofemoral problems after anterior cruciate ligament reconstruction. *Am J Sports Med.* 1989;17:760-765.
44. Safran MR, Fu FH. Uncommon causes of knee pain in the athlete. *Orthop Clin North Am.* 1995;26:547-559.
45. Sanchis-Alfonso V. *Cirugía de la rodilla. Conceptos actuales y controversias.* Madrid: Editorial Médica Panamericana; 1995.
46. Sanchis-Alfonso V, Fernandez CI, Sanchez C, et al. Hemangioma intramuscular (Aportación de 6 casos y revisión de la literatura). *Rev Esp de Cir Ost.* 1990;25:367-378.
47. Sanchis-Alfonso V, Roselló-Sastre E, Martinez-SanJuan V, et al. Occult localized osteonecrosis of the patella. Case report. *Am J Knee Surg.* 1997;10:166-170.
48. Sanchis-Alfonso V, Tintó-Pedrerol M. Femoral interferente screw divergente after anterior cruciate ligament reconstruction provoking severe anterior knee pain. *Arthroscopy.* 2004;20:528-531.
49. Schmitz MC, Schaefer B, Bruns J. A ganglion of the anterior horn of the medial meniscus invading the infrapatellar fat pad. Case report. *Knee Surg Sports Traumatol Arthrosc.* 1996;4:97-99.
50. Shelbourne KD, Trumper RV. Preventing anterior knee pain after anterior cruciate ligament reconstruction. *Am J Sports Med.* 1997;25:41-47.
51. Strobel MJ, Castillo RJ, Weiler A. Reflex extension loss after anterior cruciate ligament reconstruction due to femoral "High Noon" graft placement. *Arthroscopy.* 2001;17:408-411.
52. Tapper EM, Hoover NW. Late results after meniscectomy. *J Bone Joint Surg.* 1969;51-A:517-526.
53. Teitz CC, Harrington RM. Patellar stress fracture. *Am J Sports Med.* 1992;20:761-765.
54. Tennent TD, Birch NC, Holmes MJ, et al. Knee pain and the infrapatellar branch of the saphenous nerve. *J R Soc Med.* 1998;91:573-575.
55. Williams AM, Myers PT. Localized pigmented villonodular synovitis. A rare cause of locking of the knee. *Arthroscopy.* 1997;13:515-516.
56. Yilmaz E, Karakurt L, Ozercan I, et al. A ganglion cyst that developed from the infrapatellar fat pad of the knee. *Arthroscopy.* 2004;20:e65-e68.

# Risk Factors and Prevention of Anterior Knee Pain

11

Erik Witvrouw, Damien Van Tiggelen, and Tine Willems

## 11.1 Introduction

Anterior knee pain is known as a very common problem in the sporting population.[1,5,15,16,30] Many of the patients with anterior knee pain need conservative treatment to be able to return to sport or their daily activities. On the other hand, because of this high incidence of anterior knee pain, prevention of this pathology has been an important goal for many sports medicine practitioners for some years. However, before a scientific approach in planning and carrying out prevention and treatment of anterior knee pain can be set up, a thorough understanding of the etiology of anterior knee pain seems essential. This understanding refers to information on why a particular individual develops anterior knee pain and another individual, exposed to more or less the same exercise load, does not. In addition, it seems important to understand why some patients benefit from a treatment program while others do not, or not as well. To answer these important issues, risk factors for the development of anterior knee pain need to be identified.

General consensus exists about the fact that myriad factors may contribute to the development of anterior knee pain. Anterior knee pain can be considered as a multi-risk phenomenon with various risk factors interacting at a given time.[32] Risk factors are traditionally divided into two main categories: intrinsic (or internal) and extrinsic (or external) risk factors. The extrinsic risk factors relate to environmental variables, for example, exercise load, exercise intensity, exercise type, amount of physical activity, equipment, weather conditions, and playing field conditions. In contrast, intrinsic risk factors relate to the individual physical and psychological characteristics such as age, joint instability, gender, muscle strength, muscle flexibility, conditioning, and so forth.

Focusing on injury prevention requires the use of a dynamic model that accounts for the multifactorial nature of anterior knee pain. One such model is described by Meeuwisse.[32] This model describes how multiple factors interact to produce an injury (Fig. 11.1). It can be seen in this model that numerous intrinsic factors theoretically may predispose an individual to anterior knee pain. This model also shows very well the interaction of both intrinsic and extrinsic factors, in the way that the extrinsic risk factors act on the predisposed athlete from outside. Consequently, knowledge of both the intrinsic and extrinsic risk factors of anterior knee pain seems essential in our understanding of the etiology, and thus in creating prevention and conservative treatment programs.

## 11.2 The Role of Extrinsic Risk Factors in the Development of Anterior Knee Pain

The association between clinical overload (external risk factors) and the development of anterior knee pain is well known.[14,34] Recently, Dye[11] stated that the function of the patellofemoral joint (and any other joint) could be characterized by a load/frequency distribution (the envelope of function) that

E. Witvrouw (✉)
Department of Rehabilitation Sciences
and Physical Therapy, Faculty of Medicine,
Ghent University, Ghent, Belgium
e-mail: erik.witvrouw@ugent.be

V. Sanchis-Alfonso (ed.), *Anterior Knee Pain and Patellar Instability*,
DOI: 10.1007/978-0-85729-507-1_11, © Springer-Verlag London Limited 2011

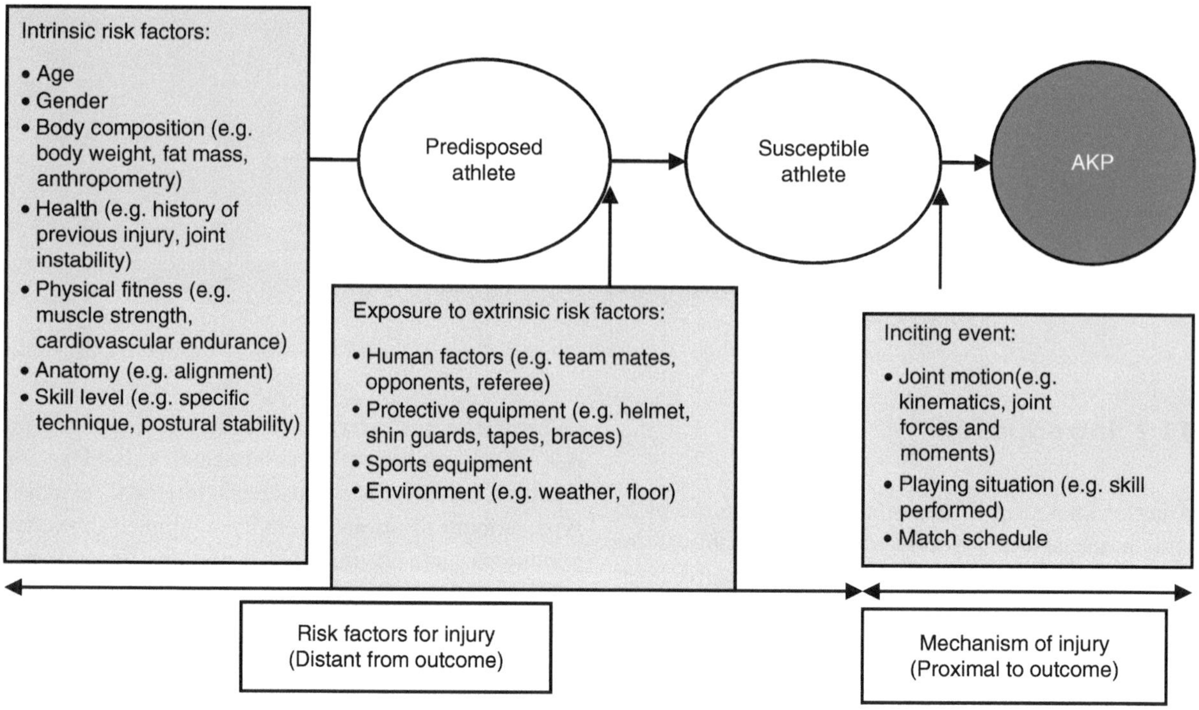


**Fig. 11.1** A dynamic, multifactorial model of sports injury etiology (Adapted from Meeuwisse[32])

defines a range of painless loading that is compatible with homeostasis of the joint tissues. If excessive loading is placed across the joint, loss of tissue homeostasis can occur, resulting in pain and other dysfunctions. Excessive loading on the PF joint can simply cause the source of loss of homeostasis. This supraphysiological loading can be a consequence of a single event (overload) or repetitive loading (overuse), but indicates the important association between extrinsic risk factors (amount of loading) and the etiology of anterior knee pain. An athlete who has sustained an overuse injury must have exceeded his or her limits in such way that the negative remodeling of the injured structure predominates over the repair process due to the stresses placed on the structure.[24] The goal of the conservative treatment is, therefore, to restore the homeostasis of the patellofemoral joint.[11] Repeated applied stresses below the tensile limit of a structure lead to a positive remodeling if sufficient time between stress applications is provided.[20,24] Consequently, this principle should be used in the construction of a conservative and a preventive program for anterior knee pain.

## 11.3 Importance and Identification of Intrinsic Risk Factors of Anterior Knee Pain

In the literature, several studies are available focusing on the relationship between the intrinsic risk factors and anterior knee pain. However, the majority of these studies are retrospective and/or lacking a control group. In the latter, it is impossible to deduce a causative relation between the examined intrinsic risk factors and anterior knee pain. Hence, to identify this causative relationship, prospective studies are needed. Looking in the available literature, the amount of prospective research in the area of anterior knee pain, focusing on the relationship between the intrinsic risk factors and anterior knee pain, is very scarce.

The first prospective study focusing on the anterior knee pain and intrinsic risk factors was performed by Milgrom and colleagues.[34] They prospectively examined 390 infantry recruits and revealed that an increased medial tibial intercondylar distance and an increased isometric strength of the quadriceps, tested at 85° of knee flexion, had a statistically significant correlation with the incidence of anterior knee pain caused by overactivity. Recruits in that study who could generate higher patellofemoral contact forces because of stronger extensor muscle strength, or the presence of more genu varum, had a higher rate of anterior knee pain related to overactivity. The authors, therefore, concluded that anterior knee pain due to overactivity is caused by an overload of patellofemoral contact forces. In our own study[50] on 282 students in physical education, we prospectively examined a broad variety of presumed intrinsic risk factors. Of this broad variety of parameters, only a shortened quadriceps muscle, an altered vastus medialis obliquus muscle reflex response time, a decreased explosive strength, and a hypermobile patella had a significant correlation with the incidence of anterior knee pain. Very conspicuous in this study was the finding that statistical analyses did not identify any of the clinically measured lower leg alignment characteristics (leg length difference, height, weight, Q angle, genu varum/valgum and recurvatum, foot alignment) as predisposing factors of anterior knee pain. This suggests that these parameters seem less important in the development of anterior knee pain, in contrast to what is frequently stated on the basis of theoretical models and/or retrospective studies. The results of our study are in agreement with the results of Milgrom and colleagues[34] in that they indicate that from a broad variety of parameters only a few contribute significantly to the development of anterior knee pain. In a recent prospective study on recreational runners,[29] this conclusion was confirmed. Lun and colleagues[29] found that of the examined static biomechanical lower leg alignment parameters (genu varum/valgum and recurvatum, height, weight, leg length difference, Q angle, hip internal and external range of motion, ankle dorsiflexion and plantar flexion, rearfoot and forefoot valgus, standing longitudinal arch), only a smaller right ankle dorsiflexion ROM, a greater genu varum, and a greater left forefoot varus was significantly different between the runners who developed anterior knee pain and the uninjured runners. In a more recent prospective study in male military recruits, Van Tiggelen and colleagues[47] identified a significant smaller peak torque at low concentric isokinetic speed as an intrinsic risk factor of anterior knee pain. This emphasizes the importance of the reinforcement of quadriceps strength in the treatment and prevention of anterior knee pain, as in other overuse injuries of the lower limb.[22]

Conclusions drawn on the basis of relatively few data should always be warranted. However, on the basis of the few existing prospective data on anterior knee pain, some trends can be identified. First, these studies have shown that clinically measured lower leg alignment characteristics such as leg length difference, height, weight, Q angle, genu varum/valgum and recurvatum, and foot alignment seem not to be very important in the development of anterior knee pain. This could be explained in different ways. First, it could be that these clinically measured parameters cannot be considered as intrinsic risk factors of anterior knee pain. Second, it could be that measuring these parameters clinically is not precise enough. For instance, small interindividual differences, which might be important in the etiology of anterior knee pain, might not be identified since the measurement error is too large. Therefore, prospective studies should be set up using more precise measuring techniques (two- or three-dimensional measurements in movement analysis labs). Third, it must be mentioned that all the available prospective studies were performed on a young sportive population (military recruits or students in physical education). This implies that this population is rather homogeneous and very select. Probably, measuring these parameters in the general population should give more interindividual variation. In addition, subjects with large "abnormalities" in these clinically measured lower leg alignment characteristics could already have developed anterior knee pain and would, therefore, decide not to start such a physically high demanding training program. Consequently, one must be very careful when applying these results to the general population of anterior knee pain patients. Clinical experience and retrospective data show us that patients with anterior knee pain show significantly more alterations of their lower leg alignment characteristics, compared to a control group. These findings let us believe that "large" deviations in lower leg alignment characteristics are probably important in the development of anterior knee pain. Yet, on the basis of the available studies, it also seems that "small" deviations in lower leg alignment characteristics probably do not play a significant role in the genesis of anterior knee pain (unless the clinical measurements are not able to evaluate these small alterations with the necessary precision).

In contrast to the findings of the lower leg alignment characteristics, the prospective data on muscular characteristics show that the extensor muscle plays a vital role in the development of anterior knee pain. Lack of agreement between the different studies in the methods used to measure these muscular parameters limits the possibility of concluding which of the muscular parameters (strength, VMO/VL speed of contraction, flexibility) are more important than the others. However, today we can state that several muscular parameters are identified as intrinsic risk factors of anterior knee pain. Consequently, these parameters will probably play a vital role in the construction of a preventive and a conservative treatment program.

## 11.4 Constructing a Scientific Prevention Program for Anterior Knee Pain

Once intrinsic and extrinsic risk factors of anterior knee pain are identified, the next step in "the sequence of prevention" can be undertaken. Van Mechelen and colleagues[46] suggest a strategy of four stages that should be followed in order to scientifically have an impact on the incidence of anterior knee pain (prevention), and on the success rate of a conservative treatment program (Fig. 11.2). After establishing the incidence and severity of anterior knee pain in the sports population (which has been done by several researchers), the risk factors and the mechanisms of the occurrence of anterior knee pain must be identified (cf. above). The next step is to introduce measures that are likely to reduce the risk of developing anterior knee pain. These measures should be based on the information about the intrinsic and extrinsic risk factors. However, as mentioned by Reider,[43] after a correct identification of the risk factors, before a preventive program can be introduced, it should be clear (1) whether the identified risk factors can be influenced, and (2) which program is best in altering these identified risk factors.

In order to examine this for anterior knee pain, we set up a randomized clinical trial to investigate which of the frequently used conservative programs (open versus closed kinetic chain programs) is best in altering the identified risk factors of anterior knee pain. Sixty patients with anterior knee pain were randomized into a 5 week program that consisted of only closed kinetic chain exercises or only open kinetic chain exercises. In this study, the evaluation focused on those parameters that (1) were previously identified as intrinsic risk factors of anterior knee pain in prospective studies, and (2) can be influenced by a conservative program. Only four parameters met these criteria at that time: namely, muscle length of the quadriceps, explosive functional strength of the quadriceps (measured by the triple jump test), reflex response time of the VMO and VL, and mediolateral patellar mobility.

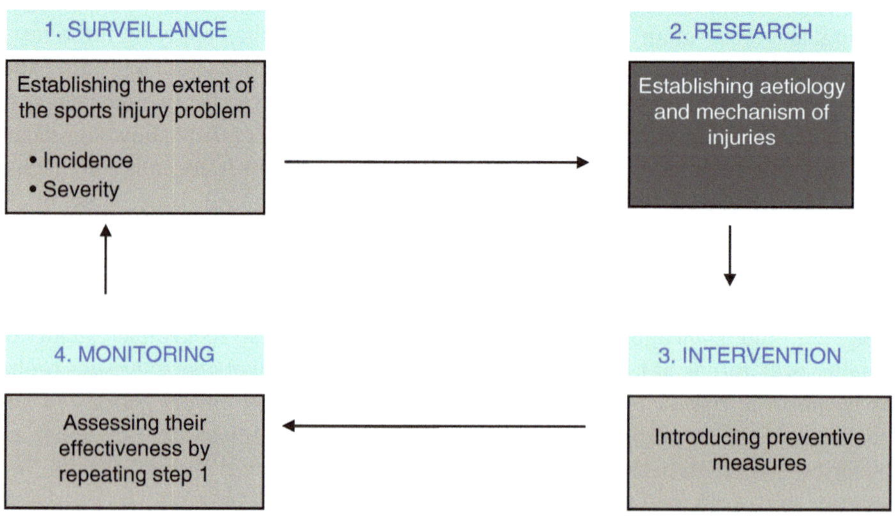


**Fig. 11.2** The sequence of prevention of sports injuries (Adapted from Van Mechelen, with permission from Adis International, Wolters Kluwer Health[46])

Concerning the muscle length measurements of the quadriceps, this study revealed significant increases in range of knee motion in both groups. However, since both training programs used the same stretching program, it was not surprising that no significant difference between both groups was observed (nor was it expected). The results of the study showed that only the closed kinetic chain group revealed a significant increase in explosive strength (jumping distance) during this study. This can be explained by the specificity of training, but favors the use of closed kinetic exercises for improving explosive functional strength. Looking at the reflex response times of VMO and VL in anterior knee pain patients, we found no significant alterations in this parameter either after an open or a closed kinetic chain program. This finding suggests that anterior knee pain patients still have an insufficient reflex response time of the VMO and VL after these training programs. Based on these findings, we are making an attempt to state that if the primary objective of a conservative or preventive treatment protocol is to modify this neuromuscular parameter, the use of these two exercise programs is not to be advised. In addition, these findings emphasize the need for studies analyzing the effect of specifically designed "VMO timing" programs. Relating to the mediolateral patellar mobility, the study did not show any significant changes after a 5 week treatment period in any of the two exercise groups.

The next step in the sequence of prevention is to construct a prevention program on the basis of the research findings described above. Until today, no such studies have been set up. Only some studies have been undertaken to evaluate the effectiveness of preventive strategies in sports medicine in general, and lower limb injuries specifically. This research has generally revealed that strategies designed to prevent sports injuries can be effective. These studies generally examined the effectiveness of a multifactorial program consisting of different items like correction of training, sport-specific cardiovascular conditioning, strength training, flexibility, and proprioceptive exercises. Therefore, it remains unclear which parts of the program were effective and which were not. However, some studies have examined the effect of solitary regular ankle disc training as a preventive measure. Although these studies were not performed to evaluate its effect on the incidence of anterior knee pain, this training seems to be promising to prevent both ankle and traumatic knee injuries.[49]

## 11.5 Constructing a Prevention Program for Anterior Knee Pain

### 11.5.1 *Influencing the Intrinsic Risk Factors of Anterior Knee Pain by Exercises*

On the basis of the available results in the literature, we made an attempt to describe where the emphasis of a prevention program of anterior knee pain to influence intrinsic risk factors should lie.

First, some literature reveals that a decreased flexibility of the hamstrings and quadriceps can be considered as risk factors of anterior knee pain. Consequently, it can be concluded that stretching of the hamstring and quadriceps should be considered as an important aspect of a preventive (and conservative) treatment program in anterior knee pain patients, and should preferably be incorporated in these treatment programs.

Regarding the use of an open or closed kinetic chain exercise program, it should be mentioned that these programs were not able to alter two of the four examined intrinsic risk factors. In addition, only the closed kinetic chain program was able to alter significantly the explosive strength. This seems to be an important issue, since several investigators have found a strong association between quadriceps strength increase and locomotor function in patients with anterior knee pain.[41,45] Natri and colleagues[35] not only observed that this association was important in the short-term outcome, but identified a strong correlation between restoration of quadriceps muscle strength and the long-term (7-year) final outcome in anterior knee pain patients. This, and the several clinical studies that show good-to-excellent results in anterior knee pain patients when emphasizing quadriceps strengthening point to the importance of a good functional quadriceps strength.[8] This implies that it can be stated that functional quadriceps strengthening should be an important aspect of a prevention program of anterior knee pain. The fact that a functional strength deficit, and not an analytical strength deficit, was identified as a risk factor of anterior knee pain leads us to conclude that the use of functional strength training as a preventive measure should be advised. To identify subjects with a low explosive strength, we advice the use of a single leg hop test or a triple jump test (Fig. 11.3).

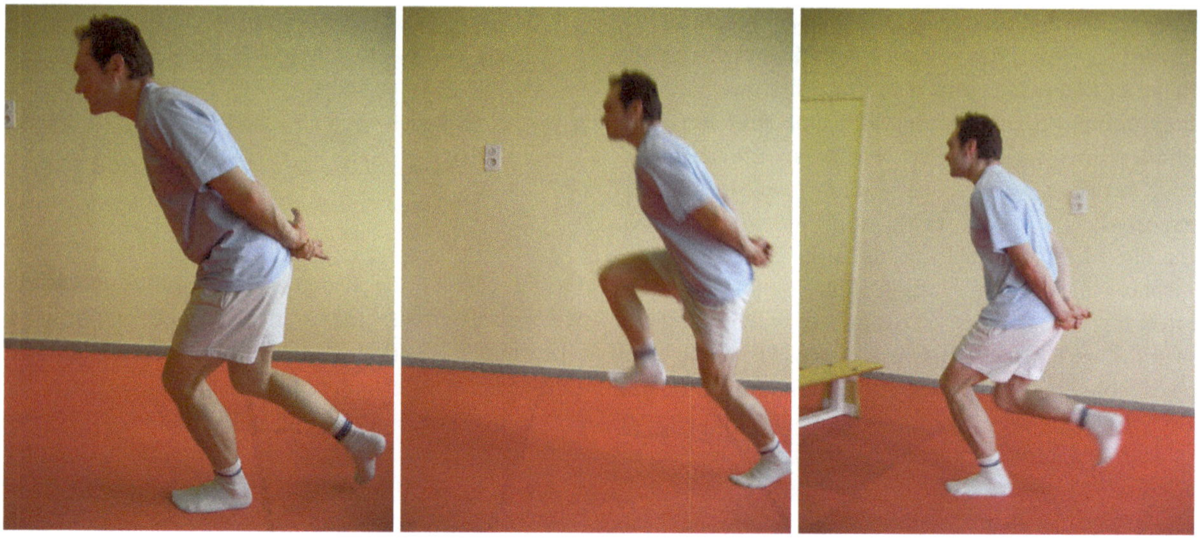

**Fig. 11.3** Performance of the single leg hop test. The arms stay at the back during the entire test

### 11.5.2 Influencing the Intrinsic Risk Factors of Anterior Knee Pain by External Devices

#### 11.5.2.1 Using Foot Orthoses in the Prevention of Anterior Knee Pain

Identification of Alterations in Foot Alignment in Anterior Knee Pain

Lun and colleagues[29] identified forefoot varus as a potential risk factor of anterior knee pain in recreational runners. On the basis of this prospective study, it is our opinion that it is necessary to evaluate the foot alignment of subjects in regard to a preventive treatment approach. It has been shown that the proper choice of adapted footwear has a positive influence on all overuse injuries of the lower limb by diminishing the deleterious impact forces.[9,10,20,23,24]

Prior to describing the effect of foot orthoses, it seems important to understand what is considered as a "normal" foot. According to Livingston and Mandigo,[28] the subtalar joint pronation accompanied by the eversion of the calcaneum, knee flexion, and the internal rotation of the tibia play an important role in the shock absorption at heel contact. The subtalar joint continues to pronate until the end of the foot flat phase. Thereafter, the subtalar joint starts to supinate combined with a knee extension and external rotation of the tibia. A delayed subtalar supination and external rotation of the tibial bone results in a compensatory reaction in the knee joint and patellofemoral joint. For both pes planus and pes cavus, a higher risk of injury has been reported among physically active people.

Duffey and colleagues[10] demonstrated that as the foot collides with the ground during the first 10% of the support phase, the runner's weight, magnified by the acceleration of gravity, increases the load on the lower extremity. Concurrently, the support foot pronates, which serves to assist in absorbing the shock impact. In their study, anterior knee pain patients had 25% less pronation during this critical phase (5.1° vs. 6.4°), although the maximum pronation and rearfoot motion was not significantly different from a control group. They hypothesize that this action might have made a more rigid landing, thereby increasing the shock to the lower limb and patellofemoral joint. Duffey and colleagues[10] also recorded higher foot arches in the anterior knee pain group, which is consistent with the report of Cowan and colleagues[7] wherein an increase of activity-related injuries correlates with increased high arch height in army recruits. Nigg and colleagues[38] demonstrated that the transfer of foot inversion to internal leg rotation was found to increase significantly with increasing arch height.

Kaufmann and colleagues[26] performed a prospective study on the effect of foot structure and range of motion on anterior knee pain in approximately 140 recruits. They did not find any significant differences in the foot structure or rearfoot motion. They evaluated static and dynamic values but only in a total range of motion. The different phases of the gait were not analyzed as in the study of Duffey and colleagues,[10] which might be the origin of these inconsistencies.

By evaluating other kinetic variables of the rearfoot, Messier and colleagues[33] did not find significant differences between runners with anterior knee pain and a control group regarding the rearfoot motion in their study. Regarding the literature on the relation between the rearfoot motion and anterior knee pain, many contradictions can be found. The methodological differences and the multifactorial nature of the conducted studies could explain parts of these discrepancies.

#### Effects of Foot Orthoses

The effects of foot orthoses have been biomechanically investigated through kinematics and pressure pattern of the foot. Orthoses have been reported to reduce maximum pronation velocity, time to maximal pronation, and total rearfoot motion during walking and running activities.[42] They also appear to limit the internal rotation of the tibia and the Q-angle at the patellofemoral joint. This latter effect will reduce the laterally directed resultant forces of the soft tissues and would theoretically reduce the contact pressure of the patella on the femoral condyles.[18]

Eng and Pierrynowski[13] studied the effect of soft foot orthotics on 3D lower limb kinematics during walking and running activities. The analysis of ten adolescent female subjects suffering from anterior knee pain and having a forefoot varus and calcaneal valgus greater than 6° showed small changes (1–3°) in the transverse and frontal plane motion of the talocrural/subtalar joint and knee during both walking and running. These very small changes were sufficient to influence the symptoms of the subjects.[12]

According to several authors,[25,27,36,37] orthoses have no influence on the quadriceps muscle function (VMO-VL), but they contribute to the alignment of the patellofemoral joint by minor changes in the patellar position (medial glide). In a recently published study, Hertel and colleagues[21] contradict these earlier findings. During slow single-leg squat and lateral step down, the EMG recordings of the VM, VL, and gluteus medius muscle differed in the foot orthotic conditions. The most surprising finding in their study was that all foot types react in the same, positive way to four different orthoses. These changes were not significant when performing explosive exercises like vertical jumps.

Sutlive and colleagues[44] conducted challenging research on the identification of anterior knee pain patients whose pain and symptoms improved after a combined program of orthoses and activity modification. Due to the multifactorial character of the impairment, not all anterior knee pain patients need orthoses. The identification of the risk factors in a primary prevention setting would be even more challenging.

We can conclude by assuming that the foot mechanics indirectly and subtly influences the patellofemoral joint, although the exact mechanisms are not fully understood. Anterior knee pain patients with altered foot alignment characteristics or running biomechanics might benefit from foot orthoses as demonstrated by some researchers. The use of orthoses as a preventive measure makes sense on a theoretical basis, but regarding the subtle biomechanical modifications caused by orthoses on anterior knee pain patients,[13,18] it is doubtful that clear clinical guidelines could be fine-tuned. Striking is the finding that no prospective studies on the use of orthoses as preventive measure for anterior knee pain are yet performed. Therefore, today no substantial evidence exists on the preventive use of foot orthoses for anterior knee pain.

### 11.5.2.2 Patellofemoral Bracing

The malalignment of the patella and lower limb is widely accepted as an important etiological factor of anterior knee pain.[15] Despite the fact that prospective studies have minimized the importance of "minor" alterations in the clinically measured lower leg alignment characteristics, mediolateral patellar hypermobility was identified as an intrinsic risk factor of anterior knee pain. Since this parameter seems to play an important role in the genesis of anterior knee pain, prevention programs should attempt to decrease this parameter in subjects with a hypermobile patella. Our study, however, failed to influence this characteristic after a 5-week training program with open or closed kinetic chain exercises. Interestingly, the function of patellofemoral knee braces is to improve the patellar tracking and maintain the patellofemoral alignment. Besides this mechanical function, some authors suggest other mechanisms (thermal effect, an increased sensory feedback, an altered circulation of the knee region) by which the brace may be effective.[4] Preventive patellofemoral bracing may be viewed as a method to help maintain an ideal biomechanical environment in order to avoid irritation of the surrounding tissues.

To our knowledge, only two prospective studies have been published on the effectiveness of braces in the prevention of anterior knee pain.[2,48] BenGal and colleagues[2] studied the efficacy of the knee brace with supportive ring as a means of preventing anterior knee pain in 60 young athletes. They found a significant reduction in the incidence of anterior knee pain at the end of the study in the braced group compared to the control group. Van Tiggelen and colleagues[48] used a different brace: the On-Track (DJ-Orthopedics) dynamic patellofemoral brace (Fig. 11.4). This brace consists of knee patches with Velcro (Velcro USA Inc., Manchester, NH) and a neoprene sleeve. The design of the brace is based on the correction of the position of the patella as described by McConnell.[30] The little plastic button (activator) foreseen to stimulate the vastus medialis obliquus (VMO) muscle was not used in this study. They performed their prospective study on 167 recruits (54 braced and 113 controls) undergoing basic military training. A smaller number of recruits in the brace group appeared to develop anterior knee pain compared to the recruits in the control group ($p=0.02$). Out of the 54 recruits in the brace group, 10 (18.5%) developed anterior knee pain during this study. In the control group ($n=113$), 42 recruits (37%) developed anterior knee pain. Hence, the results of both studies seem to scientifically support the effectiveness of a knee brace in the prevention of anterior knee pain. Nonetheless, the mechanism by which bracing seems to influence the prevention or the treatment of anterior knee pain remains enigmatic.[41] In the literature, in addition to a pure mechanical mechanism,[39] an increased sensory feedback is proposed. By using the term "increased sensory feedback," an alteration in

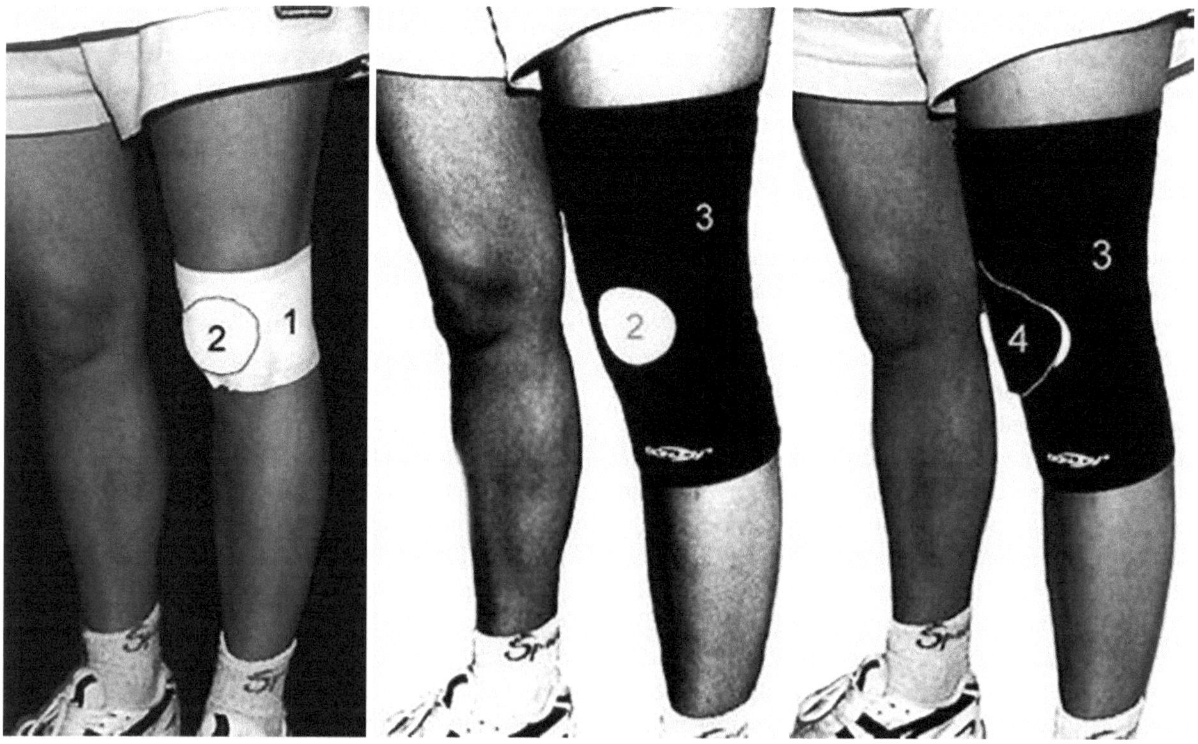


**Fig. 11.4** The On-Track brace (Donjoy) in three parts. A self-adhesive patch (*1*) is applied on the knee with the loop circle (*2*) on the patella. The neoprene cuff (*3*) is pulled onto the leg so the loop circle shows through the opening of the cuff. The hook circle (*4*) is attached to the loop circle on the patch (Reproduced from Van Tiggelen et al.[48] with kind permission of Springer Science+Business Media)

proprioception[3,31,40] and an altered muscular recruitment are proposed.[6,17,19,39] In a yet unpublished report, we were interested in the long-term effects (6 weeks) of continuous bracing. In this study, we analyzed, on an isokinetic device, the quadriceps muscle peak torque of the braced and non-braced recruits who didn't develop anterior knee pain in our previous study,[48] before and after the strenuous training in non-braced test conditions. After the 6 week vigorous basic military training program, we observed a significantly higher quadriceps peak torque in the braced group compared to the non-braced group. Since both groups showed equal strength prior to the basic military training program, the results suggest that 6 weeks of knee bracing has a positive effect on the quadriceps muscle strength. This suggests that besides the possible mechanical effect of bracing in controlling the mediolateral patellar mobility, knee bracing might prevent anterior knee pain by some way of facilitating muscular quadriceps activity.

Irrespective of the exact underlying mechanism of bracing, studies showed its significant preventive effect on the development of anterior knee pain during strenuous training. Therefore, the results of these studies support the use of prophylactic patellofemoral bracing in subjects undergoing vigorous activities. However, further research is needed to improve our insight in the underlying working mechanisms of prophylactic bracing on anterior knee pain.

Kneepads can also be used as a protective measure for anterior knee pain due to a direct blow. These are often used by athletes in volleyball, skating, and hockey, but also by plumbers, carpenters, welders, and even soldiers.

## 11.6 Conclusions

The etiopathogenic basis of anterior knee pain must be considered as multifactorial. Consequently, before any prevention program can be constructed, knowledge of the intrinsic and extrinsic risk factors of anterior knee pain is needed. The association between clinical overload of the patellofemoral joint (extrinsic risk factors) and anterior knee pain is well known. However, since only very few prospective studies are performed, the importance and identification of the different intrinsic risk factors of anterior knee pain remains enigmatic.

However, determination of these intrinsic risk factors of anterior knee pain is the first step in the sequence of injury prevention. Trying to interpret the few existing prospective and follow-up studies, it seems clear that the quadriceps muscle can be considered as an important characteristic in the genesis of anterior knee pain. Consequently, training of this muscle seems the cornerstone in the prevention of anterior knee pain. Data on the quadriceps muscle seem to show that the flexibility and the functional strength are important. Accordingly, it can be postulated that stretching of the hamstring and quadriceps should be considered as an important aspect of a preventive (and conservative) treatment program in anterior knee pain patients, and should preferably be incorporated in these treatment programs.

Concerning the muscle strength of the quadriceps, it seems that especially a lack of "functional" quadriceps strength is an important aspect in the development of anterior knee pain. This leads us to conclude that the use of functional strength training (closed kinetic chain exercises) as a preventive measure should be advised.

Striking, and not in agreement with common practice, these very few prospective data seem to indicate that clinically measured lower leg alignment characteristics such as leg length difference, height, weight, Q angle, genu varum/valgum, and recurvatum seem not to be that important in the development of anterior knee pain.

Although some studies have shown the beneficial effect of the use of orthotics in the treatment of anterior knee pain, no prospective studies on the use of orthoses as preventive measure for AKP are yet performed. Therefore, today no substantial evidence exists on the preventive use of foot orthoses for anterior knee pain.

On the other hand, two prospective studies have shown that patellofemoral bracing does help to prevent anterior knee pain in subjects undergoing a strenuous training program. The exact underlying mechanism remains obscure, but one study showed that bracing is able to facilitate quadriceps strength.

However, it must be remembered that conclusions drawn in this chapter are based on the results of relatively few prospective data and should therefore always be warranted. Accordingly, it seems obvious that a lot of research is still needed before a scientific prevention program for anterior knee pain can be composed.

## References


1. Almeida SA, Williams KM, Shaffer RA, et al. Epidemiological patterns of musculoskeletal injuries and physical training. *Med Sci Sports Exerc.* 1999;31:1176-1182.
2. BenGal S, Lowe J, Mann G, et al. The role of the knee brace in the prevention of anterior knee pain syndrome. *Am J Sports Med.* 1997;25:118-122.
3. Birmingham TB, Inglis JT, Kramer JF, et al. Effect of a neoprene sleeve on knee joint kinesthesis: influence of different testing procedures. *Med Sci Sports Exerc.* 2000;32:304-308.
4. Cherf J, Paulos LE. Bracing for patellar instability. *Clin Sports Med.* 1990;9:813-821.
5. Clement DB, Taunton JE, Smart GW, et al. A survey of overuse running injuries. *Phys Sports Med.* 1981;9:47-58.
6. Cowan SM, Bennell KL, Hodges PW. Therapeutic patellar taping changes the timing of vasti muscle activation in people with patellofemoral pain syndrome. *Clin J Sport Med.* 2002;12:339-347.
7. Cowan DN, Jones BH, Robinson JR. Foot morphologic characteristics and risk of exercise-related injury. *Arch Fam Med.* 1993;2:773-777.
8. Crossley K, Bennell K, Green S, et al. Physical therapy for patellofemoral pain: a randomized, double-blinded, placebo-controlled trial. *Am J Sports Med.* 2002;30:857-865.
9. Dixon SJ, Waterworth C, Smith CV, et al. Biomechanical analysis of running in military boots with new and degraded insoles. *Med Sci Sports Exerc.* 2003;35:472-479.
10. Duffey MJ, Martin DF, Cannon DW, et al. Etiologic factors associated with anterior knee pain in distance runners. *Med Sci Sports Exerc.* 2000;32:1825-1832.
11. Dye SF. Therapeutic implications of a tissue homeostasis approach to patellofemoral pain syndrome. *Sports Med Arthrosc.* 2001;9:306-311.
12. Eng JJ, Pierrynowski MR. Evaluation of soft foot orthotics in the treatment of patellofemoral pain syndrome. *Phys Ther.* 1993;73:62-68; discussion 68-70.
13. Eng JJ, Pierrynowski MR. The effect of soft foot orthotics on three-dimensional lower-limb kinematics during walking and running. *Phys Ther.* 1994;74:836-844.
14. Fairbank JC, Pynsent PB, Van Poortvliet JA. Mechanical factors in the incidence of knee pain in adolescents and young adults. *J Bone Joint Surg Br.* 1984;66:685-693.
15. Fulkerson JP, Arendt EA. Anterior knee pain in females. *Clin Orthop Relat Res.* 2000;372:69-73.
16. Fulkerson JP, Shea KP. Current concepts review. Disorders of patellofemoral alignment. *J Bone Joint Surg.* 1990; 72-A:1424-1429.
17. Gilleard W, McConnell J, Parsons D. The effect of patellar taping on the onset of vastus medialis obliquus and vastus lateralis muscle activity in persons with patellofemoral pain. *Phys Ther.* 1998;78:25-32.
18. Gross MT, Foxworth JL. The role of foot orthoses as an intervention for patellofemoral pain. *J Orthop Sports Phys Ther.* 2003;33:661-670.
19. Gulling LK, Lephart SM, Stone DA, et al. The effect of patellar bracing on quadriceps EMG activity during isokinetic exercise. *Isokinet Exerc Sci.* 1996;6:133-138.
20. Hardin EC, van den Bogert AJ, Hamill J. Kinematic adaptations during running: effects of footwear, surface, and duration. *Med Sci Sports Exerc.* 2004;36:838-844.
21. Hertel J, Sloss BR, Earl JE. Effect of foot orthotics on quadriceps and gluteus medius electromyographic activity during selected exercises. *Arch Phys Med Rehabil.* 2005;86:26-30.
22. Hoffman JR, Chapnik L, Shamis A, et al. The effect of leg strength on the incidence of lower extremity overuse injuries during military training. *Mil Med.* 1999;164:153-156.
23. House CM, Waterworth C, Allsopp AJ, et al. The influence of simulated wear upon the ability of insoles to reduce peak pressures during running when wearing military boots. *Gait Posture.* 2002;16:297-303.
24. Hreljac A. Impact and overuse injuries in runners. *Med Sci Sports Exerc.* 2004;36:845-849.
25. Hung YJ, Gross MT. Effect of foot position on electromyographic activity of the vastus medialis oblique and vastus lateralis during lower-extremity weight-bearing activities. *J Orthop Sports Phys Ther.* 1999;29:93-102; discussion 103–105.
26. Kaufman KR, Brodine SK, Shaffer RA, et al. The effect of foot structure and range of motion on musculoskeletal overuse injuries. *Am J Sports Med.* 1999;27:585-593.
27. Klingman RE. Foot pronation and patellofemoral joint function. *J Orthop Sports Phys Ther.* 1999;29:421.
28. Livingston LA, Mandigo JL. Bilateral rearfoot asymmetry and anterior knee pain syndrome. *J Orthop Sports Phys Ther.* 2003;33:48-55.
29. Lun V, Meeuwisse WH, Stergiou P, et al. Relation between running injury and static lower limb alignment in recreational runners. *Br J Sports Med.* 2004;38:576-580.
30. McConnell J. The management of chondromalacia patellae: a long-term solution. *Aust J Physiotheraphy.* 1986;32:215-223.
31. McNair PJ, Stanley SN, Strauss GR. Knee bracing: effects on proprioception. *Arch Phys Med Rehabil.* 1996;77: 287-289.
32. Meeuwisse WH. Assessing causation in sport injury: a multifactorial model. *Clin J Sport Med.* 1994;4:166-170.
33. Messier SP, Davis SE, Curl WW, et al. Etiologic factors associated with patellofemoral pain in runners. *Med Sci Sports Exerc.* 1991;23:1008-1015.
34. Milgrom C, Finestone A, Shlamkovitch N, et al. Anterior knee pain caused by overactivity: a long term prospective followup. *Clin Orthop Relat Res.* 1996;331:256-260.
35. Natri A, Kannus P, Järvinen M. Which factors predict the long-term outcome in chronic patellofemoral pain? *Med Sci Sports Exerc.* 1998;30:1572-1577.
36. Nawoczenski DA, Ludewig PM. Electromyographic effects of foot orthotics on selected lower extremity muscles during running. *Arch Phys Med Rehabil.* 1999;80:540-544.
37. Neptune RR, Wright IC, van den Bogert AJ. The influence of orthotic devices and vastus medialis strength and timing on patellofemoral loads during running. *Clin Biomech (Bristol, Avon).* 2000;15:611-618.
38. Nigg BM, Cole GK, Nachbauer W. Effects of arch height of the foot on angular motion of the lower extremities in running. *J Biomech.* 1993;26:909-916.
39. Parsons D, Gilleard W. The effect of patellar taping on quadriceps activity onset in the absence of pain. *J Appl Biomech.* 1999;15:373-380.

40. Perlau R, Frank C, Fick G. The effect of elastic bandages on human knee proprioception in the uninjured population. *Am J Sports Med.* 1995;23:251-255.
41. Powers CM. Rehabilitation of the patellofemoral joint disorders: a critical review. *J Orthop Sports Phys Ther.* 1998;28: 345-354.
42. Razeghi M, Batt ME. Biomechanical analysis of the effect of orthotic shoe inserts: a review of the literature. *Sports Med.* 2000;29:425-438.
43. Reider B. An ounce of prevention. *Am J Sports Med.* 2004; 32:1383-1384.
44. Sutlive TG, Mitchell SD, Maxfield SN, et al. Identification of individuals with patellofemoral pain whose symptoms improved after a combined program of foot orthoses use and modified activity: a preliminary investigation. *Phys Ther.* 2004;84:49-61.
45. Thomee R, Augustsson J, Karlsson J. Patellofemoral pain syndrome: a review of current issues. *Sports Med.* 1999;28: 245-262.
46. Van Mechelen W, Hlobil H, Kemper HC, et al. Incidence, aetiology and prevention of sports injuries: a review of concepts. *Sports Med.* 1992;14:82-89.
47. Van Tiggelen D, Witvrouw E, Coorevits P, et al. Analysis of isokinetic parameters in the development of anterior knee pain syndrome: a prospective study in a military setting. *Isokinet Exerc Sci.* 2004;12:223-228.
48. Van Tiggelen D, Witvrouw E, Roget Ph, et al. Effect of bracing on the prevention of anterior knee pain: a prospective randomized study. *Knee Surg Sports Traumatol Arthrosc.* 2004;12:434-439.
49. Wedderkopp N, Kaltoft M, Lundgaard B. Prevention of injuries in young female players in European team handball: a prospective intervention study. *Scand J Med Sci Sports.* 1999;9:41-47.
50. Witvrouw E, Lysens R, Bellemans J, et al. Intrinsic risk factors for the development of anterior knee pain in an athletic population: a two-year prospective study. *Am J Sports Med.* 2000;28:480-489.

# Non-operative Treatment of Athletes with Anterior Knee Pain: Science, Classical, and New Ideas

12

Suzanne Werner

## 12.1 Introduction

Anterior knee pain (AKP) is one of the most common knee disorders in physically active individuals.[29,34,95] The definition of AKP and the pathophysiological background are disputed. Despite several scientific studies through the years, the reason for AKP is still unclear. Grana and Kriegshauser maintain that the cause of AKP is multifactorial.[50] Some authors mean that anatomical patella abnormalities could be causative factors (e.g., ref.[48]), while others mean that it is an extensor mechanism disorder, resulting in patellar malalignment during flexion and extension of the knee joint.[47,52,60,118] Why this extensor mechanism disorder has developed is, however, not reported. There are also those authors maintaining that overuse is the most dominating reason for AKP, especially in youths.[34,115]

## 12.2 Symptoms

Typical symptoms are pain and/or problems during stair climbing, mostly when descending stairs and squatting as well as during prolonged sitting with flexed knees, the so-called movie sign.[42,95] AKP is often described as dull and aching with occasional episodes of acute sharp pain.[35] Giving way is another common symptom due to a sudden reflex inhibition of the quadriceps muscle, often while performing some movement with the knee flexing or extending under load, e.g., during stair climbing. Patients sometimes report locking of the knee, which usually only is a catching sensation on an attempt to extend the knee joint under load. However, the AKP patients commonly are able to actively unlock the knee and therefore this type of locking should not be mixed up with the one experienced by patients with meniscal lesions.[42] A few AKP patients present with mild swelling due to synovial irritation.[41] The different symptoms in patients with AKP are frequently related to sports[1,38,47] and usually become aggravated by physical activity with knee loading characteristics.[61]

## 12.3 Patellar Pain Versus Patellar Instability Problems

Some patients with AKP mostly complain of nonspecific knee pain localized peripatellarly, often anteromedially and/or retropatellarly,[1,38,47,61] while others complain of a feeling of patellar instability.[1,38,43] Patients that mostly complain of pain usually have a normal patellar mobility and they mainly report the symptoms to occur after physical activity, while those with patellar instability often present with a patellar hypermobility with noticeable tracking problems and they rather complain of knee problems during physical activity.[63] This means that the AKP patients should be divided into two treatment groups, one where the treatment mainly should be based on pain limitation and another one on stabilization of the patella.

S. Werner
Stockholm Sports Trauma Research Center,
Karolinska institutet, Stockholm, Sweden Capio Artro Clinic,
Stockholm, Sweden
e-mail: suzanne.werner@ki.se

V. Sanchis-Alfonso (ed.), *Anterior Knee Pain and Patellar Instability*,
DOI: 10.1007/978-0-85729-507-1_12, © Springer-Verlag London Limited 2011

## 12.4 Personality: Psychological Factors

Many authors have studied the relationship between personality and chronic pain (e.g., ref.[14]). Fritz et al. reported presence of psychological factors associated with knee pain in adolescence complaining of different types of knee pain.[39] Some studies on patients with AKP show a bad correlation between the patients' clinical symptoms and the clinicians objective findings (e.g., ref.[8]). Jacobson and Flandry reported that some of the patients that came to visit the doctor for AKP problems at a Sport Medicine Clinic were having both chronic AKP and psychological problems.[63] Thomeé et al. studied the coping strategies for pain that AKP patients use.[116] They found that their degree of well-being is in agreement with other patient groups with chronic pain. However, some concerns could be raised in terms of the high scores that AKP patients reported for the coping strategy "catastrophizing."[116] Carlsson et al. used the Rorschach test and found elevations in psychological parameters such as hostility, dependency, and depression in AKP patients compared with healthy controls, matched for gender and age, as well as with three other reference groups.[15] However, these problems are not always evident for the patient himself or herself, and their character may also vary.[15] In such cases, a psychological evaluation is often advisable and therefore, collaboration with a pain clinic with psychological expertise may be beneficial.

## 12.5 Clinical Evaluation

The clinical examination establishes the diagnosis and tries to determine the underlying causative factors of the patient's symptoms and based on this, the appropriate treatment program can be designed.[81,134] A thorough clinical examination is the key for optimal treatment of patients with AKP. This is due to that this category of patients present with a myriad of symptoms and complaints. Since we still do not know the pathophysiological reason for AKP, we concentrate our treatment on the patient's symptoms and on the clinician's findings.

### *12.5.1 Risk Factors*

A few studies on risk factors for AKP have been published. Milgrom et al. reported presence of genu varum and high isometric quadriceps strength to be risk factors for developing AKP.[85] Witvrouw et al. found that a shortened vastus medialis obliquus (VMO) reflex response time, a decreased flexibility of the quadriceps muscle, an increased medial patellar mobility, and a reduction of vertical jump performance were significantly correlated with the incidence of AKP.[132] Recently, Thijs et al. prospectively evaluated possible gait-related risk factors for AKP in officer cadets entering a Military Academy without a history of any knee or lower leg complaints.[113] After a 6-week basic military training period, they found that a heel strike in a less pronated position and roll over more on the lateral side was a risk factor for developing AKP.[113]

### *12.5.2 History*

It is important to obtain an accurate and thorough subjective history from the patient. Paying attention to this history will greatly aid the clinician in making an accurate assessment of the patient's condition and design an appropriate treatment program.[5,16]

### *12.5.3 Differential Diagnosis*

The careful objective evaluation must include screening to rule out other pathology than patellofemoral problems.[5] The differential diagnosis of AKP should primarily be based on localization of the pain. The patient with a "true" AKP syndrome is usually recognized by having a distinct palpable tenderness peripatellarly, mostly anteromedially and/or retropatellarly (e.g., refs.[1,38,47,61]). We cannot rule out that patients complaining of retropatellar pain have pain of other reasons than chondromalacia patellae, unless we examine this with arthroscopy or magnetic resonance imaging. However, chondromalacia patients usually present with the same variations of symptoms and findings as AKP patients without chondromalacia patellae. Nowadays, both AKP patients with and without chondromalacia patellae are mainly receiving the same nonoperative treatment, based on each patient's symptoms and findings. Furthermore, tenderness in the lateral retinaculum, which might be tight,[126] and the insertion of the vastus lateralis (VL) is relatively common in patients with AKP.[40]

Fairbank's sign, a passive movement of the patella laterally, is an apprehension test and a classical examination that can be used to differentiate AKP from two other diagnoses that should be treated differently, patellar subluxation and patellar dislocation. A positive Fairbank's sign is associated with a giving-way feeling of the patella laterally and tenderness at the medial margin of the patella.[38] When considering the possible differential diagnosis, one should also be aware of that the lumbar spine and the hip can refer symptoms to the knee.[81]

### 12.5.4 Alignment of the Lower Extremity

The clinical examination should consist of a careful control of the entire lower extremity. This should be performed in a standing position when determining the alignment of the lower extremity. Possible prevalence of increased internal femoral rotation that can be observed clinically, which often causes a squinting of the patella, and compensatory external tibial torsion should be noted as well as genu recurvatum, genu valgum, and hyperpronation of the subtalar joint (e.g., refs.[16,63,81,108]). Furthermore, it is important to control the patient's foot position during weightbearing, e.g., walking and running, and check how his/her shoes, especially sport shoes, are worn.

### 12.5.5 Quadriceps Angle

Measurement of the quadriceps angle (Q-angle) belongs to the classical examination protocol in AKP patients; despite that, the correlation between an increased Q-angle and the patient's symptoms can be questioned (e.g., ref.[34]). The Q-angle itself is not a reliable indicator of patellar alignment. However, it should be regarded as one bit of information, which might correlate with other clinical findings in order to understand a malalignment problem as fully as possible.[42] The measurement of the Q-angle has a good intra- and interreliability when performed with the patient in a supine position with relaxed quadriceps muscles[17] and the patella localized in the trochlea and approximately in 30° of knee flexion.[42] A normal Q-angle is reported to be 12° in males and 15° in females.[81]

### 12.5.6 Patellar Position

Assessing the orientation of the patella relative to the femur and controlling the patellar position within the patellofemoral joint should be done. An optimal patellar position is when the patella is parallel to the femur in the frontal and the sagittal planes, and when the patella is midway between the two condyles during 20° of knee flexion.[81] Possible anatomical variations such as patella alta, patella infera, tilted patella, and rotated patella should be checked for. One should be aware of that a high-riding patella (patella alta) is reported to be a risk factor for patellar subluxation or dislocation,[62] while patients with patella infera rather seem to complain of patellar pain at the area of apex patellae. Tilted patella with a medial "opening", a lateral tilt, seems to be relatively common in AKP patients. The reason for this depends on tightness of the lateral retinaculum, which will tilt the patella so that the medial border of the patella is higher than the lateral border.[81] Furthermore, a hypotrophy of the VMO may aid in creating lateral patellar tilt. There are some patients presenting with an externally rotated patella, when the inferior pole of the patella is sitting lateral to the long axis of the femur, indicating tightness of the lateral retinaculum. Very few patients present with the opposite, an internally rotated patella. The ideal patellar position is when the long axis of the femur is parallel to the long axis of the patella.[81]

### 12.5.7 Patellar Mobility

Patellar mobility should also be checked.[16,43,63,111] "Patellar tracking test" is performed by clinically observing patellar movement by manual resistance against concentric as well as eccentric open kinetic chain knee extension, and during closed kinetic chain in knee loading conditions, e.g., single-leg squat. A number of patients complain mostly of patellar instability problems.[1,38,43] This patellar instability feeling is the second most common symptom in patients with imbalance of the muscles around the patellofemoral joint, which probably depends on a sudden inhibition of the quadriceps due to pain.[1] The patella can be unstable laterally, medially, or multidirectionally.[59,111,118] Clinically, those patients often have a hypermobile patella and an observable tracking disorder.[125] Assessment of patellar mobility belongs to a complete knee examination. Manually produced passive medial and lateral displacement is a reproducible method for checking passive patellar motion.[105] The patella is surrounded by a rather mobile structure, which means that in full extension, the patella can be passively moved about 20 mm both laterally and medially.[38] However, as the knee flexes, the patellar mobility decreases and it should be checked in a slight knee flexion (approximately 30° of knee flexion), when the patella has a better congruency in the patellofemoral joint. Osborne and Farquharson-Roberts suggest that a passive deviation of 10 mm as well laterally as medially should be diagnosed as normal patellar mobility,[91] and this should be judged in the slightly flexed knee.

### 12.5.8 Quadriceps Muscle Strength

The quadriceps muscle is often weakened in patients with AKP.[122] Manual muscle testing performed as a side-to-side comparison gives a rough awareness of quadriceps strength. If possible, isokinetic measurement of the quadriceps torque is recommended. However, isokinetic testing must be used cautiously[41] and patients with patellar hypermobility should not be measured eccentrically during fast angular velocities (>90°/s) due to risk of subluxation or even dislocation.[121] During the isokinetic measurements, it is preferable to evaluate whether pain inhibition might interfere with the "true" result of muscle torques. This could nicely be done with twitch interpolation technique,[83] but also to some extent by evaluating possible pain with Borg's pain scale[10] or the visual analogue scale (VAS).[20,37,99]

### 12.5.9 Hamstring/Quadriceps Ratio

Imbalance between the hamstring and quadriceps muscles is frequently shown in patients with AKP. This usually depends on a weakened quadriceps muscle but a normal strength of the hamstrings, which subsequently results in a higher hamstring/quadriceps ratio compared to healthy subjects.[122] The hamstring/quadriceps ratio in patients with AKP is reported to be between 0.65 and 0.70, while the corresponding values in healthy subjects is about 0.50, when measurements have been performed with an isokinetic dynamometer, where torque values were corrected for gravitational force.[122]

### 12.5.10 Vastus Medialis Versus Vastus Lateralis

Hypotrophy of the vastus medialis (VM) is common in AKP patients (e.g., refs.[51,78]), and VM is the weakest and most vulnerable muscle of the extensor mechanism.[38] VL comprises the largest muscle mass and extensor power of the quadriceps muscle group. This is probably the reason why VM hypotrophy is a common finding in AKP patients,[16,51] and that the patients also often present with a reduced electromyography (EMG) activity of the VM in their symptomatic leg compared to their contralateral healthy leg (e.g., refs.[16,78]). VMO:VL ratio has also been reported to be lower in AKP patients compared with healthy subjects.[12,18,86] The lower activity of VM and the higher activity of VL could lead to an imbalance between VM and VL.[78,96] Unbalanced actions of the quadriceps components are closely linked to patellar maltracking and AKP. During knee extension, VM pulls the patella first medially and then proximally, while VL pulls the patella first proximally and then laterally. VMO pulls the patella mainly medially and vastus medialis longus (VML) more proximally.[74] It has also been reported that the onset of the VL contraction occurs before that of the VMO, indicating a difference in motor control in AKP patients compared to asymptomatic controls.[23,25,26] Furthermore, it is postulated that the VMO needs time to develop force, relative to the VL, for optimal patellar tracking.[49] Since VL has a larger cross-sectional area than the VMO, there is a tendency for the patella to track laterally. In a controlled laboratory EMG study, maximum voluntary knee extensions during concentric as well as eccentric actions were evaluated in AKP patients and asymptomatic controls.[92] The result showed that the activation amplitude of the VMO and VL in AKP patients was mostly altered during eccentric contractions and differed significantly from the controls. The authors conclude that the activation amplitudes of the VMO and VL in AKP patients are consistent with a lateral tracking of the patella during eccentric contractions.[92] Furthermore, there are authors reporting that the time to activation often is disturbed in AKP patients.[120,133] Therefore, it is important to improve the onset of muscle activity of the VMO in many patients with AKP. Using EMG in a randomized double-blind, placebo-controlled trial, Cowan et al. reported that at baseline, the EMG onset of VL occurred prior to that of VMO in AKP patients.[25] Following a physical therapy intervention for 6 weeks, there was a significant change in the time of onset of EMG of VMO compared to VL with the onsets occurring simultaneously. This change was also associated with a reduction in symptoms.[25] In another controlled study, the same research group also showed that after six treatment sessions of physical therapy over a 6 week period, the onset of VMO preceded VL in the eccentric phase and occurred at the same time in the concentric phase of a stair-stepping task.[23] Several authors maintain that the primary role of VMO is to enhance patellar stabilization within the patellofemoral joint and to prevent lateral patellar subluxation by pulling the patella medially during knee extension and flexion.[38,78,80,96,100] Portney et al. maintain that VM, especially VMO, is important for optimal patellar movement within the patellofemoral joint during knee extension.[96] Almost 50 years ago, Brewerton,[13] followed by Lieb and Perry,[73] Martin and Londeree[79] and Bose et al.[11] reported VMO to be active during the full range of knee extension. Mariani et al. found the EMG activity of both VM and VL to be of similar degree and mostly pronounced during the last 30° of knee extension in healthy subjects.[78] Werner found that the two vasti muscles, however, were active throughout the range of motion of 90–10° of knee extension in healthy subjects. Furthermore, most healthy individuals present with higher EMG activity of the VL compared to VM, but there are also those that show higher EMG activity of the VM than VL and there is also a third group of healthy individuals that have about the same EMG activity of both vasti muscles (unpublished data). This means that it is important to check the muscle activity pattern between VM and VL of the patient's asymptomatic leg as well as his/her symptomatic leg when designing an optimal treatment protocol for patients with AKP. When bilateral problems exist, I suggest that one relies on the EMG activity pattern of the less symptomatic leg.

### 12.5.11 Flexibility

Soft tissue or muscle length is essential to musculoskeletal evaluation and have specific implications in patients with AKP. Smith et al. found poor hamstring and quadriceps flexibility to be correlated with AKP.[106] Tightness of the lateral muscle structures such as the tensor fascia lata and iliotibial band is associated with AKP.[31] All the above-mentioned muscle structures are relatively common and could have negative effects at the patellofemoral joint and should, therefore, be controlled. A tight iliotibial band will result in deviation of the patella laterally, lateral tracking and lateral tilting, and usually, also weakening of the medial retinaculum.[117] Tight hamstrings and gastrocnemius may lead to an increase in foot pronation of the subtalar joint, resulting in an increased valgus vector force at the knee, which can cause AKP problems.[32,67,82] Dorsiflexion of the talocrural joint will also decrease if the gastrocnemius is tight,[82] indicating biomechanical limitations and possible knee problems during walking and running. Furthermore, AKP patients sometimes show tightness of the lateral retinaculum, which might lead to an "opening" of the patella on the medial side, a lateral patellar tilt.

### 12.5.12 Knee-Related Functional Performance Tests

Dynamic evaluation with knee-related functional performance tests could be preferably used to reproduce the patient's symptoms and to make comparisons before and after a treatment period. There are different types of pain provocation tests that comprise knee function. Except for walking, there are more stressful activities such as stair climbing (up and down), steps up and down on different heights, double-leg and single-leg squat, and raise from a chair and sit down using one leg. These tests could be used to evaluate both quadriceps muscle function and the patient's subjective knee pain. Loudon et al. reported a good intrarater reliability of the following four functional performance tests: anteromedial lunge, step-down, single-leg press, and balance and reach.[76] Single-leg tests are very good indicators of controlling the extensor mechanism and thereby the patient's symptoms. Since the AKP patients often report symptoms during eccentric quadriceps work, walking downstairs is a good knee-related functional test for eccentric control of the quadriceps muscle. When the aim is to evaluate muscle function, those tests should be performed slowly, which makes it easier to observe possible patellar maltracking. However, those tests can also be evaluated according to the patient's subjective pain rating, which could be done by using Borg's pain scale[10] or the visual analogue scale.[20,37,99] Future research is needed to study intrarater reliability as well as interrater reliability, validity, and sensitivity of functional performance tests.[27]

### 12.5.13 Functional Knee Scores

During the last decade, many knee scoring systems for subjective evaluations have been utilized (e.g., ref.[70]). While signs such as, e.g., effusion, muscle hypotrophy, and muscle tightness are identified by the examining clinician, a knee score is built on the patient's own subjective evaluation of his/her knee function. Each functional score should be tested for reproducibility, meaning that the score is reliable for repeated measurements under the same conditions. Furthermore, the most optimal functional score should be tested for validity or sensitivity and thereby tailored for a specific diagnosis.

A knee score for functional evaluation of patients with AKP should consist of different categories of symptoms that are common in these patients. The Werner functional knee score (Table 12.1) is modified from an earlier published version.[123] A test–retest of this score has revealed a very good reproducibility, and to some extent we have also tested the sensitivity of the score, which reveals a good sensitivity to AKP patients (unpublished data). Fifty points at this particular knee score means lack of AKP, and subsequently, 0 means maximal knee problems. Due to the good reliability and sensitivity results, we can recommend the use of the Werner functional knee score for evaluating patients with AKP syndrome.

In order to investigate a possible prevalence of AKP following anterior cruciate ligament reconstruction, we have modified the above-mentioned functional knee score and tailored it for anterior cruciate ligament reconstructed patients (Table 12.2). This score has shown a good reproducibility when tested three times

**Table 12.1** Werner functional knee score for anterior knee pain (*Please, circle what usually applies to your knee problem(s)!*)

| | | | |
|---|---|---|---|
| *Pain* | | *Sitting with flexed knees >30 min* | |
| None | 5 | No problems | 5 |
| Slight and infrequent | 3 | Slightly impaired | 4 |
| Constant pain | 0 | Difficulties | 2 |
| | | Unable | 0 |
| *Occurrence of pain* | | *Squatting* | |
| No activity-related pain | 15 | No problems | 5 |
| During or after running | 12 | Slightly impaired | 4 |
| After >2-km walk | 9 | Difficulties | 2 |
| After <2-km walk | 6 | Unable | 0 |
| During normal walk | 3 | | |
| During rest | 0 | | |
| *Feeling of patellar instability* | | *Walking upstairs* | |
| Never | 5 | No problems | 5 |
| Sometimes | 3 | Slightly impaired | 4 |
| Frequently | 0 | Difficulties | 2 |
| | | Unable | 0 |
| *Arretations–catching* | | *Walking downstairs* | |
| Never | 5 | No problems | 5 |
| Sometimes | 3 | Slightly impaired | 4 |
| Frequently | 0 | Difficulties | 2 |
| | | Unable | 0 |
| Sum of points: ________ | | | |

**Table 12.2** Werner functional knee score for anterior knee pain after ACL reconstruction (*Please, circle what usually applies to your knee problem(s)!*)

| | | | |
|---|---|---|---|
| *Pain* | | *Sitting with flexed knees >30 min* | |
| None | 5 | No problems | 5 |
| Slight and infrequent | 3 | Slightly impaired | 4 |
| Constant pain | 0 | Difficulties | 2 |
| | | Unable | 0 |
| *Occurrence of pain* | | *Squatting* | |
| No activity-related pain | 15 | No problems | 5 |
| During or after running | 12 | Slightly impaired | 4 |
| After >2-km walk | 9 | Difficulties | 2 |
| After <2-km walk | 6 | Unable | 0 |
| During normal walk | 3 | | |
| During rest | 0 | | |
| *Kneeling* | | *Walking upstairs* | |
| No problems | 5 | No problems | 5 |
| Slightly impaired | 4 | Slightly impaired | 4 |
| Difficulties | 2 | Difficulties | 2 |
| Unable | 0 | Unable | 0 |
| *Arretations–catching* | | *Walking downstairs* | |
| Never | 5 | No problems | 5 |
| Sometimes | 3 | Slightly impaired | 4 |
| Frequently | 0 | Difficulties | 2 |
| | | Unable | 0 |
| Sum of points: ________ | | | |

in the same group of subjects. Furthermore, it has been shown to be most sensitive for patients with anterior cruciate ligament injuries (unpublished data).

## 12.6 Treatment

Nowadays, most orthopedic surgeons agree that patients with AKP and without any malalignment should be treated nonoperatively.[29,43,65,108] Only, if a careful long-term physical therapy program has failed, one might consider surgery.[33,47] The treatment protocol should be based on findings from the patient's history, clinical examination, and functional assessment.[112,129,134] A comprehensive treatment approach is often required to treat AKP patients successfully. When designing a treatment program, it is important to realize that each patient is specific and will present with different symptoms and signs, which makes it necessary to have a flexible treatment approach.[5] A thorough evaluation and assessment will reveal each patient's unique set of clinical signs, and the treatment protocol should be tailored to that patient.

Patient education is one of the key factors in the management of AKP. The patient must have a clear understanding of why the symptoms have occurred and what needs to be done to reduce the symptoms. Therefore, the patient should be informed already from the very start that the treatment period sometimes can last several months. This is due to the gradually progressive treatment protocol, often including a combination of different methods that is needed to restore good muscle activity and muscle strength, improve balance and coordination, and end up in a normal knee functional movement pattern.

The cause of AKP varies between patients. Each patient is unique, which means that the same treatment in different patients may lead to different effects. Therefore, it is important with a thorough clinical examination based on control of patellar mobility, muscle function and each patient's specific functional problem. Furthermore, the patient's history should be included in order to design an individual treatment program based on each patient's specific symptoms and findings.

If patellar hypermobility exists, the patella could initially be supported by a patellar stabilizing brace or patellar taping during the physical therapy treatment. However, it is of most importance to check in what direction the patella is hypermobile, laterally, medially or both. I recommend either taping or bracing in patients with a lateral or a medial hypermobility, and bracing in patients with both a lateral and medial hypermobility. The external patella supports, irrespective of what type, bracing or taping, should then gradually be removed, when the patient improves and his/her symptoms are reduced. This means that the last step in the rehabilitation protocol will be to remove the patient's patella support during dynamic heavy knee loading exercises that put great demands on stability of the patella.

Toward the end of the treatment period, it is recommended to stimulate the patient either to return to some kind of sport/physical activity or to start with a suitable regular physical exercise, where long walks could be an alternative. The reason for this is that the improved muscle function and balance that have been gained through the rehabilitation need to be maintained by physical exercises. We have found that patients, who start or continue with some kind of physical training following a treatment program, were the ones with good long-term results of knee function.[123,124]

### *12.6.1 Extensor Mechanism: Quadriceps Strengthening*

Several authors have emphasized the importance of quadriceps training in patients with AKP in order to improve the extensor mechanism (e.g., refs.[43,61,108]). Powers et al. reported functional ability to be associated with increased ability to generate quadriceps muscle torque.[98] However, the main objective is to strengthen the VM,[19] since appropriate timing and intensity of VMO activation relative to VL has been promoted as a key aspect in patients with AKP.[130,133] Therefore, the balance between VMO and VL should be restored before starting to train the entire quadriceps muscle group.

### *12.6.2 Training of Vastus Medialis Obliquus*

Muscular hypotrophy and a reduced and/or delayed EMG activity of the VM is very common in patients with AKP (e.g., refs.[19,51,78]). This will often result in an imbalance between the VM and the VL. Therefore, the initial treatment should consist of restoring the function of VMO in an attempt to enhance patellar stabilization.[9,18,38,78,80,107] The VMO is a stabilizing muscle, which means that endurance training is the ultimate goal and therefore, the patient should increase the number of repetitions rather than load.[101] The importance of this initial stage of treatment is further magnified by the fact that the rate of strength development for the VM has been shown to be slower than for the VL and the rectus femoris,[38,50,73] which might create the potential for patellar tracking dysfunction and the accompanying knee problems.

In the literature, there have been many suggestions to improve the VM by different exercises. Hanten and Schulthies reported significantly greater activity of the VM compared to VL by performing isometric hip adduction exercises.[53] Later, Karst and Jewett performed a similar study, where they combined straight leg raises with hip adduction, but they could not repeat the beneficial results from Hanten and Schulthies and therefore suggest isometric quadriceps exercises without hip adduction.[66] Laprade et al. also studied EMG activity of VM and VL during different exercises and they did not find a greater recruitment of the VM compared with VL during hip adduction or a combination of hip adduction and knee extension.[71] Nor could Cerny find increased activity of the VM over that of VL in commonly prescribed exercises.[18] Only terminal knee extension with the hip medially rotated resulted in a somewhat higher VM/VL activity.[18] Sczepanski et al. suggested isokinetic concentric knee extension exercises at 120°/s angular velocity within 60–85° of knee flexion in order to selectively activate the VMO and improve the balance between the two vasti muscles.[102] McConnell suggested patellar taping with a medial glide in order to prevent lateral tracking of the patella.[80] With the patella taped, the patient is instructed to tighten the medial portion of the quadriceps by isometrically contracting the hip adductors.[80] This exercise should be performed in a weightbearing position, walk stance with the symptomatic leg forward and the knee flexed to 30°.[80] Activation of adductor magnus has been reported to improve the contraction of the VMO during weightbearing.[57]

However, transcutaneous electrical muscle stimulation is the most optimal way proven to selectively contract and improve the function of VM.[123] Steadman proposed electrical muscle stimulation of VM in order to keep the patella in a proper position within the patellofemoral joint.[108] With the help of computer tomography, Werner et al. reported a significantly increased area of the VM after transcutaneous electrical stimulation of this muscle, while the VL was unchanged.[123] Two-thirds of those patients also improved from a functional point of view directly after 10 weeks of daily electrical stimulation, and at the follow-ups 1 year and 3.5 years later, the same patients still were improved.[123] Those patients have also been followed prospectively on average 13 years later and more than half of the patients reported to be symptom-free (unpublished data). The rest of the patients reported to have minor AKP occurring mostly during physical activities such as running. Only one-fourth of the patients have received another type of treatment during those years. Three-fourth of those patients reported to be physically active, whereas the remaining one-fourth is not, mainly depending on lack of interest in sporting activities.

### 12.6.3 Isometric Training

Reports from earlier studies suggested isometric quadriceps exercises or training in a short arc motion toward the end of knee extension in order to decrease the knee pain by a reduced patellofemoral compression.[128,135] Based on the amount of electrical muscle activity, Boucher et al.[12] and Signorile et al.[104] reported that the most effective angle for isometric quadriceps training would be with the knee at 90° of flexion and the foot held in a neutral position. However, isometric exercises are time consuming, since one mostly gains strength at a fixed position (knee joint angle).[2,75] Furthermore, isometric training does not improve functional performance and could therefore be questioned in AKP patients, since their knee problems most often result in a quadriceps mechanism disorder, which very likely should be treated during functional exercises. Therefore, in my opinion, isometric quadriceps training is only indicated in patients, who present with such a "severe" pain inhibition, that they are not able to perform dynamic exercises. Fortunately, these AKP patients are rare.

### 12.6.4 Isokinetic Training

During the last decade, isokinetic quadriceps training has been suggested as a possible treatment for quadriceps strengthening.[7,58,95,124] In an intervention study on males with and without AKP, isokinetic training for 6 weeks led to positive effects on knee joint position sense as well as increased quadriceps and hamstring muscle torques.[54] The term "isokinetic" is defined as a dynamic muscular contraction, when the velocity of the movement is controlled and maintained constant by a special device.[114] Isokinetic training therefore provides optimal loading of the muscles and allows muscular performance at different velocities.[3] There are less compressive forces on the joint surfaces during high angular velocity. This means that isokinetic training at high angular velocity (≥120°/s) should be preferred in AKP patients during concentric actions. However, eccentric actions are more difficult to perform due to unfamiliarity with the decelerating type of movement and problems to coordinate the different portions of the quadriceps muscles during decelerated knee extensions.[122,124] My suggestion is, therefore, that patients with AKP should perform isokinetic eccentric contractions at 90°/s or lower angular velocities. After improvement of muscle coordination, some patients might be able to increase the angular velocity. There is a need for eccentric training, particularly among AKP patients,[122] and it should be pointed out that isokinetic quadriceps training is an outstanding method in order to improve eccentric muscle torque and should therefore be included in the rehabilitation protocol (if possible). However, those patients that show maltracking of the patella at the "patellar tracking test" should not perform isokinetic training at high angular velocities during eccentric action due to risk for possible patellar subluxation or even dislocation.[121] The advantage with isokinetic training in AKP patients is, except for rapid muscular effect also a possibility of specific eccentric loading, training without body weightbearing and the exercise can be adjusted to possible knee pain and therefore diminish the risk for overload. However, there are also other exercises of a more functional character that improve the eccentric muscle strength, e.g., walking downstairs and stepping or jumping down from a height.

### 12.6.5 Closed and Open Kinetic Chain Training

Quadriceps can be strengthened during closed kinetic chain (CKC) as well as open kinetic chain (OKC) exercises. Palmitier et al. suggest that rehabilitation in a weightbearing position, such as during CKC exercises, may have a greater carryover to functional activities, as lower extremity function in daily weightbearing activities involves multiple muscle groups acting in synergy.[93] Stiene et al. found CKC to be more effective than OKC exercises in restoring perceived function in patients with AKP syndrome.[110] However, their CKC exercises, lateral step-ups, retro step-ups, double-leg squats, and StairMaster exercise are solely performed at the final knee extension and in my opinion, quadriceps performance should be improved during the entire range of knee flexion. Souza and Gross reported greater VMO/VL ratio during step-up/step-down exercises.[107] This might suggest that the stabilizing function of the VMO is increased during CKC exercises. McConnell advocates performing CKC exercises with the hip in external rotation to improve VMO activity.[80] In conflict with this, Ninos et al. could not demonstrate any difference in either VMO or VL with the hip externally rotated.[89] However, for optimal functional quadriceps' performance, my suggestion is that the quadriceps muscle group should be strengthened during CKC as well as OKC. This is also in agreement with other authors (e.g., refs.[55,131]). In order to reduce the patellofemoral joint reaction forces, CKC exercises, such as leg press and step exercises, should be trained during the last 30° of knee extension, while OKC exercises, such as sitting knee extensions, should rather be trained between 90° and 40° of knee flexion.[30,109]

### 12.6.6 Stretching

A number of patients with AKP show tightness mostly of the iliotibial band and other lateral muscle structures, the quadriceps muscle and, sometimes, also of the hamstrings and the gastrocnemius. Most of the stretching procedures could be performed by the patients themselves; therefore, they should be instructed in how to stretch their tight muscle structures. Static stretching in periods of 30 seconds should preferably be performed.[4,44] The lateral retinaculum might also be tight, which could interfere with a normal patellar tracking, and should, therefore, be treated with medial patellar glide. With the patient in a sidelying position on the opposite side with the symptomatic knee in approximately 30° of knee flexion, the clinician moves the patella medially, tilts the medial border of the patella posteriorly and stretches the lateral retinaculum.[82] Friction and massage of the lateral retinacular tissue can also be recommended in order to improve a tight lateral retinaculum.

### 12.6.7 Balance and Coordination Training

AKP patients often have a reduced balance of their lower extremities, measured as postural sway, as well of their symptomatic as their asymptomatic leg (unpublished data). This indicates that balance and coordination training should be included in the treatment program. Physical training causes changes within the nervous system that leads to improved coordination between muscle groups, and practice will result in automatics, which indicates a change and improvement in the motor program.[96,103] When the activity and the function of VM have improved, balance and coordination training of the lower extremity should be started. Balance and coordination exercises should preferably be performed during knee loading conditions and with slightly flexed knees in order to try to direct the training to the knee joint.

### 12.6.8 Knee-Related Functional Training

When the quadriceps muscle has improved and a good balance exists within the extensor mechanism, functional training with gradual increase of knee loading exercises could begin. The patient should practice slowly, stepping on and off a step with adequate pelvic control. Initially, a small step height should be used and the patient is recommended to train in front of a mirror to be able to observe muscle function. The pelvis must remain parallel with the floor and the hip, knee, and foot should be aligned.[82] There is a wide variation of functional knee loading exercises that makes different heavy demands upon the knee, e.g., walking, jogging, running, stair climbing, jumping, and bicycling.

### 12.6.9 Sport-Specific Exercises

Those athletic patients that have improved, i.e., good quadriceps strength, good muscle flexibility, and a proper movement pattern during functional heavy knee loading activities performed without pain or swelling are encouraged to start sport-specific training.

### 12.6.10 Bracing and Taping

Supportive devices such as patellar stabilizing braces and patellar taping are aimed to improve patellar tracking problems.[36,77,94] Some authors suggest that AKP patients should be treated with patellar stabilizing orthoses,[56,61,77,87] although there is no evidence of any major alteration of patellar tracking.[42] Palumbo reported decreased symptoms in 92% when a patella stabilizing brace was used in AKP patients.[94] Sega et al. reported that an orthosis with a medial support gave a good pain reduction in patients with patellar instability.[103] We have found improvements in balance of the lower extremity, when patients with patellar hypermobility were supported with brace, i.e., patients with a lateral patellar hypermobility improved when the patella had a lateral support and patients with a medial patellar hypermobility improved when the patella had a medial support (unpublished data). In military recruits with AKP, Finestone et al. reported better response without a brace or with a simple sleeve compared with the use of a brace during physical exercise.[35] However, some authors suggest that bracing may play a role in patients with AKP that participate in strenuous physical exercise. BenGal et al. performed a prospective investigation of the efficacy of knee brace on preventing AKP in young healthy subjects undergoing strenuous physical training.[6] Their data indicate that the use of a brace with a silicon patellar support ring might be effective to prevent the development of AKP in individuals participating in intensive physical exercise.[6] Van Tiggelen et al. reported a considerably lower number of military recruits with AKP after a 6 week strenuous training program if they wore a dynamic patellofemoral brace when compared with recruits that were unbraced.[119] They concluded that the use of a dynamic patellofemoral brace is an effective way to prevent AKP in subjects undergoing strenuous physical exercises.[119]

Other authors recommend an elastic strap or taping in order to improve patellar tracking and thereby reduce patellar instability problems.[80,103] McConnell reported a success rate of 92% maintaining that patellar taping with a medial glide technique can modify patellar tracking and therefore act as pain relief.[80] Gilleard et al. found that the onset of VMO activity occurred earlier, when the patella was taped compared to untaped, during step-up and step-down tasks, while the activity of VL was unchanged during the step-up task and delayed during the step-down task with taping.[46] Gerrard reported a pain-free success rate of 96% after only five treatments using the McConnell taping technique.[45] Bockrath et al.[9] studied the effect of patella taping on patellar position (Merchant's x-ray view) and knee pain (VAS). They found a reduced perceived pain during a step-down task, when the patella was taped according to McConnell, but no significant changes occurred in patellar position.[9] Using a radiographic technique in a partial weightbearing position with the knee flexed 40°, Larsen et al. indicated that the McConnell medial glide taping technique was effective in significantly moving the patella medially.[72] However, the taping was ineffective in maintaining this patellar position after a 15 min exercise program, including forward sprint, side shuffling, back peddling, figure of eight running, and mini-squats.[72] Powers et al. studied the effect of patellar taping according to McConnell on functional outcomes.[97] With the patella taped, they reported an average pain reduction of 78% using the VAS. No significant differences were found in gait velocity or cadence between taped and untaped trials. A small increase in stride length during ascending a ramp was the only significant effect that improved with taping. However, patellar taping also resulted in a small increase in loading response knee flexion, which the authors believe demonstrates more willingness to load the knee joint.[97] Whether this finding depends on patellar taping or the effect of reduced pain is, however, not known. Kowall et al. performed a prospective study comparing two similar groups of anterior knee pain patients that were treated during 4 weeks.[69] Both groups received the same physical therapy program, one group with the patella taped and the other group without taping. Both groups improved; however, no beneficial effect of adding patellar taping was found.[69] In contrast, Whittingham et al. reported that a combination of patellar taping and exercise was superior to exercise alone in terms of reduction of knee pain and improved knee function.[127] In another EMG study, AKP patients and asymptomatic controls performed a stair-stepping task during three experimental conditions: therapeutic patellar tape, placebo tape, and no tape.[24] They reported that therapeutic patellar tape was found to alter the temporal characteristics of VMO and VL activation in AKP patients, whereas placebo tape had no effect. No change of onset of VMO and VL with either placebo or therapeutic tape was found in asymptomatic controls. The authors conclude that the use of patellar taping is an adjunct to rehabilitation of AKP patients.[24] Christou reported increased VMO activity and decreased VL activity in AKP patients when the patella was taped medially.[21] In a recent pilot EMG study, AKP patients performed a posteroanterior knee perturbation test under the following three conditions: real taping, placebo taping, and no taping of the patella.[88] The test was carried out before as well as after quadriceps muscle fatigue. No significant difference in electromyographic onset timing of VMO and VL was found between testing conditions. Furthermore, the amplitude of VMO was significantly higher in the no taping compared to the real taping condition irrespective of the state of muscle fatigue. The authors concluded that patellar taping may not enhance activation of VMO in patients with AKP neither before nor after muscle fatigue of the quadriceps. They also concluded that contraction of the VMO might be inhibited by patellar taping.[88] The benefits of patellar taping are not due to a change in patellar position but rather due to enhanced support of the patellofemoral ligaments and/or pain modulation via cutaneous stimulation.[21] Werner et al. reported that patients with patellar hypermobility (≥15 mm deviation laterally or medially) improved their quadriceps muscle torque and agonist EMG activity during isokinetic knee extensions, when the patella was stabilized by taping, while patients with a normal patellar mobility did not benefit from taping.[125] However, we also found that in order to optimize the treatment for supporting the patella with tape, it is important to check the direction of the patient's patellar hypermobility, which can be laterally, medially, or both.[125] Furthermore, in order to control whether the patient needs a patellar support, orthosis or taping, it is important to check patellar tracking within the patellofemoral joint during both concentric and eccentric knee extension ("patellar tracking"-test). In my opinion, patellar taping can be recommended only if patellar hypermobility exists and as a temporary treatment to facilitate physical therapy exercises, especially quadriceps training.

Foot orthotics to control excessive pronation of the subtalar joint have also been advocated to improve patellar tracking and lead to a decrease in AKP.[32,67,117] D'Amico and Rubin found that foot orthotics could reduce the Q-angle and, therefore, suggested that this foot–knee relationship might be an indication for using foot orthotics in AKP patients with malalignment.[28] Furthermore, footwear should be closely evaluated for quality and fit, and the use of arch supports should be considered.[64] However, it should be pointed out that in a recent prospective, single-blind, randomized study on 179 patients with AKP, Collins et al. found no significant differences between foot orthoses and physiotherapy or between physiotherapy and a combination of physiotherapy and foot orthoses.[22]

## 12.7 Appendix: A Step-By-Step Treatment Protocol for AKP Patients

### *12.7.1 Phase 1*

#### 12.7.1.1 Goals

Reduce pain and swelling, improve VMO:VL balance and thereby patellar tracking, improve flexibility, restore normal gait, and decrease loading of the patellofemoral joint.

#### 12.7.1.2 Treatment

- Cryotherapy – after the physical therapy exercise and daily activities that exacerbate symptoms to reduce pain and edema.[68,84]
- Transcutaneous electrical stimulation of VMO to restore the function of VMO and improve VMO:VL balance (Fig. 12.1). This could be done according to our specific protocol (Table 12.3).
- Flexibility training. Stretching of tight muscle structures, usually the tensor fascia lata and the iliotibial band (Fig. 12.2), the quadriceps, in particular rectus femoris (Fig. 12.3), the hamstrings (Fig. 12.4), and the gastrocnemius. Tight lateral retinaculum can, except for stretching, be treated with medial patellar glide, friction, and massage.
- If gait has been altered, the patient should be instructed in proper gait mechanics, which preferably could be done in front of a mirror.
- Instruct the patient to change postural habits such as, e.g., standing in genu recurvatum.
- If patellar hypermobility exists, it is recommended to either tape the patella or to use a patellar stabilizing brace during the physical therapy exercises. However, patellar supporting devices should only be used temporarily until exercises and functional activities can be performed without knee pain.
- If increased pronation of the subtalar joint exists, treat the patient with foot orthotics or arch taping. Foot orthotics can be used temporarily or may be needed indefinitely to improve patellar tracking and alignment of the lower extremity.
- Check the patient's shoe wear, in particular sport shoes, and if needed, suggest shock absorptive shoes.
- Modify daily activity level to temporarily reduce the load on the patellofemoral joint.

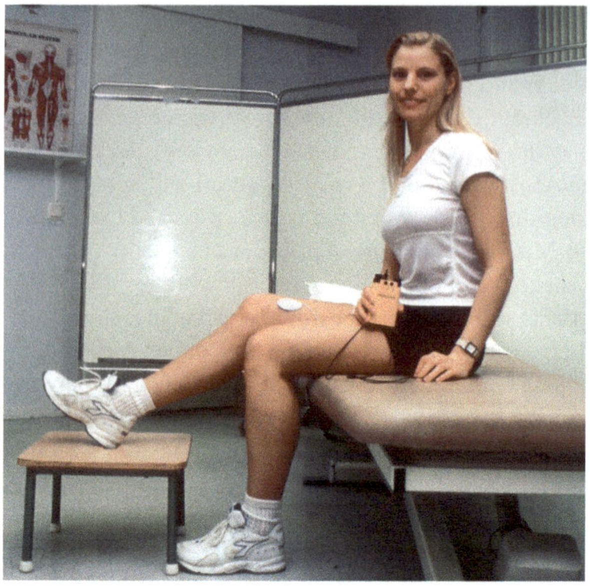

**Fig. 12.1** Transcutaneous electrical stimulation of VMO

**Table 12.3** Transcutaneous electrical stimulation protocol of VMO in patients with anterior knee pain syndrome

| Stimulation type | Constant pulse |
|---|---|
| Pulse width | 300 μs |
| Frequency | 40 Hz |
| Rise time | 4 s |
| On time | 18 s |
| Fall time | 2 s |
| Off time | 25 s |

Keep the knee joint in approximately 30° of knee flexion. Stimulate passively without any activation of the quadriceps muscle

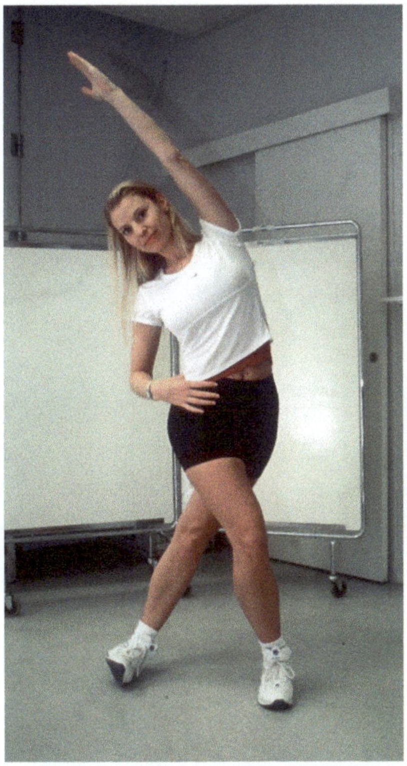

**Fig. 12.2** Stretching of lateral muscle structures, the tensor fascia lata, and the iliotibial band

### 12.7.2 Phase 2

#### 12.7.2.1 Goals

Improve balance of the lower extremity, increase quadriceps strength, and restore good knee function.

#### 12.7.2.2 Additional Treatment

- Balance and coordination training with gradual increase of difficulty and loading on the patellofemoral joint. In order to try to mainly train the knee joint stabilizers, I suggest that these exercises should be performed in a standing position with a slightly flexed knee joint. Balance training on a balance board can initially be performed standing on one leg with addition of electrical stimulation of VMO to facilitate a proper balance between VMO and VL (Fig. 12.5). When good muscle control is achieved, the patient can continue the balance exercise standing on one leg without electrical muscle stimulation (Fig. 12.6) or standing on both legs on two balance boards (Fig. 12.7).
- Stationary bicycle training with a high seat aimed to reduce a big knee flexion angle and thereby compression forces within the patellofemoral joint (Fig. 12.8).[90]

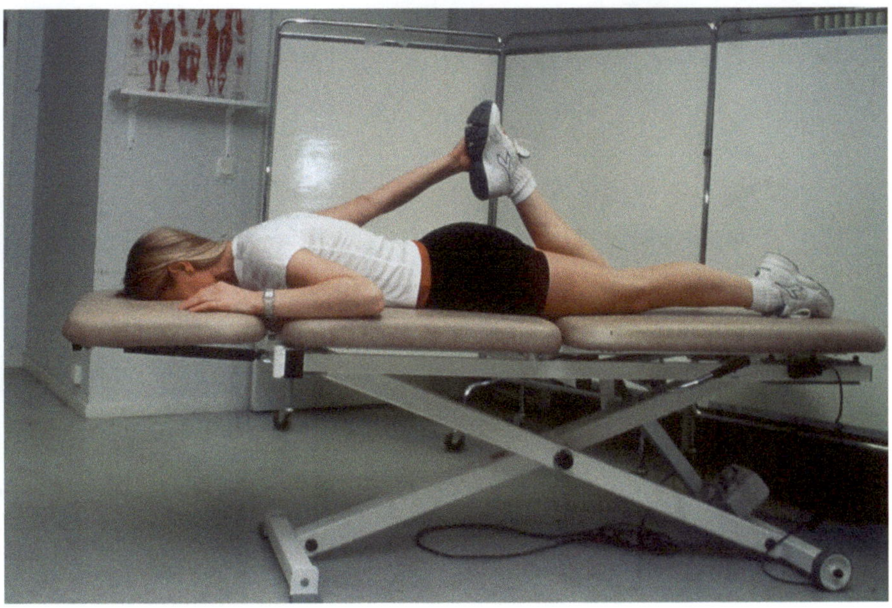

**Fig. 12.3** Stretching of rectus femoris

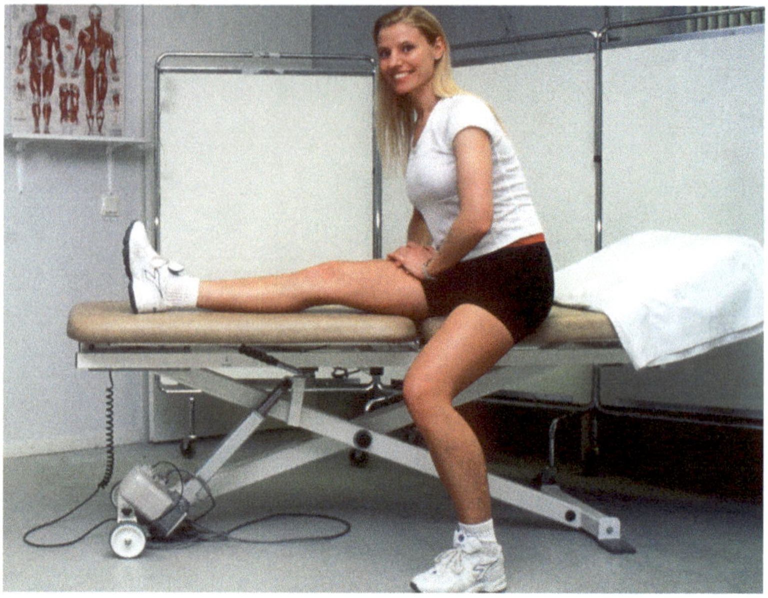

**Fig. 12.4** Stretching of hamstrings

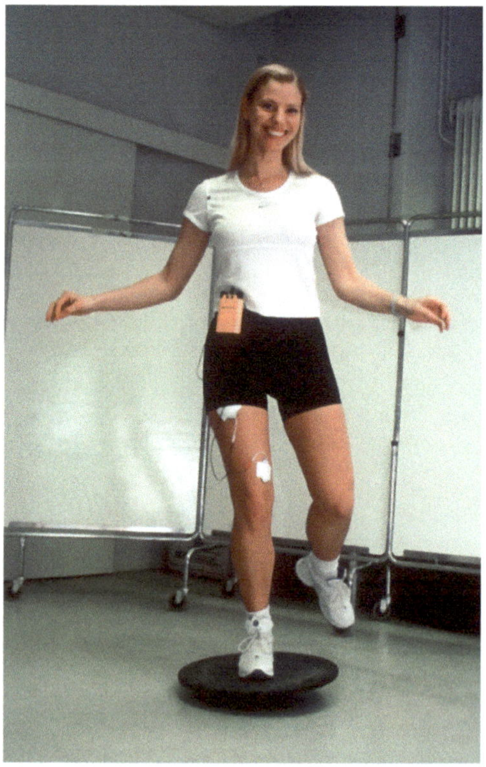

**Fig. 12.5** Single-leg standing balance board training with addition of electrical stimulation of VMO

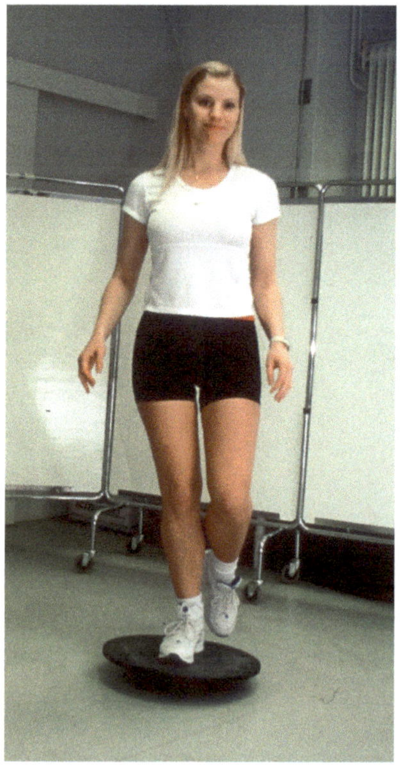

**Fig. 12.6** Single-leg standing balance board training

This type of exercise might improve both physical conditioning and thigh muscle strength.

- Functional knee exercises. Start with shallow squats, and proceed with deeper ones. Squatting can initially be performed with addition of electrical stimulation of VMO to improve the VMO:VL balance (Fig. 12.9). Stepping down can also be started with addition of electrical muscle stimulation (Fig. 12.10), and gradually be performed without (Fig. 12.11).

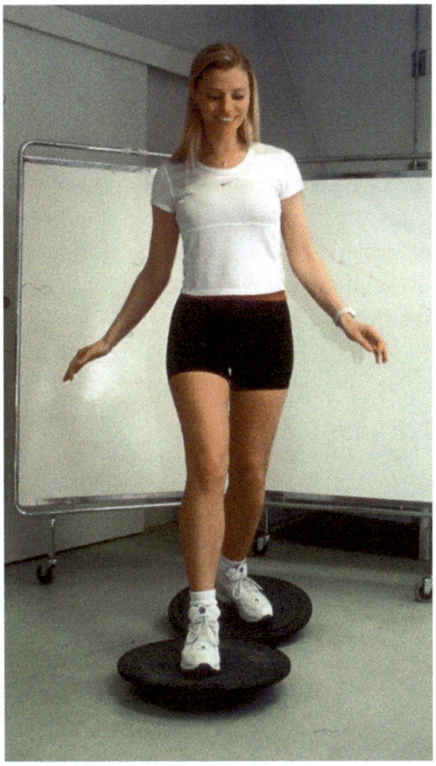

**Fig. 12.7** Balance board training standing on two legs on two balance boards

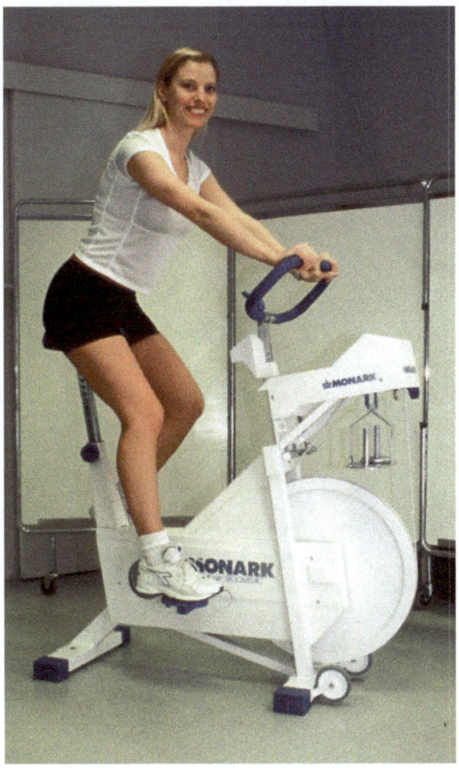


**Fig. 12.8** Stationary bicycle training with a high seat

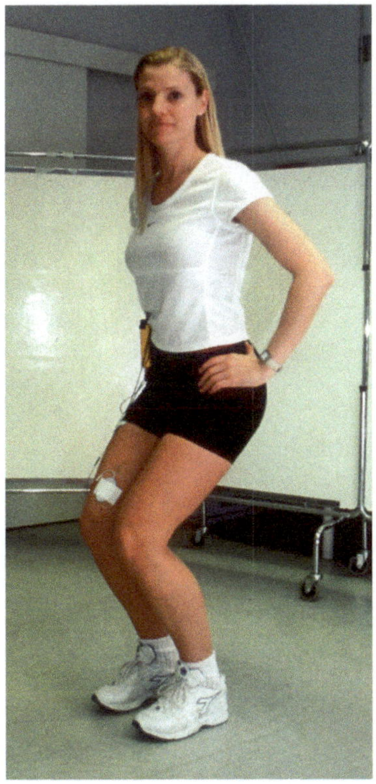

**Fig. 12.9** Squatting with addition of electrical stimulation of VMO

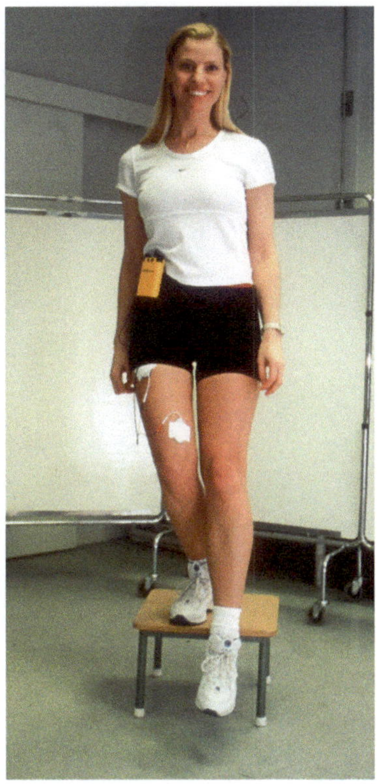

**Fig. 12.10** Stepping down with addition of electrical stimulation of VMO

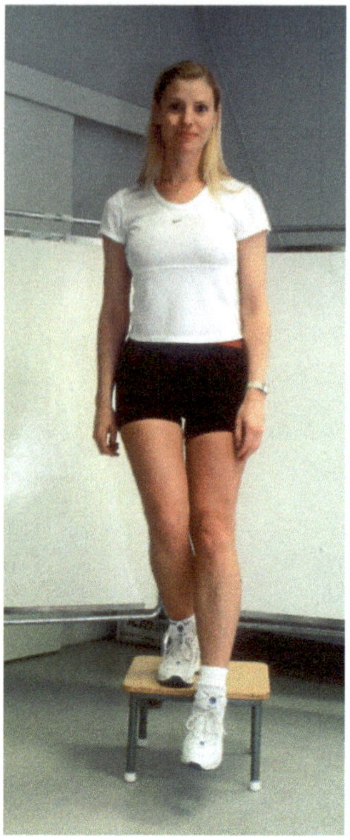

Fig. 12.11 Stepping down

- Quadriceps strengthening is recommended to be started when a good balance between VMO and VL exists. Closed kinetic chain exercises should be performed during terminal knee extension, approximately between 30–0° of knee flexion, and open kinetic chain between approximately 90–40° of knee flexion. Isokinetic training should preferably be performed at 120°/s or higher during concentric actions and at 90°/s or lower during eccentric actions (Fig. 12.12).

## 12.7.3 Phase 3

### 12.7.3.1 Goal

Return to previous physical activity level.

### 12.7.3.2 Additional Treatment

- Functional training with a gradual increase of knee loading activities can begin after improved quadriceps strength. Walking, jogging, and different types

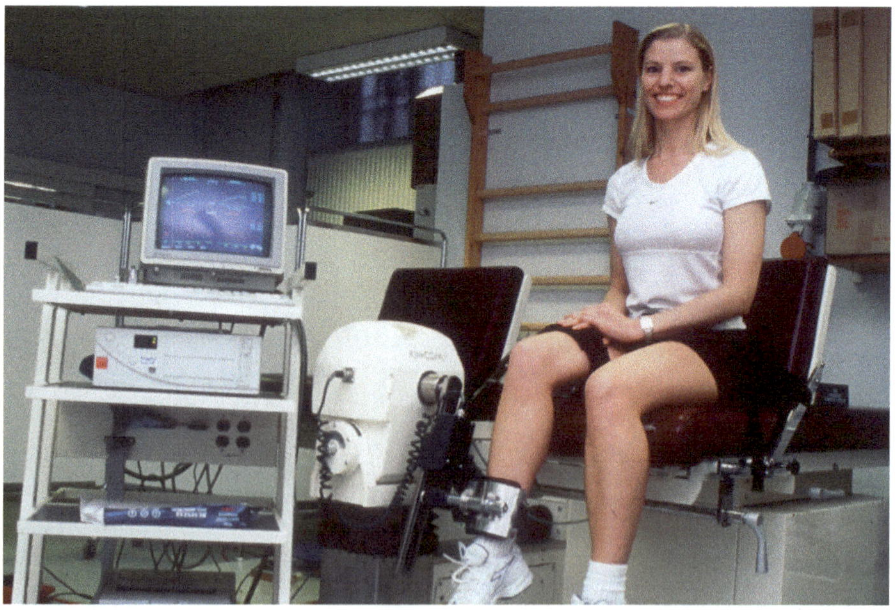

Fig. 12.12 Isokinetic quadriceps training

of jumping exercises are recommended during this phase. However, proceeding to a higher knee loading activity or exercise should only be allowed, if there is no knee pain and no swelling.

- Sport-specific exercises with a gradual increase of intensity can start as soon as the athletic patient is pain-free, has a good muscle function, and a proper movement pattern during functional knee exercises.
- It is recommended to give the patient individual guidelines for physical activity and exercises regarding, e.g., number of repetitions, duration, intensity, and frequency.
- Patient education is also recommended in order to try to prevent recurrence of knee symptoms.

## References


1. Aglietti P, Buzzi R, Pisaneschi A. Patella pain. *J Sports Trauma Rel Res*. 1990;12:131-150.
2. Åstrand PO, Rodahl K. *Textbook of Work Physiology*. New York: McGraw-Hill; 1977.
3. Baltzopoulos V, Brodie DA. Isokinetic dynamometry. Applications and limitations. *Sports Med*. 1989;8:101-116.
4. Bandy WD, Irion JM. The effect of time on static stretch on the flexibility of the hamstring muscles. *Phys Ther*. 1994;74:845-852.
5. Beckman M, Craig R, Lehman RC. Rehabilitation of patellofemoral dysfunction in the athlete. *Clin Sports Med*. 1989;8:841-860.
6. BenGal S, Lowe J, Mann G, et al. The role of the knee brace in the prevention of anterior knee pain syndrome. *Am J Sports Med*. 1997;25:118-122.
7. Bennett JG, Stauber WT. Evaluation and treatment of anterior knee pain using eccentric exercise. *Med Sci Sports Exerc*. 1986;18:526-530.
8. Bentley G, Dowd G. Current concepts of etiology and treatment of chondromalacia patellae. *Clin Orthop Relat Res*. 1984;189:209-228.
9. Bockrath K, Wooden C, Worrel T, et al. Effects of patella taping on patella position and perceived pain. *Med Sci Sports Exerc*. 1993;25:989-992.
10. Borg G, Holmgren A, Lindblad I. Quantitative evaluation of chest pain. *Acta Med Scand Suppl*. 1981;644:43-45.
11. Bose K, Kanagasuntherum R, Osman M. Vastus medialis oblique: an anatomical and physiologic study. *Orthopedics*. 1980;3:880-883.
12. Boucher JP, King MA, Lefebvre R, et al. Quadriceps femoris muscle activity in patellofemoral pain syndrome. *Am J Sports Med*. 1992;20:527-532.
13. Brewerton DA. The function of the vastus medialis muscle. *Ann Phys Med*. 1955;2:164-168.
14. Carlsson AM. *Studies on Pain Assessment and Egopsychological Analysis of Personality in Chronic Pain Patients* [thesis]. Stockholm: Karolinska Institute; 1987.
15. Carlsson AM, Werner S, Mattlar CE, et al. Personality in patients with long-term patellofemoral pain syndrome. *Knee Surg Sports Traumatol Arthrosc*. 1993;1:178-183.
16. Carson WG. Diagnosis of extensor mechanism disorders. *Clin Sports Med*. 1985;4:231-246.
17. Caylor D, Fites R, Worrell TW. The relationship between quadriceps angle and anterior knee pain syndrome. *J Orthop Sports Phys Ther*. 1993;17:11-16.
18. Cerny K. Vastus medialis oblique/vastus lateralis muscle activity ratios for selected exercises in persons with and without patellofemoral pain syndrome. *Phys Ther*. 1995; 75:672-683.
19. Cesarelli M, Bifulco P, Bracale M. Study of the control strategy of the quadriceps muscles in anterior knee pain. *IEEE Trans Rehabil Eng*. 2000;8:330-341.
20. Chesworth BM, Culham EG, Tata GE, et al. Validation of outcome measures in patients with patellofemoral syndrome. *J Orthop Sports Phys Ther*. 1989;10:302-309.
21. Christou EA. Patellar taping increases vastus medialis oblique activity in the presence of patellofemoral pain. *J Electromyogr Kinesiol*. 2004;14:495-504.
22. Collins N, Crossley K, Beller E, et al. Foot orthoses and physiotherapy in the treatment of patellofemoral pain syndrome: randomised clinical trial. *Br J Sports Med*. 2009;43:169-171.
23. Cowan SM, Bennell KL, Crossley KM, et al. Physical therapy alters recruitment of the vasti in patellofemoral pain syndrome. *Med Sci Sports Exerc*. 2002;34:1879-1885.
24. Cowan SM, Bennell KL, Hodges PW. Therapeutic patellar taping changes the timing of the vasti muscle activation in people with patellofemoral pain syndrome. *Clin J Sport Med*. 2002;12:339-347.
25. Cowan SM, Bennell KL, Hodges PW, et al. Simultaneous feedforward recruitment of the vasti in untrained postural tasks can be restored by physical therapy. *J Orthop Res*. 2003;21:553-558.
26. Cowan SM, Hodges PW, Bennell KL, et al. Altered vastii recruitment when people with patellofemoral pain syndrome complete a postural task. *Arch Phys Med Rehabil*. 2002;83:989-995.
27. Crossley KM, Bennell KL, Cowan SM, et al. Analysis of outcome measures for persons with patellofemoral pain: which are reliable and valid? *Arch Phys Med Rehabil*. 2004;85:815-822.
28. D'Amico JC, Rubin M. The influence of foot orthoses on the quadriceps angle. *J Am Podiatry Assoc*. 1986;76:337-340.
29. DeHaven KE, Dolan WA, Mayer PJ. Chondromalacia patellae in athletes. *Am J Sports Med*. 1979;7:5-11.
30. Doucette SA, Child DP. The effect of open and closed chain exercise and knee joint position on patellar tracking in lateral patellar compression syndrome. *J Orthop Sports Phys Ther*. 1996;23:104-110.
31. Doucette SA, Goble EM. The effect of exercise on patellar tracking in lateral patellar compression syndrome. *Am J Sports Med*. 1992;20:434-440.

32. Eng JJ, Pierrynowski MR. Evaluation of soft foot orthotics in the treatment of patellofemoral pain syndrome. *Phys Ther.* 1993;73:62-70.
33. Engebretsen L, Arendt E. Patellofemorale smerter: diagnostikk og behandling. *Tidsskr Nor Laegeforen.* 1991;111:1949-1952.
34. Fairbank J, Pynsent P, van Poortvliet J, et al. Mechanical factors in the incidence of knee pain in adolescents and young adults. *J Bone Joint Surg.* 1984;66-B:685-693.
35. Finestone A, Radin EL, Lev B, et al. Treatment of overuse patellofemoral pain. Prospective randomized controlled clinical trial in a military setting. *Clin Orthop Relat Res.* 1991;293:208-210.
36. Fisher RL. Conservative treatment of patellofemoral pain. *Orthop Clin North Am.* 1986;17:269-271.
37. Flandry F, Hunt JP, Terry GC, et al. Analysis of subjective knee complaints using visual analog scales. *Am J Sports Med.* 1991;19:112-118.
38. Fox TA. Dysplasia of the quadriceps mechanism, hypoplasia of the vastus medialis as related to the hypermobile patella syndrome. *Surg Clin North Am.* 1975;55:199-226.
39. Fritz GK, Bleck EE, Dahl IS. Functional versus organic knee pain in adolescents. *Am J Sports Med.* 1981;9:247-249.
40. Fulkerson JP. Awareness of the retinaculum in evaluating patellofemoral pain. *Am J Sports Med.* 1982;10:147.
41. Fulkerson JP, Hungerford DS. Biomechanics of the patellofemoral joint. In: Fulkerson JP, Hungerford DS, eds. *Disorders of the Patellofemoral Joint.* 2nd ed. Baltimore: Williams & Wilkins; 1990:25-41.
42. Fulkerson JP, Hungerford DS. Evaluation and rehabilitation of nonarthritic anterior knee pain. In: Fulkerson JP, Hungerford DS, eds. *Disorders of the Patellofemoral Joint.* 2nd ed. Baltimore: Williams & Wilkins; 1990:86-101.
43. Fulkerson JP, Shea KP. Current concepts review disorders of patellofemoral alignment. *J Bone Joint Surg.* 1990;72-A:1424-1429.
44. Gajdosik RL. Effects of static stretching on the maximal length and resistance to passive stretch of short hamstring muscles. *J Orthop Sports Phys Ther.* 1991;14:250-255.
45. Gerrard B. The patello-femoral pain syndrome: a clinical trial of the McConnell programme. *Aust J Physiother.* 1989;35:71-80.
46. Gilleard W, McConnell J, Parsons D. The effect of patellar taping on the onset of vastus medialis obliquus and vastus lateralis muscle activity in persons with patellofemoral pain. *Phys Ther.* 1998;78:25-32.
47. Goldberg B. Chronic anterior knee pain in the adolescent. *Pediatr Ann.* 1991;20:186-193.
48. Goodfellow J, Hungerford DS, Zindel M. Patello-femoral joint mechanics and pathology. 1. Functional anatomy of the patello-femoral joint. *J Bone Joint Surg.* 1976;58-B:287-290.
49. Grabiner MD, Koh TJ, Draganich LF. Neuromechanics of the patellofemoral joint. *Med Sci Sports Exerc.* 1994;26:10-21.
50. Grana WA, Kriegshauser LA. Scientific basis of extensor mechanism disorders. *Clin Sports Med.* 1985;4:247-257.
51. Gruber MA. The conservative treatment of chondromalacia patellae. *Orthop Clin North Am.* 1979;10:105-115.
52. Gunther KP, Thielemann F, Bottesi M. Anterior knee pain in children and adolescents. Diagnosis and conservative treatment. *Orthopade.* 2003;32:110-118.
53. Hanten WP, Schulthies SS. Exercise effect on electromyographic activity of the vastus medialis oblique and vastus lateralis muscles. *Phys Ther.* 1990;70:561-565.
54. Hazneci B, Yildiz Y, Sekir U, et al. Efficacy of isokinetic exercise on joint position sense and muscle strength in patellofemoral pain syndrome. *Am J Phys Med Rehabil.* 2005;84:521-527.
55. Heintjes E, Berger MY, Bierma-Zeinstra SM, et al. Exercise therapy for patellofemoral pain syndrome. *Cochrane Database Syst Rev.* 2003;4:CD003472.
56. Henry JH, Crosland JW. Conservative treatment of patellofemoral subluxation. *Am J Sports Med.* 1979;7:12-14.
57. Hodges P, Richardson C. An investigation into the effectiveness of hip adduction in the optimization of the vastus medialis oblique contraction. *Scand J Rehabil Med.* 1993; 25: 57-62.
58. Hoke B, Howell D, Stack M. The relationship between isokinetic testing and dynamic patellofemoral compression. *J Orthop Sports Phys Ther.* 1983;4:150-153.
59. Hughston JC, Deese M. Medial subluxation of the patella as a complication of a lateral retinacular release. *Am J Sports Med.* 1988;16:383-388.
60. Hungerford DS, Barry M. Biomechanics of the patello-femoral joint. *Clin Orthop Relat Res.* 1979;144:9-15.
61. Insall J. Current concepts review, patellar pain. *J Bone Joint Surg.* 1982;64-A:147-152.
62. Insall J, Goldberg V, Salvati E. Recurrent dislocation and the high-riding patella. *Clin Orthop Relat Res.* 1972;88:67-69.
63. Jacobson KE, Flandry FC. Diagnosis of anterior knee pain. *Clin Sports Med.* 1989;8:179-195.
64. Juhn MS. Patellofemoral pain syndrome: a review and guidelines for treatment. *Am Fam Physician.* 1999;60: 2012-2222.
65. Karlsson J, Thomeé R, Swärd L. Eleven year follow-up of patello-femoral pain syndrome. *Clin J Sport Med.* 1996;6: 22-26.
66. Karst GM, Jewett PD. Electromyographic analysis of exercises proposed for differential activation of medial and lateral quadriceps femoris muscle components. *Phys Ther.* 1993;73:286-295.
67. Klingman RE, Liaos SM, Hardin KM. The effect of subtalar joint position on patellar glide position in subjects with excessive rearfoot pronation. *J Orthop Sports Phys Ther.* 1997;25:185-191.
68. Kowal MA. Review of physiological effects of cryotherapy. *J Orthop Sports Phys Ther.* 1983;5:66-73.
69. Kowall MG, Kolk G, Nuber GW, et al. Patellar taping in the treatment of patellofemoral pain. A prospective randomized study. *Am J Sports Med.* 1996;24:61-66.
70. Laprade JA, Culham EG. A self-administered pain severity scale for patellofemoral pain syndrome. *Clin Rehabil.* 2002;16:780-788.
71. Laprade J, Culham E, Brouwer B. Comparison of five isometric exercises in the recruitment of the vastus medialis oblique in persons with and without patellofemoral pain syndrome. *J Orthop Sports Phys Ther.* 1998;27:197-204.
72. Larsen B, Andreasen E, Urfer A, et al. Patellar taping: a radiographic examination of the medial glide technique. *Am J Sports Med.* 1995;23:465-471.
73. Lieb F, Perry J. Quadriceps function. *J Bone Joint Surg.* 1968;50-A:1535-1548.

74. Lin F, Wang G, Koh JL, et al. In vivo and non-invasive three-dimensional patellar tracking induced by individual heads of quadriceps. *Med Sci Sports Exerc.* 2004;36:93-101.
75. Lindh M. Increase of muscle strength from isometric quadriceps exercise at different angles. *Scand J Rehabil Med.* 1979;11:33-36.
76. Loudon JK, Wiesner D, Goist-Foley HL, et al. Intrarater reliability of functional performance tests for subjects with patellofemoral pain syndrome. *J Athl Train.* 2002; 37:256-261.
77. Lysholm J, Nordin M, Ekstrand J, et al. The effect of a patella brace on performance in knee extension strength test in patients with patellar pain. *Am J Sports Med.* 1984;12: 110-112.
78. Mariani PP, Caruso I. An electromyographic investigation of subluxation of the patella. *J Bone Joint Surg.* 1989;61-B: 169-171.
79. Martin JA, Londeree BR. EMG comparison of quadriceps femoris activity during knee extension and straight leg raises. *Am J Phys Med.* 1979;58:57-69.
80. McConnell J. The management of chondromalacia patellae: a long term solution. *Aust J Physiother.* 1986;32:215-223.
81. McConnell J. Examination of the patellofemoral joint: the physical therapist's perspective. In: Grelsamer RP, McConnell J, eds. *The Patella. A Team Approach.* Gaithersburg, Maryland: Aspen Publishers Inc.; 1998:109-118.
82. McConnell J. Conservative management of patellofemoral problems. In: Grelsamer RP, McConnell J, eds. *The Patella. A Team Approach.* Gaithersburg Maryland: Aspen Publishers Inc; 1998:119-136.
83. McKenzie DK, Bigeland-Ritchie B, Gorman RB, et al. Central and peripheral fatigue of human diaphragm and limb muscles assessed by twitch interpolation. *J Physiol.* 1992; 454:643-656.
84. Michlovitz SL. Cryotherapy: the use of cold as a therapeutic agent. In: Michlovitz SL, ed. *Thermal Agents in Rehabilitation.* 2nd ed. Philadelphia: FA Davis Company; 1990: 63-86.
85. Milgrom C, Kerem E, Finestone A, et al. Patellofemoral pain caused by overactivity. A prospective study of risk factors in infantry recruits. *J Bone Joint Surg.* 1991;73-A:1041-1043.
86. Miller JP, Sedory D, Croce RV. Vastus medialis obliquus and vastus lateralis activity in patients with and without patellofemoral pain syndrome. *J Sport Rehabil.* 1997;6:1-10.
87. Möller RN, Krebs B. Dynamic knee brace in the treatment of patellofemoral disorders. *Arch Orthop Trauma Surg.* 1986;104:377-379.
88. Ng GY, Wong PY. Patellar taping affects vastus medialis obliquus activation in subjects with patellofemoral pain before and after quadriceps muscle fatigue. *Clin Rehabil.* 2009;23:705-713.
89. Ninos JC, Irrgang JJ, Burdett R, et al. Electromyographic analysis of the squat performed in self-selected lower extremity neutral rotation and 30° of lower extremity turn-out from the self-selected neutral position. *J Orthop Sports Phys Ther.* 1997;25:307-315.
90. Nisell R, Ekholm J. Patellar forces during knee extension. *Scand J Rehabil Med.* 1985;17:63-74.
91. Osborne AH, Farquharson-Roberts MA. The aetiology of patello-femoral pain. *J Roy Nav Med Serv.* 1983;69: 97-103.
92. Owings TM, Grabiner MD. Motor control of the vastus medialis oblique and vastus lateralis muscles is disrupted during eccentric contractions in subjects with patellofemoral pain. *Am J Sports Med.* 2002;30:483-487.
93. Palmitier RA, An K-N, Scott SG, et al. Kinetic chain exercise in knee rehabilitation. *Sports Med.* 1991;11:404-413.
94. Palumbo PM. Dynamic patellar brace: patellofemoral disorders. A preliminary report. *Am J Sports Med.* 1981;9: 45-49.
95. Percy EC, Strother RT. Patellalgia. *Phys Sports Med.* 1985; 13:43-59.
96. Portney LG, Sullivan PE, Daniell JL. EMG activity of vastus medialis obliquus and vastus lateralis in normals and patients with patellofemoral arthralgia. *Phys Ther.* 1986; 66:808.
97. Powers CM, Landel R, Sosnick T, et al. The effects of patellar taping on stride characteristics and joint motion in subjects with patellofemoral pain. *J Orthop Sports Phys Ther.* 1997;26:286-291.
98. Powers CM, Perry J, Hislop HJ. Are patellofemoral pain and quadriceps femoris muscle torque associated with locomotor function? *Phys Ther.* 1997;77:1063-1075.
99. Price DD, McGrath PA, Rafii A, et al. The validation of visual analog scale measures for chronic and experimental pain. *Pain.* 1983;17:45-56.
100. Reynolds L, Levin T, Medeiros J, et al. EMG activity of the vastus medialis oblique and the vastus lateralis in their role in patellar alignment. *Am J Phys Med.* 1983;62:61-70.
101. Richardson CA, Bullock MI. Changes in muscle activity during fast alternating flexion and extension movements of the knee. *Scand J Rehabil Med.* 1986;18:51-58.
102. Sczepanski TL, Gross MT, Duncan PW, et al. Effect of contraction type, angular velocity, and arc of motion on VMO:VL EMG ratio. *J Orthop Sports Phys Ther.* 1991; 14:256-262.
103. Sega L, Galante M, Fortina A, et al. Association of dynamic bandage with kinesitherapy in the treatment of patellar instability. *Ital J Sports Traum.* 1988;10:89-94.
104. Signorile JF, Kacsik D, Perry A, et al. The effect of knee and foot position on the electromyographical activity of the superficial quadriceps. *J Orthop Sports Phys Ther.* 1995;-22:2-9.
105. Skalley TC, Terry GC, Teitge RA. The quantitative measurement of normal passive medial and lateral patellar motion. *Am J Sports Med.* 1993;21:728-732.
106. Smith AD, Stroud L, McQueen C. Flexibility and anterior knee pain in adolescent elite figure skaters. *J Pediatr Orthop.* 1991;11:77-82.
107. Souza DR, Gross MT. Comparison of vastus medialis obliquus: vastus lateralis muscle integrated electromyographic ratios between healthy subjects and patients with patellofemoral pain. *Phys Ther.* 1991;71:310-320.
108. Steadman JR. Nonoperative measures for patellofemoral problems. *Am J Sports Med.* 1979;7:374-375.
109. Steinkamp LA, Dillingham MF, Markel MD, et al. Biomechanical considerations in patellofemoral joint rehabilitation. *Am J Sports Med.* 1993;21:438-444.
110. Stiene HA, Brosky T, Reinking MF, et al. A comparison of closed kinetic chain and isokinetic joint isolation exercise in patients with patellofemoral dysfunction. *J Orthop Sports Phys Ther.* 1996;24:136-141.

111. Teitge RA. Iatrogenic medial dislocation of the patella. *Orthop Trans.* 1991;15:747.
112. Thein Brody L, Thein JM. Nonoperative treatment for patellofemoral pain. *J Orthop Sports Phys Ther.* 1998; 28:336-344.
113. Thijs Y, Van Tiggelen D, Roosen P, et al. A prospective study on gait-related intrinsic risk factors for patellofemoral pain. *Clin J Sport Med.* 2007;17:437-445.
114. Thistle HG, Hislop HJ, Moffroid M, et al. Isokinetic contraction: a new concept of resistive exercise. *Arch Phys Med Rehabil.* 1967;48:279-282.
115. Thomeé R *Patellofemoral Pain Syndrome in Young Women. Studies on Alignment, Pain Assessment and Muscle Function, with a Model for Treatment* [thesis]. Göteborg university, Göteborg, Sweden;1995.
116. Thomeé P, Thomeé R, Karlsson J. patellofemoral pain syndrome: pain, coping strategies and degree of well-being. *Scand J Med Sci Sports.* 2002;12:276-281.
117. Tiberio D. The effect of excessive subtalar joint pronation on patellofemoral mechanics: a theoretical model. *J Orthop Sports Phys Ther.* 1987;9:160-165.
118. Van Kampen A. *The Three Dimensional Tracking Pattern of the Patella: In vitro Analysis* [thesis]. Nijmegen, Holland; 1987.
119. Van Tiggelen D, Witvrouw E, Roget PM, et al. Effect of bracing on the prevention of anterior knee pain – a prospective randomized study. *Knee Surg Sports Traumatol Arthrosc.* 2004;12:434-439.
120. Voight ML, Wieder DL. Comparative reflex response times of vastus medialis obliquus and vastus lateralis in normal subjects and subjects with extensor mechanism dysfunction. An electromyographic study. *Am J Sports Med.* 1991; 19:131-137.
121. Werner S. *Patello-Femoral Pain Syndrome – An Experimental Clinical Investigation* [thesis]. Stockholm: Karolinska Institutet, Sweden; 1993.
122. Werner S. An evaluation of knee extensor and knee flexor torques and EMGs in patients with patellofemoral pain syndrome in comparison with matched controls. *Knee Surg Sports Traumatol Arthrosc.* 1995;3:89-94.
123. Werner S, Arvidsson H, Arvidsson I, et al. Electrical stimulation of vastus medialis and stretching of lateral thigh muscles in patients with patello-femoral symptoms. *Knee Surg Sports Traumatol Arthrosc.* 1993;1:85-92.
124. Werner S, Eriksson E. Isokinetic quadriceps training in patients with patellofemoral pain syndrome. *Knee Surg Sports Traumatol Arthrosc.* 1993;1:162-168.
125. Werner S, Knutsson E, Eriksson E. Effect of taping the patella on concentric and eccentric torque and EMG of the knee extensor and flexor muscles in patients with patellofemoral pain syndrome. *Knee Surg Sports Traumatol Arthrosc.* 1993;1:169-177.
126. Westfall DC, Worrell TW. Anterior knee pain syndrome: role of vastus medialis oblique. *J Sport Rehabil.* 1992;1:317-325.
127. Whittingham M, Palmer S, Macmillan F. Effects of taping on pain and function in patellofemoral pain syndrome: a randomized controlled trial. *J Orthop Sports Phys Ther.* 2004;34:504-510.
128. Wild JJ, Franklin TD, Woods GW. Patellar pain and quadriceps rehabilitation. An EMG study. *Am J Sports Med.* 1982;10:12-15.
129. Wilk KE, Davies GJ, Mangine RE, et al. Patellofemoral disorders: a classification system and clinical guidelines for nonoperative rehabilitation. *J Orthop Sports Phys Ther.* 1998;28:307-321.
130. Willett GM, Karst GM. Patellofemoral disorders: is timing or magnitude of vastus medialis obliquus and vastus lateralis muscle activity affected by conservative treatment? [abstract]. *J Orthop Sports Phys Ther.* 1995;21:61.
131. Witvrouw E, Danneels L, Van Tiggelen D, et al. Open versus closed kinetic chain exercises in patellofemoral pain: a 5-year prospective randomized study. *Am J Sports Med.* 2004;32:1122-1130.
132. Witvrouw E, Lysens R, Bellemans J, et al. Intrinsic risk factors for the development of anterior knee pain in an athletic population. A two year prospective study. *Am J Sports Med.* 2000;28:480-489.
133. Witvrouw E, Sneyers C, Lysens R, et al. Reflex response times of vastus medialis oblique and vastus lateralis in normal subjects and in subjects with patellofemoral pain syndrome. *J Orthop Sports Phys Ther.* 1996;24: 160-165.
134. Witvrouw E, Werner S, Mikkelsen C, et al. Clinical classification of patellofemoral pain syndrome: guidelines for non-operative treatment. *Knee Surg Sports Traumatol Arthrosc.* 2005;13:122-130.
135. Yates C, Grana WA. Patellofemoral pain - a prospective study. *Orthopedics.* 1986;9:663-667.

# Conservative Management of Anterior Knee Pain: The McConnell Program

13

Jenny McConnell and Kim Bennell

## 13.1 Introduction

Traditionally, conservative management of patellofemoral pain syndrome (PFPS) involved pain-relieving techniques and standard quadriceps strengthening in non-weight bearing positions. In 1986, an Australian physiotherapist, Jenny McConnell, proposed an innovative management program based on the premise that abnormal patellar tracking plays a key role in the etiology of PFPS.[63] Passive, active, and neural factors predisposing to abnormal patellar tracking were to be identified via a thorough assessment of the patient. Based on the assessment findings, the treatment program aimed first to unload abnormally stressed soft tissue around the patellofemoral joint by optimizing the patellar position and second, to improve the lower limb mechanics. The program included vastus medialis obliquus (VMO) retraining in functional weight-bearing positions combined with patellar taping, patellar mobilization, correction of foot and lower limb mechanics, and stretching to reduce pain and enhance VMO activation. This chapter will focus on the McConnell program for conservatively managing PFPS. It will describe factors predisposing to PFPS as a theoretical rationale for the program and include details of assessment and treatment.

K. Bennell (✉)
Centre for Health, Exercise and Sports Medicine, Physiotherapy, School of Health Sciences, The University of Melbourne, Victoria, VIC, Australia
e-mail: k.bennell@unimelb.edu.au

## 13.2 Factors Predisposing to Patellofemoral Pain

Individuals with patellofemoral pain tend to demonstrate a failure of the intricate balance of the soft tissue structures around the joint. This may alter the pressure distribution from the patella to the femur. However, the mechanism of pain production in patellofemoral pain is not fully understood. Patellofemoral pain is most likely due to either tension or compression of the soft tissue structures. Patellofemoral pain may, therefore, be classified by the area of pain, as this usually indicates the compromised structure and the possible mechanism for the compromise. For example, lateral pain may be indicative of adaptive shortening of the lateral retinaculum. Those with lateral pain will have chronically tilted patellae (excessive lateral pressure syndrome) and there is often evidence of small nerve injury in the lateral retinaculum when the retinaculum is sectioned histologically.[34] Inferior patellar pain is likely to implicate the infrapatellar fat pad, one of the most pain sensitive structures in the knee.[4,28] A patient with a recurrently subluxing patella often presents with medial patellofemoral pain because the medial retinaculum is chronically overstretched. It is unusual for this type of patient to have tight lateral structures as the patella is generally mobile in all directions and the VMO is poorly developed.

It is postulated that in individuals who complain of a deep ache in the knee, the articular cartilage has failed such that the load is now borne on the richly innervated underlying subchondral bone.[34] These patients often have the classic chondromalacia patellae where softening and fissuring is present on the undersurface of the patella.

V. Sanchis-Alfonso (ed.), *Anterior Knee Pain and Patellar Instability*,
DOI: 10.1007/978-0-85729-507-1_13, © Springer-Verlag London Limited 2011

### 13.2.1 Biomechanical Faults

Although a direct blow or a traumatic dislocation of the patella may precipitate patellofemoral pain, suboptimal mechanics of the patella from biomechanical faults is thought to be the major contributory factor.[102] The biomechanical faults may be divided into structural and non-structural. Structural causes of malalignment may be divided into intrinsic and extrinsic causes and may be quite subtle. The extrinsic factors are more common and magnify the effect of the non-structural faults.

Intrinsic structural factors relate to dysplasia of the patella or femoral trochlea and the position of the patella relative to the trochlea. Although uncommon, developmental abnormalities such as patellar or trochlea dysplasia will create patellofemoral incongruence with resultant instability of the patella and pain.[32,52,80,98] Extrinsic structural faults are reported to cause a lateral tracking of the patella.[48,54,58] The extrinsic factors include increased Q angle[68] and tightness of the hamstrings and gastrocnemius muscles.

The Q angle has been used to estimate the angle of pull of the quadriceps muscle group.[58] It forms a valgus vector, particularly in extension. The outer limit of Q angle for females is 15°, for males 12°[54,58] The Q angle varies dynamically, decreasing with knee flexion and increasing with knee extension due to the external rotation of the tibia, which occurs during the screw home mechanism to allow full extension to occur.[34,54] Increased femoral anteversion, external tibial torsion, or a lateral displacement of the tibial tubercle can cause an increase in Q angle.[61] Often, individuals with an increased Q angle have "squinting" patellae. These individuals usually present with an anteversion of the femur.[61] Its clinical usefulness, however, is questionable with a recent systematic review finding considerable disagreement on the reliability and validity of the clinical Q-angle measurement.[87]

### 13.2.2 Soft Tissue Tightness

Soft tissue tightness is particularly prevalent during the adolescent growth spurt where the long bones are growing faster than the surrounding soft tissues.[67] This leads not only to problems with lack of flexibility and alteration of stress through joints but also to muscle control problems where the motor program is no longer able to appropriately control the limb. A decrease in extensibility of the lateral retinaculum, a reduction in the flexibility of the tensor fasciae latae, hamstrings, gastrocnemius, or rectus femoris, as well as the anterior hip structures will adversely affect patellar tracking.

When the knee flexes, a shortened lateral retinaculum will come under excessive stress as the patella is drawn into the trochlea and the iliotibial band pulls posteriorly on the already shortened lateral retinaculum.[33,34] This will cause a lateral tracking and tilting of the patella.[66] Additionally, a tight TFL, through its attachment into the iliotibial band, will cause a lateral tracking of the patella, particularly at 20° of knee flexion when the band is at its shortest. There is evidence that people with patellofemoral pain do have tighter iliotibial bands than matched controls.[47]

Hamstrings and gastrocnemius tightness also cause a lateral tracking of the patella, by increasing the dynamic Q angle.[7,82,93] During running, tight hamstrings will lead to increased knee flexion when the foot lands. Because the knee cannot straighten, an increased amount of dorsiflexion is required to position the body over the planted foot. If the range of full dorsiflexion has already occurred at the talocrural joint, further range is achieved by pronating the foot, particularly at the subtalar joint. This causes an increase in the valgus vector force and hence increases the dynamic Q angle.[93]

### 13.2.3 Muscle Imbalance

#### 13.2.3.1 Quadriceps

While it would seem that the control and timing of the lower limb muscles, in particular VMO and vastus lateralis (VL), are critical to the smooth functioning of the patellofemoral joint, this is still a controversial area. Voight and Weider[100] found that the reflex response time of the VMO was earlier than the VL in an asymptomatic group, but in a symptomatic patellofemoral group there was a reversal of the pattern. These findings were recently confirmed by Witvrouw and colleagues,[105] but curiously these investigators found that there was a shorter reflex response time in the PF group relative to the control group.[105] Dynamically, this issue has been supported by the work of Koh and colleagues,[53] who examined isokinetic knee extension at 250°s$^{-1}$, following hamstrings preactivation, finding that the VMO activated 5.6 ms earlier than VL. Even though this finding was statistically significant, these authors questioned the functional relevance. Our research group has shown that the EMG onset of VMO is delayed relative to VL during both stair stepping[16] and postural perturbation tasks[18] in patients with patellofemoral pain compared with asymptomatic controls. However, in the asymptomatic group, VMO onset occurred at the same time as VL and not before. Others have found that the VMO did not fire earlier than the VL in the asymptomatic group and that the VMO was not delayed in the symptomatic group.[35,49,74,76]

Not only is the relative timing of the vastii considered to be a causative factor in the development of PF pain, but so too is weakness of the VMO relative to the VL, causing increased lateral patellar translation and lateral patellar spin.[103] Recently, Wilson and colleagues investigated[104] the VMO and VL tendon lengths in symptomatic and asymptomatic individuals using real-time ultrasonography. The PFP subjects showed significantly less VMO tendon strain than control subjects but there was no difference in VL tendon strain. The authors concluded that relative weakness of the VMO was the most likely cause of the decreased tendon strain seen in subjects with PFP and felt that PF pain may be due to increased lateral subchondral bone loading caused by the VMO weakness.

There is also contention about whether there is a difference in the ratio of VMO and VL activity.[62,74] Part of the conflict might relate to the problem of normalization of EMG data. Normalization involves obtaining a ratio of the recorded muscle activity and muscle activity from the maximal voluntary contraction (MVC), which then enables comparison of the ratio of one muscle relative to its maximal with another muscle relative to its maximal. There has been some discussion that normalization is affected by the presence of pain, which will mask differences as there may be error in the MVC, which may appear in the error of the recorded EMG.[89] Furthermore, there is debate about the reliability of the maximal contraction throwing some concern on the normalization process.[46,106] However, Hodges and colleagues[43] found after inducing pain in asymptomatic individuals, by injecting the fat pad with hypotonic saline that there was a decrease in both the VMO and VL activity during a squat maneuver, whereas random intermittent application of an electric shock across the knee, provoking fear of pain, only reduced VMO, not VL, activity. VMO would seem to be more greatly affected than VL by pain and swelling.[43,91]

#### 13.2.3.2 Hip Muscle Weakness

There is increasing evidence that hip muscle weakness, particularly in abduction, external rotation, and extension is a common finding in PF pain patients.[79] Although the studies are limited and the strength testing has often used handheld dynamometry, which has not consistently been shown to be reliable,[8,70,85] the influence of the hip muscles on dynamic femoral position as a causative factor in PF pain must be considered when rehabilitating patients with PF pain.[90]

### *13.2.4 Altered Foot Biomechanics*

Altered foot biomechanics such as excessive, prolonged, or late pronation will alter the tibial rotation at varying times through range, thus having an effect on patellofemoral joint mechanics.[82,93] However, studies investigating abnormal foot biomechanics and patellofemoral pain have found inconsistent results.[24,56,97]

It is essential for the therapist to realize that the foot may be mobile or stiff and that if a foot problem is discovered, orthotics may not necessarily be the only course of action – joint mobilization and muscle training can be extremely effective, particularly if the foot is stiff.

## 13.3 Clinical Examination

In the history taking, the clinician needs to elicit the location of the pain, the aggravating activities, the history of the pain, its behavior, and any other associated symptoms such as giving way or swelling. Simple outcome measures that are valid and reliable should also be obtained from the patient so that the effectiveness of treatment can be evaluated. These measures include a visual analogue scale for overall usual or worst pain in the past week or the anterior knee pain scale.[20] A change of more than 2 cm out of 10 on the visual analogue scale is needed to represent a clinically important change.

The clinical examination is important to establish the diagnosis and to determine the underlying causative factors of the patient's symptoms so the appropriate treatment can be implemented. The patient is initially examined in standing for assessment of lower extremity alignment. Biomechanical faults are noted so that the clinician has a reasonable indication of how the patient will move. Of particular interest is femoral position, which is easier to see when the patient has the feet together. Internal femoral rotation is a common finding in patients with patellofemoral pain (Fig. 13.1). The term internal femoral rotation is preferred to femoral anteversion, because the term rotation implies not only the bony position, but also the soft tissue adaptation that occurs as a result of the femoral anteversion. The soft tissue changes are quite amenable to change by conservative management.

The internal femoral rotation often causes a squinting of the patellae but if the lateral structures of the patellofemoral joint are tight, the patella may appear straight. The clinician is interested in the presence of an enlarged fat pad, which indicates that the patient is standing in hyperextension or a "locked back" knee position. The muscle bulk of the VMO is observed and compared with the other side. The VL and ITB are palpated to determine the resting tension. Presence of varus /valgus and/or torsion of the tibia is noted. The talus is palpated on the medial and lateral sides to check for symmetry of position. In relaxed standing, the patient should be in mid-stance position, so ideally, the subtalar joint should be in mid position.[57,82] If the talus is more prominent medially, then the patient's subtalar joint is pronated. The shape of medial and lateral longitudinal arches is noted. If, for example, the medial longitudinal arch is flattened, then the patient will exhibit a prolonged amount of pronation during walking. The great toe and first metatarsal are examined for callus formation as well as position. If the patient has callus on the medial aspect of the first metatarsal or the great toe, or has a hallux valgus, then the therapist should expect the patient to have an unstable push off in gait. When examined prone, this patient will have a forefoot deformity.

From the side, the clinician can check pelvic position, to determine whether there is an anterior tilt, posterior tilt, or a sway back posture.[50] Position of hyperextension or lock back knees can be verified looking from the side. From behind, the level of the

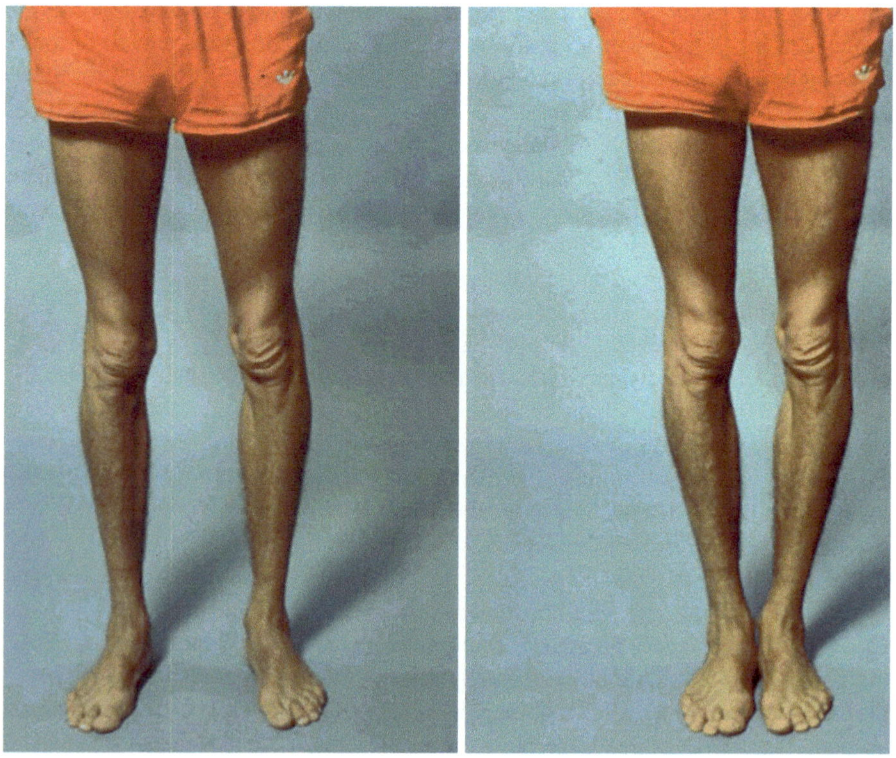

**Fig. 13.1** Common biomechanical presentation – internal rotation of the femurs

PSIS is checked, gluteal bulk is assessed, and the position of the calcaneum is observed. If the therapist finds that the calcaneum is in a relatively neutral or inverted position and the talus is more prominent on the medial side, then the therapist could probably expect that the patient would have a stiff subtalar joint. Thus, from a person's static alignment, the clinician can have a reasonable idea of the dynamic picture. Any deviations from the anticipated gives a great deal of information about the muscle control of the activity.

### 13.3.1 Dynamic Examination

The aim of the dynamic examination is not only to evaluate the effect of muscle action on the static mechanics, but also to reproduce the patient's symptoms so the clinician has an objective reassessment activity to evaluate the effectiveness of the treatment. The least stressful activity of walking is examined first. For example, individuals with patellofemoral pain who stand in hyperextension, will not exhibit the necessary shock absorption at the knee, at heel strike. Consequently, the femur will internally rotate and the quadriceps will not function well in inner range due to lack of practice. If the patient's symptoms are not provoked in walking, then evaluation of more stressful activities such as stair climbing, are performed. If symptoms are still not provoked, then squat and one leg squat may be examined and used as a reassessment activity. For the athlete, the clinician will, in many cases, be evaluating the control of the one leg squat as symptom production in the clinic may be difficult.

### 13.3.2 Supine Lying Examination

With the patient in supine lying, the clinician gains an appreciation of the soft tissue structures and begins to confirm the diagnosis. Gentle, but careful palpation should be performed on the soft tissue structures around the patella. First, the joint lines are palpated to exclude obvious intra-articular pathology. Second, palpation of the retinacular tissues determine which parts of the retinaculum are under chronic recurrent stress. If pain is elicited in the infrapatellar region on palpation, the clinician should shorten the fat pad by lifting it towards the patella. If on further palpation, the pain is gone, then the clinician can be relatively certain that the patient has a fat pad irritation. If the pain remains, then patellar tendinosis is the most likely diagnosis. The knee is passively flexed and extended with overpressure applied so the clinician has an appreciation of the quality of the end feel. If any of these maneuvers reproduce pain, they can be used as a reassessment sign[60]; for example, the symptoms of fat pad irritation can often be produced with an extension overpressure maneuver.

The hamstrings, iliopsoas, rectus femoris, tensor fascia latae, gastrocnemius, and soleus muscles are tested for length. Tightness of any of these muscles has an adverse effect on patellofemoral joint mechanics and will have to be addressed in treatment. The iliopsoas, rectus femoris, and tensor fascia latae may be tested using the Thomas test.[45,51] Hamstrings flexibility may be examined by a passive straight leg raise, once the lumbar spine is flattened on the plinth and the pelvis is stable.[51] Normal length hamstrings should allow 80–85° of hip flexion, when the knee is extended and the lumbar spine is flattened.[51]

An essential part of patellofemoral evaluation in supine is assessment of the orientation of the patella relative to the femur. In order to maximize the area of contact of the patella with the femur, the patellar position should be optimal before the patella enters the trochlea. The clinician needs to consider the patellar position not with respect to the normal, but with respect to the optimal, because articular cartilage is nourished and maintained by evenly distributed, intermittent compression.[6,39,69]

An optimal patellar position is one where the patella is parallel to the femur in the frontal and the sagittal planes, and the patella is midway between the two condyles when the knee is flexed to 20°[63,65] The position of the patella is determined by examining four discrete components: glide, lateral tilt, anteroposterior tilt, and rotation, in a static and dynamic manner. Determination of the glide component involves measuring the distance from the midpole of the patella to the medial and lateral femoral epicondyles (Fig. 13.2). The patella should be sitting equidistant (±5 mm) from each epicondyle when the knee is flexed 20°. A 5 mm lateral displacement of the patella causes a 50% decrease in VMO tension.[2] In some instances, the patella may sit equidistant to the condyles, but moves lateral, out of the line of the femur, when the quadriceps contracts,

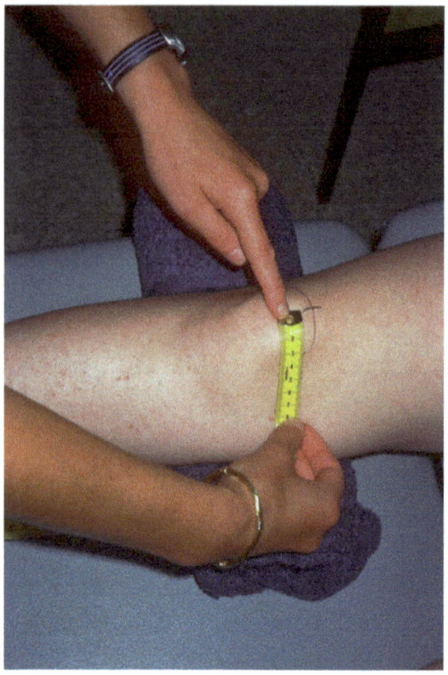

**Fig. 13.2** Assessment of patellar glide

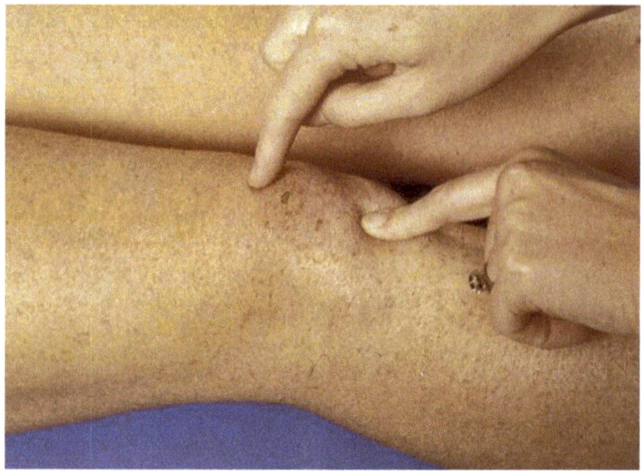

**Fig. 13.3** Assessment of posterior tilt of the inferior pole of the patella

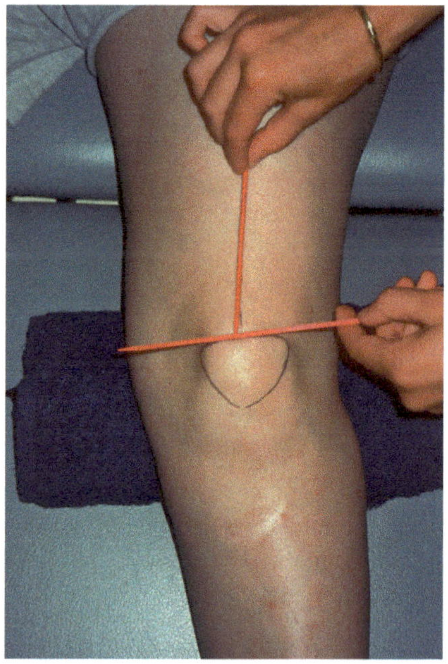

**Fig. 13.4** Assessment of rotation of the patella

indicating a dynamic problem. A recent systematic review found that the intra-tester reliability of assessing mediolateral patellar position is good, but that inter-tester reliability is variable.[86] The dynamic glide examines both the effect of the quadriceps contraction on patellar position as well as the timing of the activity of the different heads of quadriceps. If the passive lateral structures are too tight, then the patella will tilt so that the medial border of the patella will be higher than the lateral border and the posterior edge of the lateral border will be difficult to palpate. This is a lateral tilt and if severe, can lead to excessive lateral pressure syndrome.[34] When the patella is moved in a medial direction, it should initially remain parallel to the femur. If the medial border rides anteriorly, the patella has a dynamic tilt problem, which indicates that the deep lateral retinacular fibers are too tight, affecting the seating of the patella in the trochlea.

An optimal position also involves the patella being parallel to the femur in the sagittal plane. A most common finding is a posterior displacement of the inferior pole of the patella (Fig. 13.3). This will result in fat pad irritation and often manifests itself as inferior patella pain that is exacerbated by extension manoeuvres of the knee.[64] A dynamic posterior tilt problem can be determined during an active contraction of the quadriceps muscle as the inferior pole is pulled posteriorly, particularly in patients who hyperextend.

To complete the ideal position, the long axis of the patella should be parallel to the long axis of the femur. In other words, if a line was drawn between the most medial and most lateral aspects of the patella, it should be perpendicular to the long axis of the femur (Fig. 13.4). If the inferior pole is sitting lateral to the long axis of the femur, the patient has an externally rotated patella. If the inferior pole is sitting medial to the long axis of the femur, then the patient has an internally rotated patella. The presence of a rotation component indicates that a particular part of the retinaculum is tight. Tightness in the retinacular tissue compromises the tissue and can be a potent source of the symptoms.[34]

### 13.3.3 Side Lying

The retinacular tissue can be specifically tested for tightness with the patient in side lying and the knee flexed to 20°. The therapist moves the patella in a medial direction, so the lateral femoral condyle is readily exposed. If the lateral femoral condyle is not readily exposed, the superficial retinacular fibers are tight. To test the deep fibers, the therapist places his/her hand on the middle of the patella, takes up the slack of the glide and applies an anterior-posterior pressure on the medial border of the patella. The lateral should move freely away from the femur and on palpation, the tension in the retinacular fibers should be similar along the length of the patella. This test procedure can also be used as a treatment technique. Iliotibial band tightness may be confirmed further by Ober's test.[45]

### 13.3.4 Prone

In prone, the clinician may examine the foot to determine whether the patient has a primary foot deformity that is contributing to the patient's patellofemoral symptoms. The deformity will need to be addressed with orthotics or specific muscle training. In the prone position, the clinician is also able to evaluate the flexibility of the anterior hip structures, by examining the patient in a figure of four position, with the underneath foot at the level of the tibial tubercle (Fig. 13.5). This position tests the available extension and external rotation at the hip, which is often limited because of chronic adaptive shortening of the anterior structures as a result of the underlying femoral anteversion. The distance of the ASIS from the plinth is measured, so the clinician has an objective measure of change. A modification of the test position can also be used as a treatment technique. A lumbar spine palpation can be

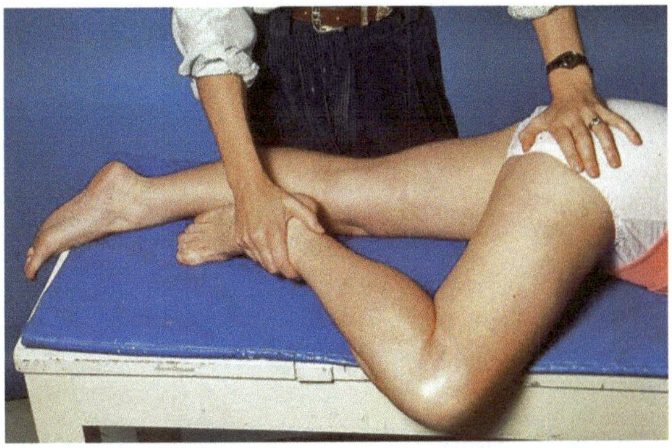

**Fig. 13.5** Assessment of the flexibility of the anterior hip structures

performed at this stage of the examination, if the clinician feels that the knee symptoms have been referred from a primary pathology in the lumbar spine. A summary of the examination process is listed in Table 13.1. Once the patellofemoral joint has been thoroughly examined, and the primary problems have been identified, appropriate treatment can be instigated.

## 13.4 Treatment

### 13.4.1 Conservative

Most patellofemoral conditions may be successfully managed with physical therapy. Treatment aims to optimize the patellar position and improve lower limb mechanics and thus decrease the patient's symptoms.

Stretching the tight lateral structures and changing the activation pattern of the VMO may decrease the tendency for the patella to track laterally and should enhance the position of the patella. Stretching the tight lateral structures can be facilitated passively by the therapist mobilizing and massaging the lateral retinaculum and the iliotibial band, as well as the patient performing a self-stretch on the retinacular tissue. However, the most effective stretch to the adaptively shortened retinacular tissue may be obtained by a sustained low load, using tape, to facilitate a permanent elongation of the tissues. This utilizes the creep phenomenon that occurs in viscoelastic material when a constant low load is applied. It has been widely documented that the length of soft tissues can be increased

**Table 13.1** Examination checklist

| |
|---|
| *PATIENT STANDING* – examine for biomechanical abnormalities<br>Observe Alignment from :<br>1. In front<br>• Normal standing<br>– Position of the feet with respect to the legs<br>– Q angle<br>– Tibial valgum/varum<br>– Tibial torsion<br>– Talar dome position<br>– Navicular position<br>– Morton's toe<br>– Hallux valgus<br>• Feet together<br>– Squinting patellae<br>– VMO bulk<br>– VL tension<br>2. Side<br>• Pelvic position – tilt<br>• Hyperextension of the knees<br>3. Behind<br>• PSIS position<br>• Gluteal bulk<br>• Calf bulk<br>• Calcaneal position |
| *DYNAMIC EVALUATION* – evaluate the the effect of the bony alignment and soft tissue on dynamic activities<br>1. Walking, if no pain<br>2. Steps, if no pain<br>3. Squat, if no pain<br>4. One leg squat |
| *ASSESSMENT IN SUPINE LYING POSITION* – determine the causative factors of the symptoms and formulate a diagnosis<br>1. Palpation of the tibiofemoral joint line and soft tissue structures of the patellofemoral joint<br>2. Tibiofemoral tests<br>3. Meniscal tests<br>4. Ligament tests<br>5. Thomas' test – psoas, rectus femoris, tensor fascia lata<br>6. Tests for hamstrings, gastrocs<br>7. Slump test for dural length, particularly indicated if the patient complains of lateral knee pain when sitting with their legs out straight.<br>8. Hip tests (if applicable)<br>9. Orientation of the patella<br>• Glide, dynamic glide<br>• Lateral tilt<br>• Anteroposterior tilt<br>• Rotation |
| *ASSESSMENT IN SIDE LYING POSITION*:<br>Tests for tightness of the lateral structures:<br>1. Medial glide – tests superficial lateral structures<br>2. Medial tilt – tests deep lateral structures<br>3. Ober's test for iliotibial band tightness |
| *ASSESSMENT IN THE PRONE POSITION*:<br>Lumbar spine palpation (only if applicable, i.e., if dural test positive)<br>Foot assessment<br>Hip rotation<br>Femoral nerve mobility |

with sustained stretching.[31,40,44,59,96] The magnitude of the increase in displacement is dependent on the duration of the applied stretch.[59,96] If the tape can be maintained for a prolonged period of time, then this, plus training of the VMO to actively change the patellar position, should have a significant effect on patellofemoral mechanics. However, there is some debate as to whether tape actually changes the position of the patella. Some investigators have found that tape changes PF angle and lateral patellar displacement, but congruence angle is not changed.[81] Others have concurred, finding no change in congruence angle when the patella is taped, but congruence angle is measured at 45° knee flexion so subtle changes in patellar position may have occurred before this.[13] A study of asymptomatic subjects found that medial glide tape was effective in moving the patella medially but ineffective in maintaining the position after vigorous exercise. However, tape seems to prevent the lateral shift of the patella that occurred with exercise.[5] The issue for a therapist, however, is not whether the tape changes the patellar position on x-ray, but whether the therapist can decrease the patient's symptoms by at least 50%, so the patient can exercise and train in a pain-free manner.

### 13.4.2 Patellar Taping

Patellar taping is based on the assessment of the patellar position. The component/s corrected, the order of correction, and the tension of the tape is tailored for each individual (Figs. 13.6 and 13.7). After each piece of tape is applied, the symptom producing activity should be reassessed. The tape should always immediately improve a patient's symptoms by at least 50%. If it does not, then the order in which the tape has been applied or the components corrected should be reexamined. In most cases, hypoallergenic tape is placed

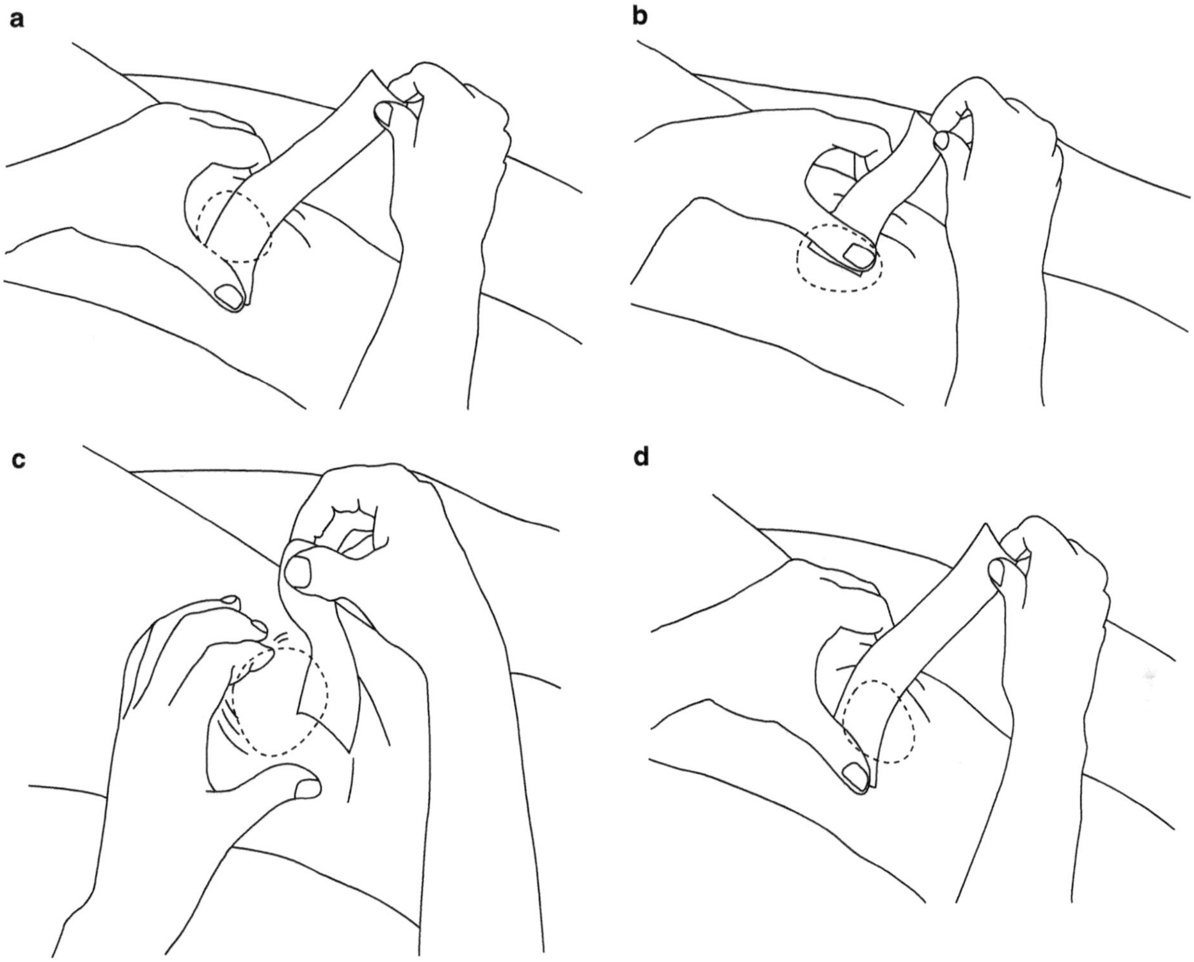


**Fig. 13.6** Taping components: (**a**) medial glide, (**b**) Medial tilt, (**c**) Internal rotation, (**d**) Anterior tilt

underneath the rigid sports tape to provide a protective layer for the skin and if there seems to be additional skin problems a plastic coating, either a spray or a roll-on may be applied to the skin prior to the tape application. The patient must be taught how to position the tape on him/herself. The patient should be in long sitting with the leg out straight and the quadriceps relaxed.

If a posterior tilt problem has been ascertained on assessment, it must be corrected first, as taping over the inferior pole of the patella will aggravate the fat pad and exacerbate the patient's pain. The posterior component is corrected together with a glide or a lateral tilt with the non-stretch tape being placed on the superior aspect of the patella, either on the lateral border to correct lateral glide or in the middle of the patella to correct lateral tilt. This positioning of the tape will lift the inferior pole out of the fat pad and prevent irritation of the fat pad.

If there is no posterior tilt problem, the glide may be corrected by placing tape from the lateral patellar border to the medial femoral condyle. At the same time, the soft tissue on the medial aspect of the knee is lifted towards the patella to create a tuck or fold in the skin. The skin lift helps anchor the tape more effectively and minimizes the friction rub (friction between the tape and the skin), which can occur when a patient has extremely tight lateral structures.

The mediolateral tilt component is corrected by placing a piece of tape firmly from the middle of the

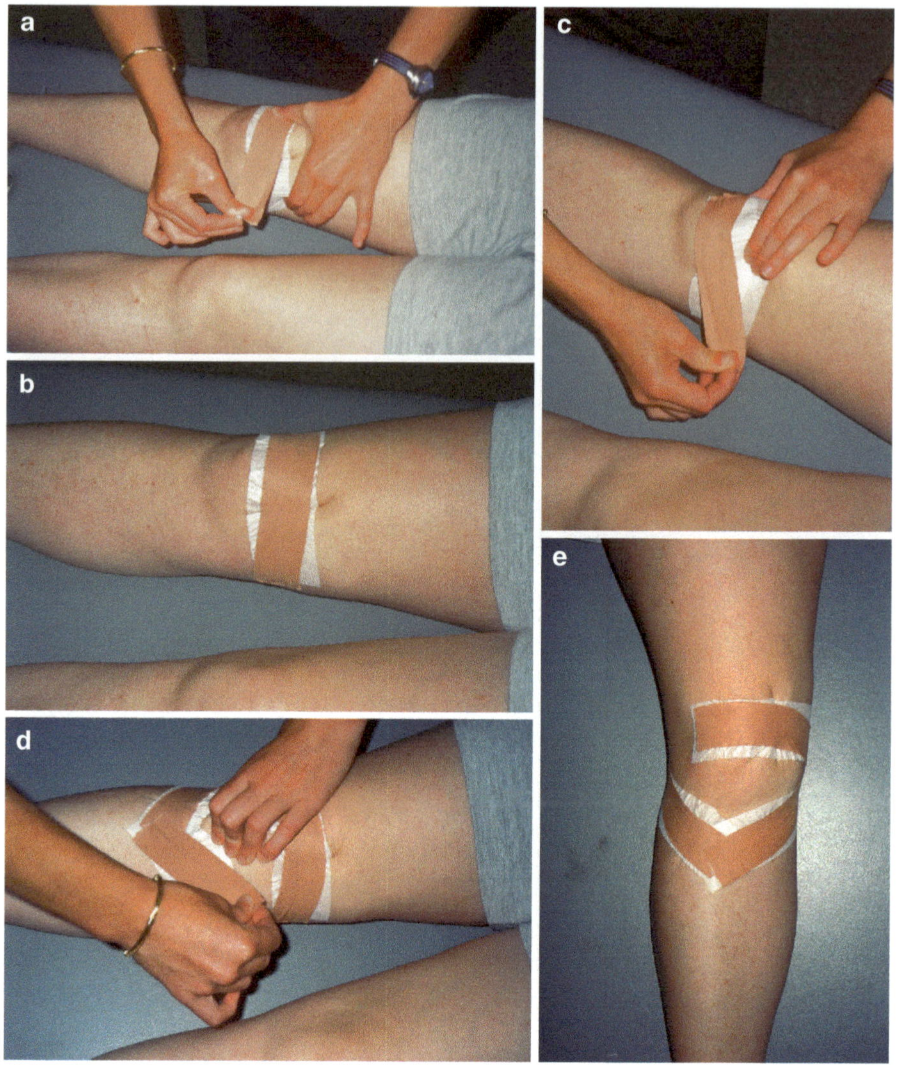


**Fig. 13.7** (**a**) Tape to correct lateral glide. (**b**) Tuck or fold in the skin. (**c**) Tape in internal rotation to correct external rotation of the patella. (**d** and **e**) Unloading fat pad with tape, lift the soft tissue towards the patella

patella to the medial femoral condyle. The object is to shift the lateral border away from the femur so that the patella becomes parallel with the femur in the frontal plane. Again, the soft tissue on the medial aspect of the knee is lifted towards the patella.

External rotation is the most common rotation problem and to correct this, the tape is positioned at the inferior pole and pulled upwards and medially towards the opposite shoulder while the superior pole is rotated laterally. Care must be taken so that the inferior pole is not displaced into the fat pad. Internal rotation, on the other hand, is corrected by taping from the superior pole downwards and medially.

#### 13.4.2.1 Unloading

The principle of unloading is based on the premise that inflamed soft tissue does not respond well to stretch. For example, if a patient presents with a sprained medial collateral ligament, applying a valgus stress to the knee will aggravate the condition, whereas a varus stress will decrease the symptoms. The same principle applies for patients with an inflamed fat pad, an irritated iliotibial band, or a pes anserinus bursitis. The inflamed tissue needs to be shortened or unloaded. To unload an inflamed fat pad, for example, a "V" tape is placed below the fat pad, with the point of the "V" at the tibial tubercle coming wide to the medial and lateral joint lines (Fig. 13.7d, e). As the tape is being pulled towards the joint line, the skin is lifted towards the patella, thus shortening the fat pad.

#### 13.4.2.2 Principles of Using Tape to Correct the Patella

The tape is kept on all day everyday until the patient has learnt how to activate his/her VMO at the right time, that is, the tape is like trainer wheels on a bicycle and can be discontinued once the skill is established. The tape is removed with care in the evening allowing the skin time to recover. The tape can cause a breakdown in the skin either through a friction rub or as a consequence of an allergic reaction. Preparation of the skin and skin care advice is essential.

The patient should never train with or through pain or effusion as it has been shown quite conclusively in the literature that pain and effusion have an inhibitory effect on muscle activity.[23,43,73,91,92] If the patient experiences a return of the pain, the tape should be readjusted. If the activity is still painful, the patient must cease the activity immediately. The tape will loosen quickly if the lateral structures are extremely tight or the patient's job or sport requires extreme amounts of knee flexion.

#### 13.4.2.3 Studies Investigating the Effects of Tape

A recent meta-analysis concluded that there was evidence that tape applied to exert a medially directed force on the patella produces a clinically meaningful change in chronic knee pain[101] but the mechanism of the effect is still being debated in the literature. As mentioned previously, there is some evidence to show that taping can improve the position of the patella[41,55,81,88] although improvements do not seem to be maintained after exercise.[75] Others have assessed the effect of tape on quadriceps function.[1,13,84] Using isokinetic dynamometry, studies have found that tape significantly increases the quadriceps torque.[1,13] However, the increase in muscle torque with tape does not necessarily correlate with pain reduction. Ernst and colleagues[30] showed greater knee extensor moments and power during a vertical jump and lateral step up in a taped condition compared with placebo and no tape conditions in PFPS subjects. It has also been found that during gait, individuals with PFPS decrease the amount of knee flexion in early stance to reduce the patellofemoral joint reaction force.[22,25,37,78] Patellar taping results in small but significant increases in loading response knee flexion in a variety of gait conditions indicating a greater ability to load the knee joint with confidence.[77]

It has been suggested that patellar tape could influence the magnitude of VMO and VL activation although most studies do not necessarily support this contention.[9,10,19,42,72,84] Similarly, there is conflict with regards to the effect of tape on onset timing of VMO and VL with some showing earlier timing of VMO. Taping the patella of symptomatic individuals such that the pain was decreased by 50%, resulted in an earlier activation of the VMO relative to the VL, on both step up and step down.[35] Our research group has also found that tape leads to a change in the onset timing of VMO relative to VL compared with placebo tape and no tape.[15] This effect seems to be related to pain reduction with tape because similar onset timing changes with tape were not seen in asymptomatic individuals with a VMO-VL timing deficit.[3]

### *13.4.3 Muscle Training*

There is currently debate about the best type of quadriceps strengthening for rehabilitating the patellofemoral joint. We have demonstrated that a "McConnell" based physiotherapy treatment regime (taping, functional training with biofeedback on VMO and VL) for PFPS alters the motor control of VMO relative to VL in both a functional task[18] and a postural perturbation task.[17] However, Powers concludes that because there is no difference in the activation pattern of the VMO and VL in symptomatic individuals and the ratio of the two muscles is the same, generalized quadriceps strengthening is all that is required.[76] Only one study has directly compared generalized quadriceps strengthening with VMO selective retraining.[94] This clinical trial involved 69 patients randomized to either of the exercise groups or to a no treatment control group for

8 weeks. The results showed that both the general and selective exercise groups demonstrated statistically significant and "moderate" to "large" effect size reductions in pain and improvements in function and quality of life when compared to the control group. Whilst this study did not measure VMO-VL imbalance, we have shown that a VMO retraining program is more effective in improving VMO-VL timing deficits than a generalized quadriceps strengthening program (unpublished data). Given the recurrent nature of PFPS, and the results of a recent prospective study showing that a VMO timing deficit was related to the occurrence of PFPS,[99] it would be interesting to see whether both types of programs are equally effective in the longer term.

What types of exercises are most appropriate in training? From the current evidence available, it seems that closed chain exercise (when the foot is on the ground) is the preferred method of training, not only because closed kinetic training has been shown to improve patellar congruence, but muscle training has been found to be specific to limb position.[26] In a group of patients with lateral patellar compression syndrome, it was found that open chain exercise with isometric quadriceps sets at 10° intervals with 3-kg weight resulted in more lateral patellar tilt and glide from 0° to 20° on CT scan. Closed chain exercise by pushing a foot-plate with resistance cords attached to provide 18-kg resistance led to improved congruence from 0° to 20°[26] Another study showed that in closed chain exercises, there is more selective VMO activation than in open chain exercises.[95] However, there is still debate in the literature. A 5-year follow-up of patients in a clinical trial found good maintenance of subjective and functional outcomes in both the open and closed kinetic chain exercise groups.[95]

#### 13.4.3.1 Specificity of Training

Before examining the issue of exercise prescription for the PFPS patient, some discussion on the different philosophies of strength training is required. The traditional strengthening view holds that strength gained in non-specific muscle training can be harnessed for use in performance, that is, the engine (muscles) is built in the strength training room; learning how to turn the engine on (neural control) is acquired on the field.[83] Strength is, therefore, increased by utilizing the overload principle, meaning exercising at least 60% of maximal.[36] However, the muscles around the patellofemoral joint are stabilizing muscles and need to be endurance trained, so working at 20–30% of maximal is more appropriate. A more recent interpretation of how to facilitate strength is based on the premise that the engine (muscles) and how it is turned on (neural control) should both be built in the strength training room.[83] Training should, therefore, simulate movement in terms of anatomical movement pattern, velocity, type, and force of contraction. Thus, with training, the neuromuscular system will tend to become better at generating tension for actions that resemble the muscle actions employed in training, but not necessarily for actions that are dissimilar to those used in training. If the desired outcome of treatment is for the patient to be pain-free on weight bearing activities, then the therapist must give the patient appropriate weight bearing training. At no stage should the patient's recovery be compromised by training into pain.

A useful starting exercise is small range knee flexion and extension movements (the first 30°) with the patient in stance position, where the feet are facing forward and positioned at the width of the pelvis. It is preferable that the patient has a dual channel biofeedback with electrodes on the VMO and the VL so the patient can monitor the timing of the contraction and the amount of activity. This is particularly important for those patients who have trouble activating the VMO. The patient is instructed to squeeze the gluteals and slowly flex the knees to 30° and slowly return to full extension without locking the knees back. The patient is aiming for the VMO to be activated before the VL and remain more than the VL during the activity. This clinical interpretation of the use of EMG biofeedback is at odds with the research application, in so far as the activity of the VMO and the VL has not been normalized. However, there is some evidence from a few randomized trials that the incorporation of EMG biofeedback into a physiotherapy exercise program improves the magnitude of activation of VMO and VL in patients with anterior knee pain.[27,107]

Progression of training involves simulation of the knee during the stance phase of walking, so the patient is in a walk stance position. In this position, VMO recruitment is usually poor and the seating of the patella in the trochlea is critical. Again, small amplitude movements need to be practiced. Again, emphasis should be given to the timing and intensity of the VMO contraction relative to the VL. For a patient who is having difficulty contracting the VMO, muscle stimulation may be used to facilitate the contraction. Further progression of treatment can be implemented by introducing step training. The patients need to practice stepping down from a small height initially. This should be performed slowly, in front of a mirror, so that changes in limb alignment can be observed and deviations can be corrected (Fig. 13.8). Specific work on the hip musculature may be necessary to improve the limb alignment. Some patients may only be able to do one repetition before the leg deviates. This is sufficient for them to start with, as inappropriate practice can be detrimental to learning. The number of repetitions should be increased as the skill level improves. It is therefore preferable for the therapist to emphasize quality not quantity. Initially, small number of exercises should be performed frequently throughout the day. The aim is to achieve a carryover from functional exercises to functional activities. Later, the patient can move to a larger step, initially decreasing the number of contractions and slowly increasing them again. As the control improves, the patient can alter the speed of their stepping activity and vary the place on descent where the stepping action is stopped. Weights may be introduced in the hands or in a backpack. Again, the number of repetitions and the speed of the movement should be decreased, initially and built back up again.

Training should be applicable to the patient's activities/sport, so a jumping athlete, for example, should have jumping incorporated in his program. Figure of eight running, bounding jumping off boxes, jumping and turning, and other plyometric routines are particularly appropriate for the high-performance athlete. However, the patient's VMO needs to be monitored at all times for timing and level of contraction relative to the VL. The number of repetitions performed by the patient at a training session will depend upon the onset of muscle fatigue. The aim would be to increase the number of repetitions before

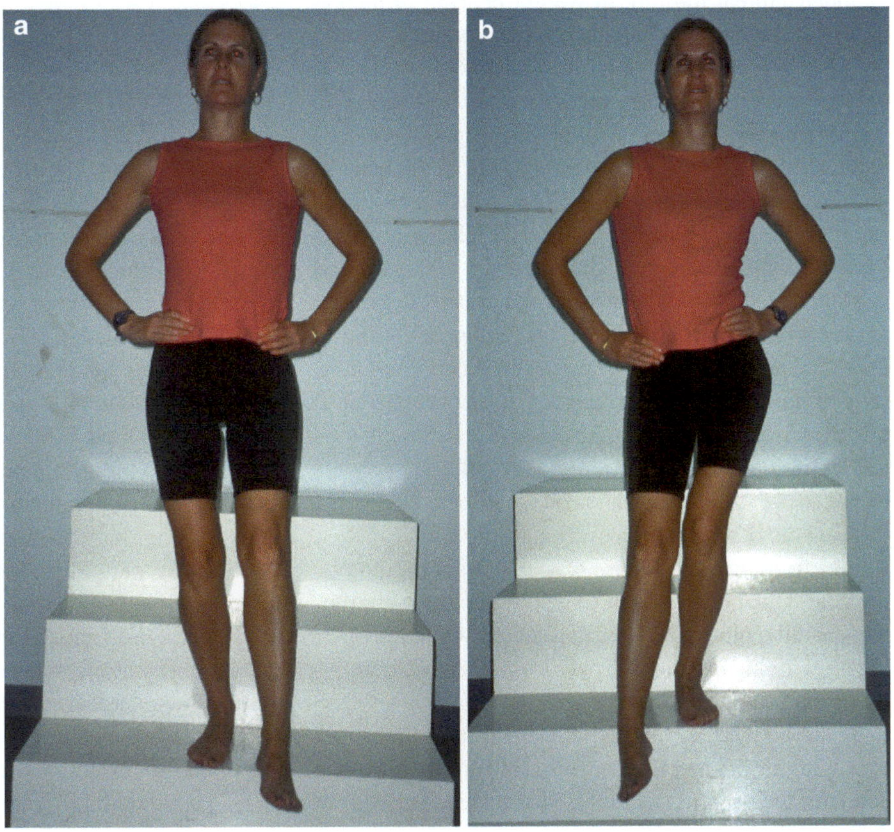


**Fig. 13.8** (**a**) Stepping down with correct limb alignment. (**b**) Stepping down with incorrect limb alignment

the onset of fatigue. Patients should be taught to recognize muscle fatigue or quivering, so that they do not train through the fatigue and risk exacerbating their symptoms.

### 13.4.4 Improving Lower Limb Mechanics

A stable pelvis will minimize unnecessary stress on the knee. Training of the gluteus medius (posterior fibers) to decrease hip internal rotation and the consequent valgus vector force that occurs at the knee is necessary to improve pelvic stability. Weakness of the hip abductors and external rotators has been documented in people with patellofemoral pain compared with pain-free controls.[79] Furthermore, a pilot study showed that adding strengthening of hip abductor and external rotator muscles to a quadriceps exercise program provided additional benefits with respect to the perceived pain symptoms during functional activities after 6 weeks of treatment.[71] Our research group showed that a comprehensive muscle training program which included gluteal training in weight bearing (which is described below) was superior to placebo treatment in the management of patellofemoral pain.[21]

The posterior gluteus medius may be trained in weight bearing with the patient standing side-on to a wall. The leg closest to the wall is flexed at the knee so the foot is off the ground. The hip is in line with the standing hip. The patient should have all their weight back through the heel of the standing leg, which is slightly flexed. The patient externally rotates the standing leg without turning the foot, the pelvis, or the shoulders. The patient should sustain the contraction for 20 s, so a burning can be felt in the gluteus medius region. If this exercise is difficult for a patient to coordinate, then rubber tubing may be used around the ankles to provide resistance as the patient stands on the affected leg while pushing the other leg back diagonally at 45°.

The training may be progressed to standing on one leg where the pelvis is kept level and the lower abdominals and the glutei are worked together while the other leg is swinging back and forward, simulating the activity of the stance phase of gait.

If the patient has marked internal femoral rotation, stretching of the anterior hip structures to increase the available external rotation may be required. The patient lies prone with the hip to be stretched in an abducted, externally rotated, and extended position. The other leg is extended and lies on top of the bent leg. The malleolus of the underneath leg is at the level of the tibial tubercle. The patient attempts to flatten the abducted and rotated hip by pushing along the length of the thigh and holding the stretch for 5 s. This action activates gluteals in inner range. Although it is not functional, it may facilitate gluteus medius activity in someone who is finding it difficult to activate the muscle in weight bearing.

### 13.4.5 Muscle Stretching

Appropriate flexibility exercises must be included in the treatment regime. The involved muscles may include hamstrings, gastrocnemius, rectus femoris, and TFL/ITB. A tight gastrocnemius will increase the amount of subtalar joint pronation exhibited in mid-stance phase of gait, so after the stretching, appropriate foot muscle training will be required.

### 13.4.6 Consideration of Foot Problems

The supinators of the foot, specifically tibialis posterior, should be trained if the patient demonstrates prolonged pronation during the mid-stance in gait. With the foot supinated, the base of the first metatarsal is higher than the cuboid, which will allow the peroneus longus to work more efficiently to increase the stability of the first metatarsal complex for push off. The therapist can train this action to improve the efficiency of push off. The position of training is in mid-stance, the patient is instructed to lift the arch while keeping the first metatarsal head on the floor, and then pushing the first metatarsal and great toe into the floor. If the patient is unable to keep the first metatarso- phalangeal joint on the ground when the arch is lifted, then the foot deformity is too large to correct with training alone and orthotics will be necessary to control the excessive pronation.

The effectiveness of prefabricated commercially available foot orthotics with and without a McConnell-based physiotherapy program was recently assessed in a randomized controlled trial involving 179 participants with PFPS.[12] The results showed that foot orthoses are superior to flat inserts according to participants' overall perception, but they have similar effects to physiotherapy and do not improve outcomes when added to physiotherapy in the short term. The authors also developed a clinical prediction rule for identifying patients with PFPS who are likely to benefit from foot orthoses and found age (>25 years), height (<165 cm), worst pain visual analogue scale (<53.25 mm) and a difference in mid-foot width from non-weight bearing to weight bearing (>10.96 mm) as possible predictors. Further research is needed to validate this clinical prediction rule.

### 13.4.7 Evaluation of the McConnell Program

Few clinical trials have evaluated the effectiveness of a "McConnell" type program for PFPS.[11,29,38] Harrison and colleagues[38] performed a randomized, blinded, controlled trial investigating three physiotherapy treatment options, one of which best reflects the protocol designed by McConnell.[63] At the end of the 1 month intervention period, the participants in the McConnell-based program showed significant improvements in pain and function compared with a group who had supervised exercises, but did not differ from the group given a home exercises program only. However, the sample size was only sufficient to detect a large effect between the groups. The large dropout rate (up to 48%) at 12 months may have affected the results at this time point, especially since a significantly greater number of subjects in the intervention group who showed substantial improvement were lost to follow-up. The authors concluded that any of the treatments could provide long-term improvements in pain and function.

Clark and colleagues[11] found that proprioceptive muscle stretching and strengthening aspects of physiotherapy have a beneficial effect at 3 months sufficient to permit discharge from physiotherapy. These benefits were maintained at 3 months. While they noted that taping did not influence the outcome, the numbers in each group may not have been large enough to detect independent effects of taping.

We conducted a randomized, double-blind, placebo-controlled trial of the McConnell program in 71 PFPS patients.[14,21] Standardized treatment consisted of six treatment sessions, once weekly for both the physiotherapy and placebo groups. Sixty seven (33 physiotherapy; 34 placebo) participants completed the trial. The physiotherapy group demonstrated significantly better response to treatment and greater improvements in pain and functional activities than the placebo group. The physiotherapy treatment also changed the onset timing of VMO relative to VL measured using surface electromyography during stair stepping and postural perturbation tasks. At baseline in both groups, VMO came on significantly later than VL. Following treatment, there was no change in muscle onset timing of the placebo group. However, in the physiotherapy group, the onset of VMO and VL occurred simultaneously (concentric) or VMO actually preceded VL (eccentric).[14,17] This study demonstrates that a McConnell-based physiotherapy program significantly improves pain and function and can alter EMG onset of VMO relative to VL compared with placebo treatment.

More recently, as described previously, Syme and colleagues[94] conducted a randomized controlled trial in 69 patients and found that both general quadriceps strengthening and selective VMO retraining were equally effective in reducing pain and improving function compared with a no treatment control.

## 13.5 Conclusion

Management of patellofemoral pain is no longer a conundrum if the therapist can determine the underlying causative factors and address those factors in treatment. It is imperative that the patient's symptoms are significantly reduced. This is often achieved by taping the patella, which not only decreases the pain, but also promotes an earlier activation of the VMO and increases quadriceps torque. Management will need to include specific VMO training, gluteal control work, stretching tight hip and lateral patellar structures and appropriate advice regarding the foot, be it orthotics, training, or taping.

## References


1. Handfield T, Kramer J. Effect of McConnell taping on perceived pain and knee extensor torques during isokinetic exercise performed by pateients with patellofemoral pain. *Physioth Can*. 2000; Winter:39-44.
2. Ahmed A, Shi S, Hyder A, et al. The effect of quadriceps tension characteristics on the patellar tracking pattern. *Transactions of the 34th Orthopaedic Research Society*; 1988; Atlanta:280.
3. Bennell K, Duncan M, Cowan S. Effect of patellar taping on vasti onset timing, knee kinematics, and kinetics in asymptomatic individuals with a delayed onset of vastus medialis oblique. *J Orthop Res*. 2006;24:1854-1860.
4. Bennell K, Hodges P, Mellor R, et al. The nature of anterior knee pain following injection of hypertonic saline into the infrapatellar fat pad. *J Orthop Res*. 2004;22:116-121.
5. Bockrath K, Wooden C, Worrell T, et al. Effects of patella taping on patella position and perceived pain. *Med Sci Sports Exerc*. 1993;25:989-992.
6. Brandt K. Pathogenesis of osteoarthritis. In: Kelley WN, Harris ED, Ruddy S, Sledge CB, eds. *Textbook of Rheumatology*. Philadelphia: W.B. Saunders Co; 1981.
7. Buchbinder R, Naparo N, Bizzo E. The relationship of abnormal pronation to chondromalacia patellae in distance runners. *J Am Podiatry Assoc*. 1979;69:159-161.
8. Burnham RS, Bell G, Olenik L, et al. Shoulder abduction strength measurement in football players: reliability and validity of two field tests. *Clin J Sport Med*. 1995;5:90-94.
9. Cerny K. Vastus medialis oblique/vastus lateralis muscle activity ratios for selected exercises in persons with and without patellofemoral pain syndrome. *Phys Ther*. 1995; 75:672-683.
10. Christou EA. Patellar taping increases vastus medialis oblique activity in the presence of patellofemoral pain. *J Electromyogr Kinesiol*. 2004;14:495-504.
11. Clark DI, Downing N, Mitchell J, et al. Physiotherapy for anterior knee pain: a randomised controlled trial. *Ann Rheum Dis*. 2000;59:700-704.
12. Collins N, Crossley K, Beller E, et al. Foot orthoses and physiotherapy in the treatment of patellofemoral pain syndrome: randomised clinical trial. *BMJ*. 2008;337:a1735.
13. Conway A, Malone T, Conway P. Patellar alignment/ tracking alteration: effect on force output and perceived pain. *Isokinet Exerc Sci*. 1992;2:9-17.
14. Cowan SM, Bennell KL, Crossley KM, et al. Physical therapy alters recruitment of the vasti in patellofemoral pain syndrome. *Med Sci Sports Exerc*. 2002;34:1879-1885.
15. Cowan SM, Bennell KL, Hodges PW. Therapeutic patellar taping changes the timing of vasti muscle activation in people with patellofemoral pain syndrome. *Clin J Sport Med*. 2002;12:339-347.
16. Cowan SM, Bennell KL, Hodges PW, et al. Delayed onset of electromyographic activity of vastus medialis obliquus relative to vastus lateralis in subjects with patellofemoral pain syndrome. *Arch Phys Med Rehabil*. 2001;82:183-189.
17. Cowan SM, Bennell KL, Hodges PW, et al. Simultaneous feedforward recruitment of the vasti in untrained postural tasks can be restored by physical therapy. *J Orthop Res*. 2003;21:553-558.
18. Cowan SM, Hodges PW, Bennell KL, et al. Altered vastii recruitment when people with patellofemoral pain syndrome complete a postural task. *Arch Phys Med Rehabil*. 2002;83:989-995.
19. Cowan SM, Hodges PW, Crossley KM, et al. Patellar taping does not change the amplitude of electromyographic activity of the vasti in a stair stepping task. *Br J Sports Med*. 2006;40:30-34.
20. Crossley KM, Bennell KL, Cowan SM, et al. Analysis of outcome measures for persons with patellofemoral pain: which are reliable and valid? *Arch Phys Med Rehabil*. 2004;85:815-822.
21. Crossley K, Bennell K, Green S, et al. Physical therapy for patellofemoral pain: a randomized, double-blinded, placebo-controlled trial. *Am J Sports Med*. 2002;30:857-865.
22. Crossley KM, Cowan SM, Bennell KL, et al. Knee flexion during stair ambulation is altered in individuals with patellofemoral pain. *J Orthop Res*. 2004;22:267-274.
23. Deandrade JR, Grant C, Dixon AS. Joint distension and reflex muscle inhibition in the knee. *J Bone Joint Surg Am*. 1965;47:313-322.
24. Dierks TA, Manal KT, Hamill J, et al. Proximal and distal influences on hip and knee kinematics in runners with patellofemoral pain during a prolonged run. *J Orthop Sports Phys Ther*. 2008;38:448-456.
25. Dillon PZ, Updyke WF, Allen WC. Gait analysis with reference to chondromalacia patellae. *J Orthop Sports Phys Ther*. 1983;5:127-131.
26. Doucette SA, Child DD. The effect of open and closed chain exercise and knee joint position on patellar tracking in lateral patellar compression syndrome. *J Orthop Sports Phys Ther*. 1996;23:104-110.
27. Dursun N, Dursun E, Kilic Z. Electromyographic biofeedback-controlled exercise versus conservative care for patellofemoral pain syndrome. *Arch Phys Med Rehabil*. 2001;82:1692-1695.
28. Dye SF. The knee as a biologic transmission with an envelope of function: a theory. *Clin Orthop Relat Res*. 1996; 325:10-18.
29. Eburne J, Bannister G. The McConnell regimen versus isometric quadriceps exercises in the management of anterior knee pain. A randomised prospective controlled trial. *Knee*. 1996;3:151-153.
30. Ernst GP, Kawaguchi J, Saliba E. Effect of patellar taping on knee kinetics of patients with patellofemoral pain syndrome. *J Orthop Sports Phys Ther*. 1999;29:661-667.
31. Frankel VH, Nordin M. *Basic Biomechanics of the Skeletal System*. Philadelphia: Lea and Febiger; 1980.
32. Fucentese SF, von Roll A, Koch PP, et al. The patella morphology in trochlear dysplasia – a comparative MRI study. *Knee*. 2006;13:145-150.
33. Fulkerson JP. Awareness of the retinaculum in evaluating patellofemoral pain. *Am J Sports Med*. 1982;10:147-149.
34. Fulkerson J, Hungerford D. *Disorders of the Patellofemoral Joint*. 2nd ed. Baltimore: Williams & Wilkins; 1990.
35. Gilleard W, McConnell J, Parsons D. The effect of patellar taping on the onset of vastus medialis obliquus and vastus lateralis muscle activity in persons with patellofemoral pain. *Phys Ther*. 1998;78:25-32.
36. Grabiner MD, Koh TJ, Draganich LF. Neuromechanics of the patellofemoral joint. *Med Sci Sports Exerc*. 1994;26: 10-21.

37. Greenwald AE, Bagley AM, France EP, et al. A biomechanical and clinical evaluation of a patellofemoral knee brace. *Clin Orthop Relat Res*. 1996;324:187-195.
38. Harrison EL, Sheppard MS, McQuarrie AM. A randomized controlled trial of physical therapy treatment programs in patellofemoral pain syndrome. *Physiother Can.* 1999; Spring:93-106.
39. Helminen H, Kiviranta I, Tammi M, et al. *Joint Loading: Biology and Health of Articular Structures*. London: Butterworth & Co Ltd; 1987.
40. Herbert R. Preventing and treating stiff joints. In: Crosbie J, McConnell J, eds. *Key issues in Musculoskeletal Physiotherapy*. Oxford: Butterworth – Heinemann; 1993.
41. Herrington L. The effect of corrective taping of the patella on patella position as defined by MRI. *Res Sports Med.* 2006;14:215-223.
42. Herrington L, Payton CJ. Effects of corrective taping of the patella on patients with patellofemoral pain. *Physiotherapy*. 1997;83:566-572.
43. Hodges PW, Mellor R, Crossley K, et al. Pain induced by injection of hypertonic saline into the infrapatellar fat pad and effect on coordination of the quadriceps muscles. *Arthritis Rheum*. 2009;61:70-77.
44. Hooley CJ, McCrum NG, Cohen RE. The viscoelastic deformation of tendon. *J Biomech*. 1980;13:521-528.
45. Hoppenfeld S. *Physical Examination of the Spine and Extremities*. New York: Appleton; 1976.
46. Howard JD, Enoka RM. Maximum bilateral contractions are modified by neurally mediated interlimb effects. *J Appl Physiol*. 1991;70:306-316.
47. Hudson Z, Darthuy E. Iliotibial band tightness and patellofemoral pain syndrome: a case-control study. *Man Ther.* 2009;14:147-151.
48. Insall J. "Chondromalacia patellae": patellar malalignment syndrome. *Orthop Clin North Am*. 1979;10:117-127.
49. Karst GM, Willett GM. Onset timing of electromyographic activity in the vastus medialis oblique and vastus lateralis muscles in subjects with and without patellofemoral pain syndrome. *Phys Ther*. 1995;75:813-823.
50. Kendall HD, Kendall FP, Boynton DA. *Posture and Pain*. Baltimore: Williams & Wilkinson Co; 1952.
51. Kendall F, McCreary L. *Muscle Testing and Function*. Baltimore: Williams & Wilkins; 1983.
52. Keser S, Savranlar A, Bayar A, et al. Is there a relationship between anterior knee pain and femoral trochlear dysplasia? Assessment of lateral trochlear inclination by magnetic resonance imaging. *Knee Surg Sports Traumatol Arthrosc*. 2008;16:911-915.
53. Koh TJ, Grabiner MD, De Swart RJ. In vivo tracking of the human patella. *J Biomech*. 1992;25:637-643.
54. Kramer PG. Patella malalignment syndrome: rationale to reduce excessive lateral pressure. *J Orthop Sports Phys Ther*. 1986;8:301-309.
55. Larsen B, Andreasen E, Urfer A, et al. Patellar taping: a radiographic examination of the medial glide technique. *Am J Sports Med*. 1995;23:465-471.
56. Levinger P, Gilleard W. Tibia and rearfoot motion and ground reaction forces in subjects with patellofemoral pain syndrome during walking. *Gait Posture*. 2007;25:2-8.
57. Lutter LD. The knee and running. *Clin Sports Med*. 1985; 4:685-698.
58. Lyon LK, Benz LN, Johnson KK, et al. Q-angle: a factor in peak torque occurrence in isokinetic knee extension. *J Orthop Sports Phys Ther*. 1988;9:250-253.
59. MacKay-Lyons M. Low-load, prolonged stretch in treatment of elbow flexion contractures secondary to head trauma: a case report. *Phys Ther*. 1989;69:292-296.
60. Maitland GD. *Vertebral Manipulation*. London: Butterworths; 1986.
61. Malek MM, Mangine RE. Patellofemoral pain syndromes: a comprehensive and conservative approach. *J Orthop Sports Phys Ther*. 1981;2:108-116.
62. Mariani PP, Caruso I. An electromyographic investigation of subluxation of the patella. *J Bone Joint Surg Br*. 1979;61: 169-171.
63. McConnell J. The management of chondromalacia patellae: a long term solution. *Aust J Physiother*. 1986;32:215-223.
64. McConnell J. Fat pad irritation: a mistaken patellar tendonitis. *Sport Health*. 1991;9:79.
65. McConnell J. Training the vastus medialis oblique in the management of patellofemoral pain. In: *Tenth Congress of the World Confederation for Physical Therapy*; 1987; Sydney.
66. Merican AM, Amis AA. Iliotibial band tension affects patellofemoral and tibiofemoral kinematics. *J Biomech*. 2009;42: 1539-1546.
67. Micheli LJ, Slater JA, Woods E, et al. Patella alta and the adolescent growth spurt. *Clin Orthop Relat Res*. 1986;213:159-162.
68. Mizuno Y, Kumagai M, Mattessich SM, et al. Q-angle influences tibiofemoral and patellofemoral kinematics. *J Orthop Res*. 2001;19:834-840.
69. Mow VC, Lai WM, Eisenfeld J, et al. Some surface characteristics of articular cartilage. II. On the stability of articular surface and a possible biomechanical factor in etiology of chondrodegeneration. *J Biomech*. 1974;7:457-468.
70. Nadler SF, DePrince ML, Hauesien N, et al. Portable dynamometer anchoring station for measuring strength of the hip extensors and abductors. *Arch Phys Med Rehabil*. 2000;81:1072-1076.
71. Nakagawa TH, Muniz TB, Baldon Rde M, et al. The effect of additional strengthening of hip abductor and lateral rotator muscles in patellofemoral pain syndrome: a randomized controlled pilot study. *Clin Rehabil*. 2008;22: 1051-1060.
72. Ng GY, Cheng JM. The effects of patellar taping on pain and neuromuscular performance in subjects with patellofemoral pain syndrome. *Clin Rehabil*. 2002;16:821-827.
73. On AY, Uludag B, Taskiran E, et al. Differential corticomotor control of a muscle adjacent to a painful joint. *Neurorehabil Neural Repair*. 2004;18:127-133.
74. Owings TM, Grabiner MD. Motor control of the vastus medialis oblique and vastus lateralis muscles is disrupted during eccentric contractions in subjects with patellofemoral pain. *Am J Sports Med*. 2002;30:483-487.
75. Pfeiffer RP, DeBeliso M, Shea KG, et al. Kinematic MRI assessment of McConnell taping before and after exercise. *Am J Sports Med*. 2004;32:621-628.
76. Powers CM, Landel R, Perry J. Timing and intensity of vastus muscle activity during functional activities in subjects with and without patellofemoral pain. *Phys Ther*. 1996; 76:946-955; discussion 956-967.

77. Powers CM, Landel R, Sosnick T, et al. The effects of patellar taping on stride characteristics and joint motion in subjects with patellofemoral pain. *J Orthop Sports Phys Ther.* 1997;26:286-291.
78. Powers CM, Mortenson S, Nishimoto D, et al. Criterion-related validity of a clinical measurement to determine the medial/lateral component of patellar orientation. *J Orthop Sports Phys Ther.* 1999;29:372-377.
79. Prins MR, van der Wurff P. Females with patellofemoral pain syndrome have weak hip muscles: a systematic review. *Aust J Physiother.* 2009;55:9-15.
80. Radin EL. A rational approach to the treatment of patellofemoral pain. *Clin Orthop Relat Res.* 1979;144:107-109.
81. Roberts JM. The effect of taping on patellofemoral alignment a radiological pilot study. In: *Sixth Biennial Conference of the Manipulative Therapists Association of Australia.* 1989:146-151.
82. Root M, Orien W, Weed J. *Clinical Biomechanics*, vol. II. Los Angeles: Clinical Biomechanics Corp; 1977.
83. Sale D, MacDougall D. Specificity in strength training: a review for the coach and athlete. *Can J Appl Sport Sci.* 1981;6:87-92.
84. Salsich GB, Brechter JH, Farwell D, et al. The effects of patellar taping on knee kinetics, kinematics, and vastus lateralis muscle activity during stair ambulation in individuals with patellofemoral pain. *J Orthop Sports Phys Ther.* 2002; 32:3-10.
85. Scott DA, Bond EQ, Sisto SA, et al. The intra- and interrater reliability of hip muscle strength assessments using a hand-held versus a portable dynamometer anchoring station. *Arch Phys Med Rehabil.* 2004;85:598-603.
86. Smith TO, Davies L, Donell ST. The reliability and validity of assessing medio-lateral patellar position: a systematic review. *Man Ther.* 2009;14:355-362.
87. Smith TO, Hunt NJ, Donell ST. The reliability and validity of the Q-angle: a systematic review. *Knee Surg Sports Traumatol Arthrosc.* 2008;16:1068-1079.
88. Somes S, Worrell TW, Corey B, et al. Effects of patellar taping on patellar position in the open and closed kinetic chain: a preliminary study. *J Sport Rehabil.* 1997;6:299-308.
89. Souza DR, Gross MT. Comparison of vastus medialis obliquus: vastus lateralis muscle integrated electromyographic ratios between healthy subjects and patients with patellofemoral pain. *Phys Ther.* 1991;71(4):310-316; discussion 317-320.
90. Souza RB, Powers CM. Predictors of hip internal rotation during running: an evaluation of hip strength and femoral structure in women with and without patellofemoral pain. *Am J Sports Med.* 2009;37:579-587.
91. Spencer JD, Hayes KC, Alexander IJ. Knee joint effusion and quadriceps reflex inhibition in man. *Arch Phys Med Rehabil.* 1984;65:171-177.
92. Stokes M, Young A. Investigations of quadriceps inhibition: implications for clinical practice. *Physiotherapy.* 1984;70: 425-428.
93. Subotnick SI. The foot and its relationship to gait: a series of articles and editorial comments. *J Orthop Sports Phys Ther.* 1980;2:48-54.
94. Syme G, Rowe P, Martin D, et al. Disability in patients with chronic patellofemoral pain syndrome: a randomised controlled trial of VMO selective training versus general quadriceps strengthening. *Man Ther.* 2009;14:252-263.
95. Tang SF, Chen CK, Hsu R, et al. Vastus medialis obliquus and vastus lateralis activity in open and closed kinetic chain exercises in patients with patellofemoral pain syndrome: an electromyographic study. *Arch Phys Med Rehabil.* 2001;82:1441-1445.
96. Taylor DC, Dalton JD Jr, Seaber AV, et al. Viscoelastic properties of muscle-tendon units. The biomechanical effects of stretching. *Am J Sports Med.* 1990;18:300-309.
97. Thijs Y, De Clercq D, Roosen P. Gait-related intrinsic risk factors for patellofemoral pain in novice recreational runners. *Br J Sports Med.* 2008;42:466-471.
98. Townsend PR, Rose RM, Radin EL, et al. The biomechanics of the human patella and its implications for chondromalacia. *J Biomech.* 1977;10:403-407.
99. Van Tiggelen D, Cowan S, Coorevits P, et al. Delayed vastus medialis obliquus to vastus lateralis onset timing contributes to the development of patellofemoral pain in previously healthy men: a prospective study. *Am J Sports Med.* 2009;37: 1099-1105.
100. Voight ML, Wieder DL. Comparative reflex response times of vastus medialis obliquus and vastus lateralis in normal subjects and subjects with extensor mechanism dysfunction. An electromyographic study. *Am J Sports Med.* 1991;19:131-137.
101. Warden SJ, Hinman RS, Watson MA, et al. Patellar taping and bracing for the treatment of chronic knee pain: a systematic review and meta-analysis. *Arthritis Rheum.* 2008; 59:73-83.
102. Waryasz GR, McDermott AY. Patellofemoral pain syndrome (PFPS): a systematic review of anatomy and potential risk factors. *Dyn Med.* 2008;7:9.
103. Wilson NA, Press JM, Koh JL, et al. In vivo noninvasive evaluation of abnormal patellar tracking during squatting in patients with patellofemoral pain. *J Bone Joint Surg Am.* 2009;91:558-566.
104. Wilson NA, Press JM, Zhang LQ. In vivo strain of the medial versus lateral quadriceps tendon in patellofemoral pain syndrome. *J Appl Physiol.* 2009;107:422-428.
105. Witvrouw E, Sneyers C, Lysens R, et al. Reflex response times of vastus medialis oblique and vastus lateralis in normal subjects and in subjects with patellofemoral pain syndrome. *J Orthop Sports Phys Ther.* 1996;24:160-165.
106. Yang JF, Winter DA. Electromyography reliability in maximal and submaximal isometric contractions. *Arch Phys Med Rehabil.* 1983;64:417-420.
107. Yip SL, Ng GY. Biofeedback supplementation to physiotherapy exercise programme for rehabilitation of patellofemoral pain syndrome: a randomized controlled pilot study. *Clin Rehabil.* 2006;20:1050-1057.

# Skeletal Malalignment and Anterior Knee Pain: Rationale, Diagnosis, and Management

# 14

Robert A. Teitge and Roger Torga-Spak

## 14.1 Introduction

Any variation from optimal skeletal alignment may increase the vector forces acting on the patellofemoral joint causing either ligament failure with subsequent subluxation or cartilage failure as in chondromalacia or arthrosis or both ligament and cartilage failure (Fig. 14.1). Anterior knee pain may result from these abnormal forces or their consequences.

The mechanical disadvantage provided by a skeleton with a geometrical or architectural flaw distributes abnormal stresses to both the ligaments and the joints of the misaligned limb. Ligament overload and subsequently failure (insufficiency) may occur with a single traumatic episode as well as repetitive episodes of minor trauma or chronic overload. Skeletal malalignment may cause chondromalacia patella and subsequently osteoarthritis by creating an increased mechanical leverage on the patellofemoral joint, which can exceed the load capacity of the articular cartilage. A reduction in contact surface area such as a small patella or a high patella or a subluxed patella may also increase the unit area loading beyond the load capacity of the articular cartilage leading to cartilage failure (osteoarthritis).

Anterior knee pain in association with bony malalignment may be the result of the abnormal tension or compression placed on the capsule, ligaments, synovium, or subchondral bone.

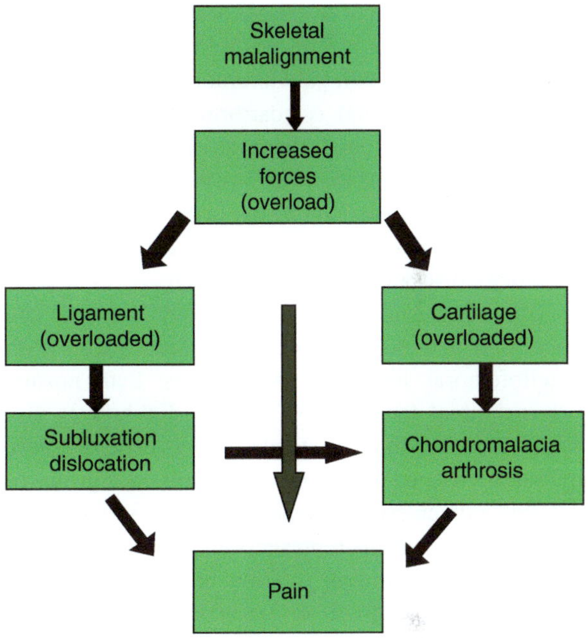


**Fig. 14.1** Pathogenesis of anterior knee pain

## 14.2 Association of Skeletal Malalignment and Patellofemoral Joint Pathology

Abnormal skeletal alignment of the lower extremity has been associated with various patellofemoral syndromes and biomechanical abnormalities. Our understanding of these associations continues to develop as many references consider only one aspect of the analysis.

In the frontal plane, malalignment has been shown to influence the progression of patellofemoral joint arthritis.[4,12] Varus alignment increases the likelihood of medial patellofemoral osteoarthrosis progression

R. Torga-Spak (✉)
Faculty of Orthopaedics and Traumatology,
Department of Surgery, Instituto Universitario CEMIC,
Buenos Aires, Argentina
e-mail: rtorgaspak@gmail.com

V. Sanchis-Alfonso (ed.), *Anterior Knee Pain and Patellar Instability*,
DOI: 10.1007/978-0-85729-507-1_14, © Springer-Verlag London Limited 2011

while valgus alignment increases the likelihood of lateral patellofemoral osteoarthrosis progression. Fujikawa[13] in a cadaveric study found a marked alteration of patellar and femoral contact areas with the introduction of increased varus alignment produced by a varus osteotomy.

Lerat et al.[29] noted a statistically significant correlation between increased femoral internal torsion and both patellar chondropathy and instability. Janssen[22] also found patellar dislocation was most commonly combined with increased medial torsion of the femur and speculated that this medial torsion was responsible for the development of dysplasia of the trochlea and of the patella. Takai et al.[41] measured femoral and tibial torsion in patients with patellofemoral medial and lateral unicompartmental osteoarthrosis and noted that the correlation of patellofemoral osteoarthritis with increased femoral torsion (23° vs 9° in controls) was statistically their most significant observation and suggested that excessive femoral torsion is one of the contributory causes of patellofemoral wear.

Turner[43] studied the association of tibial torsion and knee joint pathology and observed that patients with patellofemoral instability had greater than normal external tibial torsion (25° vs 19°). Eckhoff et al.[11] found the tibia in the extended knee to be 6° more externally rotated than normal controls in a group of patients with anterior knee pain. This was termed knee version. Whether this represents an abnormal skeletal torsion or an abnormal rotation of the tibia on the femur due to knee joint soft tissue laxity or abnormal muscle pull is unknown.

These studies and many others clearly show the importance of abnormal skeletal alignment of the lower extremity in the pathogenesis of various disorders of the patellofemoral joint.

### 14.2.1 Q-Angle and Skeletal Malalignment

The Q-angle has been implicated as a major source of patellofemoral pathology, but it must be emphasized that the Q-angle is a normal and necessary anatomic fact responsible to balance the tibiofemoral force transmission. Hvid et al.[19] demonstrated a significant relation between the Q-angle measurement and increased hip internal rotation, thus supporting the existence of a torsional malalignment syndrome of the patellofemoral joint. Insall[20] called an increased Q-angle "patellar malalignment" and noted that it was usually associated with increased femoral anteversion and external tibial torsion so that the motion of the knee occurred about an axis, which is rotated medially compared with the axes of the hip and ankle joints producing "squinting" patella. This type of knee he stated is prone to chondromalacia (clinically "a diffuse aching pain on the anteromedial aspect of the knee"). It should be noted, however, that an increased Q-angle was present in only 40 of 83 (48%) knees in which surgical realignment for chondromalacia was performed. Thus, the problem is not the value of the Q-angle; the problem is that the Q-angle rotates around the coronal plane of the lower extremity.

Finally, it should be perhaps mentioned that Greene et al.[15] showed the reliability of the Q-angle measurement to be poor.

## 14.3 Definitions: Patellofemoral Alignment

There are two common uses for the term alignment: (a) malposition of the patella on the femur, and (b) malposition of the knee joint between the body and the foot with the subsequent effect on the patellofemoral mechanics. While it is more common to consider the position of the patella in the trochlea (i.e., subluxation), this view inhibits the more important consideration of what the position of the knee in space relative to the center of gravity of the body has in developing the force, which the patellofemoral joint will experience. Tracking is the change in position of patella relative to the femur during knee flexion and extension and while it is obviously important, no clinically useful tracking measurement systems exist and the loading characteristics of the patellofemoral joint are largely unrelated to tracking.

The relationship of the patella to the femur (patellar malalignment) must be viewed in all three planes (Table 14.1). In the coronal plane, one can measure Q-angle and patellar spin. In the sagittal plane, one can measure patellar flexion and height; in the horizontal plane, one can measure patellar tilt or shift. Lauren[25] noted that shift and mini-tilt may both be manifestations of decreased lateral facet cartilage.

It is a common mistake to consider alignment as referring only to the position of the patella on the

**Table 14.1** Classification of patellar malalignment

| Frontal plane | | Sagittal plane | | Horizontal plane | |
|---|---|---|---|---|---|
| Internal rotation (spun) | External rotation (spun) | Flexion | Extension | Medial tilt | Lateral tilt |
| High Q-angle | Low Q-angle | Alta | Baja | Medial shift (translation) | Lateral shift (translation) |

**Table 14.2** Classification of skeletal malalignment

| Frontal plane | | Sagittal plane | | Horizontal plane | |
|---|---|---|---|---|---|
| | Location | | Location | | Location |
| Varus | Femur<br>Tibia<br>Ligaments | Prominent trochlea | Femur | Inward pointing knee | Femur (internal torsion)<br>Tibia (external torsion)<br>Subtalar joint complex (hyperpronation) |
| Valgus | Femur<br>Tibia<br>Ligaments | Shallow trochlear<br>Aplasic tuberosity | Femur<br>Tibia | Outward pointing knee<br>Increased TT-TG > 20 mm<br>Decreased TT-TG | Femur (external torsion)<br>Tibia (internal torsion)<br>Subtalar joint complex<br>Tibia |

femoral trochlea. Alignment refers to the changing relationship of all the bones of the lower extremity and might best be considered as the relationship of the patellofemoral joint to the body. Mechanical alignment is the sum total of the bony architecture of the entire lower extremity from sacrum (center of gravity) to the foot (ground). The position and orientation of patellofemoral joint to the weight bearing line determines the direction and magnitude of forces, which will cross the patellofemoral joint. The relationship of the patellofemoral joint to the body must be defined in all three planes (Table 14.2). In the frontal plane, one can measure varus or valgus and patellar height. In the sagittal plane, one can measure the patellar height, distance from the knee joint axis to the patella, depth of the trochlea, and height of the tibial tubercle. In the horizontal plane, one can measure the torsion of the acetabulum, femur, tibia and foot, the version of the knee, the position of the tibial tubercle relative to the trochlear groove, and the depth of the groove as well as the "patellofemoral alignment."

## 14.4 Diagnosis of Skeletal Alignment

Malalignment refers to a variation from the normal anatomy; normal is that which is biomechanically optimal. In order to detect and understand deformities of the lower extremity, it is important to establish the limits and parameters of normal alignment based on average values for the general population.

### 14.4.1 Frontal Plane Alignment

Frontal plane alignment is best determined using long-standing AP radiographs including hip, knee, and ankle joint. To determine the mechanical axis, a line is drawn from the center of the femoral head to the center of the ankle joint (Fig. 14.2). Typically, normal alignment is defined as the mechanical axis passing just medial to the center of the knee.[33] Valgus alignment refers to the mechanical axis passing lateral to the center of the knee while varus refers to the mechanical axis passing medial to the center of the knee.

Two commonly measured angles are the mechanical tibiofemoral angle (center of femoral head to center of knee to center of talus) and the anatomic tibiofemoral angle (line down center of femoral shaft and line down center of tibial shaft). The mechanical tibiofemoral angle is the angle between the mechanical axis of the femur and the tibia. An angle of $1.2° \pm 2°$ is considered normal (i.e., the limb mechanical axis falls just medial to the center of the knee joint).[5,6,18,33] The anatomic tibiofemoral angle is the angle between the femur shaft and tibia shaft and is usually $5.5° \pm 2°$. Different investigators found no difference between males and females in these angles.[18,45,46]

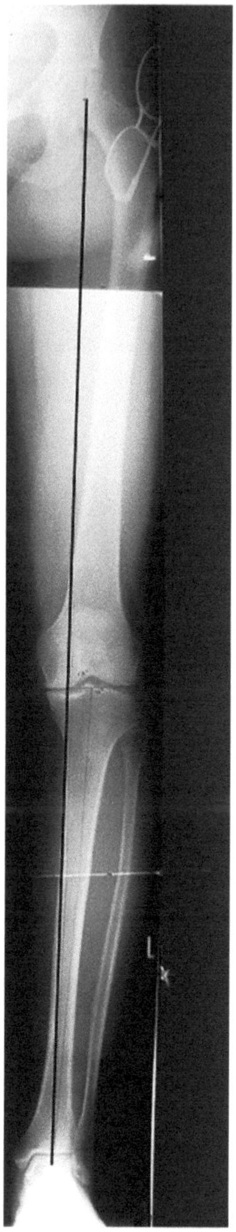

Fig. 14.2 Whole limb standing radiograph with mechanical axis added showing varus

### 14.4.2 Rotational (Horizontal or Transverse) Plane Alignment

Rotational plane alignment can be determined accurately with the use of axial computed tomography. Common measurements are the torsion of the femur, torsion of the tibia, version or the relationship of the distal femur and proximal tibia, and the relationship between the femur and the tibial tuberosity (TT-TG).

#### 14.4.2.1 Bone Torsion

Femoral torsion is defined as the angle formed between the axis of the femoral neck and distal femur and is measured in degrees. To assess femoral torsion with CT scan, a line from the center point of the femoral head to the center point of the base of the femoral neck is created. This second point is more easily selected by locating the center of the femoral shaft at the level of the base of the neck where the shaft becomes round. Based on the classic tabletop method, the condylar axis is defined as the line between the two most posterior aspects of the femoral condyles. Alternatively, a line connecting the epicondyles can be used. Then, the angle formed by the intersection of these two tangents is measured (Fig. 14.3).

For assessment of tibial torsion, a line is drawn across the center of the tibial plateau. As this line is not easy to locate, some authors use the tangent formed by the posterior cortical margin of the tibial plateau. The femoral epicondylar axis might also be selected as it is easier to locate and would appear to be valid because it is the relationship of the knee joint axis to the ankle joint axis, which is of concern. Next, a line connecting the center point of the medial malleolus with the center point of the lateral malleolus is produced. The angle

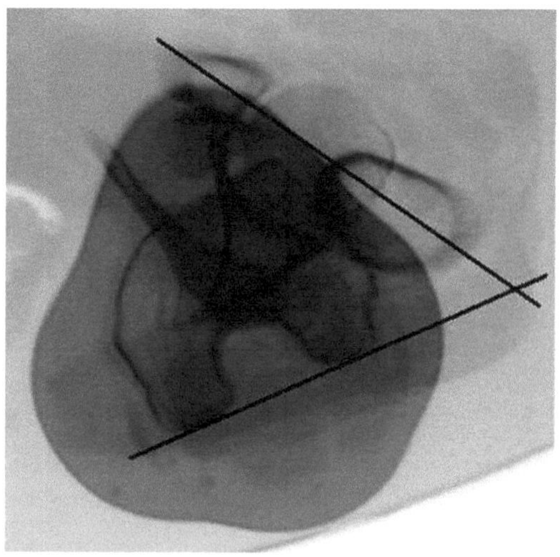

Fig. 14.3 Femoral torsion can be seen with an overlay of proximal and distal femur

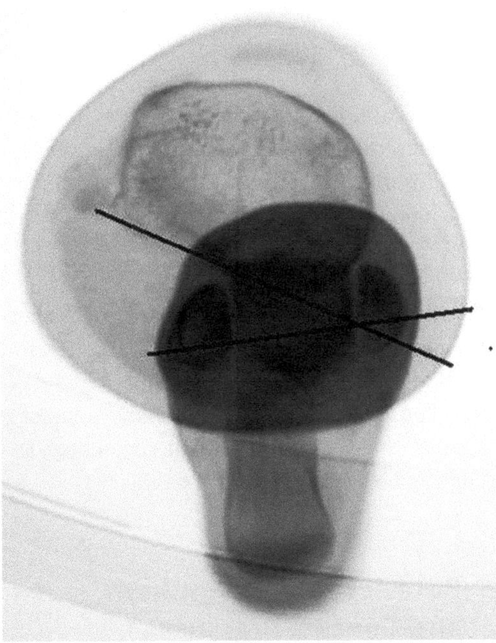

**Fig. 14.4** Tibial torsion can be seen with an overlay of the proximal tibia and distal tibia

formed by the intersection of these two lines is measured to determine the tibial torsion (Fig. 14.4).

Strecker et al.[39,40] reported the largest series of torsion determinations in normal individuals using CT scan. The authors measured torsion in 505 femurs and 504 tibia and found femoral anteversion of 24.1° ± 17.4° and external tibial torsion of 34.85° ± 17.4°. No correlation to sex could be established. Yoshioka[44] made direct skeletal measurements of femur and tibia and found femoral anteversion to average 13° measuring off the tangent of the distal femoral condyles and 7° measuring off the epicondylar axis (SD 8°). His values generally agree with those reviewed in the literature, which he tabulated. There was no significant difference between males and females. Conversely, lateral tibial torsion averaged 24° with a significant difference between males and females at 21° (SD 5°) vs 27° (SD 11°). Furthermore, even greater differences were noted in the outward foot rotation (−5° vs. 11°), which must reflect increases in subtalar position although this was not mentioned in their paper. These gender differences would explain the higher incidence of patellofemoral disease in females as well as the higher incidence of ACL tears in female athletes. Although this hypothesis is attractive, his findings have not been corroborated by other authors.[34,35]

#### 14.4.2.2 TT-TG (Tibial Tuberosity–Trochlear Groove)

The relationship of the position of the tibial tuberosity to the trochlear groove will determine the lateralization force acting on the patella through quadriceps contraction. This relationship can be evaluated and quantified by the measurement of the TT-TG. The TT-TG is the distance measured in mm between two perpendiculars to the bicondylar axis.[1] One perpendicular passes through the center of the tibial tuberosity and the other through the center of the trochlear groove. The measurements are taken by superposing two CT scans cuts, one cut at the level of the proximal third of the trochlear groove and the other at the superior part of the tibial tuberosity (Fig. 14.5). A TT-TG distance of less than 20 mm is considered normal.[14]

### *14.4.3 Sagittal Plane Alignment*

In the sagittal plane, the osseous factors to be evaluated include the trochlea, the tibial tuberosity, the patellar height, flexion, and length of the radius of curvature for the trochlea.

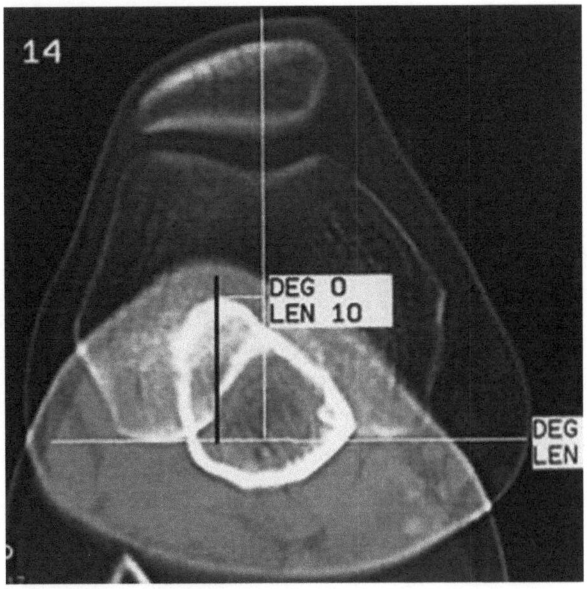


**Fig. 14.5** CT scan shows measurement of the distance TT-TG. Tibial Tubercle- Trochlear Groove is seen with overlay of distal femur and tibia at the level of tibial tuberosity. Also note trochlear shape, patellar shift, patellar tilt, patellar and trochlear subchondral bone sclerosis

Femoral trochlear dysplasia is an abnormality of the shape and depth of the trochlear groove mainly at its cranial part and has been associated with patellar instability and anterior knee pain. Brattström in 1964[2] studied trochlear geometry in recurrent dislocation of the patella and concluded that a shallow femoral groove (i.e., femoral dysplasia) was the most common cause. Trochlear dysplasia can be diagnosed by using a true lateral conventional radiograph of the knee[16,31] (Fig. 14.6).

Dejour suggested three criteria to diagnose trochlear dysplasia on the lateral view radiograph: the crossing sign, the trochlear boss or prominence, and the depth of the trochlea. The crossing sign is present when the line representing the floor of the trochlea, as it moves proximally, crosses the outline of the lateral femoral condyle.[8,9] Dejour's second criterion occurs when the proximal extent of the trochlear floor extends anterior to the anterior femoral cortex. A prominence or boss of greater than 3 mm is considered as a type of trochlear dysplasia.[8,9] This may be a variant of the ridge described by Outerbridge. Dejour's third criterion is the actual distance of the floor of the trochlea below the femoral condyles measured at a point in the proximal trochlea. In controls this measured 7.8 mm, while in patients with objective patellar instability it measured 2.3 mm.

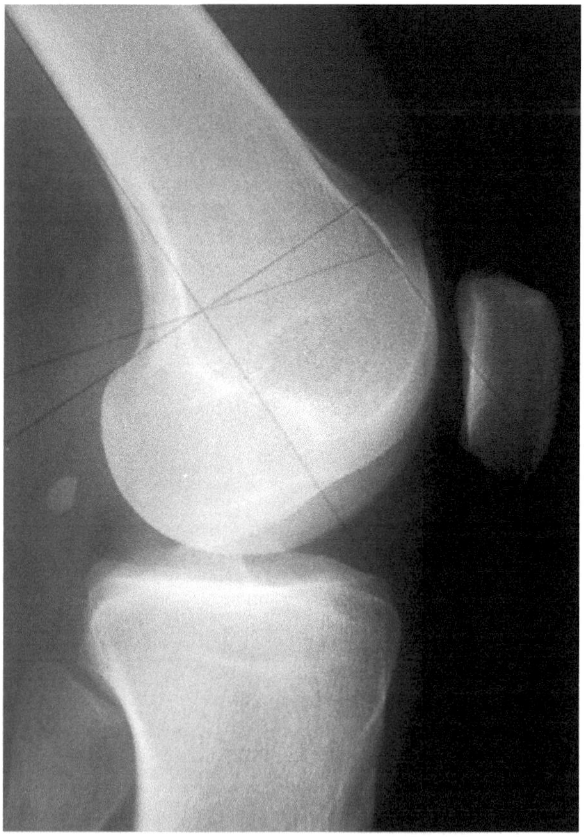

**Fig. 14.6** True lateral view shows trochlear dysplasia. The trochlear line crosses the contour of the condyles (*crossing sign*) and a trochlear boss or prominence is present

The shape of the tibial tuberosity is best seen on the lateral radiograph and a hypoplasic tibial tuberosity may be identified. The prominence of the tibial tuberosity will alter the angle of patellar flexion and consequently change compressive forces and contact areas in a manner not yet quantified but speculated as contributing to chondromalacia and pain.

## 14.5 Rotational Malalignment and Contact Pressures in the Patellofemoral Joint

Fixed rotation of either the femur or tibia has been shown to have a significant influence on the patellofemoral joint contact areas and pressures. Lee et al.[26-28] investigated the effects of rotational deformities of the lower extremity on patellofemoral contact pressures in a cadaver model. They simulated various types of rotational deformities of the femur by internally and externally rotated the cadaver knees about the axis representing the distal third of the femur. They found that 30° of both internal and external rotation of the femur in their cadaver knee model created a significantly greater peak contact pressure on the contralateral facet of the patella. External rotational deformities of the femur were associated with greater peak contact forces on the medial facet of the patella, while internal rotational deformities were associated with higher peak contact pressures on the lateral facet of the patella.

A study performed in our institution by Kijowski et al.[24] on specimens including the femoral head and foot confirmed the Lee's observations (Fig. 14.7). When the distal femur was internally rotated about an osteotomy, which increased femoral anteversion, there was increased contact pressure on the lateral aspect of the patellofemoral joint and decreased contact pressure on the medial aspect of the joint. When femoral torsion was decreased by external rotation osteotomy, there was increased contact pressure on the medial

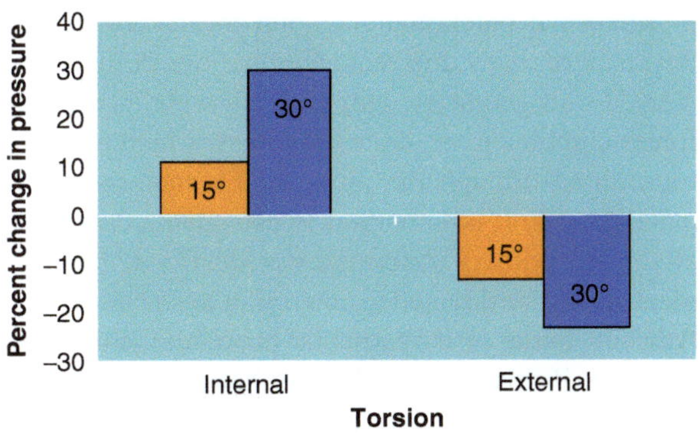


**Fig. 14.7** Lateral facet pressure change with femoral rotational osteotomy

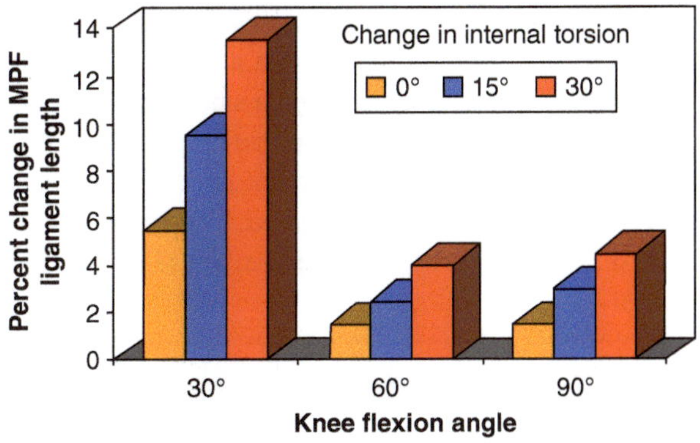


**Fig. 14.8** Change in length of the medial patellofemoral ligament with increased femoral torsion

side and decreased contact pressure on the lateral side of the patellofemoral joint.

## 14.6 Rotational Malalignment and Medial Patellofemoral Ligament Strain

Our study also found that internal rotation osteotomy of the femur of 30° results in a significant increase in the strain in all areas of the medial patellofemoral ligament (Fig. 14.8). The results of this study show that variations in femoral torsion (anteversion–retroversion) caused alterations in the patterns of force transmission across the patellofemoral joint and in the strain present in the medial patellofemoral ligament. The increased strain present in the medial patellofemoral ligament during quadriceps activity in individuals with an internally rotated femur may first result in pain over the medial aspect of the knee joint. The medial patellofemoral ligament may fail as a result of this increase in strain, leading to instability of the patellofemoral joint.

Hefzy et al.[17] used a cadaveric model to study the effects of tibial rotation on the patellofemoral contact pressures and areas. The authors found that internal tibial rotation increases medial patellofemoral contact areas while external tibial rotation increases lateral patellofemoral contact areas at all flexion angles. Lee et al.[27,28] corroborated their findings and they also determine the strain in the peripatellar retinaculum at different tibial rotations. They showed that with increased knee flexion, once the patella is engaged in the trochlea, the function of the peripatellar retinaculum is minimal and less affected by tibial rotation.

## 14.7 Effect of Rotational Malalignment on Patellofemoral Joint Position in Space

Maximum gait efficiency with minimal stress is affected by normal limb alignment. Any deviation from normal limb alignment in any plane may also give the same conditions as twisting of the knee. These include femoral anteversion or retroversion, excess internal or external tibial torsion, genu valgum or varus, hyperpronation, Achilles contracture, and so on.

Twisting of the knee away from the limb mechanical axis (inward or outward) will change the direction and magnitude of the patellofemoral compression force and will also add a side-directed vector to the patella. This side-directed vector is resisted by the soft tissue (both the medial and the lateral patellofemoral ligaments) and by the depth and shape of the trochlea. With a more dysplastic trochlea, the ligament stress is increased and with a more normal trochlea, the trochlear stress is increased.

The foot progression angle (FPA) is generally defined as the angle between the long axis of the foot and the direction of body progression and varies from 10° to 20°.[30] It has been shown that despite congenital or acquired (after fracture) torsional deformities in the lower limb bones, the FPA remains similar.[21,36,42] It is hypothesized that the hip musculature plays a role to accommodate for these deformities during gait. For example, in the presence of an internal femoral or external tibial rotational deformity with a normal FPA, the knee joint axis rotates inward and a side force vector is produced acting on the patella so that both the strain on the medial patellofemoral ligament and the compression on the lateral facet are increased. The opposite situation is present with opposite deformities (Fig. 14.9).

## 14.8 Treatment

Treatments are best based on an accurate diagnosis and analysis of the above predisposing factors (Table 14.3). However, we remain limited by the inability to quantify all of the contributing factors. In the history of the treatment of the anterior knee pain, efforts have been made to try to correlate one predisposing factor or one cause as responsible of the pathogenesis of the anterior knee pain. Likewise, different authors have proposed different operations to treat patellofemoral pain in a standardized fashion. This approach has lead to a high incidence of failure in patellofemoral surgery and a bad reputation.

Abnormal patellofemoral joint mechanics can be the result of many different abnormalities of the alignment. Limb geometry, length, body weight, muscles forces combine to generate the forces, which are to be transmitted through the joint. In the analysis of the pathogenesis, it is important to establish a cause and effect. If a primary abnormality is identified, the treatment should be directed to correcting this abnormality. Any soft tissue or intraarticular procedure is destined to failure if this causality has not been determined. In the vast majority of cases, a combination of predisposing factors exists. James,[38] in 1978, described a "miserable malalignment syndrome," a combination of femoral anteversion, squinting patellae, genu varum, patella alta, increased Q-angle, external tibial rotation, tibia varum, and compensatory feet pronation. A single common surgical procedure such as lateral release or tibial tubercle transfer is not likely to cure anterior knee pain in this setting. It is essential to try and detect all of the bony and soft tissue factors that exist, but when multiple contributors are present, the relative contribution of each is not yet quantifiable. In a case with only one variable believed to be responsible for the pathogenesis, that variable, when possible, is

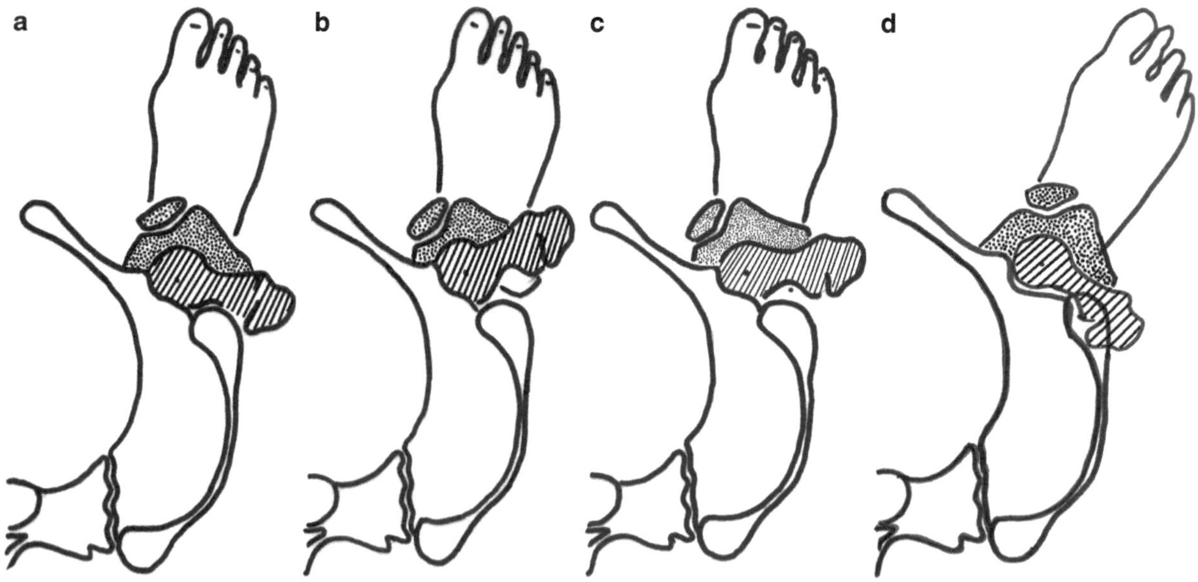


**Fig. 14.9** (**a**) Drawing shows 20° excess femoral anteversion. With the foot forward, the knee joint points inward. (**b**) Drawing shows 20° excess tibial external torsion. With the foot forward, the knee joint points inward, but the hip is also excessively internally rotated. (**c**) Combined excess external tibial torsion (20°) and excess femoral anteversion (20°) with the foot forward. The inward pointing of the knee is the sum of the increase in femoral anteversion plus the excess of external tibial torsion. The hip in this position gains abduction leverage. (**d**) Combined 20° excess external tibial torsion and 20° excess femoral anteversion. With the knee joint pointing forward, the foot points outward and the hip is in a position of abductor weakness

**Table 14.3** Correction of skeletal malalignment associated to patellofemoral pathology

| Deformity | Procedure |
|---|---|
| *Frontal plane* | |
| Genu valgum | Femoral osteotomy (supracondylar) |
| Genu varum | Tibial osteotomy (infratuberosity) |
| *Sagittal plane* | |
| Prominent trochlea | Trochleoplasty |
| Shallow trochlea | Lateral condyle osteotomy |
| Patella alta | Distal tubercle transfer |
| Aplasic tuberosity | Maquet osteotomy (maintain normal Q-angle) |
| *Horizontal plane* | |
| Increased femoral anteversion (>25°) | Proximal femoral external rotation osteotomy (intertrochanteric) |
| Tibial external torsion (>40°) | Proximal tibial internal rotation (infratuberosity) |
| Increased AG-TG (>20 mm) | Tibial tubercle medialization |
| Decreased TT-TG | Lateral tibial tubercle transfer |
| *Combined deformities* | |
| Valgus + femoral anteversion | Distal femoral varus external rotation osteotomy |
| Varus + femoral anteversion | Distal femoral valgus external rotation osteotomy |
| Tibial torsion + increased TT-TG | Proximal tibial osteotomy (supratuberosity) |
| Femoral anteversion + tibial torsion("miserable malalignment") | Proximal femoral external rotation osteotomy + proximal tibial internal rotation osteotomy |

corrected. For the cases with multiple abnormalities (i.e., femoral anteversion, tibial torsion, genu valgum, and patellar subluxation), our approach is either to correct the deformity that is most abnormal or to correct the factor that we believe contributes most to the symptoms. Multiplane osteotomy is useful when bone geometry is abnormal.

It is important to recognize that with a mechanical overload, the most prudent treatment should be a reduction of loading conditions by activity restriction or modification, weight loss, flexibility, and strength training. It might seem too aggressive in some cases to perform a femoral or tibial osteotomy to treat anterior knee pain; however, it has to be understood that the patellofemoral pain is often the expression of a complex problem of skeletal geometry. We have seen patients that experienced not only an improvement of the pain after a corrective femoral osteotomy, but also improvement in the gait pattern, disappearance of compensatory foot pronation and bunions, disappearance of muscle tightness in the thigh and calf, and even improvement in the posture and lumbar pain (Fig. 14.10).

It has not been uncommon that the asymptomatic knee becomes symptomatic by comparison to the improved side after correction of deformity. Some patients come to us after five or six unsuccessful procedures around the patella, these patients presenting with severe instability and chondropathy often have an underlying skeletal malalignment that has gone unrecognized. In such cases, it is clear to us that a successful corrective osteotomy performed earlier in the evolution of the disease would not have been too aggressive. In some cases, with deformities in two bones, we opt to operate on the more altered bone first and wait for the evolution instead of correcting both bones in the same procedure. It is not unusual that the patient experiences some improvement after recovering from the first operation and asks for the second bone to be corrected or alternatively, considers the improvement sufficient to defer other procedures. As Brattström[2] stated in 1964:"…osteotomy is a big operation."

### 14.8.1 Level of the Osteotomy

With excessive external torsion of the tibia and the foot moving in the line of a normal foot progression angle, the patella is pulled laterally in the trochlear groove, thus increasing the displacement or subluxation force and the lateral articular compression force, while internal torsion of the tibia moves the patella medially within the femoral sulcus. If the TT-TG angle is normal, the derotational osteotomy should be performed below the tibial tubercle (Fig. 14.11).

An osteotomy above the tibial tubercle will change this normal relationship, leading to a reduction in the normal lateral vector with, subsequently, overload of the medial compartment and the addition of an external rotation vector to the tibial femoral joint. Kelman[23] found that a medial transfer of the tibial tubercle in a knee with normal TT-TG did not pull the patella medially as much as it may pull the tibia into external rotation.

On the femoral side, the goal is to create a normal skeletal geometry. With an excessive increase in

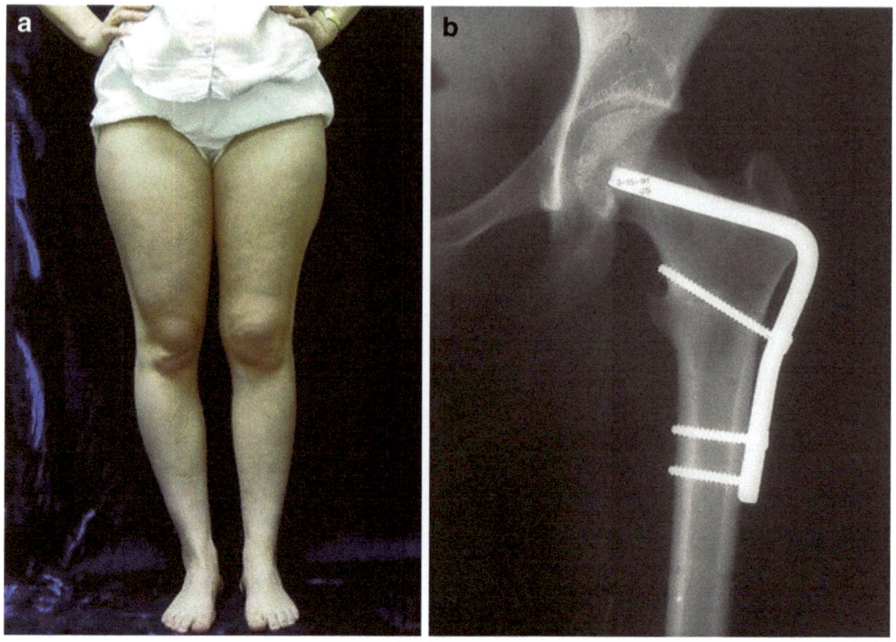

**Fig. 14.10** (**a**) Picture shows a patient with excess femoral anteversion. On the left side, a proximal intertrochanteric femoral derotational osteotomy was performed, the right lower extremity had no surgery. Observe the difference between right and left in the alignment of the extremity. On the right, the patella points inward, the calf muscles are more prominent given a pseudovarus appearance and the foot is more pronated. (**b**) Postoperative x-rays after proximal femur derotational osteotomy

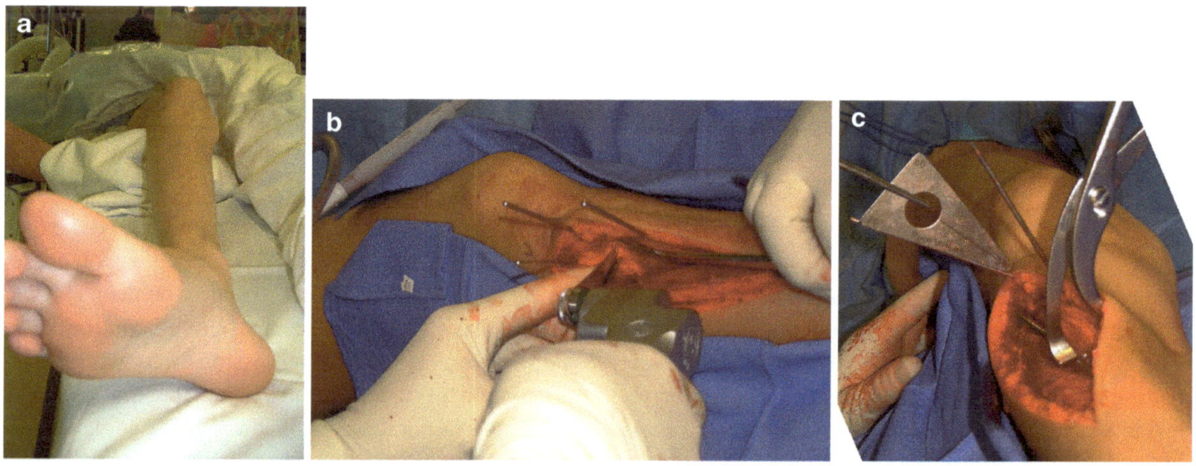

**Fig. 14.11** (**a**) Patient with excess tibial external torsion (55°) and normal TT-TG, the foot points outward while the patella points to the front. (**b**) A proximal tibial internal rotation osteotomy is performed below the tibial tubercle. (**c**). K-wires show a 30° correction. A blade plate is used for fixation

femoral anteversion, we prefer to perform rotational osteotomy at the intertrochanteric femur to reduce the sudden change in direction the quadriceps muscle must make when the osteotomy is located supratrochlear. If two planes need to be corrected, the restoration of a normal tibiofemoral angle usually requires that osteotomy be performed at the distal femur (Fig. 14.12). We have not noted any difference in patients undergoing rotation osteotomy at the proximal, mid, or distal femur.

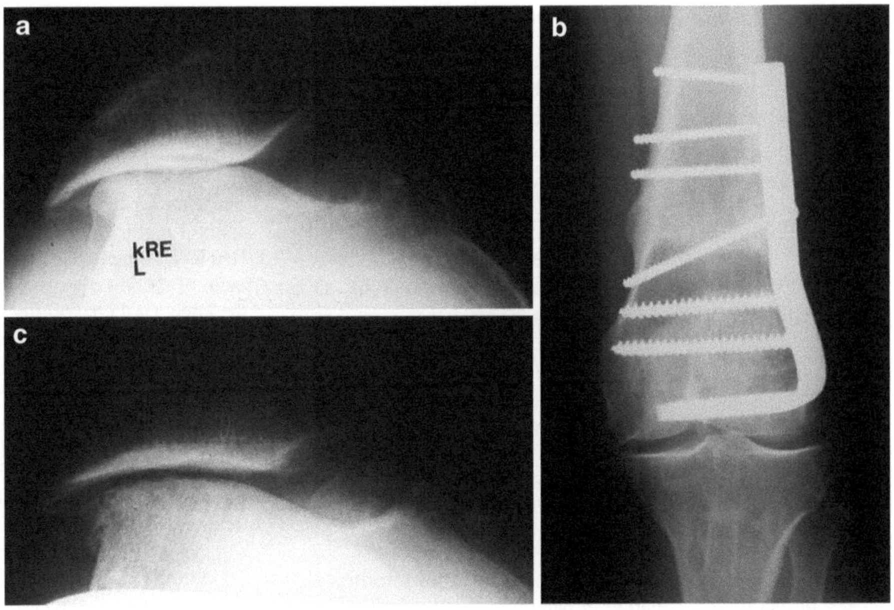


**Fig. 14.12** (**a**) Preoperative axial view of a 28-year-old female with history of pain and instability shows collapse of the lateral patellofemoral joint. The patient had valgus and increased femoral anteversion (43°). (**b**) AP Postoperative x-rays after distal femoral varus and external rotation osteotomy. (**c**) Axial view taken 5 years postoperative shows widening of the lateral patellofemoral space

### 14.8.2 Clinical Experience

Cooke et al.[7] operated on nine knees in seven patients with inwardly pointing knees and patellofemoral complaints. The authors found this group of patients to have a combined abnormal varus and external torsion of the tibia. The operation performed was derotation valgus Maquet osteotomy with associated lateral release. After a 3-year follow-up period, the outcome assessments were excellent for all the cases.

Meister and James[32] reported on eight knees in seven patients with severe rotational malalignment of the lower extremities associated with debilitating anterior knee pain. The rotational deformity consisted of mild femoral anteversion, severe external tibial torsion, and mild tibia vara and pes planovalgus. Internal rotation tibial osteotomy was performed proximal to the tibial tubercle with an average correction of 19.7°. At 10 years average follow-up, all but one patient obtained a subjective good or excellent result while functionally all of them had a good or excellent result.

Server et al.[37] performed 35 tibial rotational osteotomies in 25 patients with patellofemoral subluxation secondary to lateral tibial torsion. At 4.3 years follow-up, the results were good or excellent in 88.5% of the patients and all the patients but two were not satisfied with the procedure.

Delgado et al.[10] treated operatively nine patients with 13 affected extremities with patellofemoral pathology related to torsional malalignment. The procedures performed were femoral external rotation osteotomy, tibial internal rotation osteotomy, or both. No additional soft tissue procedure that would alter patellar tracking was carried out. At 2.6 years average follow-up, all the patients had an improvement in gait pattern, extremity appearance, and a marked decrease in knee pain.

In a recent publication, Bruce and Stevens[3] reviewed the results of correction of miserable malalignment syndrome in 14 patients with 27 limbs. The patients presented significant patellofemoral pain in association with increased femoral anteversion and tibia external rotation. Ipsilateral femoral external rotational osteotomy and tibia internal rotation osteotomy were performed in all the cases. At an average 5.2 years follow-up, all of the patients reported full satisfaction with their surgery and outcomes.

## 14.9 Conclusions

- Bony architecture dictates where the force vectors acting on the patella will be directed.
- Abnormal skeletal alignment may increase the displacement forces acting on both the ligaments and articular surface of the patella causing either

ligament failure with subsequent instability or cartilage overload with subsequent arthrosis.

- Treatment depends on what the primary pathology is; with large displacement force, the best treatment might be osteotomy of long bones.
- Procedures intended to repair soft tissues often fail if the forces directed by the skeletal malalignment are unrecognized or not addressed.
- Osteotomy for patellofemoral arthrosis may be as logical as HTO for varus gonarthrosis.

## References


1. Bernageau J, Goutallier D. La mesure de la distance TA-GT. In: *Le scanner ostéo-articulation*. Le genou, Paris, Vigot; 1991:132-144.
2. Brattström H. Shape of the intercondylar groove normally and in recurrent dislocation of patella. A clinical and x-ray anatomical investigation. *Acta Orthop Scand*. 1964;68(suppl 68):1-148.
3. Bruce WD, Stevens PM. Surgical correction of miserable malalignment syndrome. *J Pediatr Orthop*. 2004;24:392-396.
4. Cahue S, Dunlop D, Hayes K, et al. Varus-valgus alignment in the progression of patellofemoral osteoarthritis. *Arthritis Rheum*. 2004;50:2184-2190.
5. Chao EY, Neluheni EV, Hsu RW, et al. Biomechanics of malalignment. *Orthop Clin North Am*. 1994;25:379-386.
6. Cooke TD, Li J, Scudamore RA. Radiographic assessment of bony contributions to knee deformity. *Orthop Clin North Am*. 1994;25:387-393.
7. Cooke TD, Price N, Fisher B, et al. The inwardly pointing knee. An unrecognized problem of external rotational malalignment. *Clin Orthop Relat Res*. 1990;260:56-60.
8. Dejour H, Walch G, Neyret P, et al. La dysplasie de la trochlee femorale. *Rev Chir Orthop Reparatrice Appar Mot*. 1990;76:45-54.
9. Dejour H, Walch G, Nove-Josserand L, et al. Factors of patellar instability: an anatomic radiographic study. *Knee Surg Sports Traumatol Arthrosc*. 1994;2:19-26.
10. Delgado ED, Schoenecker PL, Rich MM, et al. Treatment of severe torsional malalignment syndrome. *J Pediatr Orthop*. 1996;16:484-488.
11. Eckhoff DG, Brown AW, Kilcoyne RF, et al. Knee version associated with anterior knee pain. *Clin Orthop Relat Res*. 1997;339:152-155.
12. Elahi S, Cahue S, Felson DT, et al. The association between varus-valgus alignment and patellofemoral osteoarthritis. *Arthritis Rheum*. 2000;43:1874-1880.
13. Fujikawa K, Seedhom BB, Wright V. Biomechanics of the patello-femoral joint. Part II: a study of the effect of simulated femoro-tibial varus deformity on the congruity of the patello-femoral compartment and movement of the patella. *Eng Med*. 1983;12:13-21.
14. Goutallier D, Bernageau J, Lecudonnec B. Mesure de l'écart tubérosité tibiale antérieure-gorge de la trochlée (T.A.-G.T.). *Rev Chir Orthop*. 1978;64:423-428.
15. Greene CG, Edwards TB, Wade MR, et al. Reliability of the quadriceps angle measurement. *Am J Knee Surg*. 2001;14: 97-103.
16. Grelsamer RP, Tedder JL. The lateral trochlear sign: femoral trochlear dysplasia as seen on a lateral view roentgenograph. *Clin Orthop Relat Res*. 1992;281:159-162.
17. Hefzy MS, Jackson WT, Saddemi SR, et al. Effects of tibial rotations on patellar tracking and patello-femoral contact areas. *J Biomed Eng*. 1992;14:329-343.
18. Hsu RW, Himeno S, Coventry MB, et al. Normal axial alignment of the lower extremity and load-bearing distribution at the knee. *Clin Orthop Relat Res*. 1990;255:215-227.
19. Hvid I, Andersen LI, Schmidt H. Chondromalacia patellae. The relation to abnormal patellofemoral joint mechanics. *Acta Orthop Scand*. 1981;52:661-666.
20. Insall J, Falvo KA, Wise DW. Chondromalacia patellae. A prospective study. *J Bone Joint Surg Am*. 1976;58:1-8.
21. Jaarsma RL, Ongkiehong BF, Gruneberg C, et al. Compensation for rotational malalignment after intramedullary nailing for femoral shaft fractures. An analysis by plantar pressure measurements during gait. *Injury*. 2004;35: 1270-1278.
22. Janssen G. Increased medial torsion of the knee joint producing chondromalacia patella. In: Trickey E, Hertel P, eds. *Surgery and Arthroscopy of the Knee, 2nd Congress*. Berlin: Springer-Verlag;1986:263-267.
23. Kelman GJ, Focht L, Krakauer JD, et al. A cadaveric study of patellofemoral kinematics using a biomechanical testing ring and gait laboratory motion analysis. *Orthop Trans*. 1989;13:248-249.
24. Kijowski R, Plagens D, Shaeh SJ, et al. The effects of rotational deformities of the femur on contact pressure and contact area in the patellofemoral joint and on strain in the medial patellofemoral ligament. Presented at: the annual meeting "Interational Patellofemoral Study Group"; 1999; Napa Valley, San Francisco.
25. Lauren CA, Dussault R, Levesque HP. The tangential x-ray Investigation of the patellofemoral joint: x-ray technique, diagnostic criteria and their interpretation. *Clin Orthop Relat Res*. 1979;144:16-26.
26. Lee TQ, Anzel SH, Bennett KA, et al. The influence of fixed rotational deformities of the femur on the patellofemoral contact pressures in human cadaver knees. *Clin Orthop Relat Res*. 1994;302:69-74.
27. Lee TQ, Morris G, Csintalan RP. The influence of tibial and femoral rotation on patellofemoral contact area and pressure. *J Orthop Sports Phys Ther*. 2003;33:686-693.
28. Lee TQ, Yang BY, Sandusky MD, et al. The effects of tibial rotation on the patellofemoral joint: assessment of the changes in in situ strain in the peripatellar retinaculum and the patellofemoral contact pressures and areas. *J Rehabil Res Dev*. 2001;38:463-469.
29. Lerat JL, Moyen B. Morphological types of the lower limbs in femoro-patellar disequilibrium. Analysis in 3 planes. *Acta Orthop Belg*. 1989;55:347-355.
30. Lösel S, Burgess-Milliron MJ, Micheli LJ, et al. A simplified technique for determining foot progression angle in children 4 to 16 years of age. *J Pediatr Orthop*. 1996;16: 570-574.
31. Malghem J, Maldague B. Depth insufficiency of the proximal trochlear groove on lateral radiographs of the knee: relation to patellar dislocation. *Radiology*. 1989;170:507-510.

32. Meister K, James SL. Proximal tibial derotation osteotomy for anterior knee pain in the miserably malaligned extremity. *Am J Orthop*. 1995;24:149-155.
33. Moreland JR, Bassett LW, Hanker GJ. Radiographic analysis of the axial alignment of the lower extremity. *J Bone Joint Surg Am*. 1987;69:745-749.
34. Reikeras O, Hoiseth A. Torsion of the leg determined by computed tomography. *Acta Orthop Scand*. 1989;60:330-333.
35. Sayli U, Bolukbasi S, Atik OS, et al. Determination of tibial torsion by computed tomography. *J Foot Ankle Surg*. 1994;33:144-147.
36. Seber S, Hazer B, Kose N, et al. Rotational profile of the lower extremity and foot progression angle: computerized tomographic examination of 50 male adults. *Arch Orthop Trauma Surg*. 2000;120:255-258.
37. Server F, Miralles RC, Garcia E, et al. Medial rotational tibial osteotomy for patellar instability secondary to lateral tibial torsion. *Int Orthop*. 1996;20:153-158.
38. Sl J, Bates BT, Ostering LR. Injuries to runners. *Am J Sports Med*. 1978;6:40-50.
39. Strecker W, Franzreb M, Pfeiffer T, et al. Computerized tomography measurement of torsion angle of the lower extremities. *Unfallchirurg*. 1994;97:609.
40. Strecker W, Keppler P, Gebhard F, et al. Length and torsion of the lower limb. *J Bone Joint Surg Br*. 1997;79:1019-1023.
41. Takai S, Sakakida K, Yamashita F, et al. Rotational alignment of the lower limb in osteoarthritis of the knee. *Int Orthop*. 1985;9:209-215.
42. Tornetta P, Ritz G, Kantor A. Femoral torsion after interlocked nailing of unstable femoral fractures. *J Trauma*. 1995;38:213-219.
43. Turner MS. The association between tibial torsion and knee joint pathology. *Clin Orthop Relat Res*. 1994;302:47-51.
44. Yoshioka Y, Cooke TDV. Femoral anteversion: assessment based on function axes. *J Orthop Res*. 1987;5:86-91.
45. Yoshioka Y, Siu D, Cooke TDV. The anatomy and functional axes of the femur. *J Bone Joint Surg Am*. 1987;69:873-880.
46. Yoshioka Y, Siu DW, Scudamore RA, et al. Tibial anatomy and functional axes. *J Orthop Res*. 1989;7:132-137.

# Patellar Tendinopathy: Where Does the Pain Come From?

15

Jill L. Cook and Karim M. Khan

## 15.1 Introduction

The aim of this chapter is to address the question: Where is the pain coming from in patellar tendinopathy? The biochemical sources of pain will be discussed in Patrik Danielson and Alex Scott's chapter, so this chapter will focus on the potential inflammatory, mechanical, and structural sources in the tendon and surrounding tissues.

## 15.2 Inflammatory Models of Pain in Tendinopathy

The inflammatory basis of patellar tendinopathy has been questioned, despite the link between pain and inflammation. As long ago as 1976, Giancarlo Puddu of Rome documented that the pathology in what was clinically known as "Achilles tendinitis" was separation and fragmentation of collagen, which he labeled "tendinosis."[36] Since then, numerous authors have shown that tendinosis, a noninflammatory pathology involving the cells and matrix, is the predominant pathology in patellar tendinopathy.[23] Although classic inflammation is not thought to have a key role in chronic patellar tendinopathy, we shall see later in this chapter that nonclassical models of inflammation may influence tendon pain and pathology.

It is thought by some that a tendon might transition to tendinosis through a stage of inflammation. There is no doubt that ruptured or surgically lacerated tendon has an inflammatory stage; however, overuse tendinopathy seems to follow a different pathway. Experiments to detect a significant interim phase of "tendinitis" in overuse tendinopathy in humans are difficult and experiments in animals have not yielded great evidence of inflammation.[39]

There are no animal models of patellar tendinopathy, but experiments causing overuse tendinopathy of the plantaris tendon and Achilles tendon provide important histopathological specimens of tendon tissue soon after injury. This provides insight as to the length of any inflammatory process that might precede collagen degeneration.

In a rat plantaris tendinopathy model,[47] overloaded tendons were examined at 1 and 2 weeks. At both these times, there was no evidence of inflammation but there was strong evidence of a tendon response, as quiescent fibroblasts had transformed into rounded, active cells. Similarly, in a rabbit model of overuse Achilles tendinopathy, collagen changes and neovascularization, together with some inflammatory cells in the adipose tissue close to the paratenon were seen.[8] These changes in animal models are identical to those found in human overuse tendinopathy.

Some human studies have demonstrated the presence of a few inflammatory cells, both in the acute and chronic stages of tendinopathy.[40] The presence of inflammatory cells in human tissue is variable and dependent on many experimental and individual factors. Although there may be a period of inflammation for a few days after certain tendon injuries, symptoms may not be present and symptoms that are present for any extended time must arise from a noninflammatory mechanism. Based on this, it seems reasonable that

J.L. Cook (✉)
School of Primary Health Care,
Monash University, Melbourne, Australia
e-mail: jill.cook@monash.edu

V. Sanchis-Alfonso (ed.), *Anterior Knee Pain and Patellar Instability*,
DOI: 10.1007/978-0-85729-507-1_15, © Springer-Verlag London Limited 2011

inflammation is not a consistent feature of tendon pathology and pain.

Despite this evidence, there are ways in which non-classical inflammation may be associated with pathology and possibly pain. Neurogenic inflammation, growth factors, cytokines and mast cells have been implicated; in addition, the role of inflammation in the peritendon cannot be excluded.

Cytokines that have a potential inflammatory role have been with tendon pathology. In particular, TNFa is directly linked with bone–tendon pathology in rheumatological diseases[6]; these conditions affect similar areas of the tendon to that of overuse disease. Other growth factors such as IGF-1,[39] interleukins 1, and 6[43] have been known to be an upstream modulator of cell activity and matrix structure.

Mast cells are present in tendon pathology in greater numbers than normal tendon, and aside from their usual role in releasing histamines and heparin, they may modulate cytokine expression. More interestingly, the number of mast cells has been correlated with the duration of pain.[40]

Neurogenic inflammation refers to tissue responses initiated by neuropeptides such as substance P, CGRP, and glutamate. These substances have been demonstrated in overuse tendon tissue and they have the potential to induce cell and matrix changes.[29] Changes in tendon structure mediated through spinal cord connections and driven by neuropeptides are possible, as overload to one tendon induces changes in the contralateral tendon.[15] The exact role neuropeptides play in initiating or sustaining tendon pathology has not been fully elucidated.

These three possible sources of inflammation in tendons may be closely linked. The proximity between neural elements and tissue mast cells in tendon would permit the mast cell–neurite "unit" to stimulate neurogenic inflammation.[16] Neurotransmitters such as substance P can influence mast cell degranulation and secretory activity. Neural activity could be amplified, via a feedback mechanism, when mast cells release a panel of biologically active molecules, which impact on vascular elements and fibroblasts. Theoretically, the mediators contained in mast cells such as cytokines and growth factors could influence a number of potentially pain-producing factors such as cellular edema and chemotaxis for inflammatory cells. This type of "neurogenic inflammation" has been seen in various body tissues, although not established in tendon. This is an "endogenous inflammatory system," in contrast to the "exogenous inflammatory system" composed of blood-borne cells generally associated with inflammation.[16] One criticism of this model as it stands is that mast cells are not prevalent and consistent in tendon tissue. Nevertheless, the model may apply to paratenonitis, and it may explain the process of neovascularization in tendinosis.

Do any of these potential inflammatory mechanisms explain the positive clinical effect of corticosteroid injections? Both clinical experience and randomized studies[17,44] have shown these medications provide, at least, short-term pain relief.

There are several potential mechanisms through which corticosteroids may work. Based on the biochemical model reviewed in the next chapter, it seems likely that the capacity of corticosteroids to damp down cell proliferation and activity may, in turn, dampen pain. This may be linked to the theory that a chemical agent (e.g., corticosteroids) may alter the composition of the matrix.[27] Alternatively, fenestration of an area of tendinosis with needling may promote beneficial bleeding into new channels created through degenerated mucoid tissue. This mechanical disruption may transform a failed intrinsic healing response to a therapeutic extrinsic one.[41]

## 15.3 Mechanical and Structural Models of Pain in Tendinopathy

Mechanical models of patellar tendon pain include those that attribute pain to damage within the tendon structure, specifically the collagen fibers. Other mechanical causes are attributed to structures around the tendon causing pain or impinging on the tendon tissue itself. Before we consider mechanical models, we have to consider the relationship between pain and structural change.

### *15.3.1 Dissociation Between Tendon Pain and Pathology*

In patients with patellar tendon pain, size of collagen abnormality as measured on ultrasound does not correspond with pain, either in cross-sectional studies[11,28] or in longitudinal observational studies.[24] Patients with patellar tendinopathy can also have a normal MR scan[42] and US scan.[31] This is seen in clinical practice where a patient may have a very small, or no, morphological abnormality, yet have significant symptoms.

In studies of large number of asymptomatic athletes, ultrasonographic hypoechoic regions (abnormal collagen) were common, even in subjects with no past history of jumper's knee.[10,11,28] Magnetic resonance imaging in asymptomatic controls confirmed this, which found an abnormal signal consistent with collagen degeneration.[42] These examples demonstrate that there is more to tendon pain than discontinuity of collagen.

However, the most compelling evidence of the dissociation between pain and pathology comes from the seminal paper of Kannus and Jozsa, which reported that two thirds of tendons that rupture, all of which had pathological change, were not painful.[20]

### 15.3.2 Collagen Fiber Disruption and Patellar Tendon Pain

The evidence of dissociation between pain and pathology makes the collagen tearing model, where collagen fibers are pain free when intact and painful when disrupted, somewhat tenuous. While nobody would deny that acute tearing of collagen causes pain (e.g., acute ligament tears), tendons without intact collagen can remain pain free.

A clear example that collagen disruption does not equate to pain comes from two types of surgery performed on the patellar tendon – ACL autograft reconstruction and tenotomy for painful jumper's knee. In autograft ACL reconstruction, there is minimal donor site knee pain, yet collagen has been excised. Significant histologic abnormality persists for years, yet remains pain free.[21,33]

Clinical observations in athletes undergoing surgery for jumper's knee also suggest that collagen and pain are not strongly linked. Athletes recovering from open patellar tenotomy had abnormal imaging for 12 months, but this correlated poorly with pain.[22] This study confirms that even substantial degrees of collagen insult do not automatically produce tendon pain.

Jumper's knee can also be treated by arthroscopic debridement of the posterior border of the patellar tendon,[9] where the surgeon first debrides the adherent fat pad to expose the posterior aspect of the tendon and then removes the tendinosic tissue itself. The body of the tendon, however, remains largely untouched and postoperative ultrasonography reveals that the intratendinous hypoechoic region (so often considered pathognomonic of this condition) is still evident, yet pain is significantly reduced.

Lastly, longitudinal tenotomy is a treatment for patellar tendinopathy.[46] This causes new injury to tendon and the collagen is disrupted. Nevertheless, the procedure is often therapeutic rather than deleterious. This phenomenon cannot be explained by invoking a pure mechanical model of pain in tendinopathy.

### 15.3.3 Tissue Impingement Causing Patellar Tendon Pain

Impingement is a form of mechanical load, and adds compressive or shearing load to the tendon's normal tensile load. Although tensile load is clearly implicated in tendinopathy, there is increasing interest in the role of compressive loads and some evidence that alteration of compressive loads can ameliorate pain.[19] Whatever the load type, it seems that the pathological response is the same.

Johnson and colleagues[18] proposed that the pain and the lesion of jumper's knee was due to impingement of the inferior pole of the patella on the patellar tendon during knee flexion. However, a dynamic magnetic resonance study showed no difference in patellar movement between symptomatic tendons and those tendons without pain and pathology, suggesting that impingement was not a causative factor.[38]

Clinical observations are also inconsistent with deep knee flexion (and impingement), causing jumper's knee pain. Athletes with severe jumper's knee have pain on muscle contraction even when the knee is fully extended and unloaded, whereas patients with impingement syndromes generally obtain substantial relief when the joint is moved away from the impinging direction. Also, the pain of jumper's knee does not disappear and may actually increase when palpation is performed with the knee in full extension.

### 15.3.4 *Underloading Tendons or Stress Shielding*

Another theory proposed is the "stress-shielding" theory.[4,5] The stress-shielding theory considers tendinopathy to be a combined overuse–underuse injury, where the superficial portion of the tendon bears too much of the tensile load, whilst the deep portion of the tendon bears too little of the same load. Further investigation is required; however, it is clear that critical etiological questions such as the nature of tendon load must be answered quickly, as it is the essence of adequate management.

### 15.3.5 *Structural Sources of Tendon Pain*

Peritendinous pathology is common in tendons with a substantial peritendinous structures and is rarely reported in tendons with undifferentiated peritendon. Although it might seem that peritendon pathology is solely inflammatory, changes associated with a noninflammatory response such as an increase in fibroblasts and myofibroblasts are also seen. Suffice to say that changes in the peritendon must impact on the tendon as peritendon tissue is structurally continuous with the endotendon and fascial structures.[14] These fascial structures have the potential in other tendons to cause pathology, but the extent of the effect on the tendon of pathology in the peritendon is unknown, although the evidence is that it can induce tendon changes[26]

The fat pad is classically impinged between the tibia and femur in knee hyperextension, although it is considered clinically that it could be pinched between the patella and the proximal tibia as described in the patellofemoral literature,[32] something similar to the condition referred to as Hoffa's syndrome, when presenting with acute trauma to the anterior knee. As it is highly vascular and neural, and is implicitly linked to the patellar tendon, it has potential to cause the pain of patellar tendinopathy.[13,37]

However, surgical management of the main body of the patellar tendon in athletes revealed no macroscopic abnormality of the fat pad.[46] Intuitively, one would be loath to attribute tendon symptoms to a structure found only at one or two anatomical sites (i.e., the patellar fat pad, Kager's triangle) when tendinopathy occurs at various sites. On the other hand, the fat pad may be a specific form of the nociceptive peritendinous tissue that is sensitive to biochemical irritants. That is, the fat pad in the patellar tendon may play the same role as the paratenon in Achilles tendinopathy and the subacromial bursa in rotator cuff tendinopathy.

#### 15.3.5.1 Neural and Vascular Sources of Pain in Tendinopathy

Normal tendons have a low vascularity, but have sufficient supply for their metabolic needs. In the pathological tendon, increases in vascularity (neovascularization) have been demonstrated histopathologically,[27] with imaging on Doppler ultrasound,[1,35,45] and with laser flowmetry.[7] Further investigations have demonstrated that neovascularization has been associated with pain and furthermore, the use of sclerosants on the neovascularization decreases tendon pain.[34] Paradoxically, injections with vascular sclerosants leads to an increase in vessels,[3] and it is thought that the sclerosant has its pain-relieving effect through its analgesic and neurotoxic effects.

Neovascularization is associated with nerve fibers,[2] including those immunoreactive to substance P and CGRP.[30] The association between pain and neovascularization is not absolute, as some studies demonstrate that tendons with neovascularization are not painful.[25,48] Conversely, pathological tendons without neovascularization may also be painful. However, there is evidence that there is more pain in pathological tendons with neovascularization compared to pathological tendons without neovascularization.[12] Longitudinal studies demonstrate that neovascularization may come and go, and the stimulus for this and the relation to pain is currently undefined.[12] Most importantly, the presence of vessels in a tendon do not predict clinical outcome; that is, a highly vascular tendon may recover as well as a nonvascular tendon. It is also important to realize that Doppler ultrasound detects blood flow in tendons and this can be affected by a range of factors such as activity prior to imaging and environmental temperature. Therefore, the absence of flow does not mean that vessels are not present, just that they have no flow at that particular time.[12]

## 15.4 Conclusions

Any model of pain in patellar tendinopathy must be consistent with the following observations:

- The pathology underlying tendinopathy is tendinosis.
- Abnormal tendon morphology on imaging confers a risk, but not a guarantee, of symptoms.
- Various surgical treatments including longitudinal tenotomy and arthroscopic tendon debridement can alleviate pain without directly affecting pathological tissue.
- Medical treatment such as corticosteroid injection can relieve the pain quickly, but not necessarily permanently.

Currently, the cause of tendon pathology and pain is unclear. Experimental and clinical research is clarifying aspects of the etiology of tendon pain and pathology, but the relationship between them is still unclear. Until we discover the cause of patellar tendon pain, options for ameliorating tendon pain will remain limited.

## References


1. Alfredson H. Chronic midportion Achilles tendinopathy: an update on research and treatment. *Clin Sports Med.* 2003; 22:727-741.
2. Alfredson H, Forsgren S, Thorsen K, et al. Glutamate NMDAR1 receptors localised to nerves in human Achilles tendons. Implications for treatment? *Knee Surg Sports Traumatol Arthrosc.* 2001;9:123-126.
3. Alfredson H, Ohberg L. Increased intratendinous vascularity in the early period after sclerosing injection treatment in Achilles tendinosis: a healing response? *Knee Surg Sports Traumatol Arthrosc.* 2006;14:399-401.
4. Almekinders LC, Vellema JH, Weinhold PS. Strain patterns in the patellar tendon and the implications for patellar tendinopathy. *Knee Surg Sports Traumatol Arthrosc.* 2002;10:2-5.
5. Almekinders LC, Weinhold PS, Maffulli N. Compression etiology in tendinopathy. *Clin Sports Med.* 2003;22:703-710.
6. Al-Shukaili AK, Al-Jabri AA. Rheumatoid arthritis, cytokines and hypoxia. What is the link? *Saudi Med J.* 2006;27:1642-1649.
7. Astrom M, Westlin N. Blood flow in the normal Achilles tendon assessed by laser Doppler flowmetry. *J Orthop Res.* 1994;12:246-252.
8. Backman C, Boquist L, Friden J, et al. Chronic Achilles paratenonitis with tendinosis: an experimental model in the rabbit. *J Orthop Res.* 1990;8:541-547.
9. Coleman BD, Khan KM, Kiss ZS, et al. Open and arthroscopic patellar tenotomy for chronic patellar tendinopathy: a retrospective outcome study. *Am J Sports Med.* 2000;28:183-190.
10. Cook JL, Khan KM, Harcourt PR, et al. Patellar tendon ultrasonography in asymptomatic active athletes reveals hypoechoic regions: a study of 320 tendons. Victorian Institute of Sport Tendon Study Group. *Clin J Sport Med.* 1998;8:73-77.
11. Cook JL, Khan KM, Kiss ZS, et al. Patellar tendinopathy in junior basketball players: a controlled clinical and ultrasonographic study of 268 tendons in players aged 14–18 years. *Scand J Med Sci Sports.* 2000;10:216-220.
12. Cook JL, Malliaras P, De Luca J, et al. Vascularity and pain in the patellar tendon of adult jumping athletes: a five-month longitudinal study. *Br J Sports Med.* 2005;39:458-461.
13. Dye SF, Vaupel GL, Dye CC. Conscious neurosensory mapping of the internal structures of the human knee without intraarticular anesthesia. *Am J Sports Med.* 1998;26:773-777.
14. Franklyn-Miller A, Falvey E, McCrory P. Fasciitis first before tendinopathy: does the anatomy hold the key? *Br J Sports Med.* 2009;43:887-889.
15. Friedrich T, Schmidt W, Jungmichel D, et al. Histopathology in rabbit Achilles tendon after operative tenolysis (longitudinal fiber incisions). *Scand J Med Sci Sports.* 2001;11:4-8.
16. Hart DA, Frank CB, Bray RC. Inflammatory processes in repetitive motion and overuse syndromes: potential role of neurogenic mechanisms in tendons and ligaments. In: Gordon SL, Blair SJ, Fine LJ, eds. *Repetitive Motion Disorders of the Upper Extremity.* Park Ridge: American Academy of Orthopaedic Surgeons; 1995:247-262.
17. Hay EM, Thomas E, Paterson SM, et al. A pragmatic randomised controlled trial of local corticosteroid injection and physiotherapy for the treatment of new episodes of unilateral shoulder pain in primary care. *Ann Rheum Dis.* 2003;62: 394-399.
18. Johnson DP, Wakeley CJ, Watt I. Magnetic resonance imaging of patellar tendonitis. *J Bone Joint Surg.* 1996;78-B:452-457.
19. Jonsson P, Alfredson H, Sunding K, et al. New regimen for eccentric calf muscle training in patients with chronic insertional Achilles tendinopathy: results of a pilot-study. *Br J Sports Med.* 2008;42:746-749.
20. Kannus P, Jozsa L. Histopathological changes preceding spontaneous rupture of a tendon. A controlled study of 891 patients. *J Bone Joint Surg.* 1991;73-A:1507-1525.
21. Kartus J, Rostgard-Christensen L, Movin T, et al. Evaluation of harvested and normal patellar tendons: a reliability analyses of magnetic resonance imaging and ultrasonography. *Knee Surg Sports Traumatol Arthrosc.* 2000;8:275-280.
22. Khan KM, Bonar F, Desmond PM, et al. Patellar tendinosis (jumper's knee): findings at histopathologic examination, US, and MR imaging. Victorian Institute of Sport Tendon Study Group. *Radiology.* 1996;200:821-827.
23. Khan KM, Cook JL, Bonar F, et al. Histopathology of common overuse tendon conditions: update and implications for clinical management. *Sports Med.* 1999;6:393-408.
24. Khan KM, Cook JL, Kiss ZS, et al. Patellar tendon ultrasonography and jumper's knee in female basketball players: a longitudinal study. *Clin J Sport Med.* 1997;7:199-206.

25. Khan KM, Forster BB, Robinson J, et al. Are ultrasound and magnetic resonance imaging of value in assessment of Achilles tendon disorders? A two year prospective study. *Br J Sports Med.* 2003;37:149-153.
26. Khan MH, Li Z, Wang J. Repeated exposure of tendon to prostoglandin-E2 leads to localised tendon degeneration. *Clin J Sport Med.* 2005;15:28-33.
27. Kraushaar B, Nirschl R. Tendinosis of the elbow (tennis elbow). Clinical features and findings of histological, immunohistochemical, and electron microscopy studies. *J Bone Joint Surg.* 1999;81-A:259-278.
28. Lian O, Holen KJ, Engebretsen L, et al. Relationship between symptoms of jumper's knee and the ultrasound characteristics of the patellar tendon among high level male volleyball players. *Scand J Med Sci Sports.* 1996;6:291-296.
29. Ljung B, Alfredson H, Forsgren S. Neurokinin 1-receptors and sensory neuropeptides in tendon insertions at the medial and lateral epicondyles of the humerus. Studies on tennis elbow ad medial epicondylalgia. *J Orthop Res.* 2004;22:321-327.
30. Ljung B, Forsgren S, Friden J. Substance P and calcitonin gene-related peptide expression at the extensor carpi radialis brevis muscle origin: implications for the etiology of tennis elbow. *J Orthop Res.* 1999;17:554-559.
31. Malliaras P, Cook JL. Patellar tendons with normal imaging and pain: change in imaging and pain status over a volleyball season. *Clin J Sport Med.* 2006;16:388-391.
32. McConnell J. The management of chondromalacia patellae: a long term solution. *Aust J Physiother.* 1986;32:215-223.
33. Nixon RG, SeGall GK, Sax SL, et al. Reconstitution of the patellar tendon donor site after graft harvest. *Clin Orthop Relat Res.* 1995;317:162-171.
34. Ohberg L, Alfredson H. Ultrasound guided sclerosis of neovessels in painful chronic Achilles tendinosis: pilot study of a new treatment. *Br J Sports Med.* 2002;36:173-177.
35. Ohberg L, Lorentzon R, Alfredson H. Neovascularisation in Achilles tendons with painful tendinosis but not in normal tendons: an ultrasonographic investigation. *Knee Surg Sports Traumatol Arthrosc.* 2001;9:233-238.
36. Puddu G, Ippolito E, Postacchini F. A classification of Achilles tendon disease. *Am J Sports Med.* 1976;4:145-150.
37. Sanchis-Alfonso V, Rosello-Sastre E. Anterior knee pain in the young patient – what causes the pain? "Neural model". *Acta Orthop Scand.* 2003;74:697-703.
38. Schmid MR, Hodler J, Cathrein P, et al. Is impingement the cause of jumper's knee? Dynamic and static magnetic resonance imaging of patellar tendinitis in an open-configuration system. *Am J Sports Med.* 2002;30:388-395.
39. Scott A, Cook JL, Hart DA, et al. Tenocyte responses to mechanical loading in vivo: a role for local insulin-like growth factor 1 signaling in early tendinosis in rats. *Arthritis Rheum.* 2007;56:871-881.
40. Scott A, Lian O, Bahr R, et al. Increased mast cell numbers in human patellar tendinosis: correlation with symptom duration and vascular hyperplasia. *Br J Sports Med.* 2008; 42:753-757.
41. Shalabi A, Svensson L, Kristoffersen-Wiberg M, et al. Tendon injury and repair after core biopsies in chronic Achilles tendinosis evaluated by serial magnetic resonance imaging. *Br J Sports Med.* 2004;38:606-612.
42. Shalaby M, Almekinders LC. Patellar tendinitis: the significance of magnetic resonance imaging findings. *Am J Sports Med.* 1999;27:345-349.
43. Skutek M, van Griensven M, Zeichen J, et al. Cyclic mechanical stretching enhances secretion of interleukin 6 in human tendon fibroblasts. *Knee Surg Sports Traumatol Arthrosc.* 2001;9:322-326.
44. Stahl S, Kaufman T. The efficacy of an injection of steroids for medial epicondylitis. A prospective study of sixty elbows. *J Bone Joint Surg.* 1997;79-A:1648-1652.
45. Terslev L, Qvistgaard E, Torp-Pedersen S, et al. Ultrasound and power Doppler findings in jumper's knee – preliminary findings. *Eur J Ultrasound.* 2001;13:183-189.
46. Testa V, Capasso G, Maffulli N, et al. Ultrasound-guided percutaneous longitudinal tenotomy for the management of patellar tendinopathy. *Med Sci Sports Exerc.* 1999;31: 1509-1515.
47. Zamora AJ, Marini JF. Tendon and myotendinous junction in an overloaded skeletal muscle of the rat. *Anat Embryol.* 1988;179:89-96.
48. Zanetti M, Metzdorf A, Kundert HP, et al. Achilles tendons: clinical relevance of neovascularization diagnosed with power Doppler US. *Radiology.* 2003;227:556-560.

# 16 Biochemical Causes of Patellar Tendinopathy?

Patrik Danielson and Alexander Scott

## 16.1 Introduction

During recent years, increasing attention has been devoted to the biochemical milieu of human tendons. Prompted by the lack of evident causality in the aetiology of tendinopathy, much contemporary research is focused on the possible roles of biochemical agents in the development of tendon symptoms and tissue changes. Although further experiments testing the functional importance of such biochemical mediators in tendinopathy are greatly needed, evidence of a dramatic metamorphosis in local cell signalling within chronically painful tendons exists. The evidence for biochemical aspects of tendinopathy that has consequently emerged might complement, rather than replace, existing theories on pathogenesis (see Chap. 15). It furthermore fits a theoretical model in which tendon pathology exists on a continuum which, at various points, involves abnormalities in blood vessels, nerves, tenocytes, and extracellular matrix.[14] The aim of this chapter is to present the evidence that supports this biochemical model of patellar tendinopathy.

P. Danielson (✉)
Department of Integrative Medical Biology,
Section for Anatomy, Faculty of Medicine,
Umeå University, Umeå, Sweden
e-mail: patrik.danielson@anatomy.umu.se

## 16.2 Original Ideas on Biochemical Causes of Tendinopathy Pain, and Early Evidence of Changes in the Intratendinous Production of Signal Substances

Early ideas of a biochemical, rather than a directly structural, origin of pain in tendinopathy were minted as early as 2000, by Khan, Cook, and collaborators.[31] They hypothesized that biochemical mediators in the tendon tissue might influence nociceptors in or around the tendon, thus causing pain. The rationale for exploring new theories of tendinopathy was that older models in which inflammatory agents and/or collagen separation were primary sources of pain were heavily contradicted by clinical observations, not to mention a growing body of research. Chapter 15 reviews the basis for discarding collagen separation as a major source of pain, and also discusses the abandonment of the problematic "tendinitis" nomenclature. As the previous chapter furthermore highlights, there is frequently a disconnect between histology (tendinosis) and clinical symptoms (tendinopathy). Still, it is now commonly accepted that the underlying histology of patellar tendinopathy is usually "tendinosis" – a condition characterized by the proliferation of tenocytes and vascular tissue and the disruption of collagen fibers.[29,30] However, the possibility of inflammatory processes somewhere along the continuum of the pathology has gained increasing interest. Nevertheless, classic prostaglandin-mediated inflammation can be ruled out as the explanation for pain and tissue derangement in chronic stages of tendinopathy. Microdialysis studies on patellar tendinopathy demonstrated no elevation of

V. Sanchis-Alfonso (ed.), *Anterior Knee Pain and Patellar Instability*,
DOI: 10.1007/978-0-85729-507-1_16, © Springer-Verlag London Limited 2011

prostaglandin $E_2$ levels in tendons of patients with Jumper's knee as compared to tendons of asymptomatic individuals,[2] and no inflammatory cells are detected in microscopic examination of patellar tendon tissue from patients suffering from tendinopathy.[29]

It was in these same microdialysis studies that the earliest signs of changes in intratendinous biosynthesis were detected in patellar tendinopathy.[29] It was shown that the level of an excitatory nerve transmitter – glutamate – was significantly higher in chronically painful patellar tendons as compared to normal tendons.[2] Glutamate, apart from being a well-known transmitter in the central nervous system, has been shown to be able to evoke pain and vasomotor responses in peripheral tissue of humans.[23] Experimental studies have also shown that glutamate can induce a proapoptotic response in cultured tendon cells, and it has been suggested that this plays a role in the degeneration seen in tendinosis.[34] It is known that advanced stages of tendinosis are associated with apoptotic events (e.g.,[41,42,49]). Therefore, glutamate may be playing several roles at different points along the continuum of pathology. These findings stressed the possibility that an increase in the intratendinous production of classically neuronal signal substances may not only contribute to pain in tendinopathy, but also to tissue changes and vascular events associated with tendon pathology.

## 16.3 The Paradox of Few Nerves and Substantial Pain: Can It Be Explained by an Increase in Biochemical Mediators?

The most prominent clinical symptoms of patellar tendinopathy are chronic tendon pain, tenderness in the painful area, onset or increase of pain during tendon-loading activity, and impaired tendon function.[1]

Interesting findings in recent years have suggested that there may be an increase in the number of sensory nerve fibers in patellar tendinopathy,[32] which seems to correspond to observations in Achilles tendinopathy of sprouting of sensory afferents.[39] However, results are not conclusive in this regard. The referred studies show statistically insignificant results, or were conducted by comparing tendinopathic to ruptured tendons. Other studies have been unable to show any evident difference in the occurrence of sensory nerves in patellar[15] or Achilles[7] tendinopathy when compared to appropriate controls. All the studies, nevertheless, stress an important point; that tendon tissue, traditionally considered to be hyponeural, actually does contain sensory nerves, and consequently hold the capacity to transmit pain signals. It is, however, demonstrated that this innervation is very sparse in deep parts of the patellar tendon, i.e., the actual tendon tissue proper, and most nerves are instead situated in the loose paratendinous connective tissue surrounding the tendon.[15]

Of further interest is the fact that the nerve fascicles containing sensory afferents within and around the patellar tendon express receptors for different signal substances of the cholinergic,[16] sympathetic,[18] and peptidergic[22] systems, and also glutamate receptors have been found on nerves in patellar tendons.[2] These findings provide a morphological basis whereby biochemical mediators such as acetylcholine, catecholamines, substance P, and glutamate could affect pain signalling from the patellar tendon. Theoretically, such substances might be produced in other parts of the peripheral nervous system, or speculatively by the tendon tissue itself. Studies of recent years give support for both theories, as will be discussed in the following section.

## 16.4 Potential Origins of Biochemical Mediators

### *16.4.1 Sympathetic Neurons and the Possibility of Sympathetically Maintained Pain*

There is a phenomenon called sympathetically maintained pain (SMP) that is rather widely discussed in the literature in relation to symptoms in the extremities (e.g.,[33]). The idea of SMP is that sympathetic peripheral nerves can generate or enhance pain (e.g.,[6]), and that this is performed by means of functional interactions with sensory counterparts in a pathological way.[48] These interactions have been postulated to occur when catecholamines released from sympathetic nerves bind to adrenergic receptors on sensory nerves.[5] In patellar tendinopathy, it has been shown that sympathetic efferent nerves coexist within the same fascicles as sensory afferent nerves.[18] It is therefore tempting to speculate that adrenergic receptors found in these fascicles[18] are located on the membranes of sensory neurons, and may be susceptible to catecholamines released from sympathetic neurons.

### 16.4.2 Production in Nonneuronal Cells of Signal Substances Traditionally Associated with Neurons: A Widespread Phenomenon of Increasing Interest

Research of recent years has demonstrated the occurrence of signal substances traditionally associated with neurons in nonneuronal cells in a variety of tissues throughout the human body. Particular attention has been devoted to the classical neurotransmitter acetylcholine (ACh). Several nonneuronal human cells, such as epithelial cells of airways and skin, endothelial cells, muscle cells, and different kind of immune cells, have been demonstrated to produce ACh.[28,46] The possible role of such nonneuronal ACh in the pathogenesis of various diseases has been discussed,[46] and the mere existence of this ACh has been proposed to explain why ACh receptors are so widespread in tissues not innervated by cholinergic neurons.[47] In addition to nonneuronal ACh, glutamate[27] and catecholamines[35] have also been found to be produced outside the nervous system in mammalians.

Of interest in the discussion of patellar tendon pathology are observations that ACh and catecholamines can affect the properties of fibrogenic cells, i.e., cells that are analogous to tenocytes in several tissues. Fibrogenic cells in the liver are known to respond to ACh,[37] as well as to catecholamines,[36] by increased cellular proliferation and collagen gene expression, and even by promoting hepatic fibrosis, a histological condition with several similarities to tendinosis.

### 16.4.3 Nonneuronal Production of Biochemical Mediators in Tenocytes

Given the very sparse innervation in deep parts of the patellar tendon,[15] and also the fact that cells closely related to tenocytes have been shown to produce signal substances[35] that promote histopathology similar to tendinosis (see previous text), one might ask whether tenocytes themselves are a source of neurotransmitters and/or neuropeptides, which then target receptors present on the sensory nerves that are predominantly seen in the paratendinous tissue. With this rationale, studies have recently been performed at the tissue level comparing human patellar tendinosis tendons with healthy tendons, with analytic methods for both protein and mRNA detection.[16-19,40] Parallel studies have been performed on the human Achilles tendon.[4,8-10]

These studies have demonstrated that there are indeed signs of neurotransmitter production by tenocytes in patellar tendinopathy. The tenocytes of tendinosis patellar tendons have been shown to harbor enzymes involved in ACh synthesis and transport. The ACh synthesizing enzyme choline acetyltransferase (ChAT), as well as vesicular ACh transporter (VAChT; Fig. 16.1) – an enzyme known to shuffle ACh from an intracellular site of synthesis into vesicles in nerve terminals[21] – have been detected intracellularly in the tenocytes of patellar tendons from tendinopathy patients, but not in control tendons.[16] These findings strongly suggest that tenocytes in chronically painful patellar tendons are capable of production and release of ACh. In addition, this phenomenon was most apparent in patients with severe, therapy-resistant, tendinopathy.[19]

The studies have furthermore shown that human patellar tendon cells not only contain enzymes related to production/transport of ACh, but also of catecholamines and glutamate. Human tenocytes of patellar tendons were found to contain tyrosine hydroxylase (TH), the rate-limiting enzyme in catecholamine synthesis[17,18] (Fig. 16.2), as well as vesicular glutamate transporter 2 (VGluT2),[40] an indirect marker for glutamate release; these findings again being most evident in tendons from patients with patellar tendinopathy.

The findings of locally produced ACh, catecholamines, and glutamate, in tenocytes, have been shown at both protein (via immunohistochemistry) and mRNA (via in situ hybridization) levels.[16-19,40]

## 16.5 Potential Targets and Effects of Locally Produced Biochemical Mediators

### 16.5.1 Receptors on Sensory Nerves: Potential Role in Chronic Tendon Pain

As previously stated, nerve fascicles within and especially adjacent to human patellar tendons contain sensory neurons (e.g.,[15,32]), and the nerves also express receptors

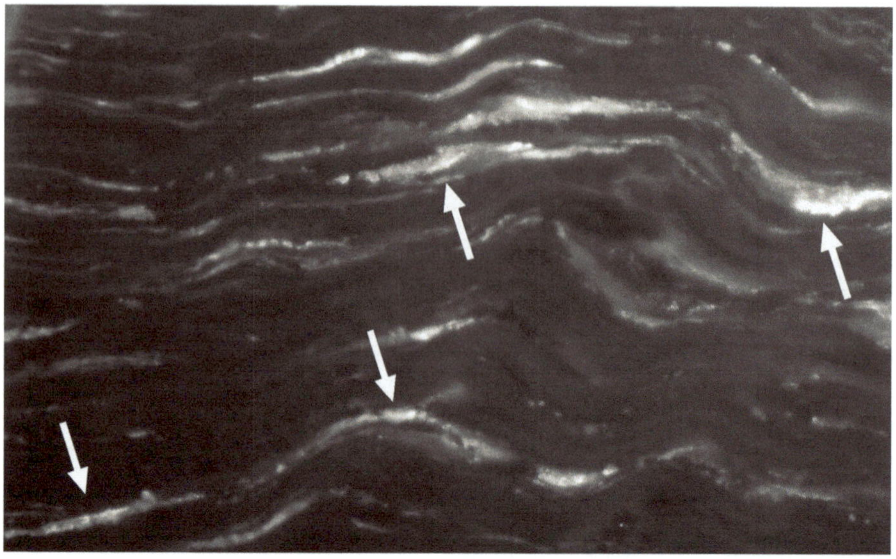

**Fig. 16.1** Evidence of intratendinous ACh production. Tenocytes of patellar tendon tissue have been shown to harbor enzymes related to acetylcholine (ACh) production in tendinopathy patients. The ACh synthesizing enzyme choline acetyltransferase (ChAT), as well as its mRNA, have been found at intracellular locations. Furthermore, vesicular acetylcholine transporter (VAChT) – an enzyme that shuffles ACh from an intracellular site of synthesis into vesicles – has also been detected inside tenocytes as shown by this picture. Immunohistochemical staining (immunofluorescence method, TRITC) show specific immunoreactions inside the tenocytes, some indicated with *arrows*

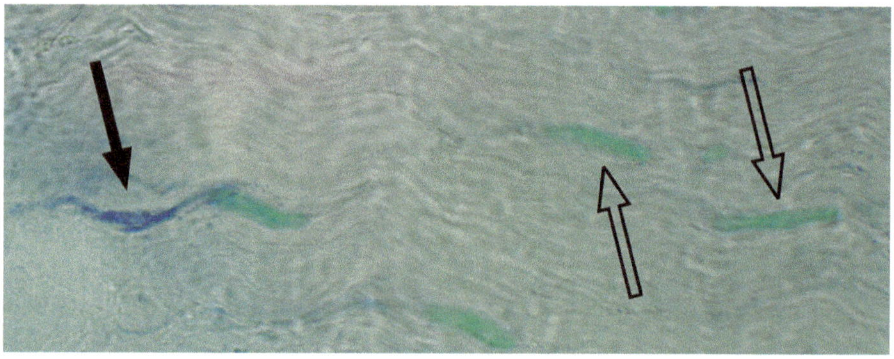

**Fig. 16.2** Evidence of intratendinous catecholamine production. In-situ hybridization method shows reactions for tyrosine hydroxylase (TH) mRNA within some tenocytes (*filled arrow*) in patellar tendon tissue from a patient with tendinopathy. Other tenocytes (*unfilled arrows*) are negative in this regard. TH is the rate-limiting enzyme in the synthesis of catecholamines

for ACh ($M_2$ muscarinic ACh receptors),[16] catecholamines ($\alpha_1$-, $\alpha_{2A}$-, and $\beta_1$-adrenoreceptors),[18] and glutamate (N-methyl-D-aspartate [NMDA] receptors).[2]

In light of this, it is interesting to note that cholinergic stimulation has been shown to induce pain in vivo,[45] and to stimulate excitation of nociceptive C-fibers in vitro.[44] Such excitatory effects on sensory afferents seen by stimulation with ACh, or its analogues, might be, at least partly, mediated by the activation of $M_2$ receptors, as these have also previously been demonstrated to be localized to sensory nerve fibers.[25] However, in sharp contrast, other studies have shown that stimulation of $M_2$ receptors on sensory neurons may inhibit nociception.[20] The role of ACh and its receptors in tendinopathy must be subjected to experimental research in the future to elucidate these questions.

As already mentioned (see previous sections), catecholamines[5] and glutamate[23] are also known to elicit pain.

In summary, one could ask whether locally produced ACh, catecholamines, and/or glutamate in patellar tendinopathy are involved in the pain mechanisms of this condition.

### 16.5.2 Receptors in Blood Vessel Walls: Potential Role in Tendinopathy Angiogenesis and Abnormalities of Vascular Flow

Tendinopathy is associated with vascular abnormalities, both in terms of capillary proliferation[29] and increased vascularity (measured as augmented blood flow using ultrasound and color/power Doppler technique). This increased blood flow is seen in close relation to the area with structural changes in tendinopathy (e.g.,[3,12,24]). In addition, a link has been noted between the degree of such pathological vascularity and the level of pain in tendinopathy patients.[13]

In view of this, it is interesting to note that blood vessels of patellar tendon tissue express receptors for ACh[16] and catecholamines.[18] It is thus tempting to speculate whether biochemical mediators produced in tenocytes might exert cholinergic and adrenergic effects on tendon blood vessels, which contribute to the pathological vascular phenomena of patellar tendinopathy. Both ACh and catecholamines are well known for their effects on blood vessel regulation. Furthermore, stimulation of certain ACh receptors leads to angiogenesis during wound healing.[26]

### 16.5.3 Receptors on Tenocytes: Potential Role in Tendinosis Tissue Changes

As previously stated, it is now commonly accepted that the underlying histopathology of chronically painful patellar tendons are of a degenerative, rather than acute inflammatory, nature, i.e., tendinosis. The tendon tissue changes seen include hypercellularity, hypervascularity, and derangement of collagen and other extracellular matrix components,[29,30] and also apoptosis.[41,42,49]

The recent studies of nonneuronal signalling pathways in tendinosis tissue of patellar tendons have revealed evidence of cholinergic and adrenergic receptors not only on nerves and blood vessels, but also on the tenocytes themselves (adrenergic[18]; cholinergic[16,19]). These findings, together with the findings of biosynthetic enzymes for ACh and catecholamines, provide a morphological basis for autocrine/paracrine cholinergic and catecholaminergic effects in tendinosis tissue. It is possible that tenocytes influence themselves via such signalling, thereby promoting tissue changes as a response to injury, either in a pathological degenerative/apoptotic fashion or in an attempt of self-healing. In favor of the former suggestion, stimulation in vivo of catecholamine receptors has been shown to induce apoptosis of cardiac muscle cells in the rat heart.[11] However, contradicting this and endorsing a proliferative/healing role of ACh/catecholamines in tendon tissue, studies already mentioned have shown that ACh[37] and norepinephrine[38] stimulate the proliferation of fibrogenic cells in the liver and induce collagen gene expression in these cells. Also, stimulation of receptors for catecholamines on rat fibroblasts induces proliferation,[50] and stimulation of ACh receptors on pulmonary fibroblasts may augment collagen accumulation.[43] This may be particularly relevant given the close similarity between tenocytes and fibroblasts elsewhere in the body.

## 16.6 Conclusions and Potential Clinical Implications

In conclusion, evidence points in a new direction: that biochemical mediators, deriving from nerves in or around the patellar tendon or from the tendon tissue itself, may profoundly influence the nerves, blood vessels, and tenocytes in patellar tendon tissue (Fig. 16.3). The findings furthermore suggest that these phenomena arise or increase in response to patellar tendinopathy, or even precede/elicit the condition, as they are only rarely or very moderately seen in normal patellar tendons. Thus, the ramifications of neuronal or nonneuronal biochemical mediators in patellar tendinopathy include effects on tendon tissue (tendinosis changes), vascular regulation, and/or pain signalling. Clinical use of this knowledge in the future might be of potentially high impact. If the model of biochemical pathogenesis/pathology in patellar tendinopathy proves to have some validity, it would mean that clinical management would aim to modify the biochemical milieu, rather than just focusing on collagen repair. Eccentric training regimens and surgery would probably still have their uses, but researchers would be encouraged to pursue a pharmaceutical approach focused on reducing the irritant biochemical compounds in or around the tendon, if proven to be a causative factor in tendinopathy. This would actually mean

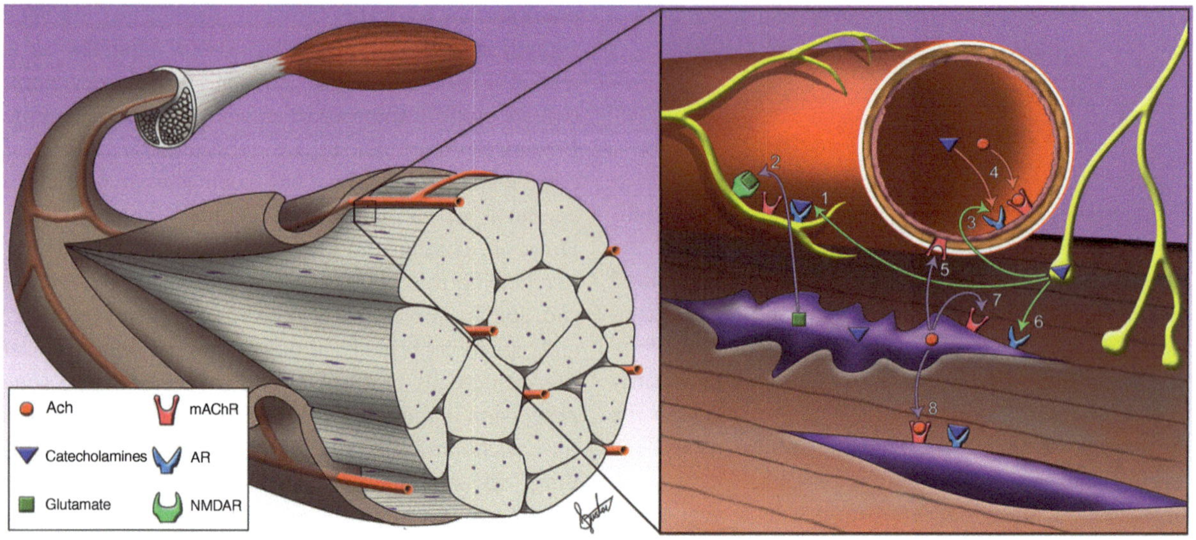


**Fig. 16.3** The biochemical model for patellar tendinopathy. Schematic figure of patellar tendon tissue, showing the possible roles of biochemical mediators. The microscopic milieu is depicted in the frame to the right. Afferent sensory nerve fibers, here seen to the left in close association with a blood vessel, express muscarinic acetylcholine receptors (mAChR), *N*-methyl-D-aspartate receptors (NMDA R), and adrenergic receptors (AR). The sensory nerves are hereby susceptible to stimulation by the neurotransmitters acetylcholine (ACh) and glutamate, as well as by catecholamines. All these substances might thus theoretically affect pain signalling from the tendon. The adrenergic receptors might be influenced by catecholamines produced by neighboring efferent sympathetic nerves (*1*) "sympathetically maintained pain"). However, the mAChRs, the NMDA Rs, and the adrenergic receptors on the sensory nerves might also be stimulated by acetylcholine (ACh), glutamate, and catecholamines, respectively, which are produced by the tenocytes themselves (*2*) since these principal tendon cells have been shown to express biosynthetic enzymes for the substances in question when tendinopathy occurs. This phenomenon has been noted for the morphologically disfigured tenocytes that are frequently seen in tendinosis tissue (upper tenocyte in picture). Such tenocytes lack the slender, spindle-shaped, appearance of normal tenocytes (lower tenocyte in picture). The efferent sympathetic nerves are furthermore likely to affect blood vessel regulation, via stimulation of adrenergic receptors in the blood vessel walls (*3*). Such receptors, alongside mAChRs in the blood vessel walls, are moreover expected to be stimulated by circulating catecholamines and ACh, respectively (*4*). A third possible source of catecholamines and ACh affecting blood vessel regulation is the tenocytes of the tendon tissue (*5*). The tenocytes, in addition to producing the signal substances in question, express adrenergic receptors and mAChRs, making them receptive to catecholaminergic and cholinergic effects (proliferation, changes in collagen production, and/or degeneration/apoptosis). The receptors on the tenocytes might, in the case of adrenergic receptors, be influenced by signal substances (catecholamines) produced by efferent nerves (*6*), or by signal substances (ACh and catecholamines) produced by the tenocytes themselves. In the latter case, autocrine (*7*) as well as paracrine (*8*) loops are suggested to occur. In summary, receptors on sensory nerves, blood vessels, and tenocytes in patellar tendons, might be affected by substances from efferent nerves (*green arrows*), the blood circulation (*red arrows*), and/or the tendon tissue itself (*purple arrows*) Copyright with artist: Gustav Andersson

that treatments might challenge the cause, rather than only the symptoms or consequences, of tendinopathy development.

However, first experimental studies must follow, to bring clarity to the actual role of the biochemical mediators produced in tendinosis tissue. Which substances inflict or enhance pain and tissue degeneration, and which substances promote tissue healing? Animal and cell culture models are currently being used to capture the dynamic events of tendinosis and answer these questions.

## References

1. Alfredson H. The chronic painful Achilles and patellar tendon: research on basic biology and treatment. *Scand J Med Sci Sports*. 2005;15:252-259.
2. Alfredson H, Forsgren S, Thorsen K, et al. In vivo microdialysis and immunohistochemical analyses of tendon tissue demonstrated high amounts of free glutamate and glutamate NMDAR1 receptors, but no signs of inflammation, in Jumper's knee. *J Orthop Res*. 2001;19:881-886.
3. Alfredson H, Ohberg L. Neovascularisation in chronic painful patellar tendinosis – promising results after sclerosing neovessels outside the tendon challenge the need for

surgery. *Knee Surg Sports Traumatol Arthrosc*. 2005;13: 74-80.

4. Andersson G, Danielson P, Alfredson H, et al. Presence of substance P and the neurokinin-1 receptor in tenocytes of the human Achilles tendon. *Regul Pept*. 2008;150:81-87.
5. Baron R. Peripheral neuropathic pain: from mechanisms to symptoms. *Clin J Pain*. 2000;16:S12-S20.
6. Baron R, Levine JD, Fields HL. Causalgia and reflex sympathetic dystrophy: does the sympathetic nervous system contribute to the generation of pain? *Muscle Nerve*. 1999;22:678-695.
7. Bjur D, Alfredson H, Forsgren S. The innervation pattern of the human Achilles tendon: studies of the normal and tendinosis tendon with markers for general and sensory innervation. *Cell Tissue Res*. 2005;320:201-206.
8. Bjur DK, Alfredson HK, Forsgren SK. Presence of the neuropeptide Y 1 receptor in tenocytes and blood vessel walls in the human Achilles tendon. *Br J Sports Med*. 2009;43(14): 1136-1142.
9. Bjur D, Danielson P, Alfredson H, et al. Immunohistochemical and in situ hybridization observations favor a local catecholamine production in the human Achilles tendon. *Histol Histopathol*. 2008;23:197-208.
10. Bjur D, Danielson P, Alfredson H, et al. Presence of a non-neuronal cholinergic system and occurrence of up- and down-regulation in expression of M2 muscarinic acetylcholine receptors: new aspects of importance regarding Achilles tendon tendinosis (tendinopathy). *Cell Tissue Res*. 2008;331: 385-400.
11. Burniston JG, Tan LB, Goldspink DF. Beta2-Adrenergic receptor stimulation in vivo induces apoptosis in the rat heart and soleus muscle. *J Appl Physiol*. 2005;98:1379-1386.
12. Cook JL, Malliaras P, De Luca J, et al. Neovascularization and pain in abnormal patellar tendons of active jumping athletes. *Clin J Sport Med*. 2004;14:296-299.
13. Cook JL, Malliaras P, De Luca J, et al. Vascularity and pain in the patellar tendon of adult jumping athletes: a 5 month longitudinal study. *Br J Sports Med*. 2005;39:458-461.
14. Cook JL, Purdam CR. Is tendon pathology a continuum? A pathology model to explain the clinical presentation of load-induced tendinopathy. *Br J Sports Med*. 2009;43: 409-416.
15. Danielson P, Alfredson H, Forsgren S. Distribution of general (PGP 9.5) and sensory (substance P/CGRP) innervations in the human patellar tendon. *Knee Surg Sports Traumatol Arthrosc*. 2006;14:125-132.
16. Danielson P, Alfredson H, Forsgren S. Immunohistochemical and histochemical findings favoring the occurrence of autocrine/paracrine as well as nerve-related cholinergic effects in chronic painful patellar tendon tendinosis. *Microsc Res Tech*. 2006;69:808-819.
17. Danielson P, Alfredson H, Forsgren S. In situ hybridization studies confirming recent findings of the existence of a local nonneuronal catecholamine production in human patellar tendinosis. *Microsc Res Tech*. 2007;70:908-911.
18. Danielson P, Alfredson H, Forsgren S. Studies on the importance of sympathetic innervation, adrenergic receptors, and a possible local catecholamine production in the development of patellar tendinopathy (tendinosis) in man. *Microsc Res Tech*. 2007;70:310-324.
19. Danielson P, Andersson G, Alfredson H, et al. Extensive expression of markers for acetylcholine synthesis and of M2 receptors in tenocytes in therapy-resistant chronic painful patellar tendon tendinosis – a pilot study. *Life Sci*. 2007;80:2235-2238.
20. Dussor GO, Helesic G, Hargreaves KM, et al. Cholinergic modulation of nociceptive responses in vivo and neuropeptide release in vitro at the level of the primary sensory neuron. *Pain*. 2004;107:22-32.
21. Eiden LE. The cholinergic gene locus. *J Neurochem*. 1998;70:2227-2240.
22. Forsgren S, Danielson P, Alfredson H. Vascular NK-1 receptor occurrence in normal and chronic painful Achilles and patellar tendons: studies on chemically unfixed as well as fixed specimens. *Regul Pept*. 2005;126:173-181.
23. Gazerani P, Wang K, Cairns BE, et al. Effects of subcutaneous administration of glutamate on pain, sensitization and vasomotor responses in healthy men and women. *Pain*. 2006;124:338-348.
24. Gisslen K, Alfredson H. Neovascularisation and pain in jumper's knee: a prospective clinical and sonographic study in elite junior volleyball players. *Br J Sports Med*. 2005;39: 423-428.
25. Haberberger RV, Bodenbenner M. Immunohistochemical localization of muscarinic receptors (M2) in the rat skin. *Cell Tissue Res*. 2000;300:389-396.
26. Jacobi J, Jang JJ, Sundram U, et al. Nicotine accelerates angiogenesis and wound healing in genetically diabetic mice. *Am J Pathol*. 2002;161:97-104.
27. Kalariti N, Pissimissis N, Koutsilieris M. The glutamatergic system outside the CNS and in cancer biology. *Expert Opin Investig Drugs*. 2005;14:1487-1496.
28. Kawashima K, Fujii T. The lymphocytic cholinergic system and its contribution to the regulation of immune activity. *Life Sci*. 2003;74:675-696.
29. Khan KM, Bonar F, Desmond PM, et al. Patellar tendinosis (jumper's knee): findings at histopathologic examination, US, and MR imaging. Victorian Institute of Sport Tendon Study Group. *Radiology*. 1996;200:821-827.
30. Khan KM, Cook JL, Bonar F, et al. Histopathology of common tendinopathies. Update and implications for clinical management. *Sports Med*. 1999;27:393-408.
31. Khan KM, Cook JL, Maffulli N, et al. Where is the pain coming from in tendinopathy? It may be biochemical, not only structural, in origin. *Br J Sports Med*. 2000;34:81-83.
32. Lian O, Dahl J, Ackermann PW, et al. Pronociceptive and antinociceptive neuromediators in patellar tendinopathy. *Am J Sports Med*. 2006;34:1801-1808.
33. McMahon SB. Mechanisms of sympathetic pain. *Br Med Bull*. 1991;47:584-600.
34. Molloy TJ, Kemp MW, Wang Y, et al. Microarray analysis of the tendinopathic rat supraspinatus tendon: glutamate signaling and its potential role in tendon degeneration. *J Appl Physiol*. 2006;101:1702-1709.
35. Oben JA, Diehl AM. Sympathetic nervous system regulation of liver repair. *Anat Rec A Discov Mol Cell Evol Biol*. 2004; 280:874-883.
36. Oben JA, Roskams T, Yang S, et al. Hepatic fibrogenesis requires sympathetic neurotransmitters. *Gut*. 2004;53: 438-445.

37. Oben JA, Yang S, Lin H, et al. Acetylcholine promotes the proliferation and collagen gene expression of myofibroblastic hepatic stellate cells. *Biochem Biophys Res Commun*. 2003;300:172-177.
38. Oben JA, Yang S, Lin H, et al. Norepinephrine and neuropeptide Y promote proliferation and collagen gene expression of hepatic myofibroblastic stellate cells. *Biochem Biophys Res Commun*. 2003;302:685-690.
39. Schubert TE, Weidler C, Lerch K, et al. Achilles tendinosis is associated with sprouting of substance P positive nerve fibres. *Ann Rheum Dis*. 2005;64:1083-1086.
40. Scott A, Alfredson H, Forsgren S. VGluT2 expression in painful Achilles and patellar tendinosis: evidence of local glutamate release by tenocytes. *J Orthop Res*. 2008;26: 685-692.
41. Scott A, Khan KM, Duronio V. IGF-I activates PKB and prevents anoxic apoptosis in Achilles tendon cells. *J Orthop Res*. 2005;23:1219-1225.
42. Scott A, Khan KM, Heer J, et al. High strain mechanical loading rapidly induces tendon apoptosis: an ex vivo rat tibialis anterior model. *Br J Sports Med*. 2005;39:e25.
43. Sekhon HS, Keller JA, Proskocil BJ, et al. Maternal nicotine exposure upregulates collagen gene expression in fetal monkey lung. Association with alpha7 nicotinic acetylcholine receptors. *Am J Respir Cell Mol Biol*. 2002;26:31-41.
44. Steen KH, Reeh PW. Actions of cholinergic agonists and antagonists on sensory nerve endings in rat skin, in vitro. *J Neurophysiol*. 1993;70:397-405.
45. Vogelsang M, Heyer G, Hornstein OP. Acetylcholine induces different cutaneous sensations in atopic and non-atopic subjects. *Acta Derm Venereol*. 1995;75:434-436.
46. Wessler I, Kilbinger H, Bittinger F, et al. The biological role of non-neuronal acetylcholine in plants and humans. *Jpn J Pharmacol*. 2001;85:2-10.
47. Wessler I, Kirkpatrick CJ, Racke K. Non-neuronal acetylcholine, a locally acting molecule, widely distributed in biological systems: expression and function in humans. *Pharmacol Ther*. 1998;77:59-79.
48. Wong HY. Neural mechanisms of joint pain. *Ann Acad Med Singapore*. 1993;22:646-650.
49. Yuan J, Wang MX, Murrell GA. Cell death and tendinopathy. *Clin Sports Med*. 2003;22:693-701.
50. Zhang H, Faber JE. Trophic effect of norepinephrine on arterial intima-media and adventitia is augmented by injury and mediated by different alpha1-adrenoceptor subtypes. *Circ Res*. 2001;89:815-822.

# The Pathophysiology of Patellofemoral Arthritis

17

Ronald P. Grelsamer and Jason Gould

## 17.1 Introduction

Faced with a patient suffering from patellofemoral (PF) arthritis, the surgeon should determine the pathophysiology of the arthritis, as different etiologies will demand different treatments. The surgeon must specifically, to the best of his/her ability, determine whether the patellofemoral arthritis is truly isolated to the patellofemoral compartment. If so, will it remain isolated?

The articular cartilage of the patella, like all other articular cartilage, consists of a fluid phase and a solid phase made up mostly of collagen and glycosaminoglycans. The solid phase is permeable, and when a load is applied to the articular surface, the fluid gradually redistributes itself within the solid matrix.[22,23] The pressure within the fluid is largely responsible for the cushioning effect of articular cartilage. Disruption of the articular surface by way of cracks, fissures, crevices, and the like leads to a loss of pressure within the fluid phase. Abnormal stresses are then borne by the collagen fibers which become prone to breaking down.[3] The articular cartilage of the patella is thicker, softer and more permeable than any other articular cartilage including that of the trochlea.

Some etiologies are associated with *isolated* patellofemoral arthritis, while others are more likely to be a reflection of a generalized knee condition.

Causes of isolated PF arthritis include malalignment (abnormal tilt, abnormal Q angle, abnormal torsion), dysplasia (trochlear and patellar), instability, and trauma.

R.P. Grelsamer (✉)
Mount Sinai Medical Center, New York, NY, USA
e-mail: ronald.grelsamer@mountsinai.org

## 17.2 Malalignment

Malalignment is a general term encompassing conditions that lead to abnormal positioning and tracking of the patella. An improper fit of the mating surfaces leads to anomalous pressure distributions, which in turn can lead to arthritis. Merchant[21] in California and Ficat[11] in France were the first to postulate that a tilted patella (lateral side down), in association with a tight lateral retinaculum, would lead to excessive pressures over the lateral aspect of the patellofemoral joint. Eckstein and colleagues[10] demonstrated CT scan evidence of lateral hyper-pressure on the subchondral bone of tilted patellae.

No prospective study verifying that patients with malalignment have a greater predisposition to arthritis has been undertaken, but patients with patellofemoral arthritis are often noted to demonstrate malalignment. Iwano and colleagues[16] reviewed 108 knees in 61 women and 5 men with patellofemoral arthritis (with or without concomitant femorotibial arthritis). 28% of patients with isolated patellofemoral arthritis (9/32) had a history of patellar instability. In 59 of the 64 knees (92%) with isolated patellofemoral arthritis, the arthritis was located at the lateral half of the patella.

A greatly increased (or decreased) Q angle would be expected to lead to increased pressures between the patella and the lateral (or medial) wall of the trochlea. Goutallier and colleagues[12] have found increased pain in patients whose normally positioned tibial tuberosity is transposed medially. They have studied the Q angle – trochlear angle relationship: A patient with a steep trochlea will be susceptible to increased patellar-trochlear pressures if the Q angle is significantly high or low. In their study, patients with the greatest pain following tibial tuberosity transfers had steep trochleas (<140°) and low Q angles.

V. Sanchis-Alfonso (ed.), *Anterior Knee Pain and Patellar Instability*,
DOI: 10.1007/978-0-85729-507-1_17, © Springer-Verlag London Limited 2011

Distal femoral torsion – usually internal – will lead to excessive pressure on the lateral aspect of the patellofemoral compartment and is functionally the equivalent of patellar tilt.

Patients whose isolated patellofemoral arthritis is secondary to malalignment are good candidates for surgery on the extensor mechanism, as the arthritis is not likely to progress to the other compartments.

## 17.3 Patellofemoral Dysplasia

The patellofemoral articulation varies significantly from person to person. Wiberg studied the variability of the patella in the axial plane, Grelsamer studied the patella in the sagittal plane,[14] and Henri Dejour,[9] and then David Dejour,[7] have studied the various forms of trochlear dysplasia.

The patellofemoral articulation is well suited to its function and does not usually breakdown – despite the fact that in the sagittal plane, it is incongruent. (only a small portion of the patella contacts the trochlea at any given time[15]). When inspected closely, the articular cartilage of the patella is noted to be shaped by multiple facets arrayed in patterns that are unique to each patient.[17] The trochlea is generally U-shaped. The U begins at the proximal portion of the trochlea and becomes progressively steeper and deeper distally. On an axial radiograph taken with the knee flexed 30°–40°, the trochlea has an angle of approximately 140°.

The normal functioning of the patellofemoral joint is dependent on the smooth interplay of these complex geometries. When a variation occurs at the patella that is well matched by the trochlea, one can imagine that the forces will remain well distributed and that the stresses will remain within tolerable range. Thus, if the trochlea is slightly steeper or more shallow than usual, this will be tolerated, as long as the patella features the corresponding variation.

Some trochlear variations are so significant, however, that even a matching patella may not adequately compensate for them. These would include unusually steep or shallow trochleas, or trochleas featuring a proximal convexity.

There exists a high correlation between the presence of patellofemoral dysplasia and that of patellofemoral arthritis.[8] The diagnosis of trochlear dysplasia is made on a true lateral x-ray, where, ideally, the two femoral condyles appear superimposed posteriorly.[26] The characteristic feature of dysplasia is the so-called crossing sign, a convergence of the trochlea and of the lateral femoral condyle – on a normal trochlea, the two lines remain distinct up to the origin of the trochlea.[13] The more distal the crossing, the more extensive the dysplasia.

In more severe forms of dysplasia, the trochlea is elevated anteriorly relative to the anterior cortex of the femur. This is easily judged by prolonging the anterior cortex distally on the lateral x-ray and by judging the position of the trochlea relative to this projection.

Dejour and Tecklenburg have classified trochlear dysplasia into four categories.[7,27]

The dysplastic process can include patella alta, as reflected by the various parameters of patellar height.[4,14]

In a study of 367 patients with isolated patellofemoral arthritis, Dejour found that patellofemoral dysplasia was the most common predisposing factor.[8] Seventy-eight percent of patients had a positive crossing sign on the lateral x-ray.

Dysplasia represents the link between patellar instability and patellofemoral arthritis. Patients in whom the proximal trochlea is anterior to the distal femoral cortex and/or patients featuring a spur at the proximal trochlea are at greatest risk.[7] The lesions that we see at the patellofemoral articulation in patients with history of patellar dislocation most likely represent precursors to the eventual arthritis.

The prominence of the proximal trochlea presumably has a reverse Maquet effect by increasing the patellofemoral pressures. Patella alta as an isolated factor does not predispose to arthritis.[15]

## 17.4 Instability (Symptomatic Medial–Lateral Displacement)

Although the patellofemoral compartment is not congruent in the sagittal plane, it is very congruent in the axial plane. Thus any medial–lateral displacement of the patella will come at the expense of abnormal shear stresses at the level of the articular surface.

The association between subluxation of the patella (partial loss of congruence in the axial plane) and arthritis has not been formally studied, but arthritis following frank patellar dislocation has been the object of studies, many of which have come out of Finland.[18,19,24] Patients suffering from a single dislocation exhibit a higher rate of arthritis than patients with multiple dislocations. The anatomy of patients with recurrent dislocations is likely to facilitate these episodes of instability. Thus, less force is required to dislocate the patella than in patients who suffer just one dislocation. The situation is somewhat analogous to shoulder instability.

A study of patients who have undergone surgical treatment for their instability has demonstrated a higher rate of arthritis than patients treated nonoperatively.[18] However, the spectrum of surgical procedures in these patients include procedures no longer performed with any frequency.

## 17.5 Trauma

Direct blunt trauma onto articular cartilage can lead to arthritis, but no study has determined the threshold of trauma applied to the front of the knee that is required to cause lasting damage to the patellofemoral cartilage.

Articular fractures of the patella and trochlea, on the other hand, can be expected to pose the same risk of arthritis as other intra-articular fractures. In their 1995 study, Argenson and colleagues[2] found that trauma was the etiology of the arthritis in 20 out of 66 patients who were candidates for the patellofemoral arthroplasty.

As with malalignment and dysplasia, traumatic arthritis lends itself to isolated patellofemoral procedures, because the arthritis is not likely to progress to the other compartments.

## 17.6 Obesity

Climbing stairs, getting out of a chair, or performing any other closed chain activity, a person experiences pressures across the patellofemoral articulation in proportion to his or her weight. It stands to reason that obesity is a risk factor for patellofemoral arthritis. The Body Mass Index (BMI) is the yardstick by which obesity is determined. It is calculated as a subject's weight divided by the square of his/her height. A BMI greater than 30 reflects obesity.

Obesity has been found to predispose to knee pain,[1,28] to knee arthritis,[6] and to patellofemoral arthritis.[5,20]

## 17.7 Osteoarthritis and Inflammatory Arthritis

A number of patients with seemingly isolated patellofemoral arthritis, in fact, suffer from osteoarthritis or inflammatory arthritis that happens to have afflicted the patellofemoral compartment first. In time, the other compartments can be expected to deteriorate. Such patients are naturally more likely to obtain only short-term relief from a patellofemoral procedure.

## 17.8 Genetic Factors

As we gradually discover new causes for our physical afflictions, the "idiopathic" category of human diseases will eventually disappear, and patellofemoral arthritis will be no exception. Articular cartilage most likely exhibits a genetic predisposition to deterioration in select patients. Spector and MacGregor, for example, have noted that the ability of collagen to withstand high stresses has a genetic component.[25] This probably accounts for the wide range of clinical response to a given set of joint loads.

## 17.9 Summary

It is important for the surgeon contemplating patellofemoral surgery to consider the etiology of the patient's arthritis. If malalignment, instability, or trauma are at the root of the problem, the surgeon can feel more confident that his patellofemoral surgery will have lasting results.

## References

1. Andersen RE, Crespo CJ, Bartlett SJ, et al. Relationship between body weight gain and significant knee, hip, and back pain in older Americans. *Obes Res*. 2003;11: 1159-1162.

2. Argenson JN, Guillaume JM, Aubaniac JM. Is there a place for patellofemoral arthroplasty? *Clin Orthop Relat Res.* 1995;321:162-167.
3. Ateshian GA, Hung CT. Patellofemoral joint biomechanics and tissue engineering. *Clin Orthop Relat Res.* 2005;436: 81-90.
4. Caton J, Deschamps G, Chambat P, et al. Patella infera. Apropos of 128 cases. *Rev Chir Orthop Reparatrice Appar Mot.* 1982;68:317-325.
5. Cooper C, McAlindon T, Snow S, et al. Mechanical and constitutional risk factors for symptomatic knee osteoarthritis: differences between medial tibiofemoral and patellofemoral disease. *J Rheumatol.* 1994;21:307-313.
6. Dawson J, Juszczak E, Thorogood M, et al. An investigation of risk factors for symptomatic osteoarthritis of the knee in women using a life course approach. *J Epidemiol Community Health.* 2003;57:823-830.
7. Dejour D, Le Coultre B. Osteotomies in patello-femoral instabilities. *Sports Med Arthrosc.* 2007;15:39-46.
8. Dejour D, Allain J. Histoire naturelle de l'arthrose fémoro-patellaire isolée. *Rev Chir Orthop.* 2004;90(Suppl 5): 1S69-1S129.
9. Dejour H, Walch G, Nove-Josserand L, et al. Factors of patellar instability: an anatomic radiographic study. *Knee Surg Sports Traumatol Arthrosc.* 1994;2:19-26.
10. Eckstein F, Muller-Gerbl M, Putz R. The distribution of cartilage degeneration of the human patella in relation to individual subchondral mineralization. *Z Orthop Ihre Grenzgeb.* 1994;132:405-411.
11. Ficat P, Ficat C, Bailleux A. External hypertension syndrome of the patella. Its significance in the recognition of arthrosis. *Rev Chir Orthop Reparatrice Appar Mot.* 1975;61:39-59.
12. Goutallier D, Bernageau J. Le point sur la TA-GT. In: Goutallier D, ed. *La pathologie femoro-patellaire*, vol. 71. Paris: Expansion scientifique publications; 1999:175-182.
13. Grelsamer RP, Tedder JL. The lateral trochlear sign. Femoral trochlear dysplasia as seen on a lateral view roentgenograph. *Clin Orthop Relat Res.* 1992;281:159-162.
14. Grelsamer RP, Meadows S. The modified Insall-Salvati ratio for assessment of patellar height. *Clin Orthop Relat Res.* 1992;282:170-176.
15. Grelsamer R, Weinstein C. The biomechanics of the patellofemoral joint. *Clin Orthop Relat Res.* 2001;389:9-14.
16. Iwano T, Kurosawa H, Tokuyama H, et al. Roentgenographic and clinical findings of patellofemoral osteoarthrosis. With special reference to its relationship to femorotibial osteoarthrosis and etiologic factors. *Clin Orthop Relat Res.* 1990; 252:190-197.
17. Kwak SD, Colman WW, Ateshian GA, et al. Anatomy of the human patellofemoral joint articular cartilage: surface curvature analysis. *J Orthop Res.* 1997;15:468-472.
18. Maenpaa H, Lehto MU. Patellofemoral osteoarthritis after patellar dislocation. *Clin Orthop Relat Res.* 1997;339: 156-162.
19. Maenpaa H, Lehto MU. Patellar dislocation. The long-term results of nonoperative management in 100 patients. *Am J Sports Med.* 1997;25:213-217.
20. McAlindon T, Zhang Y, Hannan M, et al. Are risk factors for patellofemoral and tibiofemoral knee osteoarthritis different? *J Rheumatol.* 1996;23:332-337.
21. Merchant AC, Mercer RL. Lateral release of the patella. A preliminary report. *Clin Orthop Relat Res.* 1974;139: 40-45.
22. Mow VC, Hayes WC. *Basic Orthopaedic Biomechanics.* 3rd ed. New York: Lippincott Raven; 2004.
23. Mow VC, Kuei SC, Lai WM, et al. Biphasic creep and stress relaxation of articular cartilage in compression? Theory and experiments. *J Biomech Eng.* 1980;102:73-84.
24. Nikku R, Nietosvaara Y, Kallio PE, et al. Operative versus closed treatment of primary dislocation of the patella. Similar 2-year results in 125 randomized patients. *Acta Orthop Scand.* 1997;68:419-423.
25. Spector TD, MacGregor AJ. Risk factors for osteoarthritis: genetics. *Osteoarthritis Cartilage.* 2004;12(Suppl A): S39-44.
26. Tavernier T, Dejour D. Knee imaging: what is the best modality. *J Radiol.* 2001;82:407-388.
27. Tecklenburg K, Dejour D, Hoser C, et al. Bony and cartilaginous anatomy of the patellofemoral joint. *Knee Surg Sports Traumatol Arthrosc.* 2006;14:235-240.
28. Webb R, Brammah T, Lunt M, et al. Opportunities for prevention of 'clinically significant' knee pain: results from a population-based cross sectional survey. *J Public Health (Oxf).* 2004;26:277-284.

# Prevention of Anterior Knee Pain After Anterior Cruciate Ligament Reconstruction

**18**

K. Donald Shelbourne, Scott E. Urch, and Heather Freeman

## 18.1 Introduction

Anterior knee pain is a poorly understood entity that has not been well studied in the literature. One reason for this is because "anterior knee pain" is not specific, and the underlying cause of this symptom may encompass many different etiologies. Studies vary with their own particular definitions, and thus comparisons and conclusions are difficult to interpret. It is, therefore, important when one discusses anterior knee pain that a specific definition be initially offered. This chapter will describe anterior knee pain after anterior cruciate ligament (ACL) reconstructive surgery. After a definition is made, discussions will include incidence and possible etiologies. Prevention of anterior knee pain will be addressed, including preoperative, intraoperative, and postoperative concerns. Finally, treatment options will be offered. It has been the practice in our clinic to evaluate patients carefully with regular, long-term follow-up, scrutinizing their results so that we may learn from them and continually improve our techniques and outcomes. Through the course of the chapter, we will interject our findings where appropriate, in an effort to shed light on this complicated subject.

K.D. Shelbourne (✉)
Shelbourne Knee Center at Methodist Hospital, Indiana University School of Medicine, Indianapolis, IN, USA
e-mail: acldoc@aclmd.com

## 18.2 Definition

Anterior knee pain after reconstruction of the ACL has been documented as a frequent complaint of patients in many studies in the literature.[2-5,7,14,20] It is important, however, to differentiate pain in the knee into two broad categories. A knee that functions well until a specific injury causes a change can be understood by the patient as being broken, as opposed to when the knee gradually becomes painful or sore from overuse. Patients can easily distinguish between these two entities, and this distinction becomes helpful during history taking for narrowing a differential diagnosis. Both of these entities can occur after ACL reconstruction surgery. The former encompasses all of the different injuries that can occur in any knee regardless of previous surgery. These injuries must be identified and treated, but are not within the scope of this chapter. Knee soreness after surgery is more commonly the complaint of the patient. This pain is often vague and cannot be specifically localized with one finger. The patient, when asked to point to where it hurts, will often sweep his fingers along both sides of the patellar tendon, from the sides of the patella to the tibia tubercle. Often, the patient will think of this as "kneecap" symptoms.

## 18.3 Etiology

A review of the literature offers many possible factors leading to anterior knee pain in patients who have not had surgery. These include malalignment, muscular weakness, improper training mechanics and overuse, biochemical substance changes, and psychological

V. Sanchis-Alfonso (ed.), *Anterior Knee Pain and Patellar Instability*,
DOI: 10.1007/978-0-85729-507-1_18, © Springer-Verlag London Limited 2011

issues.[10] The speculation that these factors are involved in the cause of postoperative pain has altered operative and rehabilitation protocols at some institutions.

Alignment of the lower extremity has been implicated in the literature as a possible cause of anterior knee pain.[10] The Quadriceps angle (Q-angle) in particular has been thought to be a significant issue. It is defined as the angle created by drawing lines from the anterior superior iliac spine to the middle of the patella to the tibia tubercle. The average Q-angle is 10–15° with the knee extended. An increased Q-angle theoretically places more stress on the lateral portion of the patella as the knee is flexed as the contact area decreases. This may result in tilting, subluxation, or even frank dislocation. Of these, tilting is most common, especially in women, and may cause poor patella tracking and excess wear. Some surgeons will perform a lateral retinacular release in conjunction with ACL reconstruction if tilting of the patella is present. Because patella tilt is usually asymptomatic in these patients before injury, it has been our experience that a lateral release is usually not necessary and we no longer perform it unless properly indicated.

Muscle imbalance has also been proposed as a cause of tilt and subluxation.[10] A relative weakness of the vastus medialis muscle has often been taught to be a key component of muscle imbalance, and physical therapy protocols have been designed to selectively strengthen this muscle. However, it has recently been shown by EMG analysis that it is difficult, if not impossible, to isolate the vastus medialis using the proposed exercises, and in reality the entire quadriceps muscle group is being rehabilitated together.[6,11] After injury to the ACL, swelling in the knee causes a temporary shutdown of the quadriceps muscles causing them to be weak. While many preoperative protocols stress regaining quadriceps strength before surgery, we mainly emphasize swelling control, the return of full range of motion (ROM), and quadriceps muscle control in the injured knee.[1,12] Since 1998, we have been routinely harvesting the graft from the contralateral extremity, which has allowed us to focus the preoperative and postoperative rehabilitation on regaining ROM and quadriceps muscle control without an immediate concern for gaining strength in the ACL reconstructed knee.[21] Strengthening exercises for the graft-donor site can begin immediately after surgery without a concern for loss of ROM or an effusion. Separating the postoperative rehabilitation between knees allows for an earlier return of ROM in the ACL reconstructed knee and a quicker return of strength in graft-donor knee. Ultimately, patients are able to return to normal activities and sports sooner.

Overuse of any muscle or tendon may cause soreness, and this is no exception after ACL reconstruction. Although we believe that this is a completely different entity from the anterior knee pain that we are discussing in this chapter, it should be included in the differential diagnosis when a bone–patellar tendon–bone autograft technique is utilized, especially for pain that arises during the return to sport phase.

The prevalence of pain due to overuse during the return to sport phase became apparent after observing our patients who underwent ACL reconstruction with a contralateral graft. Some of our patients who have undergone the contralateral graft procedure have complained of soreness in the graft-donor knee after completing a few successive "two-a-day" practices. The soreness in this setting is simply overuse-related patella tendon pain. We reached this conclusion by realizing that the graft-donor knee does not share many of the same concerns as the ACL reconstructed knee, which therefore excludes many possible sources of pain. Assuming the graft-donor leg is normal (no previous injuries or congenital abnormalities), there are no other associated pathologies such as cartilage damage or meniscus tears that could cause anterior knee pain. Harvesting the graft is an extra-articular procedure; therefore, iatrogenic intra-articular damage that may cause pain is excluded. Given that the graft knee ROM and strength are normal preoperatively, and are easily regained postoperatively, the contributions by these factors to pain are minimized. Furthermore, the athletes do not complain of pain during the first few days of the new practice week, but only after many successive practices, and rest, usually, alleviates their symptoms.

We realized that we were overworking the tendon and not allowing it to recuperate between workouts. For the same reason that weightlifters alternate which body region they concentrate on each day, the patella tendon and quadriceps muscle need a day to rest between heavy workouts during the return to sport phase. Consequently, we advise our athletes to participate in impact activities (involving running/jumping) on an every-other-day basis while transitioning back into full sports participation. We believe that repetitive impact activities that load the patella tendon are a more likely cause of anterior knee pain than the graft harvest itself. This factor can be mediated with appropriate rehabilitation providing gradual, progressive stress to the healing patella tendon.

Of much lesser prevalence is a psychosomatic basis for this pain.[23] This should be low on the differential diagnosis list, but should not be dismissed altogether if an organic cause for the pain cannot be found. Sustaining an ACL injury, while not as career threatening and ominous as it may have been several years ago, can have a very strong effect on an athlete's mental state. We must remember that we are treating the patient and not just the knee injury.

Although the factors discussed above may have some role in causing anterior knee pain after ACL reconstructive surgery, other factors have much greater implications. First and foremost, the most important contributor to this syndrome is a lack of regaining full hyperextension as compared with the pre-injured state. Related to this concept are poor tunnel placement and graft-notch mismatch.

Also, previous underlying patellofemoral disease has been implicated as a source of anterior knee pain, as is other intra-articular pathology such as meniscus tears and articular surface chondral lesions. Lastly, tibia hardware may also cause pain and may need to be addressed.

By far, the most important issue is the lack of regaining full hyperextension.[14,15,20] After ACL rupture, an intra-articular hemarthrosis usually occurs acutely. The resulting pain and swelling cause the patient to keep the affected knee bent for comfort. Upon initial evaluation, patients will have limited knee extension, even if they are seen quickly after injury. Most uninjured knees will hyperextend past 0° (Fig. 18.1) and it is from this hyperextended position that lack of extension must be measured.[18] Because it is impossible to know what the full hyperextension on the injured knee was before injury, we compare the injured knee to the normal, contralateral knee. Caution must be observed if the patient has had any previous injury or condition affecting the other knee because the injury can lead to an inaccurate assessment of full hyperextension, which in turn can lead to erroneous operative planning. Without normal hyperextension, the graft may be tensioned too tightly in an attempt to match the other leg, resulting in permanent loss of hyperextension. Even a small amount of knee extension loss can greatly impact function and performance, especially for athletes who require full knee extension to jump and run well. In the nonathlete, these changes can also have a significant effect on future lifestyle issues.

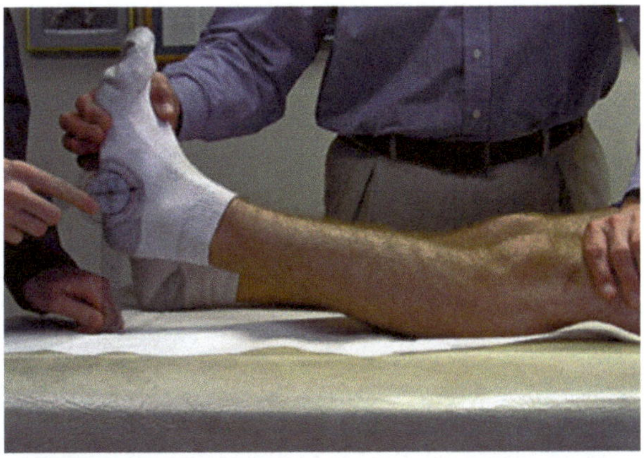

**Fig. 18.1** Most patients' knees have some degree of hyperextension. To evaluate the amount of hyperextension, place one hand above the knee to hold the thigh and place the other hand on the patient's foot to lift the heel off of the examination table

We extensively reviewed 602 patients from 1987 to 1992 regarding anterior knee pain after ACL reconstruction.[20] All knees were reconstructed using a standard ipsilateral bone–patellar tendon–bone autograft with a mini-arthrotomy technique. We observed an apparent association between limited knee extension and anterior knee pain, and this observation was similar to reports published by Sachs and colleagues.[9]

Based on these findings, we implemented a perioperative rehabilitation protocol that emphasized regaining full hyperextension before surgery and during the first week, postoperatively. Physical therapy programs used by others during the same time period had concerns regarding the extension of the reconstructed knee beyond 30° of flexion as it was thought that full extension unduly stressed the graft before it healed.[15,17] However, we have shown in another study that if the graft is placed properly in its isometric position with the appropriate amount of tension, the graft can withstand the forces applied with an aggressive rehabilitation program.[8] In fact, side-to-side KT-1000 arthrometer testing showed no significant loss of stability in patients who underwent this protocol. These patients all returned an anterior knee pain questionnaire with an average follow-up of 3.6 years. Their results were compared with those of a control group, which consisted of 122 young, healthy, asymptomatic athletes with an average age of 20.3 years. Out of a possible 100 points on the anterior knee pain questionnaire, the ACL-reconstructed patients scored 89.5 points, which was not significantly different from the control group (90.2 points). Full hyperextension was achieved in all patients and the average loss of flexion was 5° at a mean of 2.3 years after surgery. Out of 602 patients, 21 required arthroscopic lysis of adhesions at an average of 6.8 months after surgery because of lack of full hyperextension, but all of these patients eventually regained full extension symmetrical to the non-injured knee. We concluded from these results that regaining hyperextension was the key to decreasing the incidence of anterior knee pain.[20]

Regaining full hyperextension begins with obtaining the proper fit of the graft within the notch intraoperatively. When proper graft placement, appropriate tensioning, and adequate notchplasty are simultaneously performed, full hyperextension should be achievable if it was obtained preoperatively (Fig. 18.2). If full extension is not maintained postoperatively, the graft will hypertrophy and block full knee extension. When the graft fits properly within the notch with the leg in full hyperextension, it will conform to this space during its healing stages and therefore allow normal motion.

Previously existing patellofemoral chondromalacia has been thought by some orthopedic surgeons to be a relative contraindication to harvesting a bone–patellar tendon–bone autograft. The existence of patellofemoral chondromalacia can be diagnosed with history, physical examination, radiographs, and MRI. Some have tried other types of screening studies such as bone scan and thermography.[22] These special tests (other than history and physical) can be costly, invasive, and inaccurate. Furthermore, some surgeons will perform an initial diagnostic arthroscopy to evaluate the patellofemoral joint and then use this information as a basis of choosing a different graft source, such as a hamstring graft or allograft. Both of these grafts are inferior choices as they do not allow for an accelerated rehabilitation program, which may result in longer return to sport intervals.[8] In our experience, we have not found chondromalacia of the patellofemoral joint to be of any significance in postoperative performance or symptoms other than a mild increased incidence of pain with sports and kneeling. In the previously mentioned study, we noticed that only 4 out of 49 patients who reported anterior knee pain preoperatively were found to have grade III or IV chondromalacia when inspected intraoperatively.[20] Therefore, even history is inaccurate in assessing the extent of disease in this area. We did not alter our operative technique based on patellofemoral chondromalacia. Postoperatively, patients with patellofemoral disease did not have significantly different anterior knee pain scores from other patients without any patellofemoral disease or from the control group of young athletes without any disease. We believe that choosing a different source for the graft based on patellofemoral chondromalacia is unwarranted. The advantages of the bone–patellar tendon–bone autograft far outweigh the slightly increased risk of symptoms with kneeling and sports.

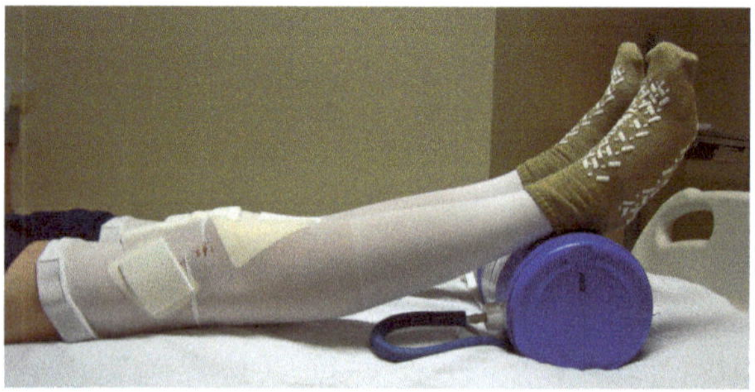

**Fig. 18.2** Immediately after surgery, patients should be able to obtain full hyperextension in the ACL-reconstructed knee equal to the normal knee. The heel prop exercise shown in this figure is an easy method for achieving full hyperextension

Associated pathology found during surgery most often includes meniscus damage and chondromalacia of the articular surfaces. Less commonly, it can also include other ligament damage and osteochondral defects. Meniscus lesions are addressed during surgery either with trephination and left in situ, partial resection, or repair. A meniscus tear is most often in the posterior horn and should not produce the type of symptoms seen with anterior knee pain. Rather, the pain is usually localized posteriorly, or is perceived by the patient to be deep in the joint. Physical findings are more specific with joint line tenderness posteriorly and a positive McMurray test. Because meniscus lesions are addressed intraoperatively, theoretically they should not cause any pain postoperatively. However, an iatrogenic source of pain after meniscus repair can occur, especially with placement of devices such as absorbable arrows, which can over-penetrate the capsule and cause sharp pain. However, meniscus arrows do not usually cause vague anterior pain, and the pain can usually be localized.

Proposed treatment of articular cartilage lesions vary greatly in aggressiveness. Debridement using an arthroscopic shaver or a thermal probe (coblation) is very popular. The long-term effects of the latter have yet to be shown, and the viability of cartilage cells has come into question. More invasive treatments including mosaicplasty and cartilage cell transfers have also been suggested, but it is unclear if these procedures produce an outcome favorable to less invasive treatments. While large, loose flaps should be debrided, it has been our experience that the remainder of the lesion does not need to be addressed surgically. Shelbourne and colleagues[13] studied the outcome of untreated articular cartilage defects in conjunction with ACL reconstruction. From 1987 to 1999, 125 patients met the study criteria of having an articular cartilage defect rated as Outerbridge grade III or IV, but had both menisci intact. The mean defect size was 1.7 $cm^2$. The objective and subjective results of the study group were compared with a matched control group of patients who had intact menisci and no articular cartilage damage. At a mean follow-up time of 8.7 years after surgery, the mean subjective score was 92.8 points in the study group versus 95.9 in the control group. This difference was statistically significantly different, but both scores represent a good outcome. The radiographic results were not statistically significantly different between the study group and the control group. The study by Shelbourne and colleagues[13] provides baseline information that can be used to compare the results of procedures designed to treat articular cartilage defects.

Retained tibia hardware can also be a source of anterior knee pain after surgery. Many fixation devices, including screws with washers, interference screws, staples, and buttons, have been used depending on graft technique. Recent design improvements, such as low-profile head-on screws, have been made in an effort to minimize irritation that can become symptomatic. In addition, careful technique in covering the device with soft tissue should be performed when possible because even suture knots may become symptomatic. Despite these advances and precautions, these hardware devices can still be a problem and may necessitate a second operation to remove the device once the graft is fully incorporated and healed. This pain, however, can also be localized over the device by palpation and usually results in a distinct pain pattern.

## 18.4 Prevention

Prevention of anterior knee pain following ACL reconstruction is an essential key to success. These measures can be subdivided into preoperative, intraoperative, and postoperative concerns.

### *18.4.1 Preoperative*

Preoperative prevention begins with proper history and physical evaluation. Pre-injury knee pain or dysfunction should be elicited from the patient. If the patient complains of preexisting pain, the cause should be explored and proper planning of surgery can then be performed. The overall alignment of the leg should be checked. Patella tracking through full ROM can be quickly evaluated, and a "J" sign can be elicited if present. Direct palpation of the articular surface of the patella as well as mobility, tilt, and apprehension are checked. Range of motion of the knee is compared with the contralateral extremity. If the knee is still markedly swollen, cold/compression (Cryo/Cuff, DJO, LLC. Vista, CA) and elevation have been shown to reduce the swelling effectively in a short period of time. Any lack of hyperextension must be regained before proceeding with surgery. Physical therapy exercises consisting of heel props, towel stretch extension exercises (Fig. 18.3) prone leg hangs, and the use of a

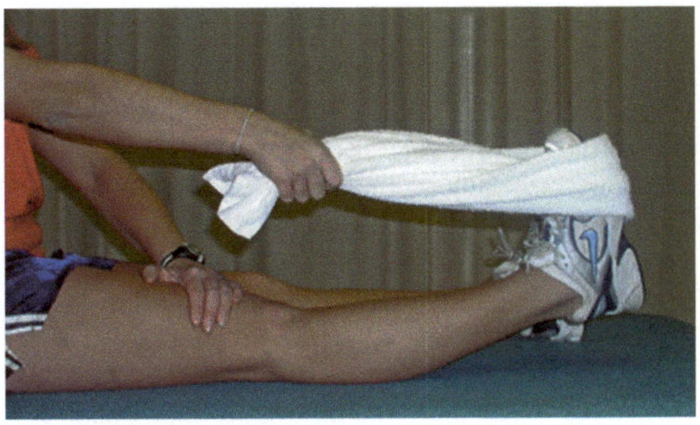

**Fig. 18.3** Towel stretch extension exercise: A towel is looped around the arch of the foot and the patient holds onto both ends of the towel with one hand. The other hand pushes down on the top of the thigh while using the towel to pull up on the foot. The maneuver allows the patient to bring the knee into hyperextension passively

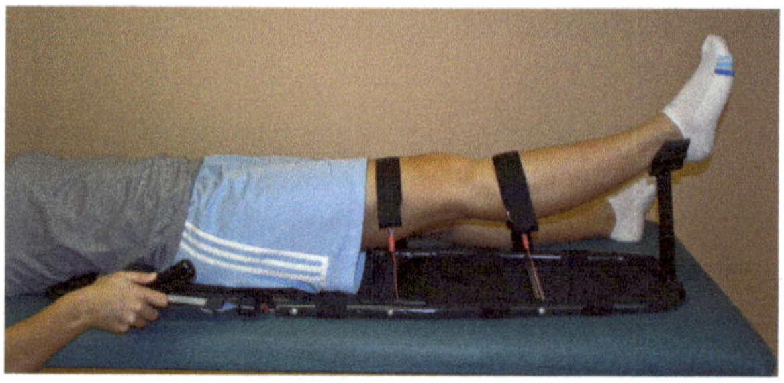

**Fig. 18.4** Patients can use a hyperextension device for 10 min several times a day to regain the natural hyperextension in their knee. The patient controls the amount of stretch applied to the knee

hyperextension device (Fig. 18.4) (Kneebourne Therapeutics, Noblesville, IN) can also be added to regain full hyperextension. In addition to therapeutic exercises, patients must be educated about how to maintain full extension throughout the day. Extension habits, including sitting with the heel propped and standing on the involved extremity with the knee locked-out and forced into full hyperextension by an active quadriceps contraction, are performed by the patient whenever they are sitting or standing. Once full hyperextension has been achieved preoperatively, surgery can then be performed with the best chance for obtaining full hyperextension and preventing anterior knee pain postoperatively.

### 18.4.2 Intraoperative

Intraoperative concerns are easily dealt with as long as the surgeon is aware of them and proficient in his craft. Graft choice is the first consideration. When using hamstring grafts, it has been recommended to avoid full hyperextension in the early postoperative period because the stress may stretch the graft. If full hyperextension is not obtained in the early postoperative period, it can be difficult to regain it later. Given that the lack of full hyperextension causes anterior knee pain after ACL reconstruction, choosing a bone–patellar tendon–bone graft which allows immediate full hyperextension after surgery should reduce the incidence of anterior knee pain postoperatively.

Placement of the incision is a subject that is not often addressed. We use an offset incision medial to the patella tendon as opposed to directly over the tendon. This location not only aids in visualization, but avoids a scar and subcutaneous scar tissue directly where patients kneel. Furthermore, by using a contralateral graft and a mini-arthrotomy approach, extensive subcutaneous dissection anterior to the ipsilateral tendon can be avoided. This again should decrease scar formation in this region, which may allow more motion and less pain.

Proper placement of the tunnels and fit of the graft in the intercondylar notch are important aspects of successful ACL reconstruction surgery. Precise placement of the tibial tunnel will prevent superior roof impingement, thereby alleviating the need for superior notchplasty. As seen on a lateral radiograph taken with the knee in full hyperextension, the anterior portion of the tibial tunnel should be parallel to Blumensaat's line. Preoperative evaluation of x-rays can help the surgeon visualize the proper orientation of the tibial tunnel and help him evaluate placement of his guide wire. Proper placement of the tibial tunnel also minimizes the amount of lateral wall resection that is needed to allow for the proper fit of the new 10-mm graft. The amount of lateral notch resection that is necessary is accurately measured with a caliper, and the appropriate amount of bone is removed to accommodate a 10-mm graft. Proper placement of the femoral tunnel is equally important. Placement of the femoral tunnel that is too far anterior will result in impingement and decreased knee ROM. The femoral tunnel should leave a 1-mm posterior cortical rim and slightly overlap the lateral border of the posterior cruciate ligament.

Impingement should be checked with the knee in full hyperextension, and any correction should be made before surgery is completed. When the graft fits properly within the notch, it remodels to fit that space as it heals. Improper placement of either tunnel or an inadequate notchplasty can result in impingement, which blocks knee extension. If the graft does not sit in the notch correctly, it hypertrophies as it heals, further preventing full hyperextension.[3] The result is a flexion contracture, which can cause anterior knee pain. In addition, pain may also occur due to the actual impingement itself.

The next issue of great importance is properly tensioning the graft. Many orthopedic surgeons try to put the graft in as tight as possible. Securing the graft too tightly does not allow full hyperextension, which results in a stiff knee that can be painful.[8] If the tension in the graft is not set with the knee in full hyperextension, then full hyperextension should be forced after graft fixation to allow the graft tension to adjust and allow full hyperextension. It is preferable to have a slightly lax knee with full ROM than an overly tight knee, because a stiff, stable knee is painful. Our operative technique incorporates a press fit technique, placing both bone blocks from the inside out and securing the graft on both sides with buttons. We are able to make subtle adjustments on the graft tension as we test for full motion and stability intraoperatively. The result is a stable knee with full hyperextension and flexion.

Another issue is repairing the tendon defect and bone plug defects. As previously described, repairing the tendon together with the paratendon should eliminate the patellar tendon defect as a source of pain. It decreases the amount of fibrous scar tissue filling the defect as well as the surrounding subcutaneous tissue. Leaving the defect unrepaired allows excessive scar formation that can persist up to the patella and displace it, as shown on postoperative CT scans.[7] Bone grafting the bone plug defect sites allows for quicker and more uniform healing of these areas. While not proven, leaving defects in the patella and tibia may act as stress risers, as can the defect in the patellar tendon. While bone grafting the bone plug defect sites may decrease the incidence of patella and tibia fractures, it has been shown to have no effect on the incidence of anterior knee pain.[2]

### 18.4.3 Postoperative

Postoperatively, the most important issue is retaining full hyperextension. While regaining full flexion also needs to be addressed, obtaining full hyperextension immediately after surgery will prevent anterior knee pain and afford the patient the best opportunity to return to their pre-injury level of play. A postoperative program can be set up to attain this goal.

The first step is to discuss with the patient and family members step by step what is to occur after surgery on a daily basis, and what is expected of them and why. Immediately after surgery, a Cryo/Cuff is applied to the knee and the leg is placed in a continuous passive motion (CPM) machine. The Cryo/Cuff is used to minimize swelling, which would otherwise restrict motion, cause pain, and inhibit wound healing. Patients remain in the hospital overnight for administration of intravenous ketorolac,[16] patient education, and supervision of the postoperative exercises. Range of motion exercises are done four times daily for the first postoperative week. Extension exercises are performed as described previously, including towel stretches and heel props with a light weight. For patients with tight knee extension, prone hangs or a hyperextension device may be needed. Flexion exercises begin with holding the knee in maximal flexion in a CPM machine for 3 min. Next, a heel slide is performed to maximal flexion. This can be easily measured using a yard stick to help patients monitor their progress. The yard stick is set with the knee fully extended so that the end of the yard stick is lined up with the heel. A measurement is taken when maximal flexion is reached by recording the number of centimeters the heel has traveled. If the patient demonstrates any restriction in full extension ROM, all flexion exercises should be stopped until full extension returns.

During the first postoperative week, the patient remains lying down with their leg elevated in a CPM and a Cryo/Cuff on their knee. This is done to keep swelling to a minimum by maintaining compression and keeping the knee above the heart. Ambulation is restricted to bathroom privileges only for the first postoperative week, but patients may place full weight on both legs and only need to use crutches if needed for balance. The patients are given the following goals for their 1 week follow-up appointment: full terminal hyperextension, flexion greater than or equal to 110°, normal gait pattern, minimal swelling, and good quadriceps muscle control.

During the second week of rehabilitation, towel extensions and heel props are continued, and prone leg hangs and/or a hyperextension device may be added if necessary. Extension habits are again reviewed and reinforced for use when both sitting and standing. Once full ROM and normal gait are achieved, strengthening exercises can be added. When a contralateral graft is used, the graft leg is started on step-down exercises after the first postoperative week as long as full motion is maintained. Our 2-week goals for the reconstructed knee now include full hyperextension, 120° of flexion, and good quadriceps control. The patient should be able to contract their quadriceps muscle strongly enough to perform an active heel lift by this visit (Fig. 18.5). When a contralateral graft is used, single leg press and single knee extension exercises are added after the second postoperative week. This program allows for greater independence by the patient,

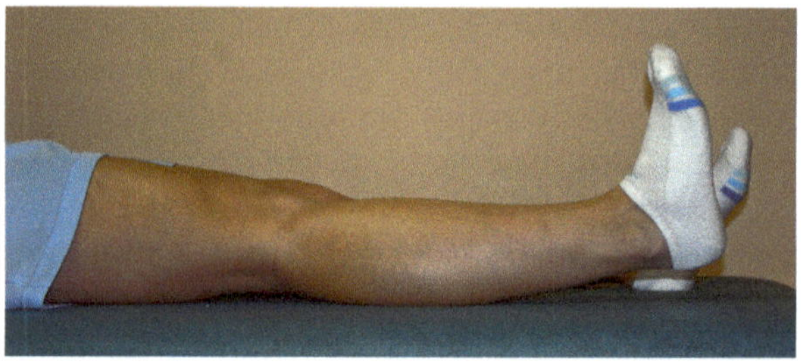

**Fig. 18.5** Active heel lift: The patient actively lifts the heel off of the table by simultaneously contracting the quadriceps muscle and dorsiflexing the ankle

and formal physical therapy visits are needed less frequently. Patients are usually seen every 1–2 weeks during the first month after surgery, then monthly thereafter. The remainder of our rehabilitation program maintains the full hyperextension while progressing with strengthening and sport-specific exercises, and is beyond the scope of this chapter.[12,21]

## 18.5 Treatment

Loss of full hyperextension is the key component for developing anterior knee pain after ACL reconstruction. Arthrofibrosis is an abnormal proliferation of scar tissue that limits knee ROM and is associated with anterior knee pain.[19] Arthrofibrosis is graded as Types 1–4 based on the degree of ROM limitations and the positioning and mobility of the patella. Type 1 arthrofibrosis is defined as less than 10° loss of knee extension with normal flexion, and Type 2 is defined as greater than 10° loss of knee extension with normal flexion.[19] Type 3 arthrofibrosis is defined as greater than 10° loss of knee extension with at least 25° loss of knee flexion, while Type 4 arthrofibrosis involves at least 30° of flexion loss and patella infera.[19]

Treatment of arthrofibrosis begins with a thorough history and physical examination. The length of time since surgery should be noted. Was the patient compliant with the postoperative protocol? Was there a re-injury to the knee? All these questions are important to ask, even if you were the operating surgeon on this patient. Proper radiographs should be done to evaluate the bone tunnels and graft placement. Possible impingement can be inferred from these studies. If the tunnels were appropriately placed and surgery was recent, it is usually easier to regain hyperextension than if the tunnel placement is incorrect or the ROM loss has become chronic. If full hyperextension is regained early, the graft will conform to the intercondylar space as it continues to heal, allowing full ROM and preventing further anterior knee pain. A lateral radiograph view of the knee can be used to evaluate for patella tendon contracture by measuring the distance between the tendinous attachment sites on the inferior patella and tibial tubercle and comparing this measurement to the opposite knee. For patients who demonstrate a patella tendon contracture, decreased flexion will be observed and the patient will have Type 3 or 4 arthrofibrosis. This loss of flexion is likely the result of the contracted patella tendon.

When arthrofibrosis is suspected, nonoperative treatment should be instituted as soon as possible. The longer a ROM deficit exists, the more difficult it is to overcome. Early management includes formal evaluation by a physical therapist and implementation of a therapeutic exercise program designed to maximize the amount of knee hyperextension. Towel extension exercises, prone leg hangs, emphasis of both sitting and standing extension habits (described above), and the use of a hyperextension device should all be implemented. The hyperextension device (Fig. 18.4) allows the patient to independently apply a long-duration stretch to the posterior knee several times throughout the day. Another advantage of this device is that the tension is controlled by the patient and the patient can progressively add tension during the treatment. Since the patient is controlling the amount of stretch applied to the knee, they are able to relax the musculature around the knee, making the stretch from the device more effective. The hyperextension stretch should be held for 10–12 min at a time. This routine of using the hyperextension device and performing therapeutic exercises should be done three to five times throughout the day to fully maximize the patients' extension ROM. If the patient is suffering from a chronic loss of knee extension, correction will take a prolonged course and the patient should be properly educated about goals. The longer the loss of motion has existed, the longer it will take to correct. It is important that the patient maintain a positive mental attitude during this long process.

Often, patients with arthrofibrosis have been to several medical providers that offer little to no help with their condition. This can easily lead to patients' frustration with the whole process. Consistent communication of goals and feedback on improvement will help focus the patient and motivate them strive to attain their goal of full ROM. Often these patients do not only complain of pain and stiffness, but also of loss of strength. However, it is only after full motion is regained that the knee can be strengthened and strengthening exercises should be avoided until full ROM can be demonstrated. This is simply due to the biomechanical disadvantages that exist when the knee cannot fully extend. Attempting to work on strengthening a stiff knee will only slow the progress toward achieving full ROM.

Occasionally, nonoperative means fail for patients with arthrofibrosis, and surgical intervention must be offered. This is considered only after the patient has failed an appropriate therapy program as described above. Patients should only proceed with surgical treatment once forced extension produces anterior pain only. If posterior pain is present, then posterior structures need to be addressed and more improvement may be possible with rehabilitation.

Surgical intervention is most often performed with an arthroscopic procedure. Type 1 arthrofibrosis is treated by excising the cyclops lesion from the graft, which allows the graft to fit properly within the notch with the knee in full hyperextension. Type 2 arthrofibrosis requires resection of anterior scar tissue that forms in front of the graft and proximal tibia. If impingement persists with extension, a notchplasty is also performed. Type 3 arthrofibrosis requires resection of scar tissue that forms between the patella tendon and fat pad. Type 4 arthrofibrosis requires capsular release to free the patella and patella tendon completely. Patients are kept overnight in the hospital for a 1–2 nights to prevent postoperative hemarthrosis, allow for continuous intravenous ketorolac infusion, and to start postoperative rehabilitation immediately. Full weightbearing is immediately allowed. No casting is performed at this time because this can lead to problems with hemarthrosis, decreased knee flexion, and most importantly, decreased quadriceps control. Instead, patients use the hyperextension device followed by towel stretches three to five times throughout the day to focus on maximizing extension. The patient remains on bed rest with bathroom privileges only, and their leg is elevated in a CPM machine moving from 0° to 30°. Patients remain in a supine position with their knee elevated above the level of their heart to avoid a hemarthrosis. Additionally, the Cryo/Cuff is worn continuously to provide cold and compression to the knee joint. Anti-embolism stockings are worn to prevent problems with postoperative blood clot and provide further knee joint compression. While the patient is in the hospital, daily visits are made by the physical therapist to ensure consistent improvement and to answer any questions the patient may have. Patients are discharged home when they can demonstrate full hyperextension equal to the opposite knee and appropriate independence with their exercises. Patients are instructed to continue with the same exercise routine and should remain supine with their leg elevated in the CPM machine for the entire first postoperative week. Even while at home, activity is restricted to bathroom privileges only. Consistent, daily follow-up by phone is important to ensure continued maintenance of full hyperextension and is helpful in keeping the patient motivated during the postoperative process. Patients are seen by a physical therapist at least once a week until hyperextension can be maintained actively.

Once full passive hyperextension is maintained, the next goal is to maintain full extension actively with a quadriceps contraction (Fig. 18.5). Leg control exercises are initiated when the patient demonstrates full hyperextension, and exercises focusing on leg control include: terminal knee extension with rubber tubing, step-ups onto a box, single leg knee extensions, and step-downs. Continued focus should be maintained on hyperextension exercises during this phase. When the patient can demonstrate a full, symmetric active heel lift equal to the opposite side, then exercises for flexion can be added as long as full hyperextension is maintained. If there is any loss of hyperextension, flexion exercises should be decreased until full hyperextension returns. Gentle strengthening exercises can be added once the patient demonstrates full hyperextension and flexion ROM. Strengthening exercises include leg press, step-downs, knee extensions, and low-impact conditioning exercise such as a stationary bicycle, Stairmaster, or elliptical cross trainer. Consistent follow-up is maintained until the patient regains full motion and strength equal to the opposite side.

## 18.6 Summary

Anterior knee pain following reconstruction of the ACL is a problem that has plagued many patients. After extensively studying patients with this problem and comparing them to those that do not suffer from this entity, we have concluded that loss of full hyperextension is the most frequent cause of anterior knee pain after ACL reconstruction. This can be prevented with proper preoperative, intraoperative, and postoperative management. Prevention should be the number-one concern. If anterior knee pain after ACL reconstruction does occur, the symptoms can usually be alleviated through nonoperative means. Occasionally, surgical intervention may become necessary. Other causes for this pain syndrome are rare, but with proper evaluation can easily be differentiated and treated.

## References


1. Arnold T, Shelbourne KD. A perioperative rehabilitation program for anterior cruciate ligament surgery. *Phys Sports Med.* 2000;28:31-44.
2. Baszotta H, Prunner K. Refilling of removal defects: impact on extensor mechanism complaints after use of a bone-tendon-bone graft for anterior cruciate ligament reconstruction. *Arthroscopy.* 2000;16:160-164.
3. Fisher SE, Shelbourne KD. Arthroscopic treatment of symptomatic extension block complicating anterior cruciate ligament reconstruction. *Am J Sports Med.* 1993;21:558-564.
4. Kartus J, Magnusson L, Stener S, et al. Complications following arthroscopic anterior cruciate ligament reconstruction: a 2–5 year follow-up of 604 patients with special emphasis on anterior knee pain. *Knee Surg Sports Traumatol Arthrosc.* 1999;7:2-8.
5. Kleipool AE, van Loon T, Marti RK. Pain after use of the central third of the patellar tendon for cruciate ligament reconstruction: 33 patients followed 2–3 years. *Acta Orthop Scand.* 1994;65:62-66.
6. Laprade J, Culham E, Brouwer B. Comparison of five isometric exercises in the recruitment of the vastus medialis oblique in persons with and without patellofemoral pain syndrome. *J Orthop Sports Phys Ther.* 1998;27:197-204.
7. Rosenberg TD, Franklin JL, Baldwin GN, et al. Extensor mechanism function after patellar tendon graft harvest for anterior cruciate ligament reconstruction. *Am J Sports Med.* 1992;20:519-525.
8. Rubinstein RA Jr, Shelbourne KD. Graft selection, placement, fixation, and tensioning for anterior cruciate ligament reconstruction. *Oper Tech Sports Med.* 1993;1:10-15.
9. Sachs RA, Daniel DM, Stone ML, et al. Patellofemoral problems after anterior cruciate ligament reconstruction. *Am J Sports Med.* 1989;17:760-765.
10. Sanchis-Alfonso V, Rosello-Sastre E, Martinez-Sanjuan V. Pathogenesis of anterior knee pain syndrome and functional patellofemoral instability in the active young. *Am J Knee Surg.* 1999;12:29-40.
11. Sheehy P, Burdett RG, Irrgang JJ, et al. An electromyographic study of vastus medialis oblique and vastus lateralis activity while ascending and descending steps. *J Orthop Sports Phys Ther.* 1998;27:423-429.
12. Shelbourne KD, Gray T. Anterior cruciate ligament reconstruction with autogenous patellar tendon graft followed by accelerated rehabilitation: a two- to nine-year follow-up. *Am J Sports Med.* 1997;25:786-795.
13. Shelbourne KD, Jari S, Gray T. Outcome of untreated traumatic articular cartilage defects of the knee: a natural history study. *J Bone Joint Surg Am.* 2003;85-A(suppl):8-16.
14. Shelbourne KD, Johnson GE. Outpatient surgical management of arthrofibrosis after anterior cruciate ligament surgery. *Am J Sports Med.* 1994;22:192-197.
15. Shelbourne KD, Klootwyk TE, Wilckens JH, et al. Ligament stability two to six years after anterior cruciate ligament reconstruction with autogenous patellar tendon graft and participation in accelerated rehabilitation. *Am J Sports Med.* 1995;23:575-579.
16. Shelbourne KD, Liotta FJ. ACL reconstruction utilizing an abnormally thick autogenous patellar tendon graft. *Am J Knee Surg.* 1999;12:79-81.
17. Shelbourne KD, Nitz P. Accelerated rehabilitation after anterior cruciate ligament reconstruction. *Am J Sports Med.* 1990;18:292-299.
18. Shelbourne KD, Patel DV. Treatment of limited motion after anterior cruciate ligament reconstruction. *Knee Surg Sports Traumatol Arthrosc.* 1999;7:85-92.
19. Shelbourne KD, Patel KV, Martini DJ. Classification and management of arthrofibrosis of the knee after anterior cruciate ligament reconstruction. *Am J Sports Med.* 1996;24(6):857-862.
20. Shelbourne KD, Trumper RV. Preventing anterior knee pain after anterior cruciate ligament reconstruction. *Am J Sports Med.* 1997;25:41-47.
21. Shelbourne KD, Urch SE. Primary anterior cruciate ligament reconstruction using the contralateral autogenous patellar tendon. *Am J Sports Med.* 2000;28:651-658.
22. Siegel MG, Siqueland KA, Noyes FR. The use of computerized thermography in the evaluation of non-traumatic anterior knee pain. *Orthopedics.* 1987;10:825-830.
23. Witonski D. Anterior knee pain syndrome. *Int Orthop.* 1999;23:341-344.

# 19 Anterior Knee Pain with Special Emphasis on the Clinical, Radiographic, Histological, Ultrastructural, and Biochemical Aspects After Anterior Cruciate Ligament Reconstruction Using Autografts

Jüri Kartus, Lars Ejerhed, and Tomas Movin

## 19.1 Introduction

At the present time, arthroscopic ACL reconstruction is one of the most common surgical procedures in sports medicine. Every year, approximately 150,000 procedures are performed in the USA and 3,500 in Sweden (www.aclregister.nu). After the introduction of the arthroscopic technique and the opportunity to perform reproducible replacements of the ruptured ACL, the results in terms of restored laxity and a return to sports activities have generally been found to be good.[10,11,25] However, persistent donor-site morbidity such as tenderness, anterior knee pain, disturbance in anterior knee sensitivity and the inability to kneel and knee walk is still a problem and is present in approximately 40–60%, at least in patients who have undergone arthroscopic ACL reconstruction using patellar tendon autografts.[21,54,79,85,102,112,119,124] Despite efforts to utilize synthetic materials[35,40] and allografts,[65,109] the use of autografts probably remains the best option for the replacement of the torn ACL. Common autograft alternatives for reconstruction or augmentation of the ACL include the use of the iliotibial band,[12,39,88,105,106] hamstring tendons,[5,22,56,110,115,125] the patellar tendon[6,11,31,41,67,68,96], and the quadriceps tendon.[28,36,49,53,89,108]

The amount of information about the donor site after the use of patellar tendon autografts is fairly extensive. Recently, the amount of information about donor-site problems following the use of hamstring autografts has increased. The information describing the problems, which can occur after ACL reconstruction using quadriceps tendon autografts, has also increased recently.[36,53,90] However, there is very little information available after using fascia lata autografts.

The purpose of this chapter is to make an overview of the clinical, radiographical, histological, ultrastructural, and biochemical aspects of the donor site and its problems after ACL reconstruction using patellar tendon, hamstring tendon, quadriceps tendon and fascia lata autografts.

## 19.2 Postoperative Restriction in Range of Motion and Loss of Strength

There appears to be agreement in the literature that the restoration of full extension compared with the non-injured side after ACL reconstruction is essential in order to avoid postoperative discomfort in the anterior knee region. Irrgang and Harner,[64] Harner et al.,[58] Sachs et al.,[119] and Kartus et al.[76] have all stated that the loss of extension contributes to anterior knee pain. Shelbourne and Trumper[124] have stated that the restoration of full hyperextension is of major importance when it comes to avoiding anterior knee pain. Recently, Steadman et al.[130] reported that anterior scarring and flexion contracture after ACL reconstruction and other procedures caused anterior knee pain and could be successfully treated with arthroscopic release.

The influence of loss of flexion on anterior knee pain is controversial. Stapleton[129] and Kartus et al.[76]

J. Kartus (✉)
Orthopaedic Department, University of Gothenburg,
NU-Hospital Organization, Trollhättan/Uddevalla, Sweden
e-mail: juri.kartus@vgregion.se

V. Sanchis-Alfonso (ed.), *Anterior Knee Pain and Patellar Instability*,
DOI: 10.1007/978-0-85729-507-1_19, © Springer-Verlag London Limited 2011

have stated that the loss of flexion causes significantly more anterior knee pain than the loss of extension and Aglietti et al.[4] reported that a loss of flexion exceeding 10° might be correlated with anterior knee pain. However, Irrgang and Harner[64] found that a loss of flexion rarely matters, unless the knee flexion is less than 110°.

Although these reports are all concerned with the use of patellar tendon autografts or allografts,[64] we can generalize and state that the return of full range of motion (ROM) including full hyperextension is essential to reduce anterior knee problems after ACL reconstruction using any type of graft. However, the return of full range of motion might not always be possible. Kartus et al.[78] reported more pain and loss of motion both in flexion and extension after ACL reconstruction using both patellar tendon and hamstring tendon autografts if the patients underwent concomitant meniscal resection, than if the patients had intact menisci.

In line with this information, we recommend that it is essential to regain normal strength in the lower extremity to avoid future pain in the anterior knee region. Risberg et al.[116] have reported that pain and strength are the most important variables, which affect the results after ACL reconstruction using patellar tendon autografts. The corresponding can be said about regaining the proprioception and the neuromuscular control.[143]

Several reports on strength deficits after ACL reconstruction using autografts are found in the literature. Muneta et al.[104] reported that the patients' subjective evaluation of the results after ACL reconstruction using either hamstring or patellar tendon autografts was worse if the quadriceps or hamstring strength was decreased compared with the contralateral side. Hiemstra et al.[59] reported that at 1 year, the patients had substantial strength deficits in extension both after reconstruction using patellar tendon and hamstring tendon autografts. Feller et al.[47] reported a larger quadriceps peak torque strength deficit up to 1 year postoperative after harvesting the patellar tendon compared with harvesting the hamstring tendons. Adachi et al.[2] reported that the harvest of both semitendinosus and gracilis tendons causes more loss of active flexion angle and peak torque than the harvest of semitendinosus alone. Correspondingly, Tashiro et al.[136] recommended sparing the gracilis due to less loss of hamstring muscle strength at high knee flexion angles compared with harvesting both the semitendinosus and gracilis tendons.

After using quadriceps tendon autografts, Lee et al.[89] reported a loss of quadriceps strength of 13% compared with the contralateral side at 1 year after surgery. At 3 years, Lee et al.[90] reported approximately 10% decrease of the peak torque compared with the contralateral side.

After using ileotibial band augumentation for open primary ACL repair, Natri et al.[105] reported a peak torque loss of 14% in extension and 6% in flexion 2–5 years after surgery.

## 19.3 Dissection Studies in the Knee Region

Arthornthurasook and Gaew-Im,[9] Horner and Dellon,[60] Hunter et al.[63] and Kartus et al.[72] (Fig. 19.1) have shown in dissection studies that the infrapatellar nerve is in danger when incisions are made close to or above the tibial tubercle and the medial side of the knee joint. Kartus et al. dissected 60 knees and found that in 52/60 specimens the infrapatellar nerve passed between the tibial tubercle and the apex of the patella as one or two branches, which could be jeopardized during patellar tendon harvest.[72] In a dissection study, Tifford et al.[138] made similar findings and further recommended that incisions in the anterior knee region should be made

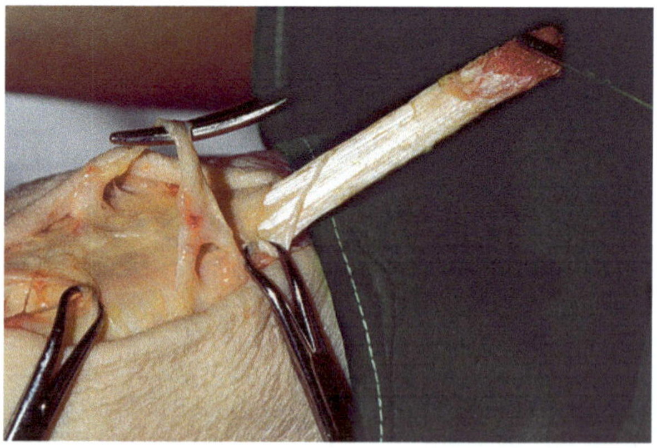

**Fig. 19.1** The infrapatellar nerve splits into two branches, right in the center of a central anterior 8 cm incision. The towel clamps indicate the paratenon. The patellar tendon autograft in this specimen was harvested using the two-incision technique with the aim of sparing the infrapatellar nerve(s) and the paratenon. In this specimen, the two incisions have subsequently been conjoined in order to examine the result of the harvesting procedure[71] (Copyright Elsevier)

with the knee in flexion in order to avoid injury to the infrapatellar nerve(s).

From anatomic descriptions of the prepatellar area, it appears that the infrapatellar nerve can be damaged when incisions are made in the anterior knee region.[1,82,141] Correspondingly, medial knee incisions even during hamstring harvest can jeopardize the saphenous nerve.[22,121] In a dissection study of 40 cadaver knees, Boon et al.[18] have recommended using oblique incisions medial to the tibial tubercle when harvesting hamstring tendons to avoid sensory nerve damage. Sanders et al.[121] dissecting 11 specimens found that the saphenous nerve was "intimately involved" with the gracilis tendon approximately 10 cm proximal to its insertion.

## 19.4 Knee Surgery and Sensory Nerve Complications

Johnson et al.,[66] Swanson[134] and Tapper and Hoover[135] have described postoperative morbidity, such as numbness and problems with kneeling, after injury to the infrapatellar branch(es) of the saphenous nerve after open medial meniscectomies. Chambers[27] explored three patients because of pain and numbness after open medial meniscectomies and found scarring or neuroma of one infrapatellar branch of the saphenous nerve. Ganzoni and Wieland[50] have shown a difference in postoperative sensory loss, depending on whether or not the infrapatellar nerve(s) were protected during medial knee arthrotomies.

Mochida and Kikuchi[101] have described the possibility of injury to the infrapatellar nerve(s) during arthroscopic surgery, and Poehling et al.[113] have described the development of reflex sympathetic dystrophy after sensory nerve injury in the knee region. The importance of the sensory nerves in the knee region was further stressed in the reports by Gordon[52] and Detenbeck[37] on prepatellar neuralgia after direct impacts to the anterior knee region, the report by House and Ahmed[62] on the entrapment of the infrapatellar nerve and the report by Worth et al.[144] on the entrapment of the saphenous nerve in the knee region. Slocum et al.[127] have discussed the possibility of damage to the nerves in the anterior knee region during a pes anserinus transplantation, which requires an incision similar to the one used for harvesting hamstring tendon autografts.

There are a few reports in the literature with regard to discomfort after injury to the infrapatellar nerve or its branches in conjunction with ACL surgery. Berg and Mjöberg[15] have reported that the difficulty in kneeling was correlated with the loss of sensitivity in the anterior knee region after open knee ligament surgery and they, therefore, recommend a lateral parapatellar skin incision. In two studies involving 90[80] and 604[76] patients, respectively, Kartus et al. have reported that the inability to kneel and knee-walk (Fig. 19.2) after arthroscopic ACL reconstruction using patellar tendon autografts harvested through a 7–8 cm vertical incision was correlated with the area of disturbed or lost anterior knee sensitivity (Fig. 19.3). Mastrokalos et al.[97] reported lost or disturbed sensitivity in 85.4% of patients after harvesting ipsilateral patellar tendon autografts.

Mishra et al.[100] have reported that the use of two horizontal incisions while harvesting the central third of the patellar tendon may offer an opportunity to protect the infrapatellar nerve(s). No results in terms of

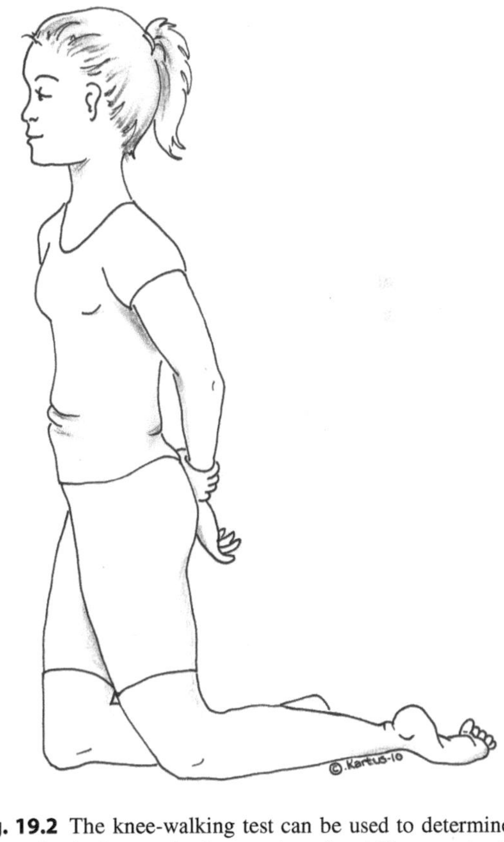


**Fig. 19.2** The knee-walking test can be used to determine the discomfort in the anterior knee region after ACL reconstruction[73] (Copyright Catarina Kartus)

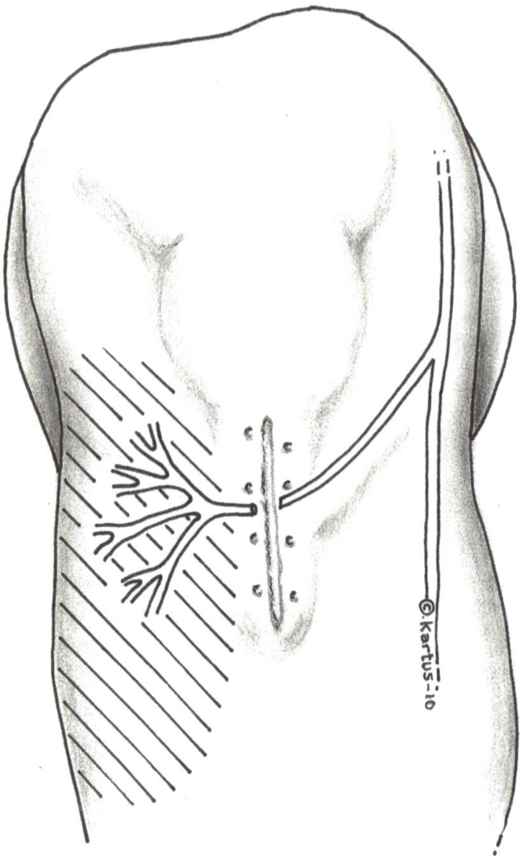


**Fig. 19.3** After the use of a central one-incision technique to harvest a patellar tendon autograft, the discomfort during the knee-walking test correlated with the area of disturbed sensitivity in the anterior knee region[73,76] (Copyright Catarina Kartus)

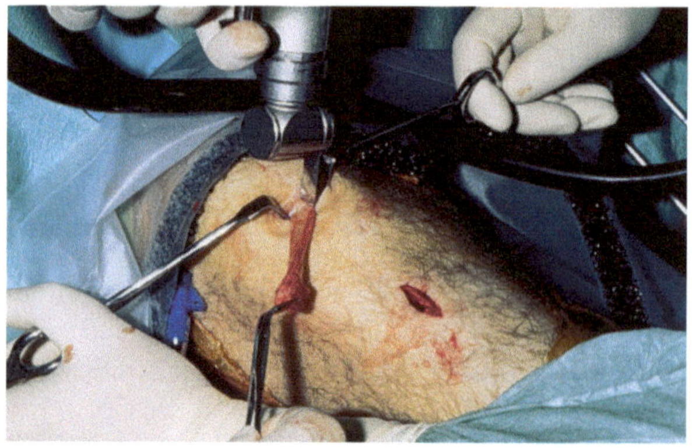

**Fig. 19.4** The use of the two-incision technique to harvest a patellar tendon autograft resulted in less discomfort during the knee-walking test than the use of the central one-incision technique (Copyright Elsevier Publication)

nerve function have, however, been presented. Kartus et al.,[70] on the other hand, presented a method using two 25-mm vertical incisions to reduce the risk of injury to the infrapatellar nerve(s) when harvesting patellar tendon autografts (Fig. 19.4). This technique was first tested in cadavers[72] and was subsequently proven in two clinical studies[73,75] to produce less loss of sensitivity and a tendency towards less knee-walking discomfort than the use of a vertical 7–8 cm incision. In a clinical study without a control group, Tsuda et al.[139] suggested patellar tendon harvest to be performed using two horizontal incisions in order to minimize postoperative anterior knee symptoms.

When hamstring tendon autografts are harvested, a branch of the infrapatellar branch of the saphenous nerve might also be jeopardized[22] and occasionally, numbness in the skin area supplied by the saphenous nerve may also occur.[48,121] Bertram et al.,[17] in a case report, described saphenous neuralgia after arthroscopically assisted ACL reconstruction using semitendinosus and gracilis tendons. Eriksson[42] as well as Ejerhed et al.[38] have shown that the area of disturbed sensitivity after harvesting either semitendinosus or patellar tendon autografts is comparable. However, both studies suggested that the area of disturbed sensitivity after harvesting semitendinosus autografts is of less clinical importance.

It appears that the same amount of disturbance in sensitivity in the knee region after harvesting hamstring tendon autografts causes fewer kneeling and knee-walking difficulties than after harvesting patellar tendon autografts. This can be due to the fact that, after patellar tendon harvest, the pressure when kneeling is applied directly on or close to the incision where the injured nerve is located as suggested by Ejerhed et al.[38] Spicer et al.[128] have reported that sensory changes in the whole anterior knee region after hamstring tendon harvest are possible and 50% of their patients reported such changes. However, this rarely limited the activity of their patients. Sanders et al.[121] reported that 74% of their patients had sensory disturbance after hamstring tendon harvest during ACL reconstruction, which is higher than previously reported.

After harvesting fascia lata and quadriceps tendon autografts, the risk of nerve injuries appears to be low and no such reports are found in the literature to our knowledge.

## 19.5 Local Discomfort in the Donor Site Region

In a prospective, randomized study, Brandsson et al.[20] have shown that suturing the patellar tendon defect and bone grafting the defect in the patella did not reduce anterior knee problems or donor-site morbidity. Boszotta and Prünner[19] also found that bone grafting the patellar defect did not reduce kneeling complaints or patellofemoral problems. It, therefore, appears that suturing and bone grafting the defects after patellar tendon harvest is of minor importance when it comes to reducing donor-site problems. Tsuda et al.,[139] on the other hand, suggested bone grafting of the defects in order to decrease donor-site problems. However, in their study, the grafts were harvested subcutaneously and no control group was available.

Kartus et al.[73] reported that 65% of the patients had difficulty or were unable to perform the knee-walking test 2 years after patellar tendon harvest using a central vertical 7–8 cm incision. The corresponding value after the use of a two-incision technique with the aim of sparing the infrapatellar nerve(s) was 47%.[73] Rubinstein et al.,[118] found that the isolated donor site morbidity was negligible after ACL surgery, when the contralateral patellar tendon was used as a graft. In contrast, Mastrokalos et al.[97] found that more than 70% of the donor knees had knee-walking problems regardless whether the patellar tendon graft was harvested from the ipsi- or contralateral side.

Preoperatively, as well as 2 years after the use of hamstring autografts, approximately 20–30% of the patients reported that they had difficulty or were unable to perform the knee-walking test as shown by Ejerhed et al.[38] in their prospective randomized trial. Corry et al.[32] reported that only 6% of patients had kneeling pain 2 years after the use of hamstring tendon autografts, compared with 31% after the use of patellar tendon autografts. However, no preoperative data were presented. Yasuda et al.[145] reported that activity-related soreness had resolved by 3 months after harvesting the contralateral hamstring tendon graft. Eriksson et al.[42-44] have, in prospective randomized studies, shown that patients operated on using semitendinosus autografts have less anterior knee problems and donor site morbidity than patients operated on using patellar tendon autografts, both in the short- and midterm. In a randomized study, Feller and Webster[47] reported that 67% of patients operated on using patellar tendon autografts and only 26% of patients operated on using hamstring tendon grafts had kneeling pain at 3 years after surgery. These findings suggest that the use of hamstring autografts causes only minor morbidity in the anterior knee region compared with the use of patellar tendon autografts. However, Liden et al.[92] in a randomized study involving 68 patients reported that in the long term, after approximately 7 years, the difference in donor site morbidity was no longer statistically significant between patellar tendon autografts and hamstring tendon autografts. It appears that in the long term, the subsequent development of degenerative changes means more than the choice of graft for anterior knee pain.

In terms of the quadriceps tendon autograft, Chen et al.[28] reported that one in 12 patients had mild harvest site tenderness after an average of 18 months, and in another study, they reported the corresponding in 3/34 patients at 4–7 years.[29] Correspondingly, Fulkerson and Langeland[49] reported no early donor site morbidity in their series of 28 patients. Lee et al. reported 12% moderate or severe anterior knee pain in their study involving 67 patients, using quadriceps tendon autograft. In another study, Lee et al.[90] reported that only 1/247 patients had moderate harvest site tenderness at approximately 3 years after the index procedure. Noronha[108] and Theut et al.[137] in their studies as well as Santori et al.[122] in a review article regarded the quadriceps tendon as a low morbidity graft.

De Angelis and Fulkerson[36] have stated that the quadriceps tendon autograft "maybe the least morbid of the currently used ACL autograft reconstruction alternatives." Gorschewsky et al.[53] and Han et al.[57] have both reported that the use of quadriceps tendon autograft for ACL reconstruction renders significantly less donor site problem than the use of patellar tendon autograft in controlled studies.

Bak et al.[12] reported that 8% of their patients complained of swelling and pain laterally on the thigh after harvesting a fascia lata autograft. Twenty per cent of their patients also expressed slight cosmetic dissatisfaction with a lateral thigh herniation. Sensory loss and nerve injuries were, however, not discussed. Natri et al.[105] reported that 84% of their patients had no or only slight anterior knee pain after harvesting iliotibial grafts.

## 19.6 Radiographic Assessments

Reports by Coupens et al.,[33] Berg[14] Nixon et al.,[107] Liu et al.,[94] Meisterling et al.,[99] Kartus et al.[80,81,132] and Svensson et al.,[132] using MRI assessments of the patellar tendon at the donor site, have all shown that the thickness of the patellar tendon increases, at least up to 6 years postoperatively, irrespective of whether or not the defect is sutured. Wiley et al.,[142] Kartus et al.[77] and Hou et al.[61] have made corresponding findings using ultrasonography 1–2 years after the harvesting procedure.

Reports in the literature on the healing of the donor site gap in the patellar tendon after harvesting its central third and leaving the defect open are contradictory. Using MRI assessments, Berg[14] and Nixon et al.[107] claimed that the defect had healed, 8 months and 2 years, respectively after the index operation. Adriani et al.[3] have used ultrasonography to show that the healing of the patellar tendon defect with tendinous-like scar tissue can be expected approximately 1 year after harvesting its central third, and Cerullo et al.[26] used CT to show that scarring of the open defect takes place within 6 months postoperatively. Rosenberg et al.[117] have demonstrated persistent defects using CT and MRI, approximately 2 years after the index operation. Kartus et al. have found persistent defects in several studies using MRI,[74,75,77,80,81] and in one study using ultrasonography[77] after leaving the defect open (Figs. 19.5 and 19.6). However, even if the defect was still present 2 years after the harvesting procedure, it showed a significant decrease over time in the prospective studies by Kartus et al.[74] and Bernicker et al.[16] using MRI and by Wiley et al.[142] using ultrasonography. Liu et al.[94] using MRI have shown that there can be a persistent donor site gap even 13 years after the harvesting procedure. After 6 years, the defect had healed in the majority of patients; however, a thinning of the central part of the tendon was still present as shown by Svensson et al.[132] in a prospective long-term study of 17 patients (Fig. 19.7). Correspondingly, Liden et al.[91] found radiographic abnormalities and a persistent defect using MRI 10 years after reharvesting the patellar tendon autograft. Koseoglu et al.[86] described that the defect after primary harvest had not healed up to 12 months after the harvesting procedure but appeared to heal in the long term. Kartus et al.[75,80] have shown that the kneeling and knee-walking problems did not correlate with any MRI findings in the patellar tendon at the donor site. The corresponding finding in terms of patellar tendon pain was made by Kiss et al.[84] using ultrasonography.

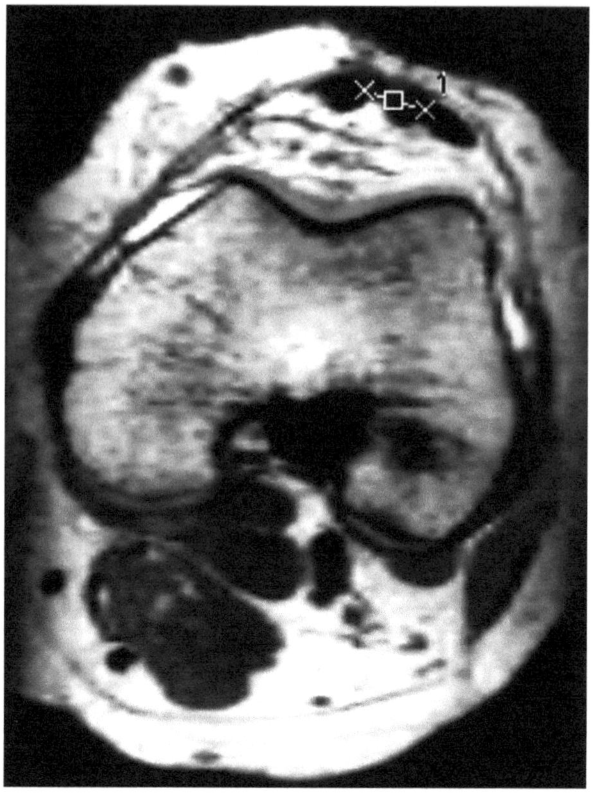

**Fig. 19.5** A persistent donor site gap is displayed on this MRI examination in the axial dimension obtained 26 months after harvesting a central third patellar tendon autograft (Copyright Jüri Kartus)

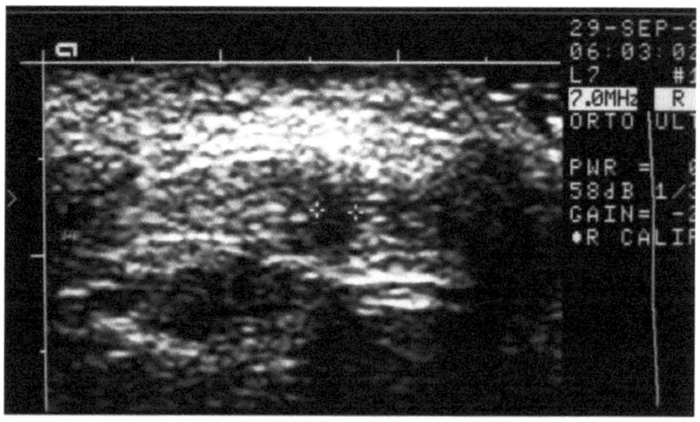

**Fig. 19.6** A persistent donor site gap is displayed on this ultrasonography examination obtained 25 months after harvesting a central third patellar tendon autograft (Copyright Jüri Kartus)

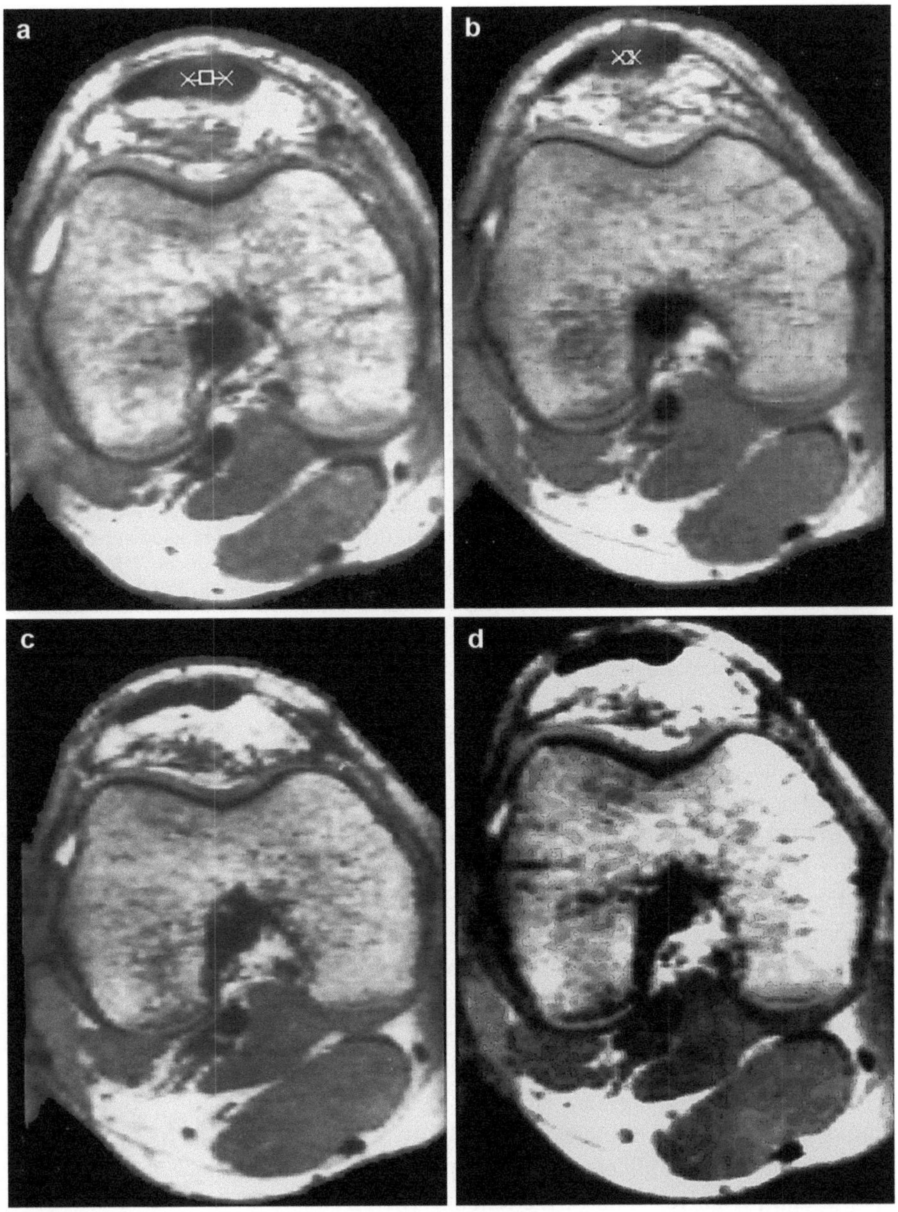


**Fig. 19.7** The serial MRI examinations demonstrate that the donor site gap was 7 mm at 6 weeks (**a**), 2 mm at 6 months (**b**) and completely healed at 27 months and 6 years (**c**) and (**d**). Furthermore, the thickness of the patellar tendon decreased over time. This is a male patient who, at the time of the index operation, was 18 years old (Copyright Jüri Kartus)

After harvesting hamstring tendon autografts, it appears that there is at least some regrowth in the semitendinosus and gracilis tendons. This has been reported in the literature by Cross et al.,[34] Simonian et al.,[126] and Eriksson et al.[42,45,46] using MRI. In their prospective ultrasonography study, Papandrea et al.[111] reported that the regrowth of the tendons appeared to be completed 2 years after the harvesting procedure. However, the insertion of the tendons was approximately 3–4 cm more proximal compared with the normal anatomic position.

Lee et al.[90] using MRI reported that the thickness of the quadriceps tendon at the donor site was significantly increased compared with the preoperative findings until 24 months postoperatively.

No radiographic data on the donor site after harvesting fascia lata autografts are available to our knowledge.

## 19.7 Histological Examinations

Reports on donor site histology in humans are few in number.[13,14,77,107] Histological descriptions of the donor site area after ACL reconstruction using central patellar tendon autografts in a goat model have been given by Proctor et al.[114] They found ill-defined fascicles, woven collagen fibrils, poorly aligned with the longitudinal axis of the patellar ligament, in the central part of the tendon 21 months after the harvesting procedure. Correspondingly, in a study of lambs, Sanchis-Alfonso et al.[120] found that the regenerated tissue in the harvest site defect did not have the histological appearance of normal patellar tendon. In a dog model, Burks et al.[24] found the entire patellar tendon involved in scar formation 3 and 6 months after harvesting its central third. In contrast, Nixon et al.[107] obtained biopsies from two patients 2 years after the harvesting procedure and found tissue that was indistinguishable from normal tendon using polarized light microscopy. In a human case report, Berg et al.[14] showed that the defect was filled with hypertrophic "tendon-like" tissue 8 months after the harvesting procedure. Battlehner et al.[13] obtained open biopsies from eight humans, a minimum of 24 months after ACL reconstruction using patellar tendon autografts and found using light microscopy that the patellar tendon did not regain the appearance of normal tendon. However, in their study, the donor site gap was closed during the ACL reconstruction. In a biopsy study of 19 patients, 27 months after harvesting the central third of the patellar tendon and leaving the defect open, Kartus et al.[77] revealed tendon-like repair tissue in the donor site. However, histological abnormalities in terms of increased cellularity, vascularity, and non-parallel fibers were present in both the central and peripheral parts of the tendon. The same patients underwent biopsies once again at 6 years after the harvesting procedure and still the same pathology was found.[131] No correlation between the histological findings and the donor site discomfort was found (Figs. 19.8 and 19.9) (Kartus et al., unpublished data).

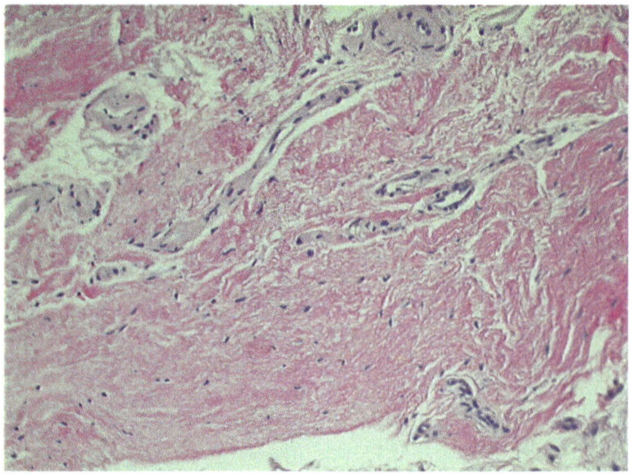

**Fig. 19.8** A high-power view of a biopsy obtained from the central part of the patellar tendon 6 years after the harvesting procedure showing increased cellularity, vascularity and non-parallel fibers.[77](Hematoxylin and eosin staining; original magnification, X200) (Copyright Springer-Verlag)

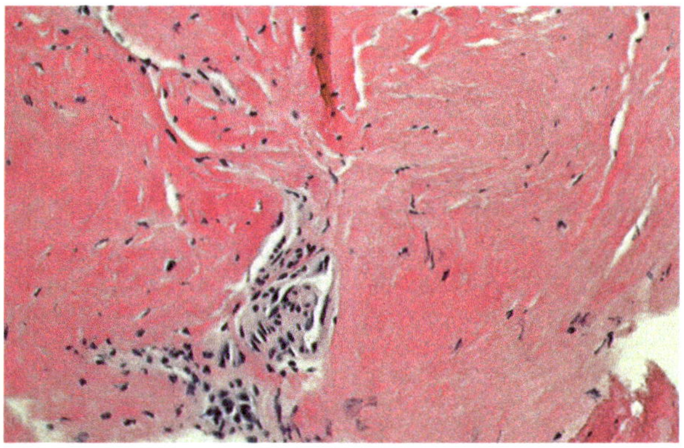

**Fig. 19.9** A high-power view of a biopsy obtained from the peripheral part of the patellar tendon 6 years after the harvesting procedure showing increased cellularity, vascularity and non-parallel fibers.[77](Hematoxylin and eosin staining; original magnification, X200) (Copyright Springer-Verlag)

The finding of histological abnormalities in the human patellar tendon up to 6 years after the primary harvest strongly suggests that reharvesting the central third of the patellar tendon cannot be recommended. This opinion is supported by the findings of LaPrade et al.,[87] who in a dog model reported inferior mechanical properties in the reharvested central third patellar tendon up to 12 months after the primary procedure, and by Scherer et al.,[123] who in a sheep model reported the corresponding finding in the remaining two-thirds of the patellar tendon. Moreover, in a clinical study by Kartus et al.,[81] patients who had undergone revision ACL reconstruction using reharvested patellar tendon autograft displayed significantly worse results, especially in terms of anterior knee problems, than patients in whom the contralateral patellar tendon autograft was used. The patients in the above study by Kartus et al.,[81] who underwent revision ACL surgery using reharvested patellar tendon autograft, were re-examined by Liden et al., both clinically[91] and histologically[93] 10 years after the reharvesting procedure. Still at 10 years, the clinical results were bad and an abnormal histology with an increased cellularity and vascularity as well as deteriorated fiber structure were found both in the central and the peripheral part of the tendon.

Eriksson[42,45] obtained open biopsies from the regenerated tendon in five humans at mean 20 months after the harvest of a semitendinosus autograft. Surprisingly, the biopsies revealed tissue resembling normal tendon. Interestingly, in a rabbit model, Gill et al.[51] found normal cellularity and collagen I, 9–12 months after harvesting the semitendinosus tendon.

No histological data from the donor site after harvesting, fascia lata, or quadriceps tendon autografts are available to our knowledge.

## 19.8 Ultrastructural Examinations

Proctor et al.[114] in a goat model reported abnormal tissue composition when biopsies were evaluated ultrastructurally in the transmission electron microscope (TEM), 21 months after the harvesting procedure. Correspondingly, Battlehner et al.[13] reported that the patellar tendon in humans does not restore *ad integrum* a minimum of 2 years after harvesting its central third. In a dog model using the electron microscope, LaPrade et al.[87] reported that the reharvested central third of the patellar tendon displayed an increased fibril size and fibril packing at 6 months compared with control tendons. However, at 12 months, no significant differences were registered.

Svensson et al.[133] reported that the patellar tendon did not regain a normal ultrastructure as seen on biopsies examined in TEM 6 years after the harvesting procedure. The fibrils were less regularly orientated and significantly more small fibrils compared with normal control tendons were found (Figs. 19.10 and 19.11). The corresponding were found by Liden et al.[93] 10 years after reharvesting the central third of the patellar tendon. Taken together, there is evidence in the literature to suggest that the patellar tendon does not regain normal ultrastructure after harvesting or reharvesting its central third in both animals and humans, at least not up to 10 years.

In a rabbit model using the electron microscope, Gill et al.[51] found "regeneration of organized collagen tissue that simulated native tendon, but with a smaller cross-sectional diameter" 9–12 months after harvesting the semitendinosus tendon.

No ultrastructural data from the donor site after harvesting quadriceps tendon and fascia lata autografts are available to our knowledge.

## 19.9 Biochemical Investigations

Sulfated glycosaminoglycans (GAGs) possess a very high water-retaining capacity and they appear in low concentrations in the normal patellar tendon.[7,8] Increasing concentrations of GAGs are seen in areas of tendons, which are subjected to compression forces, as described by Vogel et al.,[140] in pathological scar tissue in the Achilles tendon, as described by Movin et al.,[103] and in the patellar tendon in "jumper's knee" (tendinosis) disease, as described by Khan et al.[83] and Green et al.[55] Furthermore, Kannus and Jozsa[69] have reported that increasing amounts of GAGs were found in ruptured tendons compared with healthy control tendons. Kartus et al.[77] showed that there were undetectable amounts of GAGs in the biopsies obtained from the patellar tendon at 27 months after the harvesting procedure. The corresponding finding at 6 years was reported by Svensson et al.[132] This suggests that factors other than retained water contributed to the increase in the cross-sectional area of the patellar tendon. Therefore, in terms of the GAG content, the repair tissue did not display similarities with the tendon pathology that has been found in achillodynia and jumper's knee.[83,103] Correspondingly, Liden et al.[93] reported that at 10 years after reharvesting the central third of the patellar tendon, no increase in the amount of GAGs was found compared with normal control tendon.

The presence of collagen type III is associated with early collagen synthesis in a repair process in tendons, as described by Liu et al.[95] and Matsumuto et al.[98] in rat models. Collagen type III has the capacity rapidly to form cross-linked intermolecular disulphide bridges.[23,30] This capacity is supposed to be a great advantage in the development of repair tissue.[23] Collagen type III fibers are also known to be thin, with inferior mechanical properties, compared with collagen type I. Kartus et al.[77]

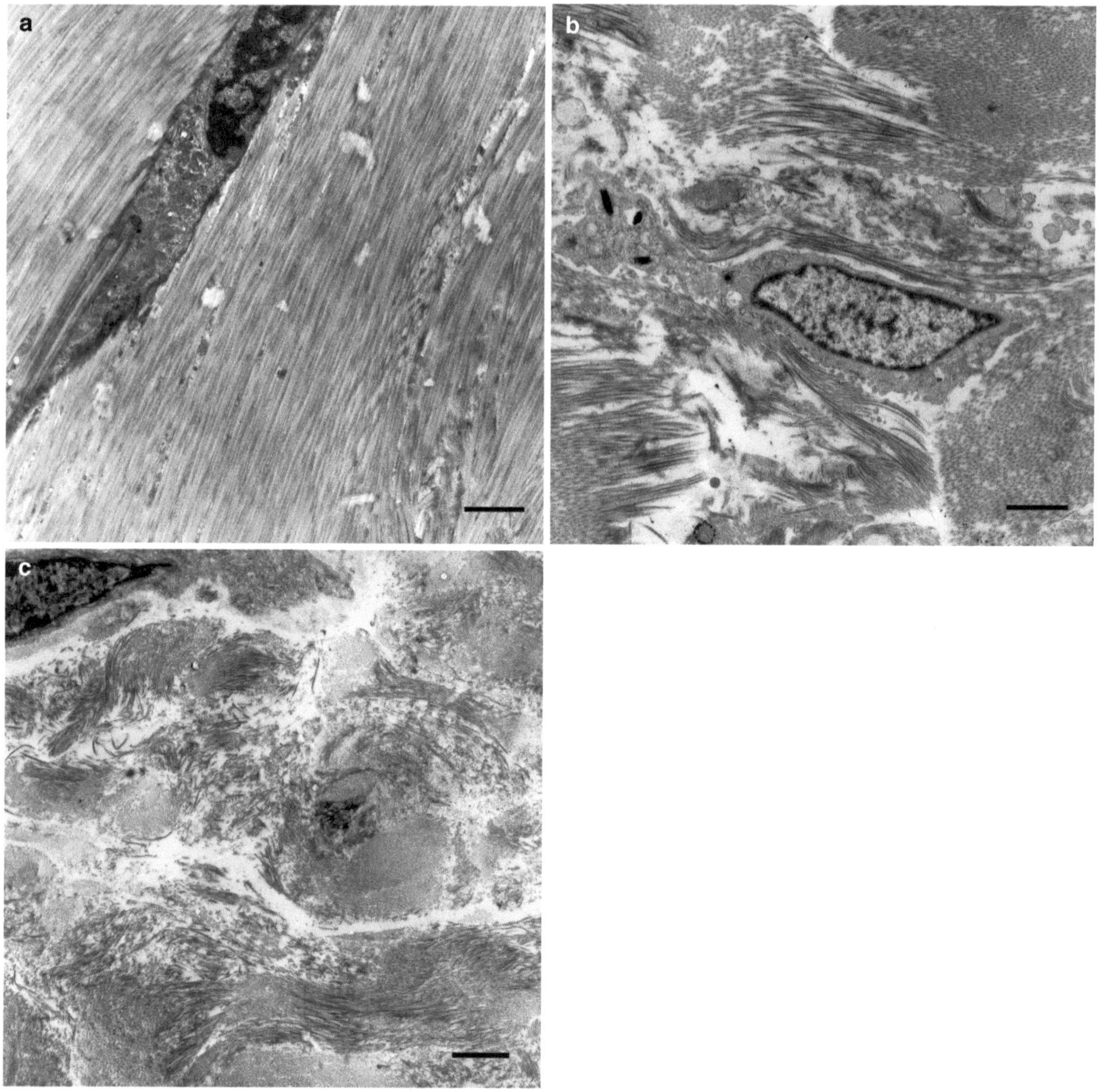


**Fig. 19.10** Transmission electron micrographs from control tendons (**a**), lateral parts (**b**), and central parts (**c**) of the tendons in the study group 6 years after the harvesting procedure. The fibrils were less regularly orientated in both the central and lateral part of the harvested tendon compared with normal tendon. (Bar = 2 μm, original magnification, ×3, 000) (Copyright Jüri Kartus)

failed to demonstrate increased amounts of collagen type III in the central and peripheral parts of the patellar tendon, which indicates that no early collagen synthesis was present 27 months after the harvesting procedure.

Eriksson has shown that the immunoreactivity for collagen types I and III in regenerated semitendinosus tendon was similar to that of normal tendon at mean 20 months after the harvesting procedure.[42,45]

## 19.10 Conclusions

- There is quite a lot of information available in the literature about the course of the donor site after using patellar tendon or hamstring tendon autografts.
- There is a gradual increase in knowledge about the course of the donor site after harvesting quadriceps tendon autografts.

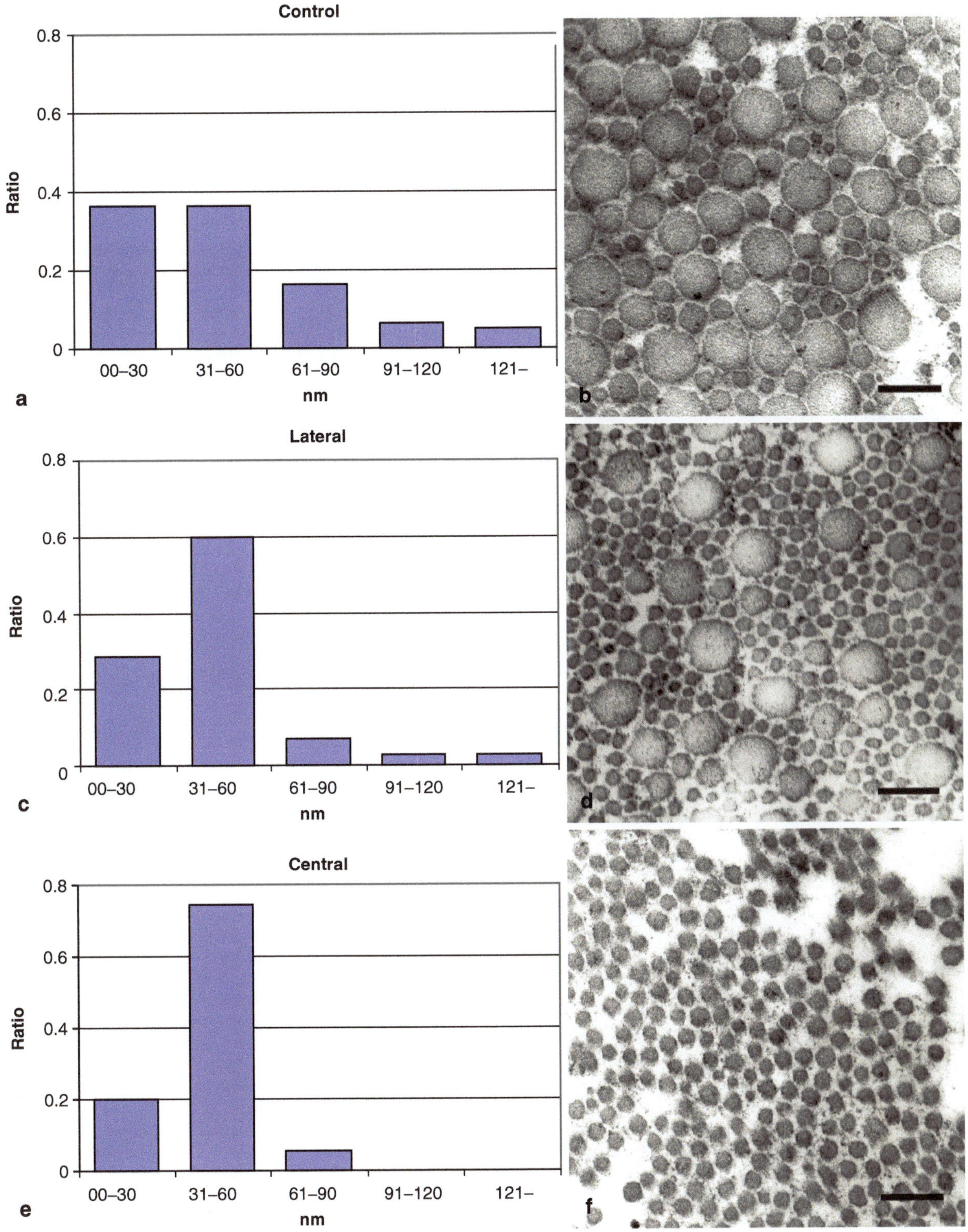


**Fig. 19.11** Relative distribution and transmission electron micrographs of the fibril diameter size in human patellar tendon from controls (**a**, **b**), lateral (**c**, **d**) and central parts (**e**, **f**) 6 years after the harvesting procedure (Bar = 200 nm, original magnification, ×101,000). These figures show that there was a significant difference in fibril size distribution between the groups[133] (Copyright Jüri Kartus)

- The quadriceps tendon autografts appears to have low harvest site morbidity.
- Reduced strength and loss of ROM are correlated with anterior knee pain after ACL reconstruction using all kinds of autografts. Efforts should be made during the surgical procedure and the rehabilitation process to regain full ROM and full strength after ACL reconstructions regardless of the type of graft used.
- Loss or disturbance of anterior knee sensitivity caused by intraoperative injury to the infrapatellar nerve(s) in conjunction with patellar tendon harvest are correlated with donor site discomfort and inability to knee-walk. A similar nerve injury after harvesting hamstring tendon grafts does not appear to cause as much knee-walking problems.
- No correlations can be found between donor site discomfort and radiographical or histological findings after the use of patellar tendon autografts.
- If the surgeon wishes to use patellar tendon autografts, efforts to spare the infrapatellar nerve(s) should be made during surgery.
- Due to radiographical, histological, and ultrastructural abnormalities in the patellar tendon after primary harvest, reharvesting cannot be recommended, at least not up to 6 years after the primary harvest.
- Since prospective randomized studies have shown that the use of hamstring tendon autografts for ACL reconstruction produce laxity restoration comparable to patellar tendon autografts, we recommend the use of hamstring tendon autografts due to fewer donor site problems.

**Acknowledgment** The authors thank Catarina Kartus for the illustrations.

## References


1. Abbott LC, Carpenter WF. Surgical approaches to the knee joint. *J Bone Joint Surg*. 1945;27-A:277-310.
2. Adachi N, Ochi M, Uchio Y, et al. Harvesting hamstring tendons for ACL reconstruction influences postoperative hamstring muscle performance. *Arch Orthop Trauma Surg*. 2003;123:460-465.
3. Adriani E, Mariani PP, Maresca G, et al. Healing of the patellar tendon after harvesting of its mid-third for anterior cruciate ligament reconstruction and evolution of the unclosed donor site defect. *Knee Surg Sports Traumatol Arthrosc*. 1995;3:138-143.
4. Aglietti P, Buzzi R, D'Andria S, et al. Patellofemoral problems after intraarticular anterior cruciate ligament reconstruction. *Clin Orthop Relat Res*. 1993;288:195-204.
5. Aglietti P, Buzzi R, Menchetti PM, et al. Arthroscopically assisted semitendinosus and gracilis tendon graft in reconstruction for acute anterior cruciate ligament injuries in athletes. *Am J Sports Med*. 1996;24:726-731.
6. Alm A, Gillquist J. Reconstruction of the anterior cruciate ligament by using the medial third of the patellar ligament. Treatment and results. *Acta Chir Scand*. 1974;140: 289-296.
7. Amiel D, Frank C, Harwood F, et al. Tendons and ligaments: a morphological and biochemical comparison. *J Orthop Res*. 1984;1:257-265.
8. Amiel D, Kleiner JB, Akeson WH. The natural history of the anterior cruciate ligament autograft of patellar tendon origin. *Am J Sports Med*. 1986;14:449-462.
9. Arthornthurasook A, Gaew-Im K. Study of the infrapatellar nerve. *Am J Sports Med*. 1988;16:57-59.
10. Bach BR Jr, Jones GT, Hager CA, et al. Arthrometric results of arthroscopically assisted anterior cruciate ligament reconstruction using autograft patellar tendon substitution. *Am J Sports Med*. 1995;23:179-185.
11. Bach BR Jr, Jones GT, Sweet FA, et al. Arthroscopy-assisted anterior cruciate ligament reconstruction using patellar tendon substitution. Two- to four-year follow-up results. *Am J Sports Med*. 1994;22:758-767.
12. Bak K, Jorgensen U, Ekstrand J, et al. Results of reconstruction of acute ruptures of the anterior cruciate ligament with an iliotibial band autograft. *Knee Surg Sports Traumatol Arthrosc*. 1999;7:111-117.
13. Battlehner CN, Carneiro Filho M, Ferreira Junior JM, et al. Histochemical and ultrastructural study of the extracellular matrix fibers in patellar tendon donor site scars and normal controls. *J Submicrosc Cytol Pathol*. 1996;28: 175-186.
14. Berg EE. Intrinsic healing of a patellar tendon donor site defect after anterior cruciate ligament reconstruction. *Clin Orthop Relat Res*. 1992;278:160-163.
15. Berg P, Mjöberg B. A lateral skin incision reduces peripatellar dysaesthesia after knee surgery. *J Bone Joint Surg*. 1991;73-B:374-376.
16. Bernicker JP, Haddad JL, Lintner DM, et al. Patellar tendon defect during the first year after anterior cruciate ligament reconstruction: appearance on serial magnetic resonance imaging. *Arthroscopy*. 1998;14:804-809.
17. Bertram C, Porsch M, Hackenbroch MH, et al. Saphenous neuralgia after arthroscopically assisted anterior cruciate ligament reconstruction with a semitendinosus and gracilis tendon graft. *Arthroscopy*. 2000;16:763-766.
18. Boon JM, Van Wyk MJ, Jordaan D. A safe area and angle for harvesting autogenous tendons for anterior cruciate ligament reconstruction. *Surg Radiol Anat*. 2004;26:167-171.
19. Boszotta H, Prunner K. Refilling of removal defects: impact on extensor mechanism complaints after use of a bone-tendon-bone graft for anterior cruciate ligament reconstruction. *Arthroscopy*. 2000;16:160-164.
20. Brandsson S, Faxen E, Eriksson BI, et al. Closing patellar tendon defects after anterior cruciate ligament reconstruction: absence of any benefit. *Knee Surg Sports Traumatol Arthrosc*. 1998;6:82-87.

21. Breitfuss H, Fröhlich R, Povacz P, et al. The tendon defect after anterior cruciate ligament reconstruction using the midthird patellar tendon – a problem for the patellofemoral joint? *Knee Surg Sports Traumatol Arthrosc*. 1996;3: 194-198.
22. Brown CH Jr, Steiner ME, Carson EW. The use of hamstring tendons for anterior cruciate ligament reconstruction. Technique and results. *Clin Sports Med*. 1993;12: 723-756.
23. Burgeson RE, Nimni ME. Collagen types. Molecular structure and tissue distribution. *Clin Orthop Relat Res*. 1992; 282:250-272.
24. Burks RT, Haut RC, Lancaster RL. Biomechanical and histological observations of the dog patellar tendon after removal of its central one-third. *Am J Sports Med*. 1990;18:146-153.
25. Buss DD, Warren RF, Wickiewicz TL, et al. Arthroscopically assisted reconstruction of the anterior cruciate ligament with use of autogenous patellar-ligament grafts. Results after twenty-four to forty-two months. *J Bone Joint Surg*. 1993; 75-A:1346-1355.
26. Cerullo G, Puddu G, Gianni E, et al. Anterior cruciate ligament patellar tendon reconstruction: it is probably better to leave the tendon defect open! *Knee Surg Sports Traumatol Arthrosc*. 1995;3:14-17.
27. Chambers GH. The prepatellar nerve. A cause of suboptimal results in knee arthrotomy. *Clin Orthop Relat Res*. 1972;82:157-159.
28. Chen CH, Chen WJ, Shih CH. Arthroscopic anterior cruciate ligament reconstruction with quadriceps tendon-patellar bone autograft. *J Trauma*. 1999;46:678-682.
29. Chen CH, Chuang TY, Wang KC, et al. Arthroscopic anterior cruciate ligament reconstruction with quadriceps tendon autograft: clinical outcome in 4-7 years. *Knee Surg Sports Traumatol Arthrosc*. 2006;14:1077-1085.
30. Cheung DT, DiCesare P, Benya PD, et al. The presence of intermolecular disulfide cross-links in type III collagen. *J Biol Chem*. 1983;258:7774-7778.
31. Clancy WG Jr, Nelson DA, Reider B, et al. Anterior cruciate ligament reconstruction using one-third of the patellar ligament, augmented by extra-articular tendon transfers. *J Bone Joint Surg*. 1982;64-A:352-359.
32. Corry IS, Webb JM, Clingeleffer AJ, et al. Arthroscopic reconstruction of the anterior cruciate ligament. A comparison of patellar tendon autograft and four-strand hamstring tendon autograft. *Am J Sports Med*. 1999;27: 444-454.
33. Coupens SD, Yates CK, Sheldon C, et al. Magnetic resonance imaging evaluation of the patellar tendon after use of its central one-third for anterior cruciate ligament reconstruction. *Am J Sports Med*. 1992;20:332-335.
34. Cross MJ, Roger G, Kujawa P, et al. Regeneration of the semitendinosus and gracilis tendons following their transection for repair of the anterior cruciate ligament. *Am J Sports Med*. 1992;20:221-223.
35. Dandy DJ, Flanagan JP, Steenmeyer V. Arthroscopy and the management of the ruptured anterior cruciate ligament. *Clin Orthop Relat Res*. 1982;167:43-49.
36. DeAngelis JP, Fulkerson JP. Quadriceps tendon – a reliable alternative for reconstruction of the anterior cruciate ligament. *Clin Sports Med*. 2007;26:587-596.
37. Detenbeck LC. Infrapatellar traumatic neuroma resulting from dashboard injury. *J Bone Joint Surg*. 1972;54-A: 170-172.
38. Ejerhed L, Kartus J, Sernert N, et al. Patellar tendon or semitendinosus tendon autografts for anterior cruciate ligament reconstruction?: a prospective randomized study with a two-year follow-up. *Am J Sports Med*. 2003;31: 19-25.
39. Ekstrand J. Reconstruction of the anterior cruciate ligament in athletes, using a fascia lata graft: a review with preliminary results of a new concept. *Int J Sports Med*. 1989;10: 225-232.
40. Engström B, Wredmark T, Westblad P. Patellar tendon or Leeds-Keio graft in the surgical treatment of anterior cruciate ligament ruptures. Intermediate results. *Clin Orthop Relat Res*. 1993;295:190-197.
41. Eriksson E. Reconstruction of the anterior cruciate ligament. *Orthop Clin North Am*. 1976;7:167-179.
42. Eriksson K. *On the Semitendinosus in Anterior Cruciate Ligament Reconstructive Surgery* [thesis]. Stockholm, Sweden: Karolinska Institutet; 2001.
43. Eriksson K, Anderberg P, Hamberg P, et al. A comparison of quadruple semitendinosus and patellar tendon grafts in reconstruction of the anterior cruciate ligament. *J Bone Joint Surg*. 2001;83-B:348-354.
44. Eriksson K, Anderberg P, Hamberg P, et al. There are differences in early morbidity after ACL reconstruction when comparing patellar tendon and semitendinosus tendon graft. A prospective randomized study of 107 patients. *Scand J Med Sci Sports*. 2001;11:170-177.
45. Eriksson K, Kindblom LG, Hamberg P, et al. The semitendinosus tendon regenerates after resection: a morphologic and MRI analysis in 6 patients after resection for anterior cruciate ligament reconstruction. *Acta Orthop Scand*. 2001;72: 379-384.
46. Eriksson K, Larsson H, Wredmark T, et al. Semitendinosus tendon regeneration after harvesting for ACL reconstruction. A prospective MRI study. *Knee Surg Sports Traumatol Arthrosc*. 1999;7:220-225.
47. Feller JA, Webster KE. A randomized comparison of patellar tendon and hamstring tendon anterior cruciate ligament reconstruction. *Am J Sports Med*. 2003;31:564-573.
48. Figueroa D, Calvo R, Vaisman A, et al. Injury to the infrapatellar branch of the saphenous nerve in ACL reconstruction with the hamstrings technique: clinical and elec-trophysiological study. *Knee*. 2008;15:360-363.
49. Fulkerson JP, Langeland R. An alternative cruciate reconstruction graft: the central quadriceps tendon. *Arthroscopy*. 1995;11:252-254.
50. Ganzoni N, Wieland K. The ramus infrapatellaris of the saphenous nerve and its importance for medial parapatellar arthrotomies of the knee. *Reconstr Surg Traumatol*. 1978; 16:95-100.
51. Gill SS, Turner MA, Battaglia TC, et al. Semitendinosus regrowth: biochemical, ultrastructural, and physiological characterization of the regenerate tendon. *Am J Sports Med*. 2004;32:1173-1181.
52. Gordon GC. Traumatic prepatellar neuralgia. *J Bone Joint Surg*. 1952;34-B:41-44.
53. Gorschewsky O, Klakow A, Putz A, et al. Clinical comparison of the autologous quadriceps tendon (BQT) and the autologous

patella tendon (BPTB) for the reconstruction of the anterior cruciate ligament. *Knee Surg Sports Traumatol Arthrosc*. 2007;15:1284-1292.
54. Graf B, Uhr F. Complications of intra-articular anterior cruciate reconstruction. *Clin Sports Med*. 1988;7:835-848.
55. Green JS, Morgan B, Lauder I, et al. Correlation of magnetic resonance imaging and histology in patellar tendinitis. *Sports Exerc Inj*. 1997;3:80-84.
56. Hamner DL, Brown CH Jr, Steiner ME, et al. Hamstring tendon grafts for reconstruction of the anterior cruciate ligament: biomechanical evaluation of the use of multiple strands and tensioning techniques. *J Bone Joint Surg*. 1999;81-A:549-557.
57. Han HS, Seong SC, Lee S, et al. Anterior cruciate ligament reconstruction: quadriceps versus patellar autograft. *Clin Orthop Relat Res*. 2008;466:198-204.
58. Harner CD, Irrgang JJ, Paul J, et al. Loss of motion after anterior cruciate ligament reconstruction. *Am J Sports Med*. 1992;20:499-506.
59. Hiemstra LA, Webber S, MacDonald PB, et al. Knee strength deficits after hamstring tendon and patellar tendon anterior cruciate ligament reconstruction. *Med Sci Sports Exerc*. 2000;32:1472-1479.
60. Horner G, Dellon AL. Innervation of the human knee joint and implications for surgery. *Clin Orthop Relat Res*. 1994; 301:221-226.
61. Hou CH, Wang CL, Lin CC. Ultrasound examination of patellar tendon after harvest for anterior cruciate ligament reconstruction. *J Formos Med Assoc*. 2001;100:315-318.
62. House JH, Ahmed K. Entrapment neuropathy of the infrapatellar branch of the saphenous nerve. *Am J Sports Med*. 1977;5:217-224.
63. Hunter LY, Louis DS, Ricciardi JR, et al. The saphenous nerve: its course and importance in medial arthrotomy. *Am J Sports Med*. 1979;7:227-230.
64. Irrgang JJ, Harner CD. Loss of motion following knee ligament reconstruction. *Sports Med*. 1995;19:150-159.
65. Jackson DW, Grood ES, Goldstein JD, et al. A comparison of patellar tendon autograft and allograft used for anterior cruciate ligament reconstruction in the goat model. *Am J Sports Med*. 1993;21:176-185.
66. Johnson RJ, Kettelkamp DB, Clark W, et al. Factors effecting late results after meniscectomy. *J Bone Joint Surg*. 1974;56-A:719-729.
67. Jones KG. Reconstruction of the anterior cruciate ligament. *J Bone Joint Surg*. 1963;45-A:925-932.
68. Jones KG. Reconstruction of the anterior cruciate ligament using the central one- third of the patellar ligament. *J Bone Joint Surg*. 1970;52:838-839.
69. Kannus P, Jozsa L. Histopathological changes preceding spontaneous rupture of a tendon. A controlled study of 891 patients. *J Bone Joint Surg*. 1991;73-A:1507-1525.
70. Karlsson J, Kartus J, Brandsson S, et al. Comparison of arthroscopic one-incision and two-incision techniques for reconstruction of the anterior cruciate ligament. *Scand J Med Sci Sports*. 1999;9:233-238.
71. Kartus J. *Donor Site Morbidity After Anterior Cruciate Ligament Reconstruction. Clinical, Anatomical, Radiographic and Histological Investigations with Special Reference to the Use of Central-Third Patellar Tendon Autografts* [thesis], Göteborg, Sweden: Göteborg University; 1999.
72. Kartus J, Ejerhed L, Eriksson BI, et al. The localization of the infrapatellar nerves in the anterior knee region with special emphasis on central third patellar tendon harvest: a dissection study on cadaver and amputated specimens. *Arthroscopy*. 1999;15:577-586.
73. Kartus J, Ejerhed L, Sernert N, et al. Comparison of traditional and subcutaneous patellar tendon harvest. A prospective study of donor site-related problems after anterior cruciate ligament reconstruction using different graft harvesting techniques. *Am J Sports Med*. 2000;28:328-335.
74. Kartus J, Lindahl S, Kohler K, et al. Serial magnetic resonance imaging of the donor site after harvesting the central third of the patellar tendon. A prospective study of 37 patients after arthroscopic anterior cruciate ligament reconstruction. *Knee Surg Sports Traumatol Arthrosc*. 1999;7: 20-24.
75. Kartus J, Lindahl S, Stener S, et al. Magnetic resonance imaging of the patellar tendon after harvesting its central third: a comparison between traditional and subcutaneous harvesting techniques. *Arthroscopy*. 1999;15:587-593.
76. Kartus J, Magnusson L, Stener S, et al. Complications following arthroscopic anterior cruciate ligament reconstruction. A 2-5-year follow-up of 604 patients with special emphasis on anterior knee pain. *Knee Surg Sports Traumatol Arthrosc*. 1999;7:2-8.
77. Kartus J, Movin T, Papadogiannakis N, et al. A radiographic and histologic evaluation of the patellar tendon after harvesting its central third. *Am J Sports Med*. 2000;28:218-226.
78. Kartus JT, Russell VJ, Salmon LJ, et al. Concomitant partial meniscectomy worsens outcome after arthroscopic anterior cruciate ligament reconstruction. *Acta Orthop Scand*. 2002;73:179-185.
79. Kartus J, Stener S, Köhler K, et al. Is bracing after anterior cruciate ligament reconstruction necessary? A 2-year follow-up of 78 consecutive patients rehabilitated with or without a brace. *Knee Surg Sports Traumatol Arthrosc*. 1997;5:157-161.
80. Kartus J, Stener S, Lindahl S, et al. Factors affecting donor-site morbidity after anterior cruciate ligament reconstruction using bone-patellar tendon-bone autografts. *Knee Surg Sports Traumatol Arthrosc*. 1997;5:222-228.
81. Kartus J, Stener S, Lindahl S, et al. Ipsi- or contralateral patellar tendon graft in anterior cruciate ligament revision surgery. A comparison of two methods. *Am J Sports Med*. 1998;26:499-504.
82. Kennedy JC, Alexander IJ, Hayes KC. Nerve supply of the human knee and its functional importance. *Am J Sports Med*. 1982;10:329-335.
83. Khan KM, Bonar F, Desmond PM, et al. Patellar tendinosis (jumper's knee): findings at histopathologic examination, US, and MR imaging. Victorian Institute of Sport Tendon Study Group. *Radiology*. 1996;200:821-827.
84. Kiss ZS, Kellaway DP, Cook JL, et al. Postoperative patellar tendon healing: an ultrasound study. VIS Tendon Study Group. *Australas Radiol*. 1998;42:28-32.
85. Kohn D, Sander-Beuermann A. Donor-site morbidity after harvest of a bone-tendon-bone patellar tendon autograft. *Knee Surg Sports Traumatol Arthrosc*. 1994;2:219-223.
86. Koseoglu K, Memis A, Argin M, et al. MRI evaluation of patellar tendon defect after harvesting its central third. *Eur J Radiol*. 2004;50:292-295.

87. LaPrade RF, Hamilton CD, Montgomery RD, et al. The reharvested central third of the patellar tendon. A histologic and biomechanical analysis. *Am J Sports Med.* 1997;25: 779-785.
88. Laupattarakasem W, Mahaisavariya B. Iliotibial band for anterior cruciate ligament reconstruction: a new technique for graft augmentation, placement and fixation. *J Med Assoc Thai.* 1994;77:343-350.
89. Lee S, Seong SC, Jo H, et al. Outcome of anterior cruciate ligament reconstruction using quadriceps tendon autograft. *Arthroscopy.* 2004;20:795-802.
90. Lee S, Seong SC, Jo CH, et al. Anterior cruciate ligament reconstruction with use of autologous quadriceps tendon graft. *J Bone Joint Surg.* 2007;89(suppl 3-A):116-126.
91. Liden M, Ejerhed L, Sernert N, et al. The course of the patellar tendon after reharvesting its central third for ACL revision surgery: a long-term clinical and radiographic study. *Knee Surg Sports Traumatol Arthrosc.* 2006;14: 1130-1138.
92. Liden M, Ejerhed L, Sernert N, et al. Patellar tendon or semitendinosus tendon autografts for anterior cruciate ligament reconstruction: a prospective, randomized study with a 7-year follow-up. *Am J Sports Med.* 2007;35:740-748.
93. Liden M, Movin T, Ejerhed L, et al. A histological and ultrastructural evaluation of the patellar tendon 10 years after reharvesting its central third. *Am J Sports Med.* 2008;36:781-788.
94. Liu SH, Hang DW, Gentili A, et al. MRI and morphology of the insertion of the patellar tendon after graft harvesting. *J Bone Joint Surg.* 1996;78-B:823-826.
95. Liu SH, Yang RS, al-Shaikh R, et al. Collagen in tendon, ligament, and bone healing. A current review. *Clin Orthop Relat Res.* 1995;318:265-278.
96. Marshall JL, Warren RF, Wickiewicz TL, et al. The anterior cruciate ligament: a technique of repair and reconstruction. *Clin Orthop Relat Res.* 1979;143:97-106.
97. Mastrokalos DS, Springer J, Siebold R, et al. Donor site morbidity and return to the preinjury activity level after anterior cruciate ligament reconstruction using ipsilateral and contralateral patellar tendon autograft: a retrospective, nonrandomized study. *Am J Sports Med.* 2005;33:85-93.
98. Matsumoto N, Horibe S, Nakamura N, et al. Effect of alignment of the transplanted graft extracellular matrix on cellular repopulation and newly synthesized collagen. *Arch Orthop Trauma Surg.* 1998;117:215-221.
99. Meisterling RC, Wadsworth T, Ardill R, et al. Morphologic changes in the human patellar tendon after bone-tendon-bone anterior cruciate ligament reconstruction. *Clin Orthop Relat Res.* 1993;289:208-212.
100. Mishra AK, Fanton GS, Dillingham MF, et al. Patellar tendon graft harvesting using horizontal incisions for anterior cruciate ligament reconstruction. *Arthroscopy.* 1995;11: 749-752.
101. Mochida H, Kikuchi S. Injury to infrapatellar branch of saphenous nerve in arthroscopic knee surgery. *Clin Orthop Relat Res.* 1995;320:88-94.
102. Mohtadi NG, Webster-Bogaert S, Fowler PJ. Limitation of motion following anterior cruciate ligament reconstruction. A case-control study. *Am J Sports Med.* 1991; 19:620-625.
103. Movin T, Gad A, Reinholt FP, et al. Tendon pathology in long-standing achillodynia. Biopsy findings in 40 patients. *Acta Orthop Scand.* 1997;68:170-175.
104. Muneta T, Sekiya I, Ogiuchi T, et al. Objective factors affecting overall subjective evaluation of recovery after anterior cruciate ligament reconstruction. *Scand J Med Sci Sports.* 1998;8:283-289.
105. Natri A, Jarvinen M, Kannus P. Primary repair plus intra-articular iliotibial band augmentation in the treatment of an acute anterior cruciate ligament rupture. A follow-up study of 70 patients. *Arch Orthop Trauma Surg.* 1996;115: 22-27.
106. Nicholas JA, Minkoff J. Iliotibial band transfer through the intercondylar notch for combined anterior instability (ITPT procedure). *Am J Sports Med.* 1978;6:341-353.
107. Nixon RG, SeGall GK, Sax SL, et al. Reconstitution of the patellar tendon donor site after graft harvest. *Clin Orthop Relat Res.* 1995;317:162-171.
108. Noronha JC. Reconstruction of the anterior cruciate ligament with quadriceps tendon. *Arthroscopy.* 2002;18:E37.
109. Noyes FR, Barber-Westin SD. Reconstruction of the anterior cruciate ligament with human allograft. Comparison of early and later results. *J Bone Joint Surg.* 1996;78-A: 524-537.
110. Otero AL, Hutcheson L. A comparison of the doubled semitendinosus/gracilis and central third of the patellar tendon autografts in arthroscopic anterior cruciate ligament reconstruction. *Arthroscopy.* 1993;9:143-148.
111. Papandrea P, Vulpiani MC, Ferretti A, et al. Regeneration of the semitendinosus tendon harvested for anterior cruciate ligament reconstruction. Evaluation using ultrasonography. *Am J Sports Med.* 2000;28:556-561.
112. Paulos LE, Rosenberg TD, Drawbert J, et al. Infrapatellar contracture syndrome. An unrecognized cause of knee stiffness with patella entrapment and patella infera. *Am J Sports Med.* 1987;15:331-341.
113. Poehling GG, Pollock FE Jr, Koman LA. Reflex sympathetic dystrophy of the knee after sensory nerve injury. *Arthroscopy.* 1988;4:31-35.
114. Proctor CS, Jackson DW, Simon TM. Characterization of the repair tissue after removal of the central one- third of the patellar ligament. An experimental study in a goat model. *J Bone Joint Surg.* 1997;79-A:997-1006.
115. Puddu G. Method for reconstruction of the anterior cruciate ligament using the semitendinosus tendon. *Am J Sports Med.* 1980;8:402-404.
116. Risberg MA, Holm I, Steen H, et al. Sensitivity to changes over time for the IKDC form, the Lysholm score, and the Cincinnati knee score. A prospective study of 120 ACL reconstructed patients with a 2-year follow-up. *Knee Surg Sports Traumatol Arthrosc.* 1999;7:152-159.
117. Rosenberg TD, Franklin JL, Baldwin GN, et al. Extensor mechanism function after patellar tendon graft harvest for anterior cruciate ligament reconstruction. *Am J Sports Med.* 1992;20:519-525.
118. Rubinstein RA Jr, Shelbourne KD, VanMeter CD, et al. Isolated autogenous bone-patellar tendon-bone graft site morbidity. *Am J Sports Med.* 1994;22:324-327.
119. Sachs RA, Daniel DM, Stone ML, et al. Patellofemoral problems after anterior cruciate ligament reconstruction. *Am J Sports Med.* 1989;17:760-765.

120. Sanchis-Alfonso V, Subias-Lopez A, Monteagudo-Castro C, et al. Healing of the patellar tendon donor defect created after central-third patellar tendon autograft harvest. A long-term histological evaluation in the lamb model. *Knee Surg Sports Traumatol Arthrosc*. 1999;7: 340-348.
121. Sanders B, Rolf R, McClelland W, et al. Prevalence of saphenous nerve injury after autogenous hamstring harvest: an anatomic and clinical study of sartorial branch injury. *Arthroscopy*. 2007;23:956-963.
122. Santori N, Adriani E, Pederzini L. ACL reconstruction using quadriceps tendon. *Orthopedics*. 2004;27:31-35.
123. Scherer MA, Fruh HJ, Ascherl R, et al. Biomechanical studies of change in the patellar tendon after transplant removal. *Aktuelle Traumatol*. 1993;23:129-132.
124. Shelbourne KD, Trumper RV. Preventing anterior knee pain after anterior cruciate ligament reconstruction. *Am J Sports Med*. 1997;25:41-47.
125. Siegel MG, Barber-Westin SD. Arthroscopic-assisted outpatient anterior cruciate ligament reconstruction using the semitendinosus and gracilis tendons. *Arthroscopy*. 1998; 14:268-277.
126. Simonian PT, Harrison SD, Cooley VJ, Larson RV, et al. Assessment of morbidity of semitendinosus and gracilis tendon harvest for ACL reconstruction. *Am J Knee Surg*. 1997;10:54-59.
127. Slocum DB, Larson RL. Pes anserinus transplantation. A surgical procedure for control of rotatory instability of the knee. *J Bone Joint Surg*. 1968;50-A:226-242.
128. Spicer DD, Blagg SE, Unwin AJ, et al. Anterior knee symptoms after four-strand hamstring tendon anterior cruciate ligament reconstruction. *Knee Surg Sports Traumatol Arthrosc*. 2000;8:286-289.
129. Stapleton TR. Complications in anterior cruciate ligament reconstructions with patellar tendon grafts. *Sports Med Arthrosc*. 1997;5:156-162.
130. Steadman JR, Dragoo JL, Hines SL, et al. Arthroscopic release for symptomatic scarring of the anterior interval of the knee. *Am J Sports Med*. 2008;36:1763-1769.
131. Svensson M, Kartus J, Christensen LR, et al. A long-term serial histological evaluation of the patellar tendon in humans after harvesting its central third. *Knee Surg Sports Traumatol Arthrosc*. 2005;13:398-404.
132. Svensson M, Kartus J, Ejerhed L, et al. Does the patellar tendon normalize after harvesting its central third?: a prospective long-term MRI study. *Am J Sports Med*. 2004; 32:34-38.
133. Svensson M, Movin T, Rostgard-Christensen L, et al. Ultrastructural collagen fibril alterations in the patellar tendon 6 years after harvesting its central third. *Am J Sports Med*. 2007;35:301-306.
134. Swanson AJ. The incidence of prepatellar neuropathy following medial meniscectomy. *Clin Orthop Relat Res*. 1983;181:151-153.
135. Tapper EM, Hoover NW. Late results after meniscectomy. *J Bone Joint Surg*. 1969;51-A:517-526.
136. Tashiro T, Kurosawa H, Kawakami A, et al. Influence of medial hamstring tendon harvest on knee flexor strength after anterior cruciate ligament reconstruction. A detailed evaluation with comparison of single- and double-tendon harvest. *Am J Sports Med*. 2003;31:522-529.
137. Theut PC, Fulkerson JP, Armour EF, et al. Anterior cruciate ligament reconstruction utilizing central quadriceps free tendon. *Orthop Clin North Am*. 2003;34:31-39.
138. Tifford CD, Spero L, Luke T, et al. The relationship of the infrapatellar branches of the saphenous nerve to arthroscopy portals and incisions for anterior cruciate ligament surgery. An anatomic study. *Am J Sports Med*. 2000;28: 562-567.
139. Tsuda E, Okamura Y, Ishibashi Y, et al. Techniques for reducing anterior knee symptoms after anterior cruciate ligament reconstruction using a bone-patellar tendon-bone autograft. *Am J Sports Med*. 2001;29:450-456.
140. Vogel KG, Ordog A, Pogany G, et al. Proteoglycans in the compressed region of human tibialis posterior tendon and in ligaments. *J Orthop Res*. 1993;11:68-77.
141. von Lantz T, Wachmuth W. *Praktische Anatomie*. Berlin: Springer; 1972.
142. Wiley JP, Bray RC, Wiseman DA, et al. Serial ultrasonographic imaging evaluation of the patellar tendon after harvesting its central one third for anterior cruciate ligament reconstruction. *J Ultrasound Med*. 1997;16: 251-255.
143. Wilk KE, Reinold MM, Hooks TR. Recent advances in the rehabilitation of isolated and combined anterior cruciate ligament injuries. *Orthop Clin North Am*. 2003;34: 107-137.
144. Worth RM, Kettelkamp DB, Defalque RJ, et al. Saphenous nerve entrapment. A cause of medial knee pain. *Am J Sports Med*. 1984;12:80-81.
145. Yasuda K, Tsujino J, Ohkoshi Y, et al. Graft site morbidity with autogenous semitendinosus and gracilis tendons. *Am J Sports Med*. 1995;23:706-714.

# Part II

# Emerging Technologies for Investigating Patellofemoral Joint. Clinical Relevance

# Imaging and Musculoskeletal Modeling to Investigate the Mechanical Etiology of Patellofemoral Pain

20

Thor F. Besier, Christine Draper, Saikat Pal, Michael Fredericson, Garry Gold, Scott Delp, and Gary Beaupré

## 20.1 Introduction

### 20.1.1 *Importance of Understanding the Underlying Mechanism of Pain*

Despite the wealth of scientific literature regarding the knee extensor mechanism and patellofemoral (PF) pain, the etiology of PF pain is still poorly understood. Accurate clinical assessment and subject-specific treatment plans for patients with PF pain remain a challenge due to the complexity of the extensor mechanism, large variation among subjects, and the multifactorial nature of the syndrome. However, only once the mechanism of pain is properly understood will we be able to develop effective intervention programs to reduce the incidence and severity of this common knee disorder. To this end, the goal of our research is to understand the etiology of PF pain using a novel combination of medical imaging and musculoskeletal modeling.

The subjective nature of pain presents a problem for researchers wishing to understand the mechanism of PF pain. Most of us appreciate that pain can be related to some physical cause and this explains the majority of PF pain research to date, which attempts to associate symptoms with some mechanical variable(s). However, despite the wealth of literature investigating the mechanical etiology of PF pain, mechanical variables remain poor predictors of symptoms. This is most likely due to our inability to accurately measure or estimate the mechanical variable(s) of interest, as well as our difficulty to quantify and standardize levels of pain.

Regardless of psychological state, it is fair to assume that the *initial onset* of PF pain has some pathophysiological origin. That is, some noxious stimulus (mechanical or chemical) produces a response from a nociceptor that elicits the sensation of pain. This point perhaps necessitates the differentiation between patients with acute symptoms and those with chronic pain, who might experience pain via different pathways (pathophysiological vs psychological). There are many tissues comprising and surrounding the PF joint that have a rich nerve supply and thus have the potential to be a source of pain. These include subchondral bone, infrapatellar fat pad, quadriceps tendon, patellar ligament, synovium, the medial and lateral retinaculum, and the medial and lateral patellar ligaments. These structures, individually, or in combination, may cause pain.[10,22,23,26,55,66,68]

One common hypothesis for the mechanical etiology of pain is that localized stresses transmitted through cartilage excite nociceptors in the subchondral bone.[24] Mineralized bone has a rich sensory and sympathetic innervation[45] and the presence of substance-P fibers (pain receptors) in the subchondral plate of human patellae[68] support this bone stress–pain relationship. However, support for this relationship in patients with PF pain has proven difficult, as neither stress nor pain can be easily quantified. Several factors can contribute to increased subchondral bone stress, as illustrated in Fig. 20.1.

The central focus of our research to date has been to determine if patients with PF pain exhibit increased cartilage stress compared to pain-free controls. We have selected stress as the mechanical variable of interest as stress is a normalized quantity of force (force/area)

T.F. Besier (✉)
Auckland Bioengineering Institute,
The University of Auckland, Auckland, New Zealand
e-mail: t.besier@auckland.ac.nz

V. Sanchis-Alfonso (ed.), *Anterior Knee Pain and Patellar Instability*,
DOI: 10.1007/978-0-85729-507-1_20, © Springer-Verlag London Limited 2011

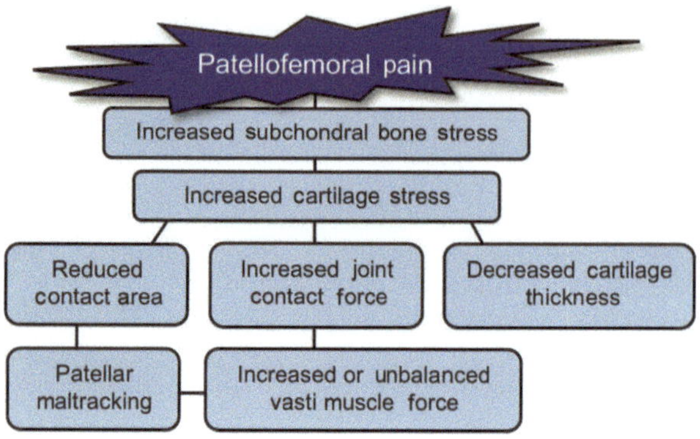


**Fig. 20.1** Factors that may contribute to increased cartilage and subchondral bone stress and patellofemoral pain

that can be compared across individuals, taking into account joint size and articulating geometry. Mechanical stress is also related to the physical stimuli imposed at the cellular level, which is responsible for maintenance and adaptation of skeletal tissues.[14] The following chapter provides an overview of our imaging and musculoskeletal modeling work to investigate factors influencing cartilage and bone stress and how these factors might contribute to PF pain.

## 20.2 Imaging the Patellofemoral Joint

### 20.2.1 *Upright Weight-Bearing Imaging of the Patellofemoral Joint*

Patellofemoral pain is typically exacerbated by activities that involve large knee extension loads such as stair climbing, squatting, and running. However, examination of the PF joint with computed tomography (CT) and magnetic resonance imaging (MRI) is commonly performed with the patient in a supine orientation with little or no load applied to the joint. To image the joint under physiologic, loaded conditions we developed MR imaging sequences for an open-bore MRI scanner (0.5T GE Signa SP), which enables volumetric scans of the knee to be taken with the patient in an upright, weight-bearing posture.[27] A custom backrest enables patients to remain still for the 2:30 min duration of the scan and the patient can squat to 60° of knee flexion with their knee at the center of the magnet (Fig. 20.2a). The volumetric images from these scans can be used to measure contact area of the PF joint (Fig. 20.2b) and determine the three-dimensional orientation of the patella with respect to the femur (Fig. 20.2c).

#### 20.2.1.1 Contact Area Measurements

Using this novel weight-bearing imaging modality, we asked several scientific questions. Firstly, what are the ranges of PF contact areas in a healthy, pain-free population of males and females? Secondly, is there a sex difference in contact area when normalizing for patella size? And third, what is the effect of upright, weight-bearing load on contact area?

To answer our first question, we measured contact areas of the PF joint at 0°, 30°, and 60° of knee flexion in eight male and eight female pain-free subjects.[6] Males displayed mean PF joint contact areas of 210, 414, and 520 mm² at 0, 30, and 60° of knee flexion, respectively in the low load condition. These values were 20–30% larger than those previously reported in the literature from non-weight bearing MR images or pressure-sensitive film in cadavers. Unloaded contact areas of female subjects were similar to males at full extension (0°), but smaller at 30° and 60°, with mean values of 269 and 396 mm², respectively. This was not surprising given that females are generally smaller than males. We therefore normalized the contact area measurements by the dimensions of the patella (height × width). After normalizing for patella area, there were no longer any sex differences in contact area between genders. Although females are more likely to develop PF pain, these data suggest that patella size is not a predisposing risk factor.

To determine the influence of load on PF joint contact area, we imaged the joint under full weight-bearing load and compared these values to a low load condition with the subject upright and resting on the seat of the backrest (~0.15 body weight through both knees). Contact areas under weight-bearing conditions increased an average of 24% compared to the low load condition (Fig. 20.3), illustrating the importance of imaging the joint in an upright weight-bearing orientation. Differences between the low load and weight-bearing load can be due to both cartilage deformation as well as altered orientation of the patella within the trochlear groove. The large standard deviations in these measures indicate that some subjects had much greater changes in contact area compared to others.

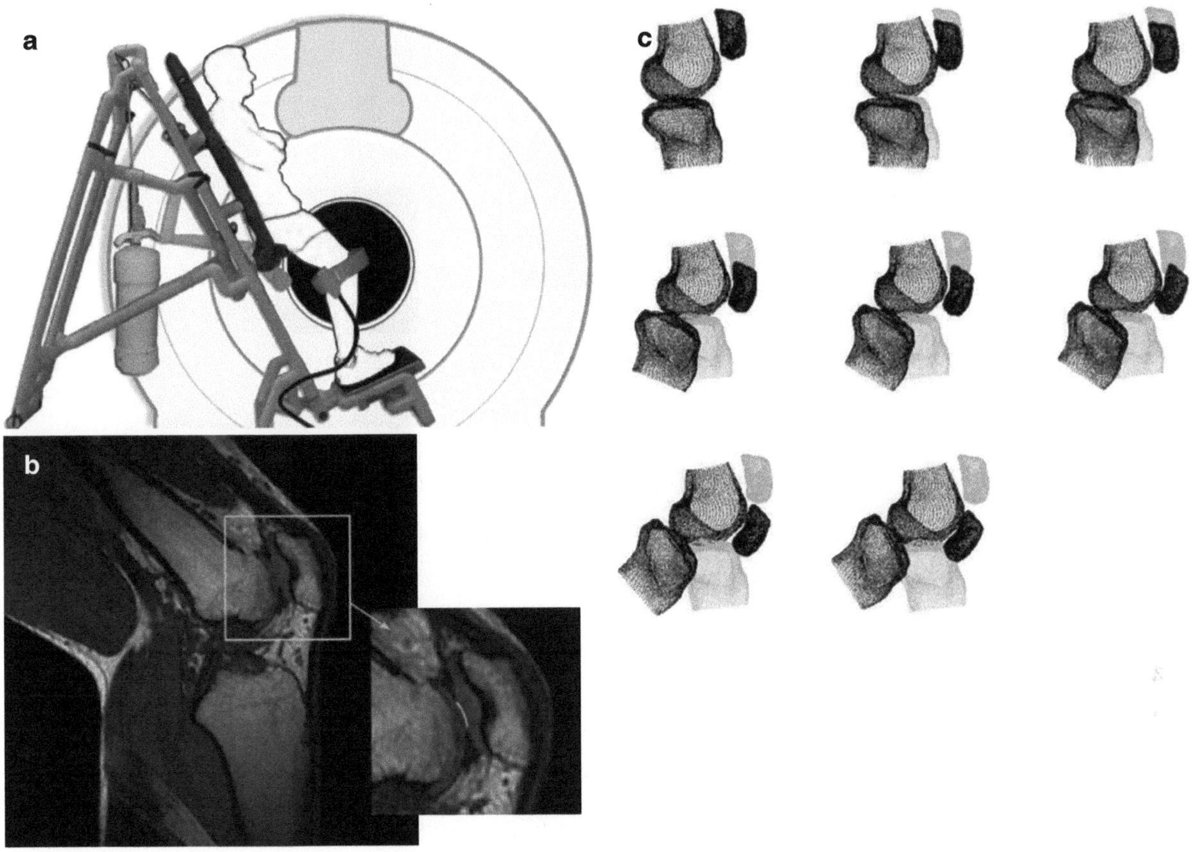


**Fig. 20.2** Upright weight-bearing imaging in the 0.5T GE Signa MRI scanner. The custom backrest (**a**) enables subjects to remain still during the scan, while supporting ~90% of their body weight. The backrest can be locked into place and a small seat can be engaged from behind to enable images to be taken under minimal load and no quadriceps activity (~0.15 body weight). Volumetric images of the knee can then be used to determine contact areas (**b**) and the three-dimensional orientation of the patellofemoral joint through different amounts of knee flexion (**c**)

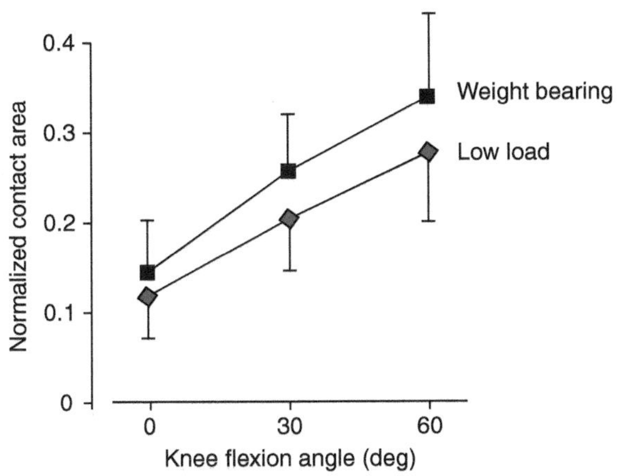


**Fig. 20.3** Normalized patellofemoral joint contact areas under loaded and unloaded conditions (Adapted from Besier et al.[5])

#### 20.2.1.2 Cartilage Morphology

High-resolution MR images of the PF joint also enable the assessment of cartilage thickness in the contacting regions of the patella and anterior femur (Fig. 20.4a). Cartilage thickness maps are relevant to tissue stress as thinner cartilage leads to increased stress[41] and it is possible that patients with PF pain have thin cartilage compared to pain-free subjects. To test this hypothesis, we compared PF joint cartilage thickness of 16 pain-free control subjects (eight males and eight females) with 34 patients with PF pain (12 males and 22 females).[19] A young subject population was chosen (28 ± 4 year) to negate any potential influences of cartilage degeneration with aging. We discretized the patella and femur surfaces into three regions of interest (Fig. 20.4c), to represent the different areas of contact

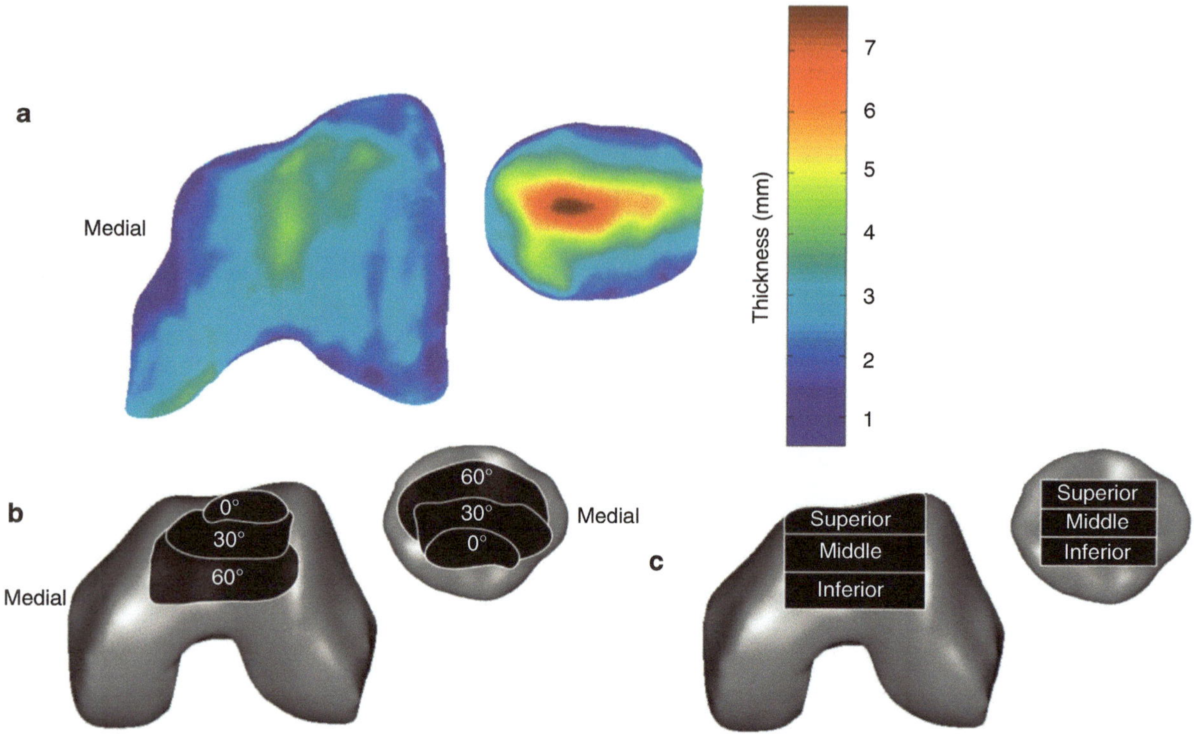


**Fig. 20.4** (**a**) Cartilage thickness map of the anterior femur and patella. (**b**) Contact areas corresponding to 0°, 30°, and 60° of knee flexion. (**c**) Discretized regions where cartilage thicknesses were examined (Adapted from Draper et al.[19])

throughout knee flexion (Fig. 20.4b). On average, males had 22% and 23% thicker cartilage than females in the patella and femur, respectively.[19] Male control subjects had 18% greater peak patellar cartilage thickness than males with PF pain; however, we did not detect differences in patellar cartilage thickness between female control subjects and females with PF pain (Fig. 20.5). Femoral cartilage thicknesses were similar between the control and pain groups. The conclusion drawn from this study was that thin patellar cartilage might be one mechanism of PF pain in male subjects, but is unlikely to be a dominant factor in the development of PF pain in females.

One question that arises from this finding is why males with PF pain might have thinner patellar cartilage. The answer to this question is difficult to ascertain, but in a young population that is devoid of degenerative changes, it is likely related to the loading history of the PF joint. The process of endochondral ossification is influenced by the local stresses within the tissue[15] and these stresses during growth and development dictate the thickness of cartilage in adulthood. Animal models also show that extended periods of inactivity can lead to continued endochondral ossification and cartilage thinning.[63] One hypothesis is that individuals who are less active during adolescence and early adulthood are predisposed to having thinner cartilage due to continued endochondral ossification. These individuals might have joints that are poorly suited to distributing large joint loads and perhaps should not take up marathon running at a later age!

### 20.2.2 Real-Time Magnetic Resonance Imaging to Measure Patellofemoral Joint Kinematics

For years, PF pain was ascribed to the presence of malalignment,[36,47] defined as abnormal patellar tracking and believed to result in overload of the lateral retinaculum and subchondral bone.[25] Malalignment continues to be the focus of many researchers and is typically defined by lateral displacement or lateral tilt

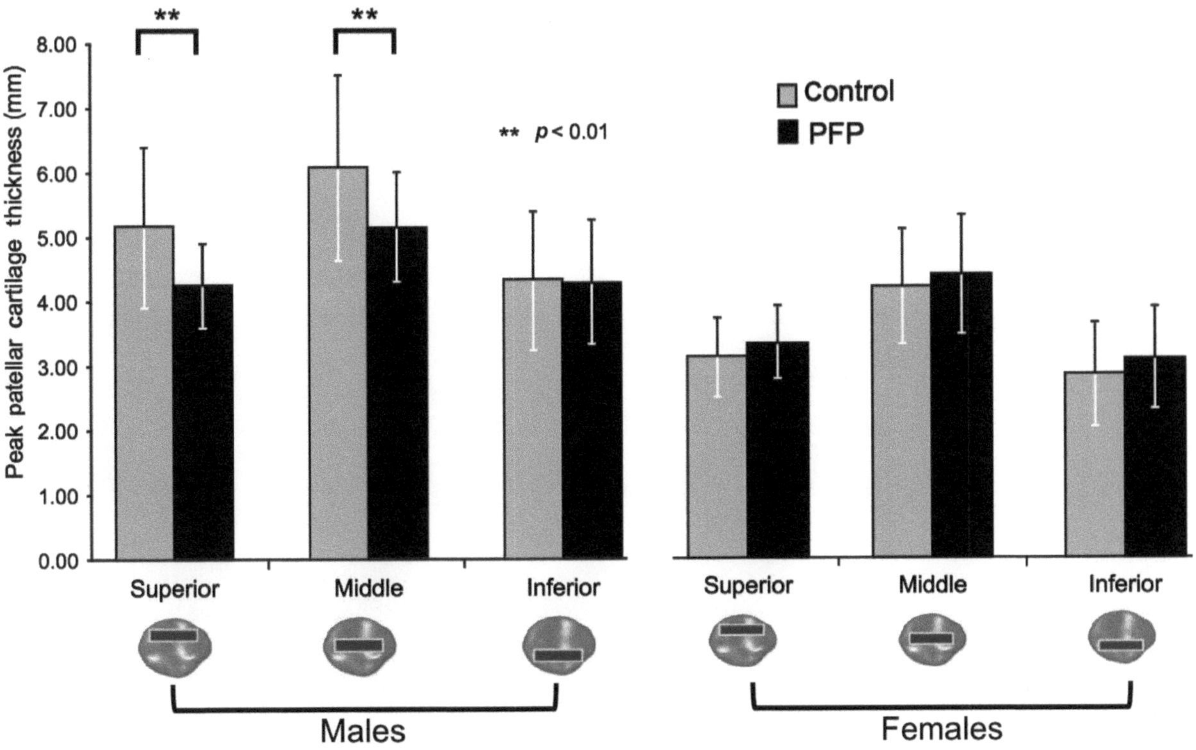


**Fig. 20.5** Peak patellar cartilage thickness of males and females with patellofemoral pain (PFP) and a group of pain-free controls. Males with patellofemoral pain had thinner cartilage compared to controls, which might lead to increased cartilage stresses, particularly at deeper angles of knee flexion when the contact is superior and middle

of the patella with respect to the femur, both being more pronounced in extension and low load conditions. Maltracking can result from altered femoral rotation,[54,58] poor joint articulation[1,65] or abnormal recruitment of the vasti muscles.[17,64,67] Recent advancements in medical imaging technologies are permitting a more accurate description of the kinematics of the patellofemoral joint in supine unloaded,[56,69] supine low load[46,53] and upright loaded configurations.[20,51,61] However, despite these recent advancements, there is no clear consensus regarding the definition of maltracking, the cause of maltracking, or the relationship between maltracking and pain. To begin exploring these relationships, we implemented real-time MR imaging in our 0.5T Signa open-bore MRI scanner to image the PF joint under dynamic upright weight-bearing motion (Fig. 20.6).

Real-time image acquisition produces a time series of single image slices.[2] The imaging plane can be continuously defined and updated in real time to follow an object if out-of-plane motion occurs. Real-time MRI can acquire a plane of image data quickly with reconstructed image display rates of 24 frames/s.[50] This high rate of image acquisition and display minimizes the risk of muscle fatigue during highly loaded motions, allowing data to be obtained under weight-bearing conditions. We first established the feasibility of using real-time MRI to measure joint motion using an MR-compatible motion phantom with a known and repeatable movement trajectory.[21] In the 0.5T open-bore MRI scanner, we measured the movement of the phantom to within 2 mm for movement speeds of up to 38 mm/s, which corresponds to ~22°/s of knee joint flexion.[21] A limitation of these real-time MR imaging acquisitions is that they cannot be used to obtain kinematic measurements during fast velocities or in three dimensions. Faster image acquisition can be achieved in scanners with greater field strengths (e.g. 1.5 or 3.0T clinical scanners); however, the closed-bore designs of these scanners do not permit upright, weight-bearing postures.

To characterize PF maltracking, we measured weight-bearing axial-plane PF joint kinematics in 13

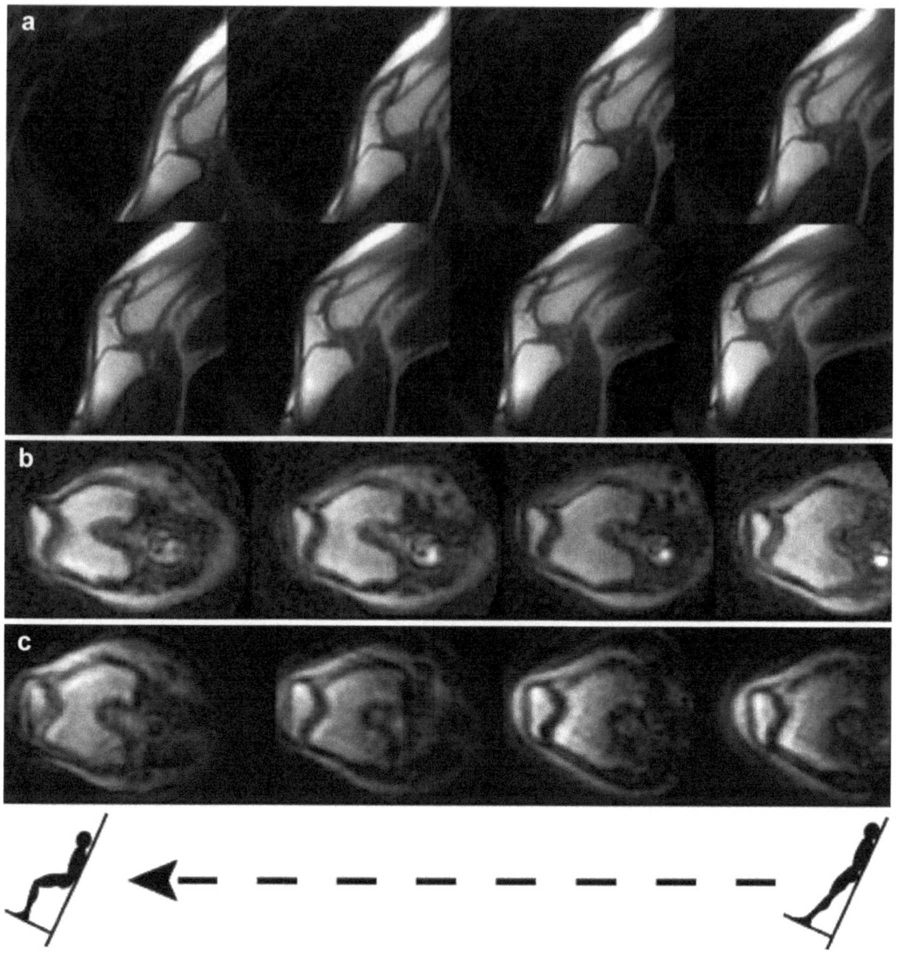


**Fig. 20.6** (**a**) Sample sagittal plane real-time MR images of patellofemoral joint during weight-bearing knee flexion. (**b**) Axial images from healthy, pain-free control and (**c**) axial images from a subject with patellofemoral pain

pain-free females and 23 females diagnosed with PF pain. We assessed the lateral displacement of the patella using a bisect offset index and the lateral rotation using a patellar tilt angle (Fig. 20.7). We found that, on average, females with PF pain exhibited a 10% increase in bisect offset and a 6° increase in patellar tilt compared to pain-free controls.[20] The greatest kinematic differences between groups occurred, as expected, near full extension. Importantly, there was a large variation in the types of maltracking in the pain subjects (Fig. 20.8), including a subset of patients ($n=5/23$, ~22%) with kinematics no different from controls. These results suggest that weight-bearing maltracking may be related to pain in some subjects, but distinct subgroups of patients with different maltracking patterns exist and it is important to recognize that the underlying mechanism of pain may be different in each subgroup. The implication of these results is that accurate classification of patients is needed for effective treatment.

If imaging modalities are going to be useful for future classification and treatment of PF patients, it is important to understand the importance of imaging under upright, weight-bearing conditions. To address this issue, we compared supine, non-weight-bearing and upright, weight-bearing patellofemoral joint kinematics in a group of 20 subjects diagnosed with PF pain. In subjects with patellar maltracking, the patella translated more laterally during upright, weight-bearing knee extension for knee flexion angles between 25 and 30°. However, in subjects without maltracking, the patella

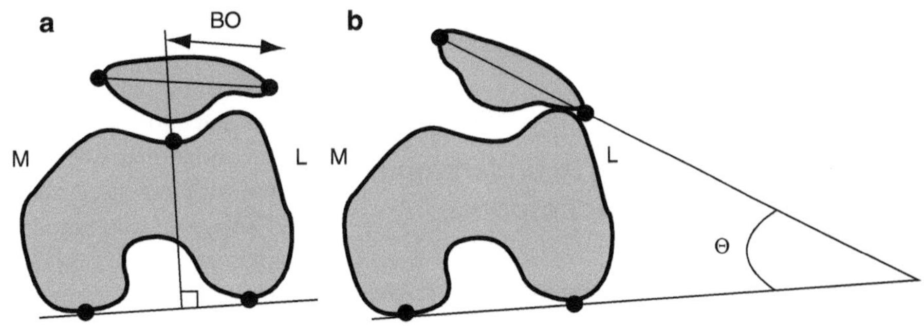


**Fig. 20.7** Axial-plane PF joint kinematics illustrating: (**a**) the Bisect Offset index (BO) - a measure of the percentage of the patellar width lateral to the midline of the femur, and (**b**) patellar tilt (theta) - the angle formed by lines joining the posterior femoral condyles and the maximum width of the patella (Adapted from Draper et al.[19])

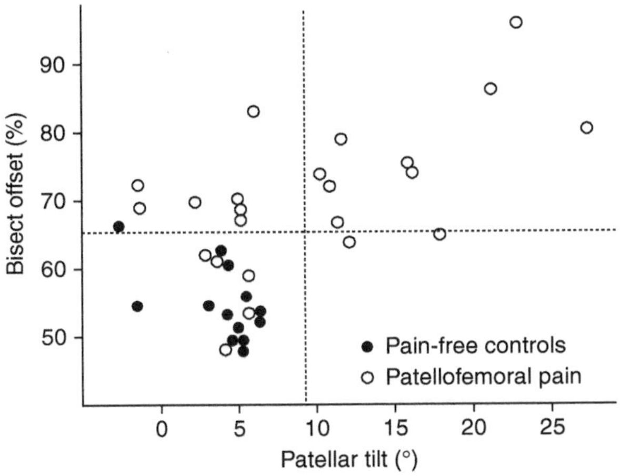


**Fig. 20.8** Relationship between bisect offset and patellar tilt at full extension in pain-free controls (*solid circles*) and patellofemoral pain subjects (*hollow circles*). The *dashed lines* represent two standard deviations above the average bisect offset and tilt of the pain-free subjects and were used as thresholds to identify subjects with abnormal patellofemoral joint kinematics (Adapted from Draper et al.[19])

translated more laterally during supine, non-weight-bearing knee extension for knee flexion angles between 0° and 8°. These results suggest that measurements of patellar tracking performed under non-weight-bearing conditions do not completely reflect weight-bearing joint motion and as a result, clinical diagnosis of patellar maltracking may be more relevant if weight-bearing joint alignment or motion is taken into account. Unfortunately, the majority of clinical MR and CT-based imaging modalities require patients to be supine with little or no load applied to the knee. In our current work, we are assessing the use of upright, static weight-bearing X-ray[11] to assess patellar maltracking and determine the ability of this accessible imaging modality to differentiate lateral maltrackers and non-lateral maltrackers.

#### 20.2.2.1 Influence of Bracing

Using our real-time MR imaging protocol, we evaluated the efficacy of a patellar stabilizing brace and a patellar sleeve in restoring normal joint kinematics. The reduction in bisect offset provided by the brace (6% at full extension) was larger than that provided by the sleeve (4% at full extension) for knee flexion angles between 0° and 60°.[20] Similarly, the brace reduced patellar tilt by 4° at full extension, while we detected no changes in patellar tilt with application of the knee sleeve. While the brace reduced abnormal patellar kinematics, it did not completely restore normal PF joint motion. An important side result that highlights the need for accurate diagnosis and subject-specific treatment was that PF pain patients with maltracking had greater decreases in both bisect offset and lateral tilt of the patella with brace and sleeve application than PF pain patients with normal PF joint motion. For instance, in patients with abnormal bisect offset, the brace and sleeve reduced bisect offset by 8% and 6%, respectively, whereas in patients with normal bisect offset, the brace and sleeve had no effect on the lateral motion of the patella. Similarly, the brace reduced patellar tilt by 5° more in patients with excessive lateral tilt compared to those with normal patellar tilt.

The clinical implications of this work are that patients with PF pain can be classified into subgroups based upon their PF joint kinematics, and these subgroups are likely to respond differently to different treatment strategies. Accurate assessment of patellar maltracking in a clinical setting would therefore be beneficial for prescribing specific treatment; however, this remains a challenge. In our previous study, the clinical assessment of 8 out of 23 subjects did not correlate with weight-bearing patellar tracking. It remains to be seen whether patients classified as having maltracking also have increased stress in the PF joint, but this will be the focus of our modeling efforts in the near future.

### 20.2.3 PET–CT Imaging to Understand Tissue Metabolic Response

Ultimately, our goal is to use computational models to predict clinical outcomes from interventions and correlate tissue-level stresses with pain and function. In mineralized bone, areas with high metabolic activity receive the richest sensory and sympathetic innervation, and therefore play an important role in the generation of skeletal pain.[45,57] Quantifying this metabolic activity with functional imaging techniques might offer us a biological metric of bone-related PF pain that we can use to compare with mechanical stresses. Positron Emission Tomography (PET) and $^{99m}$Tc-MDP bone scintigraphy (bone scans) are two functional imaging modalities that can be used to highlight areas of increased bone metabolic activity and remodeling, in response to local mechanical stresses or injury within the tissue.

While $^{99m}$Tc-MDP bone scintigraphy has provided valuable insights about potential alterations in bone remodeling activity in the PF pain population,[12,33,44,49] $^{18}$F-NaF PET/CT is a technique that offers several advantages. For example, compared to traditional bone scans, the spatial resolution of the PET scan is better, the ratio of bone uptake to soft tissue uptake is greater, and the ability to collect PET and CT data at the same time enables accurate anatomical localization of tracer uptake. Traditionally, $^{18}$F-NaF PET has been used in the field of oncology; however, recent studies have suggested that $^{18}$F-NaF PET is promising for the evaluation of orthopedic conditions, such as in the assessment of bone fracture healing[35] and the identification of sources of back pain.[42] These relationships exist as $^{18}$F localizes in areas of bone mineralization or newly exposed mineralized surface, indicating regions of both osteoblastic and osteoclastic activity.[62]

We performed a preliminary study and acquired MR and $^{18}$F-NaF PET/CT images of patients with chronic PF pain (>1 year) to assess the regions of bone metabolic activity and determine whether changes in MR signal intensity correlated to $^{18}$F uptake. We found increased bone metabolic activity in the patella and/or trochlea in 85% of the painful knees (Fig. 20.9).

The most common location of increased metabolic activity was the subchondral region on the lateral facet of the patella. In general, abnormalities in the bone and cartilage detected by MRI (e.g. subchondral cysts, bone marrow edema, cartilage damage) correlated with increased tracer uptake in the $^{18}$F-NaF PET/CT images. However, there were a number of regions of increased tracer uptake, indicating increased bone metabolic activity that did not have any structural damage detected by MRI (Fig. 20.10). These preliminary findings suggest that $^{18}$F-NaF PET/CT and MRI provide different information about the joint and perhaps $^{18}$F-NaF PET/CT can be used to detect early changes in metabolic activity prior to the development of structural damage in the bones and cartilage. We hypothesize that regions of increased metabolic activity in the bone of PF pain patients correlate to regions of increased mechanical stresses in the tissue, which are also related to the development of pain. To test this hypothesis, we have developed a musculoskeletal modeling framework for estimating the mechanical stresses throughout bone and cartilage of the PF joint.

## 20.3 Musculoskeletal Modeling of the Patellofemoral Joint

To test the hypothesis that patients with PF pain have elevated cartilage and subchondral bone stress compared to pain-free controls, one would ideally take experimental measures of cartilage and bone stresses in a patient population during various dynamic activities. However, direct measurement of in vivo tissue stresses is not feasible, so we must rely on computational methods to estimate these mechanical variables. Estimating the stresses throughout articular cartilage, bone, and surrounding soft tissues of the PF joint requires knowledge of several factors, including: the loads applied to the tissue; the articulating geometry of the joint; the orientation and position of the joint when the loads are applied; and the morphology and material properties of the different tissues. To capture these complex relationships, we use the finite element method, a numerical technique that enables the calculation of internal tissue stresses, given the joint loads, geometry, and material properties of the different tissues. The accuracy and validity of the finite element method comes from

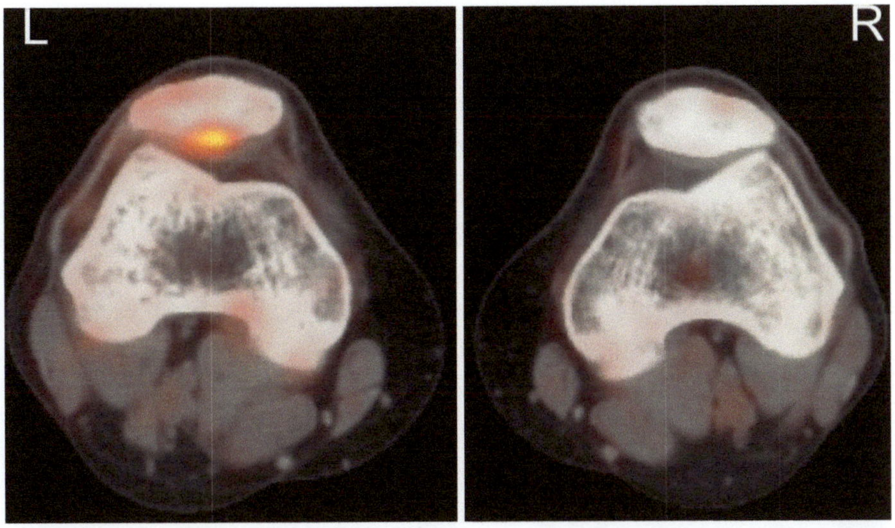


**Fig. 20.9** Co-registered axial PET/CT image of a unilateral chronic PF pain patient (Male, age 32, characterized with abnormal weight-bearing bisect offset index at full extension). The superimposed CT image enables accurate localization of the PET hotspot, in this case within the apex of the left patella, which was consistent with the area of pain

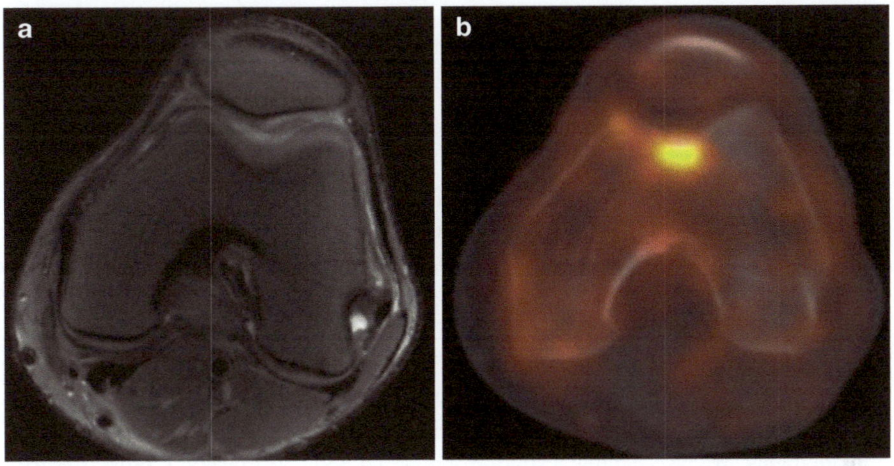


**Fig. 20.10** Axial MRI of chronic PF pain patient (**a**), showing no abnormalities within bone or cartilage of the PF joint. Corresponding PET hotspot in the same subject (**b**), indicating areas of high metabolic activity

having appropriate material properties and carefully selected loads and boundary conditions. This section briefly describes the work we have performed to create patient-specific finite element models of the PF joint to estimate in vivo cartilage and bone stresses.[8]

Our modeling framework consists of several components, each of which will be described in more detail below:

1. Defining the geometry and morphology of the various tissues
2. Defining the material properties of the tissues
3. Prescribing the joint orientation/kinematics
4. Estimating muscle forces using an EMG-driven model
5. Simulation and validation

### 20.3.1 Defining the Geometry and Morphology of the Various Tissues

To define the geometry and morphology of the various tissues of the PF joint, we take high-resolution MR images of the knee. Typically, these are sagittal plane images of the knee using a fat-suppressed spoiled gradient echo sequence in a 1.5-T or 3.0-T closed-bore MR scanner (refer to[19] for scan details, Fig. 20.11a). During this scan, the subject is supine with the knee fully extended to ensure the cartilage is imaged in an undeformed state. The MR images are then manually segmented with smooth splines to obtain a three-dimensional point cloud of the femur, tibia, and patellar, including the articular cartilage. The quadriceps tendon, patellar tendon, and suprapatellar fat

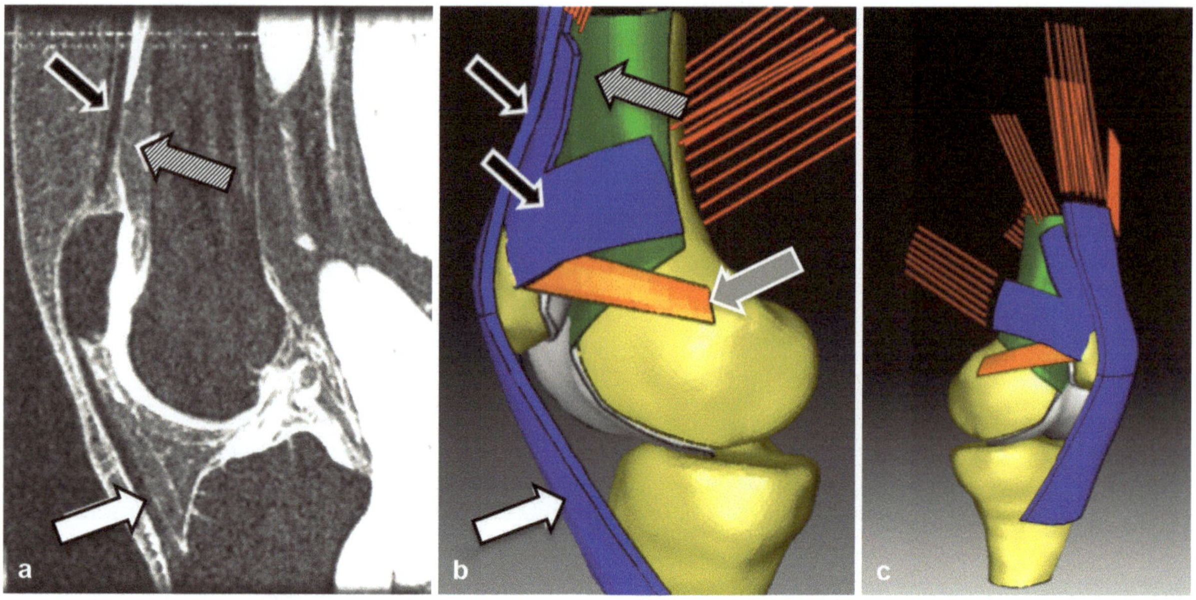


**Fig. 20.11** Sagittal MR image (**a**) and corresponding finite element model (**b**, **c**) of the patellofemoral joint. The patellar ligament (*white arrows*) and quadriceps tendon (*black arrows*) were represented as nonlinear fiber-reinforced solid elements, while the medial patellofemoral ligament (*gray arrow*) was modeled using 2D composite elements. Articular cartilage and supra-trochlear fat pad (*striped arrows*) were modeled as linear elastic solids

pad are also segmented from these images (Fig. 20.11a). Triangulated surfaces are then fit to the point clouds using a commercial software package (Geomagic, Research Triangle Park, NC). We then represent each structure as three-dimensional continuum elements with appropriate material properties (see below). To mimic the physiologic tendon lines-of-action at the patella, we represent the quadriceps and patellar tendon as hexahedral continuum elements. We also include a supra-trochlear fat pad to facilitate patella cartilage–fat pad interaction at extended knee postures (Fig. 20.11a, b, gray arrow). To replicate the physiologic medial–lateral constraint at the patella, the medial PF ligament is included as 2D composite elements. Contact is defined between the relevant structures to enable wrapping of the tendons around bone–cartilage–fat pad construct. Three-dimensional continuum element representations of the patella and the distal femur are also defined to facilitate stress calculations throughout the bone.

### 20.3.2 Defining the Material Properties of the Tissues

Describing the deformations and stresses throughout a tissue under a given load requires knowledge of the material properties of the tissue. In the finite element method, a continuum approach that describes the overall, macroscopic behavior of the tissue is typically used and these material properties are assigned to each element within the mesh. In its simplest form, each element of a discretized tissue is assigned the same material property, regardless of the direction of loading (isotropic), which includes a stiffness, or elastic modulus, and a Poisson's ratio (describing the ratio of expansion or contraction of a material under compressive or tensile load). Although most biological tissues do not behave as a linear elastic isotropic material, this simple approximation can often describe a tissue's behavior under certain loading conditions. For example, during dynamic loading scenarios such as walking and running, cartilage can be adequately modeled as a linear elastic material due to its elastic response under loads at frequencies greater than 0.1 Hz.[34] The selection of appropriate material properties is therefore dependent on the intended loading scenarios. The models presented in this chapter use a simplified linear elastic material model to describe cartilage mechanical behavior (elastic modulus of 6 MPa and Poisson ratio of 0.47).

There is tremendous focus in the medical imaging community to develop non-invasive methods to estimate material properties of biological tissues. Articular cartilage has received much of this focus in an attempt to detect early degenerative changes and characterize tissue health. Certain parameters measured from an MRI scan of cartilage are known to correlate with the microscopic constituents of the tissue (e.g. $T_1$ and $T_2$ relaxation times correlate to proteoglycan and collagen content, respectively), which in turn correlate to the macroscopic material properties.[40] Although outside the scope of this book chapter, our group has a history of developing novel MR imaging sequences for cartilage[28–32] and we are currently exploring the relationship between cartilage imaging (T1rho and sodium imaging) and cartilage mechanical properties.[37] Our aim is to estimate material properties of cartilage using MRI and assign these properties to our finite element simulations.

To describe the material properties for bone, we perform a CT scan to define a radiographic measure of density (measured in Hounsfield units), which can be converted to regional specific bone apparent density.[38,60] This information is mapped onto the finite element mesh[39] and each element in the mesh assigned an appropriate elastic modulus based on the measured bone apparent density (Fig. 20.12). In this case, we model bone as a linear elastic solid.

Describing material properties for tendinous structures is problematic, as the tensile loading response of a tendon is greatly influenced by its resting slack length, which is difficult to measure in vivo. Our approach is to model the quadriceps and patellar tendon as a non-linear hyper-elastic material based on experimental data,[59] as reported by Baldwin et al.[3] The resting tendon length and stiffness profile can then be 'tuned' to match vertical displacement data of the patella under weight-bearing load to ensure the correct displacement of the patellar tendon. A linear elastic material model adapted from tensile testing[48] is currently used to represent the medial PF ligament.

### 20.3.3 Prescribing the Joint Orientation/Kinematics

Contact force and stress calculations are extremely sensitive to changes in joint orientation and position, particularly for the PF articulation, which has complex articulating surfaces. Millimeters of translation or a degrees of rotation can substantially alter contact at the articulating surface of the PF joint. For this reason, the patella has 6 degrees of freedom in our simulations and is free to move in any direction and settle into a position that satisfies static equilibrium based upon the forces acting on it (i.e. the quadriceps and tendon force and the resulting contact forces). Because the joint is modeled with near-zero friction, the final position of the patella depends on the distribution of quadriceps muscle forces and the contacting geometry. Therefore, it is important to describe the initial orientation of the patella prior to the application of muscle forces. To determine the initial orientation of the joint, we register the bone surface mesh of the femur, tibia, and

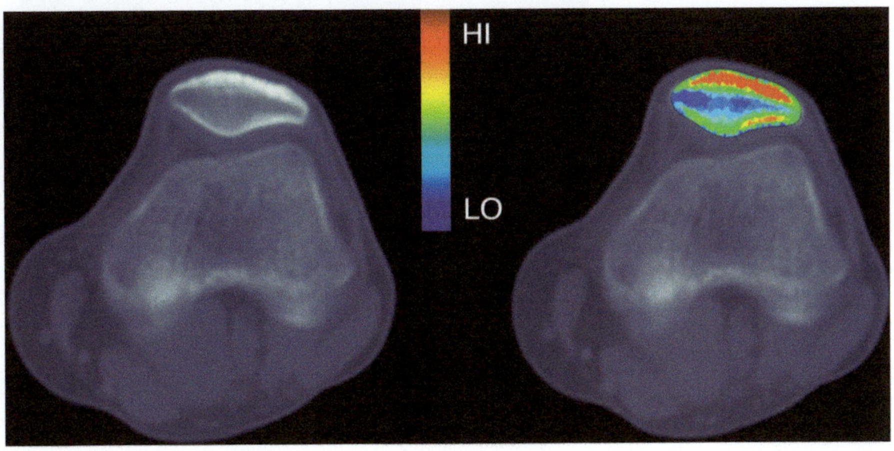


**Fig. 20.12** Axial CT image of chronic PF pain patient illustrating variation in bone mineral density. Color coding on right shows most dense bone (*red*) in the anterior aspect of the patella as well as the lateral facet of the patella

patella to our three-dimensional weight-bearing MR data sets (Fig. 20.13). This registration is performed using a closest iterative point algorithm, which minimizes the distance between points manually selected on the boundary of the bone ($n = 20$ to 30) and the surface of the bone mesh. A visual comparison of the model within the image data ensures a close registration of the mesh to the image (Fig. 20.13).

Using this registration technique, we can prescribe the initial configuration of the patellofemoral and tibiofemoral joints for each posture that was imaged (typically 0°, 30°, and 60° of knee flexion in our open-bore MR scanner). Describing the tibiofemoral joint orientation is important to ensure an accurate orientation of the patellar tendon and quadriceps tendon. For quasi-static analyses, the tibia and femur remain fixed throughout the simulation as the quadriceps muscle forces are applied. For dynamic analyses, the femur remains fixed and the tibia motion is prescribed. The simulation results presented in this chapter were performed as quasi-static analyses.

### 20.3.4 Estimating Muscle Forces Using an EMG-Driven Model

Quadriceps muscle forces influence the motion of the patella within the trochlear groove, and therefore influence the stress within the cartilage and bone. Accounting for individual muscle activation strategies is important when estimating the distribution of muscle forces across the knee joint, particularly in a pathological case when altered muscle recruitment patterns are expected. Therefore, we use a musculoskeletal modeling method to estimate muscle forces based

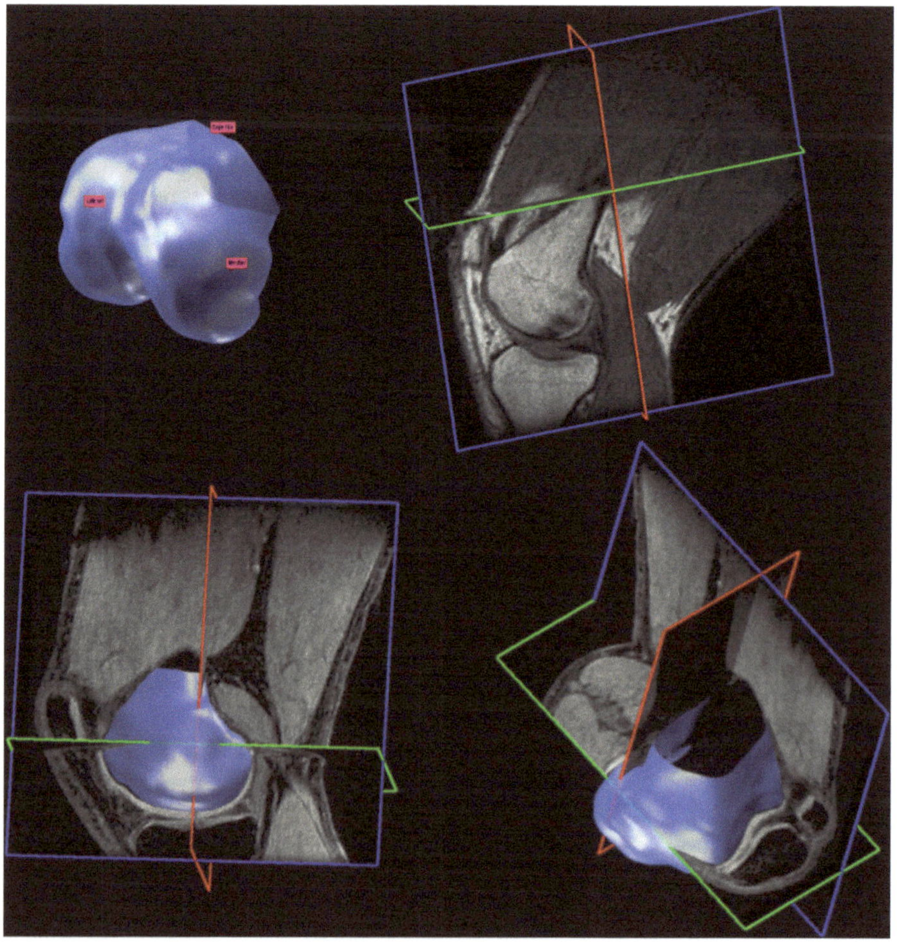

**Fig. 20.13** Registration of femur finite element mesh (*upper left*) into upright weight-bearing MR imaging volume (*upper right*). Selecting edges of the bone within the imaging data set ensures a close match between the model and MR images (*lower images*)

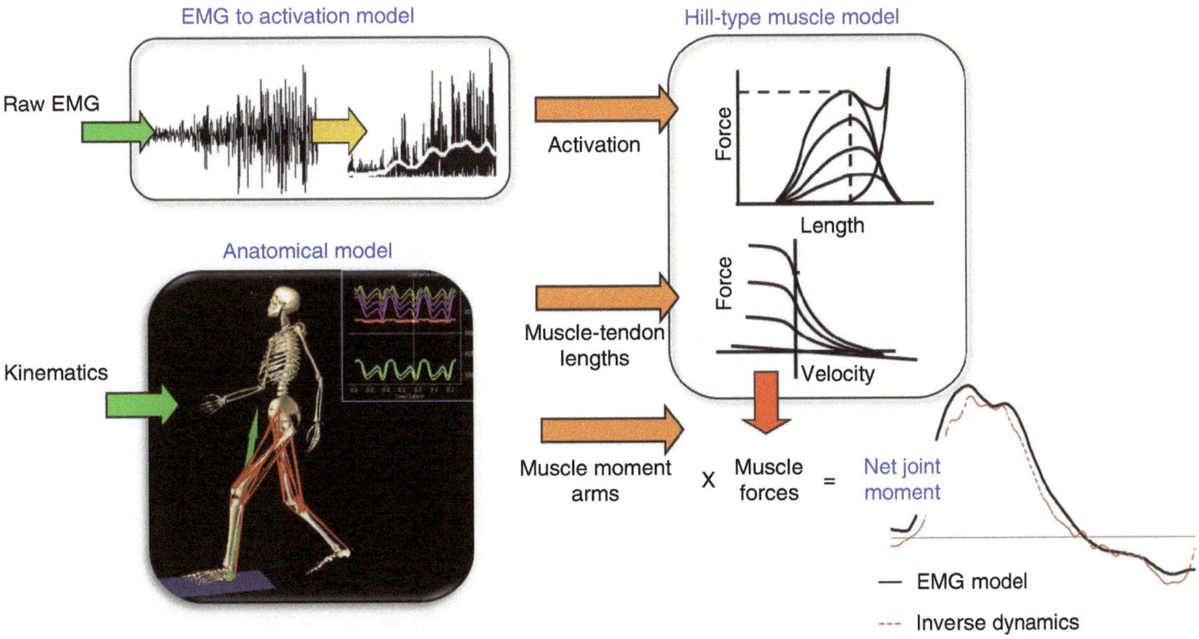


**Fig. 20.14** EMG-driven musculoskeletal model overview. Raw EMG and joint kinematics are used to estimate activation and muscle tendon lengths, which are input into a Hill-type muscle model to estimate muscle force. Muscle moment arms calculated from the anatomical model (OpenSIM) are multiplied by the muscle forces to obtain the net joint moment. The net joint moment from the model is compared to the moment calculated from inverse dynamics in a calibration/validation procedure

on electromyographic (EMG) signals[4,13,43] (Fig. 20.14). Briefly, this method takes EMG and joint kinematics (from a standard motion capture experiment) as input to estimate muscle activation and muscle contraction dynamics, respectively. An EMG-to-activation process takes raw EMG and estimates an activation time series, which represents the summed activation of the underlying motor units. This process takes into account the non-linear transfer from EMG to activation as well as the potential non-linearity between muscle force and EMG. The end result of this transfer function is an activation time series, scaled to a maximum voluntary isometric contraction.

We then scale a musculoskeletal model of each individual to match the anthropometry of each subject (from motion capture data). This process is performed using an open-source modeling platform called OpenSim.[18] This scaled anatomical model reproduces the motions of each subject from motion capture data and provides individual muscle tendon lengths and moment arms for each muscle crossing the knee joint. Muscle activation and muscle tendon length are then input to a modified Hill-type muscle model,[43] which estimates individual muscle force, taking into account muscle fiber force-length and force-velocity relationships (Fig. 20.14). The resulting muscle forces are multiplied by their respective moment arms in flexion–extension and the summed muscle moments can be compared to the net joint moment estimated using traditional inverse dynamics analysis. Although muscle forces cannot be measured in vivo, a comparison to the joint moment from inverse dynamics provides a means of indirectly validating the predicted muscle forces. Various parameters in the model are expected to differ among individuals (such as muscle cross-sectional area and non-linear EMG–force relationships) and these parameters can be altered in a calibration process to improve the prediction of the net joint moment. Importantly, this calibration process only occurs on a few select trials. Following calibration, the parameters in the model are not altered and muscle forces and joint moments are predicted equally well for other dynamic tasks, providing some confidence in the predicted muscle forces.[43]

An obvious application of this EMG-driven approach is to investigate the quadriceps muscle force distribution in patients with PF pain during functional activities, such as walking and running. Of particular interest is the relationship between the medial and lateral components of the vastii, as muscle force imbalance is often cited as a cause of patellar maltracking and PF pain. Based on previous literature,[16,64,67] one might hypothesize the relative contribution of the vastus medialis muscle would be less in the patellofemoral pain group compared to pain-free controls during walking and running. To answer this hypothesis, we estimated lower limb muscle forces during walking and running in a group of male and female patients with PF pain ($n=27$, 16 female; 11 male) and compared the peak quadriceps forces to a group of pain-free controls ($n=16$, 8 female; 8 male).[7] Surface EMG were collected from seven major muscles crossing the knee joint, including: vastus medialis, vastus lateralis, rectus femoris, biceps femoris, semimembranosus, medial gastrocnemius, and lateral gastrocnemius. We found that subjects with PF pain produced a knee extension moment using the same distribution of quadriceps forces as pain-free individuals during walking and running, which did not support our hypothesis. However, compared to controls, PF pain patients had greater co-contraction of quadriceps and hamstring muscles and greater normalized quadriceps muscle forces during walking. Muscle forces during running were similar between groups, but the net knee extension moment was less in the PF pain group compared to controls. These data suggest that some PF pain patients might experience greater joint contact forces and joint stresses than pain-free subjects by virtue of increased overall quadriceps muscle forces. It is not known whether these muscle force distributions are an adaptation to pain or if they are causative, but one could argue that increased co-contraction around heel strike might improve knee joint stability and help to align the patella within the trochlear groove. On the other hand, increased muscle forces during peak push off would have a detrimental effect of increasing joint contact forces. Whether or not these increased muscle forces lead to increased cartilage or bone stress in these patients remains to be seen, although these data provide valuable input to our finite element simulations, which are capable of answering such questions.

### 20.3.5 Simulation and Validation

The final stage in our modeling pipeline is to run the finite element simulation and validate the results. As stated previously, during quasi-static analyses the femur and tibia are fixed and the patella is constrained only by the forces of the quadriceps muscles and patellar tendon and the contact forces from the femur. The quadriceps muscle forces from the EMG-driven model are applied to the quadriceps tendons during the simulation, causing the patella to settle into the trochlear groove until reaching static equilibrium. All our simulations are run using a non-linear finite element solver (ABAQUS, Pawtucket, RI).

One of the most important aspects of using a computational model to investigate a clinical problem is validation. Although we cannot directly validate the model stresses to experimental measures, there are other variables that can be used to validate each simulation. Firstly, contact areas measured from weight-bearing MR images can be compared to those predicted by the simulation. Our initial models generated for 16 healthy, pain-free controls had PF contact areas within 5% of those measured from MRI for 10 of the 16 subjects.[9] Secondly, we can compare the final orientation of the patella to that obtained from the weight-bearing MRI. On average, the patella orientation during the simulation was within $3.7° \pm 5.98°$ of tilt and $4.7° \pm 7.68°$ of rotation of the measured orientation.[9] Discrepancies in contact area and patella orientation can be due to; incorrect estimation of muscle forces, errors in the line of action of the muscles (these simulations did not include wrapping of the quadriceps tendon), and/or the prescribed material properties of the tissue. Our current framework introduces an optimization/calibration scheme to make subtle alterations to the muscle forces and cartilage material properties to enable a closer match between the measured contact areas and patella orientation over a range of squatting postures.

### 20.3.6 Cartilage and Bone Stresses in the Patellofemoral Joint

The driving question behind much of this work is whether patients with PF pain exhibit cartilage and bone stresses that are greater than pain-free controls. Our final dataset includes 57 PF pain patients and 16 pain-free controls. Of these patients, 22 have undergone PET/CT imaging, so we have the capability of estimating bone stresses and comparing these stresses to metabolic activity. For the other 51 subjects, we will estimate the cartilage stress distributions at the layer of cartilage closest to the subchondral bone and compare stress distributions between PF pain patients and pain-free controls. We would like to conclude this chapter with some interesting findings from our preliminary modeling studies.

Firstly, we have found that cartilage stresses are not intuitively predicted based upon joint kinematics alone,[9] which may seem to contradict conventional wisdom relating to PF biomechanics. The stresses developed throughout the cartilage of the patellofemoral joint are a result of complex interactions between the articulating geometry of the patella and femur, cartilage morphology, cartilage material properties, and the distribution of forces acting on the patella. Variations in each of these parameters may be responsible for the different stress responses that resulted from these simulations. Figure 20.15 illustrates a range of different cartilage stress distributions from five patients with PF pain performing a static squat at 60° of knee flexion. These stress distributions show that peak stress locations are not always located on the lateral facet of the PF joint and are often located on the medial facet. These peak stress locations do not necessarily reflect the orientation of the bone, which is typically what we measure when we discuss PF joint kinematics and maltracking. To highlight this point, we performed a series of simulations with our pain-free control data set to determine what effect internal and external rotation of the femur would have on cartilage stress.[9] Some individuals responded to femoral internal rotation with large changes in cartilage stresses, whereas others show little or no change with the same degree of femoral rotation. This insight has clinical relevance, particularly when considering treatment strategies to reduce stress. Assuming that cartilage stresses are related to pain from increased stresses transmitted through the cartilage into the subchondral bone, individuals who are more sensitive to changes in femoral rotation might respond positively to therapies or intervention strategies that focus on controlling femoral rotation. However, subjects who are relatively insensitive to changes in femoral rotation may not respond to any intervention that is designed to alter femoral orientation, such as stretching and strengthening of hip muscles. The modeling framework presented here offers the capability to identify important variables that relate to potential changes in tissue-level stresses and how these stresses might relate to potential joint and cartilage pathology.

Preliminary comparisons between six female PF pain patients and six pain-free controls provide some support that cartilage stresses are related to PF pain. We simulated double-leg squats at 60° of knee flexion and found that peak shear stresses within the femur were 28% greater in PF pain patients compared to controls.[5] However, given the variability across subjects and the different factors that can influence cartilage stress, many more simulations are required to understand the relationship between tissue stress and pain. We are also exploring the use of statistical modeling techniques to account for known variation in model input parameters.[52] These methods will provide us with useful information regarding which parameters have the greatest influence on tissue stresses, thus guiding further interventions on a subject-specific basis.

As stated previously, one of our goals is to correlate tissue stresses to biological measures of pain and

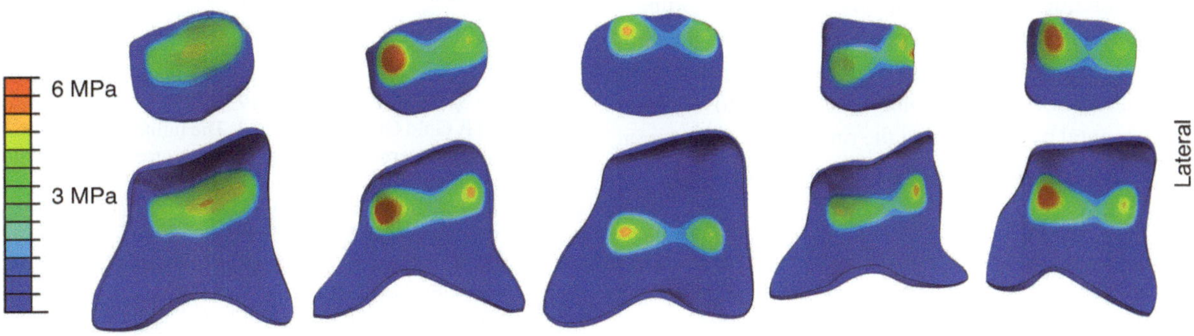


**Fig. 20.15** Example hydrostatic stresses in the layer of patellar and femoral cartilage closest to the subchondral bone in five patients with PF pain during a static squat at 60° of knee flexion. Note the varied distribution and magnitudes of peak hydrostatic pressure across this small sample. The lateral aspect of the joint is toward the right on each example. Stress "hot spots" are common on the medial aspect of the PF joint cartilage

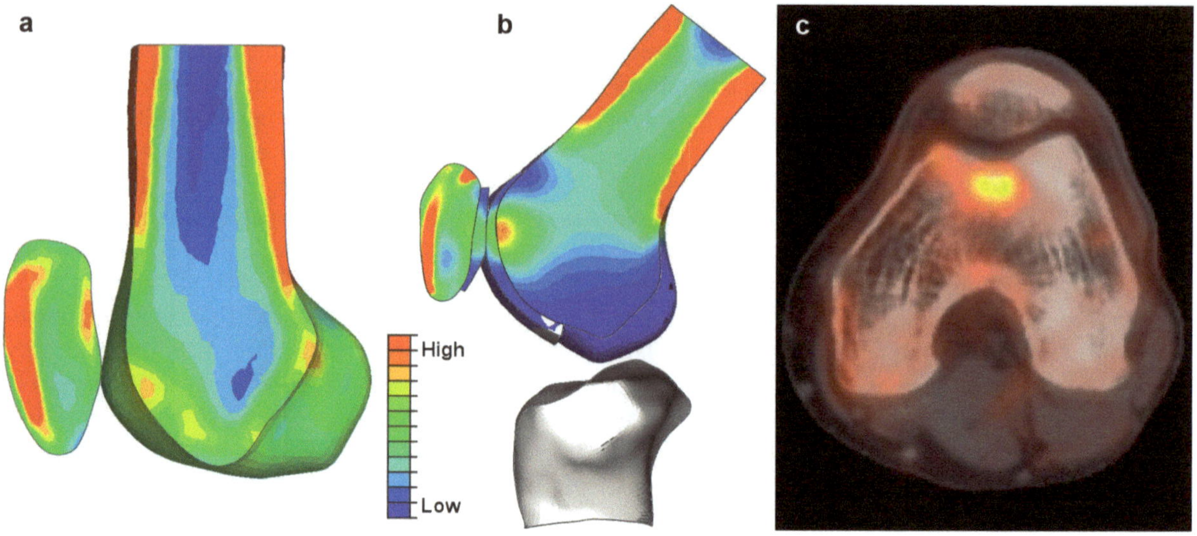


**Fig. 20.16** Bone density assignment from CT-based Hounsfield Units (**a**), and predicted bone-cartilage stress from finite element modeling (**b**) during a 60° static squat. Peak subchondral bone stresses in the trochlea of the femur correspond to the hot spot from PET scanning on the same subject (**c**)

function. To this end, we are now comparing bone stresses in the PF joint with PET image intensity, which is an indirect measure of bone metabolic activity. Preliminary findings show good qualitative comparisons between PET signal intensity and mechanical stress within the bone (Fig. 20.16). We hope this work will take us one step closer to understanding the mechanical etiology of PF pain.

## 20.4 Concluding Remarks

The combination of advanced medical imaging and musculoskeletal modeling presented here provides us with a unique set of tools to investigate the complex form and function of the PF joint. In particular, the ability to estimate patient-specific stresses throughout various tissues of the PF joint enables us to test the fundamental hypothesis that the onset and development of PF pain has an underlying mechanical etiology.

## References

1. Amis AA. Current concepts on anatomy and biomechanics of patellar stability. *Sports Med Arthrosc*. 2007;15:48-56.
2. Asakawa DS, Nayak KS, Blemker SS, et al. Real-time imaging of skeletal muscle velocity. *J Magn Reson Imaging*. 2003;18:734-739.
3. Baldwin MA, Clary C, Maletsky LP, et al. Verification of predicted specimen-specific natural and implanted patellofemoral kinematics during simulated deep knee bend. *J Biomech*. 2009;42:2341-2348.
4. Besier T, Delp S, Gold G, et al. Influence of quadriceps muscle force distributions on cartilage stresses at the patellofemoral joint during running. In: *American Society of Biomechanics*. Stanford; 2007.
5. Besier T, Delp S, Gold G, et al. Patellofemoral pain subjects display greater femoral cartilage stresses than pain-free controls. In: *Patellofemoral Pain Syndrome: International Research Retreat*. Baltimore: Elsevier; 2009.
6. Besier TF, Draper CE, Gold GE, et al. Patellofemoral joint contact area increases with knee flexion and weight-bearing. *J Orthop Res*. 2005;23:345-350.
7. Besier TF, Fredericson M, Gold GE, et al. Knee muscle forces during walking and running in patellofemoral pain patients and pain-free controls. *J Biomech*. 2009;42:898-905.
8. Besier TF, Gold GE, Beaupre GS, et al. A modeling framework to estimate patellofemoral joint cartilage stress in vivo. *Med Sci Sports Exerc*. 2005;37:1924-1930.
9. Besier TF, Gold GE, Delp SL, et al. The influence of femoral internal and external rotation on cartilage stresses within the patellofemoral joint. *J Orthop Res*. 2008;26:1627-1635.
10. Biedert RM, Sanchis-Alfonso V. Sources of anterior knee pain. *Clin Sports Med*. 2002;21:335-347.
11. Boegård T, Jonsson K. Radiography in osteoarthritis of the knee. *Skeletal Radiol*. 1999;28(11):605-615.
12. Boegard T, Rudling O, Dahlstrom J, et al. Bone scintigraphy in chronic knee pain: comparison with magnetic resonance imaging. *Ann Rheum Dis*. 1999;58:20-26.
13. Buchanan TS, Lloyd DG, Manal K, et al. Estimation of muscle forces and joint moments using a forward-inverse dynamics model. *Med Sci Sports Exerc*. 2005;37:1911-1916.

14. Carter DR, Beaupre GS. *Skeletal Function and Form. Mechanobiology of Skeletal Development, Aging and Regeneration.* Cambridge: Cambridge University Press; 2001.
15. Carter DR, Beaupre GS, Wong M, et al. The mechanobiology of articular cartilage development and degeneration. *Clin Orthop Relat Res*. 2004;427:S69-S77.
16. Cowan SM, Bennell KL, Hodges PW, et al. Delayed onset of electromyographic activity of vastus medialis obliquus relative to vastus lateralis in subjects with patellofemoral pain syndrome. *Arch Phys Med Rehabil*. 2001;82:183-189.
17. Cowan SM, Hodges PW, Bennell KL, et al. Altered vastii recruitment when people with patellofemoral pain syndrome complete a postural task. *Arch Phys Med Rehabil*. 2002;83: 989-995.
18. Delp SL, Anderson FC, Arnold AS, et al. OpenSim: open-source software to create and analyze dynamic simulations of movement. *IEEE Trans Biomed Eng*. 2007;54:1940-1950.
19. Draper CE, Besier TF, Gold GE, et al. Is cartilage thickness different in young subjects with and without patellofemoral pain? *Osteoarthritis Cartilage*. 2006;14:931-937.
20. Draper CE, Besier TF, Santos JM, et al. Using real-time MRI to quantify altered joint kinematics in subjects with patellofemoral pain and to evaluate the effects of a patellar brace or sleeve on joint motion. *J Orthop Res*. 2009;27: 571-577.
21. Draper CE, Santos JM, Kourtis LC, et al. Feasibility of using real-time MRI to measure joint kinematics in 1.5T and open-bore 0.5T systems. *J Magn Reson Imaging*. 2008;28:158-166.
22. Dye SF, Vaupel GL, Dye CC. Conscious neurosensory mapping of the internal structures of the human knee without intraarticular anesthesia. *Am J Sports Med*. 1998;26:773-777.
23. Fulkerson JP. The etiology of patellofemoral pain in young, active patients: a prospective study. *Clin Orthop Relat Res*. 1983;179:129-133.
24. Fulkerson JP. Mechanical basis for patellofemoral pain and cartilage breakdown. In: Ewing JW, ed. *Articular Cartilage and Knee Joint Function: Basic Science and Arthroscopy*. New York: Raven; 1990:93-101.
25. Fulkerson JP. Diagnosis and treatment of patients with patellofemoral pain. *Am J Sports Med*. 2002;30:447-456.
26. Fulkerson JP, Tennant R, Jaivin JS, et al. Histologic evidence of retinacular nerve injury associated with patellofemoral malalignment. *Clin Orthop Relat Res*. 1985;197:196-205.
27. Gold GE, Besier TF, Draper CE, et al. Weight-bearing MRI of patellofemoral joint cartilage contact area. *J Magn Reson Imaging*. 2004;20:526-530.
28. Gold GE, Burstein D, Dardzinski B, et al. MRI of articular cartilage in OA: novel pulse sequences and compositional/functional markers. *Osteoarthritis Cartilage*. 2006;14(suppl A): A76-A86.
29. Gold GE, Busse RF, Beehler C, et al. Isotropic MRI of the knee with 3D fast spin-echo extended echo-train acquisition (XETA): initial experience. *Am J Roentgenol*. 2007;188: 1287-1293.
30. Gold GE, Hargreaves BA, Stevens KJ, et al. Advanced magnetic resonance imaging of articular cartilage. *Orthop Clin North Am*. 2006;37:331-347.
31. Gold GE, Hargreaves BA, Vasanawala SS, et al. Articular cartilage of the knee: evaluation with fluctuating equilibrium MR imaging-initial experience in healthy volunteers. *Radiology*. 2006;238:712-718.
32. Gold GE, Reeder SB, Yu H, et al. Articular cartilage of the knee: rapid three-dimensional MR imaging at 3.0T with IDEAL balanced steady-state free precession – initial experience. *Radiology*. 2006;240:546-551.
33. Hejgaard N, Diemer H. Bone scan in the patellofemoral pain syndrome. *Int Orthop*. 1987;11:29-33.
34. Higginson GR, Snaith JE. The mechanical stiffness of articular cartilage in confined oscillating compression. *Eng Med*. 1979;8:11-14.
35. Hsu WK, Feeley BT, Krenek L, et al. The use of 18F-fluoride and 18F-FDG PET scans to assess fracture healing in a rat femur model. *Eur J Nucl Med Mol Imaging*. 2007;34:1291-1301.
36. Insall J. "Chondromalacia patellae": patellar malalignment syndrome. *Orthop Clin North Am*. 1979;10:117-127.
37. Keenan KE, Kourtis LC, Besier TF, et al. New resource for the computation of cartilage biphasic material properties with the interpolant response surface method. *Comput Methods Biomech Biomed Eng*. 2009;12:415-422.
38. Keller TS. Predicting the compressive mechanical behavior of bone. *J Biomech*. 1994;27:1159-1168.
39. Kourtis LC, Carter DR, Kesari H, et al. A new software tool (VA-BATTS) to calculate bending, axial, torsional and transverse shear stresses within bone cross sections having inhomogeneous material properties. *Comput Methods Biomech Biomed Eng*. 2008;11:463-476.
40. Kurkijarvi JE, Nissi MJ, Kiviranta I, et al. Delayed gadolinium-enhanced MRI of cartilage (dGEMRIC) and T2 characteristics of human knee articular cartilage: topographical variation and relationships to mechanical properties. *Magn Reson Med*. 2004;52:41-46.
41. Li G, Lopez O, Rubash H. Variability of a three-dimensional finite element model constructed using magnetic resonance images of a knee for joint contact stress analysis. *J Biomech Eng*. 2001;123(4):341-346.
42. Lim R, Fahey FH, Drubach LA, et al. Early experience with fluorine-18 sodium fluoride bone PET in young patients with back pain. *J Pediatr Orthop*. 2007;27:277-282.
43. Lloyd DG, Besier TF. An EMG-driven musculoskeletal model to estimate muscle forces and knee joint moments in vivo. *J Biomech*. 2003;36:765-776.
44. Lorberboym M, Ami DB, Zin D, et al. Incremental diagnostic value of 99 mTc methylene diphosphonate bone SPECT in patients with patellofemoral pain disorders. *Nucl Med Commun*. 2003;24:403-410.
45. Mach DB, Rogers SD, Sabino MC, et al. Origins of skeletal pain: sensory and sympathetic innervation of the mouse femur. *Neuroscience*. 2002;113:155-166.
46. MacIntyre NJ, Hill NA, Fellows RA, et al. Patellofemoral joint kinematics in individuals with and without patellofemoral pain syndrome. *J Bone Joint Surg*. 2006;88-A: 2596-2605.
47. Merchant AC, Mercer RL, Jacobsen RH, et al. Roentgenographic analysis of patellofemoral congruence. *J Bone Joint Surg*. 1974;56-A:1391-1396.
48. Mountney J, Senavongse W, Amis AA, et al. Tensile strength of the medial patellofemoral ligament before and after repair or reconstruction. *J Bone Joint Surg*. 2005; 87-B:36-40.
49. Naslund JE, Odenbring S, Naslund UB, et al. Diffusely increased bone scintigraphic uptake in patellofemoral pain syndrome. *Br J Sports Med*. 2005;39:162-165.

50. Nayak KS, Cunningham CH, Santos JM, et al. Real-time cardiac MRI at 3 tesla. *Magn Reson Med.* 2004;51: 655-660.
51. Nha KW, Papannagari R, Gill TJ, et al. In vivo patellar tracking: clinical motions and patellofemoral indices. *J Orthop Res.* 2008;26:1067-1074.
52. Pal S, Beaupre G, Delp S, et al. Variations in muscle forces affect patellofemoral contact areas and cartilage stresses. In: *Patellofemoral Pain Syndrome: International Research Retreat.* Baltimore: Elsevier; 2009.
53. Patel VV, Hall K, Ries M, et al. Magnetic resonance imaging of patellofemoral kinematics with weight-bearing. *J Bone Joint Surg.* 2003;85-A:2419-2424.
54. Powers CM, Ward SR, Fredericson M, et al. Patellofemoral kinematics during weight-bearing and non-weight-bearing knee extension in persons with lateral subluxation of the patella: a preliminary study. *J Orthop Sports Phys Ther.* 2003;33:677-685.
55. Sanchis-Alfonso V, Rosello-Sastre E, Martinez-Sanjuan V. Pathogenesis of anterior knee pain syndrome and functional patellofemoral instability in the active young. *Am J Knee Surg.* 1999;12:29-40.
56. Seisler AR, Sheehan FT. Normative three-dimensional patellofemoral and tibiofemoral kinematics: a dynamic, in vivo study. *IEEE Trans Biomed Eng.* 2007;54:1333-1341.
57. Sevcik MA, Luger NM, Mach DB, et al. Bone cancer pain: the effects of the bisphosphonate alendronate on pain, skeletal remodeling, tumor growth and tumor necrosis. *Pain.* 2004;111:169-180.
58. Souza RB, Powers CM. Differences in hip kinematics, muscle strength, and muscle activation between subjects with and without patellofemoral pain. *J Orthop Sports Phys Ther.* 2009;39:12-19.
59. Stäubli HU, Schatzmann L, Brunner P, et al. Mechanical tensile properties of the quadriceps tendon and patellar ligament in young adults. *Am J Sports Med.* 1999;27: 27-34.
60. Taddei F, Schileo E, Helgason B, et al. The material mapping strategy influences the accuracy of CT-based finite element models of bones: an evaluation against experimental measurements. *Med Eng Phys.* 2007;29:973-979.
61. Tennant S, Williams A, Vedi V, et al. Patello-femoral tracking in the weight-bearing knee: a study of asymptomatic volunteers utilising dynamic magnetic resonance imaging: a preliminary report. *Knee Surg Sports Traumatol Arthrosc.* 2001;9:155-162.
62. Toegel S, Hoffmann O, Wadsak W, et al. Uptake of bone-seekers is solely associated with mineralisation! A study with 99mTc-MDP, 153Sm-EDTMP and 18F-fluoride on osteoblasts. *Eur J Nucl Med Mol Imaging.* 2006;33: 491-494.
63. Tomiya M, Fujikawa K, Ichimura S, et al. Skeletal unloading induces a full-thickness patellar cartilage defect with increase of urinary collagen II CTx degradation marker in growing rats. *Bone.* 2009;44(2):295-305.
64. Van Tiggelen D, Cowan S, Coorevits P, et al. Delayed vastus medialis obliquus to vastus lateralis onset timing contributes to the development of patellofemoral pain in previously healthy men: a prospective study. *Am J Sports Med.* 2009;37:1099-1105.
65. Ward SR, Terk MR, Powers CM. Patella alta: association with patellofemoral alignment and changes in contact area during weight-bearing. *J Bone Joint Surg.* 2007;89-A: 1749-1755.
66. Witonski D, Wagrowska-Danielewicz M. Distribution of substance-P nerve fibers in the knee joint in patients with anterior knee pain syndrome. A preliminary report. *Knee Surg Sports Traumatol Arthrosc.* 1999;7:177-183.
67. Witvrouw E, Sneyers C, Lysens R, et al. Reflex response times of vastus medialis oblique and vastus lateralis in normal subjects and in subjects with patellofemoral pain syndrome. *J Orthop Sports Phys Ther.* 1996;24:160-165.
68. Wojtys EM, Beaman DN, Glover RA, et al. Innervation of the human knee joint by substance-P fibers. *Arthroscopy.* 1990;6:254-263.
69. Yamada Y, Toritsuka Y, Horibe S, et al. In vivo movement analysis of the patella using a three-dimensional computer model. *J Bone Joint Surg.* 2007;9-B:752-760.

# 21 Computational Models for Investigating the Patellofemoral Joint: Clinical Relevance

John J. Elias and Andrew J. Cosgarea

## 21.1 Biomechanical Investigation of Patellofemoral Disorders

Conservative and surgical methods for treating patellofemoral disorders are commonly focused on improving patellofemoral biomechanics by balancing the forces acting on the patella. Due to the normal valgus alignment of the knee, the resultant force and moment acting on the patella from the quadriceps muscles and the patella tendon typically act to shift and tilt the patella laterally. If the lateral force and tilt moment are not properly balanced by other forces and moments acting on the patella, the patella can maltrack. Chronic tilt can lead to adaptive shortening of the lateral retinaculum, providing an additional lateral constraint on the patella.[27] Conservative treatment options include bracing and taping to provide a medial force to resist the lateral force applied by the quadriceps muscles and the patella tendon, as well as training the vastus medialis obliquus (VMO) to counter the forces applied by other components of the quadriceps muscle group. Surgical treatment options performed to decrease the lateral force and tilt moment acting on the patella include lateral retinacular release, medialization of the tibial tuberosity, reconstruction of the medial patellofemoral ligament (MPFL), and advancement of the VMO.

Due to the clinical focus on improving patellofemoral biomechanics for patients with pain and/or instability, biomechanical studies are commonly performed to investigate patellofemoral disorders and common treatment options. For these studies, the primary output parameters are loads applied to the patella by the quadriceps muscles, the patella tendon and the retinacular structures, patellofemoral kinematics, and the pressure applied to patellofemoral cartilage. Parameters related to patellofemoral loading are studied due to their influence on kinematics and cartilage pressures. Kinematics are studied as an indicator of risk of patellofemoral subluxation or instability, but also due to the influence on the pressure applied to cartilage. Maltracking with the knee extended, lateral maltracking in particular, can return to nearly normal once the patella enters the trochlear groove with early flexion (20–30°). The return to central trochlear tracking is due to the lateral trochlear ridge constraining the patella. As the articular force required to constrain the patella increases, cartilage pressures can increase.[17] Overloading cartilage can lead to areas of degradation, or lesions.[27,45] Cartilage lesions increase the pressure applied to the surrounding normal cartilage[22,30] and can lead to pain due to overloading of the subchondral bone.[26,27,42]

Studies investigating patellofemoral loading typically focus on the strength and activation timing of the VMO. These studies are commonly performed with EMG using live subjects. Some studies have indicated that patients with patellofemoral pain generate less force through the VMO than asymptomatic subjects.[37,51] The onset of VMO activity has also been shown to be delayed in patients with patellofemoral pain.[12-15,53] Data on the relative strengths and muscle orientations of the quadriceps muscles have also been obtained by measuring physiological cross-sectional areas (PCSAs) and pennation angles, or fiber orientations, in vitro,[24,55] although this data does not account for variations in the VMO that can be related

J.J. Elias (✉)
Calhoun Research Lab, Akron General Medical Center, Akron, OH, USA
e-mail: john.elias@akrongeneral.org

V. Sanchis-Alfonso (ed.), *Anterior Knee Pain and Patellar Instability*,
DOI: 10.1007/978-0-85729-507-1_21, © Springer-Verlag London Limited 2011

to patellofemoral disorders. In addition to providing valuable information to help assess the causes of patellofemoral disorders, the studies focused on quadriceps loading also provide data that is used to set loading levels for in vitro experimental and computational studies focused on patellofemoral biomechanics. In vitro studies focusing on passive constraints are also common, with several studies focused on the stiffness of the retinacular structures[11,16] and the distance between MPFL attachments on the femur and patella as the knee flexes.[49,50] Data on the properties of the retinacular structures is also incorporated into in vitro studies and computational modeling studies.

Alterations to patellofemoral loading lead to altered patellofemoral kinematics and contact areas. Patellofemoral kinematics and contact areas can be characterized in vivo utilizing diagnostic imaging. While imaging data has been used without additional graphical reconstruction of models to characterize patellofemoral kinematics and contact areas,[17,39,46] computational modeling can be combined with diagnostic imaging to enhance measurement capabilities. Graphical reconstruction provides 3-D models that can be used to create anatomical coordinate systems, align models from separate imaging sources, and identify areas of contact (Fig. 21.1).

Studies focused on the pressure applied to patellofemoral cartilage are commonly performed using in vitro experimental models. Simulated muscle forces are applied to cadaveric specimens while measuring the pressure applied to cartilage with sensors inserted into the joint. In vitro studies have typically focused on the influence of the position of the tibial tuberosity on the patellofemoral pressure distribution.[3,31,43,44]

Computational models have been developed to characterize the pressure applied to patellofemoral cartilage in order to overcome some of the limitations of in vitro experimental models. In vitro studies do not typically represent the young patient population[37,51] that seeks treatment for patellofemoral pain. Anatomical conditions that can contribute to patellofemoral disorders, such as femoral anteversion, tibial torsion, patella alta, a hypoplastic lateral trochlear ridge or genu valgum are also not typically represented in vitro. Cartilage lesions can be created in vitro,[22] but the size and position of lesions are limited. The testing frames and condition of the cadaveric specimens commonly require application of sub-physiologic load levels.[3,44] The number of sensors that can be applied within an experimental environment is limited, and tissue degradation limits the number of parametric variations that can be performed with a single specimen. The expense and time required to perform cadaveric studies also hinders the progress of patellofemoral biomechanics studies. While computational modeling can address these limitations, inherent to computational modeling are concerns related to the accuracy and clinical relevance of the computational output.

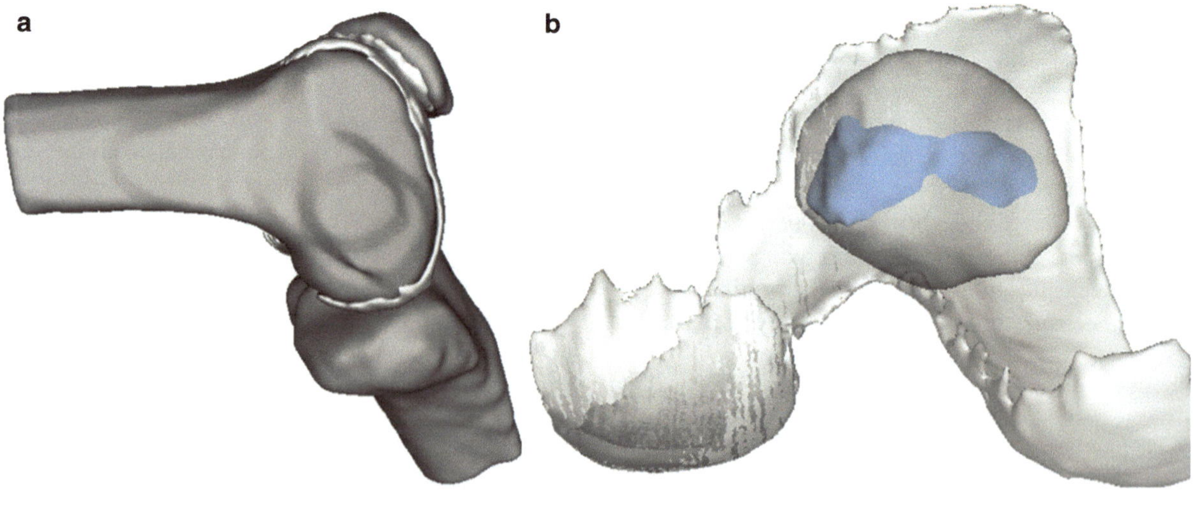


**Fig. 21.1** Graphical representation of a flexed knee, showing the femur, patella, tibia, and the cartilage on the femur and patella (**a**). Manipulating the model to remove the femur and make the cartilage on the femur transparent allows visualization of the area of patellofemoral contact (**b**)

## 21.2 Computational Modeling

A computational model of the patellofemoral joint is a graphical representation of joint anatomy that can be manipulated to reproduce or simulate joint function. Three-dimensional representations of joint anatomy are typically constructed from imaging data obtained from knees. Currently, MRI data is most commonly used to create computational models that include representations of the femur, patella, and tibia, with representation of the patellofemoral cartilage included in many models (Fig. 21.1). Computational models are frequently developed for studies focused on patellofemoral kinematics and contact areas, with the models showing 3-D representations of anatomical structures and motions that are captured during diagnostic imaging. Computational models can also be further developed to mathematically represent the mechanical characteristics of the represented anatomy. Muscle forces and passive restraints can also be applied to these models to allow computational characterization of the influence of variations in patellofemoral loading on kinematics and the pressure applied to cartilage.

The clinical relevance of a computational model is determined by the ability to investigate issues of interest to clinicians and the accuracy of the modeling technique. Developing computational models requires balancing the clinical relevance of the questions being investigated and the accuracy of the models. While a computational model showing motion of a knee from a patient in a MRI scanner can accurately reconstruct the motion, the computational models provide limited data that could not be obtained from the imaging data alone. These in vivo studies are also limited by the patient populations that can be recruited to participate. Modifications made to a computational model to provide additional output parameters require adding assumptions and mathematical representations of tissues, which can influence the accuracy of the computational output.

Characterizing the accuracy of a computational model requires experimental validation. In order to validate a computational model, computational data is compared to data that is known to be accurately measured, or a "gold standard." Validation should be performed with a test setup that allows collection of the gold standard data under the same testing conditions utilized to acquire the imaging data that is used to create the models. The validation should also be performed for test conditions that are similar to those that will be used when the model is utilized to generate clinically relevant data. In addition, the validation should compare computational to experimental data for each variable that will be utilized in future computational studies.

Methods of experimental validation vary with the function of the computational models. For models that characterize patellofemoral kinematics using diagnostic imaging, validation studies are commonly performed by simulating knee function in vitro with cadaveric knees with tantalum beads inserted into the femur, tibia, and patella.[7,25,33] Tantalum beads are considered to be rigidly fixed in the bones, and the beads are easily identifiable in MRI and CT images. With beads in place, knee motion can be reconstructed and quantified with respect to an anatomical coordinate system using Roentgen stereophotogrammetric analysis (RSA), serving as the gold standard data for models developed without considering the bead positions. For models that focus on predicting patellofemoral kinematics and cartilage pressures as a function of loading conditions, rather than computationally reproducing in vivo motion, models are generally constructed to represent knees tested in vitro for validation. Experimentally measured patellofemoral kinematics,[1,28,32] contact areas,[32] and cartilage pressures[21,23] are compared to computationally determined data to validate the models. In vivo data can also be used to evaluate a predictive computational model when a parameter such as the contact area can be measured in vivo and predicted computationally with models representing the subjects.[5]

## 21.3 Enhanced Display of Patellofemoral Kinematics

The most straightforward way to create graphical models displaying patellofemoral kinematics is to have subjects perform functional activities with their knees in a closed-bore MRI scanner (1.5T or higher). In order for the data to be clinically relevant, subjects should perform functional activities that induce realistic levels of muscle activation and cover the range of flexion angles of interest. Muscle activation is induced by creating a nonmetallic loading frame that can be placed in the MRI suite. A typical design induces simulated weight-bearing in a supine patient by allowing the patient to press against resistance at the heal, with

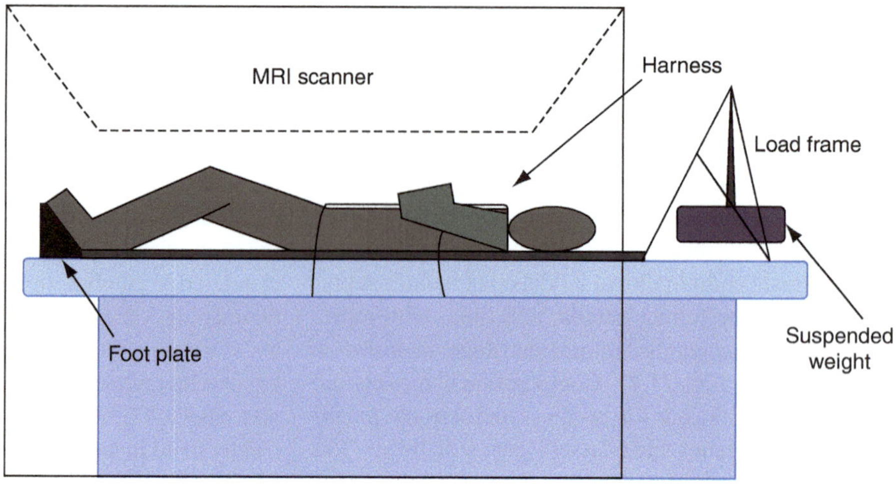


**Fig. 21.2** Representation of a subject in a MRI scanner for a study focused on enhanced visualization of patellofemoral kinematics. Muscle loading is induced by applying a force to the foot plate, which is connected to the weight outside of the scanner

support at the shoulders. The resistance is controlled by connecting weights outside of the scanner to a foot plate (Fig. 21.2).[36,41] This technique requires full scans at each flexion angle under investigation. To overcome this limitation, one high-resolution scan with the knee extended can be combined with low-resolution scans taken with the knee flexed to multiple flexion angles. Computational models are developed from each set of scans, and the bones created from the high-resolution scan are aligned with the bones created from the low-resolution scans at each flexion angle using an iterative closest point algorithm,[6] providing a representation of the knee at each flexion angle with a model reconstructed from the high-resolution images.[35,36] Because the additional computational alignment creates a potential source of error when quantifying kinematics with respect to an anatomical coordinate system, this method requires additional experimental validation. Comparison of in vitro kinematics between data based on this technique and data obtained by aligning models based on the position of implanted tantalum beads produced errors of 0.3–1.8° for the three rotations and 0.5–0.9 mm for the three translations.[25] An additional concern is that subjects can flex their knees only to about 50° in a closed-bore scanner. By 50°, only the distal patella has engaged with the trochlear groove. To allow a larger range of flexion, some studies have been performed using open coil magnets (0.2 T).[29,54] Because of the lower resolution of the open coil magnets, contact area measurements for this technique were compared to values obtained using a closed-bore magnet, with the correlation between the two depending on the sequence used for the open MRI scans.[29]

Due to the limited functional activities that can be performed in a MRI scanner, techniques have been developed to computationally replicate motions performed in a more natural environment. These techniques also utilize a combination of low resolution and high-resolution imaging. The low-resolution scans are performed using imaging modalities that provide 2-D images. High-resolution scans are also performed using CT or MRI to provide a 3-D model, and mathematical and graphical alignments of the 3-D model with the 2-D images is used to reconstruct motion in 3-D. The primary 2-D imaging modalities used for studies on patellofemoral kinematics are dual-plane fluoroscopy[40,52] and biplane X-ray.[7] For the dual-plane fluoroscopy system, subjects perform functional activities within the overlapping imaging field of two fluoroscopes, which are aligned perpendicular to one another. The experimental environment, including cameras representing the two fluoroscopes, is reproduced in a virtual environment on a computer (Fig. 21.3). At each position investigated, the two fluoroscopic images are imported into the virtual image intensifiers. Full 3-D models of joints created from MRI data are computationally aligned with the outlines from the two fluoroscopy images by adjusting all 6 degrees of freedom. For the biplane X-ray method, the 3-D model is developed from CT data, and a ray tracing algorithm is used to create digitally reconstructed radiographs for alignment with the 2-D images. Alignment takes into account the internal density features within the bones, as well as the bone outlines. For both techniques, measured kinematics have been compared to

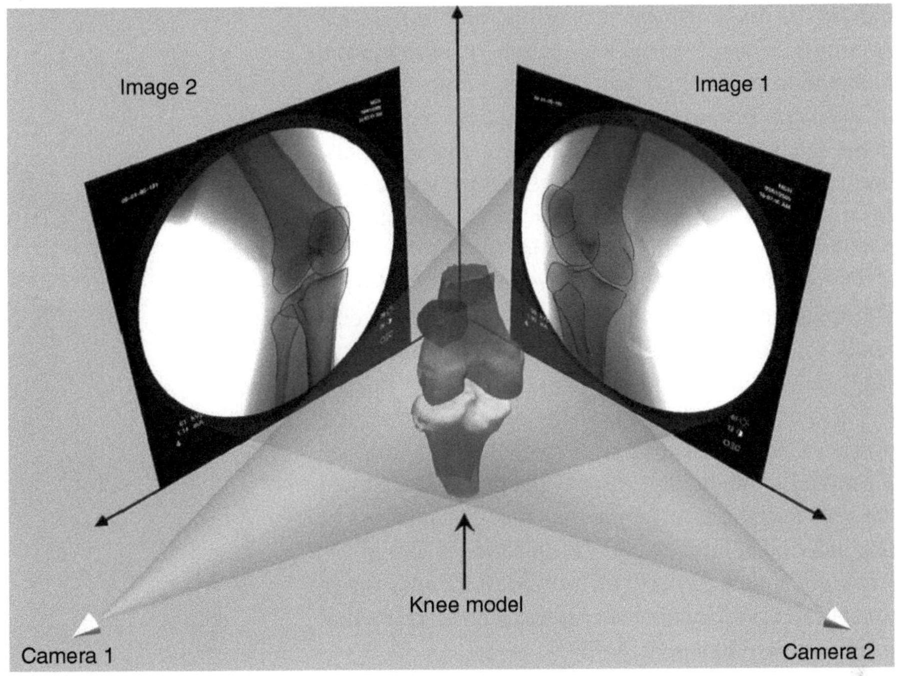


**Fig. 21.3** For the dual-orthogonal fluoroscopic image system used for enhanced visualization of patellofemoral kinematics, a virtual system is developed to align computational models of knees constructed from MRI data with the images acquired with the fluoroscopy units (From Nha et al.[40]) with permission

measurements obtained in vitro with beads within the bones.[7,33] Reported errors in kinematic measurements are less than 0.5 mm for translations and 1° for rotations.

While the methods used for enhanced display of patellofemoral kinematics produce data with sufficient accuracy to be clinically relevant, the relevant data produced to date has been limited. The detailed validation studies have been followed up with relatively few studies with subjects with patellofemoral disorders. One study showed that the overall pattern of patellar motion up to 50° of flexion was similar for subjects with patellofemoral pain with and without evidence of malalignment and asymptomatic subjects, although the patella tended to be shifted about 2 mm more laterally for the malalignment group than for the asymptomatic group at approximately 20° of flexion.[35] Another study indicated that the patellofemoral contact area is smaller for patients with patellofemoral subluxation than for asymptomatic subjects.[29] One study focused on the influence of ACL injury on patellofemoral kinematics and contact areas.[52] The study showed that ACL injury decreased patellofemoral flexion, increased the valgus rotation, and increased lateral tilt, while the contact area shifted proximally and laterally on the patella.

The limited clinically relevant data is related to the limitations of enhanced display of patellofemoral kinematics. Aside from the limited functional activities that can be performed in a closed-bore scanner, the studies are limited by the study populations. The analyses only focus on existing joint function. In order to study the influence of a disorder or treatment on kinematics, a control group is needed. For ACL injuries, an uninjured contralateral knee is commonly used as a control,[52] but the high incidence of bilateral malalignment makes this approach difficult for patellofemoral disorders. Control groups of patients without patellofemoral disorders have been utilized.[29,35] Evaluating patients before and after treatment is an approach that could be utilized in future studies to characterize the influence of treatment of kinematics.

## 21.4 Computational Prediction of Patellofemoral Kinematics and Cartilage Pressures

Predictive computational models allow direct assessment of the influence of anatomical variables and conservative and surgical treatment methods on patellofemoral biomechanics. These models are created from imaging data to replicate patellofemoral anatomy, but include mathematical representation of muscle forces, cartilage properties, and soft tissue restraints. Output variables include patellofemoral kinematics, areas of contact, and the pressure applied to cartilage. Because of the mathematical representations and approximations included in these models, there is a greater risk of inaccurate results, so the need for validation is greater than for models displaying patellofemoral kinematics of subjects.

Computational models have been constructed from CT images and MRI, although MRI is preferable currently to allow reconstruction of the bones and cartilage and eliminate exposure to radiation. MRI images can also be used to help locate the origin and insertion points of the quadriceps muscles and patella tendon on the models,[5] although previously published anatomical data is necessary to represent the orientations of the individual muscles of the quadriceps group.[15,24] Anatomical data can also be utilized to identify insertion points for retinacular structures, such as the medial patellofemoral ligament (MPFL).[20]

In engineering disciplines, finite element analysis is typically utilized to characterize the stresses and strains within structures. Finite element analysis has been applied to the patellofemoral joint to characterize kinematics, areas of contact, and pressure applied to cartilage. Each anatomical structure included in a finite element model is divided into interconnected elements (Fig. 21.4), with properties assigned to each element based on the material properties of the structure. Since finite element analysis quantifies the deformation of each element, the computational power required for models representing all structures of the patellofemoral joint can become unreasonable. Therefore, numerous simplifications are incorporated into the models. Bones are typically treated as rigid structures and cartilage is typically assumed to be linearly elastic, although a finite element model incorporating deformable bone and treating cartilage as an elastic nearly incompressible neo-Hookean material has been developed.[28] Tibiofemoral kinematics are generally prescribed, although a model incorporating tibiofemoral freedom has also been developed.[47] The patella tendon is typically modeled as a deformable element with individual fibers. As for the retinacular structures, some models ignore their influence,[5,28] while others represent the medial and lateral patellofemoral ligaments.[1,47] Even with the simplifications noted, the computational demands can limit the functionality of finite element models. Finite element analysis studies focused on the influence of muscle forces or joint anatomy on patellofemoral forces and pressures typically include only one model[4,38,47] or include analysis at only a single flexion angle.[5]

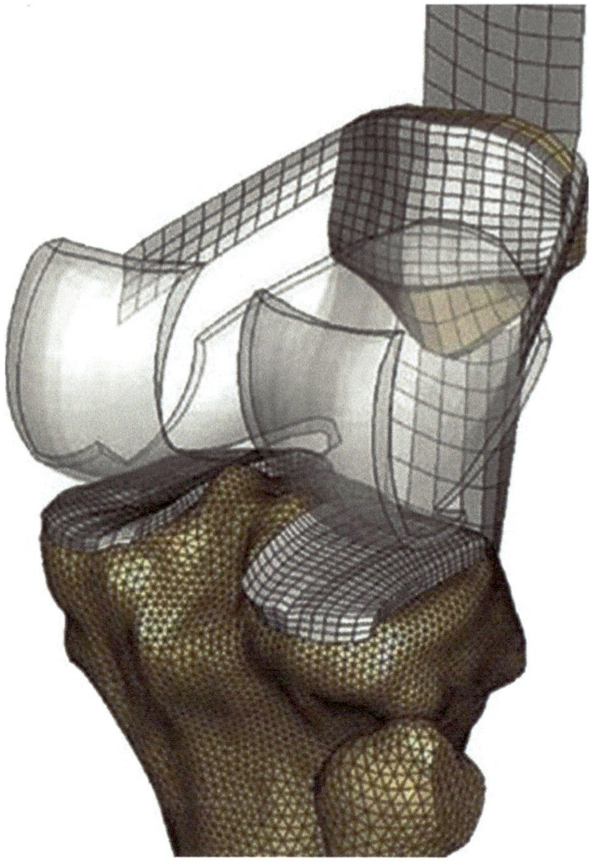

**Fig. 21.4** Representation of a fiite element model of the patellofemoral joint, showing the mesh assigned to the tibia and patella, as well as the cartilage on the tibia and patella. Meshes are also shown for the representation of the quadriceps tendon, the patella tendon, and the medial and lateral patellofemoral ligaments. The femur and mesh on the femoral cartilage have been removed for clarity (Reprinted from J Biomech 42: Baldwin et al.[1] With permission from Elsevier)

The computational power required to simulate patellofemoral function is dramatically reduced for some models by simplifying the representation of cartilage. Within a finite element model, the cartilage can be represented as a rigid surface with contact based on a linear pressure-over closure relationship.[1] Using a similar formulation for cartilage, computational programs have been created to simulate patellofemoral function without utilizing finite element analysis software.[23,32] These programs treat the cartilage as layers of springs on the femur and patella. The pressure within each spring can be represented with linear elastic theory for an isotropic material as[8]:

$$p = \frac{E(1-v)d}{(1+v)(1-2v)h}$$

where $E$ is the elastic modulus, $v$ is the Poisson's ratio, $h$ is the thickness, and $d$ is the spring deformation. The reduced computational demand also allows representation of strain hardening of the cartilage. For this case, the pressure within each spring is represented as[8,21]:

$$p = \frac{-E(1-v)\ln(1-d/h)}{(1+v)(1-2v)}$$

Models that utilize custom-written code can also be built and manipulated faster than models that are created and manipulated using finite element analysis software, allowing analysis of four or more models at multiple flexion angles for various loading conditions.[9,10,20,21] For the modeling technique developed by the authors,[18-20] the time required to flex a model of a knee, apply loading conditions, and quantify the patellofemoral force and pressure distributions is under 2 min on a multiprocessor desktop PC. At a given flexion angle, parameters such as the forces applied by the quadriceps muscles and the location of cartilage lesions can be varied and the force and pressure distributions can be recalculated in under 1 min.

For all predictive models, the primary loading inputs are the forces applied by the quadriceps muscles. The quadriceps force has typically been divided among the muscles of the quadriceps group based on the physiological cross-sectional area of each muscle.[24,55] The contribution of each muscle of the quadriceps group to the total knee extension moment derived from the combination of electrical stimulation and EMG measurements has also been utilized.[56] The quadriceps force distribution can be individualized for patients by replicating simulated activities in a laboratory while recording EMG data from the quadriceps muscles. When the EMG data is combined with kinematic data, the quadriceps muscle forces can be estimated using a modified Hill-type muscle model.[34]

The primary advantage of predictive computational modeling is the ability to manipulate the model. Parameters that are commonly manipulated include the orientation of the patella tendon, forces applied by the quadriceps muscles, and the properties of the retinacular structures. Other parameters that can be manipulated include the properties of patellofemoral cartilage, patellofemoral alignment, and tibiofemoral alignment. While the primary output is typically the force and pressure distributions within the patellofemoral cartilage, the forces applied by all soft tissues that are not input to the model can be calculated. The resultant force and moment acting on the patella due to the forces applied by the quadriceps muscles, the patella tendon, and the retinacular structures can also be calculated. Patellofemoral kinematics and the area of contact can also be quantified. Models can be created to represent knees with patellofemoral disorders or normal knees, and physiologically realistic loading levels can be applied.

The primary concern for predictive models is the accuracy of the computational output. The accuracy of the computational output is influenced by all the data input to the model. Approximated parameters that can dramatically influence computational output include the magnitude and orientation of the forces used to represent the quadriceps muscles, the stiffness and orientation of the retinacular structures and the patella tendon, and the properties assigned to the cartilage. The accuracy of the computational output is also influenced by the governing equations used to simulate knee function. Validation studies comparing in vitro or in vivo experimental data to computational data should be performed for all predictive models to assess accuracy. Ideally, the validation should be performed while varying parameters similar to those that will be varied for studies designed to produce clinically relevant data. In addition, the validation should compare computational to experimental data for each variable that will be computationally predicted. Several methods have been utilized to validate existing predictive computational models of the patellofemoral joint. Validation has been performed by comparing in vitro experimental measurements of patellofemoral kinematics to computational measurements.[1,28,32] Other models have been validated in comparison to in vitro measurements[32] and in vivo[5] measurements of contact area. The modeling technique developed by the authors was validated by comparing in vitro measurements of the influence of variations in quadriceps loading on the distribution of

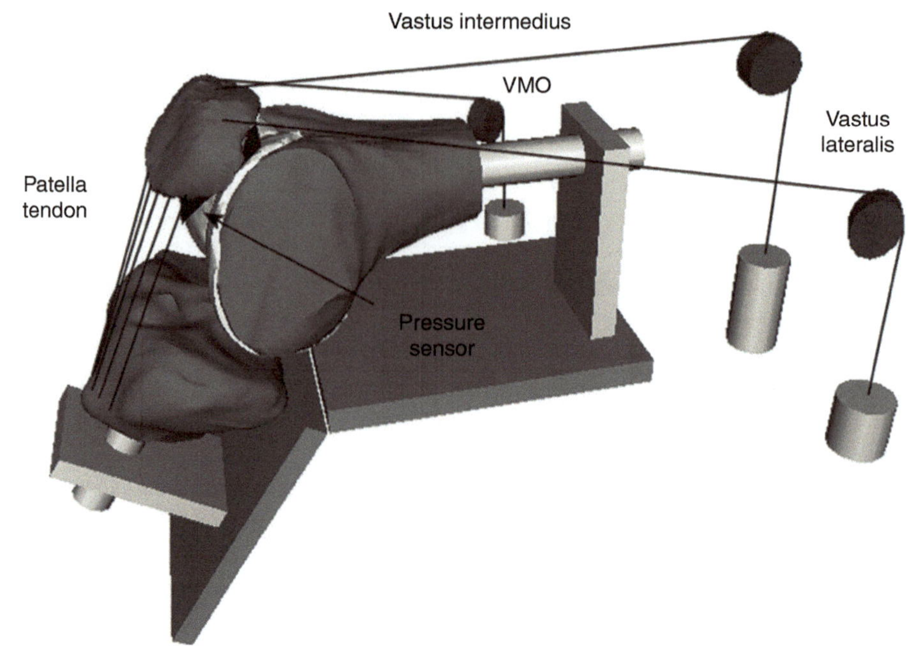


**Fig. 21.5** Computational model of a flexed knee, embedded in a graphical representation of an in vitro testing frame used to validate the computational model. The loading cables used to apply forces through the quadriceps muscles are represented, along with representations of the pulleys and weights. The line segments representing the patella tendon are also shown, along with the position of the pressure sensor used to experimentally measure patellofemoral pressures (Adapted from Elias et al.[21])

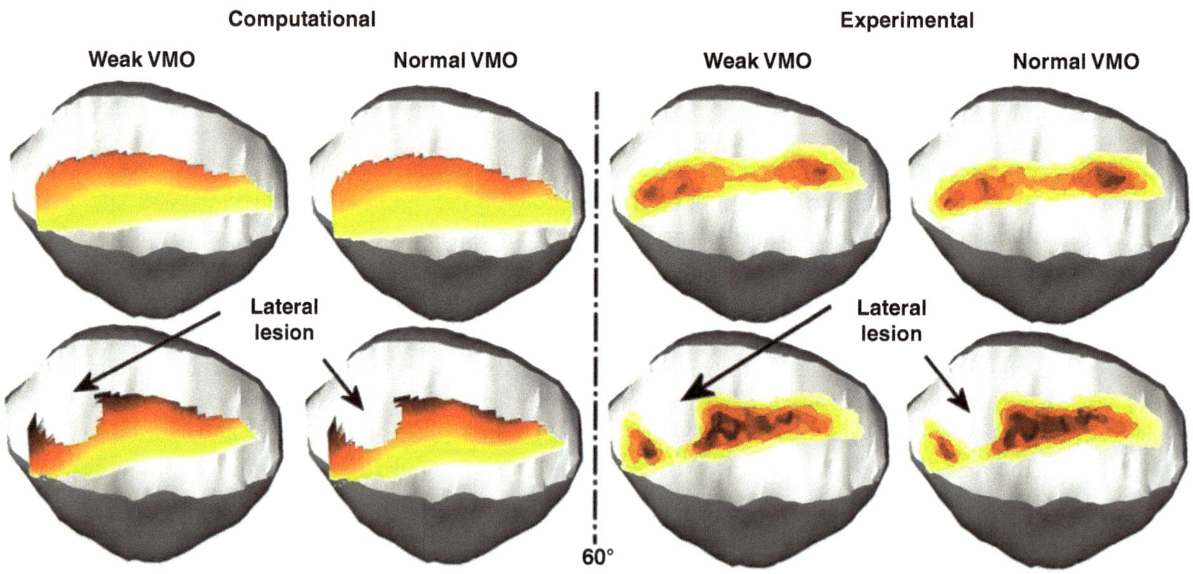


**Fig. 21.6** Computationally determined and experimentally determined pressure patterns superimposed over a graphical representation of the patella for one knee at 60° of flexion. The pressure distribution is shown for a weak VMO and a normal VMO, for intact cartilage and cartilage with a lateral lesion. Decreasing the force applied by the VMO shifts pressure laterally on the patella (Reprinted from Elias et al.[21])

force between the lateral and medial facets, the maximum lateral pressure and the maximum medial pressure to computational measurements[21,23] (Fig. 21.5). For one study, the comparisons were performed for both intact cartilage and cartilage with a lateral lesion[21] (Fig. 21.6). Data obtained from an unvalidated model or validated with test conditions or output parameters different from those used to generate clinically relevant data should be considered with care. In some cases, even unvalidated data can be beneficial if the model helps explain similar data obtained in vitro or helps explain clinical findings.

Clinically relevant data has been obtained from computational models of the patellofemoral joint. Several studies have focused on tibial tuberosity realignment and the force applied by the VMO. Tibial tuberosity anteriorization has been shown to decrease patellofemoral contact forces and pressures over the majority of the flexion angles tested, although pressure increases near 90° were noted.[4,9,47] An experimental study indicated that anteriorizing the tibial tuberosity tended to decrease contact forces and pressures for all flexion angles tested, although the changes were smallest at 90°.[44] Computational studies have shown that medialization of the tibial tuberosity tends to decrease maximum contact pressures,[9,18,19] with the maximum lateral pressure decreasing as the maximum medial pressure increases.[4] An experimental study also showed a decrease in the maximum pressure and a shift in force from lateral to medial following tibial tuberosity medialization.[43] Computational studies have also shown that decreasing the force applied to the VMO tends to produce a small increase in the maximum pressure.[18,19] An in vitro study showed that decreasing the VMO force produced a small, but significant increase in the maximum lateral pressure and a corresponding decrease in the maximum medial pressure.[22] Another computational study indicated that anatomical reconstruction of the MPFL has minimal influence on the patellofemoral pressure distribution, but using a short graft or proximal malpositioning of the graft on the femur tends to increase the maximum medial pressure, with the increase being significant at most flexion angles when the errors are combined.[20] An in vitro study indicated that the maximum medial pressure tended to increase when the tension in the reconstructed MPFL reached 10 N.[2]

## 21.5 Limitations of Computational Modeling and Future Directions

Currently, computational models still are limited in the ability to represent patellofemoral dysplasia. While muscle forces and orientations and cartilage conditions can be easily manipulated to represent pathology, varying the shape of the bone is more difficult. Models can be created from imaging data obtained from symptomatic knees to incorporate patellofemoral dysplasia, but patellofemoral dysplasia can vary markedly between symptomatic patients. A group of subjects recruited as a source for modeling could include those with a shallow trochlear groove, femoral anteverison, patella alta, or other anatomical conditions that contribute to patellofemoral disorders. Creating models from patients does not provide control of the dysplasia to determine cause and effect of a single parameter. In order to control a single parameter, manipulation of models to vary anatomy in a manner that represents dysplasia is necessary. While morphing algorithms have been created for computational models of the musculoskeletal system,[48] these can be difficult to apply to the patellofemoral joint. Shape changes related to dysplasia do not occur along a single anatomical axis or within a single plane. Also, variations in the anatomy of the patella or femur do not happen in isolation. A dysplastic condition that influences the trochlear groove also influences the forces applied to the patella, with the shape of the patella modifying during development to conform to the femur.

Computational models are also limited by the output that can be generated. The primary output obtained from computational models includes patellofemoral kinematics, contact areas, and the pressure applied to cartilage. Of these, pressure measurements are most directly related to patellofemoral pain due to the belief that overloading cartilage leads to degeneration and subsequent overloading of subchondral bone. Pain can develop within other structures of the patellofemoral joint, however. Stretching of an adaptively shortened lateral retinaculum with increasing knee flexion can be a source of pain, as can a pathologic medial plical fold. While computational models do not provide data related to all sources of pain, modeling can generate output that reflects parameters clinicians attempt to manipulate with conservative and surgical treatment.

Computational representation of instability has yet to be achieved. The mathematical methods used to simulate patellofemoral function typically require balanced forces to generate solutions. An instability episode creates mathematical instability as well, complicating attempts to computationally assess the risk of instability. The total force acting in the lateral direction or division of force between the lateral and medial facet can be used to provide some information related to the risk of instability,[18,19] although these are indirect measures.

Advancements in computational resources will lead to future improvements in computational modeling. The cost of computational power continues to decrease, which will reduce the time needed for the analysis of complex models in the future. Software approaches for automated and semi-automated segmentation of medical imaging continues to improve, which decreases the time needed to create computational models, allowing more models to be developed for research purposes. The improved techniques for model reconstruction and increased computational power could decrease the time needed for model development and analysis to the point that models could be developed to represent individual symptomatic knees and analyzed fast enough to evaluate treatment options. If modeling is used to assess treatment options for individual patients, validation will become even more important. Morphing techniques also continue to be developed, which should allow users more control of patellofemoral anatomy in the future.

Developments in diagnostic imaging will also lead to further improvements in computational modeling. Improvements in imaging include increased field strength, increased bore sizes, and improved imaging sequences for evaluating cartilage. Increased field strength improves the resolution of anatomical structures for reconstruction of models. Increased bore sizes without loss of field strength will allow more activities to be performed in a scanner. As more activities are performed in scanners, enhanced representation of patellofemoral kinematics will become more relevant. The models used for enhanced representation of kinematics can also be incorporated into predictive computational models to improve the input to these models. Combining enhanced representation of kinematics with predictive models will provide improved assessment of pathologic conditions for subjects being studied, along with parametric assessment of multiple treatment methods. Also, advances in sequences to represent cartilage, such as T1 rho and T2 mapping, will allow improved assessment of cartilage properties based on diagnostic imaging data. Improved assessment of cartilage properties will also improve the accuracy of the data input to predictive models.

## References


1. Baldwin MA, Clary C, Maletsky LP, et al. Verification of predicted specimen-specific natural and implanted patellofemoral kinematics during simulated deep knee bend. *J Biomech.* 2009;42:2341-2348.
2. Beck P, Brown NA, Greis PE, et al. Patellofemoral contact pressures and lateral patellar translation after medial patellofemoral ligament reconstruction. *Am J Sports Med.* 2007; 35:1557-1563.
3. Beck PR, Thomas AL, Farr J, et al. Trochlear contact pressures after anteromedialization of the tibial tubercle. *Am J Sports Med.* 2005;33:1710-1715.
4. Benvenuti JF, Rakotomanana L, Leyvraz PF, et al. Displacements of the tibial tuberosity. Effects of the surgical parameters. *Clin Orthop Relat Res.* 1997;343:224-234.
5. Besier TF, Gold GE, Delp SL, et al. The influence of femoral internal and external rotation on cartilage stresses within the patellofemoral joint. *J Orthop Res.* 2008;26:1627-1635.
6. Besl P, McKay N. A method for registration of 3-D shapes. *IEEE Trans Pattern Anal Mach Intell.* 1992;14:239-256.
7. Bey MJ, Kline SK, Tashman S, et al. Accuracy of biplane x-ray imaging combined with model-based tracking for measuring in-vivo patellofemoral joint motion. *J Orthop Surg.* 2008;3:38.
8. Blankevoort L, Kuiper J, Huiskes R, et al. Articular contact in a three-dimensional model of the knee. *J Biomech.* 1991;24:1019-1031.
9. Cohen ZA, Henry JH, McCarthy DM, et al. Computer simulations of patellofemoral joint surgery. Patient-specific models for tuberosity transfer. *Am J Sports Med.* 2003;31:87-98.
10. Cohen ZA, Roglic H, Grelsamer RP, et al. Patellofemoral stresses during open and closed kinetic chain exercises. An analysis using computer simulation. *Am J Sports Med.* 2001; 29:480-487.
11. Conlan T, Garth WP Jr, Lemons JE. Evaluation of the medial soft-tissue restraints of the extensor mechanism of the knee. *J Bone Joint Surg.* 1993;75-A:682-693.
12. Cowan SM, Bennell KL, Hodges PW. Therapeutic patellar taping changes the timing of vasti muscle activation in people with patellofemoral pain syndrome. *Clin J Sport Med.* 2002;12:339-347.
13. Cowan SM, Bennell KL, Hodges PW, et al. Delayed onset of electromyographic activity of vastus medialis obliquus relative to vastus lateralis in subjects with patellofemoral pain syndrome. *Arch Phys Med Rehabil.* 2001;82:183-189.
14. Cowan SM, Bennell KL, Hodges PW, et al. Simultaneous feedforward recruitment of the vasti in untrained postural tasks can be restored by physical therapy. *J Orthop Res.* 2003;21:553-558.
15. Delp SL, Loan JP, Hoy MG, et al. An interactive, graphics-based model of the lower extremity to study orthopaedic surgical procedures. *IEEE Trans Biomed Eng.* 1990;37:557-567.
16. Desio SM, Burks RT, Bachus KN. Soft tissue restraints to lateral patellar translation in the human knee. *Am J Sports Med.* 1998;26:59-65.
17. Draper CE, Besier TF, Santos JM, et al. Using real-time MRI to quantify altered joint kinematics in subjects with patellofemoral pain and to evaluate the effects of a patellar brace or sleeve on joint motion. *J Orthop Res.* 2009;27:571-577.
18. Elias JJ, Bratton DR, Weinstein DM, et al. Comparing two estimations of the quadriceps force distribution for use during patellofemoral simulation. *J Biomech.* 2006;39: 865-872.
19. Elias JJ, Cech JA, Weinstein DM, et al. Reducing the lateral force acting on the patella does not consistently decrease patellofemoral pressures. *Am J Sports Med.* 2004;32: 1202-1208.

20. Elias JJ, Cosgarea AJ. Technical errors during medial patellofemoral ligament reconstruction could overload medial patellofemoral cartilage: a computational analysis. *Am J Sports Med.* 2006;34:1478-1485.
21. Elias JJ, Kilambi S, Cosgarea AJ. Computational assessment of the influence of vastus medialis obliquus function on patellofemoral pressures: model evaluation. *J Biomech.* 2010;43(4):612-617.
22. Elias JJ, Kilambi S, Goerke DR, et al. Improving vastus medialis obliquus function reduces pressure applied to lateral patellofemoral cartilage. *J Orthop Res.* 2009;27:578-583.
23. Elias JJ, Wilson DR, Adamson R, et al. Evaluation of a computational model used to predict the patellofemoral contact pressure distribution. *J Biomech.* 2004;37:295-302.
24. Farahmand F, Senavongse W, Amis AA. Quantitative study of the quadriceps muscles and trochlear groove geometry related to instability of the patellofemoral joint. *J Orthop Res.* 1988;16:136-143.
25. Fellows RA, Hill NA, Gill HS, et al. Magnetic resonance imaging for in vivo assessment of three-dimensional patellar tracking. *J Biomech.* 2005;38:1643-1652.
26. Fulkerson JP. Diagnosis and treatment of patients with patellofemoral pain. *Am J Sports Med.* 2002;30:447-456.
27. Fulkerson JP, Shea KP. Disorders of patellofemoral alignment. *J Bone Joint Surg.* 1990;72:1424-1429.
28. Heegaard J, Leyvraz PF, Curnier A, et al. The biomechanics of the human patella during passive knee flexion. *J Biomech.* 1995;28:1265-1279.
29. Hinterwimmer S, Gotthardt M, von Eisenhart-Rothe R, et al. In vivo contact areas of the knee in patients with patellar subluxation. *J Biomech.* 2005;38:2095-2101.
30. Huberti HH, Hayes WC. Contact pressures in chondromalacia patellae and the effects of capsular reconstructive procedures. *J Orthop Res.* 1988;6:499-508.
31. Kuroda R, Kambic H, Valdevit A, et al. Articular cartilage contact pressure after tibial tuberosity transfer. A cadaveric study. *Am J Sports Med.* 2001;29:403-409.
32. Kwak SD, Blankevoort L, Ateshian GA. A mathematical formulation for 3D quasi-static multibody models of diarthrodial joints. *Comput Methods Biomech Biomed Eng.* 2000;3:41-64.
33. Li G, Van de Velde SK, Bingham JT. Validation of a noninvasive fluoroscopic imaging technique for the measurement of dynamic knee joint motion. *J Biomech.* 2008;41:1616-1622.
34. Lloyd DG, Besier TF. An EMG-driven musculoskeletal model to estimate muscle forces and knee joint moments in vivo. *J Biomech.* 2003;36:765-776.
35. MacIntyre NJ, Hill NA, Fellows RA, et al. Patellofemoral joint kinematics in individuals with and without patellofemoral pain syndrome. *J Bone Joint Surg.* 2006;88-A:2596-2605.
36. Macintyre NJ, McKnight EK, Day A, et al. Consistency of patellar spin, tilt and lateral translation side-to-side and over a 1 year period in healthy young males. *J Biomech.* 2008;41:3094-3096.
37. Makhsous M, Lin F, Koh JL, et al. In vivo and noninvasive load sharing among the vasti in patellar malalignment. *Med Sci Sports Exerc.* 2004;36:1768-1775.
38. Mesfar W, Shirazi-Adl A. Biomechanics of the knee joint in flexion under various quadriceps forces. *Knee.* 2005;12:424-434.
39. Muhle C, Brinkmann G, Skaf A, et al. Effect of a patellar realignment brace on patients with patellar subluxation and dislocation. Evaluation with kinematic magnetic resonance imaging. *Am J Sports Med.* 1999;27:350-353.
40. Nha KW, Papannagari R, Gill TJ, et al. In vivo patellar tracking: clinical motions and patellofemoral indices. *J Orthop Res.* 2008;26:1067-1074.
41. Patel VV, Hall K, Ries M, et al. Magnetic resonance imaging of patellofemoral kinematics with weight-bearing. *J Bone Joint Surg.* 2003;85-A:2419-2424.
42. Powers C. Rehabilitation of patellofemoral joint disorders: a critical review. *J Orthop Sports Phys Ther.* 1998;28:345-354.
43. Ramappa AJ, Apreleva M, Harrold FR, et al. The effects of medialization and anteromedialization of the tibial tubercle on patellofemoral mechanics and kinematics. *Am J Sports Med.* 2006;34:749-756.
44. Rue JP, Colton A, Zare SM, et al. Trochlear contact pressures after straight anteriorization of the tibial tuberosity. *Am J Sports Med.* 2008;36:1953-1959.
45. Saleh KJ, Arendt EA, Eldridge J, et al. Symposium. Operative treatment of patellofemoral arthritis. *J Bone Joint Surg.* 2005;87-A:659-671.
46. Sheehan FT, Derasari A, Brindle TJ, et al. Understanding patellofemoral pain with maltracking in the presence of joint laxity: complete 3D in vivo patellofemoral and tibiofemoral kinematics. *J Orthop Res.* 2009;27:561-570.
47. Shirazi-Adl A, Mesfar W. Effect of tibial tubercle elevation on biomechanics of the entire knee joint under muscle loads. *Clin Biomech.* 2007;22:344-351.
48. Sigal IA, Hardisty MR, Whyne CM. Mesh-morphing algorithms for specimen-specific finite element modeling. *J Biomech.* 2008;41:1381-1389.
49. Smirk C, Morris H. The anatomy and reconstruction of the medial patellofemoral ligament. *Knee.* 2003;10:221-227.
50. Steensen RN, Dopirak RM, McDonald WG 3rd. The anatomy and isometry of the medial patellofemoral ligament: implications for reconstruction. *Am J Sports Med.* 2004;32:1509-1513.
51. Tang SF, Chen CK, Hsu R, et al. Vastus medialis obliquus and vastus lateralis activity in open and closed kinetic chain exercises in patients with patellofemoral pain syndrome: an electromyographic study. *Arch Phys Med Rehabil.* 2001;82:1441-1445.
52. Van de Velde SK, Gill TJ, DeFrate LE, et al. The effect of anterior cruciate ligament deficiency and reconstruction on the patellofemoral joint. *Am J Sports Med.* 2008;36:1150-1159.
53. Voight ML, Wieder DL. Comparative reflex response times of vastus medialis obliquus and VL in normal subjects and subjects with extensor mechanism dysfunction. An electromyographic study. *Am J Sports Med.* 1991;19:131-137.
54. von Eisenhart-Rothe R, Vogl T, Englmeier KH, et al. A new in vivo technique for determination of femoro-tibial and femoro-patellar 3D kinematics in total knee arthroplasty. *J Biomech.* 2007;40:3079-3088.
55. Ward SR, Eng CM, Smallwood LH, et al. Are current measurements of lower extremity muscle architecture accurate? *Clin Orthop Relat Res.* 2009;467:1074-1082.
56. Zhang LQ, Wang G, Nuber GW, et al. In vivo load sharing among the quadriceps components. *J Orthop Res.* 2003;21:565-571.

# Kinetic Analysis: A Sensitive Outcome Objective Measurement Method in Evaluating Lateral Patellar Instability

22

## A Preliminary Study

Vicente Sanchis-Alfonso, José María Baydal-Bertomeu, Erik Montesinos-Berry, Andrea Castelli, and José David Garrido-Jaén

*While the individual man is an absolute puzzle, in the aggregate he becomes a mathematical certainty. You can, for example, never foretell what any one man will do, but you can say with precision what an average number will be up to. Individuals vary, but percentages remain constant.*

*Sherlock Holmes, The Sign of Four*

## 22.1 Introduction

There are many diagnostic clinical tests (e.g., apprehension patellar test or the moving patellar apprehension test), outcome measures (general health and knee scales [IKDC form, Kujala scale, Fulkerson scale, Lysholm knee scoring scale, Tegner activity level scale, short form-36]), and instrumented measurements of patellar mobility (static stability), to assess lateral patellar instability.[7,10,15,16] However, according to Smith and colleagues,[15] the sensitivity/specificity – reliability/validity of such tests and outcome tools remain unclear for this patient population. These authors conclude that further work is needed to assess the appropriateness of these tests and outcomes.[15] Moreover, there are many surgical techniques to treat patients with chronic lateral patellar instability, all of them based on level of evidence IV or V.[4] This is due, in part, to the lack of prospective randomized trials, and also to the lack of an objective, suitable, reliable, valid, and reproducible noninvasive in vivo method to evaluate lateral patellar instability in the clinical setting. This makes it difficult to compare different surgical treatments in order to find the best surgical technique to treat patients with chronic lateral patellar instability.

In making decisions about the best method to manage chronic lateral patellar instability, it is important to consider the concept of evidence-based practice. Evidence-based practice integrates the best research evidence with the surgeon's clinical expertise and the patient's values and wishes. Given that clinical practice modification is based on outcome studies, the ability to measure clinical results is thus vital. Because of limitations of the current methods to assess clinical outcome after lateral patellar instability surgery, new technologies are needed to measure the benefits and to compare the surgeries more precisely.

For too long, a patient who did not complain and who returned to a high level of function was considered functionally intact. Our methods of measurement have improved so that we are now able to measure restoration of the anatomic form using computed tomography scan and magnetic resonance imaging. But, we can now ask for much more, the integration into the static equation of a dynamic understanding. That is, the objective would be the measurement during dynamic activities that cause a lateral subluxation or dislocation of the

V. Sanchis-Alfonso (✉)
International Patellofemoral Study Group,
International ACL Study Group, Hospital 9 de Octubre,
Hospital Arnau de Vilanova, School of Medicine,
Catholic University of Valencia,
Valencia, Spain
e-mail: vicente.sanchis.alfonso@gmail.com

V. Sanchis-Alfonso (ed.), *Anterior Knee Pain and Patellar Instability*,
DOI: 10.1007/978-0-85729-507-1_22, © Springer-Verlag London Limited 2011

patella, under realistic loading conditions (dynamic or functional instability). We believe that this objective could be reached by means of kinetic analysis.

To the best of our knowledge, no pre- and postoperative clinical studies of lateral patellar stability using kinetic analysis have been published. With kinetic analysis, it would be possible to critically evaluate the effectiveness of different surgical techniques for restoring lateral patellar stability and preventing patellofemoral osteoarthritis associated with patellofemoral instability.[3,8,9,14] The application of kinetic analysis in the objective assessment of lateral patellar instability is discussed in this chapter. We highlight the importance of developing new methods for in vivo evaluation of patellar instability under dynamic conditions, given that during functional activities the knee is subjected to a combination of active muscular forces and dynamic physical forces (gravitational, inertial, and contact forces).

## 22.2 Kinetic Analysis in Evaluating Lateral Patellar Instability

### 22.2.1 *What Is Kinetic Analysis?*

Kinetic analysis consists of the study of forces* and moments† that produce movement.[12] There are different techniques for kinetic analysis. Our study group in the "Instituto de Biomecánica of Valencia (IBV)" has focused for many years on the use of biomechanical techniques for human movement analysis.

*A force is a vectorial magnitude that can be defined as an action that tends to produce a movement of a body, which acquires an acceleration in proportion to the magnitude of the applied force. The force is defined as the product between mass and acceleration. In order to compare curves of different subjects, with different anthropometric characteristics, the force's signals are processed normalizing the subject's weight values.

$$\vec{F}(N)=m(kg).\vec{a}\left(\frac{m}{s^2}\right)$$

†A moment or torque is a force couple that produces a rotatory effect (Fig. 22.1). The moments are normalized due to a characteristic of a rotating body, the moment of inertia. Any body that rotates around an axis has rotation inertia, which is a resistance to change the rotation speed and the direction of the spin axis. Normalization enables us to make comparisons between subjects with different anthropometric characteristics.

$$\vec{M}(N.m)=\vec{F}(N)\times\vec{d}(m)$$

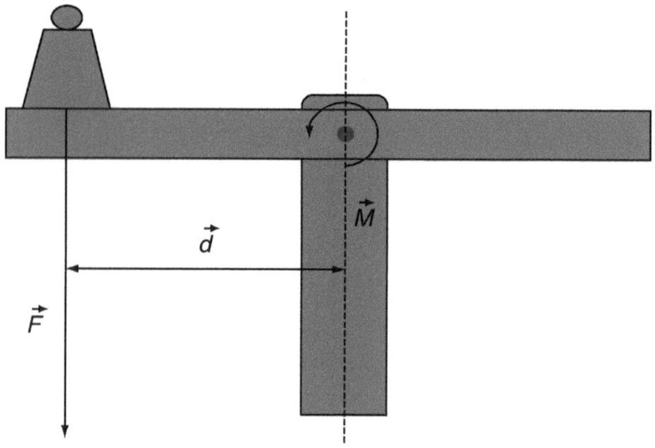


**Fig. 22.1** A moment is a force couple that produces a rotator effect

### 22.2.2 *Instruments: Dynamometric Platforms*

Currently, dynamometric platforms are the most extended technique for kinetic analysis. A dynamometric platform is an electronic instrument that measures and analyzes the reaction force that a person exerts on the ground during a certain movement or gesture.

Our kinetic analysis was performed using the dynamometric platform Dinascan/IBV (Instituto de Biomecánica de Valencia, Valencia, Spain), installed flush within the floor. The Dinascan/IBV platform has four extensometric transducers located at the four corners of the platform. Each transducer has eight extensometric sensors, four being sensitive to vertical loads and four being sensitive to horizontal loads. The arrangement of the sensors in the transducers has been established after studies with finite element models, eliminating a theoretical cross-sensitivity between both directions of the measurement. Two of the four transducers on the platform are sensitive to anteroposterior forces (as well as vertical ones) and the other two are sensitive to medial–lateral forces (as well as the vertical ones). With this information, the platform is capable of measuring the ground reaction moment. Each platform is equipped with an internal amplifier that sends high-level analog signals, protecting them from electromagnetic distortion. When a force acts on the dynamometric platform, it is distributed among these four transducers and the generated torque is also transmitted to the knee via the tibia. The platform's active area is 600 × 370 mm. The system has a measurement range from 200 to 1,500 N for vertical forces and from ±100 N to ±750 N for horizontal forces, with an accuracy of at least 98% of the highest measurement or 0.15% of the total range.

### 22.2.3 The Question Is: Is the Kinetic Analysis with Dynamometric Platforms a Good Method to Evaluate the Torsion Moments of the Knee?

The dynamometric platform registers the forces exerted by the subject against the ground and determines the exact point of application underneath the foot, which is called **c**enter **o**f **p**ressure (COP). This variable defines the projection point of our center of gravity on the platform. We consider that the moment registered with the platform could be a good estimation of the real torsional moment of the knee,[‡] because the COP nearly coincides with the vertical projection of the center of rotation of the knee joint (the differences are minimal mostly in the pivoting phase, which is the most important movement phase for our study), as we have demonstrated after stereophotogrammetry studies, during the task analyzed in our study (monopodal jumping with pivoting with external tibial rotation).

### 22.2.4 Which Is the Best "Provoking Activity" to Evaluate Lateral Patellar Instability? Task Proposed in Evaluating Lateral Patellar Instability. Clinical Rationale

Within the range of 0–30º of knee flexion, the patella is in its most unstable position. Soft tissues, mainly the medial patellofemoral ligament (MPFL), and alignment are the most important elements for the patella's stability in the range of 0–30º.[1,2] The Q-angle is largest in full extension because the tibia rotates externally in terminal knee extension (screw-home mechanism), moving the tibial tuberosity more laterally. This is the reason why in full extension, the patella is at greatest risk for dislocation.[4]

On the other hand, tibial external rotation over a planted foot produces a lateral displacement force on the patella due to the shift of the tibial tuberosity laterally that may end in dislocation or subluxation.[11]

Therefore, we believe that a maneuver of tibial external rotation over a planted foot, in the range of 0–30° of knee flexion, would be the best provoking activity to evaluate lateral patellar instability, because it mimics an actual dislocation or lateral patellar instability episode (Fig. 22.2). One way to twist the knee around a vertical axis is to twist the body while standing with the same foot planted.

Our study group, in the "Instituto de Biomecánica of Valencia (IBV)," has a great deal of experience in the evaluation of the pivot-shift phenomenon in ACL

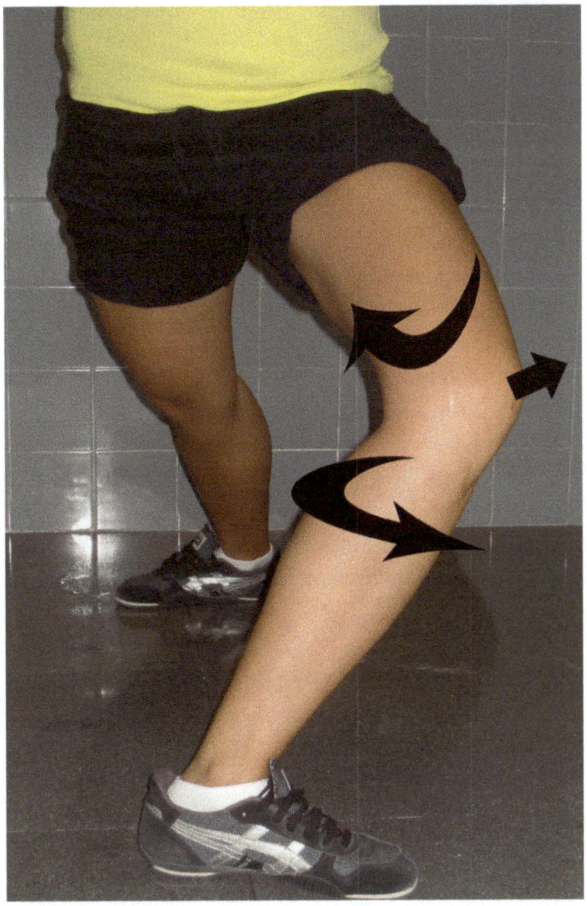

**Fig. 22.2** Mechanism of lateral patellar dislocation

[‡] The axial moment exerted by the subject on the platform is the sum of the product of the forces measured by the four sensors and their distance to the COP.

$$M_r = F_{c1} \times d_{c1\text{-}CDP} + F_{c2} \times d_{c2\text{-}CDP} + F_{c3} \times d_{c3\text{-}CDP} + F_{c4} \times d_{c4\text{-}CDP}$$

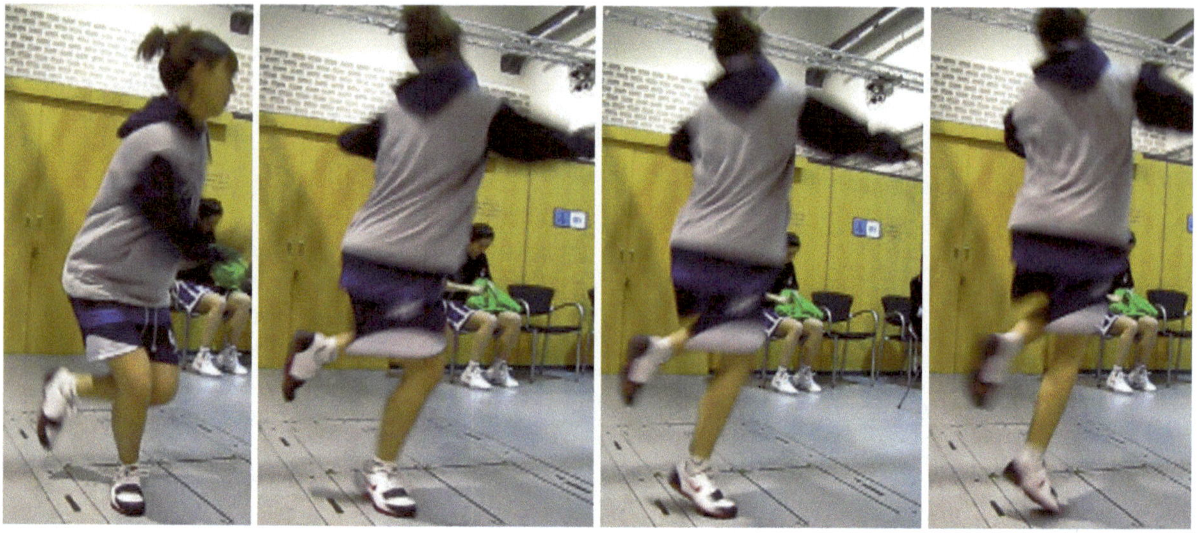

**Fig. 22.3** Image sequence of the monopodal jumping with pivoting with external tibial rotation test

deficient knees with dynamometric platforms.[13] In this patient group, we evaluate the pivot-shift phenomenon with two tests; monopodal jumping with pivoting with external tibial rotation and monopodal jumping with pivoting with internal tibial rotation.[§] The pivoting phase of the first test reproduces the pathomechanics of a lateral patellar subluxation or dislocation. The loading phase of the second test reproduces also the pathomechanics of a lateral patellar dislocation. But the pivoting phase of the first test is more demanding for the patella than the second test loading phase.

Therefore, the task proposed in evaluating lateral patellar instability is monopodal jumping with pivoting with external tibial rotation (Fig. 22.3). Subjects perform this provoking activity on dynamometric platforms with both the healthy limb as well as the injured/operated limb. The proposed task duplicate: muscle forces, weight-bearing conditions, and rotational loads caused by sports gestures (higher than the load applied to the knee during clinical test).

### 22.2.5 Laboratory Procedures

The subject is placed in a standing position on the platform facing a reference point with both arms extended alongside the body. When the examiner says, "ready," the subject lifts up the uninvolved limb and keeps the one under study in full extension. Next, the subject will flex the involved knee and rotate the body in the direction opposite to the intended spin, in order to use the full rotational path and to reach the joint's maximum contrary rotation. This is the loading phase. The second part of the movement is the pivoting phase and it begins when the loading phase is completed. The subject begins rotating in the intended spin direction while extending the knee to push himself/herself upward. For the analysis to be effective, the pivoting phase has to be fast and explosive in order to achieve maximum rotation demand of the joint.

The participants perform three practice trials prior to data collection followed by five tests using suitable sport shoes. The sequence of testing with the uninvolved and involved lower extremity is randomized in order to prevent an order effect.[6] To ensure that the task is always performed in the same fashion, we always have the same examiners next to the subject advising him or her on how to perform the task correctly and checking to see if he or she follows the instructions while performing the task. We also have a video camera recording our patients while performing the tasks to confirm that the pivoting is performed correctly.

[§] The relative motion of the tibia with respect to the femur is considered as either an internal or external rotation of the knee.

### 22.2.6 Data Analysis. Kinetic Variables

We measure the torques and forces that the patient can tolerate while stressing his or her knee actively simulating a lateral patellar dislocation mechanism, produced on the dynamometric platform by the jumping limb, during the jumping phase, immediately prior to the flying phase.

The software package to acquire and treat data, Dinascan/IBV (Instituto de Biomecánica de Valencia, Valencia, Spain) was used to graphically represent the torque and to calculate the kinetic variables.

Kinetic variables are expressed in a curve with two humps, a positive and a negative one (Fig. 22.4). The synchronizing of the video with the software used for curve elaboration shows that the segment A-B of the curve represents the loading phase, and the segment B-D of the curve represents the pivoting phase. For curves to be comparable, we have normalized the moments with the moment of inertia. Moreover, we have removed the curves obtained from gestures that did not follow the established protocol, and have recalculated a coherent average curve using a spline fitting technique, to enable curve shape comparison.

We have calculated the following kinetic variables (see Tables 22.1 and 22.2): (1) loading slope – it describes the speed with which the subject develops the torque on the platform during the loading phase; (2)

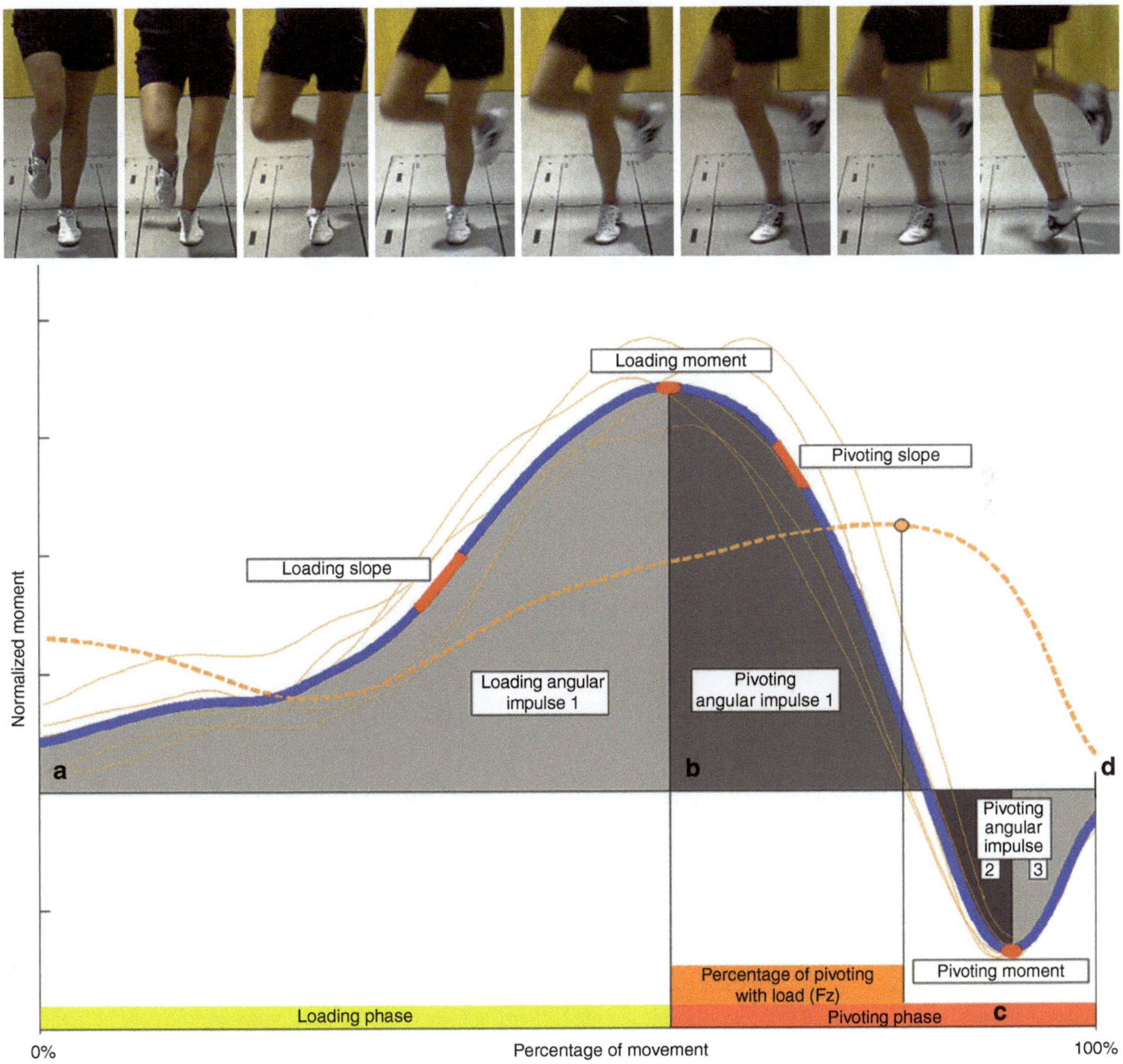


**Fig. 22.4** Curve representing the normalized moments and the vertical reaction force (Fz) registered during the jumping with pivoting with external tibial rotation test

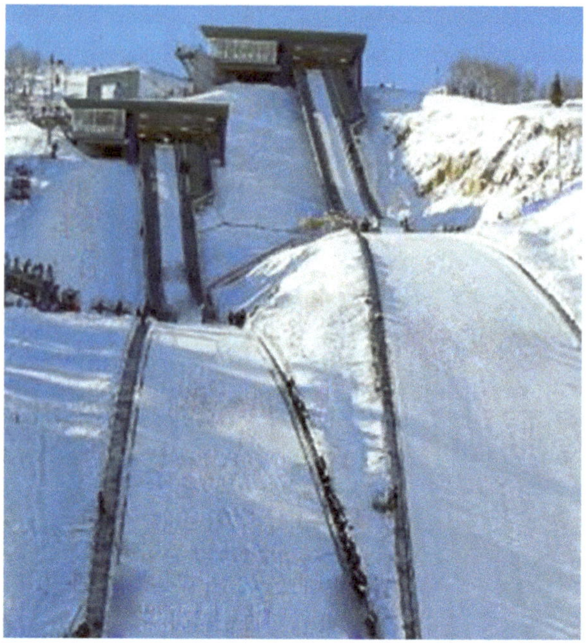

**Fig. 22.4** (continued)

loading moment[¶] – maximum torque generated by the foot standing on the dynamometric platform during the loading phase, the values are positive; (3) loading angular impulse[**] – area enclosed by the curve during the loading phase; (4) pivoting slope[††] – speed with which the torque is developed during the pivoting phase; (5) pivoting moment – torque generated during the pivoting phase, we are talking about the negative moment, defined by the direction of the rotational movement; (6) torque amplitude – range of ground reaction torque representing the difference between the loading moment and the pivoting moment; and (7) pivoting angular impulse – areas enclosed by the different sections of the curve describing the pivoting phase (total of 3).

We have also determined a variable composed of the normalized moment and the vertical force (Fz).[‡‡] The vertical force gives us information about the axial load exerted by the body's weight on the involved limb. Given that the final goal of the test we have designed is the pivoting, we have calculated the percentage of

**Table 22.1** Control Group: Dominant vs nondominant limb, external rotation: (values table)

| | Nondominant | | | | Dominant | | | |
|---|---|---|---|---|---|---|---|---|
| | Average | Standard deviation | Maximum | Minimum | Average | Standard deviation | Maximum | Minimum |
| Loading moment | 1287.73 | 243.97 | 1800.22 | 615.84 | 1471.76 | 289.03 | 2159.63 | 770.18 |
| Pivoting moment | −439.73 | 172.23 | −16.60 | −917.80 | −423.31 | 123.44 | −163.30 | −779.99 |
| Torque amplitude | 1727.46 | 293.96 | 2444.64 | 1118.45 | 1895.07 | 332.29 | 2553.50 | 1173.78 |
| Pivoting slope | −8335.80 | 2514.05 | −3652.08 | −15940.83 | −9680.04 | 3262.01 | −3167.80 | −16171.17 |
| Loading slope | 3696.50 | 1558.80 | 7804.93 | 1064.75 | 4268.29 | 1962.43 | 10292.43 | 1086.32 |
| Loading impulse | 212.32 | 42.92 | 330.73 | 117.68 | 239.96 | 44.60 | 324.92 | 112.81 |
| Pivoting impulse 1 | 141.49 | 46.96 | 285.14 | 64.10 | 155.27 | 43.72 | 291.97 | 80.42 |
| Pivoting impulse 2 | −12.91 | 10.84 | −0.06 | −85.74 | −9.96 | 3.59 | −1.84 | −19.05 |
| Pivoting impulse 3 | −12.60 | 12.87 | 2.32 | −95.89 | −10.77 | 7.09 | −2.81 | −44.27 |
| Body rotation angle | 212.23 | 47.28 | 345.56 | 75.68 | 238.46 | 43.65 | 384.83 | 128.42 |
| Percentage pivoting with load | 45.31 | 24.06 | 100.00 | 0.00 | 32.99 | 24.69 | 95.12 | 0.00 |

¶Normalized moment = moment/moment of inertia

**Angular impulse is the effect of a moment acting over a period of time. It is determined by the area under the moment–time curve. The change in the moment experienced by a body under the action of a field of forces is equal to the angular impulse of the resulting moment.

††We can compare the pivoting slope with a ski run slope (Fig. 22.4). The greater the slope inclination, the higher the skier's speed will be; and, the longer the ski run, the higher the speed reached by the skier.

‡‡Vertical force (Fz). The push produced when one object (foot) acts on another (force plate).

**Table 22.2** Control group: Dominant vs nondominant limb, external rotation

| | *t* | Sig. | Average difference | 95% confidence interval for the difference | | Statistical power (%) |
|---|---|---|---|---|---|---|
| | | | | Inferior | Superior | |
| Loading moment | 2.00 | 0.065 | 129.97 | −9.45 | 269.40 | 61 |
| Pivoting moment | 0.25 | 0.805 | 8.93 | −67.08 | 84.93 | 96 |
| Torque amplitude | 1.74 | 0.105 | 121.05 | −28.55 | 270.65 | 70 |
| Pivoting slope | −0.37 | 0.716 | −178.25 | −1206.26 | 849.76 | 95 |
| Loading slope | 0.89 | 0.387 | 398.75 | −558.56 | 1356.05 | 89 |
| Loading impulse | 1.76 | 0.1 | 18.05 | −3.96 | 40.07 | 69 |
| Pivoting impulse 1 | 2.54 | 0.024 | 24.54 | 3.78 | 45.31 | 58 |
| Pivoting impulse 2 | −0.18 | 0.858 | −0.28 | −3.61 | 3.04 | 97 |
| Pivoting impulse 3 | −0.16 | 0.873 | −0.34 | −4.80 | 4.13 | 97 |
| Body rotation angle | 2.30 | 0.038 | 27.02 | 1.77 | 52.28 | 51 |
| Percentage of pivoting with load | −2.81 | 0.014 | −10.27 | −18.13 | −2.42 | 67 |

pivoting with load (Fz). Lastly, we have estimated the maximum body rotation angle during the test by integrating the normalized moment's curve twice.

### 22.2.7 The Problem: Patellar Stability Depends on Several Factors. What Should We Compare? Healthy Knee Versus Contralateral Injured Knee

Patellofemoral instability is a multifactorial problem. Patellar stability depends on: limb alignment, articular geometry, muscle actions, and passive soft tissue restraints. The main lesion in the lateral patellar instability is the MPFL failure. The problem is the variability in pathological motion of the patella in MPFL deficient knees. It could be the result of the degree of injury to the MPFL, tissue mechanical properties, muscle strength of the knee,[§§] the patients' unique articular anatomy, patella alta, or the contribution of unrecognized additional soft tissue injury; therefore, each case is unique (individual pattern of laxity). Moreover, we must not forget that the MPFL is also a restraint to medial patellar displacement, and therefore its injury also favors, to a certain degree, patellar medial displacement, making the problem we are analyzing in this chapter more difficult (Fig. 22.5). Moreover, many anatomic factors contribute to patellar instability after patellar dislocations. In this way, bony geometry of the knee joint, especially trochlear dysplasia, strongly affects patellar mobility. Dejour and Le Coultre[5] found that 96% of patients with true patellar dislocation had trochlear dysplasia.

Given this great pathogenic variability, it seems correct to think that the best thing to do is to compare the injured knee to the healthy contralateral knee. Therefore, our study is a biomechanical in vivo study with the intact knee of the same subject serving as control.

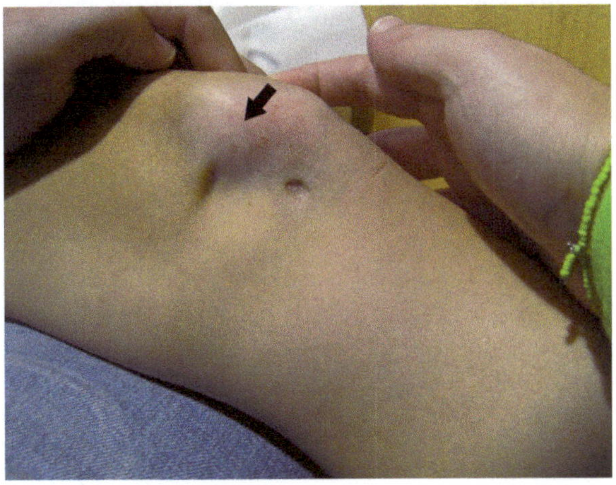

**Fig. 22.5** MPFL is a restraint to medial patellar displacement

[§§] The VMO is a dynamic medial stabilizer of the patella. The VMO's line of pull most efficiently resists lateral patellar motion when the knee is in deep flexion.

### 22.2.8 Another Problem: Limb Dominance. What Influence Does Limb Dominance Have in the Kinetic Parameters During the Proposed Task?

Prior to data collection, the participants were asked, "With which leg do you kick a ball? or With which leg do you fake, jump, or pivot?," to determine which was the dominant limb. Thus, all participants who responded that they kicked a ball (or faked, jumped, or pivoted) with their right leg were classified as right-leg dominant.

With the monopodal jumping with pivoting with external tibial rotation test, we have not observed significant differences between the dominant and nondominant limb for the following parameters¶: loading moment ($p=0.065$; $1-\beta=61\%$), loading slope ($p=0.387$; $1-\beta=89\%$), loading impulse ($p=0.100$; $1-\beta=69\%$), pivoting moment ($p=0.805$; $1-\beta=96\%$), pivoting slope ($p=0.716$; $1-\beta=95\%$), pivoting impulse 2 ($p=0.858$; $1-\beta=97\%$), pivoting impulse 3 ($p=0.873$; $1-\beta=97\%$), and torque amplitude ($p=0.105$; $1-\beta=70\%$). For the rest of parameters analyzed, there are significant differences influenced by limb dominance (see Tables 22.1 and 22.2).

### 22.2.9 Working Hypothesis

According to Strobel and Stedtfeld,[16] functional tests are designed to reproduce the subluxating or dislocating process (e.g., apprehension patellar test or the moving patellar apprehension test), or to provoke "avoidance behavior" to protect against subluxation or dislocation, which likewise is interpreted as a positive sign. Kinetic analysis, using dynamometric platforms, allows us to evaluate the avoidance behavior of the injured or operated knee under realistic loading conditions. In our case, we have developed a test (monopodal jumping with pivoting with external tibial rotation) to provoke an "avoidance behavior." Therefore, we are going to study the "avoidance behavior."

Our first hypothesis is that if there is lateral patellar instability, the patient will avoid reaching a high pivoting moment, high torque amplitude, high pivoting slope, and high pivoting impulse during the task that reproduces the mechanism for lateral patellar subluxation, generated by the foot stepping on a dynamometric platform, as a defense mechanism. Therefore, the ground reaction moment, as registered by dynamometric platforms, would be reduced ("avoidance behavior"). The patient will also perform the pivoting phase with less speed and explosiveness, less impulse, less axial load, and less body twist angle, as a defense strategy. Also, during the preparation for the pivoting phase, the loading phase, the kinetic parameters will also be reduced, so this phase would be performed with less explosiveness and less speed.

Our second hypothesis is that after successful surgical reconstruction, kinetic parameters should be similar to the contralateral healthy knee.

## 22.3 Case Studies. A "Snapshot"

We will now present some standard clinical case studies with kinetic analysis using dynamometric platforms. The graphics represent the curve for the normalized moments registered during the monopodal jumping with pivoting with external tibial rotation test. In case # 5, we represent also the graphic that corresponds to the body twist angle during the monopodal jumping with pivoting with external rotation test. In all the graphics: Right knee – red line; left knee – blue line. In each case, we are going to analyze the "avoidance behavior."

### 22.3.1 Case # 1. Volunteer with Normal Knees

Healthy subject free of injury in both limbs matched by gender, age, height, mass and activity level, and no history of traumatic injury of the lower extremities.

We have not observed significant differences between the dominant and nondominant limb for the following kinetic parameters: loading moment, loading slope, loading impulse, pivoting moment, pivoting slope, pivoting impulse, and torque amplitude (Fig. 22.6a).

¶Kinetic data from the five trials for each subject were averaged ($n=15$). Student $t$-test was performed to compare the results between two categories of the same variable, in this case one limb versus the contralateral limb. A $p<0.05$ was considered statistically significant. With the sample sizes used in our study, we obtained a statistical high power, with a significance level of 95%

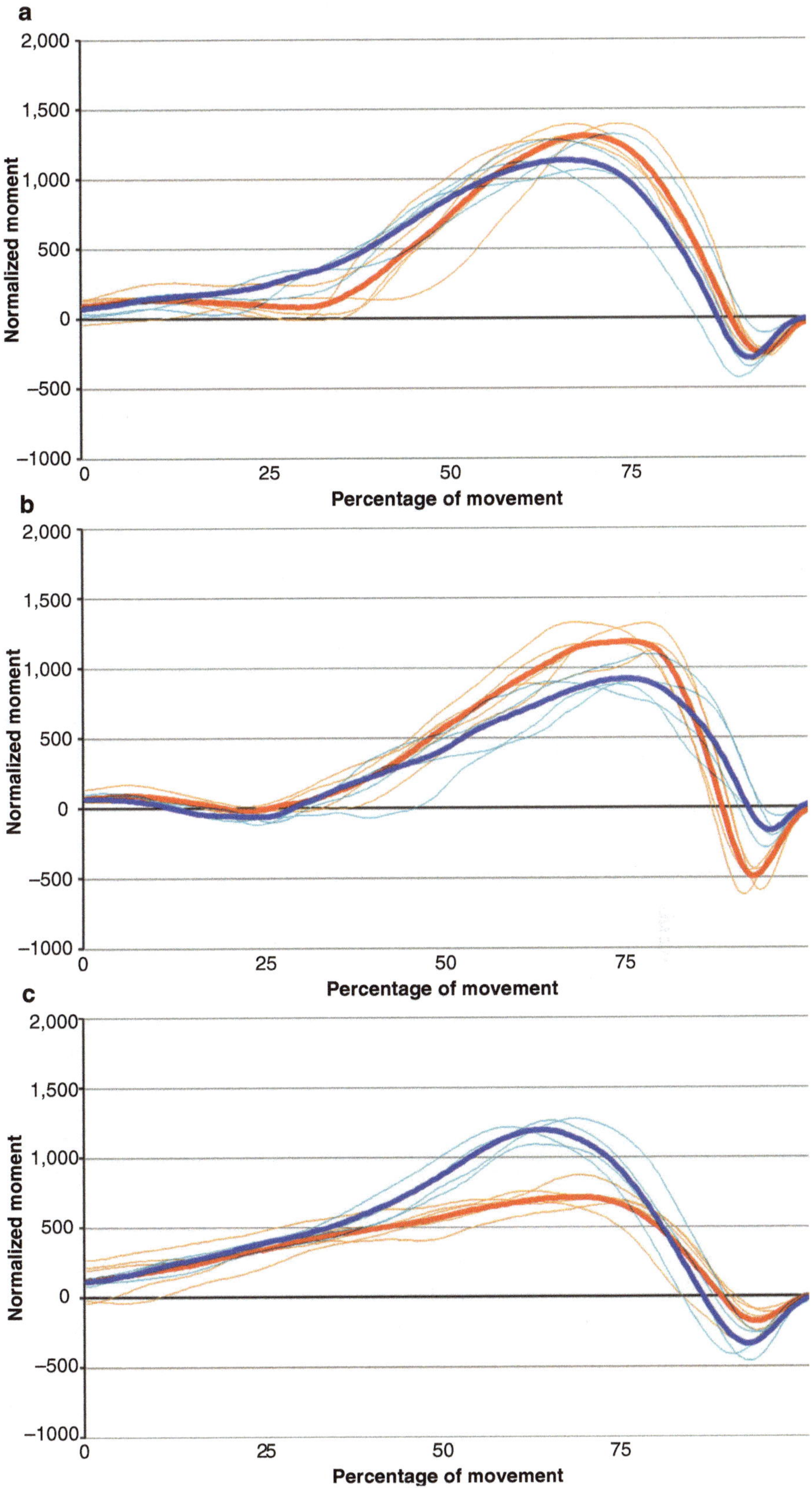


**Fig. 22.6** (**a**) Case # 1, (**b**) Case # 2, and (**c**) Case # 3 (See text)

### 22.3.2 Case # 2. Patient with an Isolated ACL Tear of the Left Knee 6-Month Follow-up

This patient had rotatory instability only playing football. Right dominant limb. Negative pivot-shift with the patient awake, and positive pivot-shift under anesthesia with an extra amount of compression applied to the lateral compartment of the knee by an assistant when the examiner performs the pivot-shift test.

The kinetic parameters were compatible with a rotatory instability: reduction of the pivoting moment, the pivoting slope, the pivoting impulse, and the torque amplitude (Fig. 22.6b).

### 22.3.3 Case # 3. Patient with Isolated Lateral Patellar Instability

Seventeen-year-old girl, right limb dominance, who does not practice sports and who was studied kinetically using dynamometric platforms 3 weeks after her first episode of right lateral patellar dislocation after an undetermined mechanism while dancing. The patellar apprehension test was negative. She had hip anteversion. A CT scan showed a TT-TG distance of 11 mm. An MRI showed the MPFL rupture and a trochlear dysplasia type B according to the classification by Dejour.[5] The left knee was completely asymptomatic.

The kinetic parameters were compatible with a rotatory instability: reduction of the pivoting moment, the pivoting slope, the pivoting impulse, and torque amplitude (Fig. 22.6c).

**Comments About Cases 1, 2, and 3**

Our results supported our first hypothesis. We have observed that in patients with lateral patellar instability, the knees used multiple defense strategies for rotational stress. One of the defense strategies is to avoid reaching high moments during the pivoting phase. We have also noticed a decrease in the pivoting slope, pivoting impulse, and torque amplitude.

Although kinetic analysis, using the jumping with pivoting with external tibial rotation test, has a high sensitivity (84.6%) to detect avoidance behaviors when the injured knee is compared to the noninjured knee in patients with a knee rotatory instability, this test is completely nonspecific.[13] So, the shape of the curve and the kinetic parameters for an ACL deficient knee (case # 2 [Fig. 22.6b]) are similar to those of a knee with lateral patellar instability (case # 3 [Fig. 22.6c]).

*So, kinetic analysis using dynamometric platforms is not a diagnostic tool for lateral patellar instability.*

### 22.3.4 Case # 4. Kinetic False Negative In a Patient with Lateral Patellar Instability

Eighteen-year-old woman, right limb dominance, who does not practice sports and has had at least 20 episodes of right lateral patellar dislocation since the age of nine. The patient cannot determine the exact mechanism of dislocation. Physical examination showed a lateral patellar subluxation clearly visible in the last 30° of flexion–extension of the knee (Fig. 22.7a, b). This was not found in the contralateral knee. The patellar apprehension test was positive. The rest of the physical examination was completely normal. She is completely asymptomatic and has no problem with her activities of daily living. She does not practice sports because she does not want to. The CT scan shows a trochlear dysplasia type D according to the classification by Dejour[5] in the right knee (Fig. 22.7c), and a type A in the left knee; and a TT-TG distance of 15 mm. The left knee was completely asymptomatic. IRM showed a patellar chondropathy.

From a kinetic standpoint, the knee is compatible with a healthy subject's knee (Fig. 22.7d).

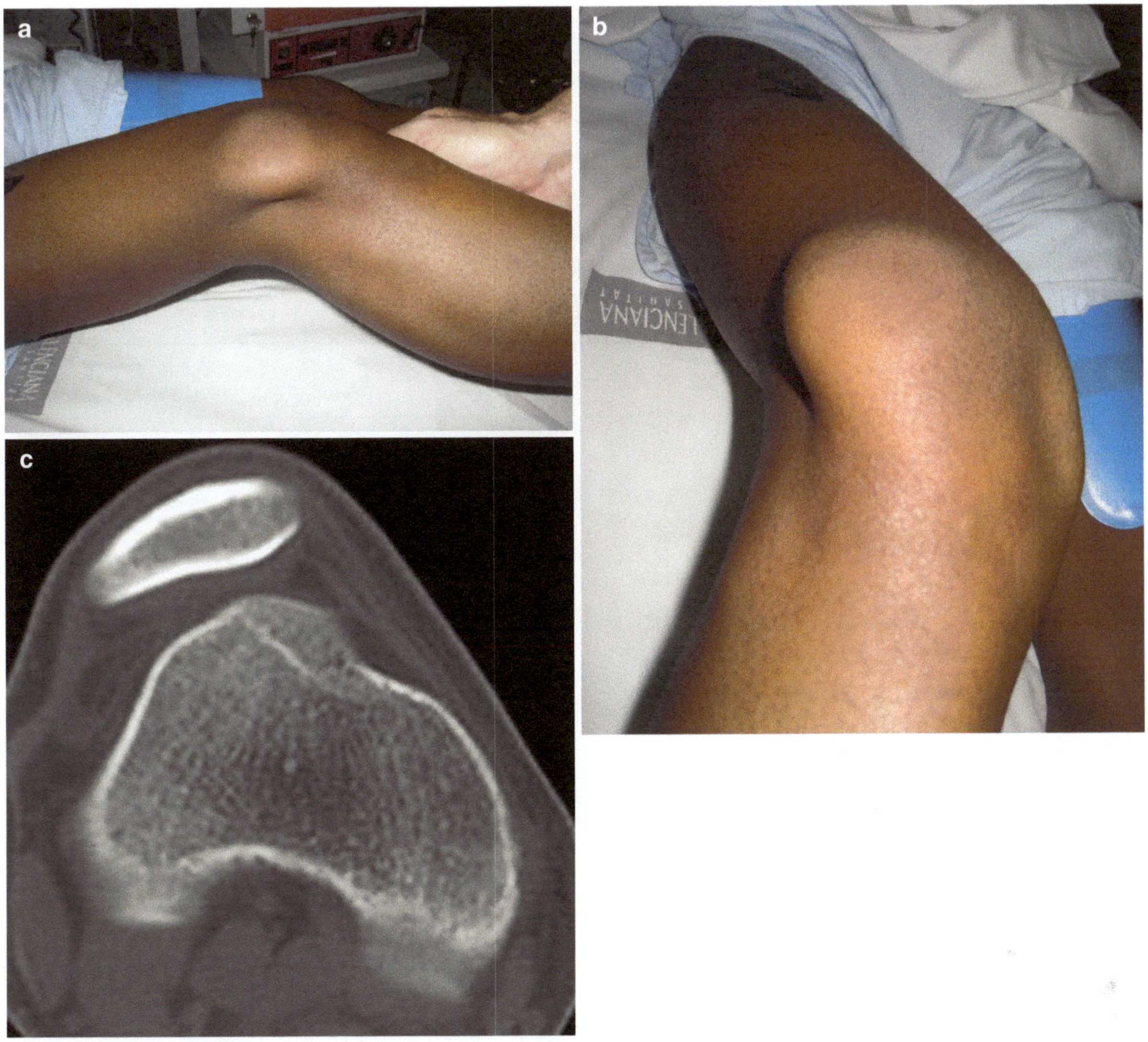

**Fig. 22.7** Case # 4. (**a**,**b**) Right lateral patellar dislocation. (**c**) CT showing trochlear dysplasia type D. (**d**) Preoperative normalized moments registered during the monopodal jumping with pivoting with external tibial rotation test

### Comment About Case 4

It is a false negative. The patient had a clear lateral patellar instability but was completely asymptomatic, and it caused no limitation in her activities of daily living. One of the reasons for surgical treatment in a patient with lateral patellar instability is the prevention of patellofemoral osteoarthritis,[3,8,9,14] which has a higher prevalence in lateral instability patients than in patients with no patellofemoral instability. However, the prevalence of patellofemoral osteoarthritis is higher in the patellofemoral instability operated group than in the nonoperated one.[3] Therefore, this does not seem to be an important argument in order to operate on a patient who is completely asymptomatic and is not demanding surgery.

*Looking at this case, the questions we ask ourselves are: What are the clinical implications of the kinetic analysis results? Would it be advisable to operate on this patient? Would it be better to perform an isolated trochleoplasty?*

**Fig. 22.7** (continued)

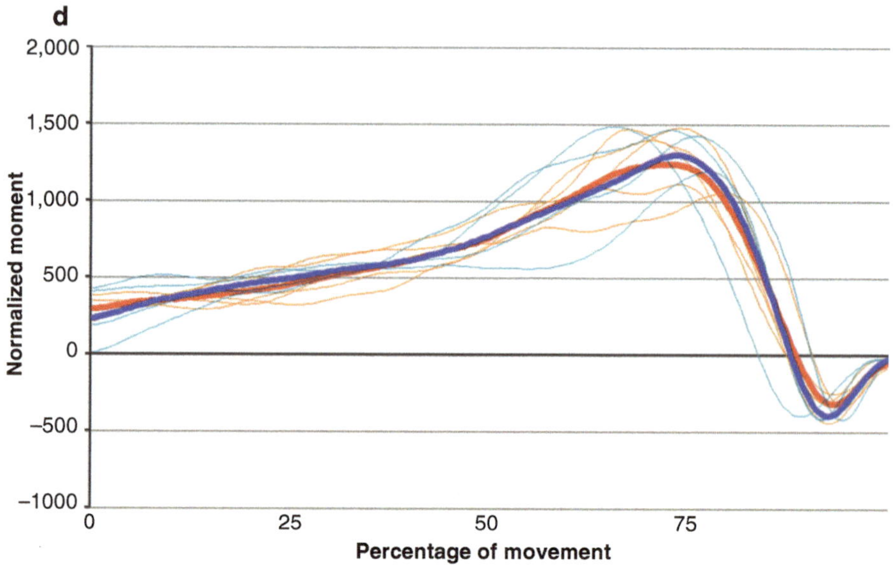


## 22.3.5 Case # 5. Reconstruction of the MPFL. Preoperative Versus Postoperative Kinetic Analysis

Sedentary 16-year-old girl, with three objective lateral patellar dislocation episodes of the left knee, with postraumatic hemarthrosis. The right knee was completely asymptomatic. The patellar apprehension test was positive. The rest of the physical examination was completely normal. The CT scan shows a trochlear dysplasia type A according to the classification by Dejour[5]; and a TT-TG distance of 13 mm. An isolated MPFL reconstruction using quadriceps tendon was performed. She was reevaluated 6 months after surgery. The patient does not complain of instability postoperatively (negative apprehension test). The subjective result was excellent. Outcome measures: Lysholm 100, Tegner (preoperative – 4/postoperative – 4), IKDC 100.

Preoperative kinetic analyses reveal a reduction of the loading moment, the loading slope, the pivoting slope, the pivoting impulse 1, the torque amplitude, and the body twist angle (Fig. 22.8a, b). Postoperatively (6 months after surgery), from a kinetic standpoint, the knee is compatible with a healthy subject's knee (Fig. 22.8c, d). Preoperatively, there was a lateral subluxation of the patella at 0° of knee flexion (Fig. 22.8e). Postoperatively, there was a correct patellofemoral congruence (Fig. 22.8f).

**Comments About Case 5**

Our results support our second hypothesis: after MPFL reconstruction, kinetic parameters should be similar to those of the contralateral healthy knee. We have observed that MPFL reconstruction restores kinetic parameters to normal levels during extreme rotation conditions such as monopodal jumping with pivoting with external tibial rotation. In this case, we have found an excellent correlation between clinical results and normalization of kinetic parameters.

*Kinetic analysis could be considered as a quality control test for a surgical technique from a kinetic standpoint. Therefore, it would be an outcome tool.*

## 22.3.6 Case # 6. Reconstruction of the MPFL in Sports

Sixteen-year-old girl that practices classical ballet and contemporary dancing. Right limb dominance. She was operated on her left knee after a second objective lateral patellar dislocation. The first episode happened while playing basketball (she cannot identify the mechanism) and the second one while doing contemporary

**Fig. 22.8** Case # 5. (**a**) Preoperative normalized moments registered during the monopodal jumping with pivoting with external tibial rotation test. (**b**) Preoperative body twist angle. (**c**) Postoperative normalized moments registered during the monopodal jumping with pivoting with external tibial rotation test. (**d**) Postoperative body twist angle. (**e**) Preoperative MRI. (**f**) Postoperative CT. TT-TG distance

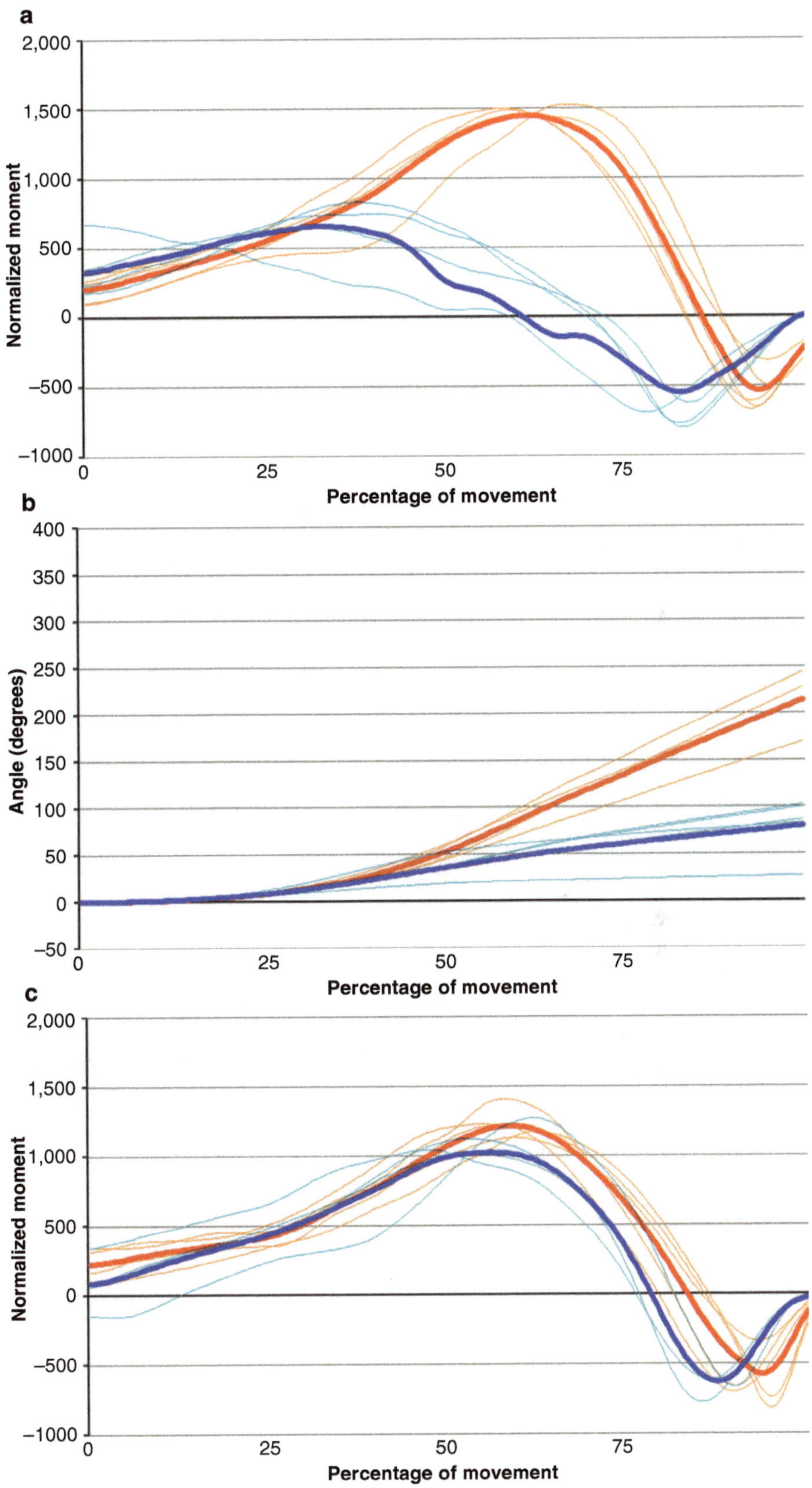

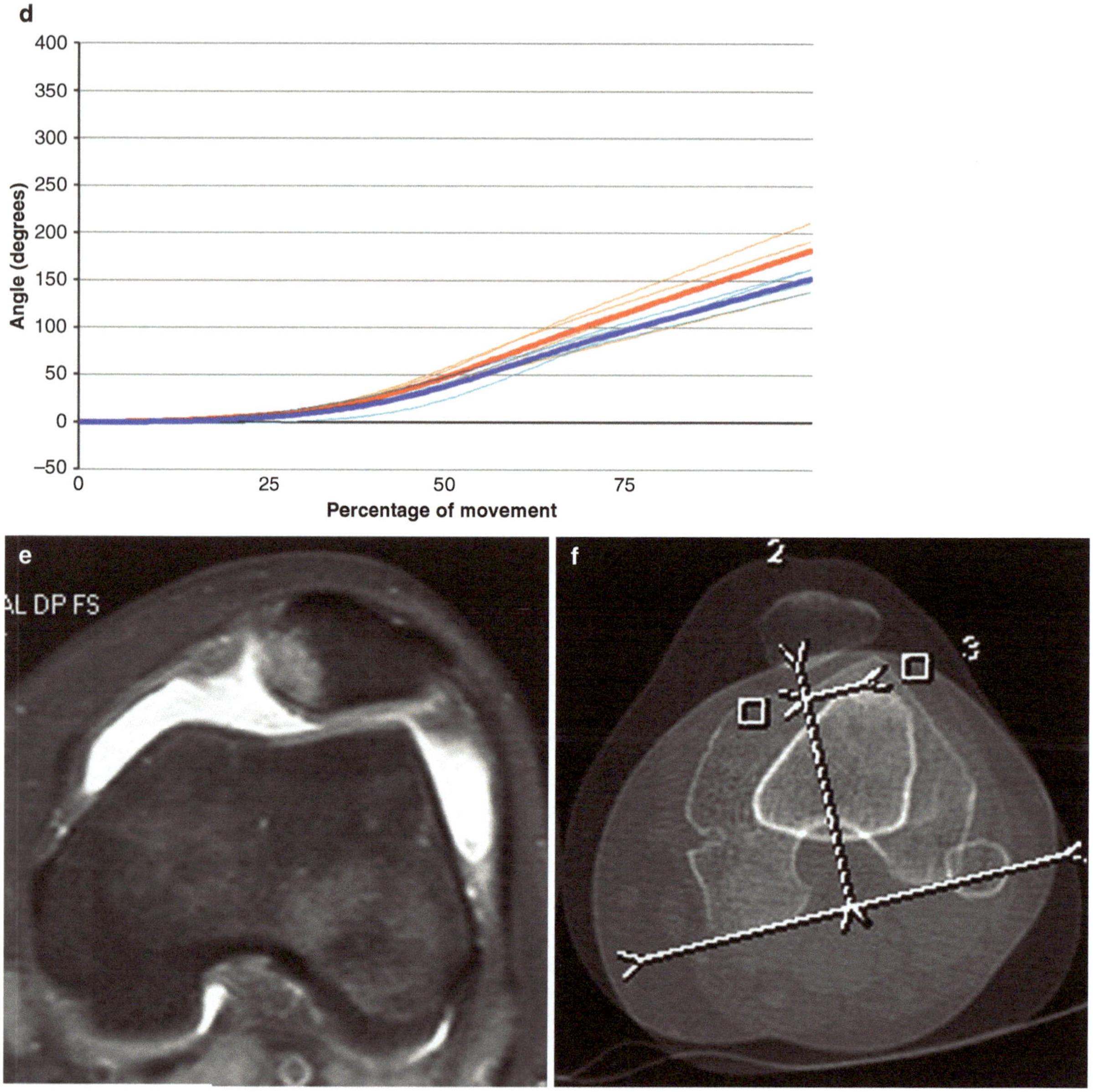


**Fig. 22.8** (continued)

dancing (sudden strong quadriceps contraction with internal rotation of the femur [Fig. 22.2]).

CT scan study revealed a trochlear dysplasia type B according to the classification by Dejour[5] (flat trochlea) (Fig. 22.9a), and a TT-TG distance of 19 mm. An isolated MPFL reconstruction was performed using double-bundle semitendinosus tendon. Postoperatively, the patient feels she is at the same sports level as before her injury, but when she finishes dancing, she complains of knee swelling, not painful, however she has to ice her knee for the swelling to resolve. Physical examination indicates that the patella is stable. Subjectively, she feels no pain and no instability when her knee is subjected to greater rotational demands during contemporary dancing or classical ballet. Imaging

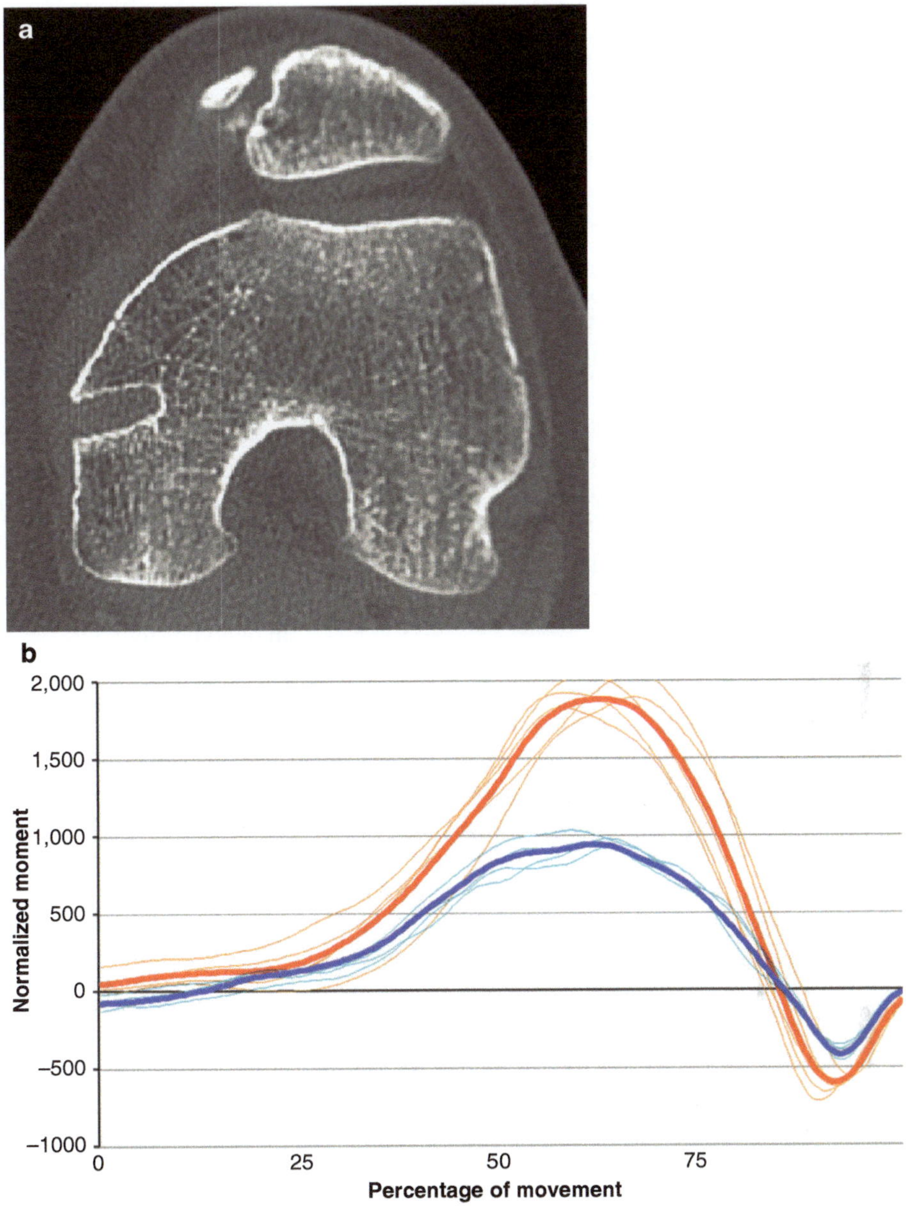


**Fig. 22.9** Case # 6. (**a**) Postoperative CT showing a flat trochlea. (**b**) Postoperative normalized moments registered during the monopodal jumping with pivoting with external tibial rotation test

studies show a correctly anchored graft and centered patella. Outcome measures: Lysholm score 96, Tegner score (preoperative – 8/postoperative – 8), IKDC score 95.

In this case, we have not found a good correlation between clinical results and normalization of kinetic parameters. Kinetic parameters are compatible with a rotatory instability: reduction of the pivoting moment, the pivoting slope, the pivoting impulse, and the torque amplitude (Fig. 22.9b).

**Comments About Case 6**

The question is: Do the people who return to a high level of function and sport level have a functionally intact knee?

Kinetic study shows avoidance behaviors. Maybe isolated MPFL reconstruction is not enough to control lateral patellar stability in highly demanding situations such as contemporary dancing and classical ballet (that can mimic a patellar dislocation event) in patients with a flat trochlea and a pathologic increase in the TT-TG distance. It is possible that, as the trochlea becomes flatter and the TT-TG index increases, the optimal tracking of the patella, as established by tibial tubercle transfer, becomes increasingly important. Therefore, we should perform "a-la carte" patellar instability surgery. Although MPFL represents the "essential lesion," there is a variability in pathological motion of the patella in MPFL deficient knees. Many anatomic factors contribute to patellar instability after patellar dislocations such as trochlear anatomy, and a high TT-TG distance. A shallow trochlea and an increment of the TT-TG distance will cause an overload of the MPFL.

For an athletic population, the ultimate outcome after lateral patellar instability is the ability to return to prior levels of sports in terms of intensity, frequency, duration, and absence of symptoms. There are many limitations to measure return to activity such as changes in lifestyle, free time, work and family obligations. On other occasions, patients go back to practicing their sport even though they might not have fully recuperated. We believe that kinetic analysis avoids these problems because the monopodal jumping with pivoting with external tibial rotation test subjects the knee to a similar demand as a sports gesture that causes a patellar dislocation or lateral subluxation.

*So, kinetic analysis using dynamometric platforms could be a good tool to compare different surgical treatments (isolated MPFL reconstruction static or dynamic vs. MPFL reconstruction plus tibial tubercle transfer vs. trochleoplasty) in order to find the best surgical technique to treat patients with chronic lateral patellar instability.*

## 22.4 Summary

Precise, repeatable, and objective outcome tools are necessary to refine surgical procedures so that short-term and long-term knee function and patient satisfaction are improved. Our study supports the fact that kinetic analysis using dynamometric platforms could be a useful tool in the objective evaluation of patients with lateral patellar instability under realistic loading conditions (evaluation of functional instability). With this task we duplicate: (1) muscle forces, (2) weight-bearing conditions, and (3) rotational loads caused by sports gestures (higher than the load applied to the knee during clinical examination).

Kinetic analysis has some limitations: (1) not useful in acute injuries, (2) in the presence of marked muscle wasting, and (3) when both knees are involved. However, our data are only a "snapshot" analysis from an ongoing study.

## References

1. Amis AA. Current concept son anatomy and biomechanics of patellar stability. *Sports Med Arthrosc*. 2007;15:48-56.
2. Amis AA, Firer P, Mountney J, et al. Anatomy and biomechanics of the medial patellofemoral ligament. *Knee*. 2003;10:215-220.
3. Arnbjornsson A, Egund N, Rydling O, et al. The natural history of recurrent dislocation of the patella: long-term results of conservative and operative treatment. *J Bone Joint Surg*. 1992;74-B:140-142.
4. Colvin AC, West RV. Patellar instability. *J Bone Joint Surg*. 2008;90-A:2751-2762.
5. Dejour D, Le Coultre B. Osteotomies in patella-femoral instabilities. *Sports Med Arthrosc*. 2007;15:40.
6. Ernst GP, Saliba E, Diduch DR, et al. Lower-extremity compensations following anterior cruciate ligament reconstruction. *Phys Ther*. 2000;80:251-260.
7. Fithian DC, Mishra DK, Balen PF, et al. Instrumented measurement of patellar mobility. *Am J Sports Med*. 1995;23:607-615.
8. Maenpaa H, Lehto MU. Patellofemoral osteoarthritis after patellar dislocation. *Clin Orthop Relat Res*. 1997;339:156-162.
9. Marcacci M, Zaffagnini S, Iacono F, et al. Results in the treatment of recurrent dislocation of the patella after 30 years follow-up. *Knee Surg Sports Traumatol Arthrosc*. 1995;3:163-166.

10. Paxton EW, Fithian DC, Stone ML, et al. The reliability and validity of knee-specific and general health instruments in assessing acute patellar dislocations outcomes. *Am J Sports Med.* 2003;31:487-492.
11. Post WR, Teitge R, Amis A. Patellofemoral malalignment: looking beyond the viewbox. *Clin Sports Med.* 2002;21:521-546.
12. Prat-Pastor JM. *Biomecánica de la marcha humana normal y patológica.* Valencia: IBV; 2005.
13. Sanchis-Alfonso V, Baydal-Bertomeu JM, Castelli A, et al. Laboratory evaluation of the pivot shift phenomenon with use of kinetic analysis. A preliminary study. J. Bone Joint Surg (Am) (In press).
14. Sillanpaa P, Mattila VM, Visuri T, et al. Ligament reconstruction versus distal realignment for patellar dislocation. *Clin Orthop Relat Res.* 2008;466:1475-1484.
15. Smith TO, Davies L, O'Driscoll ML, et al. An evaluation of the clinical tests and outcome measures used to assess patellar instability. *Knee.* 2008;15:255-256.
16. Strobel M, Stedtfeld H-W. *Diagnostic evaluation of the knee.* Berlin: Springer; 1990.

# 23 Kinetic and Kinematic Analysis in Evaluating Patients with Anterior Knee Pain

Vicente Sanchis-Alfonso, Susana Marín-Roca, Erik Montesinos-Berry, José María Baydal-Bertomeu, and María Francisca Peydro-De Moya

## 23.1 Anterior Knee Pain Is Not Always a Self-limiting Condition: "The Need for an Objective Measurement"

Anterior knee pain may lead not only to functional disability, but also to knee osteoarthritis.[5] Davies and Newman[5] carried out a comparative study to evaluate the incidence of previous adolescent anterior knee pain in patients who had a patellofemoral replacement for isolated patellofemoral osteoarthritis compared to a matched group of patients who had a unicompartmental replacement for isolated medial compartment osteoarthritis. They found that the incidence of adolescent anterior knee pain syndrome and patellar instability was higher ($p<0.001$) in the patients who had a patellofemoral replacement for isolated patellofemoral osteoarthritis (22% and 14%, respectively) than in those who had a unicompartmental replacement for isolated medial compartment osteoarthritis (6% and 1%, respectively). They conclude that anterior knee pain syndrome is not always a self-limiting condition given that it may lead to patellofemoral osteoarthritis. However, the pathogenesis of knee osteoarthritis in this group of patients is not well understood.

Given that clinical practice modification is based on outcome studies, the ability to evaluate and to quantify the effects of treatment on anterior knee pain patients is therefore vital. Due to the limitations of the current methods (Visual Analog Scale, VAS; Functional Index Questionnaire, FIQ; Kujala score; IKDC) for the assessment of clinical outcome after anterior knee pain treatment, new technologies are needed to measure the benefits of treatment and to compare different methods of treatment. The final objective should be the measurement during dynamic activities that cause or aggravate the symptoms. We believe that this objective could be achieved by means of kinetic and kinematic analysis given that both are useful in the objective measurement of lower limb function.

The application of kinetic and kinematic analysis in the objective assessment of anterior knee pain patients is discussed in this chapter. Moreover, kinetic and kinematic analysis can also be useful to help us understand the knee osteoarthritis mechanisms in this population group.

## 23.2 What Provoking Activity Is the Best to Evaluate Anterior Knee Pain? Clinical Rationale

Stair climbing is a demanding locomotor task frequently performed during daily activities. It is well-known from a functional point of view that going up and down stairs, requiring high levels of quadriceps activity, is one of the most painful and challenging activities of daily living for subjects with anterior knee pain. Moreover, it is universally accepted that going downstairs is more challenging that going upstairs due to the level of eccentric control required during step descent. In fact, Costigan and colleagues[2] have

V. Sanchis-Alfonso (✉)
International Patellofemoral Study Group,
International ACL Study Group,
Hospital 9 de Octubre, Hospital Arnau de Vilanova,
School of Medicine, Catholic University of Valencia,
Valencia, Spain
e-mail: vicente.sanchis.alfonso@gmail.com

V. Sanchis-Alfonso (ed.), *Anterior Knee Pain and Patellar Instability*,
DOI: 10.1007/978-0-85729-507-1_23, 

reported that during stair descent, there is an increment of the patellofemoral joint reaction force (PFJRF) eight times greater compared to level walking. Therefore, stair descent can be demanding enough from a biomechanical standpoint, not only to aggravate pain in those patients with anterior knee pain, but also to trigger the use of defense strategies as well. So, the dynamic test we propose in order to evaluate and to quantify the effects of both surgical and nonsurgical treatment in patients with anterior knee pain is the stair descent test. Another interesting aspect that we will analyze in this chapter are the compensating strategies, to reduce load and therefore pain, that in theory a patient with anterior knee pain may develop during the stair descent test. These strategies that can be good to reduce pain could have mid-term and long-term adverse effect for the knee joint (knee osteoarthritis).

## 23.3 Kinetic and Kinematic Analysis in Evaluating Anterior Knee Pain

To evaluate the way the stair descent is performed, we use kinematic* information, registered through photogrammetric instruments and kinetic information, registered through dynamometric platforms. Both systems are combined to determine the most relevant variables that characterize going downstairs.

### 23.3.1 *Instruments, Motion Analysis System, Dynamometric Platforms*

To perform this test, we have used a four-camera computer-aided video motion analysis system† and two independent dynamometric platforms, placed as indicated in Fig. 23.1a, that register the force exerted by the foot on the floor in the three directions of space. In order to perform the test, the following accessories were needed: (1) portable two-step wooden staircase, and (2) passive markers.‡ Three boxes with the following dimensions were used: 20 cm. high step riser and 40 cm. footprint, forming a two-step staircase (Fig. 23.1b). The box serving as the first step was built to adapt perfectly to the dynamometric platform to avoid vibrations when stepping on it with the foot (Fig. 23.1c). Sixteen reflectant markers were used, eight for each leg, that determined

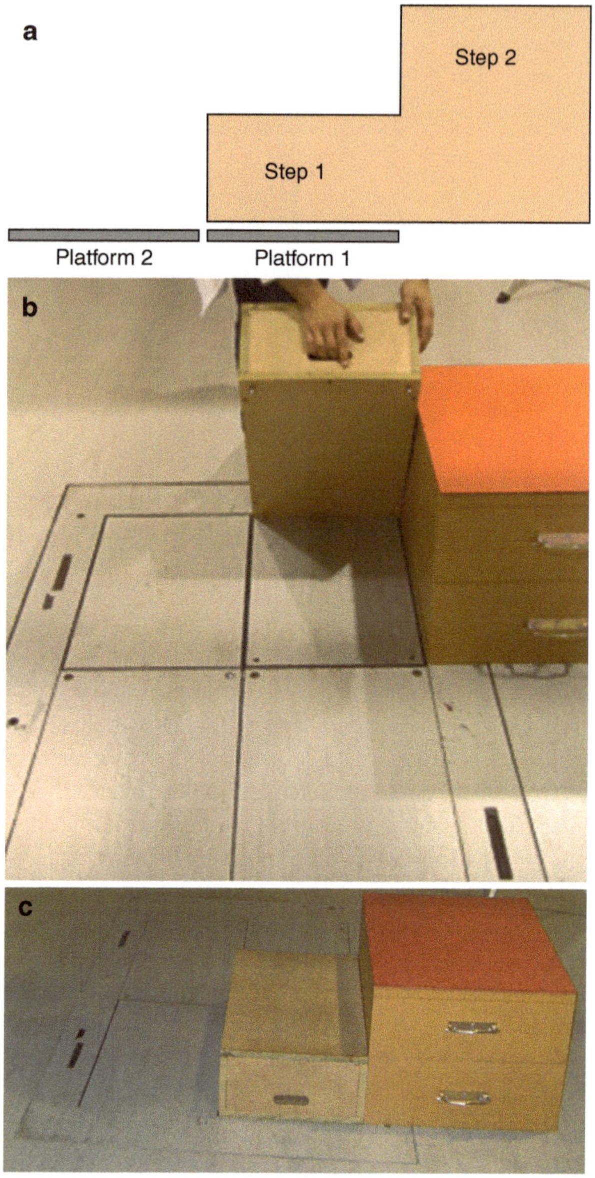


**Fig. 23.1** (**a**) Dynamometric platform disposition. (**b**) Step adaptation to the dynamometric platform. (**c**) Step disposition

*Kinematic parameters are those used in the description of movement without consideration for the causes of movement. These parameters include linear and angular displacements, velocities, and accelerations.

†Motion analysis. Interpretation of computerized data that documents an individual's lower and upper extremities, pelvis, trunk, and head motion during ambulation.

‡Passive markers. Joint and segment markers used during motion analysis that reflect visible or infrared light in contrast with active markers that emit a signal.

the spatial position of the segments of the lower limb. The markers were placed tracing two triangles in each segment (leg and thigh), with the apex in opposing directions in each of the segments (Fig. 23.2a, b). All of the markers were placed in the lateral aspect of the leg to allow for a correct visualization by the cameras. Two of the markers were placed in the lateral condyle and in the lateral malleolus, respectively, to determine the position of the knee and ankle joints.

### 23.3.2 Laboratory Procedures

To perform the test, the subject starts in a standing position with both arms crossed over the chest for the first step (Fig. 23.2c). The test involves descending the two steps of the staircase, stepping with one foot on the first step (underneath of which is one of the platforms), and the other foot on the floor (where the other platform is placed). For this analysis, the test is repeated four times (two with each leg). Participants were given a visual demonstration of the task prior to testing. Following a verbal cue, the participants performed the task (Fig. 23.3). To ensure that the task was always performed in the same fashion, we always had the same examiners next to the subject advising him or her on how to perform the task correctly and observing if he or she followed the instructions while carrying out the task. We also had a video camera recording our patients while performing the task to

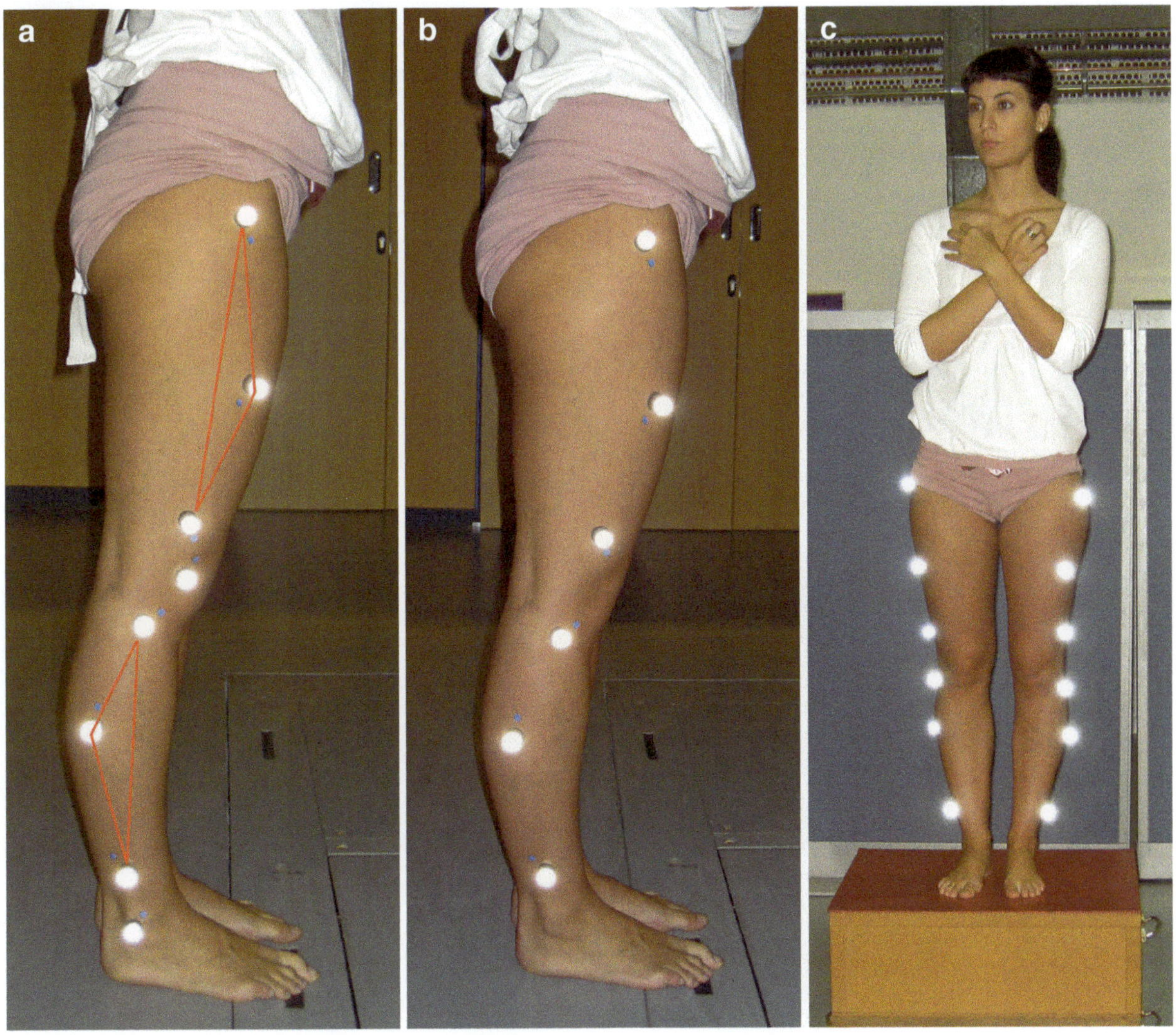


**Fig. 23.2** Marker disposition. (**a**) With calibration markers. (**b**, **c**) Without calibration markers

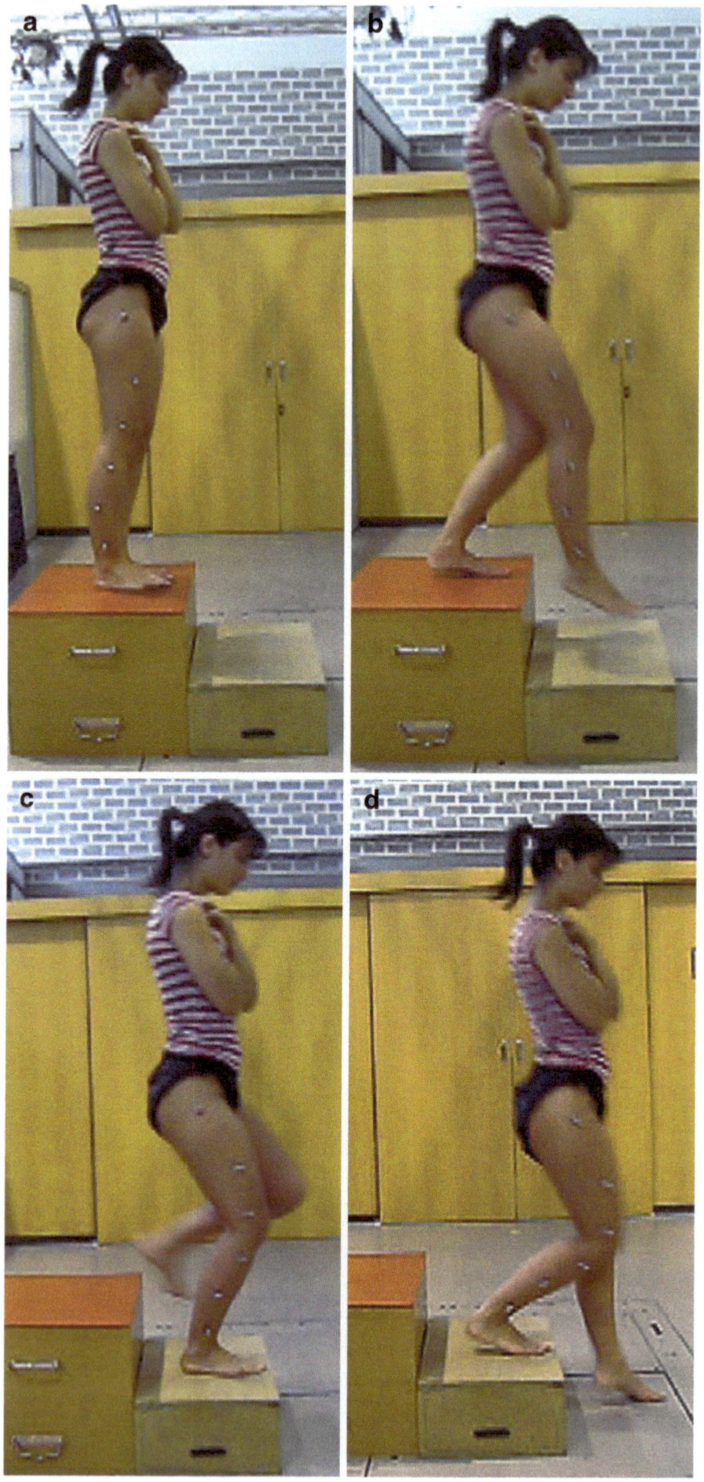


**Fig. 23.3** Photographic sequence of the stair descent test

**Table 23.1** Kinetic and kinematic variables analyzed during stair descent test

| | Control group | | | |
|---|---|---|---|---|
| | Average | SD | Max | Min |
| Knee flexion angle | 99.12 | 7.54 | 63.45 | 121.23 |
| Stance phase duration | 0.88 | 0.12 | 0.62 | 1.24 |
| Heel contact GRF | 1.45 | 0.15 | 1.16 | 1.76 |
| Oscillation GRF | 0.75 | 0.07 | 0.54 | 0.94 |
| Toe-off GRF | 0.95 | 0.08 | 0.75 | 1.14 |
| Heel contact A/A moment | 0.20 | 0.05 | 0.12 | 0.33 |
| Toe-off A/A moment | 0.16 | 0.04 | 0.08 | 0.26 |
| Heel contact F/E moment | –0.13 | 0.07 | –0.54 | –0.02 |
| Toe-off F/E moment | 0.29 | 0.05 | 0.18 | 0.42 |

confirm that it was performed correctly. To avoid the possible effects of footwear on gait when descending stairs, all subjects underwent data collection in their bare feet. Apart from standardized stair descent, the patient performed a free one, meaning going down the stairs the way he or she felt more comfortable.

### 23.3.3 Kinematic and Kinetic Variables

The video photogrammetric system provides the coordinates of the markers in a laboratory reference. From this raw data, we have computed the finite displacements from the body-reference position by using a in-house developed software based on the algorithms described by Woltring.[19] This software provides angular displacements expressed as the attitude vector. The projection of the attitude vector on the mediolateral and anteroposterior axis provides an estimation of the flexion–extension and abduction–adduction angle according with the procedure described by Page and colleagues.[15] Using the spatial position and the forces registered with the dynamometric platform, knee joint moments were calculated. We have used a smoothing technique based on a local polynomial fitting. The width of the window was optimized in each measurement for the minimum self-correlation of the residuals.[14]

The variables specific to the test are (see Table 23.1): (1) knee flexion angle – measured in degrees; (2) stance phase duration – time during which the subject is in contact with the first step and is measured in seconds; (3) normalized[§] heel contact force – ground reaction force (GRF) that appears on the platform when the heel strikes on the first step; (4) normalized oscillation force – GRF that appears on the platform when the contralateral leg is oscillating; (5) normalized toe-off peak force – GRF that appears on the platform when the foot steps off of it; (6) heel contact abduction–adduction moment[¶]– maximum torque on the coronal plane[**] that is produced during the foot's strike phase on the platform; (7) toe-off abduction–adduction moment – maximum torque on the coronal plane that is produced during the foot's take off phase on the platform; (8) heel contact flexion–extension moment – maximum torque on the sagittal plane[††] that is produced during the foot's heel strike phase on the platform; and (9) toe-off flexion–extension moment – maximum torque on the sagittal plane that is produced during the foot's take-off phase on the platform.

Kinetic and kinematic variables are expressed in a curve. In each graphic, we represent a band of normality (colored in light blue), the control group's mean value (dotted line) and our patient's mean value (black line) (Figs. 23.4–23.8).

[§]The forces are measured in N and they have been normalized for the subject's weight; therefore, it is a dimensionless magnitude.

[¶]The moment is measured in N·m, it has been normalized for subject's weight and knee height; therefore, it is a dimensionless value.

[**]Coronal plane. The plane that divides the body or body segment into anterior and posterior parts.

[††]Sagittal plane. The plane that divides the body or body segment into the right and left parts.

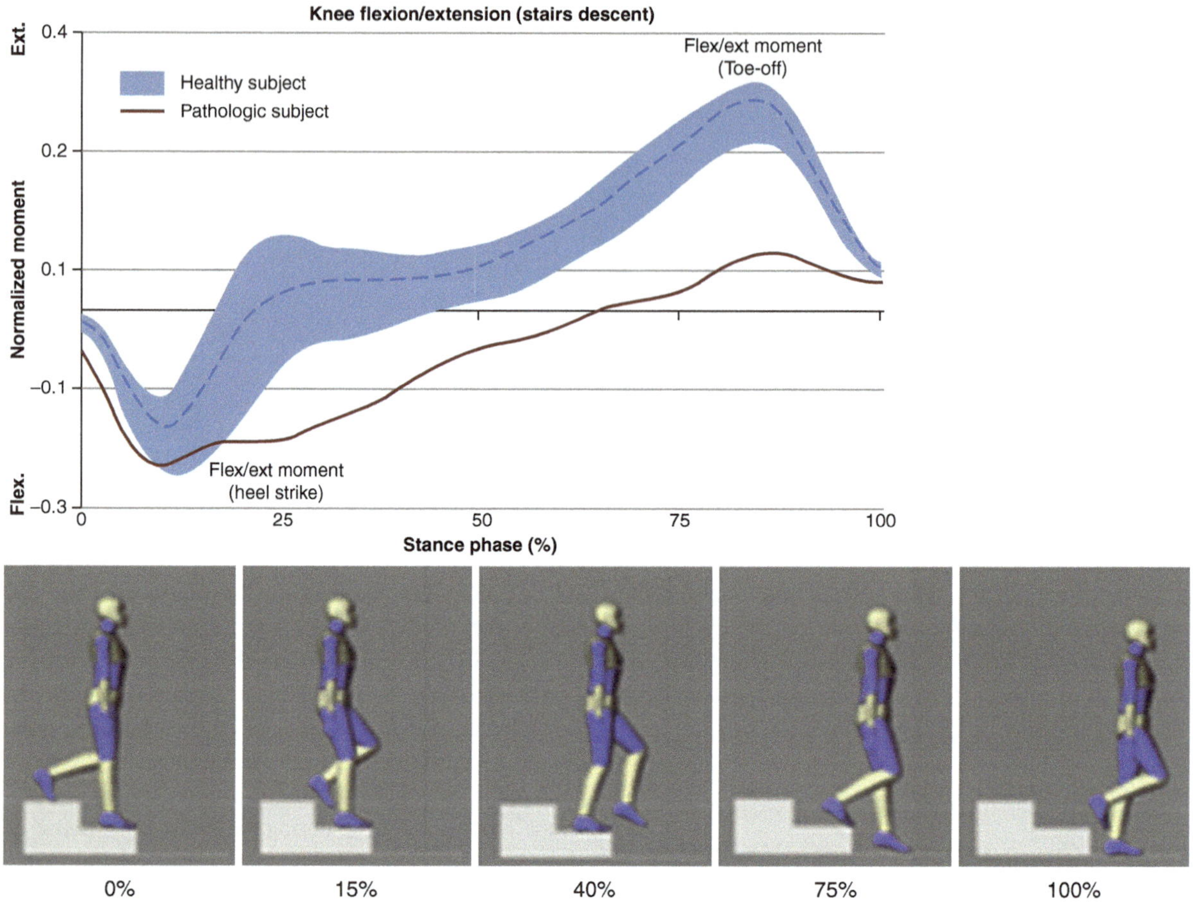


**Fig. 23.4** Knee extension moment

## 23.4 Clinical Relevance

It is well known that the moments that act upon a joint must be balanced by an equal and opposite muscle force to maintain joint equilibrium. In the healthy subject, while going downstairs, the knee joint starts from a relatively stable extended position and flexes toward an increasingly unstable position. The increased joint flexion causes a progressive increment in the external flexion moment,‡‡ which is matched by progressively increasing eccentric quadriceps contraction in order to prevent collapse. In doing so, the internal (muscle) extensor moment§§ increases during stair descent as knee flexion occurs. As the PFJRF is dependent on the magnitude of the quadriceps force and knee flexion angle,[7] the compressive force acting between the patella and femoral trochlea during stair descent would be expected to be significant. It would also increase the PFJ stress (force per unit contact area), which is a factor responsible for the patellofemoral joint cartilage degeneration. Although articular cartilage is aneural, it has been proposed that articular cartilage degeneration renders the subchondral bone susceptible to pressure variations that normally would be absorbed by healthy cartilage.

Although the knee abduction–adduction moment (valgus–varus moment) is not in the primary plane of motion (the primary plane is the sagittal plane), its magnitude should not be ignored when trying to understand the stability and function of the knee during stair climbing and the future life of the knee. Kowalk and colleagues[12] have demonstrated that coronal plane moment patterns are exclusively abductor throughout

‡‡External moment. The load applied to the human body due to the ground reaction forces, gravity, and external forces.

§§Internal joint moment. The net result of all the internal forces acting about the joint, which include moments due to the muscles, ligaments, joint friction, and structural constraints.

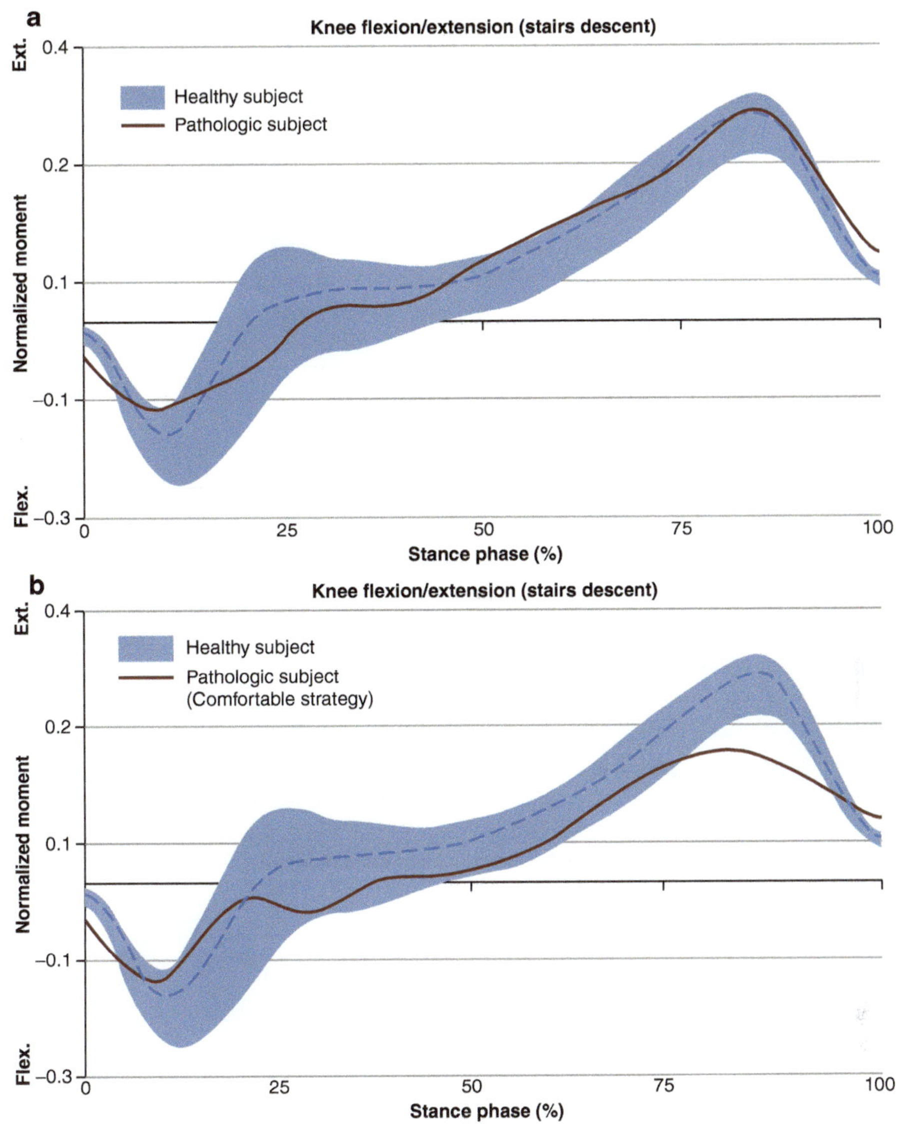


**Fig. 23.5** Knee extension moment. (**a**) Standard stair descending test. (**b**) Stair descending test following the comfort strategy

stance. When an external knee valgus moment occurs, an internal (muscle) joint moment will be generated by the medial muscles (pes anserinus) to balance the joint. An abduction moment will induce a valgus rotation of the tibia. This rotation is limited by two forces, the MCL force, a proximally oriented force at the medial aspect of the knee joint, and a joint contact force acting distally on the lateral tibial plateau.[10]

In the young patient with anterior knee pain, we have observed as other authors have,[1,18] a significant reduction in the knee extensor moment while going downstairs compared to healthy control group subjects, which generally is reversed with pain relief with physiotherapy treatment (Fig. 23.4). However, in some cases, Grenholm and colleagues[9] have demonstrated that these compensatory strategies may remain even after the pain has disappeared. This finding would go against using this test as a patient evolution control system. The reduction of the knee extensor moment, that is suggestive of quadriceps avoidance gait pattern,[16] could be a primary compensatory strategy used by patients with anterior knee pain to reduce the muscle forces acting across the PFJ, and therefore to reduce the forces acting across the PFJ to minimize pain aggravation during walking down stairs. The reduction of the knee extensor moment, with the subsequent

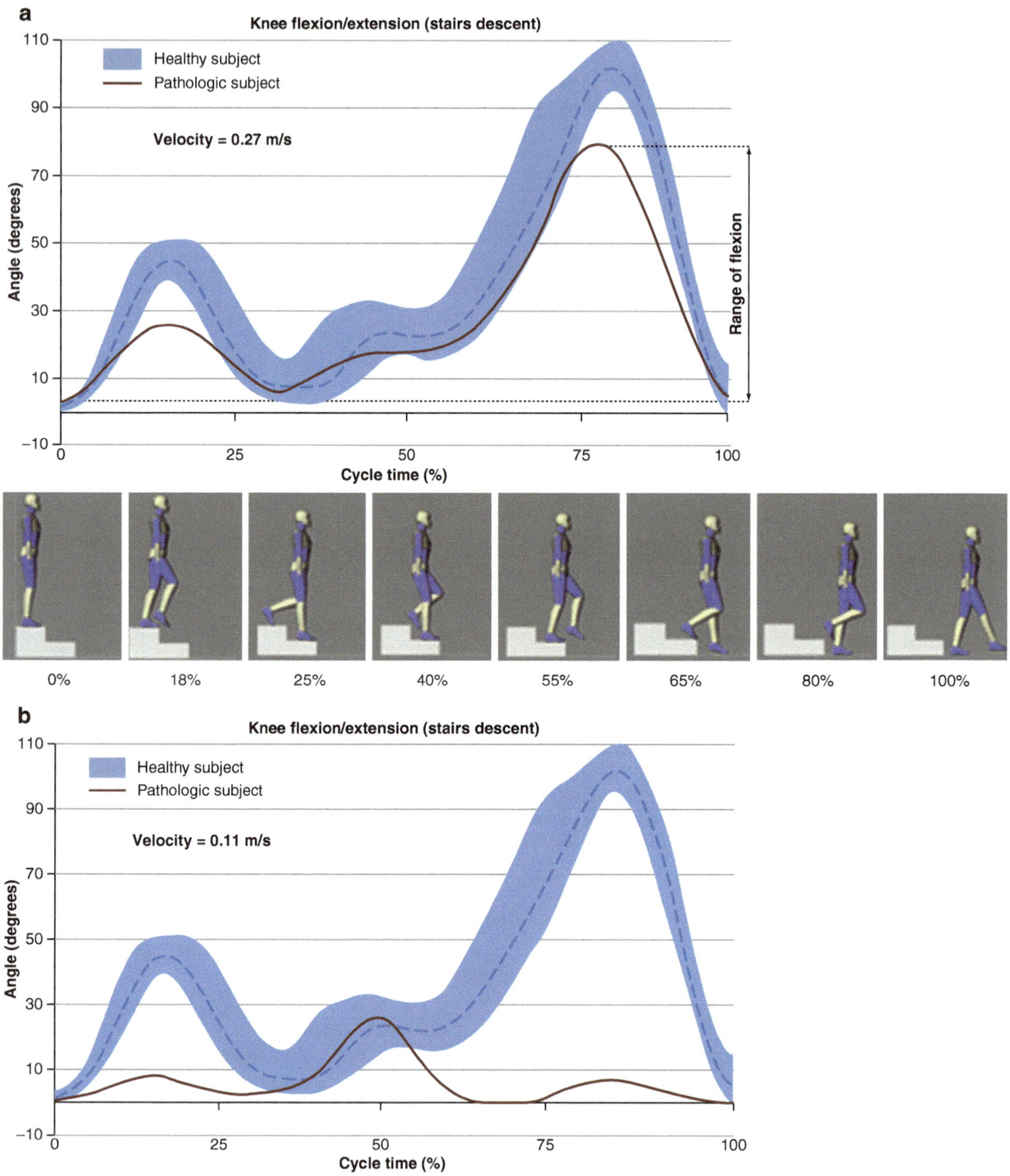


**Fig. 23.6** Knee flexion during stair descending test (**a**). (**b**) Stair descending with a severe knee extension pattern

smaller quadriceps contraction, will cause a decrease of the PFJR force and a decrease of the loading of the PFJ while going downstairs. In this sense, Brechter and Powers[1] have demonstrated that subjects with anterior knee pain did not show increased PFJ stress during stair descent compared to a pain-free control group. We have found that when a patient goes down the stairs using his or her strategy for maximum

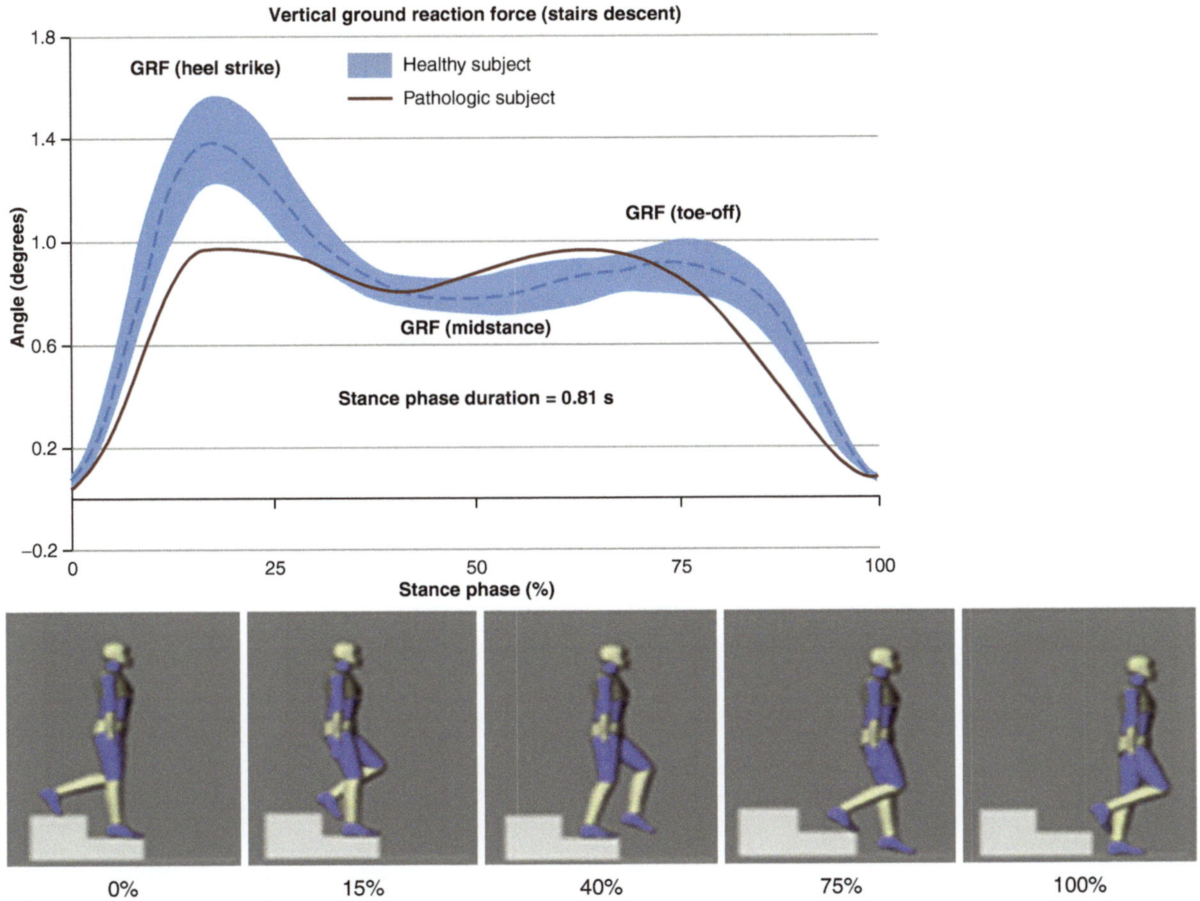


**Fig. 23.7** Vertical ground reaction force during stair descending test

comfort, the extensor moment is lower that when the stair descent is performed following standard protocol. This confirms the fact that we have discovered a defense strategy (Fig. 23.5).

One factor that could contribute to the knee extensor moment reduction is the decrease of knee flexion angle during the stance phase¶ of stair ambulation compared to control healthy subjects (Fig. 23.6). It would be a strategy to reduce the extensor moment and, therefore, pain during stair descent. With less knee flexion, the lever arm of the ground reaction force is shortened and consequently, the knee extensor moment is reduced, equilibrium being achieved by fewer quadriceps contractions. Although we have observed a decrease of the flexion angle in most of our cases, it has not been a uniform finding. In this sense, there are authors who have found a decrease of the flexion angle during stair descent,[3,8] while others have found no significant differences in the flexion angle during stair descent[1,4,9,17,18] in patients with anterior knee pain. The decrease of the knee's flexion angle during stair descent is therefore not a constant adaptive strategy or mechanism. It could be possible that the non-decrease of the flexion angle during stair descent is because, in some people, this activity may not cause enough pain so as to use compensatory strategies such as knee flexion reduction. Another possible reason for this lack of knee flexion reduction with stair descent could be the activation instant of the VMO compared to the VL. Crossley and colleagues[3] have demonstrated that those subjects with a higher deficit in the activation moment of the VMO compared with that of the VL show a higher reduction of knee flexion during stair descent because these patients show an increment

¶Stance phase. Period of time when the foot is in contact with the first step.

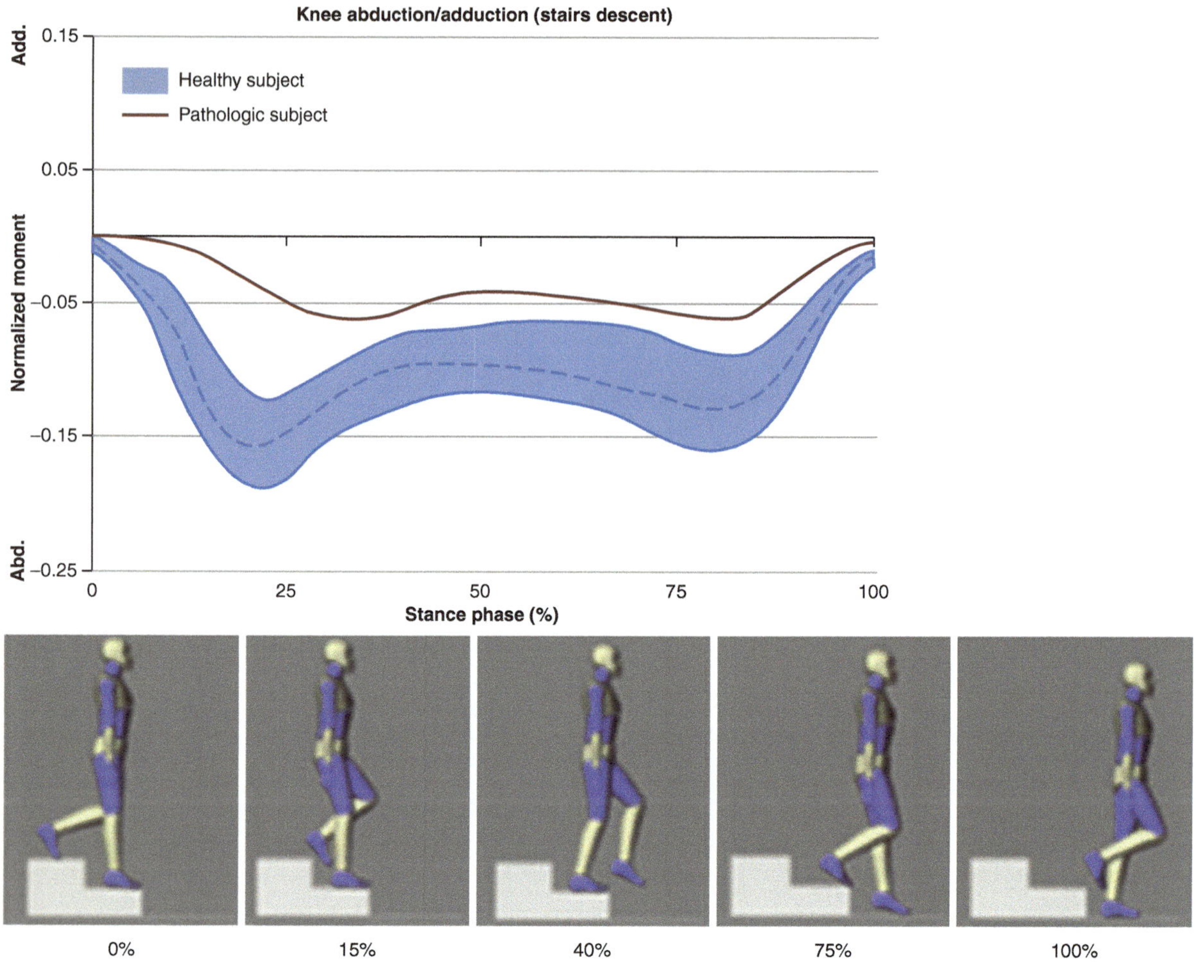


**Fig. 23.8** Knee abduction moment during stair descending test

of the PFJ stress due to the altered patellar tracking. Finally, another fact to justify not finding a decrease of the flexion angle could be how long the pain has been felt; it makes sense to think that a period of time is required for the patient to develop adaptive measures such as flexion reduction.

Other strategies, besides a decrease of knee flexion, to reduce the extensor moment would be the decrease of the vertical ground reaction force compared to the healthy limb (Fig. 23.7). This could reflect an apprehension to load the knee joint at the beginning of the stance phase. According to Salsich and colleagues,[18] other strategies for reducing knee extension moment could be the decrease of the stance time duration and the velocity of stepping. This way the decrease of the vertical ground reaction force or of the speed at which he or she performs the stair descent could contribute to the decrease of the PFJRF, and therefore the patient may not need to reduce knee flexion during stair descent.

According to Hinman and colleagues,[11] quadriceps dysfunction may be important in the development and progression of structural changes in osteoarthritis. Quadriceps dysfunction may compromise protective mechanisms of the knee. The decrease of the extensor moment that is a strategy to reduce pain can have destructive long-term effects on the knee joint. In this sense, the decrease of the active shock absorption*** during weight bearing from the eccentric quadriceps muscle contraction[3,4,7] means greater shock absorption through the bone and

***Shock absorption. The progressive damping of an applied force. Damping is a complex, generally nonlinear, phenomenon that exists whenever energy is dissipated.

cartilage that could explain tibiofemoral pain, and could be a predisposing factor to tibiofemoral osteoarthritis of the knee. There is growing evidence that subchondral bone and its turnover may play a causal role in the pathogenesis of osteoarthritis as well as its related symptoms, especially in the knee. These data support the findings by Naslund and colleagues[13] using bone scintigrams in patients suffering from anterior knee pain. They found that tracer accumulation occurred as often in the proximal tibia as in the patella.

We have been able to demonstrate a decrease of knee abduction (valgus) moment during walking downstairs compared to a healthy pain-free knee in almost all cases in patients with anterior knee pain (Fig. 23.8). The decreased abduction moments around the knee seen in the coronal plane may help to reduce joint loading, which may be a mechanism that avoids degeneration. We have found that when the patient goes down the stairs with his best comfort strategy, the abduction moment is lower than when he does it following a standard protocol, thus confirming that the decrease in the abductor moment is a defense strategy. The increment of the knee abduction moment would cause a lateral tibiofemoral overload. In this way, Elahi and colleagues[6] correlate patellofemoral osteoarthritis with increased valgus knee alignment.

## 23.5 Summary

Most assessments of anterior knee pain treatment progression are made using subjective measurements. Kinetic and kinematic analysis would be appropriate to provide the physician with an objective dynamic measurement of treatment progression (see Chap. 26, case # 2). However, we must insist that the kinetic and kinematic analysis of stair descent is not a diagnostic tool.

Our findings suggest that anterior knee pain patients use strategies to decrease PFJ loading while going downstairs compared to a pain-free control group. The problem is that compensatory strategies require some time to develop and may remain even when pain disappears, which weakens the usefulness of this measurement technique as a treatment progression evaluation method. On the contrary, this technique helps us understand some of the mechanisms behind the development of knee osteoarthritis.

## References

1. Brechter JH, Powers ChM. Patellofemoral joint stress during stair ascent and descent in persons with and without patellofemoral joint. *Gait Posture*. 2002;16:115-123.
2. Costigan PA, Deluzio KJ, Wyss UP. Knee and hip kinetics during normal stair climbing. *Gait Posture*. 2002;16:31-37.
3. Crossley KM, Cowan SM, Bennell KL, et al. Knee flexion during stair ambulation is altered in individuals with patellofemoral pain. *J Orthop Res*. 2004;22:267-274.
4. Crossley KM, Cowan SM, McConnell J, et al. Physical therapy improves knee flexion during stair ambulation in patellofemoral pain. *Med Sci Sports Exerc*. 2005;37:176-183.
5. Davies G, Newman JH. Does adolescent anterior knee pain lead to patello femoral arthritis?. *10th Congress European Society of Sports Traumatology, Knee Surgery and Arthroscopy, Rome, Book of Abstracts*. 2002:353.
6. Elahi S, Cahue S, Felson DT, et al. The association between varus-valgus alignment and patellofemoral osteoarthritis. *Arthritis Rheum*. 2000;43:1874-1880.
7. Fulkerson JP. *Disorders of the Patellofemopral Joint*. Philadelphia: Lippincott Williams & Wilkins; 2004.
8. Greenwald AE, Bagley AM, France EP, et al. A biomechanical and clinical evaluation of a patellofemoral knee brace. *Clin Orthop Relat Res*. 1996;324:187-195.
9. Grenholm A, Stensdotter AK, Hager-Ross Ch. Kinematic analyses during stair descent in young women with patellofemoral pain. *Clin Biomech*. 2009;24:88-94.
10. Grood ES, Noyes FR. Diagnosis of knee ligament injuries: biomechanical precepts. In: Feagin JA, ed. *The Crucial Ligaments*. New York: Churchill Livingstone; 1988.
11. Hinman RS, Crossley KM, McConnell J, et al. Does the application of tape influence quadriceps sensorimotor function in knee osteoarthritis? *Rheumatology*. 2004;43: 331-336.
12. Kowalk DL, Duncan JA, Vaughan CL. Abduction-adduction moments at the knee during stair ascent and descent. *J Biomech*. 1996;29:383-388.
13. Näslund J, Odenbring S, Näslund UB, et al. Diffusely increased bone scintigraphic uptake in patellofemoral pain syndrome. *Br J Sports Med*. 2005;39:162-165.
14. Page A, Candelas P, Belmar F. On the use of local fitting techniques for the analysis of physical dynamic systems. *Eur J Phys*. 2006;27:273-279.
15. Page A, De Rosario H, Mata V, et al. Effect of marker cluster desig on the accuracy of human movement analysis using stereophotogrammetry. *Med Biol Eng Comput*. 2006;44: 1113-1119.
16. Powers CM, Landel R, Perry J. Timing and intensity of vastus muscle activity during functional activities in subjects with and without patellofemoral pain. *Phys Ther*. 1996;76: 946-955.
17. Powers CM, Perry J, Hsu A, et al. Are patellofemoral pain and quadriceps femori muscle torque associated with locomotor function? *Phys Ther*. 1997;77:1063-1075.
18. Salsich GB, Brechter JH, Powers ChM. Lower extremity kinetics during stair ambulation in patients with and without patellofemoral joint. *Clin Biomech*. 2001;16: 906-912.
19. Woltring H. 3-D attitude representation: a standardization proposal. *J Biomech*. 1994;27:1399-1414.

# Part III

# Clinical Cases Commented

# Failure of Patellofemoral Surgery: Analysis of Clinical Cases

24

Robert A. Teitge and Roger Torga-Spak

## 24.1 Introduction

Malfunction of the patellofemoral joint is the result from a failure of any one or a combination of three factors:

- Alignment
- Stability
- Articular Cartilage

An analysis of patellofemoral dysfunction best proceeds with an independent analysis of each of these elements. A more clear understanding of the clinical syndrome can be made if one first looks at each factor independently and then attempts to relate the factors sequentially and causally. As yet there exists no formula, which can quantitatively determine the relative contributions of each of these components in such a way as to define the mechanics, the pathology, and the clinical picture. These three factors are not the same but are often related. It is important to think of the disease process as resulting from a combination of contributions of abnormality from each of these three components. There may be a failure of any one area individually, simultaneously, or sequentially. If the pathomechanics can be determined, then a revision surgery that first reverses the previous surgeries and then corrects the primary mechanical etiology has the best chances of success.

R. Torga-Spak (✉)
Faculty of Orthopaedics and Traumatology,
Department of Surgery, Instituto Universitario CEMIC,
Buenos Aires, Argentina
e-mail: rtorgaspak@gmail.com

## 24.2 Alignment

The first factor to analyze in patellofemoral pain is the alignment. There are two common uses for the term alignment: (1) malposition of the patella on the femur, and (2) malposition of the axis of the knee joint on the limb with the subsequent effect of that malalignment on patellofemoral mechanics. Tracking is the change in position of patella relative to the femur during knee flexion and extension.

Alignment refers to the overall anatomy, that is the lower extremity architecture, the geometrical relationship of all of its components with the result effecting patellofemoral mechanics. It is a common mistake to consider alignment as referring only to the position of the patella on the femoral trochlea. Alignment refers to the changing relationship of all the bones of the lower extremity and might best be considered as the relationship of the patella to the body. Malalignment refers to a variation from the normal anatomy considering normal that is mechanically optimal; however, normal patterns have not been fully defined or quantified.

Bones have an optimal shape and juxtaposition that create optimal functional efficiency. A deviation from optimal geometry alters mechanical loading vectors that may result in symptomatic tissue overuse. It is important to look at the lower limb skeleton in each of three planes with respect to both: geometry of the single bone and of the relative positioning of adjacent bones.

### 24.2.1 Diagnosis

X-rays, including full-length limb alignment films as well as computed axial tomography (CT) scan with determination of bone torsion, are necessary to evaluate the skeleton in three planes.

V. Sanchis-Alfonso (ed.), *Anterior Knee Pain and Patellar Instability*,
DOI: 10.1007/978-0-85729-507-1_24, © Springer-Verlag London Limited 2011

## 24.3 Stability

The second factor which can independently affect the patellofemoral joint is a failure of the normal stabilizing mechanism. It is clear that the stability is provided by a combination of bone and ligamentous restraints. Instability then must result from a failure of the patellofemoral ligaments contained within the retinaculum or the bony buttress. The contact area of bone surfaces, the total applied load, and the direction of the applied load create the friction necessary for stability. Thus, stability is the result of the restraining structures acting against the displacing forces (Table 24.1). Increasing the depth of the trochlea may convert an abnormal side-directed shearing force more perpendicular to the contact surface, thus reducing potential instability in a joint subjected to abnormal side force direction of load application; conversely, in a patient with less intrinsic bony stability (trochlear dysplasia), greater responsibility for maintaining congruent surfaces falls on the ligaments. It is clear that insufficient ligamentous tissue either constitutionally or because of injury may render a susceptible joint unstable while a joint with greater intrinsic stability through bony congruity may continue to function asymptomatically after a similar ligamentous injury.

### 24.3.1 Diagnosis

The diagnosis of instability needs to be made on the demonstration of pathologically increased sideward motion of the patella. X-rays with stress of the patellofemoral joint are needed to put in evidence ligament insufficiency. To obtain these stress x-rays, the patient is positioned as for a routine Merchant x-ray view. If there is a knee flexion angle where medial or lateral subluxation stress applied to the patella produces greater apprehension or greater sideways excursion, then this position is selected for the axial x-ray with the line tangent to the joint determined by viewing the lateral x-ray. The examiner's hand supports the knee to keep it from rotating away from the x-ray tube while stress is applied from the medial or the lateral side to the edge of the patella. A quantitative stress device had been used to standardize the displacement force (Medmetric Corp., San Diego, CA, USA) The usual stress applied is 15–18 lb depending on the patient's ability to tolerate the pressure without contracting the muscles and an equal stress is applied to both patellae. A marked increase in displacement on one side is evidence of instability with subluxation.[3]

**Table 24.1** Restraining structures acting against displacing forces

| Displacing forces | Restraining structures |
|---|---|
| Trauma | Medial patellofemoral ligament |
| Body weight | Lateral patellofemoral ligament |
| Limb malalignment<br>• Increased femoral anteversion<br>• Increased tibial external torsion<br>• Valgus knee | Trochlear depth |
| Patella alta | |
| Foot hyperpronation | |
| Tight achilles | |

## 24.4 Cartilage

Cartilage damage may result from direct trauma (acute pressure increase such as dashboard injury or fall); chronic trauma (pressure increase) secondary to the imposed stress of malalignment without ligamentous failure and subluxation or dislocation, which reduces contact pressure areas or from chronic overload on an anatomically sound knee (as weight lifting or obesity); or chronic overload from reduction in contact area and load sharing such as patella alta.[1,2] It is presumed that articular cartilage stays healthy when subjected to loads confined to a small range (3–5 MPa). A reduction of surface area or an increase in imposed load will elevate this to an unacceptable level, leading to chondromalacia and ultimately arthrosis. The presence of chondromalacia does not tell us what its etiology was.

### 24.4.1 Diagnosis

The condition of the cartilage may be seen well with double-contrast arthrography and as this also reveals the thickness of the articular cartilage over the surface of the patella, contrast CT may be preferable to arthroscopy.Good magnetic resonance images can reveal the articular cartilage but at times, lower quality studies do not, especially at the point of contact between the two surfaces.

## 24.5 Treatment

The treatment will be directed to correct the abnormality detected after the independent assessment of the three factors described above. Ideally, the treatment should address the primary mechanical factor responsible for the condition (Table 24.2). However, in most cases, the etiology is multifactorial and more than one factor or altered structure is observed during the examination. If that is the case, we generally correct the factor that is more out of what is considered normal.

## 24.6 Failed Surgery

The treatment of the complications depends on recognizing whether the complication was caused by incomplete or incorrect diagnosis or by selection of an inappropriate procedure. A common mistake that lead to failure is the local treatment of intraarticular lesions rather than the predisposing factors responsible for the pathology.

In the treatment of the patient with a failed patellofemoral surgery, a two-step approach is necessary. First, to restore to the preoperative state the anatomy and the relations of the structures, which have been incorrectly modified by the procedure. Table 24.3 shows a list of common complications and the procedures we perform to restore the preoperative anatomy. Second, to detect and correct the predisposing factors, which have lead to the preoperative symptoms (Table 24.2).

## 24.7 Clinical Cases

### *24.7.1 Case 1*

*History.* A 44-year-old woman was normal with no complaints in her knees until an automobile accident in which she was driving her car, which was struck from the side by another car. She slid underneath the seat belt striking both knees directly against the dashboard. Radiographs were negative. After physiotherapy, she

**Table 24.2** Procedures performed after independent analysis

| Alignment | | Stability | | Cartilage | |
|---|---|---|---|---|---|
| Condition | Procedure | Condition | Procedure | Condition | Procedure |
| Genu valgum | Femoral varus osteotomy | Lateral instability | MPFL reconstruction | Focal lesion | Osteotomy or biological procedure |
| Genu varum | Tibial valgus osteotomy | Medial instability | LPFL reconstruction | Generalized lesion | Allograft or prosthetic replacement |
| Increased femoral anteversion | External rotation femoral ostetomy | Multidirectional instability (medial + lateral) | MPFL + LPFL reconstruction | | |
| Increased tibial external torison | Internal rotational tibial osteotomy | Trochlear dysplasia | Trochleoplasty or MPFL reconstruction | | |
| Foot hyperpronation | Foot orthotics | | | | |
| Patella alta | Distal tubercle displacement | | | | |
| Lateral tibial tubercle (>20 mm) medial tibial tubercle | Tibial Tubercle medialization Lateral tibial tubercle transfer | | | | |

**Table 24.3** Common complications and procedures to restore preoperative anatomy

| Procedure | Complication | Treatment |
|---|---|---|
| Lateral retinacular release | Medial dislocation of the patella | Reconstruction of the lateral PF ligament |
| Medial retinacular repairs or reefings | Recurrent lateral instability | Medial PFL reconstruction |
| Lateral retinacular release | Multidirectional instability (combined medial and lateral instability) | Medial and lateral PFL reconstruction |
| Shaving chondroplasty | Patellofemoral artrosis | Osteotomy +/– allograft |
| Medial tubercle transfer with normal TT-TG distance | Pathological external rotation of tibia and medial compartment overload | Lateralization of the distal tubercle |

continued to have mild pain over the patella with no signs or symptoms of instability in the left knee. Six months after accident, she underwent arthroscopy and an arthroscopic lateral release. Anterior knee pain was much more severe after surgery. Almost immediately, she noted that a knee sleeve would push the patella out of place in the medial direction. She now had retropatellar crepitation, pain laterally, an effusion after walking for 20 min, limping, insecurity, difficulty going downstairs, a sense that the patella was out of place especially walking down hills, aching pain at night, collapsing of the knee, and inability to wear high heel shoes.

*Physical Exam.* Knee motion 0–150°, effusion, diffuse warmth, soft tissue swelling, crepitation with extension, a negative J-sign, marked increased medial and lateral mobility of the left patella compared with the non-operated right, there was considerable apprehension with pressing the patella medially and a complete medial dislocation could be demonstrated with medial stress, the Q-angle was 15°, there was significant tenderness palpating the defect in the lateral retinaculum, the Ober test was negative, collateral and cruciate ligaments were normal, limb alignment in the frontal plane was clinically normal, prone examination revealed hip rotation 65° internal and 35° external, the foot thigh axis was normal, there was moderate pronation of the foot, the Achilles tendon was tight bilaterally.

*Radiographs.* AP, lateral, and axial radiographs were normal with normal height of the patella, normal tibiofemoral axis, and normal sulcus. Stress radiographs, however, revealed a complete medial dislocation of the patella, which moved medially 24 mm more than in the normal knee, laterally 5 mm more than in the normal knee and tilted 14° more than in the normal knee. Figure 24.1 shows this abnormal displacement. Figure 24.2 shows (in another patient) clinically a medially dislocated patella.

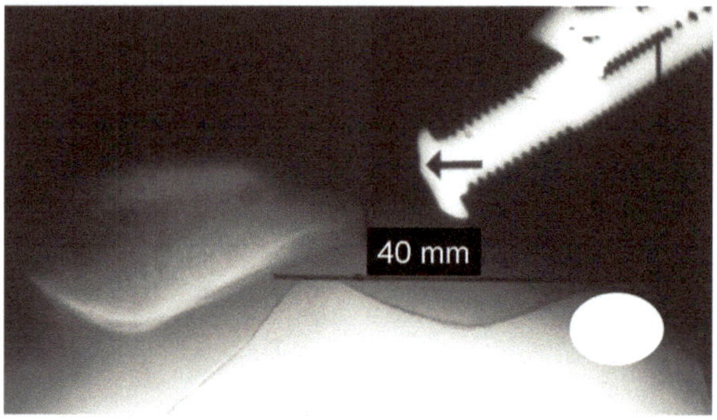


**Fig. 24.1** Medial dislocation of the patella after arthroscopic lateral patellar release

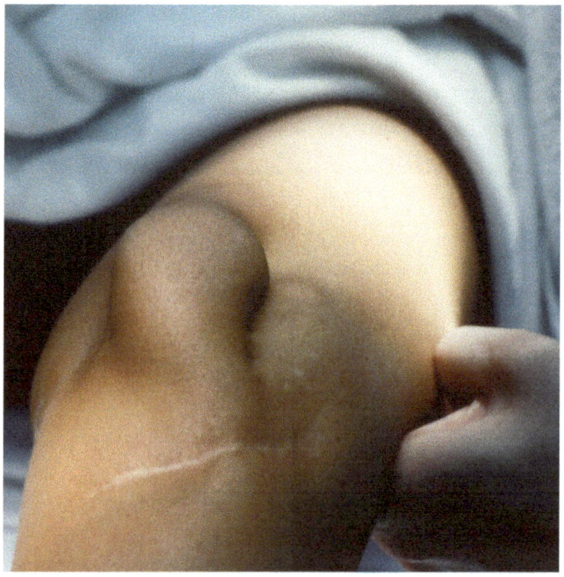

**Fig. 24.2** Example of medial dislocatable patella post realignment

*Analysis.* The complication is an iatrogenic medial patellar dislocation following an isolated arthroscopic lateral release. There is no evidence in this case to suggest that the lateral retinaculum was in any way contributing to the patient's symptoms. The normal lateral retinaculum contributes to stability in both the medial and in the lateral direction and prevents abnormal tilt.

*Treatment.* The correction was a reconstruction with quadriceps graft of the lateral patellofemoral ligament.

### 24.7.2 Case 2

*History.* A 26-year-old woman with disabling left knee pain and instability. At age 19, she was struck in the front of the knee by an opponent while playing baseball. She continued to play baseball but because of continued pain, 1 year later she underwent diagnostic arthroscopy and subcutaneous lateral release. She was somewhat worse, so 3 months later underwent a repeat arthroscopy with chondroplasty of both the patella and femur to create bleeding bone for stimulation of cartilage growth. She was definitely worse and a consultant suggested repeating the lateral release. One year later, she underwent an Insall proximal realignment, repeat lateral release, and drilling of the patella. She deteriorated further and began to experience medial dislocations of the patella. A second consultant recommended quadriceps exercises, which she performed 3 days a week for 3 years. A third consultant recommended 6 weeks of casting, which did not help. On at least four occasions, a patellar dislocation medially required manipulative reduction, twice in the hospital. Seven years after the original injury, a fourth consultant recognized medial patellar dislocation. At this point, she needed a railing to assist in going up and down the stairs, had constant aching, pain at night, and regular stiffness.

*Physical Exam.* Genu varum greater on the involved side, recurvatum, pronation of the feet and inward pointing or squinting of both patella, retropatellar crepitation with active knee extension bilaterally, a negative J-sign compared with a markedly positive J-sign on the asymptomatic side, increased medial–lateral patellar excursion, no apprehension moving the patella laterally but severe apprehension moving the patella medially, significant quadriceps atrophy, motion – 7–145°, pain at the medial joint line, pain at the lateral retinaculum, Q-angle = 20° bilaterally, negative Ober, foot thigh axis – 10°, tibia varum, no Achilles tightness, hip internal rotation 45°, external rotation 50°.

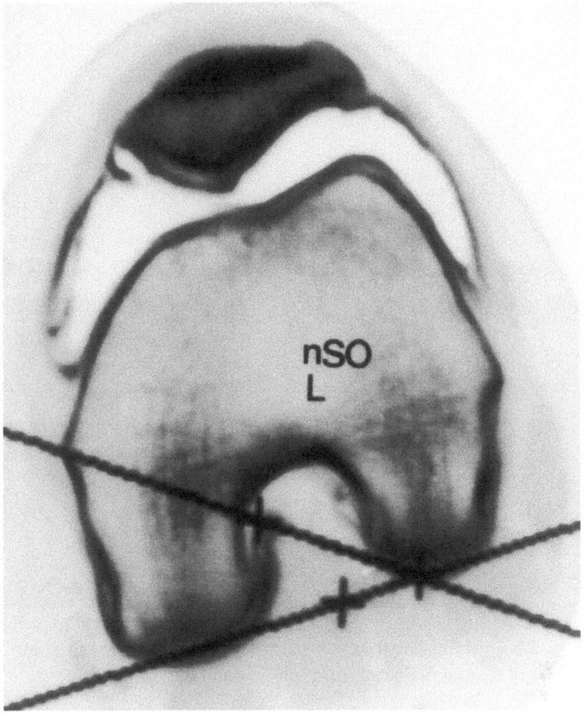


**Fig. 24.3** CT arthrogram. Loss lateral articular cartilage, shallow trochlea, post lateral release and arthroscopic chondroplasty

*Radiographs.* Narrowing of the patellofemoral joint, and a shallow sulcus, normal patellar height. CT arthrogram revealed complete loss of lateral articular cartilage with excellent preservation of medial patellar articular cartilage (Fig. 24.3). Medial stress CT revealed a complete medial dislocation of the patella. This film (Fig. 24.4) clearly shows how the lateral cartilage could be injured with good preservation of the medial cartilage during medial dislocation.

*Analysis.* The complication is iatrogenic arthrosis through removal of articular cartilage and iatrogenic medial dislocation of the patella through repeated lateral releases plus medial imbrication.

*Treatment.* Lateral patellofemoral ligament reconstruction with a quadriceps tendon graft with the result being significant improvement as the instability was treated but ultimately not the cartilage loss.

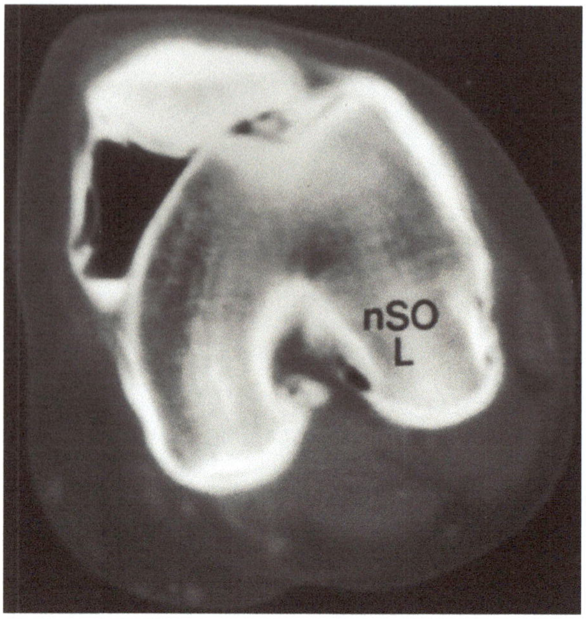


**Fig. 24.4** Medial dislocation patella post lateral release showing why medial dislocation causes lateral facet damage

### 24.7.3 Case 3

*History*. A 34-year-old woman with anterior knee pain unresponsive to arthroscopy 15 years ago. Four years prior to consultation had been injured by blunt trauma when a metal cart carrying 100 kg struck the anterior knee near the patellar tendon. One year later underwent arthroscopy, which did not improve the knee and after physiotherapy 1 year later underwent another arthroscopy. There was no change in the pain, swelling, and giving way, so she had a Maquet osteotomy with soft tissue breakdown requiring a gastrocnemius muscle flap for coverage (Fig. 24.5).

*Physical Exam*. 183-cm tall, 121 kg. Neutral alignment, pronated feet, squinting patellae, circumduction gait. Squat only 30° because of pain, motion – 5–110° bilaterally, ligaments stable, meniscal signs negative, Q-angle 15° R and 20° L, no patellofemoral crepitation but weakness of the quadriceps, moderate thigh muscle atrophy, Ober tight at 4 cm without pain, prone hip internal rotation 70°, external rotation 50°.

*Radiographs*. AP, lateral, and axial radiographs were negative except for CT study for limb rotation showing femoral anteversion 54° (vs normal 13°) (Fig. 24.6).

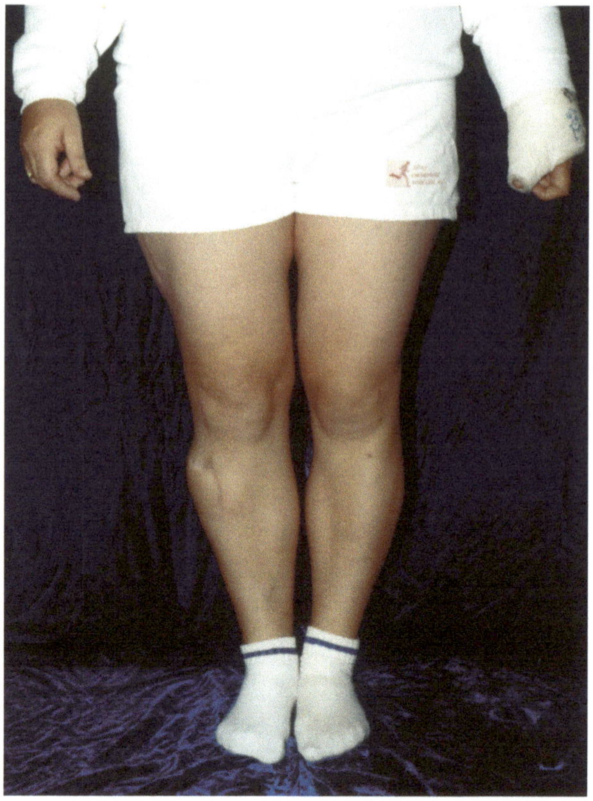

**Fig. 24.5** A 34-year-old-patient post right Maquet osteotomy with inpointing left patella. She is post-op right intertrochanteric 40° external rotation osteotomy

*Analysis*. Complication was failure to recognize limitation of external hip rotation forcing the knee joint axis to be chronically facing inward.

*Treatment*. The treatment was external rotational femoral osteotomy (intertrochanteric). The result at 4 months was she noticed the operated knee moves straight forward while in the non-operated limb the foot swings outward. The preoperative pain, which had been present for over 4 years, was gone and the operated limb now had less pain than the noninjured knee and she was anxious to have the same surgery on the noninjured limb.

### 24.7.4 Case 4

*History*. A 37-year-old woman with 6 months of constant pain, both knees requiring narcotic medication. Anterior knee pain began 19 years earlier. Two years later, 17 years ago, she underwent a medial transfer of the left tibial tubercle. Fifteen years ago, she

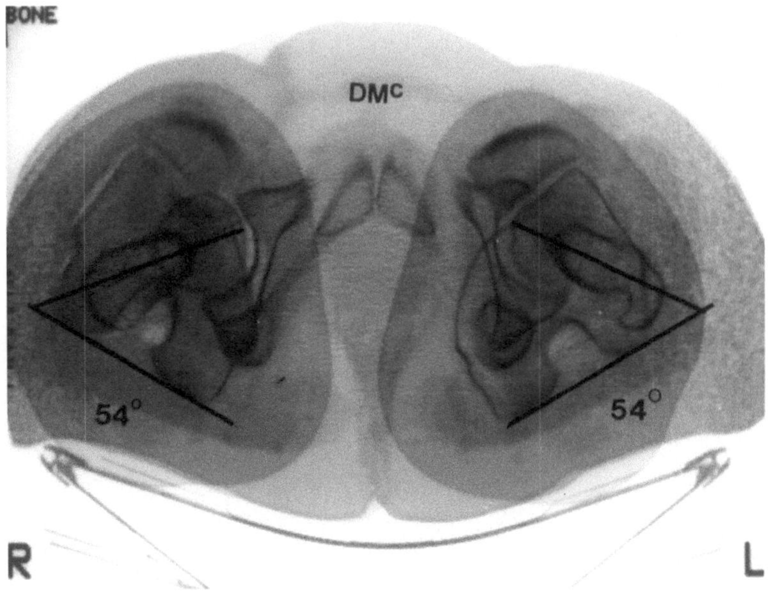


**Fig. 24.6** Preop CT rotational scan shows bilateral 54° femoral anteversion

underwent a medial transfer of the right tibial tubercle. A manipulation was required for limited motion post-op. Twelve years ago, she underwent arthroscopy with lysis of adhesions followed shortly afterward with a manipulation. Ten years ago, she had an arthroscopic synovectomy. Four years ago, she underwent right arthroscopic medial meniscectomy, patellar chondroplasty by arthroscopic shaving, and lateral release. She was much worse after that procedure. There is constant pain which keeps her awake at night, pain walking, pain going up and down the stairs, pain sitting, weakness, buckling, limping, insecurity, catching and intermittent sharp pains.

*Examination.* Slight varus, inpointing of the patella (squinting), limited squatting, motion R 0–130°, L 0–134°, L effusion, bilateral soft tissue swelling, retropatellar crepitation, increased lateral mobility bilaterally with apprehension on the right not the left, increased medial mobility on the right not the left with apprehension on the right. Q-angle :12° R and 14° L, cruciate and collateral ligaments intact, significant pain with palpation along the medial joint line on the right, prone internal hip rotation 50°, external rotation 25°. The tibial tubercles appeared to be located excessively medial and the feet were pointed outward.

*Radiographs.* The mechanical axis was neutral, flexion weight bearing showed equal joint space medial and lateral, both patellae were centered in the trochlea in the axial view, but there was narrowing with increased subchondral sclerosis of the medial patellofemoral joints. CT arthrography revealed loss of medial facet articular cartilage greater on the left (Fig. 24.7) and CT studies for torsion showing increased anteversion bilaterally at 24° and 32° (Fig. 24.8), with the tibial tubercle – trochlear groove distance 0 on the right and – 5 mm on the left.

*Analysis.* The complication is medial patellofemoral arthrosis after medial tibial tubercle transfer. In addition, the tibias are being rotated externally as a result of an external rotational pull from a medially transferred tibial tubercle, and it is felt that the medial compartments were being overloaded by the increased medial patellofemoral loading. There was no proof of subluxation or dislocation in this patient. It was assumed that lateral patellar displacement was responsible for the anterior knee pain and it was assumed that a medial transfer of the tibial tubercle would reduce this subluxation and pain. It was assumed that lateral release, chondroplasty, and medial meniscectomy would improve the symptoms. It is likely this made the situation worse.

*Treatment.* Lateral transfer of the tibial tubercles and external rotational osteotomy of the femurs. The patient remains improved at 6 years post osteotomy although she has intermittent pain along the left medial joint line, which is felt to be due to an inadequate lateral transfer of the left tibial tubercle.

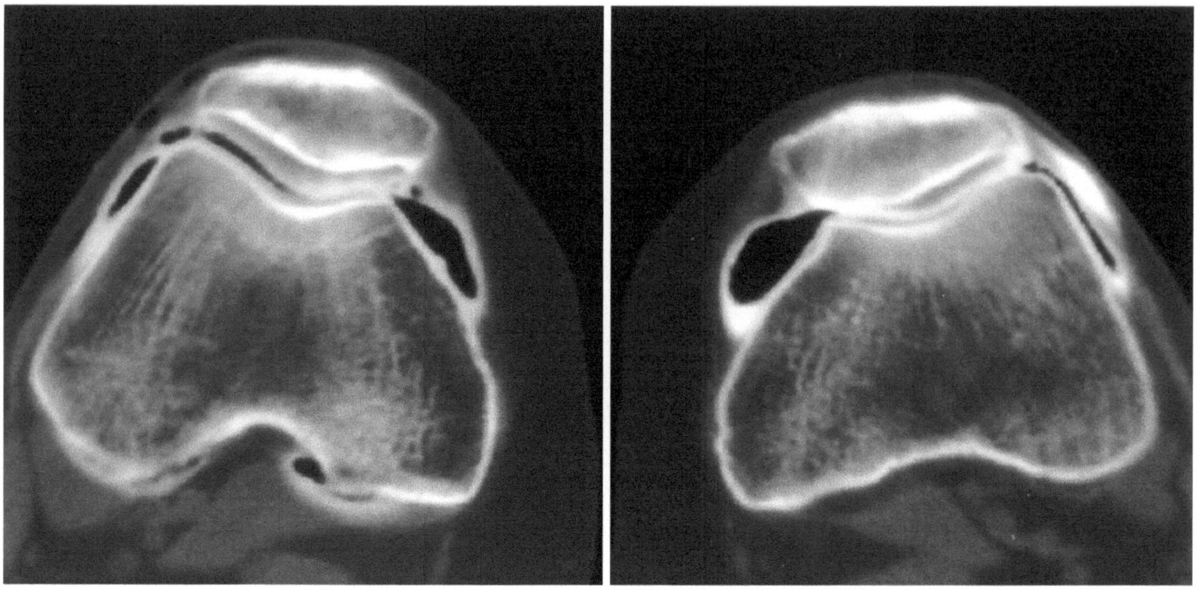

**Fig. 24.7** Double contrast CT arthrogram showing loss of medial patellofemoral cartilage bilaterally after medial tibial tubercle transfer

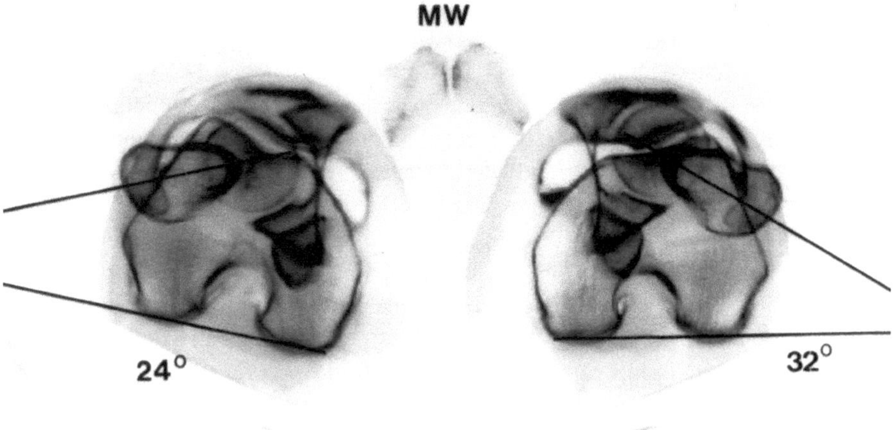


**Fig. 24.8** CT rotational study showing bilateral femoral anteversion. Treatment was lateral tibial tubercle transfer to unload medial facet and intertrochanteric external rotational osteotomy to treat rotational alignment

### 24.7.5 Case 5

*History.* A 33-year-old male hospital administrator was seen in consultation for bilateral anterior knee pain of increased severity of 3 months duration after a painful bucking episode while in church. He complained of limping, recurrent swelling, locking, buckling at least 6 times per day, pain going up and down the stairs, pain with sitting, and a feeling of the patella slipping but not requiring manipulation for relocation.

At age 20 (13 years earlier), he had realignment surgery (medial tubercle transfer, Insall-type medial imbrication, and lateral release) bilaterally. Nine years earlier, he had removal of loose bodies from the left knee.

*Physical Exam.* 193-cm tall, 119 kg, genu valgum, hyperpronation of feet, inability to squat because of pain and stiffness, motion 0–130°, there is hypermobility of both patellae, there is hypersensitivity with this motion, pain with lateral subluxation bilaterally and pain with medial subluxation of the left patella, Q-angle 0°, medial facet tenderness bilaterally, increased articular grind with side motion of the patella, patella alta, 1+ laxity to varus stress bilaterally, thigh atrophy, Ober tight at 3 cm, prone hip internal rotation 60°, external rotation 20°, tight Achilles bilaterally.

*Radiographs.* Patella alta, normal congruence angle, narrowing of the medial patellofemoral joint, stress radiographs indicated no increased lateral excursion but almost a dislocation medially. CT arthrography revealed good quality articular cartilage superiorly on the patella with marked loss of distal and, especially, medial patellar articular cartilage; CT rotation study revealed femoral anteversion 36° (normal 13°).

*Analysis.* (1) Postsurgical arthrosis, (2) medial patellar instability, (3) trochlear dysplasia, (4) increased femoral anteversion, (5) mild increased external tibial torsion, (6) hyperpronation of feet, (7) mild genu valgum, (8) contracture of Achilles tendon, and (9) post-medial tibial tubercle transfer.

*Treatment.* (1) Distal and lateral transfer tibial tubercle, (2) external rotation varus osteotomy distal femur, and (3) imbrication of both the medial and lateral retinaculum.

Postoperatively, he described "a new sensation, which is comfortable and confident" and at 1.5 years post surgery "wonderful, the knee better than he could ever remember having it been." He requested the same procedure on the opposite knee and is now 5 years post surgery on the right and 3 years post surgery on the left. He continues to remain improved over the preoperative state. However, we have not addressed the loss of articular cartilage, tibial torsion, trochlear dysplasia, Achilles contracture, or the patient's height and weight.

In each of these cases, limb alignment including varus-valgus, torsion of the femur and tibia, foot pronation, muscle contracture, trochlear dysplasia, patellar height, and patellofemoral ligament laxity need to be considered. A simple lateral release or tibial tubercle transfer fails to address the more important contributing variables.

### 24.7.6 Case 6

*History.* A 34-year-old female teacher was referred for consultation regarding recurrent dislocation of the patella starting at age 13. At age 30, because of pain and swelling, she underwent arthroscopy followed by medial transfer of tibial tubercle (Elmslie-Trillat), lateral retinacular release, and chondroplasty. She now presents with pain, swelling, weakness, and slippage of the patella.

*Physical Examination.* Straight limb alignment, bilateral foot hyperpronation, Motion 0–150°. Unable to extend against gravity, with audible crepitation as she attempts this. Q-angle = 5° compared with 20° on the opposite side. Patella is hypermobile both to the medial and the lateral direction. Gross atrophy of the quadriceps, moderate effusion, collateral and cruciate ligaments are stable, McMurray negative, Ober test negative, prone hip internal rotation 40°, external rotation 30°.

*Radiographs.* Narrowing of articular cartilage space and osteoporosis. Slight patella alta with Insall ratio = 0.8. Stress radiographs show complete dislocation of the patella medially and hypermobility laterally.

*Analysis.* The complication is iatrogenic medial patellar dislocation due to combined lateral release and medial tubercle transfer, with arthrosis aggravated by chondroplasty.

*Treatment.* Lateral transfer of the tibial tubercle and lateral retinacular repair. She improved, but at 2 years post-op, redislocated the patella medially. The lateral retinaculum is frequently not of sufficient quality to create a permanent repair. At this stage, she underwent lateral patellofemoral ligament reconstruction with a quadriceps tendon graft. This was effective in providing stability but further deterioration in the remaining articular cartilage occurred (Figs. 24.9 and 24.10).

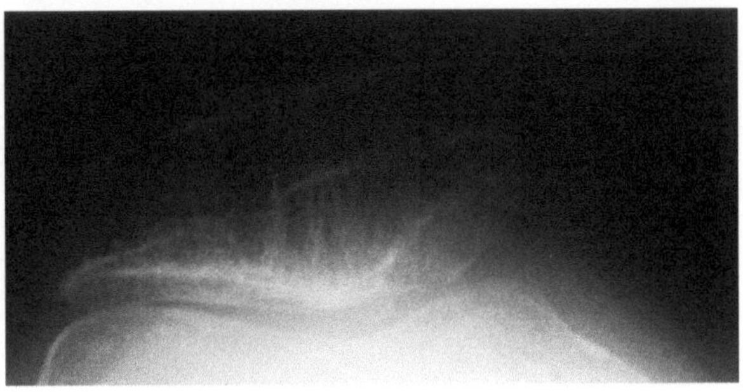

**Fig. 24.9** Post lateral PF ligament reconstruction development arthrosis PF joint

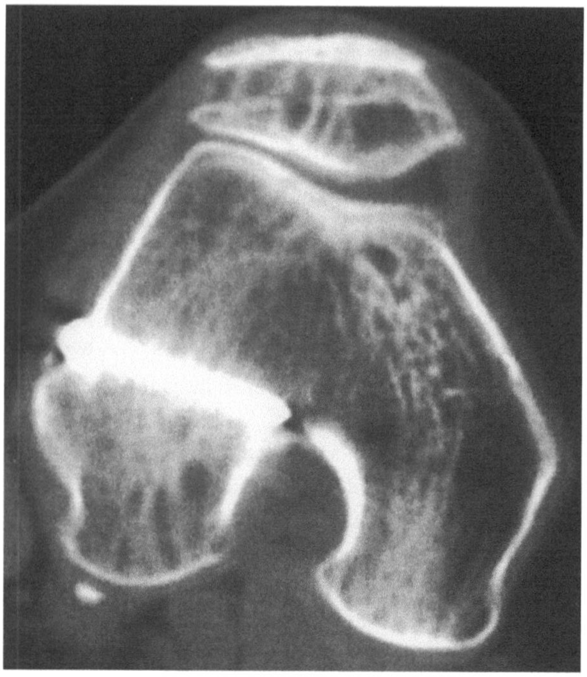

**Fig. 24.10** CT scan showing arthrosis

Three years later, she underwent patellar–trochlear fresh allograft replacement (Fig. 24.11). She is now 9 years post allograft and although the radiographs appear to show extensive abnormal bone changes, the articular space still remains widened and her symptoms are still greatly improved over her earlier treatment.

*Conclusion.* In the treatment of patellofemoral complications, the surgical treatment should address the primary pathology as well as the changes induced by the failed procedure. Cutting normal ligaments, removing articular cartilage, or transferring tendons to an abnormal position usually create new problems and should be performed cautiously.

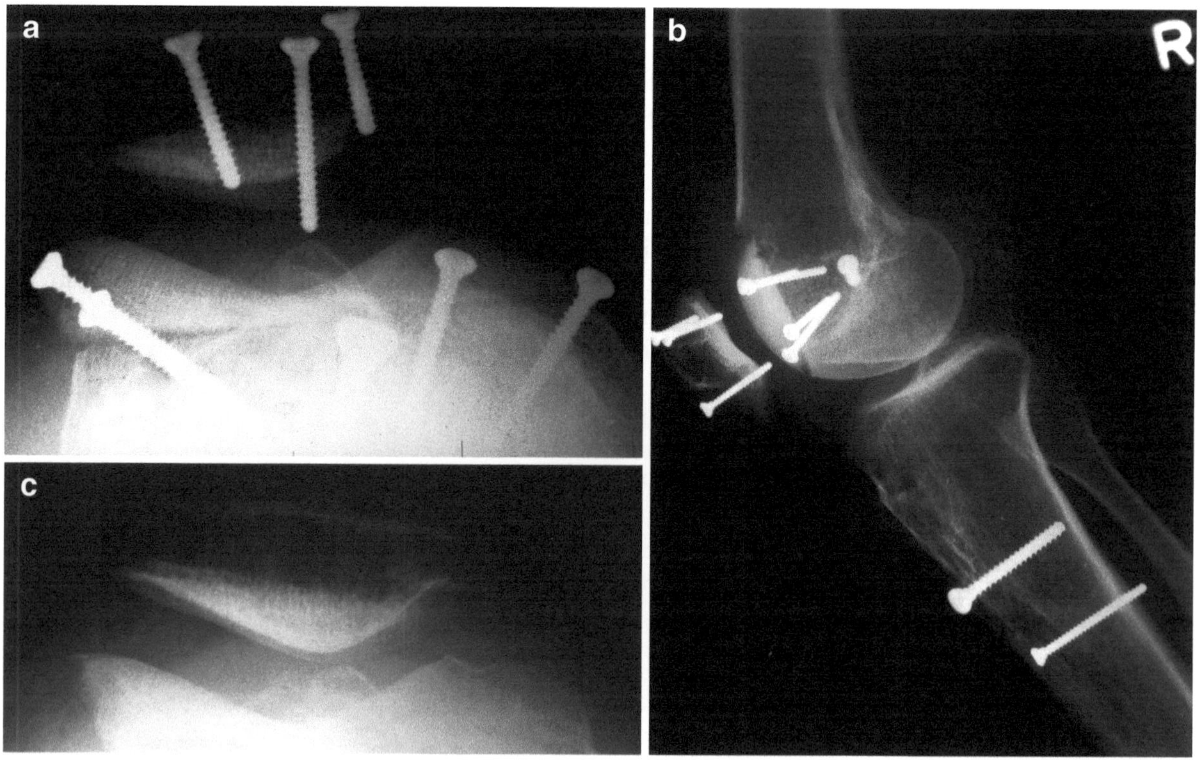


**Fig. 24.11** (**a**) Axial x-ray 2 weeks post PF fresh allograft. (**b**) Lateral x-ray 2 weeks post PF fresh allograft. (**c**) Axial x-ray 10 months post PF fresh allograft. (**d**) Lateral x-ray 10 months post PF fresh allograft. (**e**) Axial x-ray 5 years post PF fresh allograft. (**f**) CT 9 years post PF fresh allograft. Compare with Fig. 24.10

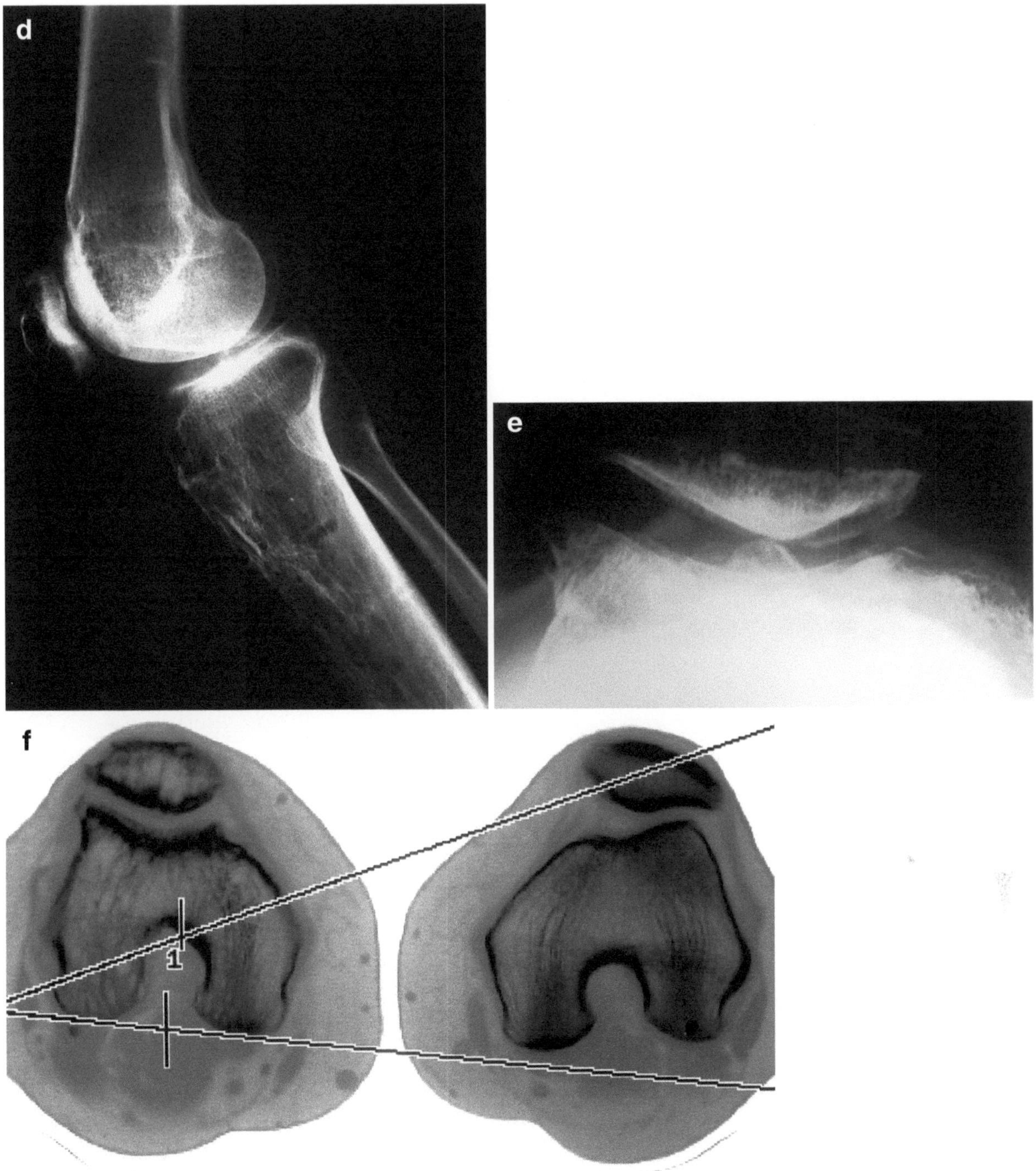


**Fig. 24.11** (continued)

## References

1. Huberti HH, Hayes WC. Patellofemoral contact pressures. The influence of q-angle and tendofemoral contact. *J Bone Joint Surg*. 1984;66-A:715-724.
2. Huberti HH, Hayes WC. Contact pressures in chondromalacia patellae and the effects of capsular reconstructive procedures. *J Orthop Res*. 1988;6:499-508.
3. Teitge RA, Faerber WW, Des Madryl P, et al. Stress radiographs of the patellofemoral joint. *J Bone Joint Surg*. 1996; 78-A:193-203.

# Neuromatous Knee Pain: Evaluation and Management

25

Maurice Y. Nahabedian

## 25.1 Introduction

The concept of selective denervation around the knee joint has received increasing attention and recognition as a legitimate treatment modality for intractable knee pain due to neuromata. Our ability to surgically manage these patients has been enhanced as our understanding of the innervation of the human knee joint has improved. Much of this is due to the pioneering work of one of my long-standing mentors, A. Lee Dellon, MD. His anatomic studies detailing the neural pathways have facilitated our understanding of the sensory mechanisms responsible for pain around the knee joint.[7] This has greatly enhanced our ability to evaluate, diagnose, and manage patients with chronic and intractable knee pain due to neuromata. Since the previous edition of the chapter, there have been very few additional reports that have focus on this treatment regimen. However, the number of surgeons interested and performing these procedures has been steadily increasing.

Denervation for chronic joint pain was initially described in 1958.[11,12] Early reports of total denervation for chronic pain about the elbow joint were not well accepted due to the untoward effects on extremity function. This is because both sensory and motor nerves were ablated. Thus, for many years, denervation was not considered a reasonable option. However, with the advent of selective denervation, the untoward sequellae have been eliminated because only the specific sensory nerves are excised and the motor nerves are preserved.[1,3]

M.Y. Nahabedian
Department of Plastic Surgery, Georgetown University, Washington, DC, USA
e-mail: drnahabedian@aol.com

Thus, in properly selected patients, a significant to complete reduction in pain is possible. It is important to realize, however, that selective denervation is primarily directed at patients with neuromatous pain. It is not recommended for chronic pain resulting from a nonneuromatous etiology.

Selective denervation for chronic neuromatous knee pain was initially described by Dellon and colleagues in 1995.[4] In his pilot study, 15 patients with persistent neuromatous pain following total knee arthroplasty were treated. All patients reported a reduction in pain. Mean follow-up was 12 months. In a subsequent study, 70 patients with chronic neuromatous knee pain following total knee arthroplasty, trauma, or osteotomy had selective denervation with a good to excellent outcome in 86% with a mean follow-up of 24 months.[5] In his most recent update, the results of 344 patients with neuromatous knee pain who were evaluated and managed with selective denervation were reported upon.[6] In the majority of patients, the etiology was total knee arthroplasty (74%) and in the rest, it was trauma (26%). Following the operation, the outcomes were reported as excellent in 70%, good in 20%, some improvement in 5%, and no improvement in 5%.

Since then, other studies evaluating the safety and efficacy of this technique have been completed. Kasim and colleagues[8] performed lateral retinacular excisions in 25 patients with anterior knee pain. Of these, 22 (88%) noted subjective improvement in the pain following surgery. Although the pain was not completely eliminated following surgery, it was reduced by 50%. Other findings included an increase in activities of daily living by 40% following surgery; whereas it was reduced by 60% prior to surgery.

Personal experience with selective denervation for chronic knee pain has demonstrated benefit in properly selected patients.[9,10] We evaluated 43 patients with

V. Sanchis-Alfonso (ed.), *Anterior Knee Pain and Patellar Instability*,
DOI: 10.1007/978-0-85729-507-1_25, 

intractable knee pain of which 25 were qualified to have and proceed to undergo selective denervation. Complete pain relief was obtained in 11 patients (44%), partial pain relief was reported in ten patients (40%), and no pain relief was reported in four patients (16%). Follow-up ranged from 1 to 4 years. Patients were satisfied with the outcome in 21/25 cases (84%).

## 25.2 Anatomic Basis for Selective Denervation

There are currently seven surgically identifiable sensory nerves around the knee joint (Fig. 25.1).[2,9] The sensory innervation around the medial aspect of the knee includes the infrapatellar branch of the saphenous nerve, the medial retinacular nerve, and the medial and anterior cutaneous nerves of the thigh. The sensory innervation to the lateral aspect of the knee includes the tibiofibular branch of the peroneal nerve, the lateral retinacular nerve, and the lateral femoral cutaneous nerve. The medial and lateral retinacular nerves provide sensation to the knee joint whereas the other five nerves provide sensation to the cutaneous surface of the knee.

The anatomic location and paths of these nerves is generally constant; however, variations and anomalies can occur, especially in the setting of prior operative procedures. The superficial nerves around the knee are located in the subcutaneous fat; whereas, the deep nerves lie deep to the medial and lateral retinaculum. These nerves are located just distal to the medial and lateral vastus lateralis muscle, respectively.

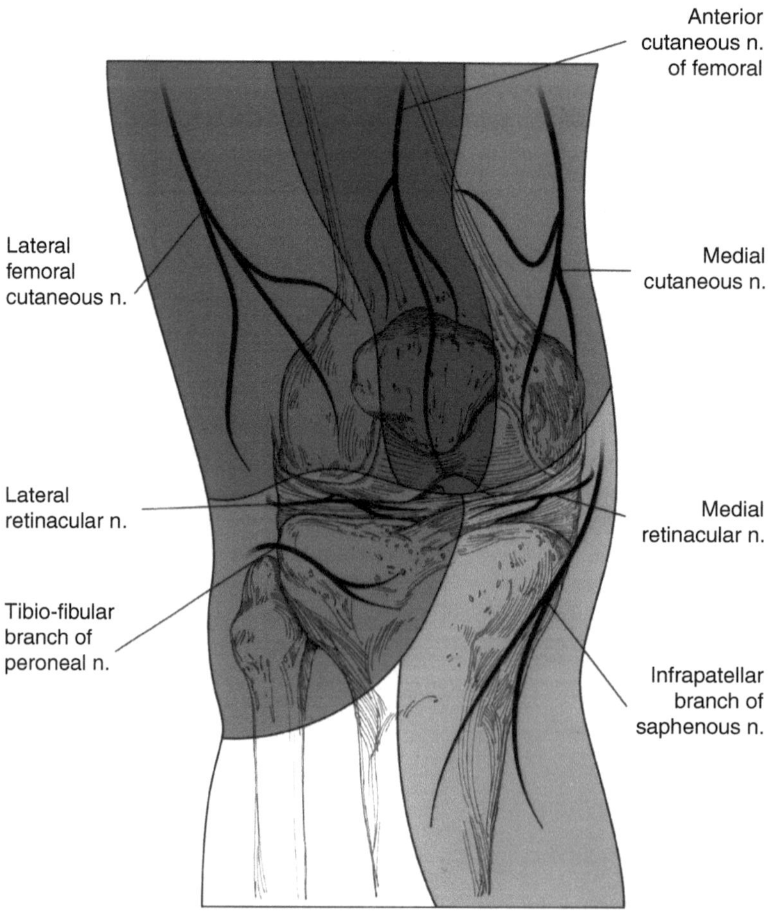


**Fig. 25.1** An illustration demonstrating the course and cutaneous territories of the seven surgically identifiable nerves about the knee

## 25.3 Technique of Selective Denervation

A critical component in the management of patients with chronic knee pain is to differentiate pain of neuromatous versus nonneuromatous origin. In general, neuromatous knee pain is characterized as sharp and localized whereas nonneuromatous knee pain is dull and diffuse. Determining whether the pain is of neuromatous origin is accomplished by obtaining a thorough history and physical examination, assessing the characteristics of the pain, and performing the appropriate diagnostic evaluation. This section will review the initial consultation, diagnostic evaluation, and operative technique.

### 25.3.1 *Initial Consultation*

At the initial consultation, patients are thoroughly questioned regarding the mechanism responsible for the knee pain. This can be secondary to chronic disease states such as arthritis or chondromalacia as well as acute events such as trauma or prior operative procedures that may include total knee arthroplasty, arthroscopy, and extirpative procedures. Chronic disease states are rarely secondary to neuromata whereas pain of acute onset can be. The date of the onset is also important because many of these painful conditions are often self-limiting and resolve by 6 months. Pain of acute origin that is persistent beyond 6 months may be secondary to neuromata.

Other factors related to the pain that are important include the nature, intensity, location, duration, aggravating factors, relieving factors, and frequency. The nature of the pain is characterized as sharp or dull, constant or intermittent, and localized or diffuse. The location of the pain is documented on the surface of the knee as well as whether it is superficial or deep. Superficial pain is usually secondary to neuromata of the five cutaneous nerves that include the anterior, medial, and lateral femoral cutaneous nerves as well as the infrapatellar branch of the saphenous nerve and the tibiofibular branch of the peroneal nerve. Deep pain may be due to neuromata of the medial or lateral retinacular nerves that innervate the capsule of the knee joint. Some patients may also experience numbness or tingling on the lateral aspect of the leg due to compression of the common peroneal nerve. The severity of the pain is graded on a visual analog scale (VAS) ranging from 0 to 10.

Important aspects of the physical examination include location of scars, assessment of knee stability, range of motion, gait assessment, and the location of the pain. It is important to rule out any infectious or inflammatory etiology. The territories of pain corresponding to the surface of the knee are delineated (Fig. 25.2). The most important finding for the diagnosis of a neuroma is the presence of a Tinels sign. This is identified by tapping on the surface of the knee and noting the response. The elicitation of a sharp pain that occasionally radiates is characteristic of neuromata (Fig. 25.3). There may be an isolated or multiple Tinels signs around the knee. It is recommended that a photograph be obtained of these markings.

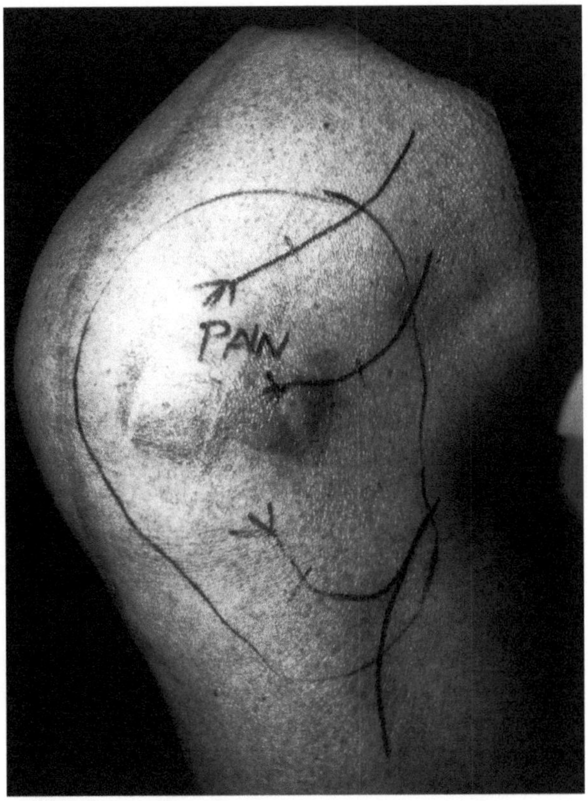


**Fig. 25.2** A photograph demonstrating the delineated territory of pain secondary to a neuroma of the infrapatellar branch of the saphenous nerve

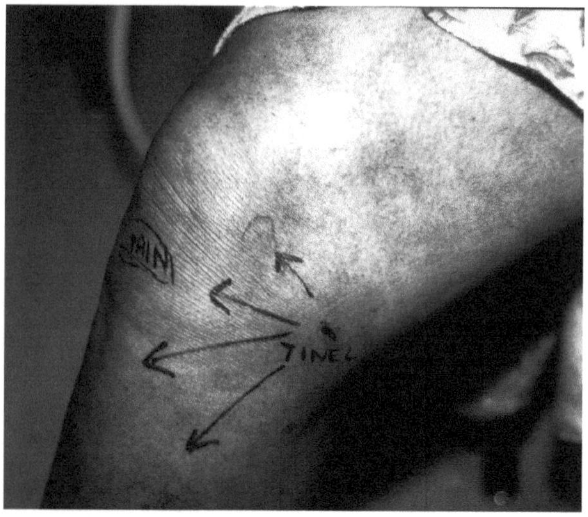


**Fig. 25.3** A photograph demonstrating the Tinels point and the paths of radiation

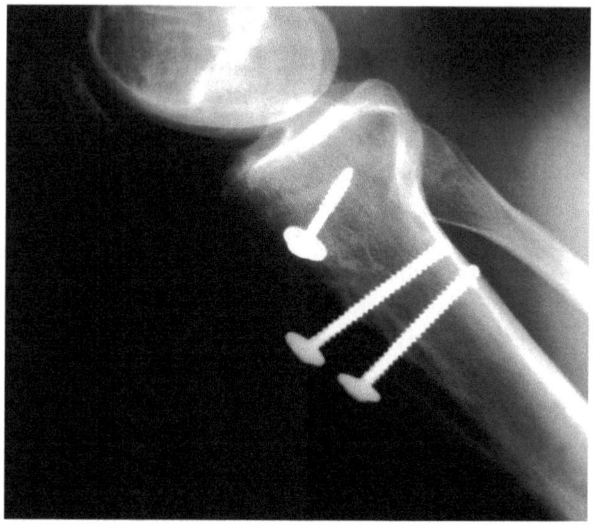

**Fig. 25.4** Radiograph demonstrating proximal tibial screws that resulted in a neuroma

### 25.3.2 Diagnostic Evaluation

The diagnosis is based on ruling out nonneuromatous causes and ruling in a neuroma. Neuromata are ruled in by a successful response to a nerve block using 1% lidocaine. Several cc's of lidocaine is injected subcutaneously at the site of the potential neuroma formation. This can range from 1 to 7 sites based on the number of potential sites that a neuroma can form. After 5–10 min, pain intensity is again charted using a VAS. Ideally, when a true neuroma is present, the pain should completely resolve following the nerve block. At least, a 5-point reduction in the VAS is recommended for a patient to be considered an appropriate candidate for selective denervation. It is important to assess gait before and after nerve blockade and document any changes. Usually, the gait is improved following successful blockade of a neuroma. Pain that is not relieved by the lidocaine injection may be related to other causes such as arthritis, ligamentous instability, misalignment of the prosthesis, aseptic loosening, and polyethylene wear. Further orthopedic evaluation is recommended in these circumstances. A plain radiograph is necessary for all prospective patients (Fig. 25.4). Electromyography and nerve conduction studies are not usually obtained for neuromatous knee pain.

For patients who are considered candidates for selective denervation, a discussion ensues regarding the risks and benefits of this operation. Candidates for this procedure understand that portions of the knee may be permanently anesthetic and rendered susceptible to other forms of trauma such as a burn. The success of the operation is variable with approximately 40–70% reporting an excellent improvement, 20–40% reporting a partial or good improvement, and 5–20% reporting no improvement. These results are based on a cumulative review of existing studies.[6,9] The response is quantitated based on the reduction in the VAS. In my personal practice, an excellent response is obtained when the VAS score is reduced to 0–1, a partial or good response is obtained when the VAS is reduced by 50%, and a poor response in obtained when there is no appreciable change in the VAS.

### 25.3.3 Operative Technique

Prior to the induction of regional or general anesthesia, the Tinels points are again marked and the bony and reticular landmarks are outlined. The incision sites and the usual course of the nerves are delineated. Following the induction of anesthesia, a proximal thigh tourniquet is applied and inflated to 300 mm of mercury. It is recommended that the tourniquet not be inflated for greater than 1 h. At least 3.5 power loupe magnification is recommended.

The techniques for excision of the various neuromata are different. The cutaneous nerves about the knee lie in the subcutaneous fat. Neuromata of the anterior, medial, and lateral cutaneous nerves as well as the infrapatellar branch of the saphenous nerve can be excised through a skin incision approximately 1–2 cm from the Tinels point along the usual course of the nerve. Dissection proceeds using fine scissors and bipolar cautery. Following identification of the nerve, traction is applied on the isolated segment to observe for skin retraction at the Tinels point. This maneuver confirms that the correct nerve has been isolated. The nerve is divided and the proximal stump of the nerve is buried in adjacent muscle to minimize the possibility of recurrence.

Neuromata of the tibiofibular branch of the common peroneal nerve are approached in a different manner (Figs. 25.5 and 25.6). The common peroneal nerve is exposed and released and the articular branches to the tibiofibular joint are isolated. It is helpful to use a nerve stimulator to ensure that motor branches to the peroneus longus muscle are not divided.

Neuromata of the deeper knee structures, i.e., medial and lateral retinacular nerves, require a different approach. Neuromata of the medial retinacular nerve are approached using a skin incision just distal to the vastus medialis muscle. The medial retinaculum is incised between the patella and the medial epicondyle of the femur. The nerve is located under the retinaculum. Neuromata of the lateral retinacular nerve are approached using a skin incision distal to the vastus lateralis muscle. The lateral retinaculum is incised between the patella and iliotibial tract. The nerve is isolated and excised.

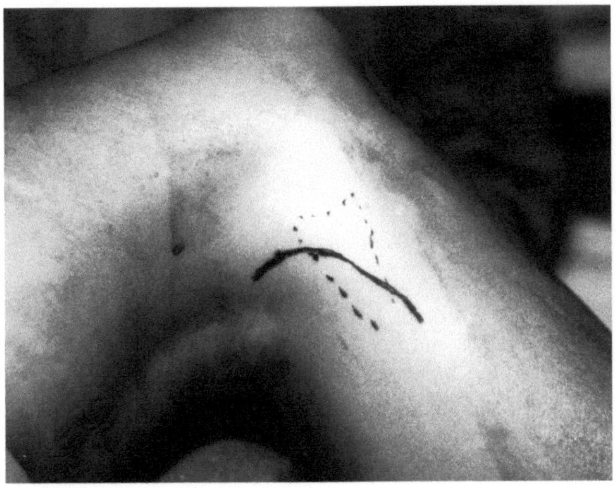

**Fig. 25.5** The incision site for exposure of the common peroneal nerve is delineated

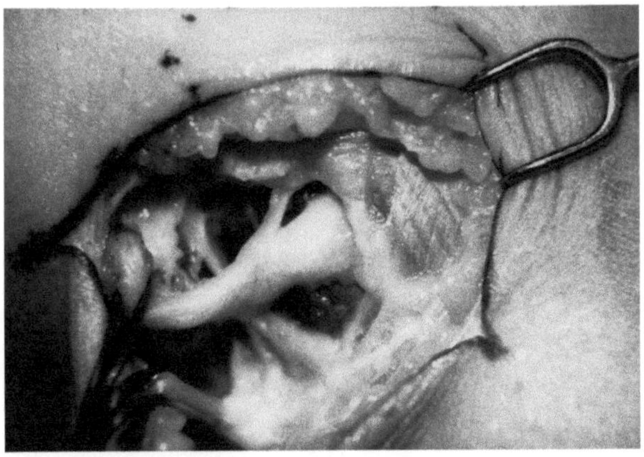

**Fig. 25.6** The common peroneal nerve is isolated and the tibiofibular branch is isolated as it traverses under the peroneus longus muscle

## 25.4 Case Examples

### *25.4.1 Case 1*

A 44-year-old man presented with 2-year history of chronic right knee pain following total knee arthroplasty. The pain was localized to the infrapatellar regions of the medial and lateral knee (Figs. 25.7 and 25.8). The pain was described as sharp and constant and was confined to the cutaneous surface and did not involve the deeper structures of the knee. It was exacerbated by knee motion. Knee stability and gait was within normal limits. The patient also described numbness and tingling on the lateral surface of the knee. Physical therapy and analgesics were unsuccessful in ameliorating the pain. Pain severity was graded on a visual analog scale as 9. Radiographs revealed well-aligned knee prosthesis.

On physical examination, a well-healed 20 cm midline knee incision was noted. There was no evidence of swelling or erythema. A Tinels sign was elicited on the infrapatellar aspect of the medial and lateral knee. In addition, there was diminished sensation along the lateral aspect of the leg extending from the fibular head to the lateral malleolus. Joint laxity or instability was not appreciated. The presumptive diagnosis was

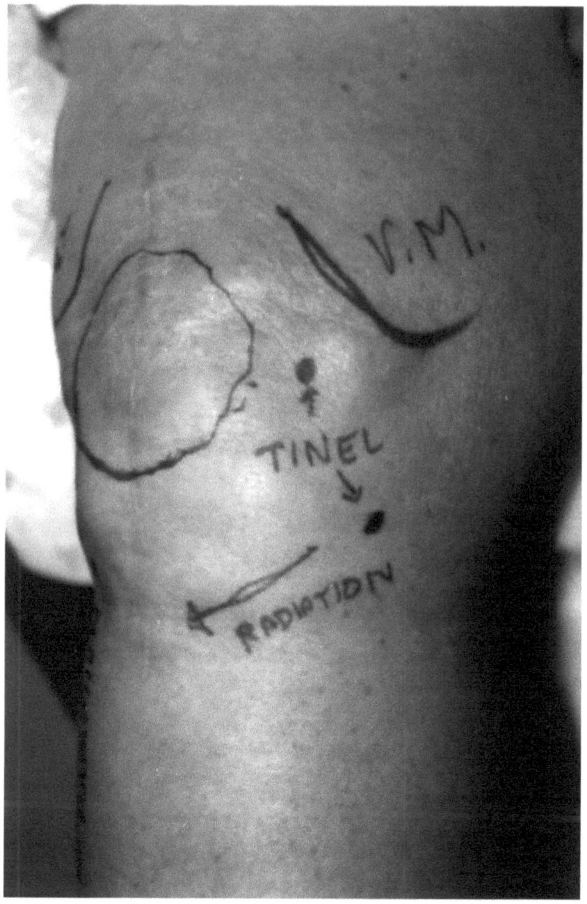


**Fig. 25.7** The medial aspect of the knee is depicted demonstrating the patella and vastus medialis muscle (*VM*). The Tinel points and path of radiation are outlined

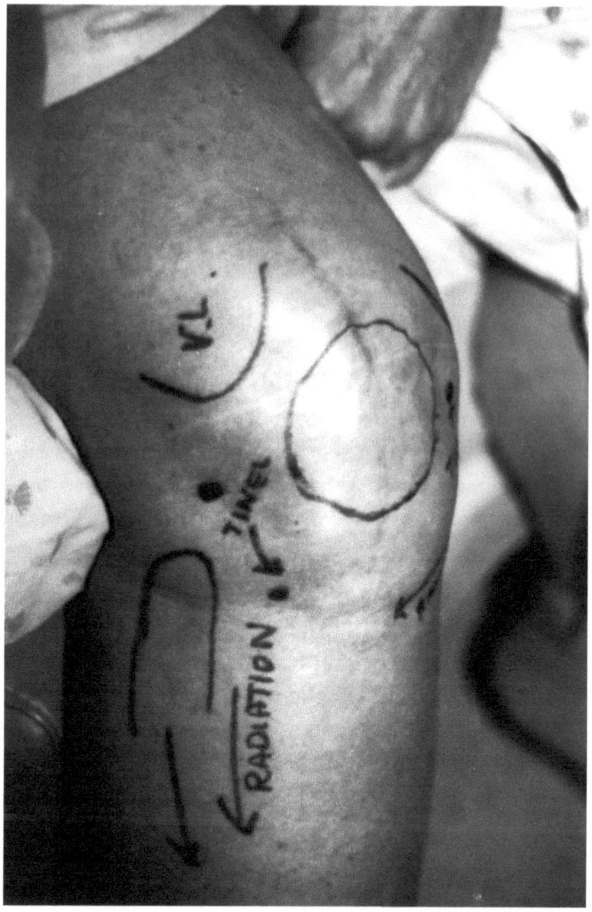


**Fig. 25.8** The lateral aspect of the knee is depicted demonstrating the fibular head and the vastus lateralis muscle (*VL*). The Tinel points are marked

a neuroma of the infrapatellar branch of the saphenous nerve and the tibiofibular branch of the common peroneal nerve as well as compression of the common peroneal nerve. A nerve block using 1% lidocaine was performed at the point of the Tinels sign with complete resolution of pain within 5 min.

In the operating room, the infrapatellar branch of the saphenous nerve and the tibiofibular branch of the common peroneal nerve were identified and resected (Fig. 25.9). The proximal nerve stump was buried in adjacent muscle. The common peroneal nerve was decompressed without incident.

Postoperatively, the pain was completely eliminated with a visual analog score of 0. The lateral leg dysesthesia resolved completely. The patient has classified this outcome as excellent with a 2-year follow-up.

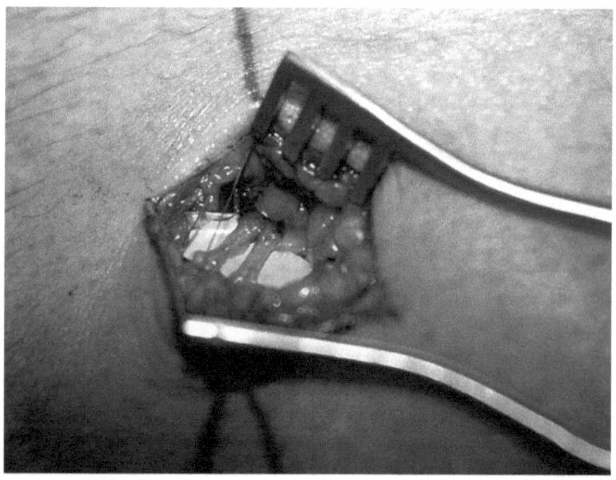

**Fig. 25.9** Two branches of the infrapatellar branch of the saphenous nerve are illustrated. These branches were excised and the proximal stumps buried in adjacent muscle

### 25.4.2 Case 2

A 28-year-old man presented with chronic knee pain of 7 years duration following a traumatic injury. In total, seven prior operations had been performed that have contributed to the chronic pain. The pain was described as sharp, constant, and located in the superficial cutaneous territory of the superior knee. Pain severity was graded as an 8 on the visual analog scale. Physical therapy and analgesics did not ameliorate the pain. Radiographs demonstrated a well-aligned knee without arthritic changes.

On physical examination, all incisions were well-healed without signs of infection or inflammation. Ligamentous laxity was not demonstrated. A Tinels sign was elicited over the medial suprapatellar region. Nerve blockade successfully eliminated the pain reducing the pain severity score to 0. A neuroma of the medial cutaneous nerve of the knee was diagnosed (Fig. 25.10). The neuroma was excised and the proximal nerve stump buried without incident.

Postoperatively, the patient reported complete resolution of pain in the medial suprapatellar territory; however, 1 week following the procedure, the patient reported new onset of anterior and lateral suprapatellar pain. This pain was described as sharp and intermittent with a visual analog score of 8 points. Nerve blockade successfully reduced the pain to 0. A second operation was performed 4 months later and the anterior and lateral femoral cutaneous neuromata were excised. Postoperatively, the patient was pain free with 2-year follow-up.

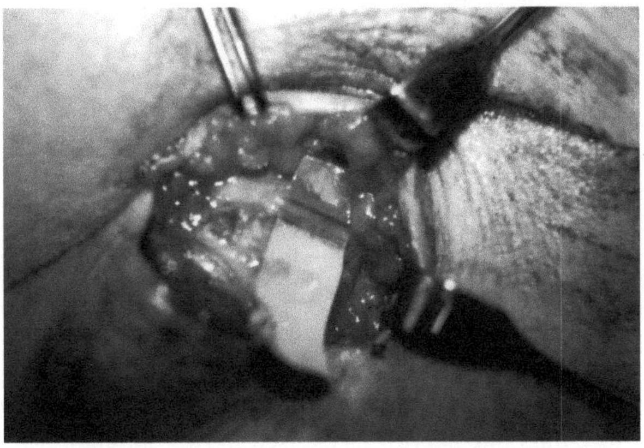

**Fig. 25.10** The medial cutaneous nerve of the knee is demonstrated

### 25.4.3 Case 3

A 70-year-old man presented with left medial infrapatellar knee pain of 2 year duration following total knee arthroplasty. The pain was described as sharp, intermittent, localized, and superficial with a visual analog score of 7 points. The pain was exacerbated by prolonged periods of sitting and knee motion. There were no complaints of mechanical dysfunction and radiographs demonstrated a knee prosthesis that was well-aligned. Physical therapy and analgesics did not alleviate the pain.

On physical examination, the midline incision was well-healed and there was no evidence of swelling, inflammation, or infection. Knee stability was intact with normal range of motion and normal gait. A Tinels sign was localized to the medial infrapatellar region of the knee. Diagnostic nerve block reduced the pain to a 2 on the visual analog scale that was suggestive of a neuroma of the infrapatellar branch of the saphenous nerve. Although there was improvement in the pain, some discomfort remained.

In the operating room, the infrapatellar branch of the saphenous nerve was isolated, resected, and proximally buried in adjacent muscle. Postoperatively, no substantial improvement in the pain was reported with a reduction in the visual analog score to 5 points. The patient graded this as a poor result at 2-year follow-up.

## 25.5 Discussion

Selective denervation for neuromatous knee pain is an excellent procedure in properly selected patients. Although considered controversial by some, its acceptance as an effective treatment modality is becoming increasingly appreciated. Some physicians feel that denervation is an extreme maneuver and that the clinical outcomes are mixed and variable. However, based on personal experience and review of the existing literature, selective denervation of the sensory nerves about the knee has been demonstrated to be safe and beneficial in the majority of properly selected patients. The three cases illustrated were selected because they represent situations and outcomes that the practicing surgeon is likely to encounter.

Case one represents a straightforward situation in which a single neuroma was responsible for the knee pain. The nerve block was effective at temporarily eliminating the pain, and the excision of the single neuroma completely eliminated the pain. Case two appeared to be straightforward with identification of a single neuroma. However, following intraoperative identification and excision of the responsible nerve, adjacent pain ensued requiring a second selective denervation procedure. This case demonstrates that additional denervation procedures, although uncommon, may be necessary. Although unclear why the subsequent pain was not demonstrated at the initial consultation, it can be postulated that the adjacent neuromata elicited a less intense signal that was masked by the primary neuroma. Case three represents a situation in which there was an equivocal response to the nerve blockade. Although, the visual analog score was reduced from 7 to 2 following the nerve block, a mild amount of pain remained. Selective denervation did not effectively relieve the pain. This incomplete resolution of pain following nerve blockade may have occurred because of adjacent nerves that were not anesthetized. The persistence of pain following denervation may have been due to nonspecific reinnervation by adjacent nerves to the denervated territory.

In order to determine the true benefit of selective denervation, prospective studies are necessary. In our previous study, 43 patients with intractable knee pain were prospectively analyzed.[6] Only patients that met the criteria for selective denervation were included in the study. Inclusion required pain of at least 1 years duration, failure of conservative management, pain localized at a Tinels point, and at least a 5-point reduction in the severity of pain based on a visual analog scale. Thirty patients met these criteria of which 25 had selective denervation. Thirteen patients did not meet the criteria. Of those that had selective denervation, the etiology of the pain was trauma in 15 patients and total knee arthroplasty in 10. The mean number of prior operations about the knee was 5.1 (range, 0–20). A single neuroma was excised in 11 patients and multiple neuromata were excised in 14. A total of 62 nerves were excised in the 25 patients that included the infrapatellar branch of the saphenous nerve ($n=24$), the tibiofibular branch of the peroneal nerve ($n=5$), the medial retinacular nerve ($n=12$), the lateral retinacular nerve ($n=8$), the medial cutaneous nerve ($n=6$), the anterior cutaneous nerve ($n=3$), and the lateral femoral cutaneous nerve ($n=4$). Pain relief was complete in 11 patients (44%), partial in ten patients (40%), and absent in four patients (16%). Follow-up ranged from 1 to 4 years. Patient satisfaction following the procedure was obtained in 21 of 25 patients (84%).

This study demonstrates that not all properly selected patients respond equally to selective denervation. Closer evaluation of the 11 patients who reported an excellent outcome reveals that the average preoperative score on the VAS was 8.5 points (range, 5–10), the average post nerve block score was 0.4 points (range, 0–1), and the average postoperative score was 0.5 points (range, 0–2). Preoperative pain was localized to the medial aspect of the knee in nine patients (82%) and to the medial and lateral aspect of the knee in two patients (18%). This outcome was obtained after a single operation in nine patients (82%) and after a second operation in two patients (18%). The nerve most commonly excised was the infrapatellar branch of the saphenous nerve that was excised in ten patients (91%). More than one nerve was excised in nine patients (82%).

A detailed evaluation of the ten patients reporting a good outcome reveals that the average preoperative score on the VAS was 8.6 points (range, 6–10), the average post nerve block score was 0.5 points (range 0–2), and the average postoperative score was 3.3 points (range, 2–5). Preoperative pain was localized to the medial aspect of the knee in five patients (50%) and to the medial and lateral aspect of the knee in five patients (50%). This outcome was obtained after a single operation in eight patients (80%) and after a second operation in two patients (20%). The nerve most commonly isolated was the infrapatellar branch of the saphenous nerve that was excised in all ten patients. More than one nerve was excised in seven patients.

Detailed evaluation of the four patients reporting a poor outcome reveals that the average preoperative score on the VAS was 8.3 points (range, 7–10), the average post nerve block score was 1.5 points (range, 0–2), and that the average postoperative score was 6.8 points (range, 5–9). Preoperative pain was localized to the medial aspect of the knee in two patients and to the medial and lateral aspect in two patients. The nerve most commonly excised was the infrapatellar branch of the saphenous nerve that was excised in four patients. More than one nerve was excised in two patients.

Outcomes that were considered less than excellent occurred in 14 of 25 patients (56%). In the group reporting a good outcome, patient complaints included new pain or migration of pain in four knees as well as persistent and deep pain in six knees. Predisposing factors to this outcome included a history of fracture or total knee arthroplasty in seven patients, arthroscopy for ligamentous injury in two patients, and soft tissue trauma in one patient. Explanations included secondary neuroma formation, persistent pain from an unrecognized neuroma, overlapping nerve territories, and persistent pain from a nonneuromatous origin.

In the group reporting a poor outcome, predisposing factors included previous bone or joint surgery in two patients and knee joint arthroscopy in two knees. All four patients reported persistent and deep joint pain. Explanations include overlapping nerve territories and unrecognized or masked neuromata. The medial retinacular nerve was excised in one of these patients and the lateral retinacular nerve was excised in no patient. This decision was made based on the preoperative evaluation and the results of the lidocaine nerve block. Subsequent denervation procedures were not performed in this group of patients.

## 25.6 Summary

In conclusion, selective denervation for neuromatous pain about the knee joint can be a beneficial procedure. Proper patient selection is a critical component that impacts the success of the operation. The salient components include pain of at least 1-year duration unrelieved by conservative measures, the presence of a Tinels sign in the painful territory, and at least a 5-point reduction in the visual analog score following nerve blockade with 1% lidocaine. This procedure is not recommended for pain on nonneuromatous origin, pain that is less than 1-year duration, and for diffuse knee pain without a Tinels sign.

## References


1. Dellon AL. Partial dorsal wrist denervation: resection of the distal posterior interosseous nerve. *J Hand Surg*. 1985;10A: 527-533.
2. Dellon AL. Partial joint denervation II: knee and ankle. *Plast Reconstr Surg*. 2009;123:208-217.
3. Dellon AL, MacKinnon SE, Daneshvar A. Terminal branch of the anterior interosseous nerve as a source of wrist pain. *J Hand Surg*. 1984;9B:316-322.
4. Dellon AL, Mont MA, Krackow KA, et al. Partial denervation for persistent neuroma pain after total knee arthroplasty. *Clin Orthop Relat Res*. 1995;316:145-150.
5. Dellon AL, Mont MA, Mullick T, et al. Partial denervation for neuromatous knee pain around the knee. *Clin Orthop Relat Res*. 1996;329:216-222.
6. Dellon AL, Mont MA, Hungerford DS. Partial denervation for the treatment of persistent neuroma pain after total knee arthroplasty. In: Insall JN, Scott WN, eds. *Surgery of the Knee*. Philadelphia: Saunders; 2000:1772-1786.
7. Horner G, Dellon AL. Innervation of the human knee joint and implications for surgery. *Clin Orthop Relat Res*. 1994;301:221-226.
8. Kasim N, Fulkerson JP. Resection of clinically localized segments of painful retinaculum in the treatment of selected patients with anterior knee pain. *Am J Sports Med*. 2000;28: 811-814.
9. Nahabedian MY, Johnson CA. Operative management of neuromatous knee pain: patient selection and outcome. *Ann Plast Surg*. 2001;46:15-22.
10. Nahabedian MY, Mont MA, Hungerford DS. Selective denervation of the knee: experience, case reports and technical notes. *Am J Knee Surg*. 1998;11:175-180.
11. Wilhelm A. Zur innervation der gelenke der oberen extremitat. *Z Anat Entwicklungs Geschechte*. 1958;120:331-371.
12. Wilhelm A. Die Gelenkdenervation und ihre anatomischen Grundlagen. Ein neues Behandlungsprinzip in der Habdchirurgie. *Hefte Unfallheilkd*. 1966;86:1-109.

# 26 Kinetic and Kinematic Analysis of Iatrogenic Medial Patellar Instability: Clinical Relevance

Vicente Sanchis-Alfonso, Erik Montesinos-Berry, Andrea Castelli, Susana Marín-Roca, and Alex Cortes

## 26.1 Introduction

Medial patellar instability is a serious well-known complication following extensor mechanism realignment surgery.[2,11,12,14,15,19-21] However, despite the fact that it is a well-known entity, with a personality of its own, we have not found publications where the kinetics and kinematics of the knee were evaluated, before and after reconstruction of the lateral retinaculum in iatrogenic medial patellar instability.

The first goal of our study is to analyze the defense mechanisms, which is the same as the avoidance behavior, that a patient with a medial patellar instability displays to reduce this instability and therefore reduce the pain. The analysis of these mechanisms will enable us to speculate about the possible origin of the pain that some patients with patellofemoral disorders have in the posterior aspect of the knee. We will also analyze the importance of retinacular structures in the genesis of pain in contrast to the role chondropathy plays in the genesis of pain in the anterior aspect of the knee. The second goal of our study is to draw attention to the importance of the retinacular structures in contrast to muscle coordination in patellar stability. To do so, we will analyze two clinical cases of iatrogenic medial patellar instability in detail.

V. Sanchis-Alfonso (✉)
International Patellofemoral Study Group,
International ACL Study Group,
Hospital 9 de Octubre, Hospital Arnau de Vilanova,
School of Medicine, Catholic University of Valencia,
Valencia, Spain
e-mail:vicente.sanchis.alfonso@gmail.com

## 26.2 Case #1

A 25-year-old female came to our institution with a history of chronic anterior right knee pain and patellofemoral instability refractory to conservative treatment, for about 5 years. The Kujala preoperative score was of 36 points. The exercise rehabilitation program performed in our institution was unsuccessful in improving her symptoms. The patient underwent an Insall's proximal realignment procedure (i.e., the advancement of the VOM and medial retinaculum into the dorsum of the patella after lateral retinaculum release), in another hospital at the age of 18 due to recurrent lateral patellar dislocation. Following surgery, the previous symptoms disappeared and she could play basketball again, but a different type of knee pain around the patella developed with time and 1 year later, she gave up playing basketball.

A physical examination of the knee revealed peripatellar and posteromedial pain, joint effusion, a positive apprehension sign upon pressing the patella medially and a positive Fulkerson's relocation test.[10] The opposite knee was asymptomatic.

Conventional radiography, including skyline views, revealed no abnormalities. A magnetic resonance imaging (MRI) examination showed lateral subluxation of the patella and joint effusion. A computed tomography (CT) examination in 0° extension with the quadriceps relaxed showed mild lateralization of the patella that increased with quadriceps contraction being greater on the right side than on the left side (Fig. 26.1), and a normal centralization of the patella in 30° of knee flexion. CT of the patellofemoral joint in extension with manual patellar pressure (stress CT), according to the technique described by Biedert,[3] revealed a concomitant medial patellar instability (Fig. 26.2).

V. Sanchis-Alfonso (ed.), *Anterior Knee Pain and Patellar Instability*,
DOI: 10.1007/978-0-85729-507-1_26, © Springer-Verlag London Limited 2011

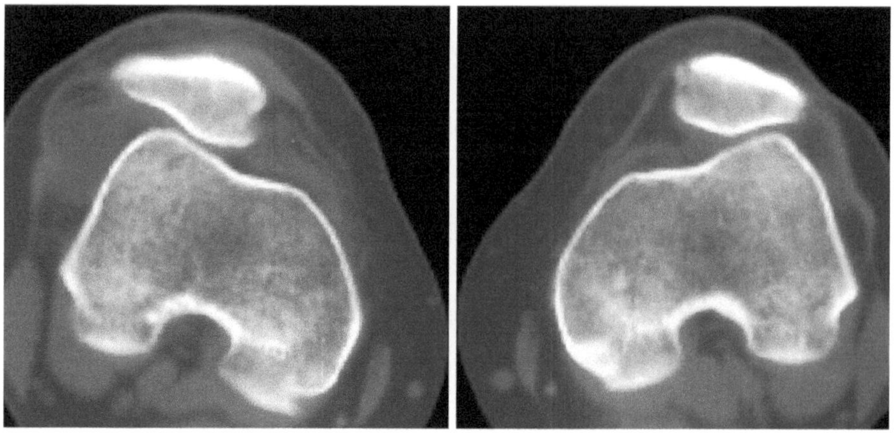

**Fig. 26.1** Computed tomography (*CT*) examination in 0° extension and quadriceps contraction shows lateralization of the patella (Reprinted from Sanchis-Alfonso et al.[23], with permission from Elsevier)

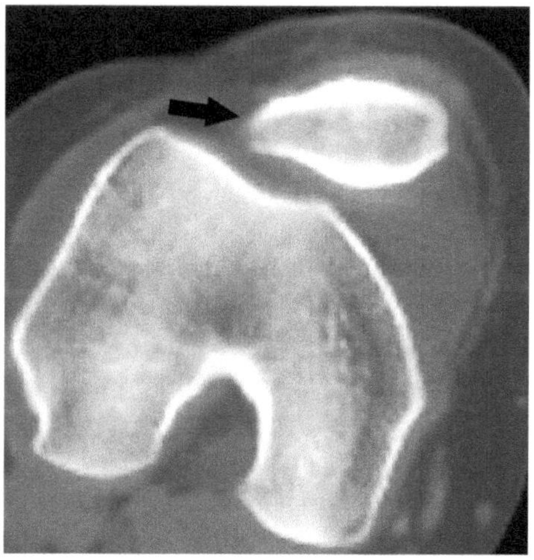

**Fig. 26.2** Documenting of medial patellar instability using manual pressure (finger on the lateral aspect of the patella *black arrow*) (Reprinted from Sanchis-Alfonso et al.[23], with permission from Elsevier)

Gait analysis was performed for documentation purposes prior to a subsequent reconstructive surgical procedure. A pathway with two extensometrics force plates on its surface was used for the analysis. The subject was asked to walk at a high cadence (140 steps/min).* Before collecting the data, the subject walked on the pathway several times until she was able to walk with a natural and constant gait. She used the same sports shoes in both pre- and postoperative sessions. Gait parameters were analyzed using the NedAMH/IBV software (Instituto de Biomecánica de Valencia, Valencia, Spain). Gait analysis revealed significant differences between the affected and the contralateral healthy limb in the following parameters: horizontal braking force (Right vs Left: 0.37 vs 0.29), vertical heel contact peak force (Right vs Left: 1.73 vs 1.28) and toe-off vertical peak force (Right vs Left: 1.40 vs 1.04) (Fig. 26.3a).

At the time of surgery, an arthroscopy of the right knee was performed. All the intraarticular structures were intact, except for a patellar chondropathy grade III, according to the Outerbridge classification, located medially, and a peripatellar synovitis. We did not perform chondroplasty or peripatellar synovectomy. After the arthroscopy, we performed an open reconstruction of the lateral patellotibial ligament[9] according to the technique described by Hughston and colleagues using the iliotibial band and the patellar tendon.[12]

Four months after surgery, she was symptom free. Gait analysis was performed at this time to evaluate the effects of surgical reconstruction of the lateral retinaculum on gait parameters. No significant differences were seen when compared to the contralateral limb, the gait pattern being normal: horizontal braking force (Right vs Left: 0.32 vs 0.34), vertical heel contact peak force (Right vs Left: 1.34 vs 1.40), and toe-off vertical

*A point of interest in gait analysis is the cadence used. The cadence has an important effect on the gait parameters.[1,16] Many authors use a spontaneous cadence in their studies. Nevertheless, when a subject is in pain, his cadence is slower than normal to make his gait more comfortable. In the present study, the subject was required to walk at the same cadence before and after the surgery. In this case, we have chosen a high frequency (140 steps/min) because the faster the subject walks, the more evident the functional impairment becomes.

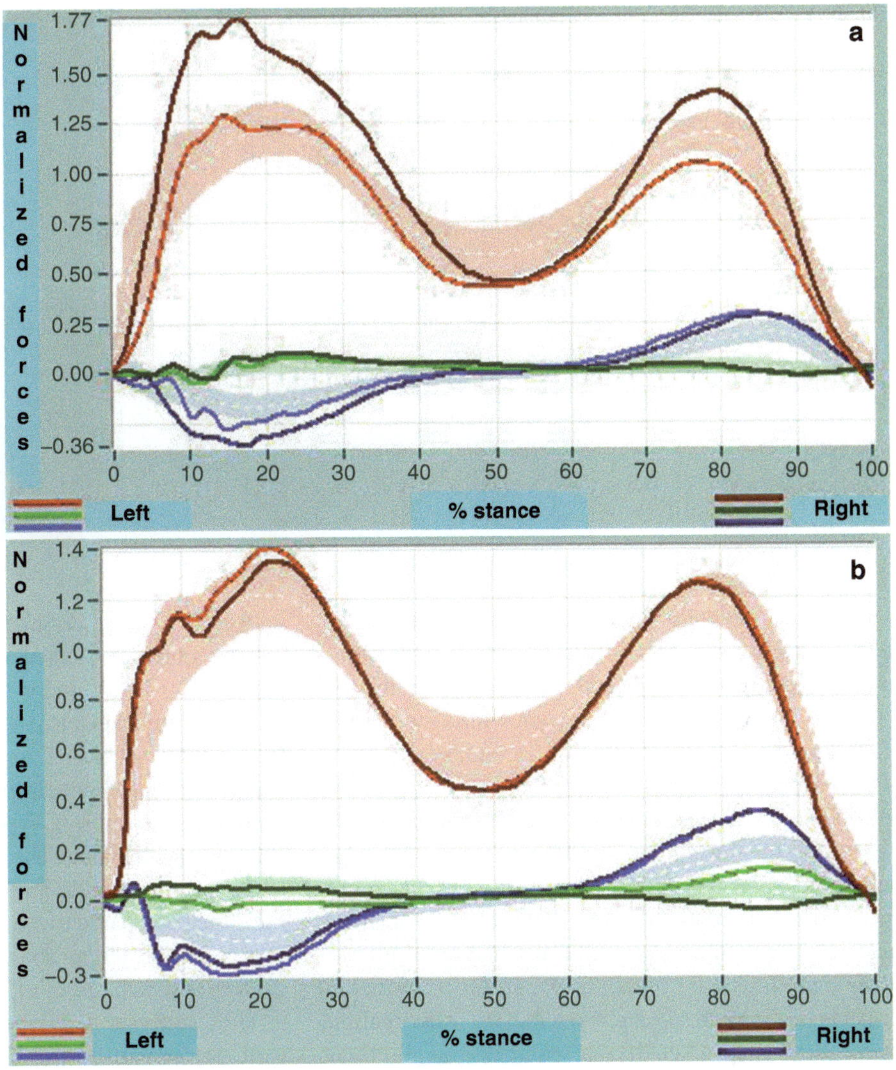


**Fig. 26.3** Gait analysis. (**a**) Preoperative. (**b**) Postoperative (Reprinted from Sanchis-Alfonso et al.[23], with permission from Elsevier)

peak force (Right vs Left: 1.26 vs 1.27)† (Fig. 26.3b). One year after surgery, she was symptom free. The follow-up Kujala score was 91 points. The follow-up CT scan at 0° extension with quadriceps contraction demonstrated a similar lateral displacement of the patella (Fig. 26.4a), and stress CT revealed medial patellar stability (Fig. 26.4b).

## 26.3 Case #2

A 41-year-old woman came to our institution complaining mainly of right patellofemoral instability, and also of right anterior knee pain that had not improved with physical therapy or symptomatic medication. The pre-op Kujala score was 24 points. The contralateral

†Preoperative left (healthy limb) vertical heel contact peak force (1.28), toe-off peak force (1.04), and horizontal braking force (0.29) are lower than the postoperative left (healthy limb) vertical heel contact peak force (1.40), toe-off peak force (1.27), and horizontal braking force (0.34) due to a phenomenon of functional compensation, as we can see in other pathologies.[22] We hypothesize that after surgery, due to the consequent recovery of the absorption mechanism in the affected knee, a redistribution of the loads between the two extremities takes place with the gait becoming more symmetrical and both extremities show gait patterns within normal limits.

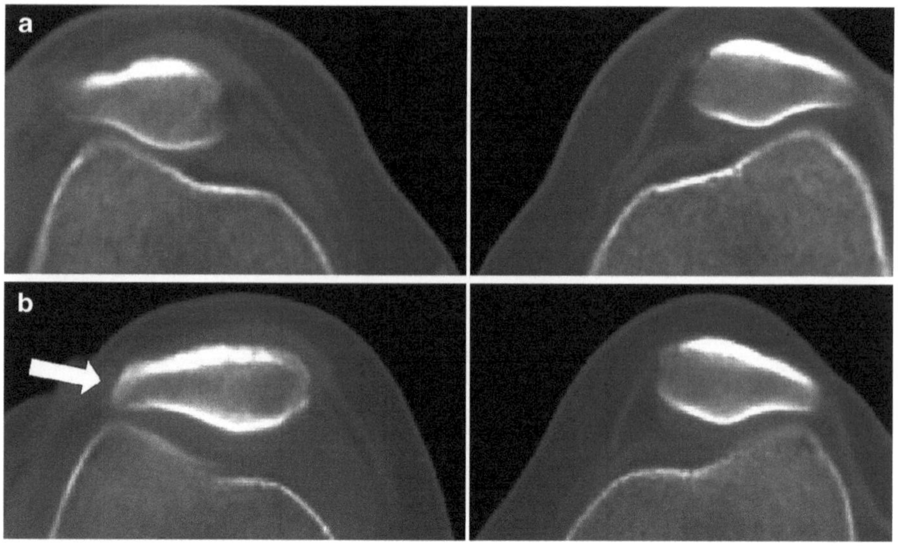

**Fig. 26.4** Follow-up CT scan at 0° extension with quadriceps contraction demonstrates similar lateral displacement of the patella in both knees (**a**), and stress CT revealed medial patellar stability (finger on the lateral aspect of the patella *white arrow*) (**b**) (Reprinted from Sanchis-Alfonso et al.[23], with permission from Elsevier)

knee was completely asymptomatic. This patient had been operated on 3 years before, with an Insall's proximal realignment for a lateral patellar instability that was the main symptom, along with mild occasional pain during physical activity as a secondary symptom. There was a deep venous thrombosis as a postoperative complication that required treatment by the hematologist. After the first surgery, as time went by, the patient mentioned that the patellar instability had increased, but it was different and more incapacitating than the pain she had before surgery. She also had more anterior knee pain. She had no pain in the posterior or medial aspects of the knee. A year and a half after her realignment surgery and given the worsening of the symptoms, another surgeon suggested a knee arthroscopy, to which the patient agreed. With this second procedure, pain worsened considerably as well as the patellar instability the patient had with activities of daily living.

A physical examination of the knee showed anterior knee pain, with a positive apprehension sign when pressing the patella medially and a positive Fulkerson's relocation test. The rest of the physical examination was completely normal, with no ligament laxity, and physical examination of the contralateral knee was also normal.

Conventional radiology showed isolated iatrogenic patellofemoral osteoarthritis (Fig. 26.5). The conventional radiology findings prior to the first surgery showed no degenerative changes. A magnetic resonance imaging (MRI) examination showed a lateral subluxation of the patella and a severe patellar chondropathy. A computed tomography (CT) examination at 0° extension and with a relaxed quadriceps showed mild lateralization of the patella. The TT-TG index was 10 mm. CT of the patellofemoral joint in extension with manual patellar pressure (stress CT), according to the technique described by Biedert,[3] revealed a medial patellar instability (Fig. 26.6a). Moreover, the stress CT of the patellofemoral joint in extension with manual lateral patellar pressure showed a lateral patellar displacement significantly greater in the right knee compared to the left knee (Fig. 26.6b). A bone scan with Tc 99 m showed an increased pathologic uptake only in the patella (Fig. 26.7).

Gait analysis and kinetic and kinematic analysis were performed during stair descent for documentation purposes prior to a subsequent reconstructive surgical procedure. The stair descent analysis was done following a standard protocol, meaning facing forward, and afterward using the strategy employed by the patient to go down the stairs with less patellar instability and therefore less pain. The strategy used was less knee flexion than the contralateral knee, with the leg in external rotation and one step at a time.

A preoperative gait analysis demonstrated a symmetric gait pattern with gait parameters within normal limits. Unlike case #1, horizontal braking force, vertical heel contact, and toe-off vertical peak forces are symmetrical and within normal limits.

The first parameter analyzed with the stair descending test was the knee flexion–extension angle (Fig. 26.8a). We observed that the angle of flexion to reach the step (following standard protocol) was 18.71°,

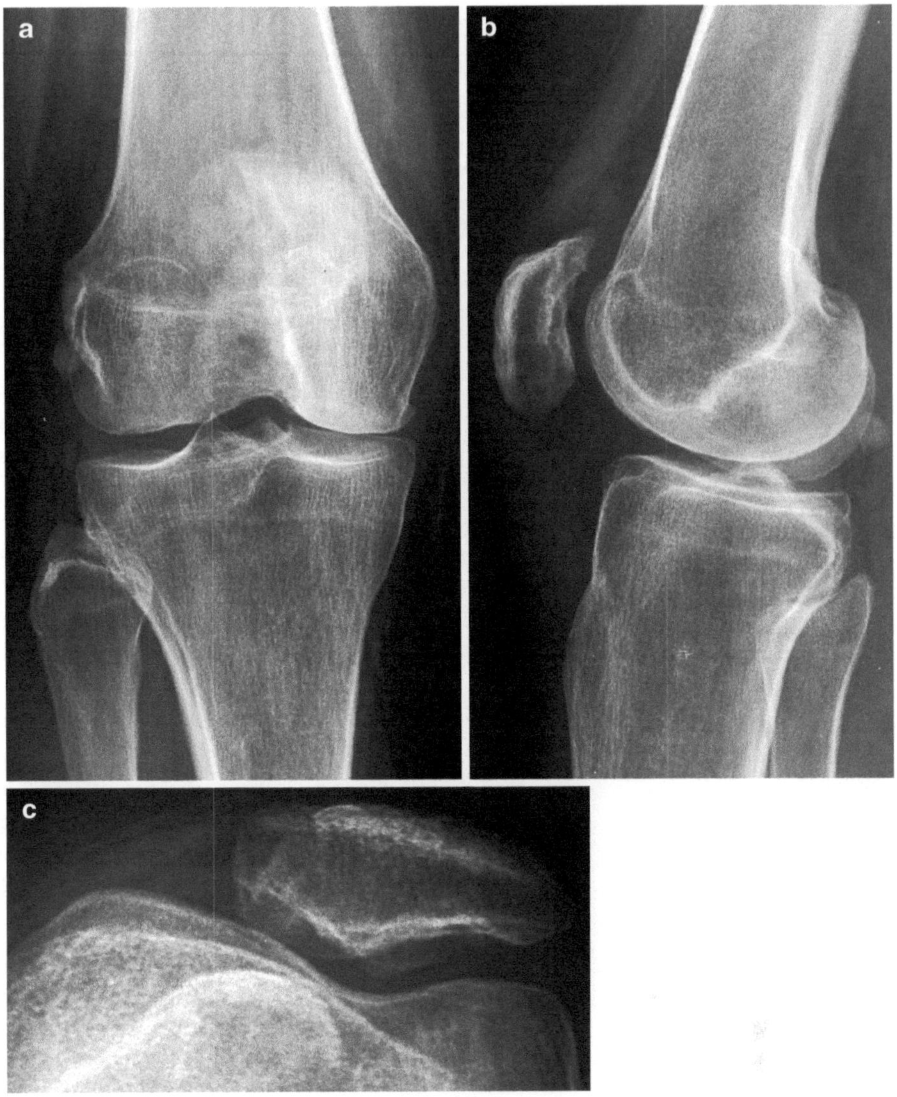

**Fig. 26.5** Conventional radiographs showing isolated patellofemoral osteoarthritis. (**a**) anteroposterior view, (**b**) lateral view (**c**) axial view

much lower than that of a healthy person (45.14º). When the patient used her defense strategies to go down the stairs more comfortably, the angle of flexion increased slightly, reaching 27.85º. In the swing phase, the flexion angle was 44.67º, approximately half of the angle reached by a healthy person, which is 101.56º. When the patient went down the stairs employing her defense strategy, the angle was 76.29º. We can conclude that the patient had a stair descent pattern with knee extension.

The second parameter analyzed with the stair descending test was the ground reaction force (GRF) that occurs when the subject steps on a platform placed underneath the step (Fig. 26.8b). The curve we obtained has two peaks, one corresponding to the heel strike and the other to the toe-off. The normalized force values for a healthy subject are 1.385 during the heel strike, 0.777 during the midstance, and 0.910 during the toe-off. The values we obtained from our patient with the standard stair descending test were: 1.356 during the heel strike, 0.783 during the midstance, and 1.078 during the toe-off. The values we obtained from our patient with the stair descending test, using her defense strategies, were: 1.292 during the heel strike, 0.798 during the midstance, and 0.828 during the toe-off. Although we observed no significant differences in the reaction forces, we did observe a decrease in the stance phase duration on the platform when the patient went down the stairs following

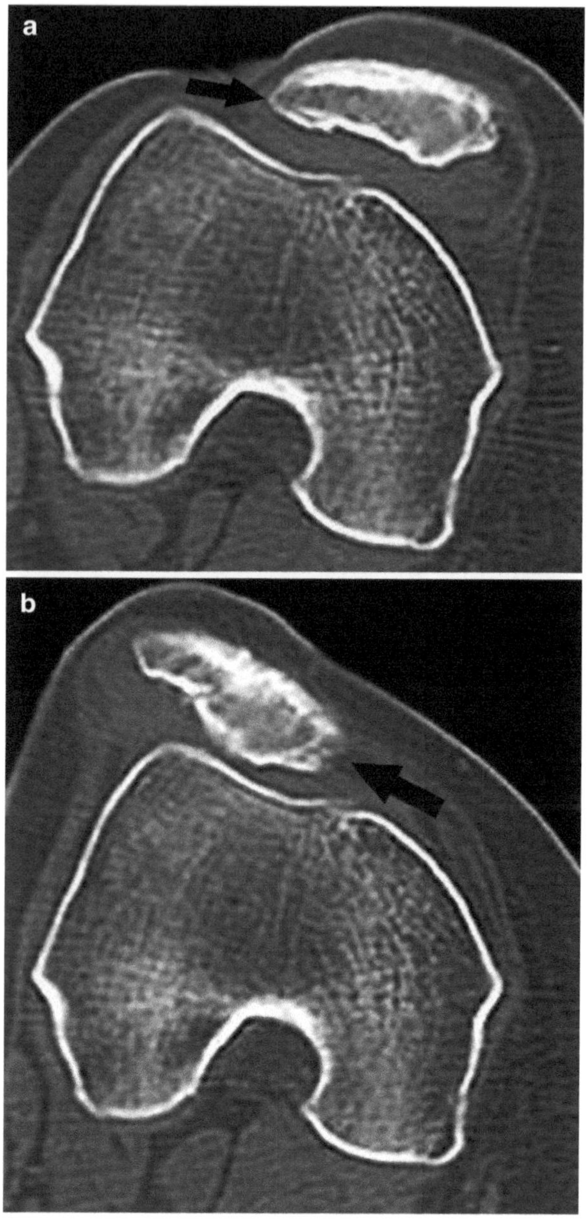


**Fig. 26.6** (**a**) Medial stress CT at 0° extension (finger on the lateral aspect of the patella *black arrow*). (**b**) Lateral stress CT at 0° extension (finger on the medial aspect of the patella *black arrow*). Note the presence of a shallow trochlea

standard protocol (0.64 s instead of 0.94±0.13 s in a healthy control subject). However, when using the more comfortable defense strategy for stair descent, the stance phase duration on the platform was 0.96 s, similar to that of a normal healthy subject.

The third parameter analyzed with the stair descending test was the flexion and extension moment (Fig. 26.8c). During stair descent, a flexion moment (negative) takes place during the heel strike and an extension moment (positive) takes place during the toe-off. In a healthy subject, we can find the normalized values of −0.145 during the heel strike and 0.265 during the toe-off. In our patient's case, by following the standard protocol, we found reduced values during the heel strike (−0.072) and most of all during the toe-off (extensor moment) with values of 0.034. When our patient used a more comfortable defense strategy, these values increased, and during the heel strike we observed normal moments of −0.174 and of 0.048 for the toe-off.

The fourth parameter analyzed using the stair descending test was the abduction–adduction moment (Fig. 26.8d). During stair descent, the moments produced are abduction moments (negative values as we can see in the graphic). On a healthy subject's curve, there are two peaks that correspond to the heel strike and toe-off. In a healthy subject, these normalized moments are −0.156 during the heel strike and −0.128 during the toe-off. In our patient's case, following standard protocol, we observed greatly reduced values compared to the normal ones: −0.062 during the heel strike and −0.061 during the toe-off. With the comfort defense strategy, the moments reached are −0.150 during the heel strike and −0.105 during the toe-off.

Before the reconstruction of the lateral patellofemoral ligament, an arthroscopy was performed. Some fibrous tissue located between the patella and the femoral trochlea was removed. A severe patellofemoral osteoarthritis was noticed; the rest of the findings were normal. Afterward, a reconstruction of the lateral patellofemoral ligament using fascia lata was performed according to the technique described by Jack Andrish, detailed in Chapter 32.

Kinetic and kinematic analysis during stair descent was performed with a 6 month follow-up (Fig. 26.8). During this period, our patient reached the following knee flexion values, 27.79° during the stance phase and 85.69° during the swing phase. The flexion–extension moments reached values of −0.174 during the heel strike and 0.071 during the toe-off, while the abduction moments were closer to normal: −0.161 during the heel strike and −0.169 during the toe-off. At 12 months

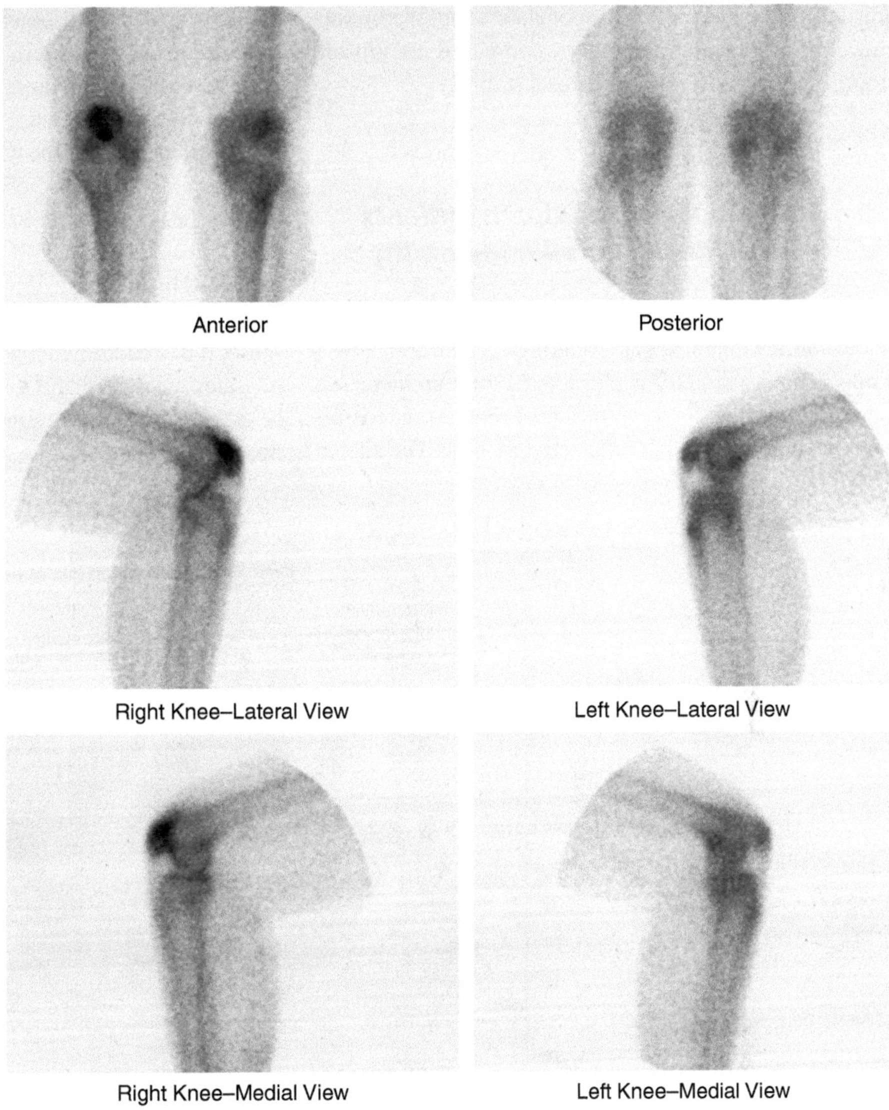


**Fig. 26.7** Standard technetium 99 methylene diphosphonate bone scan showing increased osseous metabolic activity of the patella

follow-up (Fig. 26.8), our patient reached the following knee flexion values, 30.36° during the stance phase and 82.37° during the swing phase. The flexion–extension moments reached values of −0.129 during the heel strike and 0.149 during the toe-off, while the abduction moments were closer to normal: −0.152 during the heel strike and −0.151 during the toe-off.

Twelve months after surgery, the patient is asymptomatic and could go down the stairs in a natural way without any problem. The postoperative Kujala score was 94 points.

## 26.4 Discussion

Patients with patellar disorders have pain situated behind the patella, often on the medial side of the knee, and sometimes, as in case #1, posteriorly in the popliteal fossa. The analysis of the two clinical cases we present in this chapter allows us to speculate on the possible causes of this pain in the posterior aspect of the knee, about the importance of retinacular overload in the genesis of anterior knee pain, and why certain patellofemoral chondropathies are asymptomatic.

Furthermore, it allows us to speculate about the importance of retinacular structures compared to muscle coordination in the patellofemoral stability.

### 26.4.1 Avoidance Behavior in Patients with Medial Patellar Instability

The result of the preoperative gait analysis in case #1 shows an asymmetric gait pattern between both lower limbs. This asymmetry is characterized by an increased horizontal braking force, vertical heel contact, and toe-off vertical peak forces on the affected right limb. The altered parameters could be consistent, among others, with a knee extension gait pattern that was clinically observed in our patient. Knee flexion during the stance phase is one of the determinants of gait[13], which contributes to smoothing the translation of the center of mass. In our case, the affected limb assumes more load during the stance phase than the healthy one, probably due to the fact that support comes from the rigid limb. The kinetic findings could be explained by the sense of instability and pain experienced by the patient in the first degrees of knee flexion. In this sense, it is well-known that with knee flexion, the patella migrates medially[17] and that medial displacement has to be greater if the lateral retinaculum is absent as in case #1. So, we speculate that the knee extension gait pattern in

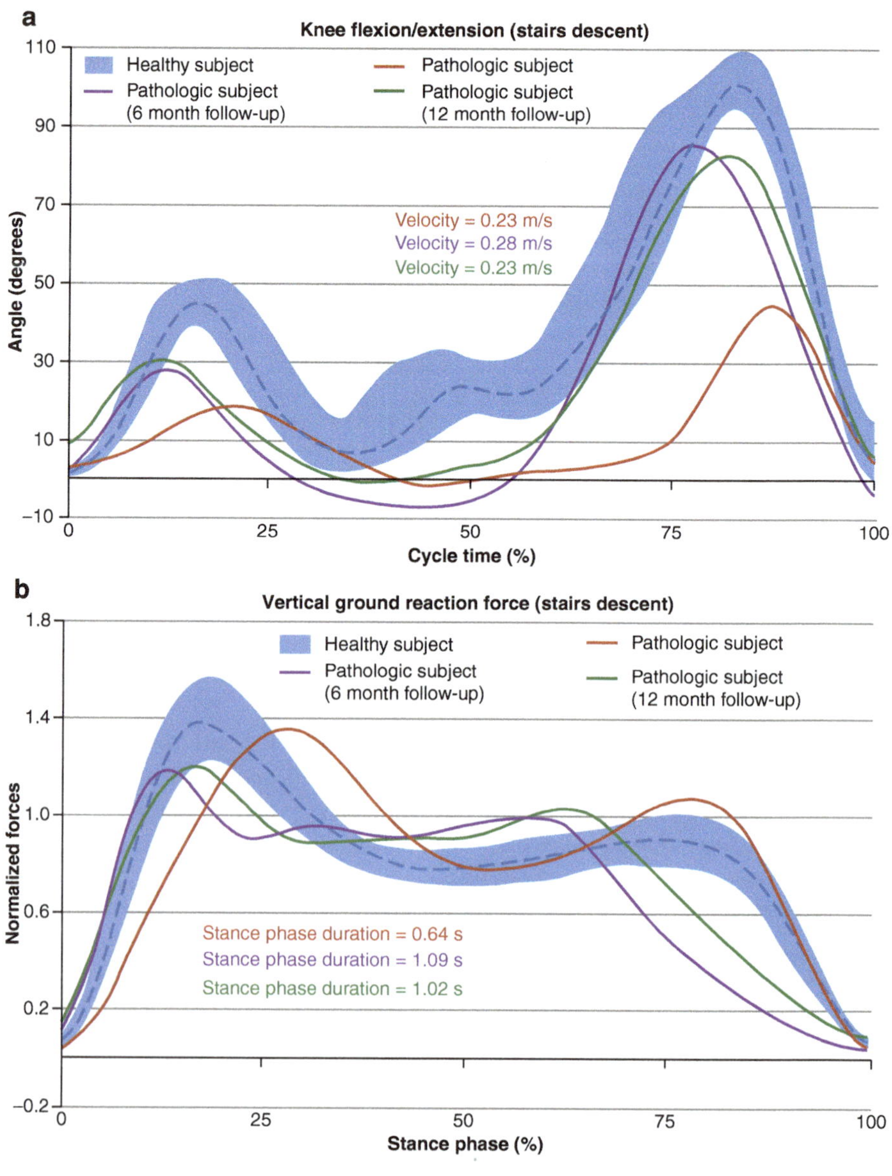


**Fig. 26.8** Knee kinetics and kinematics during stair descent in case #2. (**a**) Knee joint angle during stair descent. (**b**) Ground force reactions during stair descent. (**c**) Flexion–extension knee moments during stair descent. (**d**) Abduction–Adduction knee moments during stair descent

**Fig. 26.8** (continued)

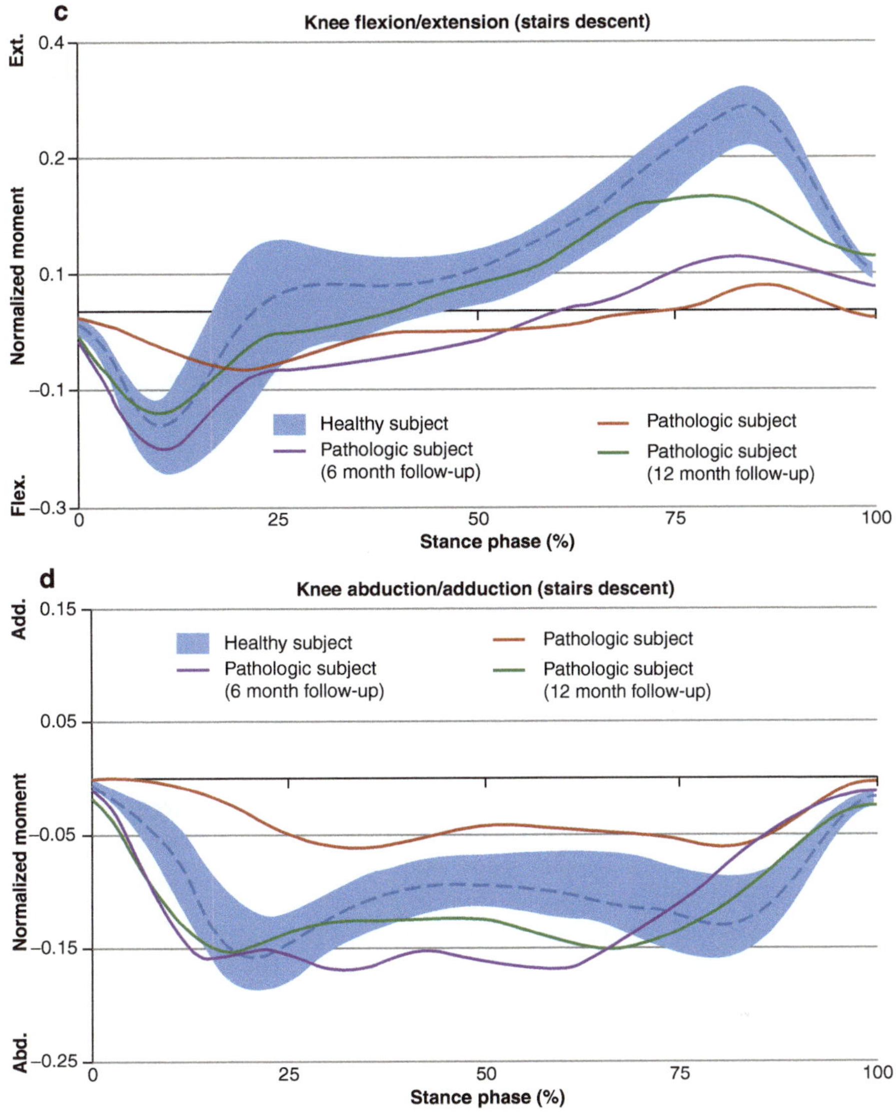


our patient is a strategy to avoid instability and therefore pain. Due to this knee extension gait pattern, the posterior muscles work in a chronic manner in an elongated eccentric condition; this situation could be responsible for the posterior knee pain. This hypothesis is similar to the one presented by Castagna and colleagues[4] to explain posterior shoulder pain in the anterior glenohumeral instability. However, the patient in case #2, although she had a medial patellar instability, she did not have a knee extension gait pattern. But she did go down the stairs with a knee extension pattern as shown in the kinematic analysis. The absence of pain in the posterior aspect of the knee in the patient in case #2 can be justified by the absence of a knee extension gait pattern and because of avoiding walking downstairs and, therefore, avoiding chronic posterior muscle chain eccentric work.

Stair descent with knee extension would be a strategy to reduce the knee extensor moment, with the subsequent smaller quadriceps contraction and the decrease of the patellofemoral joint reaction and loading during pain-provoking activities, such as going downstairs. Another factor responsible for the decrease of the knee's extensor moment is the reduction of the stance phase duration we observed when analyzing the ground reaction force during stair descent. The decrease of the abductor moment both during the heel strike and toe-off in the course of standard stair descent, compared to a healthy subject, could be a defense mechanism to reduce the valgus vector and therefore, the lateral patellar displacement. The decrease of the external abductor moment causes a decrease of the MCL force, which is oriented proximally in the medial aspect of the joint.

This decrease also causes a reduction of the joint contact forces, distally in the lateral tibial plateau. All these forces together produce an internal moment that compensates for the external moment that tends to rotate the knee into a valgus position. This would explain why our patient had no pain either in the internal or external tibiofemoral compartments. It would also be the reason for the increased uptake in the patella and none in the external or internal compartments during the bone scan. The final goal is to reduce pain.

### 26.4.2 Does Every Chondral Lesion Require Surgery?

It is also interesting to notice that the anterior knee pain subsided in the second patient despite the fact that the procedure had nothing to do with the patellofemoral osteoarthritis the patient suffered. It is a well-known fact that the patella tolerates chondral lesions well, up to a certain point. In fact, patellar chondral lesions are a frequent incidental finding in knee arthroscopies of patients without anterior knee pain that are operated on because of a meniscal lesion. Furthermore, many surgeons do not routinely perform a patellar replacement during a total knee replacement. Moreover, in our Insall's proximal realignment series, with an average follow-up period of 8 years, we can find an 8% of asymptomatic patellofemoral osteoarthritis. This should raise the questions: when is a chondral lesion the source of the pain? and what are the indications for surgical treatment in a chondral lesion? The standard bone scan test using technetium 99 methylene diphosphonate performed on the second patient showed an increased osseous metabolic activity of the patella ("hot patella"). This suggests that the patella is a source of pain in case #2. The focal overload of the subchondral bone due to patellofemoral imbalance could cause abnormal stress that might eventually lead to articular breakdown and patellofemoral osteoarthritis. In fact, our patient had no degenerative changes prior to the first surgery, and therefore we consider her patellofemoral osteoarthritis as iatrogenic. Possibly, the non-correction of the extensor moment, after our surgery, is a defense mechanism against the patellofemoral osteoarthritis.

Case #2 could show the importance that overloading the retinacular structures has in the genesis of anterior knee pain, given that the patient's symptoms disappeared with just the reconstruction of the lateral patellofemoral ligament. A CT of the patellofemoral joint in extension with manual medial patellar pressure revealed a medial patellar instability. Moreover, a stress CT applying a manual pressure pushing the patella laterally showed a lateral patellar displacement significantly greater than the contralateral healthy knee. Therefore, we can establish that case #2 is a multidirectional patellofemoral instability in the presence of an underlying shallow trochlea. Iatrogenically chronic recurrent soft tissue fatigue or overload due to patellofemoral imbalance could cause the pain in patients with multidirectional patellofemoral instability as it occurs in our case.

Finally, we can speculate that the normalization of the gait pattern after surgery in the first case, and the improvement of the kinetic and kinematic parameters of the knee during stair descent in the second case could be related to the restoration of passive stabilizers of the patellofemoral joint, in this case, the lateral retinaculum.

### 26.4.3 Retinacular Structures Versus Muscle Coordination in Patellar Stability

The lateral retinaculum is an important passive structure which, in complex interplay with the bone geometry and the dynamic structures, ensures patellofemoral stability and patellar gliding behavior in the trochlea.[2]

An interesting issue in patellar stability is the concept of passive restraints versus muscle coordination. Farahmand and colleagues[8] demonstrated in the laboratory that the quadriceps has a significant and consistent effect on lateral patellar stability across the entire range of knee flexion, the contribution of the medial retinaculum being restricted to extended knee postures. Moreover, Senavongse and colleagues[18] demonstrated that with quadriceps tension, the patella was more resistant to medial rather than lateral displacement.

However, several authors have demonstrated the contribution of the lateral retinaculum as a restraint to lateral patellar translation.[5,6] We believe that reconstruction of the lateral retinaculum would provide a restraining force to medial patellar translation and lateral patellar translation as well. Our hypothesis is based on the study performed by Desio and colleagues in 1998.[6] The authors studied the contribution of the soft tissue structures to lateral patellar translation in a cadaveric model and found that the lateral retinaculum played a significant role as a restraint to lateral patellar translation. In the same way, Christoforakis and colleagues[5] demonstrated that lateral retinacular release significantly reduced the mean force required to displace the patella 10 mm laterally, at 0°, 10°, and 20° of knee flexion, by 16–19%. Our follow-up CT scan findings support the role of lateral retinaculum as a restraint to lateral patellar displacement. Our follow-up CT scan findings also support the role of the lateral retinaculum as a restraint to medial patellar displacement.

### 26.4.4 Patellofemoral Malalignment Theory Versus Homeostasis Theory in the Genesis of Anterior Knee Pain

Our cases could be used to support the patellofemoral malalignment (PFM) theory of patellofemoral pain rather than the homeostasis theory proposed by Dye.[7] However, we believe that both theories can coexist. We look at PFM as representing internal load shifting within the patellofemoral joint that may lower the threshold (i.e., decrease of the Envelope of Function) for the initiation and persistence of loss of tissue homeostasis leading to the perception of patellofemoral pain.

## 26.5 Summary

In conclusion, we speculate that chronic recurrent soft tissue fatigue or overload due to patellofemoral imbalance could cause anterior knee pain. However, many chondropathies can be asymptomatic due to the biomechanic defense strategies used by the patients. Moreover, we emphasize the importance of the passive restraining structures in patellar stability, in contrast to the role of muscle function advocated by some authors. This could explain why an exercise rehabilitation program could be unsuccessful in improving patellar instability, as it occurred in our cases. Finally, these cases highlight the need for surgeons to be more judicious in their surgical selection for patellofemoral instability and serve as a warning for the generalized use of lateral retinacular release. The question we ask ourselves is: Is there a place for the isolated lateral retinacular release? In this sense, it would be interesting to consider the lengthening of the lateral retinaculum described by Roland Biedert as an alternative to lateral retinacular release.

## References


1. Andriachi TP, Ogle JA, Galante JO. Walking speed as a basis for normal and abnormal gait measurements. *J Biomech.* 1977;10:261-268.
2. Biedert RM, Friederich NF. Failed lateral retinacular release: clinical outcome. *J Sports Traumatol.* 1994;16:162-173.
3. Biedert RM. Computed tomography examination. In: Biedert RM, ed. *Patellofemoral Disorders. Diagnosis and Treatment.* West Sussex: Wiley; 2004:101-111.
4. Castagna A, Conti M, Borroni M, et al. Posterior shoulder pain and anterior instability: a preliminary clinical study. *Chir Organi Mov.* 2008;91:79-83.
5. Christoforakis J, Bull AM, Strachan RK, et al. Effects of lateral retinacular release on the lateral stability of the patella. *Knee Surg Sports Traumatol Arthrosc.* 2006;14:273-277.
6. Desio SM, Burks RT, Bachus KN. Soft tissue restraints to lateral patellar translation in the human knee. *Am J Sports Med.* 1998;26:59-65.
7. Dye SF, Staubli HU, Biedert RM, et al. The mosaic of pathophysiology causing patellofemoral pain: therapeutic implications. *Oper Tech Sports Med.* 1999;7:46-54.
8. Farahmand F, Naghi Tahmasbi M, Amis A. The contribution of the medial retinaculum and quadriceps muscles to patellar lateral stability—an in-vitro study. *Knee.* 2004;11:89-94.
9. Fulkerson JP, Gossling HR. Anatomy of the knee joint lateral retinaculum. *Clin Orthop.* 1980;153:183-188.
10. Fulkerson JP. A clinical test for medial patella tracking. *Tech Orthop.* 1997;12:165-169.
11. Hughston JC, Deese M. Medial subluxation of the patella as a complication of lateral retinacular release. *Am J Sports Med.* 1988;16:383-388.
12. Hughston JC, Flandry F, Brinker MR, et al. Surgical correction of medial subluxation of the patella. *Am J Sports Med.* 1996;24:486-491.
13. Inman VT, Ralston HJ, Todd F. *Human Walking*. Baltimore: Williams and Wilkins; 1981.
14. Johnson DP, Wakeley C. Reconstruction of the lateral patellar retinaculum following lateral release: a case report. *Knee Surg Sports Traumatol Arthrosc.* 2002;10:361-363.
15. Kramers-de Quervain IA, Biedert R, Stussi E. Quantitative gait analysis in patients with medial patellar instability following lateral retinacular release. *Knee Surg Sports Traumatol Arthrosc.* 1997;5:95-101.
16. Murray MP, Mollinger LA, Sepic SB, et al. Gait patterns in above-knee amputee patients: hydraulic swing control vs constant-friction knee components. *Arch Phys Med Rehabil.* 1983;64:339-345.

17. Sanchis-Alfonso V, Gastaldi-Orquin E, Martinez-San Juan V. Usefulness of computed tomography in evaluating the patellofemoral joint before and after Insall's realignment: correlation with short-term clinical results. *Am J Knee Surg*. 1994;7:65-72.
18. Senavongse W, Farahmand F, Jones J, et al. Quantitative measurement of patellofemoral joint stability: force–displacement behavior of the human patella in vitro. *J Orthop Res*. 2003;21:780-786.
19. Shellock FG, Mink JH, Deutsch A, et al. Evaluation of patients with persistent symptoms after lateral retinacular release by kinematic magnetic resonance imaging of the patellofemoral joint. *Arthroscopy*. 1990;6:226-234.
20. Small NC. An analysis of complications in lateral retinacular release procedures. *Arthroscopy*. 1989;5:282-286.
21. Teitge RA, Faerber WW, Des Madryl P, et al. Stress radiographs of the patellofemoral joint. *J Bone Joint Surg*. 1996;78-A:193-203.
22. Viosca E. *Estudio biomecánico comparativo entre el patrón de marcha humana normal y del amputado tibial* [thesis]. Valencia: Universidad Politécnica de Valencia; 1993.
23. Sanchis-Alfonso V, Torga-Spak R, Cortes A. Gait pattern normalization after lateral retinaculum reconstruction for iatrogenic medial patellar instability. *Knee*. 2007;14: 484-488.

# Part IV

# Surgical Techniques "How I Do It"

# 27 Ultrasound and Doppler-Guided Arthroscopic Shaving for the Treatment of Patellar Tendinopathy/Jumper's Knee: Biological Background and Description of Method

Håkan Alfredson, Lotta Willberg, Lars Öhberg, and Sture Forsgren

## 27.1 Background

Treatment of chronic painful patellar tendinopathy/ Jumper's knee is known to be difficult, and surgical treatment has been shown to give unreliable and, not seldom, poor clinical results.[6-8] With this in mind, there was an obvious need for studies around the pain mechanisms associated with this chronic condition.[11] We decided to use ultrasound and Doppler examinations, analyses of biopsies, and diagnostic injections of local anesthesia, to try to learn more about possible pain mechanisms. The ultrasound and Doppler findings of high blood flow in the region with structural tendon changes in the dorsal part of the tendon (blood flow coming from the fat tissue dorsal to the tendon),[13,15,16] and histological and immunohistochemical analyses of biopsies demonstrating nerves in close relation to the vessels in this area,[9,10] are cornerstones in the background to our new treatment approach for patients with patellar tendinopathy/Jumper's knee. Furthermore, small volumes of a local anesthetic in the region with neovessels and nerves (outside the tendon) temporarily cured the tendon pain in Achilles tendinosis,[1] and indicated this region as responsible for the tendon pain. In following studies on patients with Achilles[3,14] and patellar tendinosis,[2] treatment with US and color Doppler (CD)-guided injections of the sclerosing agent Polidocanol, aiming to destroy the area with neovessels and nerves, demonstrated good short-term clinical results with significantly reduced tendon pain during activity. Altogether, these findings pointed towards the vessels and nerves outside the deep tendon (dorsal to the patellar tendon and ventral to the Achilles tendon) as being responsible for the pain in chronic painful proximal patellar and midportion Achilles tendinosis. Interestingly, ultrasound and Doppler follow-ups of patients successfully treated with sclerosing Polidocanol injections outside the Achilles midportion have shown the existence of a more normal tendon (significantly reduced thickening and more normal structure), indicating a remodeling/regeneration potential.[12]

With the above-described information in mind, a new type of treatment, "arthroscopic shaving" for chronic painful patellar tendinopathy/Jumper's knee is described.

## 27.2 New Basal Findings Concerning Morphology and Innervation

In recent studies, it has been observed that there is a perivascular innervation related to the small and large blood vessels that are present in the paratendinous region dorsal to the proximal patellar tendon.[9] There was especially a pronounced sympathetic component in this innervation.[9] These observations are of interest

H. Alfredson (✉)
Sports Medicine Unit, Department of Surgical and Perioperative Sciences, Umeå University, Umeå, Sweden
e-mail: hakan.alfredson@idrott.umu.se

V. Sanchis-Alfonso (ed.), *Anterior Knee Pain and Patellar Instability*,
DOI: 10.1007/978-0-85729-507-1_27, © Springer-Verlag London Limited 2011

as these regions represent the regions that, with success, can be treated with arthroscopic shaving. In comparison, it has been observed that the ventral region of the Achilles tendon is under marked influence by the nervous system, and that the existing innervation is present in regions where there is a presence of large and small blood vessels.[5] This is the region that is targeted for treatment with Polidocanol injections[3,14] and surgical scraping.[4] The observations on innervation patterns in relation to the patellar and Achilles tendons are made via immunohistochemical analyses. They show the innervation patterns in relation to the vascularity. Consequently, the preoperative evaluation using ultrasound and color Doppler investigations to study the blood flow inside and outside the chronic painful tendon is of significant importance. This will be described below.

## 27.3 Indications for Arthroscopic Shaving

Patients with a long duration (>3 months) of pain from the proximal patellar tendon during patellar tendon loading activity, who, both clinically and with ultrasound + Doppler or MRI, are diagnosed to suffer from patellar tendinopathy/Jumper's knee.

## 27.4 Contraindications

Chronic inflammatory diseases, other systematic diseases affecting joints and/or connective tissue, previous knee injuries (ACL, menisci, cartilage, fractures).

## 27.5 Preoperative Evaluation

All patients had tried rest as treatment without any effect on the painful condition.

### *27.5.1 Gray-Scale Ultrasonography*

Ultrasound was performed with a linear transducer (Acuson Sequoia 512) with 8–13 MHz frequency. The examinations were carried out with the patients laying on their back, having the knee in a straight position. The patellar tendons were examined in the longitudinal and transverse planes. Both tendons were always examined in the same manner.

### *27.5.2 Color Doppler Examination*

Color Doppler (CD) is a sonographic method to study blood flow in the human body. We have used color Doppler velocity technique (CDV), where the color of the flow indicates the direction and velocity of the blood flow. The technique does not allow for registration of the normal circulation of the tendon because of the relatively low blood flow in normal tendons. Only high blood flows like those in chronic painful tendinosis can be registered. The Doppler registration was carried out with straight knee.

The majority of patients with Jumper's knee have structural changes and high blood flow ("neovascularization") localized to the dorsal and central parts of the proximal patellar tendon, with blood flow coming from the soft tissues dorsal to the tendon (Fig. 27.1). However, there are patients who also have structural changes and high blood flow ("neovessels") in the ventral part of the tendon, with blood flow coming from the soft tissues ventral to the tendon. Patients with changes in the ventral part of the tendon have not been

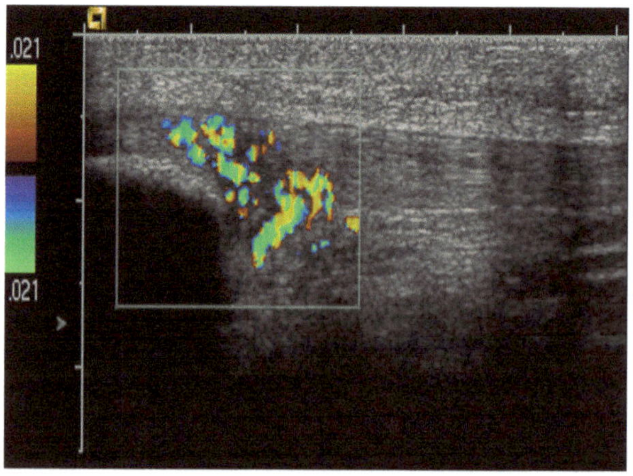


**Fig. 27.1** Gray-scale ultrasound and color Doppler examination of a patient with patellar tendinopathy/Jumper's knee, showing thickening of the proximal tendon, irregular tendon structure and hypoechoicity, and high blood flow (*color*) inside the tendon and outside the dorsal part of the tendon

included in so far performed studies, because theoretically, in these patients, there might be a vasculo-neural ingrowth also from the ventral side.

## 27.6 Surgical Technique

Before the arthroscopy is performed, ultrasound and color Doppler examination is done to characterize the region with structural tendon changes and neovessels. Thickness and length of the region with structural tendon changes and neovessels are measured. This information is used as a guide for the shaving procedure.

Arthroscopy can be done in local or general anesthesia. For local anesthesia: Altogether 40 ml 0.5% Xylocain/Adrenaline (Astra Södertälje, Sweden) is used to locally infiltrate the anteromedial and anterolateral portals, the superolateral portal, and for infiltration of the intra-articular tissues.

The patients are laying on their back with straight knee. The anteromedial and anterolateral portals are placed about 1 cm more laterally and medially, respectively, compared to the standard positioning. First, a standard arthroscopical evaluation of the whole knee joint is performed. For treatment of the patellar tendinopathy/Jumper's knee, ultrasound and arthroscopy monitors are used simultaneously (Fig. 27.2). An assistant is managing the ultrasound probe, while the surgeon is using the ultrasound and Doppler findings to guide the arthroscopic procedure. The patellar tendon insertion into the patella is identified, and careful shaving of the soft tissues on the dorsal side of the tendon is performed. For shaving, a shaver with a 4.5-mm full radius blade is used. Multiple small vessels entering the region with tendinosis in the dorsal part of the tendon is a regular finding. Shaving is done just outside the region with tendinosis in the dorsal tendon, aiming to destroy as much as possible of the region with neovessels. The tip of the patella is always visualized, and if there are osteophytes, they are removed. Calcifications in the dorsal tendinosis tissue can be removed, but is most often left without treatment. When the whole region with high blood flow ("neovessels") has been treated, the shaving procedure is stopped. The preoperative tendon thickness measurements provide valuable information minimizing the risks of shaving "too much." The portals are closed with sutures or tape. A bandage is used for 24 h.

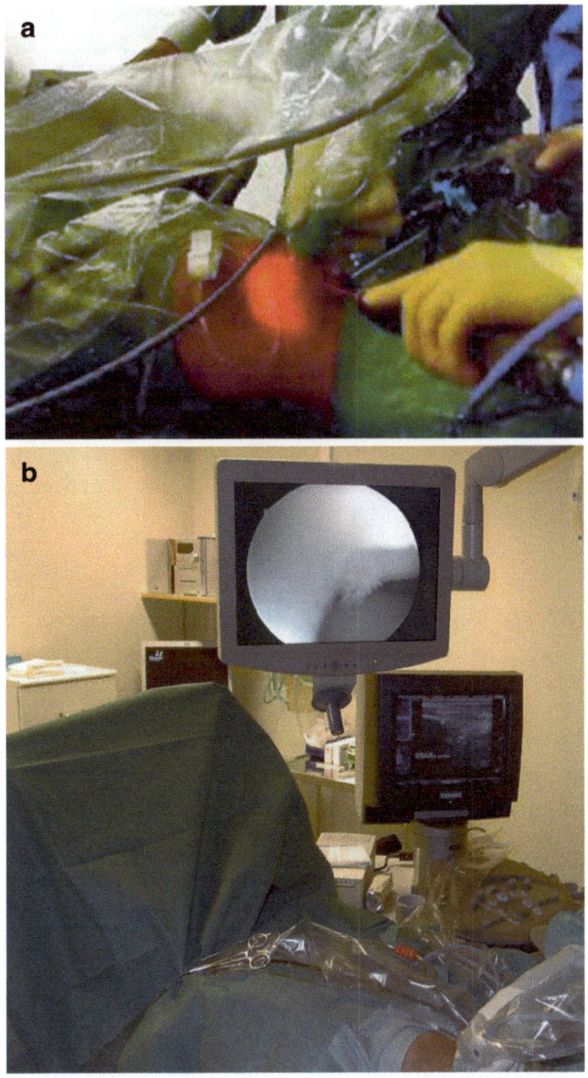


**Fig. 27.2** For treatment of the patellar tendinopathy/Jumper's knee changes, ultrasound and arthroscopy monitors are used simultaneously. An assistant is managing the ultrasound probe (draped sterile), while the surgeon is using the ultrasound and Doppler findings as a guide for the arthroscopic procedure

## 27.7 Advantage of Using Ultrasound During the Arthroscopy

A major advantage using ultrasound during the arthroscopy is that you exactly know where you have the shaver. It's not always easy to orientate the shaver in the soft tissues posterior to the patellar tendon, and because you want to minimize the trauma to the Hoffa fat pad, the ultrasound guidance provides valuable help.

## 27.8 Additional Diagnoses

We often (75% of cases) find other diagnoses in the knee during the arthroscopy. The most common findings are plicae formations and cartilage lesions in the femoro-patellar joint. This is of clinical interest, since these findings might cause pain problems similar to the patellar tendon changes.

## 27.9 Complications

We have had no serious complications related to this procedure, but of course, you need to pay attention to risks associated with knee arthroscopy.

## 27.10 Postoperative Rehabilitation Regimen

Day 1: Partial weight bearing with crutches. The patients are instructed to start full non-weight bearing range of motion exercises.

Day 2–7: Start walking and light bicycling activity. Light concentric and eccentric strength training for the quadriceps muscles is to be instituted.

Day 8–14: During the second week after treatment, the patients are told to gradually increase their tendon loading activity with more sport-specific training.

No maximum jumping-, running-, or weight training activity is allowed during the first 2 weeks.

Two weeks postoperatively: Maximum patellar tendon loading activity (back to their sport) could be started if there is no marked muscle atrophy.

## 27.11 Outcome Measures

We have decided to use the visual analogue scale (VAS) to evaluate the results of the treatment. Using a visual analogue scale (VAS) for pain, the patients record the amount of patellar tendon pain during activity (their actual sport or recreational activity) on a 100-mm long scale. The level of patellar tendon pain is recorded from 0 to 100 mm, where no pain is recorded as 0 and severe pain as 100. Patient satisfaction with treatment is also recorded. The patients hereby define if they are satisfied or not satisfied with result of treatment.

## 27.12 Results of a Pilot Study

In a pilot study,[17] 15 patients (12 men and 3 women) with the diagnosed Jumper's knee-PT, were treated with ultrasound and Doppler-guided arthroscopic shaving. At follow-up (mean 6 months) after treatment, there was a good clinical result in 13/15 tendons (6/8 elite athletes). The satisfied patients were back to previous (before injury) sport activity level, and the level of pain during tendon loading activity recorded on a VAS scale had decreased significantly (VAS from 79 to 12, $p<0.05$). A complementary telephone follow-up performed 13 months (mean) postoperatively, showed that the 13 patients with good results were still satisfied and active in their sports, and that the 2/15 poor cases were still not satisfied with the treatment. Further follow-ups (up to 3 years) of this group of patients have shown remaining good clinical results in the initially satisfied patients (unpublished material).

## 27.13 Further Analyses

After the initial pilot study described above, multiple patients have been treated with this method, some included in a large randomized study currently under final evaluation. Our impression from the results after treatment of all these patients is that the clinical results are very good, and that there are very few, if any, complications. However, before recommending this treatment method for general use, the results from scientific studies with longer term follow ups need to be presented.

## 27.14 Conclusions

Treatment with ultrasound and Doppler-guided arthroscopic shaving of the region with vessels and nerves outside the dorsal tendon has shown promising clinical results in patients with proximal patellar tendinopathy/Jumper's knee. The results concerning only a limited patient material has been published in a scientific paper. Results on larger materials are under evaluation for later publication. Proper understanding of the ultrasound and Doppler findings, to enable for a precise and minimal arthroscopic shaving procedure on the dorsal side of the tendon, are cornerstones using this new type of treatment.

## References


1. Alfredson H, Öhberg L, Forsgren S. Is vasculo-neural ingrowth the cause of pain in chronic Achilles tendinosis?- An investigation using ultrasonography and colour doppler, immunohistochemistry, and diagnostic injections. *Knee Surg Sports Traumatol Arthrosc.* 2003;11:334-338.
2. Alfredson H, Öhberg L. Neovascularisation in chronic painful patellar tendinosis promising results after sclerosing neovessels outside the tendon challenges the need for surgery. *Knee Surg Sports Traumatol Arthrosc.* 2005;13:74-80.
3. Alfredson H, Öhberg L. Sclerosing injections to areas of neovascularisation reduce pain in chronic Achilles tendinopathy: a double-blind randomized controlled trial. *Knee Surg Sports Traumatol Arthrosc.* 2005;13:338-344.
4. Alfredson H, Öhberg L, Zeisig E, et al. Treatment of mid-portion Achilles tendinosis: similar clinical results with US and CD-guided surgery outside the tendon and sclerosing polidocanol injections. *Knee Surg Sports Traumatol Arthrosc.* 2007;15:1504-1509.
5. Andersson G, Danielson P, Alfredson H, et al. Nerve-related characteristics of ventral paratendinous tissue in chronic Achilles tendinosis. *Knee Surg Sports Traumatol Arthrosc.* 2007;15:1272-1279.
6. Coleman BD, Khan KM, Maffulli N, et al. Studies of surgical outcome after patellar tendinopathy: clinical significance of methodological deficiencies and guidelines for future studies. *Scand J Med Sci Sports.* 2000;10:2-11.
7. Coleman BD, Khan KM, Kiss ZS, et al. Open and arthroscopic patellar tenotomy for chronic patellar tendinopathy. A retrospective outcome study. *Am J Sports Med.* 2000;28:183-190.
8. Cook JL. What's the appropriate treatment for patellar tendinopathy? *Br J Sports Med.* 2001;35:291-294.
9. Danielson P, Andersson G, Alfredson H, et al. Marked sympathetic component in the perivascular innervation of the dorsal paratendinous tissue of the patellar tendon in arthroscopically treated tendinosis patients. *Knee Surg Sports Traumatol Arthrosc.* 2008;16:621-626.
10. Forsgren S, Danielsson P, Alfredson H. Vascular NK-1R receptor occurrence in normal and chronic painful Achilles and patellar tendons. Studies on chemically unfixed as well as fixed specimens. *Regul Pept.* 2005;126:173-181.
11. Khan KM, Cook JL, Maffuli N, et al. Where is the pain coming from in tendinopathy? It may be biochemical, not only structural, in origin. *Br J Sports Med.* 2000;34:81-83.
12. Lind B, Öhberg L, Alfredson H. Sclerosing polidocanol injections in mid-portion Achilles tendinosis: remaining good clinical results and decreased tendon thickness at 2-year follow-up. *Knee Surg Sports Traumatol Arthrosc.* 2006;14:1327-1332.
13. Öhberg L, Lorentzon R, Alfredson H. Neovascularisation in Achilles tendons with painful tendinosis but not in normal tendons: an ultrasonographic investigation. *Knee Surg Sports Traumatol Arthrosc.* 2001;9:233-238.
14. Öhberg L, Alfredson H. Ultrasound guided sclerosis of neovessels in painful chronic Achilles tendinosis: pilot study of a new treatment. *Br J Sports Med.* 2002;36:173-177.
15. Terslev L. Ultrasound and Power Doppler findings in Jumper's knee-preliminary observations. *Eur J Ultrasound.* 2001;13:183-189.
16. Weinberg EP, Adams MJ, Hollenberg GM. Color doppler sonography of patellar tendinosis. *Am J Roentgenol.* 1998;171:743-744.
17. Willberg L, Sunding K, Öhberg L, et al. Treatment of Jumper's knee: promising short-term results in a pilot study using a new arthroscopic approach based on imaging findings. *Knee Surg Sports Traumatol Arthrosc.* 2007;15:676-681.

# Arthroscopic Patellar Denervation for Anterior Knee Pain

# 28

Jordi Vega, Pau Golanó, and Vicente Sanchis-Alfonso

## 28.1 Introduction

Pain treatment by denervation is not a new concept. The objective would be to interrupt the neural pathways that transmit the pain message. It has been applied with good clinical results in chronic spinal pain, trigeminal neuralgia, and in some cases of intractable wrist pain.[5,12,17] On the contrary, anterior knee pain (AKP) treated by selective neurotomy has obtained bad results.[8] Moller and Helming performed a medial denervation of the patella in 17 patients (20 knees) with AKP. At follow-up, only 11 knees were symptom-free or had improved, and the authors conclude that medial neurotomy is not sufficient to eliminate the pain in patients with AKP.[8]

It is well-known that innervation in the anterior knee area shows a highly variable distribution.[2,3,7] This could explain why selective neurotomy does not result in patellar desensitization in most cases.[8] The sensory innervation to the lateral aspect of the knee (see Chap. 25) includes the tibiofibular branch of the peroneal nerve, the lateral retinacular nerve (Fig. 28.1), and the lateral femoral cutaneous nerve. The sensory innervation around the medial aspect of the knee (see Chap. 25) includes the infrapatellar branch of the saphenous nerve, the medial retinacular nerve (Fig. 28.2), and the medial and anterior cutaneous nerves of the thigh. The lateral and medial retinacular nerves provide sensation to the knee joint whereas the other five nerves provide sensation to the cutaneous surface of the knee.

An alternative to selective neurotomy would be to achieve denervation by producing lesions to the nociceptive receptors located in the peripatellar soft tissue. Although the mechanism of AKP is still not fully understood, Sanchis-Alfonso et al. have demonstrated that in patients with AKP, soft tissue hyperinnervation in the peripatellar region could be the cause of pain.[1,9-11] Wojtys et al.[18] studied the final distribution of nerve fibers in the anterior knee region. He located nociceptive fibers in the peripatellar soft tissue, in the periosteum, and in the degenerative subchondral bone of the patella. Vega et al. have studied nerve fiber distribution in peripatellar soft tissue.[15] Most of the neurologic structures are distributed in a similar way. Larger nerves access the peripatellar soft tissue along with vascular structures. We located these larger structures in a deeper or capsular region of the peripatellar soft tissue. From the deeper zone of the soft tissue, neurologic fibers reach a middle zone where they undergo subdivision and concentration. It has been estimated that this middle zone is localized about 0.75 and 1.5 mm from the articular surface.[15] Most of these neurologic structures are found on a more superficial area of this middle zone. Injury caused in the peripatellar soft tissue by spherical 2 and 3.5 mm arthroscopic electrocoagulators can reach an average amplitude of 1.18 and 1.5 mm in depth.[15] Therefore, the injury caused by arthroscopic electrocoagulators could be enough to eliminate the zone where pain receptors are concentrated.

With the above-described information in mind, we designed an arthroscopic procedure, which we term "arthroscopic patellar denervation."[13,14,16] The objective is to produce, using an electrocoagulator, a thermal lesion to the peripatellar soft tissue in the region closest to the patella in order to obliterate a considerable number of nociceptive receptors.

J. Vega (✉)
Department of Orthopedic and Trauma Surgery, Hospital Asepeyo Sant Cugat, Sant Cugat del Vallés, Barcelona, Spain
e-mail: jordivega@hotmail.com

V. Sanchis-Alfonso (ed.), *Anterior Knee Pain and Patellar Instability*,
DOI: 10.1007/978-0-85729-507-1_28, © Springer-Verlag London Limited 2011

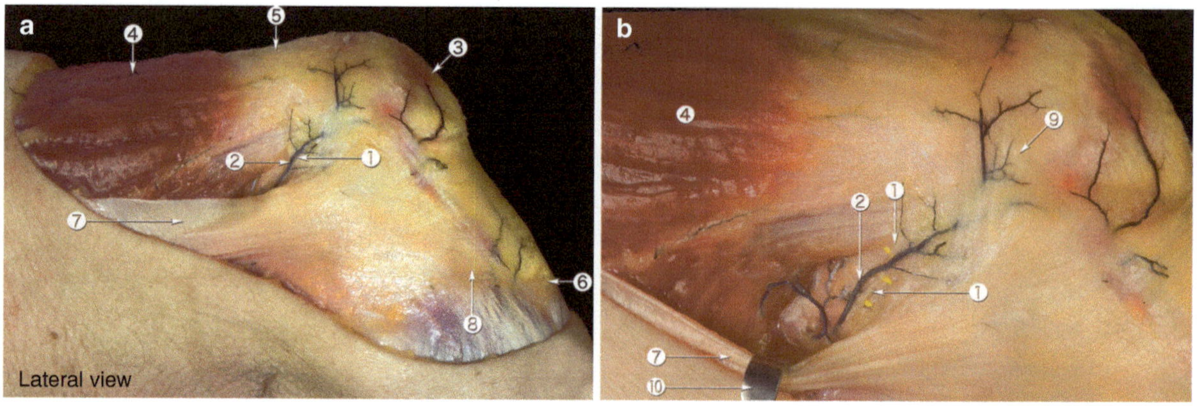


**Fig. 28.1** (**a**) Anatomic dissection of the lateral side of the right knee. (**b**) Macrophotography of the lateral patellar inervation. (*1*) Lateral retinacular nerve. (*2*) Superior lateral genicular artery. (*3*) Patella. (*4*) Vastus lateralis. (*5*) Quadriceps femoralis tendon. (*6*) Patellar tendon insertion (tibial tuberosity). (*7*) Iliotibial tract (*8*) Gerdy's tubercle. (*9*) Superior lateral angle of the patella. (*10*) Sean-Miller retracting the iliotibial tract

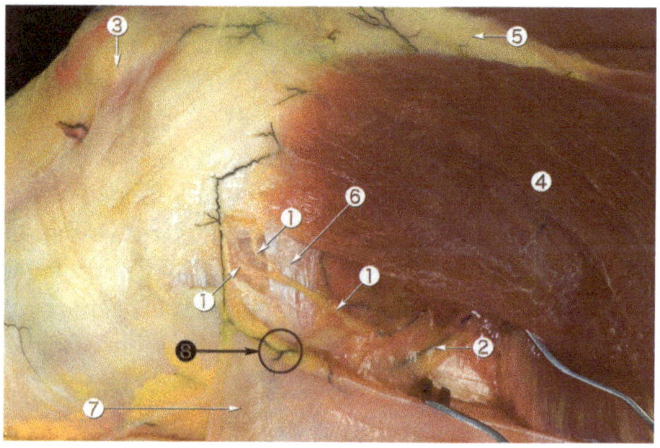

**Fig. 28.2** Anatomic dissection of the medial side of the right knee. Macrophotography. (*1*) Medial retinacular nerve and branches. (*2*) Superior medial genicular artery. (*3*) Patella (superior medial angle of the patella). (*4*) Vastus medialis. (*5*) Quadriceps femoralis tendon. (*6*) Medial patellofemoral ligament. (*7*) Fascia (rejected). (*8*) Medial epicondyle

## 28.2 Indications/Contra-Indications

Arthroscopic patellar denervation is indicated in adolescents or young adults with AKP with a long duration (>6 months), who have no apparent mechanical alterations (no or minimal malalignment) that would justify the condition, only when conservative management (medical treatment and physiotherapy) have failed. In this way, we must remember that patients with AKP often lack an easily identifiable structural abnormality to account for the symptoms.

Isolated arthroscopic patellar denervation is contraindicated in patients with Outerbridge Grade IV chondropathy. However, arthroscopic patellar denervation might become a beneficial addition to other arthroscopic methods (microfractures, chondrectomy, removal of osteophytes, and so on) for treating patellofemoral pain in patients with severe chondropathy of the patella, or a knee prosthesis without a patellar component.

## 28.3 Surgical Technique

The patient is placed in the supine position after spinal anesthesia. A tourniquet is applied for hemostasis. The knee is placed in a knee holder at the end of the operating table. The extremity is then cleansed and draped in a sterile fashion.

The knee landmarks (patella, patellar tendon, and tibial platform) are identified. A 4.5-mm 30° scope is used for the arthroscopic procedure. We routinely use a lateral suprapatellar portal for fluid inflow, joint distension, and continuous irrigation. Conventional portals, anteromedial and anterolateral portals, are used for the arthroscopic joint inspection. By using these two arthroscopic approaches, almost all the patellar joint surface can be viewed.

The knee must be in maximum extension for patellar and peripatellar access. The anterolateral or anteromedial approaches can be supplemented with external or internal suprapatellar portals. Fat tissue in the distal pole of the patella should be removed, thusly facilitating a more simple procedure. The electrocoagulator

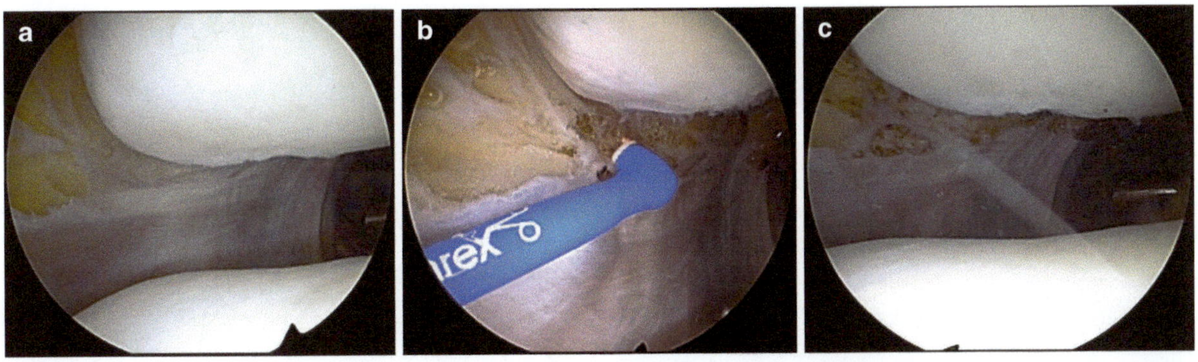


**Fig. 28.3** Arthroscopic image of thermal lesion to the peripatellar synovial tissue produced by the electrocoagulator. (**a**) Medial region of peripatellar soft tissue before denervation. (**b**) Simple thermal lesion to the peripatellar soft tissue in the region closest to the patella. (**c**) Arthroscopic view of the lesion produced by the electrocoagulator in the medial region of the peripatellar soft tissue in order to eliminate a considerable number of pain receptors

is inserted through the anterior and suprapatellar approaches to access the entire perimeter of the patella. A simple thermal lesion to the peripatellar soft tissue in the region closest to the patella will eliminate a considerable number of pain receptors (Fig. 28.3). Although cut or coagulation of the electrocoagulator can be used for performing arthroscopic patellar denervation, we recommend the use of coagulation. Meticulous hemostasis using coagulation will avoid a possible hemorrhage. Because postoperative hemarthroses is not a usual problem in arthroscopic patellar denervation, no suction drain will be necessary after the procedure.

## 28.4 Postoperative Management

All patients may be treated as day cases. An elastic bandage is applied and maintained for 3 or 4 days. Quadriceps exercises and flexion–extension of the knee are encouraged during the immediate postoperative period. Patients are allowed partial load bearing with the aid of crutches for the first 2 weeks. Antithrombotic prophylaxis is used and maintained for 10 days.

## 28.5 Pearls and Pitfalls

Some arthroscopic procedures in the anterior knee compartment are not easy to perform. This is due to multiple factors. First, the need for maximum extension of the knee in some procedures, and the insufflation of fluid to distend the joint during the arthroscopic surgery will separate the patella and the peripatellar region from the conventional portals. The anteromedial and anterolateral portals are posterior and distal to the anterior region of the knee. These circumstances can interfere with the access of the instruments, which will have to be pointed in an anterior and proximal direction. In many cases, this could be uncomfortable for the surgeon, and supplementary portals will be necessary to make the arthroscopic procedure easier. In addition, the anteromedial and anterolateral portals are located on both sides of the patellar tendon and therefore they are usually in a more central position than the region we will be working on (Fig. 28.4). Finally, the arthroscopic instruments are not specifically designed to be used in the anterior region of the knee.

A simple maneuver can expedite the arthroscopic procedure in the anterior region of the knee. With the knee in maximum extension, the placement of a hand on the anterior region of the knee, by applying selective pressure with our fingers on the patella or on the peripatellar tissue, will bring these structures to the instruments inserted through the anteromedial or anterolateral portals (Fig. 28.5). This simple maneuver allows for arthroscopic patellar denervation procedure in a safe, easy, and comfortable way without the need of supplementary portals. However, excessive external pressure will hinder the view and will increase the capacity of the arthroscopic electrocoagulator, causing a deeper undesirable injury.

Finally, the use of conventional electrocoagulators for arthroscopic procedures creates air bubbles that will disturb arthroscopic patellar denervation. New electrocoagulators with suction are useful to prevent this bubble formation.

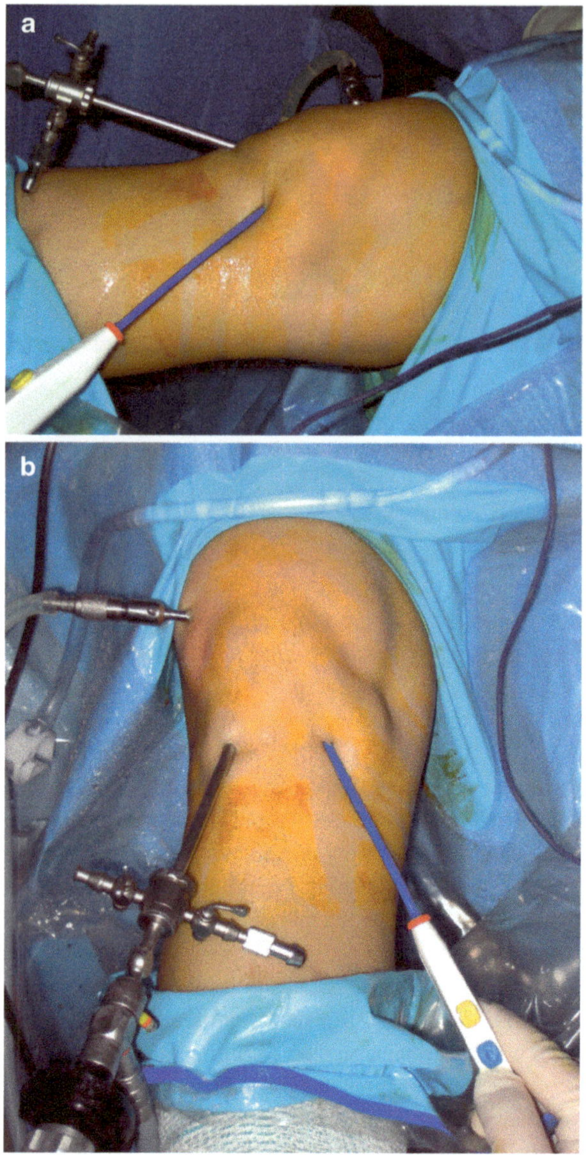

**Fig. 28.4** Maximum extension of the knee and the insufflation of fluid to distend the joint will separate the patella and the peripatellar region from the usual portals in knee arthroscopy (anteromedial and anterolateral portal). The patella and the anatomic protrusion of the distal knee region limit the electrocoagulator movement and make the procedure difficult. (**a**) Medial view of the knee with electrocoagulator inserted through the anteromedial portal, and pointed to the anterior knee area. (**b**) Anterior view of the knee with electrocoagulator inserted through the antermomedial portal, and pointed to the anterior and medial knee area

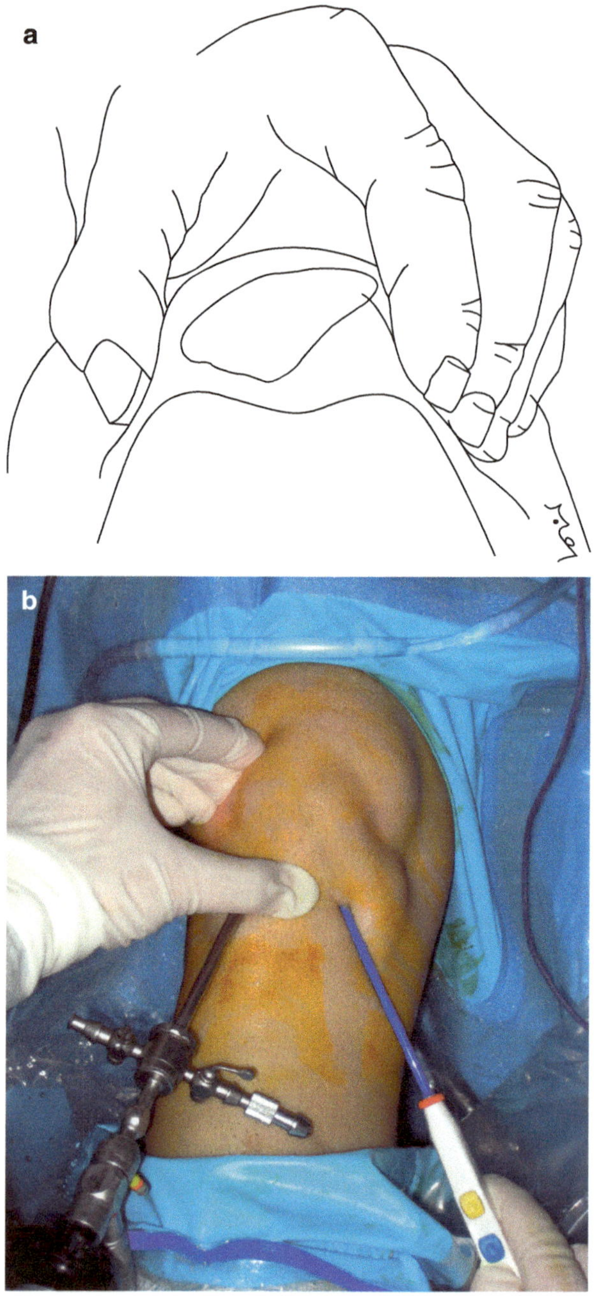

**Fig. 28.5** A selective pressure with fingers on the patella or on the peripatellar tissue will bring these structures to the instruments: Schematic view (**a**). Surgical view with the electrocoagulator inserted through the anteromedial portal (**b**)

## 28.6 Outcome Measures

The clinical outcome was evaluated by an independent surgeon who was not involved in the procedure. We have decided to use two simple scales to evaluate the results of the treatment: the Grana score and the Kujala score. The Grana score[4] is a subjective rating, which classifies the results according to limitations in the patient's activity: A (No pain or restricted activity), B (Extreme activity with non-limiting pain), C (Extreme activity with limiting pain), D (restriction in extreme activity), and E (restriction in daily activity). Knee function was assessed using the Kujala score,[6] which ranges from 0 to 100 (100 is the best possible score). These two scales allow comparison of the status before and after surgery.

## 28.7 Clinical Results of a Pilot Study

We reviewed the records of 18 patients (13 females, 5 males; average age 34, range 22–49 years) who underwent arthroscopic patellar denervation for AKP. No patient had a history of patellar instability or physical or radiographic signs of patellar malalignment. All patients had failed results after a minimum of 6 months of physical therapy before surgery.

We have analyzed a subgroup of 13 patients with a maximum follow-up of 5 years and low-grade patellofemoral chondropathy (I/II) according to the Outerbridge classification. The Kujala score improved from a mean of 72 (52–84) preoperatively to 97 (76–100) after a 2-year follow-up, and 94 (69–100) after a 5-year follow-up. In this group, preoperative assessment with the Grana score placed all patients in categories D (7 cases) and E (6 cases). Postoperative assessment after a 2-year follow-up with the Grana score was A in 10 cases, B in 2 cases, and C in 1 case, indicating satisfactory clinical outcome in 12 cases and unsatisfactory outcome in 1 case. Postoperative assessment after a 5-year follow-up with the Grana score was A in 9 cases, B in 3 cases, and D in 1 case, indicating satisfactory clinical outcome in 12 cases and unsatisfactory outcome in 1 case. Therefore, the clinical outcome of the patients treated with this technique can be considered satisfactory in almost all the cases of AKP with no or minimal malalignment and low-grade chondropathy. Moreover, the excellent clinical results observed in this group of patients after a 2-year follow-up have been maintained after a 5-year follow-up with minimal nonsignificant decrease.

In patients with a chondropathy grade III/IV (5 cases), the Kujala score improved from a mean of 61 (57–69) preoperatively to 85 (71–95) after a 2-year follow-up. A preoperative assessment with the Grana score put all patients in categories D (1 case) and E (4 cases). A postoperative assessment after a 2-year follow-up with the Grana score was B in 2 cases and C in 3 cases, indicating satisfactory clinical outcome in 2 cases and unsatisfactory outcome in 3 cases.

## 28.8 Complications

We had no serious postoperative complications related to this surgical procedure. Naturally, we need to pay attention to risks associated with knee arthroscopy: infection, deep venous thrombosis, etc.

One concern with this technique would be the possibility of developing patellofemoral osteoarthritis and avascular osteonecrosis of the patella. The objective of our technique is to obtain desensitization rather than complete denervation of the target, so that the patient does not lose proprioception. This could explain why the patient develops no neurogenic arthropathy that leads to patellofemoral osteoarthritis. Moreover, no radiologic changes in patellofemoral tracking or signs of patellar avascular necrosis were observed during follow-up.

In all cases, we have observed quadriceps atrophy after arthroscopic patellar denervation procedure. This muscle atrophy should be interpreted as a side effect of the denervation or desensitization caused by the technique. In no case did we consider the muscle atrophy, which was mild or moderate in most of the patients, to have caused a slowing or worsening of the patient evolution. In the younger patients, muscle volume and strength recovered easily with an exercise program and specific physical therapy exercises.

## 28.9 Conclusions

Arthroscopic patellar denervation has shown promising clinical results in the treatment of young patients with AKP, with or without minimal malalignment recalcitrant to conservative treatment. The substantial benefits, the considerable comfort for the patient, minimal risk, and low rates of morbidity made this technique a comfortable procedure for the patient. Therefore, arthroscopic patellar denervation might be a reasonable first surgical step in patients with AKP resistant to conservative therapy. Moreover, arthroscopic patellar denervation might become a beneficial addition to other surgical methods for treating AKP.

Moreover, the knee joint can be explored during arthroscopic procedure in order to evaluate the presence of possible causes of AKP not observed in previous complementary studies (plicae formations and cartilage lesions in the femoropatellar joint). A further advantage of the arthroscopic patellar denervation is the fact that it does not interfere with the knee kinetics and allows future surgical techniques to be performed if necessary. Finally, arthroscopic patellar denervation is a simple procedure that could be performed by surgeons with little experience in knee arthroscopy. However, before recommending this treatment method for general use, the results from randomized studies with more patients are needed.

## References


1. Biedert RM, Sanchis-Alfonso V. Sources of anterior knee pain. *Clin Sports Med.* 2002;21(3):335-347.
2. Baudet B, Durroux R, Gay R, et al. Patellar innervation. Surgical consequences. *Rev Chir Orthop Reparatrice Appar Mot.* 1982;68(Suppl 2):104-106.
3. Fontaine C. Innervation of the patella. *Acta Orthop Belg.* 1983;49(4):425-436.
4. Grana WA, Hinkley B, Hollingsworth S. Arthroscopic evaluation and treatment of patellar malalignment. *Clin Orthop Relat Res.* 1984;186:122-128.
5. Kanpolat Y, Savas A, Bekar A, et al. Percutaneous controlled radiofrequency trigeminal rhizotomy for the treatment of idiopathic trigeminal neuralgia: 25-year experience with 1600 patients. *Neurosurgery.* 2001;48:524-532.
6. Kujala UM, Jaakkola LH, Koskinen SK, et al. Scoring of the patellofemoral disorders. *Arthroscopy.* 1993;9:159-163.
7. Maralcan G, Kuru I, Issi S, et al. The innervation of patella: anatomical and clinical study. *Surg Radiol Anat.* 2005;27: 331-335.
8. Moller BN, Helming O. Patellar pain treated by neurotomy. *Arch Orthop Trauma Surg.* 1984;103:137-139.
9. Sanchis-Alfonso V, Roselló-Sastre E, Monteagudo-Castro C, et al. Quantitative analysis of nerve changes in the lateral retinaculum in patients with isolated symptomatic patellofemoral malalignment. A preliminary study. *Am J Sports Med.* 1998;26:703-709.
10. Sanchis-Alfonso V, Roselló-Sastre E. Immunohistochemical analysis for neural markers of the lateral retinaculum in patients with isolated symptomatic patellofemoral malalignment. A neuroanatomic basis for anterior knee pain in the active young patient. *Am J Sports Med.* 2000;28:725-731.
11. Sanchis-Alfonso V, Roselló-Sastre E. Anterior knee pain in the young patient – what causes the pain? "Neural model". *Acta Orthop Scand.* 2003;74(6):697-703.
12. Tzaan WC, Tasker RR. Percutaneous radiofrequency facet rhizotomy – experience with 118 procedures and reappraisal of its value. *Can J Neurol Sci.* 2000;27:125-130.
13. Vega J. Dénervation rotulienne arthroscopique pour le traitement de la douleur fémoro-patellaire. Étude anatomique. 1ère résultats cliniques. Paris: Diplôme InterUniversitaire d'Arthroscopie; 2003.
14. Vega J, Golanó P, Pérez-Carro L. Electrosurgical arthroscopic patellar denervation. *Arthroscopy.* 2006;22(9):1028.e1-1028.e3.
15. Vega J, Palacín A, Maculé F, et al. Localización de los receptores de dolor en el tejido blando perirrotuliano. Estudio inmunohistoquímico. *Cuad Artroscopia.* 2008;15(35):8-13.
16. Vega J, Marimón J, Golanó P, et al. Dolor fémoro-rotuliano. Tratamiento mediante denervación rotuliana artroscópica. *Rev Ortop Traumatol.* 2008;52:290-294.
17. Weinstein LP, Berger RA. Analgesic benefit, functional outcome, and patient satisfaction after partial wrist denervation. *J Hand Surg Am.* 2002;27:833-839.
18. Wojtys EM, Beaman DN, Glover RA, et al. Innervation of the human knee joint by substance-P fibers. *Arthroscopy.* 1990;6(4):254-263.

# Reconstruction of the Medial Patellofemoral Ligament: How I Do It

# 29

Eric W. Edmonds and Donald C. Fithian

## 29.1 Introduction

Reconstruction of the medial patellofemoral ligament (MPFL) has been described utilizing a myriad of fixation techniques. We have elected to utilize a technique that secures the graft to the femur with an interference screw and secures the graft to the patella by suturing it to itself after threading it through bone tunnels. This allows for easy tensioning of the graft while not sacrificing fixation.

## 29.2 Indications

Recurrent episodic patellofemoral instability is the primary indication for MPFL reconstruction. It is indicated for patients with at least two documented patellar dislocations and a physical examination demonstrating excessive lateral patellar motion. Examination must demonstrate excessive laxity of the medial retinacular ligaments and is evaluated by applying lateral and medial forces (about 5 lb) to the patella with the knee in 30° of flexion. In this position of flexion, in normal knees, the patella sits close to the center of the femoral groove. Increased laxity is signified by >2 quadrants of translation, or >10 mm lateral translation from the resting position. Examination under anesthesia may be necessary to accomplish this task.

E.W. Edmonds (✉)
Department of Orthopaedic Surgery, University of California, San Diego, CA, USA

Pediatric Orthopaedic and Scoliosis Center, Rady Children's Hospital San Diego, San Diego, CA, USA
e-mail: ericwedmonds@yahoo.com

## 29.3 Contraindications

Randomized studies have shown no significant benefit of surgery for first-time patellar dislocation, unless there is a loose body secondary to patella instability.[1,2] Furthermore, trochlear dysplasia (prominent or flat trochlea) may call for additional procedures to reduce joint forces, offload cartilage defects, and/or enhance patellar stability. A complete examination should evaluate the patient for associated injuries and rule out other potential causes of sudden knee pain and giving way. ACL injuries, meniscal tears, cartilage flap tears and defects, degenerative joint disease, and plica are just a few pathologies that have been mistaken for patellar instability.

## 29.4 Surgical Technique Step by Step

### *29.4.1 Positioning and EUA*

The patient is positioned supine on a standard table. A sterile bump can be placed under the knee to keep the knee slightly flexed. If a diagnostic arthroscopy is performed before MPFL reconstruction, then the limb is placed in a low profile adjustable leg holder to adjust knee flexion during the procedure. Exam under anesthesia should always be performed during positioning to confirm excessive lateral patellar mobility. This is defined as an absent checkrein sign, >2 quadrants lateral excursion, or >10 mm lateral excursion at 30° of flexion.

It is often advantageous to use image intensifier to confirm the femoral attachment sight of the MPFL radiographically and therefore patient positioning should consider convenient placement of the image intensifier.

V. Sanchis-Alfonso (ed.), *Anterior Knee Pain and Patellar Instability*,
DOI: 10.1007/978-0-85729-507-1_29, © Springer-Verlag London Limited 2011

### 29.4.2 Diagnostic Arthroscopy

Arthroscopy is used to address articular lesions and stage degenerative changes. Standard anterolateral and anteromedial portals are used. If necessary, a superolateral portal is used to facilitate additional viewing of the patellar articular surface and passive patellar tracking and mobility. At this time, the patellofemoral compartment is assessed for the severity of articular cartilage injury and the presence of degenerative changes. Unstable cartilage flaps are debrided and loose bodies addressed.

### 29.4.3 Graft Harvest

Having confirmed that the medial retinacular structures are incompetent by examination, the next step following arthroscopy is harvesting the semitendinosis autograft. Utilizing bony landmarks, the pes anserine is identified and a longitudinal incision is made in the skin of approximately 2.5 cm using a #15 blade scalpel (Fig. 29.1). Dissection is carried down to the sartorius fascia and a blunt finger sweep is performed to expose the fascia and help identify the location of the underlying gracilis and semitendinosis tendons. An incision in line with the semitendinosis is then made through the sartorius fascia to gain access to the semitendinosis tendon. Only the semitendinosis is harvested as the graft should be 240 mm to make a 120 mm-doubled graft and the gracilis is often of insufficient length.

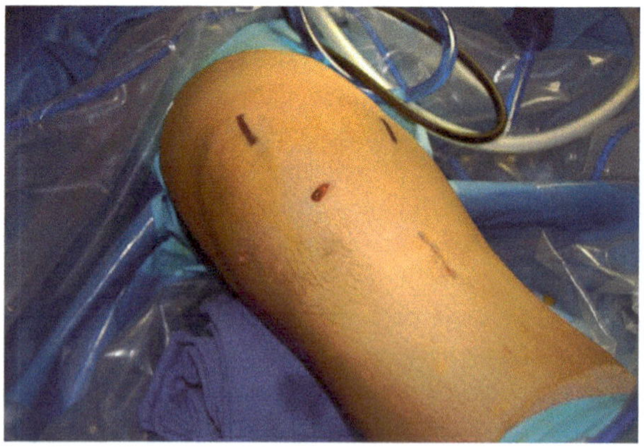

**Fig. 29.1** Intraoperative photograph demonstrating standard incisions for MPFL reconstruction, including: two anterior parapatellar arthroscopy portals, tibial incision for hamstring autograft harvest, medial patella incision, and medial distal femur incision

The semitendinosis is harvested using a closed tendon stripper after detaching the distal end from the tibia, securing the graft using 0 vicryl suture, and freeing the tendon from its fascial attachment to the medial gastrocnemius. The graft is taken to the back-table and debrided of remaining muscular tissue. The proximal end is then secured and tubularized in a similar fashion to the distal end. The graft is then doubled over and that end is whip-stitched for 20–25 mm with 0 vicryl to tubularize the graft, which is then left on the back table in a saline-soaked sponge.

### 29.4.4 Patella Exposure

A 2.5 cm incision is then made over the medial one third of the patella. The deep bursal layer is incised to expose the longitudinal fibers (layer 1) of the extensor retinaculum. The medial third of the patella, from the medial border of the patellar tendon to the insertion of the MPFL, is exposed subperiosteally. This dissection is best carried out with a sharp #15 scalpel. Care should be taken to remain subperiosteal as you turn the corner at the medial border of the patella. Continue the dissection through the MPFL fibers (layer 2), which can be identified as they course horizontally into the proximal medial two thirds of the patella. The dissection should remain extra-articular. The layer deep to the MPFL is layer 3, which is the joint capsule. After the MPFL is released, blunt dissection with a long clamp is used to develop a plane medially between the MPFL and the capsular layer.

These horizontal fibers of the MPFL are about 1-cm wide and run at a right angle to the longitudinal fibers of layer 1. This is an extra-articular plane between the medial retinaculum superficially and the joint capsule on the deep surface. The vastus medialis obliquus (VMO) tendon lies superficially. The tunnel for the MPFL graft will be placed at this level.

The plane of soft tissue dissection through the retinaculum is important. The key is to avoid dissecting too deeply into the joint, because passing the graft through the joint space is nonanatomic, can interfere with healing, and may cause joint abrasion or mechanical abrasion to the graft as it passes over the medial femur during motion and activity. It is best to dissect between layers 2 and 3. This is an easy plane to develop and allows reapproximation of the native MPFL over the graft during closure. Also acceptable is a tunnel superficial to the MPFL, between layers 1 and 2. However, the superficial surface of the MPFL is adherent to the overlying VMO insertion and layer 1, so this plane is more difficult to develop than the deeper interval.

### 29.4.5 Patella Bone Tunnels

After approaching the patella, bone tunnels in the anterior medial patella are created. Using a 3.2 or 4.5 mm drill bit, depending on graft thickness, two bone tunnels are made in the proximal half of the patella. Start by creating two anterior holes placed 5–7 mm from the medial edge of the patella. These holes are drilled approximately 10 mm in depth. Next, two medial holes aiming laterally should connect with holes just created on the anterior surface of the patella (on a right knee, these should correspond with 1 and 3 o'clock). The starting point on the medial edge of the patella for these holes corresponds with the insertion point of the MPFL, again deep to layer 2, deep to the VMO, but superficial to the joint capsule. A small angled curette is used to complete this connection and create the tunnel.

### 29.4.6 Femur Exposure

After the patella bone tunnels are prepared, a second incision 3 cm long is made centered over the medial epicondyle to approach the femoral MPFL origin. After incising the skin and subcutaneous tissue the medial epicondyle is easily palpated and blunt dissection with digital palpation confirms the relative location. The native MPFL originates on the ridge between the adductor tubercle and the medial femoral epicondyle at a point 9 mm proximal and 5 mm posterior to the medial epicondyle. The Bieth pin for the femoral tunnel will be placed at this point.

### 29.4.7 Femoral Tunnel

Placement of the femoral attachment is one of the most critical steps of the operation. The isometry and behavior of the MPFL is far more affected by the femoral insertion site than the patella site. Radiographically, the pin is placed at the junction of Blumensat's line and posterior femoral cortex. If placed at this described clinical and radiographic position, then the isometry of the MPFL should be close to physiologic (as this corresponds to its femoral origin in anatomic dissection). Fine tuning may be required and isometry should be verified by passing a suture through the tissue tunnel created with a clamp between the patellar and femoral incisions. (This same suture will be used as a shuttle to take the graft through the tissue tunnel later). The suture is looped over the femoral Bieth pin and through the patella bone tunnels (Fig. 29.2). The knee is then put through a full range of motion while holding the suture with a hemostat. If the suture tightens as you flex the knee, then keep the first Bieth pin in place and place a second pin slightly distal on the femur. If the suture tightens as you extend the knee, then keep the first Bieth pin in place and place a second pin more proximal on the femur. Recheck isometry to ensure the patella tracks smoothly in the trochlear without excess constraint throughout its range.[3-5]

With the isometric point confirmed, the femoral tunnel can now be drilled over the Bieth pin to a depth

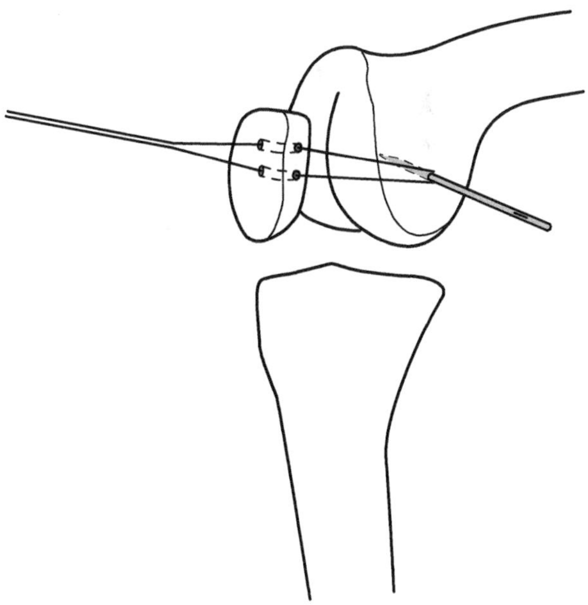

**Fig. 29.2** Line drawing demonstrating assessment of isometric point on femur utilizing Bieth pin and suture passed through patella tunnels

of 25 mm with the appropriate diameter reamer, dependent on the thickness of the doubled part of the graft (usually about 6–7 mm).

### 29.4.8 Graft Placement

Pass the doubled end of graft into the femoral tunnel by pulling the Bieth pin medially and secure it in place with an appropriately sized interference screw (Fig. 29.3). Ensure that the graft does not twist to avoid knotting the tissue on the medial femur. Pass the two free ends of the graft through the soft tissue tunnel created earlier using the shuttle suture (Fig. 29.4). Each limb is passed through a patella bone tunnel, folded over and sewn to itself with nonabsorbable suture (Fig. 29.5). This patella two bone tunnel technique

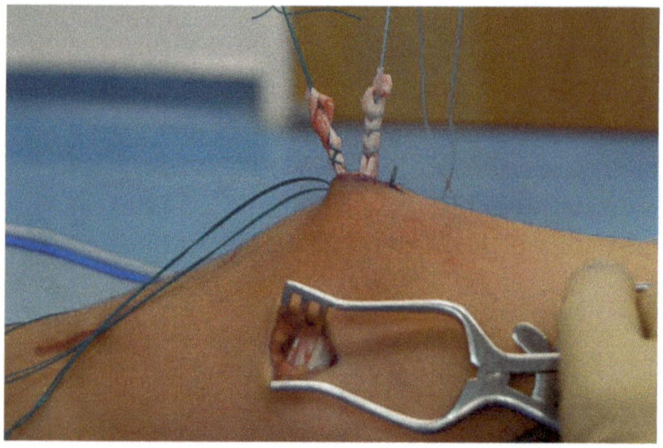

**Fig. 29.4** Intraoperative photograph demonstrating graft in place after passage between two working incisions ready for placement through patellar tunnels and tensioning

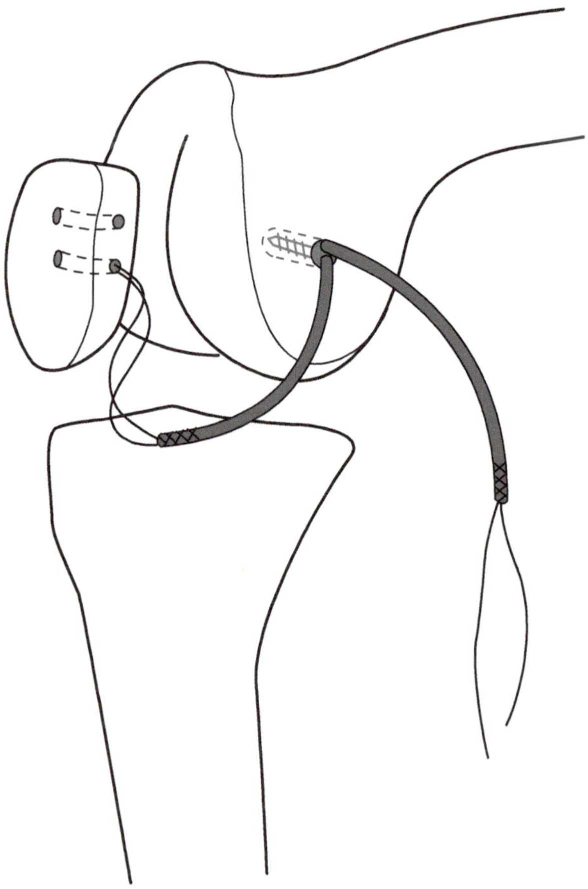

**Fig. 29.3** Line drawing demonstrating placement of graft into femoral tunnel, secured using interference screw

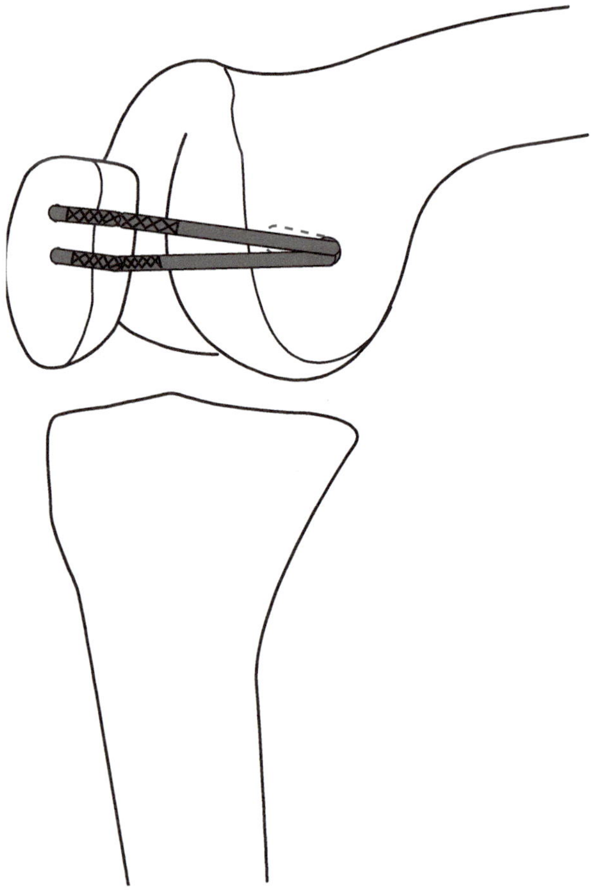

**Fig. 29.5** Line drawing demonstrating secured graft, sutured onto itself, post-tensioning, at the completion of the MPFL reconstruction

allows for titration of patellar constraint fixing the graft at the perfect length that allows no excess slack and no excess tension. Tensioning the graft is one of the most important steps in the procedure and care should be taken to avoid overtensioning the graft while obtaining adequate fixation. The length should be set such that a firm endpoint is felt as the patella is translated laterally preventing dislocation. This is done by confirming normal translation laterally (<10 mm or 2 quadrants) with a firm end point at 30° knee flexion. No tension should be felt before the end point is reached. The patella should smoothly engage the trochlea slightly on its lateral side in early flexion and track without tension throughout its range.

Incision closure is then started by first utilizing Vicryl to repair layers #2 and #1 over the top of the graft and patella. Then, absorbable skin sutures are used to perform a layered closure of the three incisions and the two arthroscopy portals.

## 29.5 Postoperative Management

Outpatient management is the norm for this procedure. A femoral nerve block placed intraoperatively and oral narcotics are used for pain control. A knee range of motion brace is used for 4–6 weeks to prevent falls. Immediate full weight bearing is allowed and gait may be progressed as soon as good muscular control has been established. Physical therapy is needed to restore quadriceps control and range of motion as quickly as possible.

The principles of rehabilitation after MPFL reconstruction are similar to those guiding rehabilitation following other ligamentous reconstructions of the knee, such as anterior cruciate ligament (ACL). The keys are to address pain control, range of motion (ROM), quadriceps strengthening, and proximal lower limb control. Return of full ROM, pain control, and protected weight-bearing are stressed in the early phases of recovery. Progression of strength training and return to functional activities follows lines of evidence regarding graft necrosis, remodeling, and tunnel ingrowth which are most commonly associated with ACL reconstruction. We emphasize early, controlled ROM to reduce pain, prevent scar formation and capsular contractions, and to re-establish full ROM (particularly extension). Proximal control is enhanced by performing nonweight-bearing exercises targeting the hip abductors, external rotators, and extensors. Patients are encouraged to return to their sport or activity once they can achieve satisfactory single limb dynamic control.

## 29.6 Pearls and Pitfalls

A pitfall to this procedure is patient selection. Remember that sudden anterior knee pain with instability is a nonspecific complaint and that this procedure should be done only to reconstruct laxity of the medial retinaculum and MPFL. Examination under anesthesia may be necessary to confirm this laxity.

A pitfall during surgery is a short graft. Inadequate graft length will not allow for proper constraint to be applied to the patella and can lead to overtensioning of the graft and subsequent failure or pain. In these rare cases, when the semitendinosis is too short, the gracilis can be harvested, as well. They are then sewn together at their insertional stumps and the joined end is fashioned as if it were the looped end of a doubled semitendinosis graft. Furthermore, an allograft semitendinosis can be used and should be prepared in the same fashion as the autograft. The pearl for allograft choice is to select a graft of sufficient length, as described.

A pitfall of tunnel placement is to make the bone bridge between the holes too narrow and fracturing the bone tunnels may occur. A pearl, if a fracture occurs, is to then place a more lateral bone tunnel. Alternatively, the graft can be fixed in the patella with an interference screw and careful graft tension applied through a transpatellar suture shuttled laterally on a Bieth pin, or secured using suture anchors if adequate fixation exists in the remaining patella.

A pearl to tunnel placement of the femoral tunnel is that this step is the most critical step of the procedure. The isometric behavior of the MPFL is far more affected by the femoral insertion site than the patella site. The native MPFL sees greatest tension in full knee extension with the quadriceps contracted. The ideal length change behavior, or isometry, for an MPFL graft has not been established. It is probably not necessary that the graft be perfectly isometric, but checking isometry will help the surgeon understand how the graft is behaving during knee motion and also verify that no untoward effect is seen. It is important to ensure that the graft is not overtightened. The graft should have no tension and no slack, acting as a passive constraint just as it does in normal physiology. An objective firm endpoint should be felt as the patella is translated about 7 mm laterally, but no tension should be felt before that point when the knee is flexed 30°.

Excessive tension will lead to early failure, pain, and medial patellar degenerative changes. Excessive laxity will not restore stability to the patella. We fix the graft to the patella with the knee at 30° flexion, with the patella centered passively in the trochlea. Care is taken to remove all slack from the graft, but the graft should be under no tension whatsoever when the patella is centered in the groove.

## 29.7 Complications

As mentioned in the section on "Pitfalls," fracturing of the patella may occur; however, in contrast to procedures that place an interference screw and require full width drilling of the patella, this technique weakens only the medial proximal quadrant of the patella and risk of fracturing is likely less. Besides this specific complication, the standard risks of operative intervention exist such as infection, blood loss, neurologic injury, and anesthetic complications, but all are very minimal risks.

Postoperatively, one of the biggest potential complications is knee stiffness. If the patient has not regained at least 0–90° of knee flexion by postoperative week 6, then the recommendation is to increase the intensity of the physical therapy program. Manipulation under anesthesia to regain that motion by week 9 may be done if the stiffness is not resolved by that time.

## References


1. Andrade A, Thomas N. Randomized comparison of operative vs. nonoperative treatment following first time dislocation. European Society for Sports, Knee and Arthroscopy, Rome. 2002.
2. Nikku R, Nietosvaara Y, Kallio PE, et al. Operative versus closed treatment of primary dislocation of the patella: similar 2-year results in 125 randomized patients. *Acta Orthop Scand.* 1997;68:419-423.
3. Nomura E, Inoue M, Osada N. Anatomical analysis of the medial patellofemoral ligament of the knee, especially at the femoral attachment. *Knee Surg Sports Traumatol Arthrosc.* 2005;13:510-515.
4. Schöttle PB, Schmeling A, Rosenstiel N, et al. Radiographic landmarks for femoral tunnel placement in medial patellofemoral ligament reconstruction. *Am J Sports Med.* 2007; 35:801-804.
5. Steensen RN, Dopirak RM, McDonald WG 3rd. The anatomy and isometry of the medial patellofemoral ligament: implications for reconstruction. *Am J Sports Med.* 2004; 32:1509-1513.

# 30 Reconstruction of the Medial Patellofemoral Ligament: How I Do It

Robert A. Teitge and Roger Torga-Spak

## 30.1 Introduction

The medial patellofemoral ligament (MPFL) has been recognized as the primary stabilizer against lateral patellar dislocation or subluxation.[2,4,5] Consequently if there is lateral patellar instability there is also an insufficient MPFL. Various reconstruction procedures of the MPFL using adductor magnus,[1,10] quadriceps tendon,[8] semitendinosus,[5] gracilis,[2,3] and synthetic tissue[6] have been recently developed.

The technique we postulate follows the same basic principles of all ligament reconstruction: (1) selection of a sufficiently strong and stiff graft, (2) isometric graft placement, (3) correct tension, (4) adequate fixation, and (5) no condylar rubbing or impingement. Adductor longus tendon was used in most of our reconstructions, whereas quadriceps tendon autograft or bone patellar tendon allograft was preferred in cases with trochlear dysplasia based on the concept that a stronger structure is needed to compensate for inadequate support provided by a flat trochlea.

## 30.2 Indications

Reconstruction of the MPFL is a very common procedure in our practice for the treatment of lateral patellar instability. We indicate the isolated reconstruction of the MPFL as the procedure of choice for three different clinical pictures: (1) when no underlying alignment or morphologic abnormality is identified; (2) when many underlying subtle alignment or morphologic abnormalities are identified (i.e., increased femoral anteversion, patella alta, trochlear dysplasia, and genu valgum), but it is not possible to detect which of these deformities contribute the most to the instability; and (3) when one underlying alignment or morphologic abnormality is identified (i.e., increased femoral anteversion or trochlear dysplasia), but the magnitude and the risks of the procedure to correct that deformity outweigh its potential benefits.

## 30.3 Surgical Technique

### *30.3.1 Graft Selection and Harvesting*

The adductor magnus with its insertion just proximal to the medial epicondyle can be conveniently used to reconstruct the MPFL. With the knee in extension a 4- to 6-cm skin incision is performed midway between the medial epicondyle and medial edge of the patella. Dissection is carried through the subcutaneous fat and fascia over the vastus medialis is opened. The vastus medialis is elevated off the intermuscular septum, which is then split longitudinally to expose the adductor tendon (Fig. 30.1). A tendon stripper is used to strip the adductor magnus tendon and a whipstitch (approximately 10 cm long) is placed in the free end. The diameter is then measured by passing it through a sizer, most conveniently a 3.5 or 4.5 drill sleeve.

R. Torga-Spak (✉)
Faculty of Orthopaedics and Traumatology, Department of Surgery, Instituto Universitario CEMIC, Buenos Aires, Argentina
e-mail: rtorgaspak@gmail.com

V. Sanchis-Alfonso (ed.), *Anterior Knee Pain and Patellar Instability*,
DOI: 10.1007/978-0-85729-507-1_30, © Springer-Verlag London Limited 2011

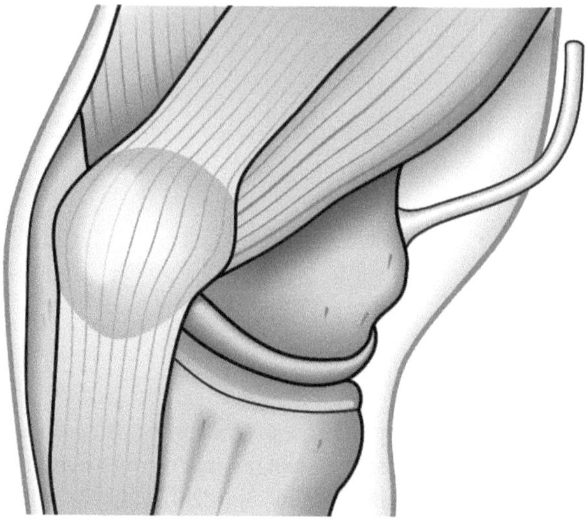

**Fig. 30.1** Harvesting of the adductor magnus tendon

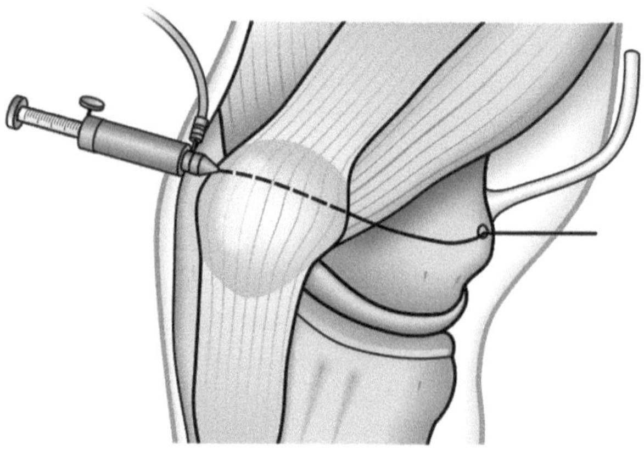

**Fig. 30.2** Location of the isometric point on the medial epicondyle

## 30.3.2 Isometric Location

The graft must be located isometrically to avoid overstretching it to failure during joint motion or overconstraining patellar motion. A transverse 2.5-mm hole is placed through the patella far anteriorly at about the junction of the proximal and mid one-third height. A 1.5-cm incision is made on the lateral side of the patella and a strand of #2 Vicryl is passed through the hole with a small loop tied on the medial aspect to pass over a 2.5-mm Kirschner wire, which is inserted into bone near the medial epicondyle. A pneumatic Isometer (Synthes, Paoli, Pa) is inserted into the hole in the lateral patella and the #2 Vicryl isometric measurement suture is passed through. The knee is placed through a full range of motion while the change in length between the medial epicondylar K-wire and the medial border of the patella is read on the isometer (Fig. 30.2). The string tension is set at 3 lb. Adjustments in the position of the K-wire around the medial epicondyle are made until no excursion is read on the isometer during the full range of knee motion. Once the isometric point is located, a tunnel is drilled from the insertion of the adductor tendon to the isometric measurement point and the graft is pulled through this tunnel. A second tunnel the diameter of the graft is drilled through the patella at the site of the 2.5-mm hole used to measure isometry. The graft is passed deep to the vastus medialis, exiting the tunnel in the medial condyle anteriorly, and then pulled into the patellar tunnel (Fig. 30.3).

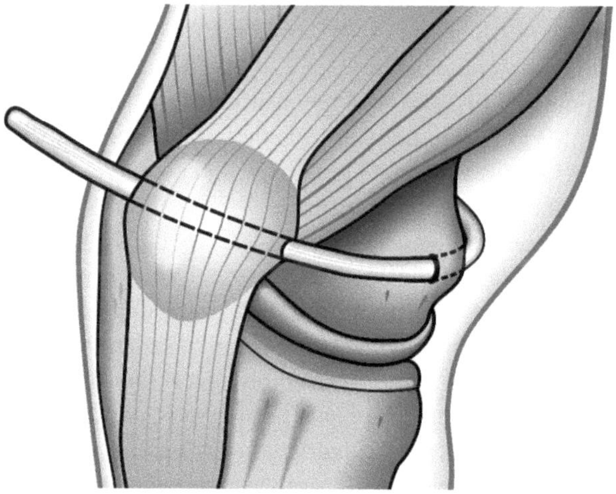

**Fig. 30.3** Graft passing through the tunnel in the medial epicondyle and through the patellar tunnel

## 30.3.3 Correct Tension

The ligament is not a dynamic structure that pulls the patella medially, but rather a static restraint that prevents is from moving too far laterally. The tension set in the graft must be enough to limit lateral excursion to an amount that approximates that of the normal contralateral knee. Tension is set with the knee flexed

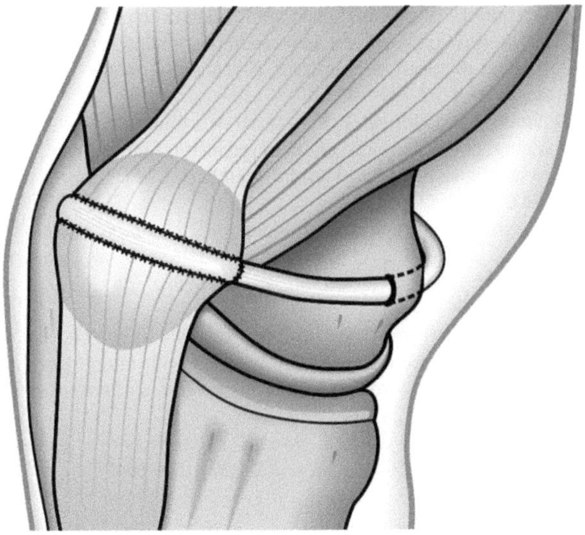

**Fig. 30.4** Graft sutured to the quadriceps expansion on the anterior aspect of the patella

60–90° to hold the patella centered in the trochlea and to avoid risk of pulling it too far medial. Tension should not be set with the knee in extension and the patella outside the trochlea, as no reference exists to determine where it is centered.

### *30.3.4 Secure Fixation*

Tendon through bone tunnel provides the greatest stable fixation, and an adequate bone tunnel can be placed transversely through the patella with 3.5-, 4.5- or 6-mm drills depending on the diameter of the graft. After passing the graft from medial to lateral it is turned superficially onto the anterior surface of the patella where it is sutured to the medial retinaculum where it enters the patella, the lateral retinaculum where it exits, and the quadriceps expansion. If the graft is long enough, extra sutures can be placed from its free end to the medial tendon before it enters the patellar tunnel (Fig. 30.4).

### *30.3.5 Avoid Impingement*

The range of motion must be tested to ensure unrestricted patellar or knee motion. The graft should not rub against the medial femoral condyle. If impingement on the medial femoral condyle wall is detected, the graft can be placed on the anterior surface of the patella and pulled into the lateral tunnel in a medial direction.

## 30.4 Postoperative Management

Postoperative treatment includes full range of motion, full weight bearing, continuous passive motion, and active exercises, with avoidance of stairs, squatting, and resistive leg extension until the tendon has healed into the tunnel. A knee brace in extension is used for ambulation during the first 3–6 weeks to protect against falling due to quadriceps inhibition

## 30.5 Our Experience

Reconstruction of the MPFL has been performed in our institution since 1982 in more than 300 patients. We have recently evaluated the clinical results of MPFL reconstruction in 34 patients with chronic patellar instability and trochlear dysplasia.[9] Patients were followed for a mean 66.5 months. There were 85.3% and 91.1% good and excellent results based on Kujala and Lysholm scores, respectively. No recurrent dislocations have occurred.

## 30.6 Complications

Patellar fracture at the transverse stress riser has occurred in the early postoperative period as a result of falling onto the flexed knee in a couple of patients. Another patient had graft advancement after loosening in a high-speed motor vehicle accident 5 months after reconstruction. Although we check isometry routinely, in a few patients the graft was found to be too tight in flexion in the early postoperative period. These patients complained of tension and pain in the medial aspect of the knee and improved immediately after arthroscopic release of the graft.

## References


1. Avikainen VJ, Nikku RK, Seppanen-Lehmonen TK. Adductor magnus tenodesis for patellar dislocation. Technique and preliminary results. *Clin Orthop Relat Res*. 1993;297:12-16.
2. Conlan T, Garth WP Jr, Lemons JE. Evaluation of the medial soft-tissue restraints of the extensor mechanism of the knee. *J Bone Joint Surg Am*. 1993;75:682-693.
3. Christiansen SE, Jacobsen BW, Lund B, et al. Reconstruction of the medial patellofemoral ligament with gracilis tendon autograft in transverse patellar drill holes. *Arthroscopy*. 2008;24:82-87.
4. Desio SM, Burks RT, Bachus KN. Soft tissue restraints to lateral patellar translation in the human knee. *Am J Sports Med*. 1998;26:59-65.
5. Hautamaa PV, Fithian DC, Kaufman KR, et al. Medial soft tissue restraints in lateral patellar instability and repair. *Clin Orthop Relat Res*. 1998;349:174-182.
6. Nomura E, Inoue M. Hybrid medial patellofemoral ligament reconstruction using the semitendinous tendon for recurrent patellar dislocation: minimum 3 years' follow-up. *Arthroscopy*. 2006;22:787-793.
7. Nomura E, Horiuchi Y, Kihara M. A mid-term follow-up of medial patellofemoral ligament reconstruction using an artificial ligament for recurrent patellar dislocation. *Knee*. 2000;7:211-215.
8. Steensen RN, Dopirak RM, Maurus PB. A simple technique for reconstruction of the medial patellofemoral ligament using a quadriceps tendon graft. *Arthroscopy*. 2005;21:365-370.
9. Steiner TM, Torga-Spak R, Teitge RA. Medial patellofemoral ligament reconstruction in patients with lateral patellar instability and trochlear dysplasia. *Am J Sports Med*. 2006;34:1254-1261.
10. Teitge R, Torga-Spak R. Medial patellofemoral ligament reconstruction. *Orthopedics*. 2004;27:1037-1040.

# MPFL Reconstruction: Principles and Complications

# 31

Pieter J. Erasmus and Mathieu Thaunat

## 31.1 Introduction

Similar to other ligamentous reconstructions around the knee, medial patellofemoral ligament (MPFL) reconstructions can lead to complications. These complications relate to a lack of understanding of the biomechanics of the MPFL ligament and technical errors made during the reconstruction.

## 31.2 Biomechanics of the MPFL

The MPFL should be seen as a checkrein in preventing abnormal lateral movement of the patella, at and near full extension; it is not suppose to pull the patella medially and is of no importance once the patella has engaged the trochlea.[14]

In the literature, on reconstruction of the MPFL, most authors suggest that the reconstructed ligament should be isometric. So-called isometric points[25,27] for the reconstruction have been suggested. However in measurements of the normal length changes in the MPFL it has repeatedly been shown to be a nonisometric ligament.[9,25,29] According to Steensen there is a 5.4 mm length change from 0° to 90° of flexion and an average of 7.2 mm length change from 0° to 120°. It is important to realize that the MPFL is a nonisometric ligament that is at its tightest at full extension and becomes more lax with flexion, as the patella engages into the trochlea.[14] Victor[33] confirmed the nonisometry of the MPFL and has suggested that there is a difference in the nonisometry of the proximal and distal fibres of the MPFL; the proximal fibres are at their tightest at full extension and the distal at 30° of flexion. In cadaveric studies it was shown that an anatomic, nonisometric, MPFL reconstruction will restore patella kinematics better than an isometric reconstruction.[22]The position of the reconstructed ligament on the patella has very little effect on the isometry of the ligament. In contrast the position on the femur has a major effect on the isometry of the ligament.[27] A more distal position increases tightness in extension and laxity in flexion; conversely a more proximal position results in a graft that is lax in extension and tight in flexion (Fig. 31.1).

In nearly all patella dislocations there are underlying causes like patella alta, trochlear dysplasia, ligamentous hyperlaxity, etc., that predisposes the patient to a patella dislocation. Patella alta seems to be the most constant predisposing factor in patella dislocations.[15] Patella height has an influence on the isometry of the MPFL, the higher the patella the bigger the nonisometry of the ligament. In unpublished cadaveric experiments we found that the average length changes in the MPFL from 0° to 90° was 4 mm. If the tibial tubercle was moved 10 mm proximally the average length change increased to 6 mm. When the tubercle was moved 10 mm distally the average length change decreased to 3 mm.[11] Considering this, it would be important to know the distance from the origin of the MPFL, at the medial epicondyle to its insertion on the patella, when the quads are fully contracted. The other important factor is the height of the patella in relation to the proximal sulcus. The so-called J-sign is seen[16] when near full extension the patella moves out of the trochlea and subluxes laterally. This subluxation can be caused by a short proximal

P.J. Erasmus (✉)
University of Stellenbosch, Mediclinic, Die Boord, Stellenbosch, South Africa
e-mail: pieter@orthoclinic.co.za

V. Sanchis-Alfonso (ed.), *Anterior Knee Pain and Patellar Instability*,
DOI: 10.1007/978-0-85729-507-1_31, © Springer-Verlag London Limited 2011

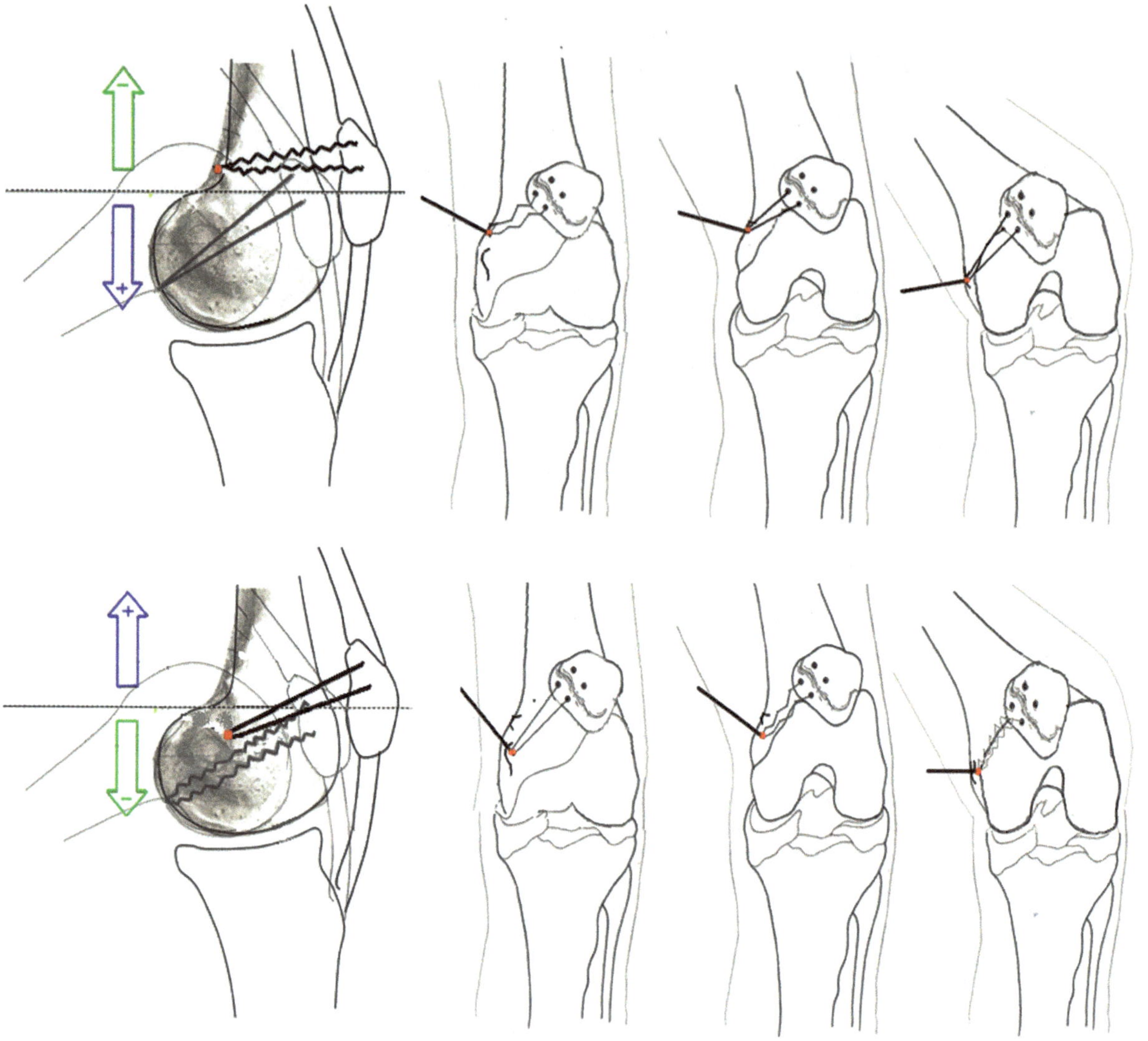

**Fig. 31.1** A proximal position on the femur will result in a graft that is loose in extension and tight in flexion. Conversely a distal femoral position will result in a graft that is tight in extension and loose in flexion

trochlea or a high patella or both. At present there is no specific imaging technique to measure the length of the MPFL. The most commonly used measurements for the patella height like, Caton-Deschamps, Blackburne-Peel, and Insall-Salvati measure patella height in relation to the tibia. However, what is more important is the height of the patella in relation to the superior border of the trochlea as suggested by Bernageau and Goutallier[3] on X-rays and Biedert on MRIs.[1,4] Patella alta is associated with a long patella tendon and patella tendon length is more sensitive than Caton-Deschamps index for patella instability.[21]

In reconstructing the ligament the aim should be to use a ligament that is stronger than the original to compensate for the underlying predisposing factors which are not corrected. The reconstructed ligament should duplicate the nonisometry. The aim of the reconstruction should be to create a "favorable anisometry"[29] that duplicates that of the original ligament before injury. Failure to create favorable nonisometry can lead to redislocation, extensor lag, and loss of flexion. Loss of flexion will also lead to overload of the patella femoral joint especially of the medial facet in flexion.

## 31.3 Complications

### 31.3.1 Loss of Motion

In a long-term follow-up in our series of more than 200 MPFL reconstructions, done from 1995 till 2008, extensor lag with full passive extension and no loss of flexion was the most common complication. There was no long-term loss of flexion. Notwithstanding slight loss of active extension these patients still had an average Kujala score of 92.7 (72–100). Smith et al.[26] did a comprehensive literature research on the clinical and radiological results of MPFL reconstructions. They could only find eight papers, involving 186 MPFL reconstructions, meeting the criteria of their scoring system. In only two of these eight papers did the authors report on the postoperative range of motion and both reported on loss of flexion compared to the nonoperated leg. None reported on loss of active knee extension or extensor lag. Only one paper in this review reported on quadriceps atrophy. In this series there was an incidence of 60% quads atrophy notwithstanding a mean Kujala score of 88.6.[7] Loss of motion after an MPFL reconstruction is directly related to the tension in the reconstructed ligament. If it is too tight in extension (femoral insertion too distal) there will be an extensor lag although passive full extension will not be affected. If it is too tight in flexion (femoral insertion too proximal) there will be loss of flexion both passive and active; in this situation the patella might still be unstable in extension (Fig. 31.1).

Both the gracilis and semitendinosis tendons, generally used for reconstructing the MPFL, are stronger and stiffer than the original MPFL.[18]The strength is a positive factor considering that the underlying predisposing factors leading to the first dislocation are not corrected. The excessive stiffness however can theoretically lead to overload in the patellofemoral joint especially in cases where the reconstructed MPFL is not in the optimal position.

In our technique of MPFL reconstruction we try to recreate the normal nonisometry of the ligament, so-called favorable anisometry.[29] This creates a ligament that is tight in extension and lax in flexion. There is however the danger that the ligament can be too tight in extension resulting in an extensor lag. Postoperative quadriceps inhibition is very common and should be distinguished from a permanent extensor lag as a result of an overtight MPFL reconstruction. At 3 months postoperative follow-up there was on average a 4° (5–15°) extensor lag, probably as a result of quads inhibition, in 45% of our patients. This extensor lag was temporary and over the long term only 4 out of the more than 200 cases had permanent loss of active full extension caused by an overtight reconstruction in extension.[31]

Elias[8] has shown experimentally that a too proximally placed femoral position for the MPLF graft will lead to increased patellofemoral load with potential overload of the articular surface in the patellofemoral joint. Loss of both active and passive flexion will also be associated with this. In techniques where the aim is to have an isometric reconstructed MPFL, the danger of having a ligament that is too tight in flexion is increased. Femoral insertions near or at the adductor tubercle, although advocated by some authors, should be avoided as this will lead to a reconstruction that is too tight in flexion and too loose in extension.[23,25,27]

In prevention of motion loss complications, special attention should be given to the technique of determining the tension in the reconstructed ligament. Too much tension in the reconstructed ligament would be more detrimental, considering possible loss of motion and late patellofemoral degeneration, than too little tension. Beck showed[2] that even when applying low loads to MPFL reconstructions, it is still possible to re-establish normal translation and patellofemoral contact pressures. The aim of the MPFL reconstruction should be to restore the tension in the MPFL to the same tension that it had before being torn, with a graft that is stronger than the original ligament. If the patella of the opposite knee is stable the amount of transverse patella movement in the reconstructed patella should be similar to that of the uninjured knee. This can be achieved intraoperatively by draping both knees and comparing the amount of transverse movement. Fithian[12] advises adjusting the graft tension in such a way that a 5 lb displacing force results in 7–9 mm of lateral displacement of the patella. We recommend that the isometry of the ligament should be tested till the "favorable anisometric point" is found by using a guide pin in the proposed femoral implantation site. The "favorable anisometric point" would be a point where the reconstructed ligament will be tight in extension and lax in flexion, with a length change of about 5 mm between extension and flexion. This can be achieved, with the knee in full extension, by pulling proximally on the patella with a bone hook in the direction of the anterior superior iliac spine. In this situation the reconstructed ligament should be tight but the tension in the reconstructed ligament should be less than in the patellar tendon. This will ensure that, with maximum quads contraction, there will be more tension in the patellar tendon than in the reconstructed MPFL (Fig. 31.2). In cases of severe patella alta a distal tibial tubercle transfer should be considered as this will decrease the nonisometry of the reconstruction, allowing easier and more precise tensioning of the reconstructed ligament[11] (Fig. 31.3). We will consider a distal tubercle transfer when the Bernageau measurement is more than 8 mm or the patella tendon length is more than 60 mm, especially if this is combined with a clinically marked positive J-Sign.[16] A distal transfer of as little as 6 mm is usually adequate in these cases. Other authors have recommended different techniques for tensioning the reconstructed MPFL, the most popular being to tension the ligament between 30° and 60° of flexion when the patella is already centered in the trochlea.[5,6,20] The major length changes in the MPFL happens after 30° of flexion[25,29] and considering this, tensioning the ligament in early flexion should prevent overtensioning provided that the correct nonisometric point has been selected on the femur.

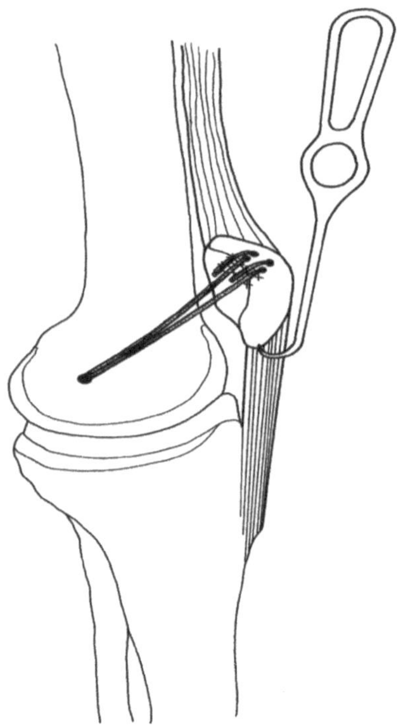

**Fig. 31.2** Tensioning the MPFL graft in full extension ensuring that the tension in the reconstruction is less than in the patellar tendon

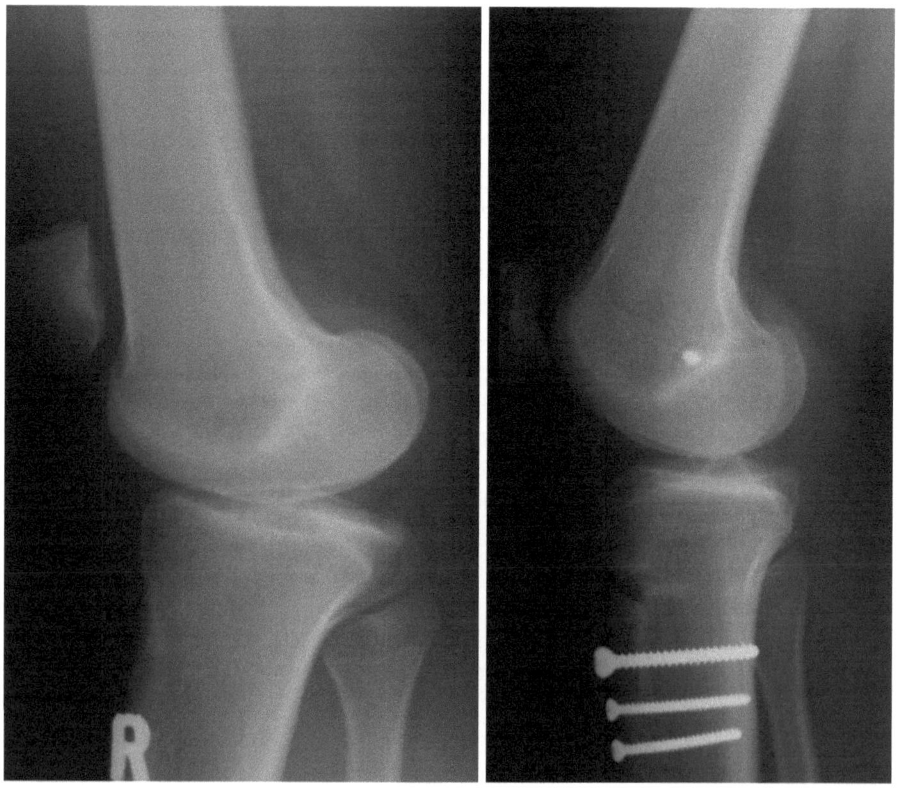

**Fig. 31.3** Distalization of the tibial tubercle combined with a MPFL reconstruction

Postoperative quadriceps inhibition, although temporary, can result in an increased rehabilitation period and a late return to sporting activities. Drez[7] reported quadriceps atrophy in more than 50% of his patients at an average follow-up of 31.5 months (24–43). In an effort to combat this we start our patients on an isometric quads contraction program preoperatively. Postoperatively no braces are used and immediate active and passive full range of motion is encouraged. Isometric quadriceps exercises are continued. Full weight bearing, with the support of one or two crutches, as necessary, is allowed. In a follow-up of 22 consecutive MPFL reconstructions at an average of 29 months (8–65) we found the average side to side difference in upper leg circumference,15 cm above the knee, to be only 0.19 cm (0–1.5 cm).[11]

Should loss of motion persist for longer than 9 months after an MPFL reconstruction, we would recommend a percutaneous sequential fish scale type of tenotomy, near the implantation of the ligament on the patella, till full range of motion is restored.[31]

### 31.3.2 Fractures

In our series we had only three redislocations, all associated with fractures of the medial rim of the patella.[30] In all these patients the fracture occurred with a definitive injury; in two this happened in contact sport, one in soccer and the other in rugby football. The third patient sustained a redislocation when she fell off a chair trying to replace a fused light bulb. The fractures occurred respectively 2, 5, and 10 years after the initial surgery. In our reconstructing technique two 3–3.5 mm drill holes, 10 mm apart, are made on the medial edge of the patella exiting the anterior cortex approximately 6–8 mm from the medial edge. These fractures were similar to that seen in acute primary patella dislocations.[32] A gracilis autograft was used for reconstructing the ligament. This reconstructed ligament is stronger than the original MPFL and as the underlying predisposing factors have not been addressed, there will at times, be high strain on the ligament. The drill holes in the patella can act as stress raisers resulting in fractures. In all three cases the fracture involved not more than 1 cm of the medial patella. The fractures were reduced and fixed with screws all resulting in a stable patella with no longstanding sequel from the fractures.

Mikashima et al.[17] reported two fractures in 12 knees. A single transverse drill hole of 4.5 mm was made from medial to lateral through the patella. These fractures all occurred within 6 weeks from the surgery resulting in a nearly 16% incidence of fractures. Both Christiansen et al.[5] using two 4.5 mm and Gomes et al.[13] using a single 7 mm transverse drill hole reported on nontraumatic patella fractures. It is possible that too large drill holes increase the possibility of a fracture especially when they transverse the patella. Fractures of the medial rim of the patella usually do not involve the articular surface of the patella as long as they do not exit too centrally on the patella and are relatively easy to treat (Fig. 31.4). However, if this drill hole exits too far laterally it can also result in a more

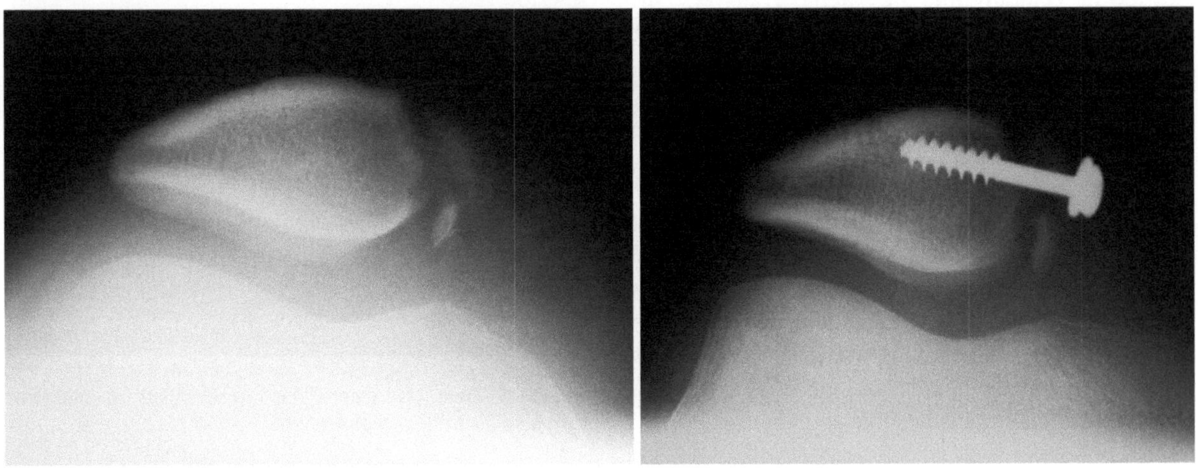

**Fig. 31.4** Redislocation after MPFL reconstruction with a fracture of the medial rim reattached with a screw and washer

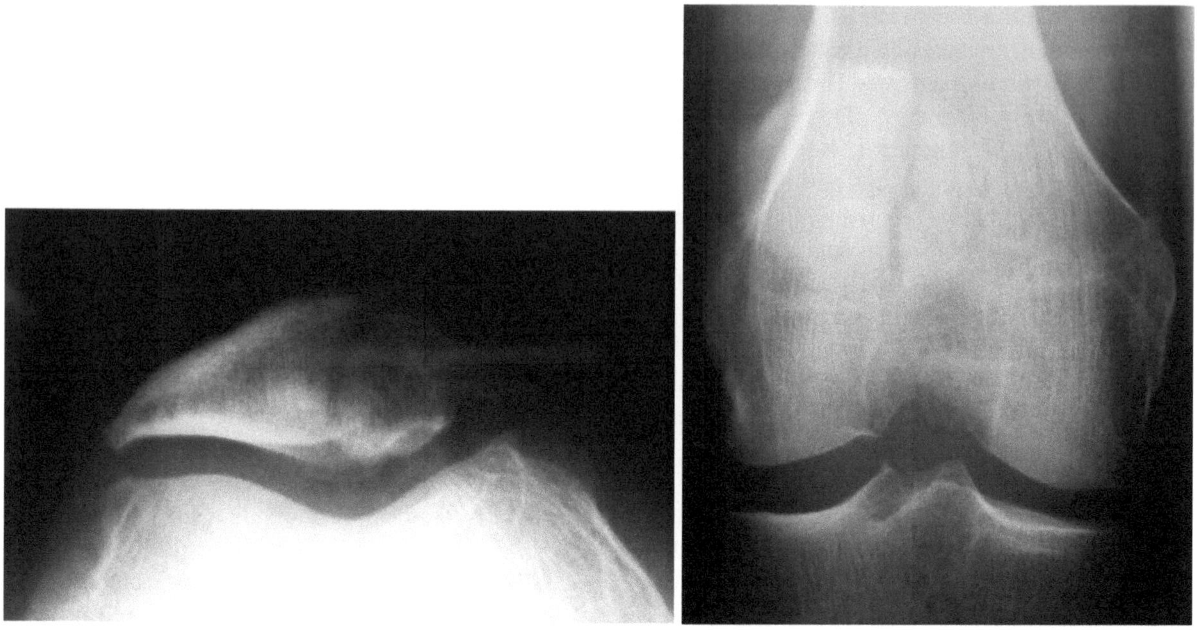

Fig. 31.5 Central patella fracture secondary to drill hole that exit too centrally on the patella

serious fracture (Fig. 31.5). In contrast transverse fractures, as a result of transverse drill holes will always involve the articular surface of the patella and in most cases are associated with fragmentation of the anterior cortex which makes it more serious and difficult to treat (Fig. 31.6). It can be expected that drill holes in the patella will act as stress raisers and might therefore predispose to fractures. Keeping this in mind the size and position of the drill holes should be carefully considered. Holes larger than 3.5 mm should probably be avoided. Drill holes through the medial rim should not exit too far centrally into the patella. Transverse drill holes through the patella will result in more serious fractures than drill holes through the medial rim.

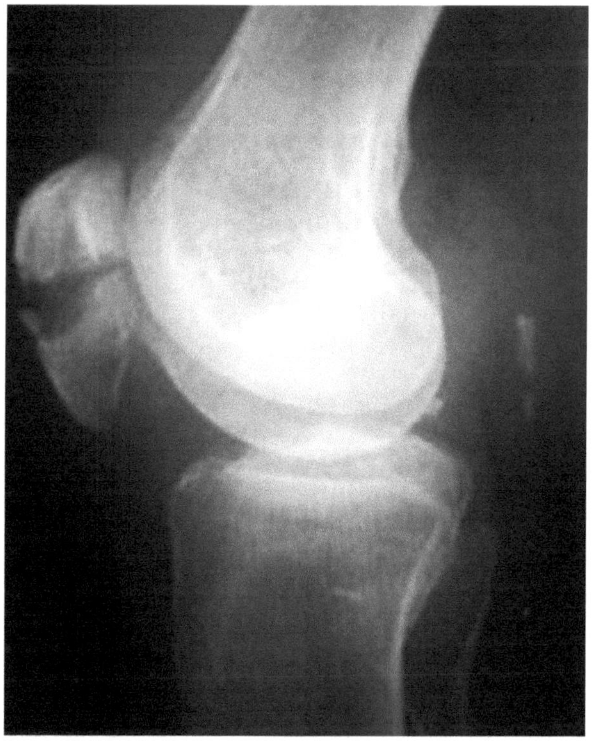

Fig. 31.6 Transverse patella fracture secondary to transverse drill hole for MPFL reconstruction

### 31.3.3 Redislocations

Redislocations are rare; in the literature it varies between 0% and 4%.[5,7,24] In our series there were only three redislocations (1.5%) all associated with a fracture of the medial rim of the patella. In Smith et al.'s[26] review article there were only two post-reconstruction patella dislocations or subluxations in 186 knees; in five patients there was a positive apprehension sign.

### 31.3.4 Localized Tenderness

Localized tenderness in the region of the medial epicondyle related to either the graft or the internal fixation used, can be an irritating complication. Nomura and Inoue[19] reported an incidence of 40% as a result of using a staple for fixation just distal to the adductor tubercle. Christiansen et al.[5] reported 50% tenderness over the medial epicondyle. Steiner et al.[28] had to remove irritating screws in 10% of his patients. We[11] use a deep seated bone anchor on the medial femur and had a 6% incidence of mild localized tenderness at the exit of the graft; no surgical intervention was required.

### 31.3.5 Patellofemoral Degeneration

In an average 7 (4.4–9.3) year follow-up of our first 29 patients[10] the Tegner (5.8), Lysholm (88.5), and IKDC (81) scores were statistically unchanged at 3, 5, and 7 years follow-up. Patellofemoral cartilage damage at the time of the MPFL reconstruction had a negative effect on the Lysholm score but no effect on the Tegner and IKDC scores. In a separate 29 (8–54) month follow-up study of 22 consecutive MPFL reconstructions[9] there was no statistical correlation between the Kujala score, trochlea dysplasia, and Caton Deschamps index. In this group of 22 patients there was a weak correlation between a lower score; a longer patella tendon and a higher patella, measured according to the Bernageau technique. There was however a statistically significant correlation between patellofemoral degeneration at the time of the reconstruction and a low Kujala score. It does seem that development of patellofemoral degeneration can be prevented by an isolated MPFL reconstruction. The effect on patellofemoral degeneration present at the time of the reconstruction is unclear. Nomura, in a 12 year follow-up, reported similar results.[20]

## 31.4 Summary

Medial patellofemoral ligament (MPFL) reconstructions have good results with few complications notwithstanding varied techniques used. Biomechanical and technical principles should be adhered to in preventing complications. The reconstructed MPFL should be tight in extension and lax in flexion. In cases of severe patella alta, a distalization of the tibial tubercle should be considered. With maximum quadriceps contraction the tension in the patellar tendon should be more than the tension in the reconstructed ligament. Drill holes in the patella should be through the medial rim preferably not exceeding 3.5 mm in diameter. Prominence of the reconstructed graft or fixation material over the medial condyle will lead to localized tenderness and is easily avoided by using nonprominent fixation devices. There seems to be no progression in patellofemoral degeneration after MPFL reconstructions, in follow-up periods of 7–12 years.

## References


1. Barnett A, Prentice M, Mandalia V. The patellotrochlear index: a more clinically relevant measurement of patella height? *J Bone Joint Surg*. 2009;91-B:413.
2. Beck P, Brown NA, Greis PE, et al. Patellofemoral contact pressures and lateral patellar translation after medial patellofemoral ligament reconstruction. *Am J Sports Med*. 2007;35:1557-1563.
3. Bernageau J, Goutallier D. Exam radiologique de l'articulationfemorale-patellaire.L'actualiterhumatologique. Paris Expansion Scientifique Francaise. 1984.
4. Biedert R, Albrecht S. The patellotrochlear index: a new index for assessing patellar height. *Knee Surg Sports Traumatol Arthrosc*. 2006;14:707-712.
5. Christiansen SE, Jacobsen BW, Lund B, et al. Reconstruction of the medial patellofemoral ligament with gracilis tendon autograft in transverse patellar drill holes. *Arthroscopy*. 2008;24:82-87.
6. Deie M, Ochi Y, Sumen M, et al. Reconstruction of the medial patellofemoral ligament for the treatment of habitual or recurrent dislocation of the patella in children. *J Bone Joint Surg*. 2003;85:887-890.
7. Drez D, Edwards TB, Williams CS. Results of medial patellofemoral ligament reconstruction in the treatment of patella dislocation. *Arthroscopy*. 2001;17:298-306.
8. Elias JJ, Cosgarea AJ. Technical errors during MPFL reconstruction could overload the medial patello femoral cartilage. *Am J Sports Med*. 2006;34:1478-1485.
9. Erasmus PJ (1998) Reconstruction of the medial patellofemoral ligament in recurrent dislocation of the patella. ISAKOS Buenos Aires May 1997 [abstract]. *Arthroscopy*. 1998;14(Suppl):S42.

10. Erasmus PJ. *Long Term Follow-up of MPFL Reconstruction.*, Washington: American Orthopedic Society for Sport Medicine (AOSS); 2005.
11. Erasmus PJ. *Influence of Patella Height on the Results of MPFL Reconstruction.* Florence: ISAKOS; 2007.
12. Fithian DC, Gupta N. Patellar instability: principles of soft tissue repair and reconstruction. *Tech Knee Surg.* 2006;5:19-26.
13. Gomes EJ, Marczyk LS, de Cesar PC, et al. Medial patellofemoral ligament reconstruction with semitendinosus autograft for chronic patellar instability: follow-up study. *Arthroscopy.* 2004;20:147-151.
14. Heegaard J, Leyvraz PF, Van Kampen A, et al. Influence of soft tissue structure on patella three dimensional tracking. *Clin Orthop Relat Res.* 1996;299:235-243.
15. Hvid I, Andersen L, Schmidt H. Patellar height and femoral trochlea development. *Acta Orthop Scand.* 1983;54:91-93.
16. Johnson JJ, van Dyk EG, Green JR, et al. Clinical assessment of asymptomatic knees: comparison of men and women. *Arthroscopy.* 1998;22:787-793.
17. Mikashima Y, Kimura M, Komayashi Y, et al. Clinical results of isolated reconstruction of the medial patellofemoral ligament for recurrent dislocation and subluxation of the patella. *Acta Orthop Belg.* 2006;72:65-71.
18. Mountney J, Senavongse W, Amis AA, et al. Tensile strength of the medial patellofemoral ligament before and after repair or reconstruction. *J Bone Joint Surg.* 2005;87:36-40.
19. Nomura E, Inoue M. Hybrid medial patellofemoral ligament reconstruction using semitendinosis tendon for recurrent patellar dislocation: minimum 3 years follow up. *Arthroscopy.* 2006;22:787-793.
20. Nomura E, Motoyasu I, Kobayashi S. Long-term follow-up and knee osteoarthritis change after medial patellofemoral ligament reconstruction for recurrent patellar dislocation. *Am J Sports Med.* 2007;35:1851-1858.
21. Neyret P, Robinson AH, Le Coultre B, et al. Patella tendon length – the factor in patella instability? *Knee.* 2002;9:3-6.
22. Parker DA, Alexander JW, Conditt MA, et al. Comparison of isometric and anatomic reconstruction of the medial patellofemoral ligament: a cadaveric study. *Orthopedics.* 2008;31:339-343.
23. Sillanpää PJ, Mäempää H, Matilla W, et al. A mini-invasive adductor magnus tendon transfer technique for medial patellofemoral ligament reconstruction: a technical note. *Knee Surg Sports Traumatol Arthrosc.* 2009;17: 508-512.
24. Schöttle PB, Fucentese SF, Romero J. Clinical and radiological outcome of medial patellofemoral ligament reconstruction with a semitendinosis autograft for patella instability. *Knee Surg Sports Traumatol Arthrosc.* 2005;13: 516-521.
25. Smirk C, Morris H. The anatomy and reconstruction of the medial patellofemoral ligament. *Knee.* 2003;10: 221-227.
26. Smith TO, Walker J, Russel N. Outcomes of medial patellofemoral ligament reconstruction for patellar instability: a systemic review. *Knee Surg Sports Traumatol Arthrosc.* 2007;15:1301-1314.
27. Steensen RN, Dopirak RM, McDonald WG. The anatomy and isometry of the medial patello femoral joint. *Am J Sports Med.* 2004;32:1509-1513.
28. Steiner TM, Torga-Spak R, Teitge RA. Medial patellofemoral ligament reconstruction in patients with lateral patella instability and trochlear dysplasia. *Am J Sports Med.* 2006;34:1254-1261.
29. Thaunat M, Erasmus PJ. The favourable anisometry: an original concept for medial patellofemoral ligament reconstruction. *Knee.* 2007;9:3-6.
30. Thaunat M, Erasmus PJ. Recurrent patella dislocation after medial patellofemoral reconstruction. *Knee Surg Sports Traumatol Arthrosc.* 2008;16:40-43.
31. Thaunat M, Erasmus PJ. Management of overtight medial patellofemoral ligament reconstruction. *Knee Surg Sports Traumatol Arthrosc.* 2009;17:480-483.
32. Toritsuka Y, Horibe S, Hiro-Oka A, et al. Medial marginal fracture of the patella following patellar dislocation. *Knee.* 2007;14:429-433.
33. Victor J, Wong P, Witvrouw E, et al. How isometric are the medial patellofemoral, superficial medial collateral, and lateral collateral ligaments of the knee? *Am J Sports Med.* 2009;37:2028-2036.

# Reconstruction of the Lateral Patellofemoral Ligament: How I Do It

# 32

Jack T. Andrish

## 32.1 Introduction

Ostensibly, reconstruction of the lateral patellofemoral ligament should be used for the treatment of medial instability of the patella.[1,6,7,15] And that it should. But in my hands, a far more frequent use of this lateral reconstruction is for the surgical reconstruction of the extensor mechanism of knee after having failed prior surgery for the treatment of *lateral* instability of the patella when a lateral retinacular release had been included in the procedure. The relative contributions of the lateral retinaculum to medial and lateral patellar stability have been well described.[3,8,12] But in brief, the lateral retinaculum contributes not only to medial restraint of the patella, but lateral restraint as well. Perhaps it is best if we remember to visualize the lateral retinaculum as exerting a sagittal force upon the patella that helps to engage and hold the patella within the femoral trochlea, rather than a predominantly horizontal force that would be implied from most illustrations.

Medial subluxation and even dislocation of the patella is a disabling condition, almost exclusively produced by an enthusiastic lateral retinacular release, often in the face of native pathoanatomies such as trochlear dysplasia or the iatrogenic pathoanatomy of a medialization of the tibial tuberosity.[10] As Fulkerson described, the hallmark of medial patellar instability is the patient that experiences pain and dysfunction out of proportion to what they were experiencing before their surgery for lateral instability.[4] That said, the objective documentation and criteria used to diagnose medial instability of the patella has not been uniform.[11] Most measures use clinical tests that elicit pain and apprehension or abnormal hypermobility of the patella. Others use radiographic demonstrations of increased medial translation under stress or kinematic demonstrations with MRI of excessive medial movement and position.[13,16] I have preferred to use the "relocation test" described by Fulkerson as an indicator of medial patellar subluxation as a cause of the patient's pain, "locking," and giving-way.[4]

## 32.2 Indications

I have three indications for lateral reconstruction of the patellar retinaculum: (1) symptomatic medial instability of the patella following lateral retinacular release, (2) failed prior surgery for lateral instability of the patella wherein a lateral retinacular release had been included, and (3) multidirectional instability of the patella, sometimes following failed prior surgery and sometimes associated with hyperelasticity syndromes such as Ehlers–Danlos Syndrome.

I cannot emphasize enough the importance and contribution to patellar stability, both medial and lateral, that is played by the lateral retinaculum. As Larson described many years ago, it is better to lengthen the lateral retinaculum rather than release, especially when treating patellar instability.[9] And when performing revision surgery for patellar instability, remember to check for competence of the lateral retinaculum and reconstruct if necessary.

J.T. Andrish
Department of Orthopaedic Surgery, Center of Sports Health, Cleveland Clinic, Cleveland, OH, USA
e-mail: andrisj@ccf.org

V. Sanchis-Alfonso (ed.), *Anterior Knee Pain and Patellar Instability*,
DOI: 10.1007/978-0-85729-507-1_32, © Springer-Verlag London Limited 2011

## 32.3 Contraindications

If for some reason the iliotibial band has been violated and used during prior surgery, then we should look for alternative methods of reconstruction, or even repair. If the patellar instability were also associated with lateral or posterolateral instability of the knee, I would not violate the integrity of the iliotibial band.

## 32.4 Surgical Technique

The purpose of this technique is to reconstruct the deep transverse layer of the lateral retinaculum and *not* technically, the lateral patellofemoral ligament. Amis has described the lateral retinaculum and noted that the true lateral patellofemoral ligaments are thickenings of the lateral capsule.[2] There is a lateral epicondylopatellar ligament described and present in some individuals, to a varying degree of frequency, but the superficial oblique and deep transverse retinacular layers are more consistent.[5,14] The superficial oblique retinaculum is quite thin. The deep transverse retinaculum is stout, oriented in an optimal direction to restrain the patella, and attached to the lateral boarder of the patella and the deep surface of the iliotibial band. To date, we do not have studies that document the relative contributions of these *individual components* of the lateral retinaculum and lateral capsule to patellar stability.[2] That said, I have chosen to try to reconstruct what appears to be the layer most suited to restrain the patella, the deep transverse lateral retinaculum.

1. The surgical incision is often dictated by the location of prior incisions, but my preferred incision is located anterolateral. It begins 2 cm proximal to the superolateral border of the patella and extends distally to the level of, and just anterior to, Gurdy's tubercle.
2. Dissection is then carried posterior to expose what is left of the lateral retinaculum and onward to expose the iliotibial band. I then will isolate the anterior half of the iliotibial band (about 1.5 cm in width) and detach this portion from its insertion onto Gurdy's tubercle (Fig. 32.1a). This strip is then reflected proximally well beyond the level of the lateral femoral epicondyle (Fig. 32.1b).
3. Often, there is only a thin layer present that represents the lateral capsule and the scar remains of the lateral retinaculum. In that case, the iliotibial band transfer is laid directly over this tissue. But if there is some manner of (superficial oblique) retinaculum present, then an interval is developed deep to this tissue and superficial to the capsule (Fig. 32.2a). The isolated strip of iliotibial band is brought forth between these layers in order to be attached to the lateral border of the patella (Fig. 32.2b).
4. When attaching and tensioning this tendon transfer, I prefer to have a bolster beneath the knee to

a

b

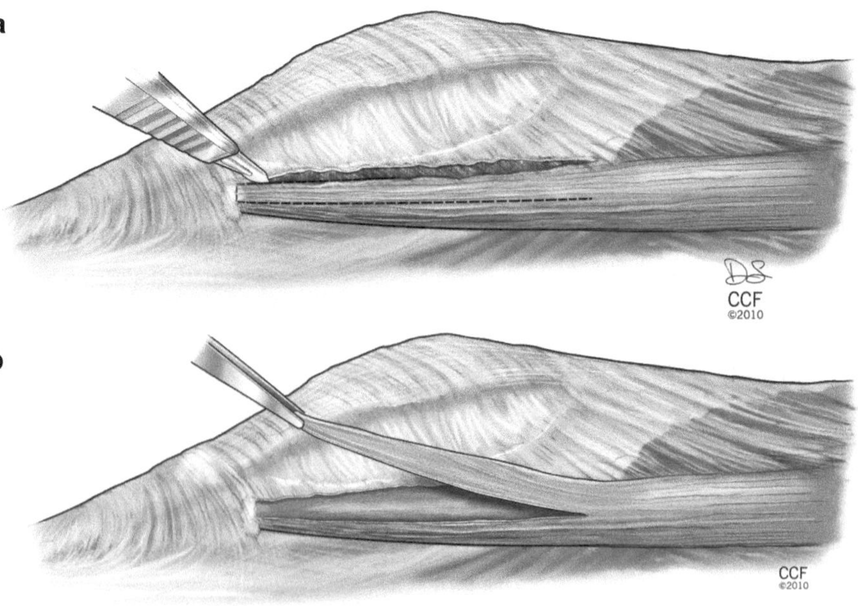


**Fig. 32.1** The lateral retinaculum is exposed to include the iliotibial band (**a**). The anterior half of the iliotibial band is detached from Gurdy's tubercle and then reflected proximally, beyond the lateral femoral epicondyle (**b**) (Copyright The Cleveland Clinic Foundation)

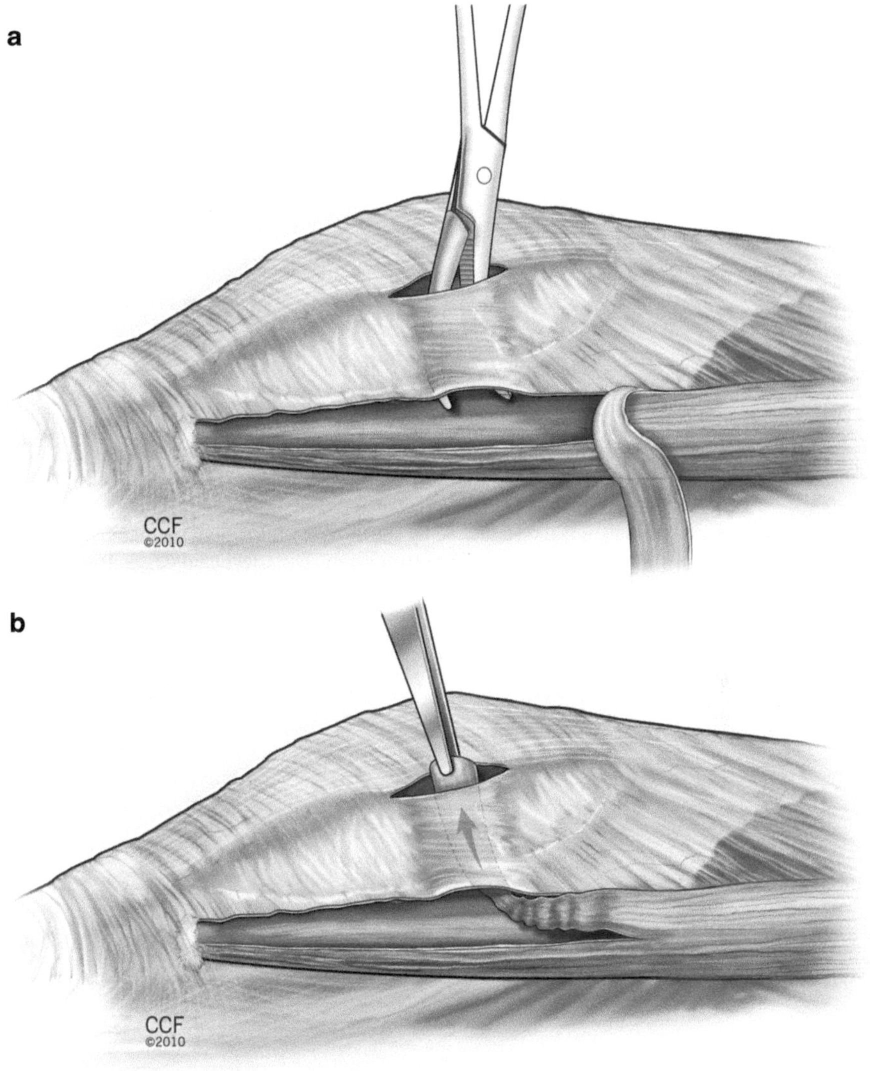


**Fig. 32.2** If there is some manner of attenuated lateral retinaculum remaining, an interval is developed between the lateral capsule and the retinaculum (**a**). The strip of iliotibial band is then brought through this interval to be attached to the lateral border of the junction of the middle and proximal third of the patella (**b**) (Copyright The Cleveland Clinic Foundation)

position the knee in about 20° of flexion. Although it could be debated about the biomechanical advisability of flexion versus extension, I prefer to have the patella engaged within the trochlea as a means of preventing overtensioning and producing an abnormal translation.

5. Attachment to the patella can be either by direct suture to the remaining pre and peripatellar retinaculum if there is adequate tissue present, or by suture anchor (Fig. 32.3). I do not prefer drill holes for this reconstruction, nor would it be easy to use a drill hole since the length available of transferred iliotibial band is just sufficient to reach the lateral border of the patella.
6. At this point, the orientation of the transferred iliotibial band is somewhat oblique to the patella. Our goal is to make it transversely oriented and "attached" to the remaining iliotibial band at the level of the lateral femoral epicondyle. In order to do this, and to adjust and establish tension, I begin a series of sutures reattaching the posterior border of the transferred tendon to the anterior border of the remaining intact iliotibial band. This begins at the proximal location of the isolation and works distally until the desired orientation and tension of the transfer has been achieved. Simple sutures work well (Fig. 32.4).
7. Often, there will appear to be a kink or wrinkle at the anterior bend of the transfer. In this case, I will place one additional suture within this fold and attach to either itself or the posterior border of the remaining lateral retinaculum to "un-kink" the fold (Fig. 32.5a, b).

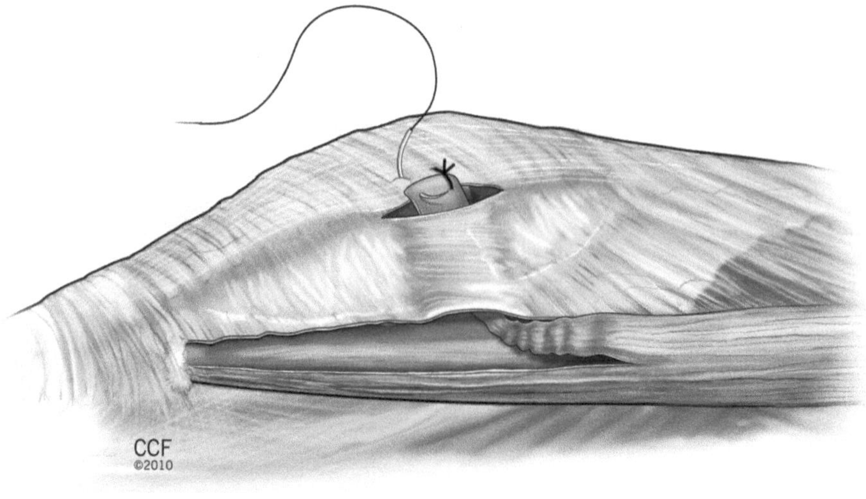


**Fig. 32.3** The transferred tendon is then attached by suture to the remaining peripatellar retinacular tissue, or by suture anchor. It is not necessary to attempt attachment by a drill hole (Copyright The Cleveland Clinic Foundation)

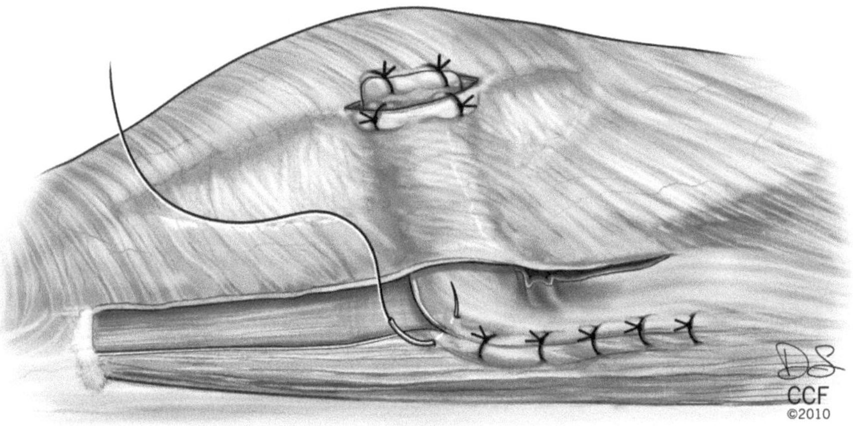


**Fig. 32.4** Our goal is to make the transferred tendon transversely oriented and "attached" to the remaining intact iliotibial band at the level of the lateral femoral epicondyle. In order to do this, and to adjust and establish tension, a series of sutures are placed reattaching the posterior border of the transferred tendon to the anterior border of the remaining intact iliotibial band. This begins at the proximal location of the isolation and works distally until the desired orientation and tension of the transfer has been achieved (Copyright The Cleveland Clinic Foundation)

8. If there is native lateral retinaculum present, then it is repaired to the lateral border of the patella, if possible, and even at times to the remaining intact iliotibial band. The deep transverse retinaculum has now been reconstructed deep to the remnants of lateral retinaculum.
9. The knee is passed through a range of motion from full extension to at least 90° of flexion to judge patellar tracking and to observe the competence of the suture attachments.
10. Wound closure is routine.

## 32.5 Postoperative Management

Since most often I use this procedure as a part of a revision surgery for lateral or multidirectional patellar instability, the postoperative care is directed by the aggregate of what was done. But for an isolated lateral reconstruction, I apply a cooling unit over an elastic dressing and then apply a double upright brace with a motion control hinge set to allow full extension but block flexion at 40°. The procedure is performed as an outpatient and the dressing left in place until

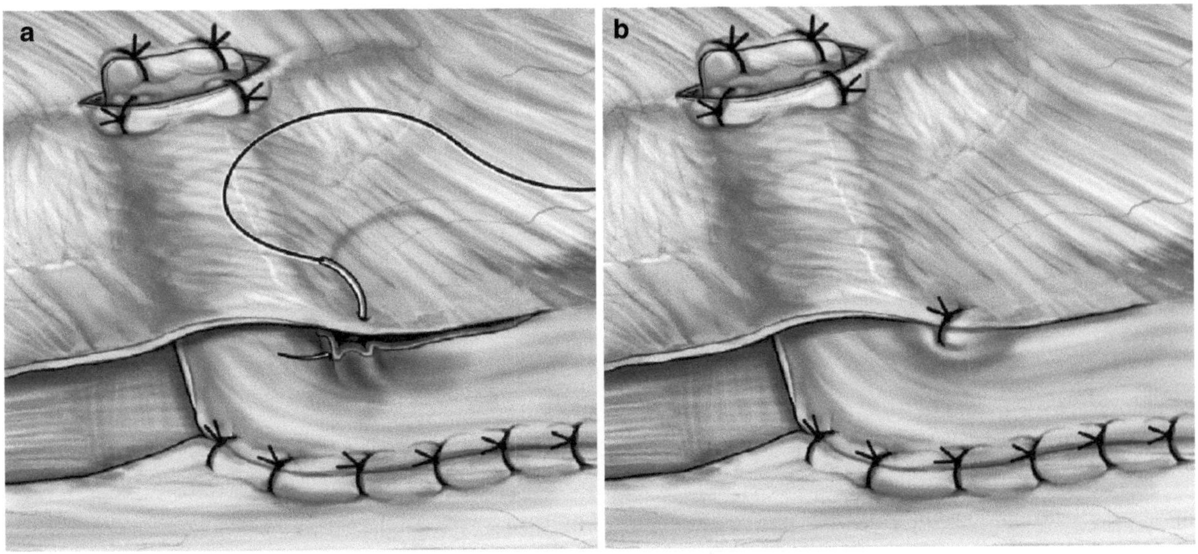


**Fig. 32.5** Often, there will be a kink at the bend of the transfer. A simple suture from the corner of the iliotibial band to remaining retinacular tissue improves the alignment (**a**). All sutures in place and properly "tensioned," the deep transverse lateral retinaculum has been reconstructed (**b**) (Copyright The Cleveland Clinic Foundation)

their first return to the office at 1 week. No drains are used. Upon the first return, the dressing is removed and the patient is instructed to use the brace only at nighttime and for community ambulation to "protect" against the odd fall. They are advised to ambulate with the use of crutches with full weight bearing as tolerated. But out of the brace, they are encouraged to move the knee as tolerated without limits. Physical therapy is begun at this time, out of the brace, for range of motion exercises and pelvifemoral conditioning. The subcuticular sutures are removed at 3 weeks and the average length of time needed for crutch support is 3–6 weeks.

## 32.6 Pearls and Pitfalls

Don't forget the importance of a competent lateral retinaculum when dealing with the surgical management of patellar instability. In the first case when performing patellar realignment and reconstructive surgery for patellar instability, it is always safer to lengthen rather than release the lateral retinaculum. And most certainly, never release the lateral retinaculum in the face of trochlear dysplasia, patella alta, or hyperelasticity. In the case of revision surgery for failed patellar realignment and reconstruction, do not forget to establish a competent lateral retinaculum, even if the only observable instability is lateral. Although not common, I have had cases of recurrent lateral patellar subluxations where the only technique required to correct the problem was a lateral reconstruction alone, not medial. It is amazing.

And what is my biggest pitfall? Making the wrong diagnosis of medial patellar instability as the primary cause of the patient's pain and mechanical symptoms. Many if not most of the patients with symptomatic iatrogenic medial patellar instability have *chronic* pain and chronic pain is multifactorial with a different pathoneurophysiology than acute pain. The mere fact that the patient can subluxate and even dislocate their patella medially is no guarantee that their pain and disability are directly due to the instability. Go with caution into that dark night.

## 32.7 Clinical Results and Complications

Since most of the patients that have this procedure have multiple mechanical and, at times, psychosocial issues involved, the clinical results cannot be isolated to the lateral reconstruction alone. My "results" of those patients with only an isolated lateral reconstruction are therefore anecdotal. I can say, however, that I have been using this technique for over 15 years and continue to use it as my primary method of lateral reconstruction. Complications and poor results, as related above, are mostly a product of misinterpreting and misunderstanding the multifactorial pathology involved in the patient.

## References


1. Abhaykumar S, Craig DM. Fascia lata sling reconstruction for recurrent medical dislocation of the patella. *Knee.* 1999; 6:55-57.
2. Amis A. Current concepts on anatomy and biomechanics of patellar stability. *Sports Med Arthrosc.* 2007;15:48-56.
3. Desio SM, Burks RT, Bachus K. Soft tissue restraints to lateral patellar translation in the human knee. *Am J Sports Med.* 1998;26:59-65.
4. Fulkerson J. Anterolateralization of the tibial tubercle. *Tech Orthop.* 1997;12:165-169.
5. Fulkerson J, Gossling H. Anatomy of the knee joint lateral retinaculum. *Clin Orthop Relat Res.* 1980;153: 183-188.
6. Hughston J, Deese M. Medial subluxation of the patella as a complication of lateral retinacular release. *Am J Sports Med.* 1988;16:383-388.
7. Hughston J, Flandry F, Brinker M, et al. Surgical correction of medial subluxation of the patella. *Am J Sports Med.* 1996;24:486-493.
8. Ishibashi Y, Okamura Y, Otsuka H, et al. Lateral patellar retinaculum tension in patellar instability. *Clin Orthop Relat Res.* 2002;397:362-369.
9. Larson R, Cabaud HE, Slocum D, et al. The patellar compression syndrome: surgical treatment by lateral retinacular release. *Clin Orthop Relat Res.* 1978;134:158-167.
10. Metcalf R. An arthroscopic method for lateral release of the subluxating or dislocating patella. *Clin Orthop Relat Res.* 1982;167:9-18.
11. Nonweiler DE, DeLee JC. The diagnosis and treatment of medial subluxation of the patella after lateral retinacular release. *Am J Sports Med.* 1994;22:680-686.
12. Senavongse W, Farahmand F, Jones J, et al. Quantitative measurement of patellofemoral joint stability: force-displacement behavior of the human patella in vitro. *J Orthop Res.* 2003;21:780-786.
13. Shellock F, Mink J, Deutsch A, et al. Evaluation of patients with persistent symptoms after lateral retinacular release by kinematic magnetic resonance imaging of the patellofemoral joint. *Arthroscopy.* 1990;6:226-234.
14. Starok M, Lenchik L, Trudell D, et al. Normal patellar retinaculum: MR and sonographic imaging with cadaveric correlation. *AJR.* 1997;168:1493-1499.
15. Teitge R, Spak R. Lateral patellofemoral ligament reconstruction. *Arthroscopy.* 2004;20:998-1002.
16. Teitge R, Faerber W, Des Madryl P, et al. Stress radiographs of the patellofemoral joint. *J Bone Joint Surg.* 1996;78-A:193-203.

# Reconstruction of the Lateral Patellofemoral Ligament: How I Do It

33

Robert A. Teitge and Roger Torga-Spak

## 33.1 Introduction

Medial dislocation or subluxation of the patella is a disabling condition that can occur after an isolated lateral release, or after lateral release in combination with tibial tubercle transfer or medial soft tissue imbrications.[2-4,6-8]

Techniques to repair the lateral retinaculum can be found in the literature,[5,6] as well as descriptions of reconstruction with local soft-tissue augmentation (fascia lata, patellar tendon).[1,4] In our experience with lateral retinacular repair and imbrication, a noticeable increase in medial excursion usually would reappear after the first postoperative year. This led us to develop a technique for lateral patellofemoral ligament (LPFL) reconstruction following the same principles of the medial patellofemoral ligament reconstruction previously described: (1) selection of a sufficiently strong and stiff graft, (2) isometric graft placement, (3) adequate fixation, (4) correct tension, and (5) no condylar rubbing or impingement.

## 33.2 Surgical Technique

### 33.2.1 Graft Selection and Harvesting

The quadriceps tendon provides a reliable graft but bone–patellar tendon–bone and Achilles allograft can also be used. With the knee in extension, a 6- to 8-cm skin incision is made midway between the lateral epicondyle and the lateral edge of the patella. A 4- to 5-mm × 1-cm partial-thickness quadriceps tendon is obtained. The posterior quadriceps tendon is left intact to avoid scar in the synovial pouch. A 1 cm² × 5-mm thick bone is removed from the superior central one third of the patella with a small oscillating saw. The graft is harvested from the quadriceps tendon, as far proximal as feasible, and generally 8–10 cm can be obtained before the muscle fibers of the vastus lateralis and vastus medialis converge (Fig. 33.1). The graft is prepared by drilling a 2.5-mm hole through the bone block and then running a No. 2 Vicryl suture from the free tendon end toward the bone block and back using the Krackow technique.

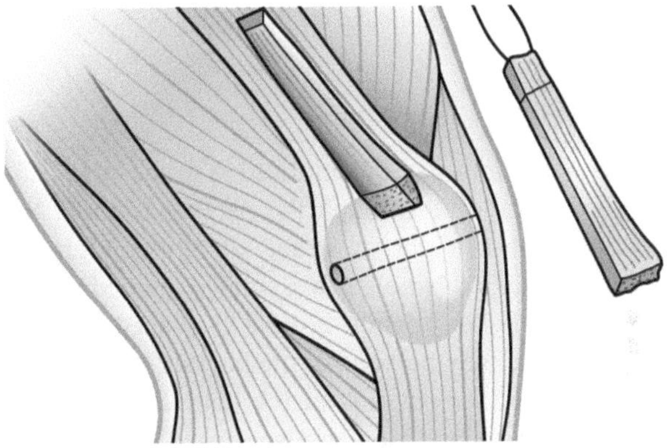

**Fig. 33.1** Harvesting of the quadriceps graft. A transversal tunnel is performed through the patella

### 33.2.2 Isometric Location

The graft must be located isometrically to avoid overstretching it to failure during joint motion or to avoid

R. Torga-Spak (✉)
Faculty of Orthopaedics and Traumatology,
Department of Surgery, Instituto Universitario CEMIC,
Buenos Aires, Argentina
e-mail: rogerts@traumatologiapenta.com.ar

V. Sanchis-Alfonso (ed.), *Anterior Knee Pain and Patellar Instability*,
DOI: 10.1007/978-0-85729-507-1_33, © Springer-Verlag London Limited 2011

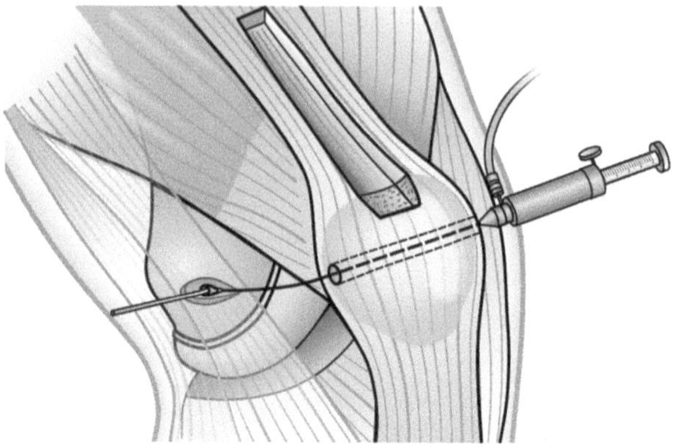

**Fig. 33.2** Isometric location of the insertion point in the lateral condyle

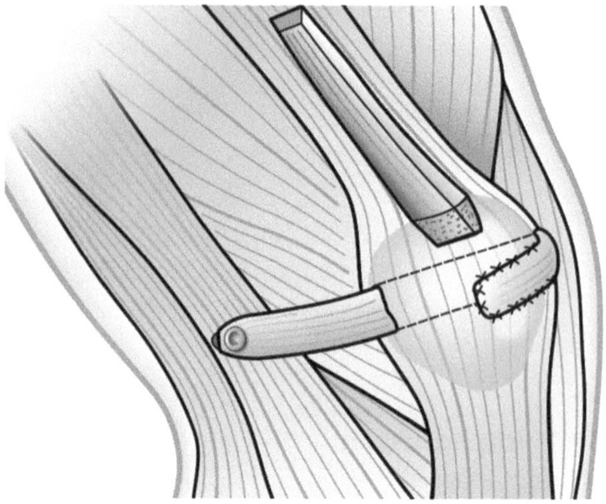

**Fig. 33.3** Quadriceps graft fixed to the lateral condyle, passed through the patellar tunnel, and sutured on the anterior aspect of the patella

overconstraining patellar motion. A transverse 2.5-mm hole is placed through the patella at about the mid one third height. A strand of No. 2 Vicryl is passed through this hole and a small loop tied on the lateral aspect. A 2.5-mm K-wire is placed through this loop and into the bone of the lateral femoral condyle at about the position of the lateral epicondyle. Next, the pneumatic Isometer is inserted into the hole in the medial patella and the No. 2 Vicryl isometric measurement suture passed into it (Fig. 33.2). The knee is then placed through a full range of motion while the change in length of the lateral suture is read in the Isometer. Adjustments in the position of the K-wire in the lateral condyle are made until no excursion is read in the isometer during the full range of motion.

### 33.2.3 Secure Fixation

The bone block is countersunk into the femur and fixed with a 4.0-mm fully threaded lag screw. To create an accurate countersunk hole for the bone block in the femur, the bone block that has the 2.5-mm diameter hole in it is slid over the K-wire, which locates the isometric site on the femur. Then the bone block lies against the femur like a template while a thin chisel outlines the bone block and penetrates the cortex of the lateral femoral condyle. Because the femoral bone is often osteoporotic from disuse, cancellous bone is impacted instead of removed to create the recess for the patellar bone block. It is then fixed with a 4.0-mm lag screw. An adequate bone tunnel can be placed transversely through the patella with two parallel 4.5- to 6-mm drills, avoiding the anterior tension trabeculae in the patella and avoiding the articular surface. Fixation of the quadriceps tendon to the patella is easily accomplished by pulling the tendon graft into the oval transverse tunnel in the patella, out the medial side, and turning it superficially onto the anterior surface of the patella, where it is sutured to the quadriceps expansion (Fig. 33.3).

### 33.2.4 Correct Tension

The tension set in the graft must be enough to limit medial excursion to an amount that approximates that of the normal contralateral knee. We set the tension with the knee flexed 60°–90° to avoid the risk of pulling too far lateral. Do not set the tension with the patella outside the trochlea. Realize that the ligament is not a dynamic structure that pulls the patella laterally, but rather a static restraint that holds the patella against moving too far medially.

### 33.2.5 Avoid Impingement

When the correct location is found, the patellar bone block is countersunk into the femur to avoid a prominence producing an iliotibial band friction syndrome. The range of motion must be tested to ensure there is no restriction of patellar or knee motion. The graft should not be rubbing against the lateral femoral condyle. If impingement on the wall of the lateral femoral condyle is detected, the graft can be placed on the anterior surface of the patella and pulled into the medial tunnel in a lateral direction.

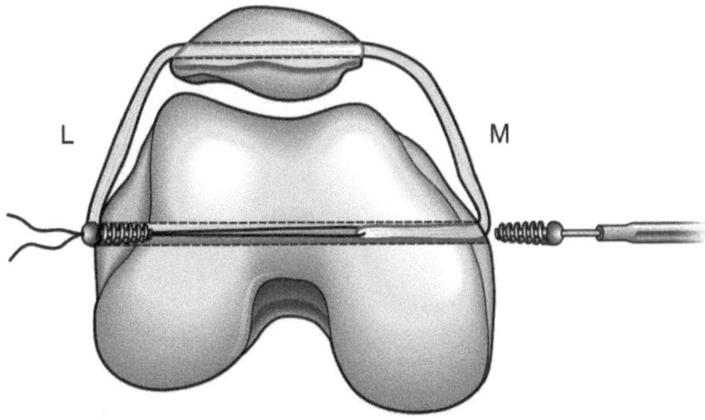


**Fig. 33.4** Combined MPFL and LPFL reconstruction passing a free graft through a transverse patellar and epicondylar tunnel

## 33.3 Postoperative Care

Postoperative treatment is to allow full range of motion, full weight bearing, continuous passive motion, active exercises, but avoiding stairs, squatting, and resistive leg extension until the patellar bone donor site has adequate time to heal.

## 33.4 Our Experience

This procedure has been performed in our institution since 1980 in 80 patients. The results have been excellent when assessed from stability standpoint and none of the knees has lost the stability obtained at surgery. Three patients have sustained a patellar fracture, which occurred with a fall in the early postoperative phase; two of them have required open reduction and internal fixation. This is a salvage procedure for repair of medial iatrogenic instability. It does not address the original source of complaint. It clearly cannot improve or reverse osteoarthrosis, chondromalacia, bony malalignment, or lateral instability caused by an insufficient medial patellofemoral ligament.

In cases with associated medial and lateral patellar instability (multidirectional instability) a combination of the techniques described to reconstruct the MPFL and LPFL can be used. An option for reconstruction of both patellofemoral ligaments during the same procedure is by means of a free semitendinosus graft passed through a transverse patellar and transepicondylar tunnel (Fig. 33.4).

## References

1. Abhaykumar S, Craig DM. Fascia Lata sling reconstruction for recurrent medial dislocation of the patella. *Knee*. 1999;6:55-57.
2. Blazina NE. Complications of the Hauser procedure. In: Kennedy JC, ed. *The Injured Adolescent Knee*. Baltimore: Williams & Wilkins; 1979:198.
3. Eppley RA. Medial patellar subluxation. In: Fox JM, Del Pizzo W, eds. *The Patellofemoral Joint*. New York: McGraw Hill; 1993:149-156.
4. Hughston JC, Deese M. Medial subluxation of the patella as a complication of lateral retinacular release. *Am J Sports Med*. 1988;16:383-388.
5. Johnson DP, Wakeley C. Reconstruction of the lateral patellar retinaculum following lateral release: a case report. *Knee Surg Sports Traumatol Arthrosc*. 2002;10:361-363.
6. Nonweiler DE, DeLee JC. The diagnosis and treatment of medial subluxation of the patella after lateral retinacular release. *Am J Sports Med*. 1994;22:680-686.
7. Shea KP, Fulkerson JP. Preoperative computed tomography scanning and arthroscopy in predicting outcome after lateral retinacular release. *Arthroscopy*. 1992;8:327-334.
8. Small NC. An analysis of complications in lateral retinacular release procedures. *Arthroscopy*. 1989;15:282-286.

# 34 Osteotomies Around the Patellofemoral Joint

Roland M. Biedert and Philippe M. Tscholl

## 34.1 Introduction

A normal patellofemoral gliding mechanism with perfect stability is guaranteed by the complex interaction of skeletal geometry, soft tissues, and neuromuscular control.[10] During knee flexion, the patella moves from a medial to a lateral tilted position as knee flexion approaches 90°.[29,32,33,51,53] Abnormal skeletal geometry – such as increased femoral anteversion, trochlear dysplasia, patella alta or infera, increased tibial external torsion, increased tibial tubercle lateralization, and variations of combined deformities – may lead to patellofemoral complaints.[10] Altered vectors and forces acting on the patellofemoral joint (PFJ) can cause cartilage failure with secondary osteoarthritis instability and musculotendinous insufficiency. Osteotomy with soft tissue balancing might be the best treatment, depending on the underlying pathology. Surgery aims to eliminate the present pathomorphology.

## 34.2 Femur

### 34.2.1 Pathologic Femoral Anteversion

Patient's complaints may appear as a diffuse knee or hip pain and even present with patellar dislocation in some cases. Others may be asymptomatic; however are bothered by the appearance of their leg axes. Typically it begins at the young age, although some may be up to 50 years of age at the onset of symptoms.

Since increased femoral anteversion (coxa antetorta) is most frequent, decreased femoral anteversion (coxa retrotorta) is not further described in this section.

#### 34.2.1.1 Physical Examination

In *supine* position, increased internal rotation of the distal femoral head is apparent with both knee caps verged internal, also known as "squinting patellae".[48] Examination of hip rotation in 90° flexion shows increased internal rotation compared to the external rotation, and may reach up to 80–90°.[16] Physical examination of the patella highlights an often tilted and rarely lateralized position. Tender points are found along the lateral patellar facet due to hypercompression on the lateral trochlea, potential soft tissue impingement, and painful lateral retinaculum.

In the *sitting* position with hanging lower extremity, the patella is well centered (with mild negative lateral patellar tilt) in the trochlear groove, and therefore the tuberculum–sulcus angle is normal.

When *standing* in a comfortable position, the feet are slightly externally rotated (10–15°), but the patellae are internally rotated on the distal femur (Fig. 34.1a). Active correction of the patella position to normal (straight to anterior) causes increased and no more comfortable external rotation of the feet (Fig. 34.1b). In some patients, coxa saltans may be seen, when the iliotibial tract skips over the greater trochanter. Additional clinical findings, such as the too many toes sign, may be observed.

R.M. Biedert (✉)
Sportclinic Villa Linde, Swiss Olympic Medical Center
Magglingen-Biel, University of Basel, Biel, Switzerland
e-mail: r.biedert@bluewin.ch

V. Sanchis-Alfonso (ed.), *Anterior Knee Pain and Patellar Instability*,
DOI: 10.1007/978-0-85729-507-1_34, © Springer-Verlag London Limited 2011

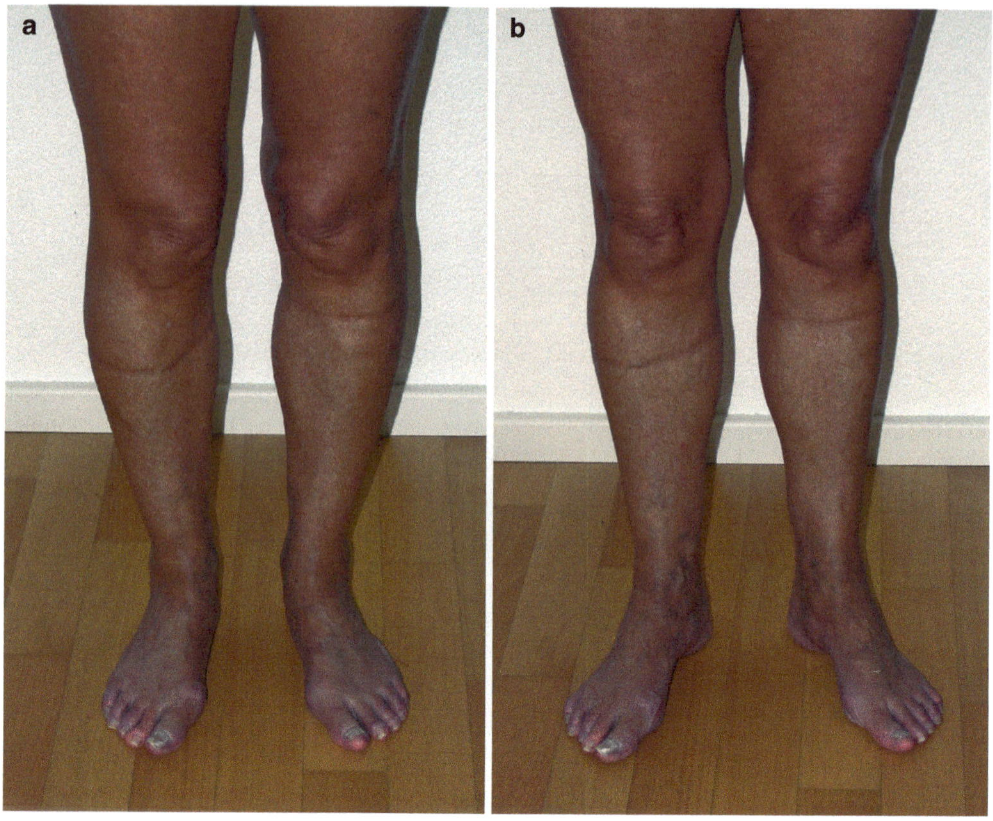


**Fig. 34.1** (**a**) Internally rotated patellae in comfortable standing position. (**b**) Active correction of the patella to normal causes increased external rotation of the feet

#### 34.2.1.2 Imaging

##### CT Evaluation

Lower extremity alignment is measured by series of 2D-CT scans. The following planes are selected: greater trochanter, distal femur, tibial head, and malleolus. Greater trochanter and distal femur are superimposed, and the angle of the femoral anteversion is measured (Fig. 34.2). Values of more than 20° are considered as pathologic.[10,39] At the same time, tibial rotation and TT-TG distance should be analyzed, since concomitant findings are frequent and crucial for successful therapy.[24]

Any other causes of patellar maltracking and its subsequent damage should be eliminated.

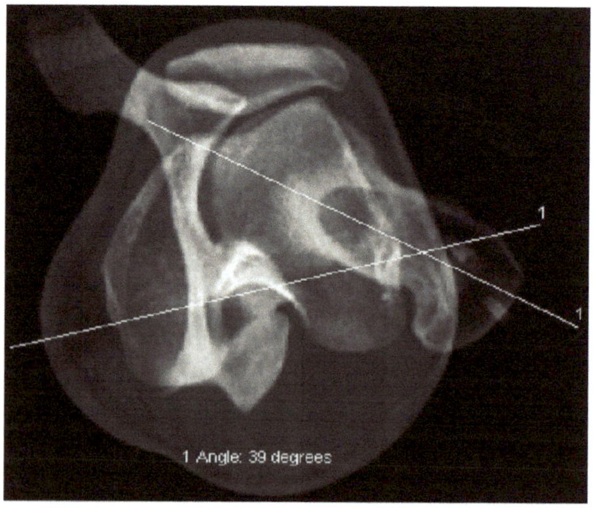


**Fig. 34.2** Axial CT evaluation of the femoral anteversion. The femoral anteversion is 39°

#### Plain Radiographs and MRI

Plain radiographs and MRI are demanded to exclude other pathologies, such as cartilage lesions and trochlear dysplasia.

### 34.2.1.3 Special Considerations

For practical understanding it is crucial to know that the underlying cause is not a malpositioning of the patella; it is a malrotation of the distal femur with regard to the knee extensor mechanism alignment.

Muscular causes, such as insufficiency or contractures, need to be ruled out. Malalignment of the tibia or biomechanical failures such as hyperpronation of the foot may clinically mimic increased femoral anteversion or may concomitantly exist described as "miserable malalignment syndrome" by James et al.[37]

Often, a tight lateral retinaculum is preexisting, and therefore soft tissue balancing should be considered in surgical therapy.

### 34.2.1.4 Conservative Treatment

Conservative approach represents the first-line treatment with enforcing external hip rotators, stretching of the internal rotators and of the lateral retinaculum. Cofindings such as hyperpronation of the foot, which causes more internal femoral rotation, may be corrected by insoles. Usually, conservative treatment does not relieve pain sufficiently, especially in younger patients. In elderly patient, retropatellar osteoarthritis on the lateral patellar facet and/or lateral trochlea may appear.

### 34.2.1.5 Surgery

The surgical treatment with rotational femur osteotomy may be performed on the intertrochanteric or supracondylar level. The authors prefer the distal femoral correction, especially when additional interventions are necessary in the knee joint at the same time.[10] The correctional procedure on the intertrochanteric level is therefore not further discussed. The physis must be closed completely.

#### Supracondylar Rotation Osteotomy

Lateral incision from the lateral epicondylus of the knee is chosen for posterolateral approach to the femur. The vastus lateralis and intermedius muscles are delaminated from the lateral supracondylar line.[35] Three to five centimeter above the metaphysis, two Kirschner wires are placed to monitor both the present and the desired rotation after correction (Fig. 34.3).

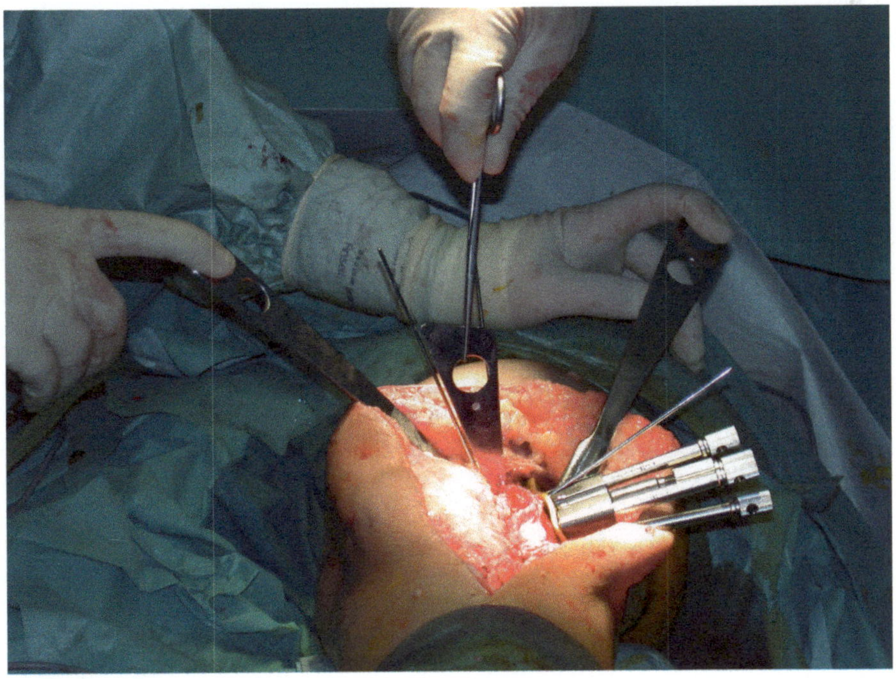

**Fig. 34.3** Two Kirschner wires indicate the angle of correction

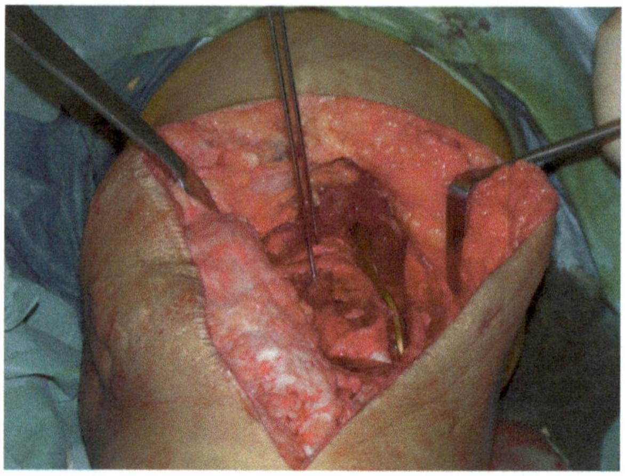

**Fig. 34.4** Fixation of the supracondylar rotation osteotomy

Always protecting the medial neurovascular bundle, the osteotomy is performed horizontally. The two Kirschner wires are rotated as the preoperative planning based on what the CT assessment has indicated. Fixation of the osteotomy is performed by locking screw osteosynthesis plate, which has at least three distal and three proximal bicortical screws for fixation (Fig. 34.4). Patellar soft tissue balancing with lengthening of the lateral retinaculum and shortening of the medial patellofemoral ligament is done at the end, if needed. Closure is performed layer by layer of the soft tissues and preventing potential muscular hernia.

#### 34.2.1.6 Postoperative Rehabilitation

Mobilization is initiated the first day after surgery with partial weight bearing of 10 kg for 6 weeks. During these first 6 weeks, healing of the osteotomy, decreasing swelling, and activation of quadriceps muscle are the main objectives. Plain radiographs verify after 6 weeks the postoperative healing of the osteotomy. If the consolidation of the osteotomy is correct, full weight bearing can be started immediately. When sufficient mobility has been regained, treadmill exercises can be started (generally 8 week after surgery). No restriction of activities is advised 6 months after osteotomy.

#### 34.2.1.7 Summary

Increased femoral anteversion is a complex biomechanical pathology which frequently includes also malalignments of the tibia and the foot. Surgical treatment with supracondylar osteotomy has shown good results in patients with patellar maltracking symptoms and (sub-)luxation when conservative treatment failed.

### 34.2.2 Trochlear Dysplasia

The femoral trochlea is important for controlling the patellofemoral gliding mechanism.[7,27] Normal articular shape of trochlea and patella allow for undisturbed patellar tracking. The normal cartilaginous surface of the trochlea consists of the lateral and medial facets of the femoral sulcus and is defined by different criteria in the proximal–distal, mediolateral, and antero-posterior direction.[10,12,51] The normal trochlea deepens from proximal to distal.[10,51] In the proximal–distal direction, it is longest laterally and shortest on the medial side (Fig. 34.5). The deepened trochlear groove separates the lateral facet from the medial part. In the antero-posterior measurements, the most anterior aspect of the lateral condyle is normally higher than the medial condyle and the deepest point is represented by the center of the trochlear groove.[12]

Trochlear dysplasia is an abnormality of shape and depth of the trochlear groove, mainly in its proximal extent.[19,52] It represents an important pathologic articular morphology that is a strong risk factor for permanent patellar instability.[4,7,10,17,19,21-23,26,41,42,50,54,55] Femoral trochlear dysplasia has been reported to occur in up to 85% of patients with recurrent patellar dislocation.[23,55] The trochlear depth may be decreased, the trochlea may be flat, or a trochlear bump is present. According to this, different classifications are described in the literature.[10,17,20] Additionally we found that also a too short lateral trochlea is a frequent cause of proximal–lateral patellar instability and noticed that there exists a widespread variability of combinations of trochlear dysplasia.[8-10,14]

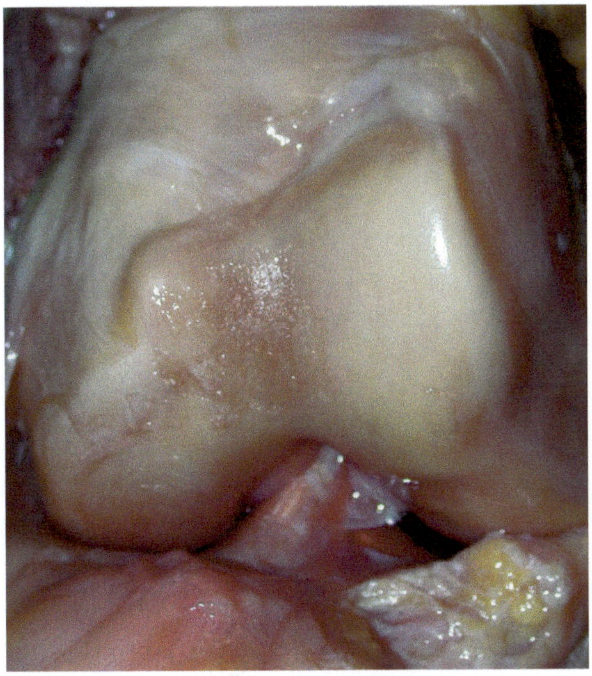

**Fig. 34.5** Shape of a normal trochlea (cadaver study)

### 34.2.3 Short Trochlea

#### 34.2.3.1 Physical Examination

The patients with a too short lateral trochlear facet suffer from patellar instability. The patella is well centered in the trochlea under relaxed conditions. But when the patient contracts the quadriceps muscle with the leg in extension, the patella is pulled to proximal out of the short trochlea because it is no more sufficiently guided and stabilized by the too short lateral facet of the trochlea. In most cases, the contraction causes also subluxation to lateral, a so-called dynamic supero-lateral patellar subluxation (Fig. 34.6a, b). In contrast to the *lateral pull sign*, described by Kolowich et al.[38], this type of patellofemoral instability is primarily not due to soft tissue abnormalities (atrophy of the vastus medialis obliquus and hypertrophy of the vastus lateralis and lateral structures), but caused by a pathologic proximal patellar tracking due to the missing osteochondral opposing force of the lateral trochlear facet.

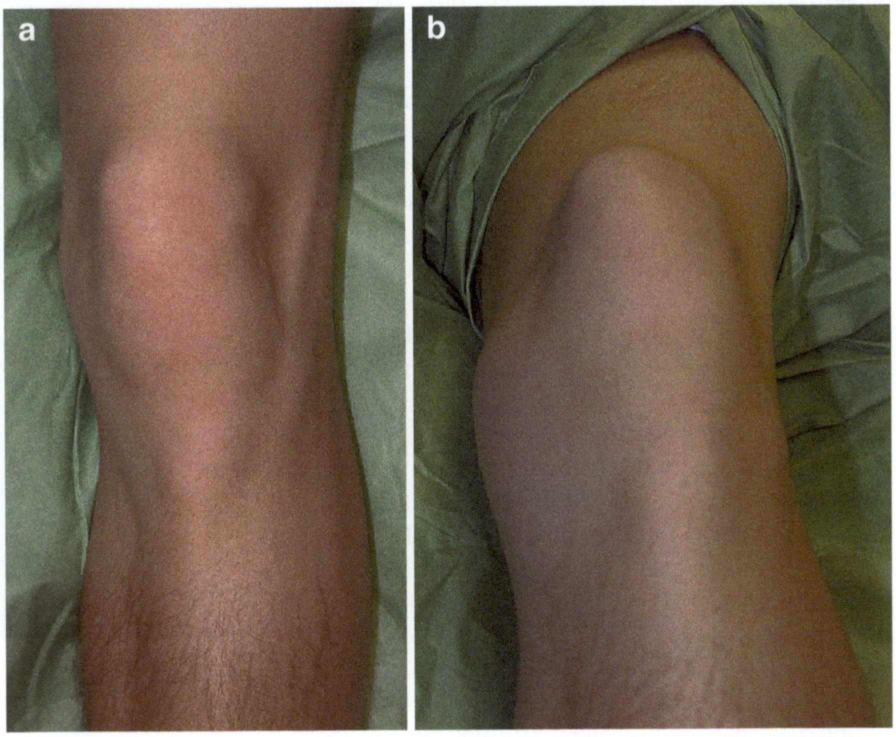

**Fig. 34.6** (**a**) Well-centered patella. (**b**) Muscle contraction causes dynamic superolateral patellar subluxation

This type of patella instability can also be depicted by manual examination in complete extension of the knee. Only minimal manual pressure to lateral causes the subluxation and discomfort to the patient. In most cases the patient feels pain and tries to resist this manoeuvre. This test in full extension must be differentiated from the *patellar apprehension test* which is performed in 20–30° of knee flexion.[7,45] With increasing knee flexion, the patella enters into the more distal and normal part of the trochlear groove and becomes therefore more and more stable. This confirms the clinical suspicion of proximal lateral patellar instability.

#### 34.2.3.2 Imaging

##### Radiographs

The radiologic examination of patients with a too short lateral facet of the trochlea do normally not show the typical findings of trochlear dysplasia in the true lateral view such as the crossing sign, supratrochlear spur, double contour[17,19,22,23],or lateral trochlear sign.[31] Radiographs can only show signs of dysplasia in combined trochlear abnormalities.[9,10,14] The different indices used for patellar height measurements are normal.

##### MR Measurements

MR measurements are performed with the knees in 0° of flexion, the foot in 15° external rotation, and the quadriceps muscle consciously relaxed. Measurements on sagittal images include different parameters.[8,9,14] First, two circles indicate the central longitudinal axis of the femoral shaft (Fig. 34.7). Second, the most lateral sagittal image on which the articular cartilage of the lateral condyle still can be analyzed is selected. A tangent line (d) on the distal femoral cartilage is drawn in 90° degrees to the femoral axis (Ca). The length to the most anterior (A) and the most posterior (P) aspect of the cartilaginous part is measured in relation to the tangent line. Its ratio ([a:p] * 100) represents the lateral condyle index in percentages. The mean lateral condyle index is 93% ± 7 (range 73–109) for patients with normal patellofemoral joints. Therefore we consider an anterior length of the lateral articular facet of the trochlea with index values of 93% or more of the length of the posterior articular cartilage as normal. Index values of less than 90% must therefore be considered as pathologic (short) and values of 84% or less confirm the presence of a too short lateral facet (Fig. 34.8).

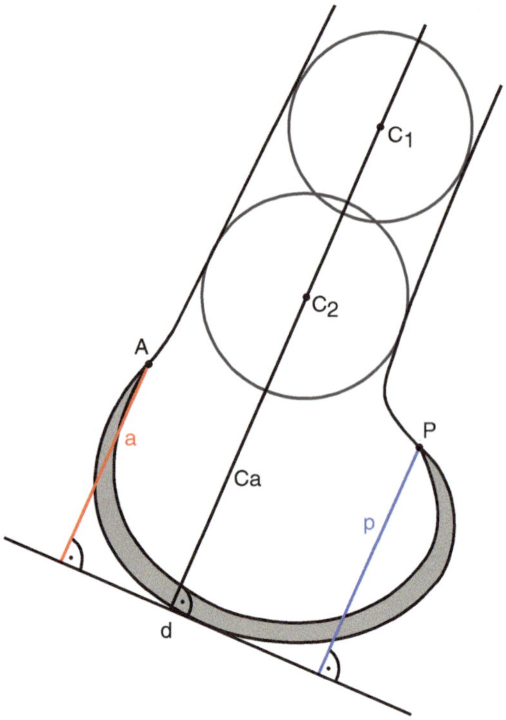


**Fig 34.7** MR measurements of the lateral condyle index

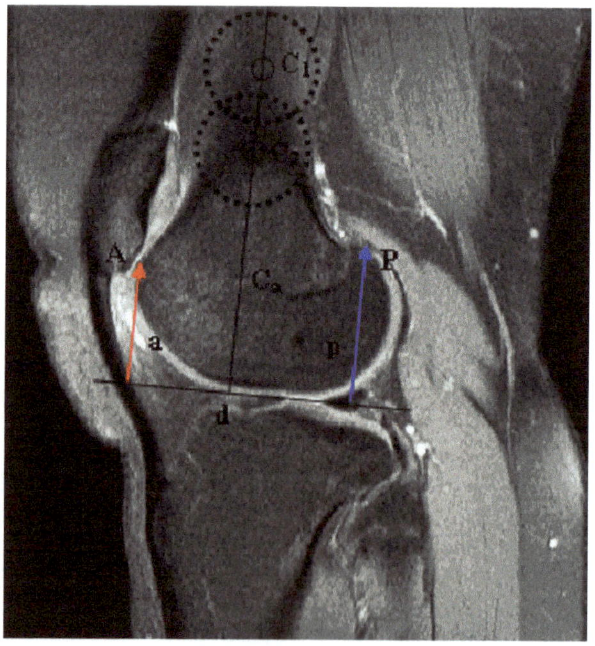


**Fig. 34.8** MR measurement shows a too short lateral condyle index of 75.2%

#### 34.2.3.3 Surgery

Surgical techniques are developed to correct the pathologic morphology. In this situation lengthening is recommended to eliminate the too short lateral trochlea.[10,11,14]

##### Lengthening

Clear indication for lengthening is given when the lateral condyle index is 84% or less. Lengthening is designed to create a longer proximal part of the lateral trochlear sulcus to improve the contact within the patellofemoral joint and with this to optimize the patellofemoral gliding mechanism. A longer lateral trochlear facet is the feature that must "capture" the patella in extension before the knee starts to flex, to ensure that it is guided into the more distal trochlear groove. Normally, the contact between the articular surface of the trochlea and the articular cartilage behind the patella is about one third of the length of the patellar cartilage (measured using the patellotrochlear index).[11] This value is very helpful both in planning (using MRI) and during surgery to determine how much lengthening to proximal should be performed.

Through a short parapatellar lateral incision the superficial retinaculum is localized. About 1 cm from the border of the patella it is longitudinally incised and carefully separated from the oblique part of the retinaculum in the posterior direction to allow at the end of surgery lengthening of the lateral retinaculum at the same time if needed.[7] Then the oblique part is cut and the patellofemoral joint is opened. The proximal shape of the lateral facet of the trochlea and the length of the articular cartilage are assessed with regard to the length of the sulcus and the medial facet of the trochlea. The presence of a too short lateral articular facet is reconfirmed. In such a case, the patellotrochlear overlap is less than one third. The present overlap allows now to determine the amount of lengthening of the lateral facet and should be about one third at the end, measured in extension (0° of flexion).[7,11] The incomplete lateral osteotomy is made at least 5 mm from the cartilage of the sulcus to prevent necrosis of the trochlea or breaking of the lateral facet. The osteotomy starts at the end of the cartilage (arrow) and is continued approximately 1–1.5 cm to distal into the femoral condyle and to proximal into the femoral shaft, always according to the aimed patellofemoral overlapping. The osteotomy is opened carefully with the use of a chisel. Fracture of the distal cartilage may occur and has no consequences; however sharp edges must be smoothed. Cancellous bone (obtained through a small cortical opening of the lateral condyle more posterior) is inserted and impacted (Fig. 34.9). Additional fixation is possible using resorbable sutures. To finish, the lateral retinaculum is reconstructed in 60° of knee flexion.

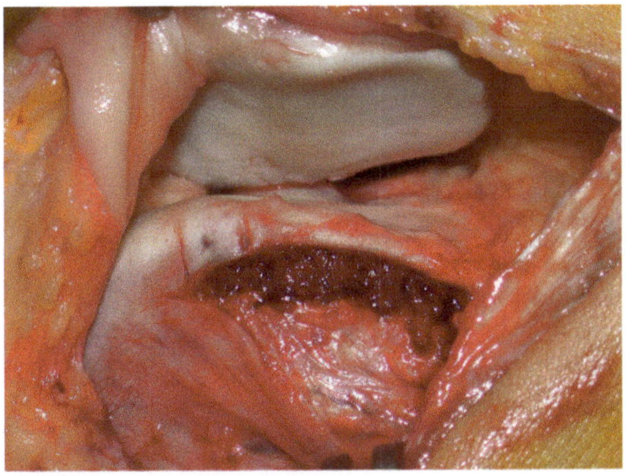

**Fig. 34.9** Lengthening osteotomy

#### 34.2.3.4 Postoperative Rehabilitation

The postoperative rehabilitation aims to center the patella in the trochlea, to balance the soft tissue structures, and to strengthen the muscle groups. Partial weight bearing is necessary for 4 weeks. The ROM starts immediately with 0° – 0° – 80° (continuous passive motion included). Full sport activities are possible after 3 months.

### 34.2.4 Flat Trochlea

#### 34.2.4.1 Physical Examination

The patella is well centered or lateralized with the quadriceps muscle relaxed. Maximum quadriceps contraction pulls the patella to lateral and causes lateral subluxation. In 30° of knee flexion, the patella is less lateralized, but the persisting overhang causes a vacuum effect on the lateral structures. The overhang is caused by tight lateral soft tissues. The apprehension test is positive and painful to lateral, negative to medial. Testing the patellar mobility to lateral, no osseous resistance is noted. Patellar mobility is decreased to medial.[7,10]

#### 34.2.4.2 Imaging

##### Radiographs

The lateral radiograph shows trochlear dysplasia. The anteroposterior radiograph reveals lateralization of the patella.

##### Axial CT Evaluation

Axial CT scans confirm trochlear dysplasia. In axial CT scans in 0° extension, the patella is subluxed to the lateral and tilted; the lateral trochlea is flat (Fig. 34.10a).

Quadriceps contraction leads to increased lateral patellar subluxation (Fig. 34.10b). In 30° of knee flexion, the patella is more centered, but still lateralized (caused by the tight lateral structures).

#### 34.2.4.3 Surgery

Conservative treatment is not successful, as it may not influence the structural failure with the trochlear dysplasia. Only surgical treatment may improve the pathomorphology.

Surgery must advise three problems: the flat lateral condyle with the dysplastic trochlea, the tight lateral soft tissues, and the insufficient medial stabilizing structures.[7,10]

##### Elevation

The surgical procedure consists of three steps: reconstruction (elevation) of the lateral condyle, lengthening of the lateral structures, and shortening and imbricating of the medial structures.[6,7,10]

Surgery starts with a parapatellar lateral arthrotomy. The flat and the trochlea are inspected. The incomplete lateral osteotomy goes from the proximal edge of the lateral trochlea to distal, always ending proximal to the sulcus terminalis (Fig. 34.11). The osteotomy is opened carefully using a chisel. Fracture of the distal cartilage may occur and has no consequence. Sharp edges must be smoothened. The lateral condyle is then lifted up[1], cancellous bone (taken from the lateral femoral condyle) inserted, and impacted. The amount of raising depends on the form of the trochlea and the femoral condyle. In most cases 5–6 mm are sufficient. Overcorrection must be avoided. Additional fixation is possible using sutures. This reconstruction improves the osseous stability. The last step consists of shortening and imbricating the MPFL and in some cases also the medial retinaculum. The lateral retinacula are adapted in about 50–60° of knee flexion to guarantee lengthening and to eliminate the preoperatively increased lateral pull. Complications are possible. They include fracturing of the lateral condyle, too much thinning of the osteochondral flap of the lateral trochlea, and loosening of the cancellous bone.

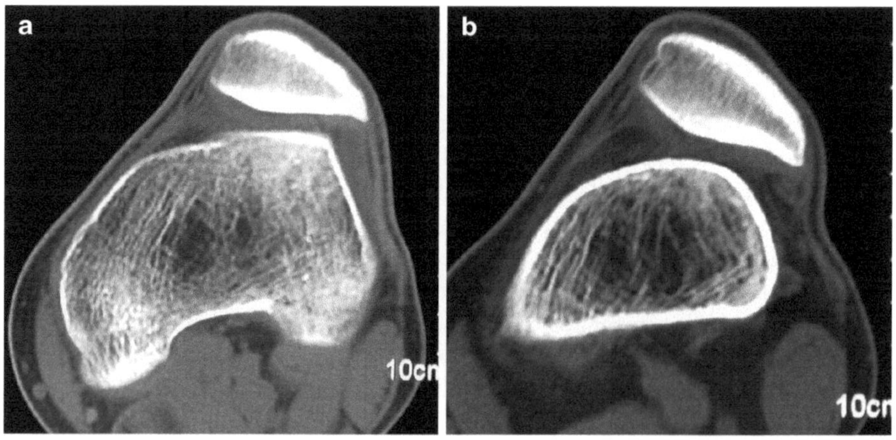


**Fig. 34.10** (**a**) Axial CT scans with flat trochlea and lateralization of the patella (*in extension*). (**b**) Increased lateral subluxation of the patella with muscle contraction (same patient as in Fig. 34.10a)

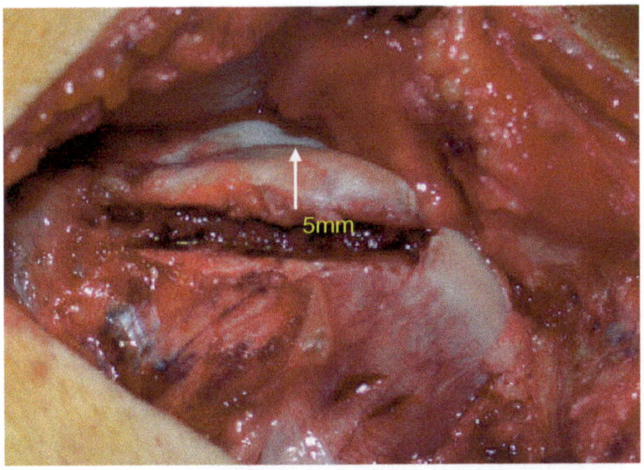


**Fig. 34.11** Intraoperative view after elevation of a flat trochlea

#### 34.2.4.4 Postoperative Rehabilitation

The postoperative rehabilitation aims to center the patella in the trochlea, to balance the soft tissue structures, and to strengthen the muscle groups. Partial weight bearing is necessary for 4 weeks. The ROM starts immediately with 0° – 0° – 80° (continuous passive motion included). Full sport activities are possible after 3 months.

### *34.2.5 Flat and Short Trochlea*

Combined pathologies with a too short, but also a flat lateral facet of the trochlea can occur.[8-10,14] This represents another type of trochlear dysplasia causing lateral patellar instability. The surgical steps consist of a lengthening osteotomy with additional elevation of the lateral facet.

#### 34.2.5.1 Lengthening and Elevation

The lateral approach is the same. The osteotomy is opened carefully and the lateral facet lifted up to the desired height and length of the trochlea. The amount of elevation and lengthening depends on the present pathomorphology. The lateral facet of the sulcus should be higher and longer than the medial facet (Fig. 34.12). The anterior cortex of the femoral shaft serves as an orientation of the necessary elevation. In most cases 5–6 mm elevation is sufficient. Overcorrection (with hypercompression) must be strictly avoided. It also has to be considered that in 5 out of 6 cases the lateral condyle is not too flat, but the floor of the trochlea too high.[12] This would be visible on preoperative axial MR images.

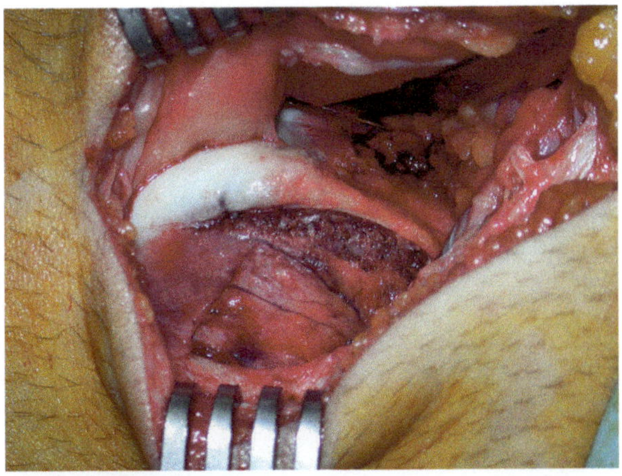

**Fig. 34.12** Lengthening and elevation of a flat and too short trochlea (*right knee*)

#### 34.2.5.2 Postoperative Rehabilitation

Partial weight bearing (10–20 kg) is recommended for 4 weeks to avoid hypercompression of the osteotomy. Range of motion is limited (0°–0°–80°) in the very beginning for some days to decrease swelling and pain. Continuous passive motion starts immediately to optimize the patellofemoral gliding mechanism and to form the reconstructed trochlea. Bicycling and swimming are the first allowed sport activities after 2–3 weeks. Sports activities without any restriction are permitted after 3 months.

### *34.2.6 Central Bump*

#### 34.2.6.1 Physical Examination

The patella is spontaneously subluxed to lateral in extension with relaxed muscles (Fig. 34.13). Contraction of the quadriceps muscle may cause complete patellar dislocation. The apprehension test is severely positive to lateral. With increased flexion, the patella moves more medially on the femur. In higher flexion, the apprehension test may become negative and the patella is better stabilized.

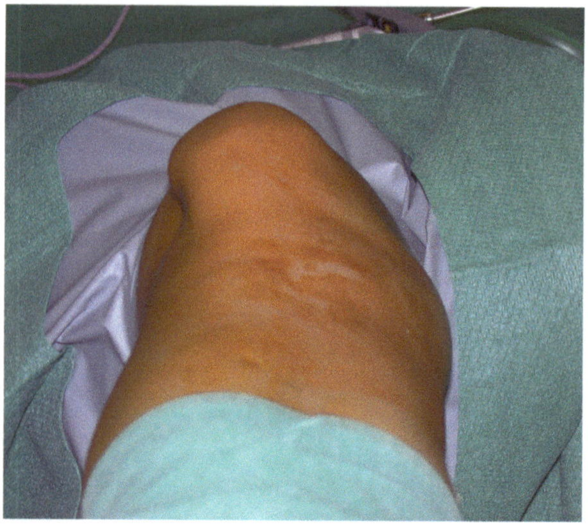

**Fig. 34.13** Subluxation of the patella (*in extension, relaxed*)

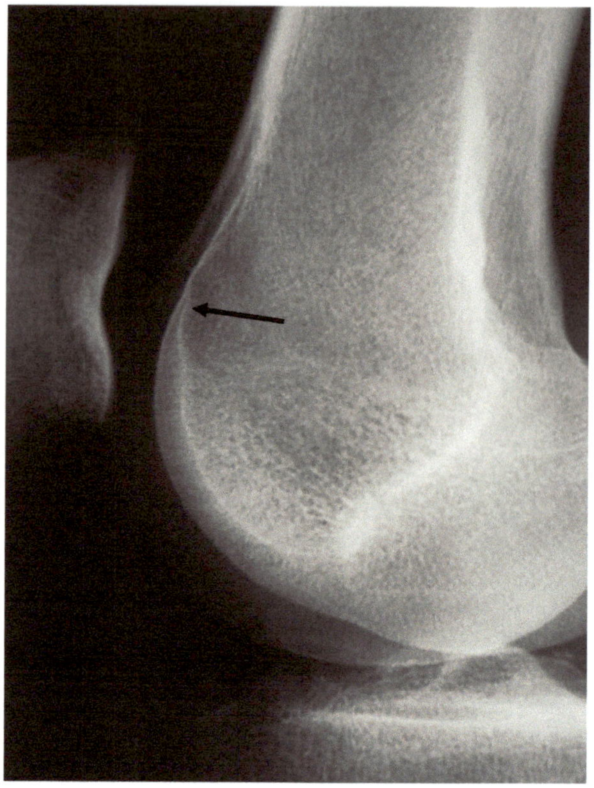

**Fig. 34.14** Crossing sign (*arrow*)

#### 34.2.6.2 Imaging

##### Radiographs

The lateral view shows a severe dysplastic trochlea with crossing sign (Fig. 34.14).[22]

##### CT Evaluation

Axial CT scans illustrate the convex-shaped dysplastic trochlea with a central bump and the severe lateral subluxation of the patella.[7,55]

##### MR Measurements

Axial MRI is the best modality to depict the articular shape of the dysplastic trochlea (Fig. 34.15). But the central bump is also visible on sagittal MRI. In addition, cartilage defects on the patella and the femur can be documented.

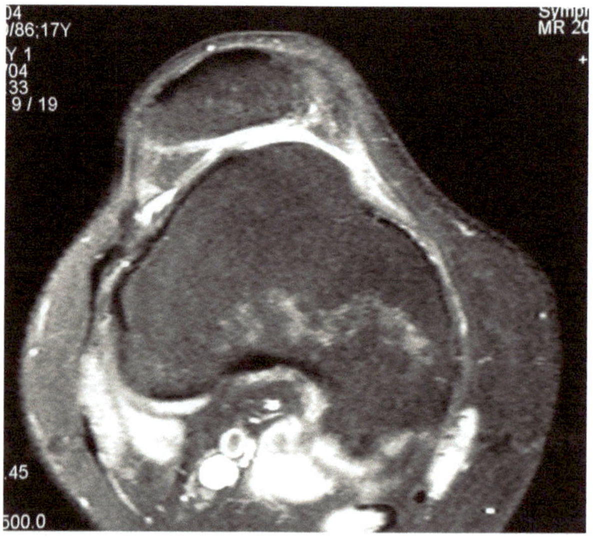


**Fig. 34.15** Central bump with severe patellar subluxation (*axial MRI*)

#### 34.2.6.3 Surgery

The treatment must eliminate the convex-shaped dysplastic trochlea. This provides osseous stability of the patella in the femoral groove, lengthening of the lateral, and doubling of the medial structures.

## Deepening Trochleoplasty

This surgical procedure consists of different steps: lengthening of the lateral retinacula, the iliotibial tract, and the vastus lateralis muscle–tendon-unit, doubling of the medial retinaculum and the medial patellofemoral ligament, and deepening of the trochlear groove (trochleoplasty).[3,4,7,19]

The surgical procedure begins with a lateral arthrotomy.[7] The inspection of the joint shows the convex shape of the trochlea with the central bump (Fig. 34.16). The lateral articular part of the trochlea is too short and too flat (even falling off) in reference to the central part. A lateral incision with the knife separates the articular cartilage from the synovial layer. Then the dysplastic trochlea is partially detached from the lateral condyle using a chisel, beginning proximally. The osteochondral flap remains attached distally (Fig. 34.17). It is extremely important not to break the distal attachment. Deepening of the cancellous femoral bone is now performed using a high-speed burr. It is important that the deepening is continued to proximal into the femoral shaft. This guarantees elimination of the central bump.[3] The correct deepening is reached when the new surface is proximally on the same plane as the anterior femoral cortical bone.[19] The detached osteochondral flap of the trochlea is now thinned with a burr without removing all bone. Thinning is completed when the osteochondral flap is

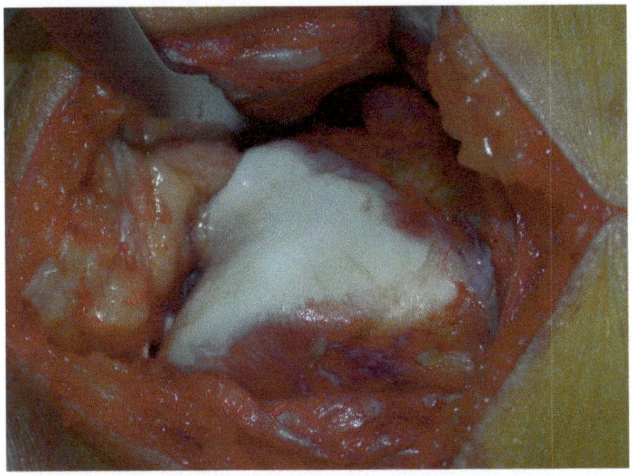

**Fig. 34.16** Convex proximal trochlea with central bump

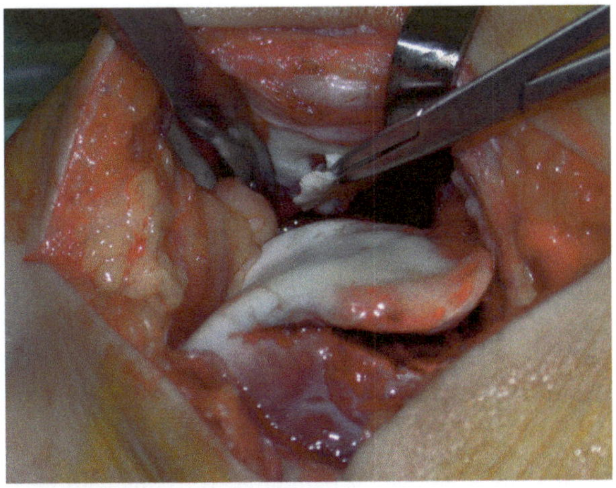

**Fig. 34.17** Osteochondral flap

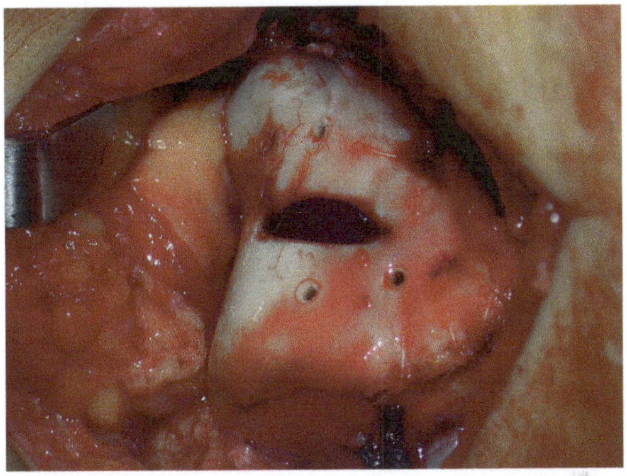

**Fig. 34.18** Deepened trochlea with refixation of the osteochondral flap

elastic and fits into the new form of the femur. This step is tested by carefully using a pestle. To keep the osteochondral flap in the new position and to guarantee deepening of the trochlea, the central part of the trochlea is fixed with a resorbable suture (Vicryl 5 mm).[7] Two lateral and two medial resorbable smart nails (length 16 mm) secure the reposition of the trochlea. The osteotomy gap is filled with the removed cancellous bone. Single sutures adapt the synovial layer to the articular cartilage (Fig. 34.18). The final step consists of doubling the medial and lengthening the lateral structures.

The risks of this technique include breaking of the osteochondral flap, distal detachment, and too much thinning of the flap, decreasing the blood supply.

#### 34.2.6.4 Postoperative Rehabilitation

Partial weight bearing is recommended for 6 weeks. The knee is placed in 20° of knee flexion to add mild compression to the refixed osteochondral flap. ROM is slowly increased during the first 6 weeks, maximal to 90° of knee flexion. The complete recovery time takes 4–6 months.

### 34.2.7 Patella Alta

Patella alta is defined as pathologic proximalization of the patella with reference to the tibia or the trochlea.[5,18,30,31,36] The patellofemoral contact surface is decreased in this position and therefore the passive osseous stabilization is low.[13,34] Improvement of patellar stability is noted during flexion. The femur rolls and glides posteriorly on the tibia during knee flexion and the patella glides in accordance into the trochlea.[29,43] This enlarges the contact area between the patella and the trochlea and improves stabilization and centralization. This biomechanical behavior is the cornerstone for the selection of the necessary treatment.

#### 34.2.7.1 Physical Examination

The patella is positioned proximal and often also lateral. Proximalization and lateralization are even increased with full contraction of the quadriceps muscle. The mobility of the patella in extension is also increased to medial and lateral indicating the instability. Manual medio-lateral movements of the patella are very loose, documenting the missing osseous stability and also a constitutional laxity. The stability is improved with higher flexion. The improved stability eliminates also the lateralization and normalizes the gliding mechanism of the patella in flexion.

#### 34.2.7.2 Imaging

Radiographs

Different measurements (Insall-Salvati, Blackburne-Peel, Caton-Deschamps ratios) of patellar height on standard sagittal radiographs are in clinical use, all with reference to the tibia.[2,5,13,15,18,31] But each of the established ratios has their own inherent problems. The definition of patella height relies heavily on the ratio used.[11,49] The patellotrochlear index (PTI) using sagittal MRI is a more functional measurement and therefore MRI is recommended.[2,11]

MR Measurement

The PTI is the best modality to depict patella alta (Fig. 34.19).[2,11] The index measures the true articular relationship between the patella and the trochlea. Normal values are around 30% ($BL_T$:$BL_P$). Index values of <10% document patella alta.[11]

#### 34.2.7.3 Surgery

Surgical treatment aims to improve the patellofemoral contact and to keep the patella in the trochlea. Excessive proximalization must be corrected. This can be achieved by distalization of the whole extensor apparatus. The amount of distalization is calculated

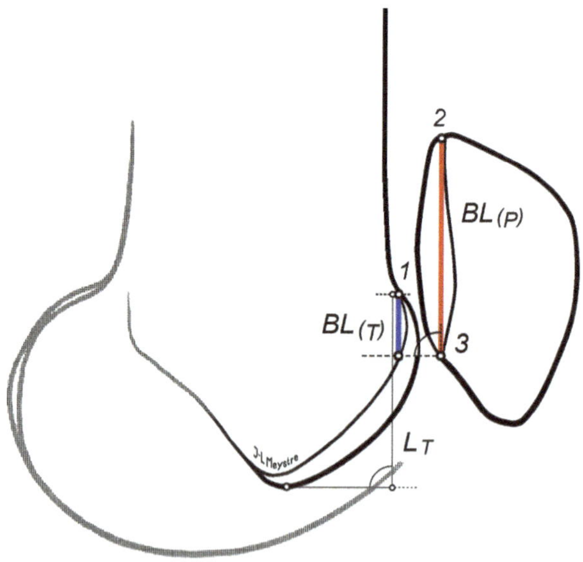


**Fig. 34.19** MR measurement for the patello-trochlear index. *1* Most anterior aspect of the trochlear cartilage, *2* Most superior aspect of the cartilage of the patella, *3* Most inferior aspect of the cartilage of the patella, $BL_P$ Baseline Patella, $BL_T$ Baseline trochlea

using the PTI. The osteotomy of the tibial tubercle is performed in the horizontal plane with a distal oblique cut. A piece of bone with the calculated length is removed after a second cut. The tibial tubercle is finally fixed with two compression screws. Imbrication or lengthening of the medial or lateral soft tissue structures may be necessary.

#### 34.2.7.4 Postoperative Rehabilitation

Partial weight bearing (15 kg) is recommended for 6 weeks. ROM is slowly increased during the first 6 weeks, maximal to 90° of knee flexion. Straight leg rising is not allowed for 6 weeks. The complete recovery time takes 4 months.

## 34.3 Tibia

### *34.3.1 Increased TT/TG*

Increased tibial tubercle–trochlear groove (TT-TG) distance is a radiographic measurement tool representing normal or increased lateralization of the tibial tuberosity. Medialization osteotomy of the tibial tubercle has often been performed in patients with patellofemoral complaints and normal TT-TG distance. Hence, tibial tubercle is transposed to a nonanatomic position. We believe that more restricted indication must be made.

#### 34.3.1.1 Physical Examination

The most obvious finding during physical examination is the lateral patellar position in extension. Lateral dynamic patellar subluxation and tilt may occur when the quadriceps muscle is contracted. The Q angle value (measured in extension without muscular contraction) is generally high. A positive patellar apprehension test to lateral may be present. In combination with other pathologies (i.e., trochlear dysplasia), the patella may almost dislocate completely. In isolated disease, the patella typically is well centered in flexion. Also, the tuberculum–sulcus angle (measured in 90° of flexion) is increased (>10° to the lateral).

#### 34.3.1.2 Imaging

Radiographs

The anteroposterior and the lateral view show mild lateral patellar subluxation. Comparative studies of plain x-rays and CT showed that localization of tibial tubercle could not be defined on plain x-rays even with the aid of markers; hence CT is needed.[56]

Axial CT Evaluation

The TT-TG distance is measured on superposed slices of the distal femur and tibial head (Fig. 34.20). First, the epicondylar line is indicated. Second, the anterior part of the tibial tubercle (star) and the trochlear groove (point) are indicated. Then perpendicular lines are drawn to the epicondylar line. The TT-TG distance corresponds to the length between these two lines (thick black line). TT-TG distances of 20 mm and more are considered as pathologic[10] Measurement error on CT-scans has been found around 3.5 mm.[40]

MRI

MRI is of valuable help to depict other patellofemoral pathology and may even measure TT-TG distance.[46,47]

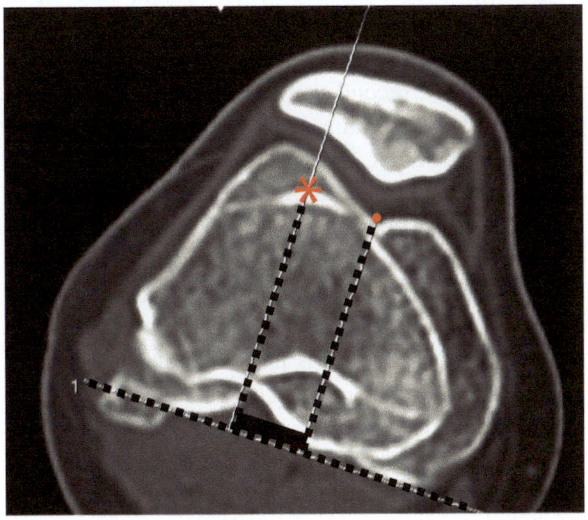


**Fig. 34.20** TT-TG distance measurements on axial CT scans

#### 34.3.1.3 Special Considerations

Differential diagnosis of clinical findings of patients with increased TT-TG distance may be vast; however pathologic tuberculum–sulcus angle is pathognomonic. Increased Q angle should not be used alone as indicator for osteotomy of tibial tubercle. Lateralization of the patella, which is found in patients with increased TT-TG distance, typically decreases the Q angle, and the cadaveric trials could not find any correlation between Q angle and patellar instability. Other biases are gynecoid pelvis, genu valgum, and internal foot rotation.

Increased lateralization of the tibial tubercle in extension can be related to the final tibial external rotation with full knee extension.[44] Therefore, tuberculum–sulcus angle is more sensitive.[7]

Concomitant findings, such as patellar dysplasia, constrained lateral retinaculum, and secondary instability due to patellar dislocation have to be taken into consideration when medial transposition of the tibial tubercle is planned, since results after osteotomy are better in lateralized patella than in unstable patellae.[25] In addition, overcorrections may lead to medial patellofemoral and/or even femorotibial medial osteoarthritis.

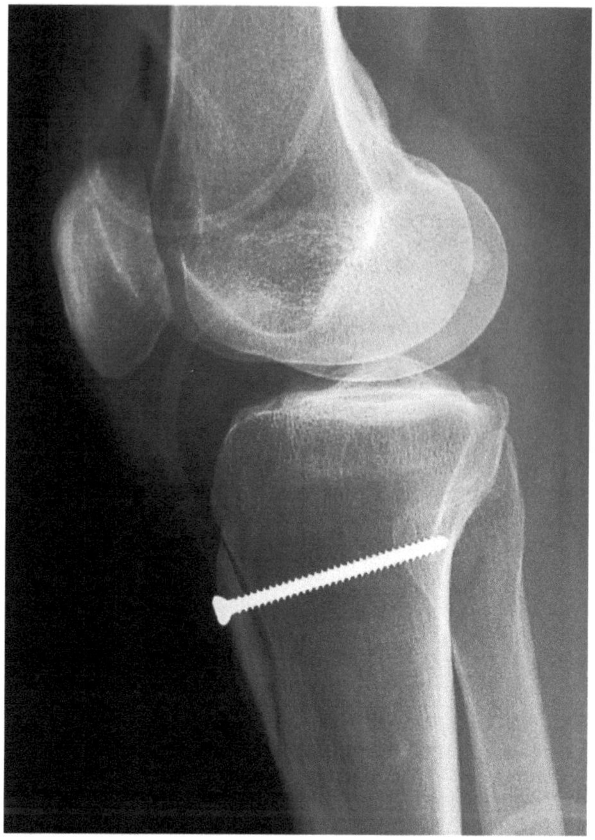

**Fig. 34.21** Screw fixation after medialization of the tibial tubercle

#### 34.3.1.4 Surgery

Treatment must eliminate the lateral patellar subluxation and tilt. The surgical intervention consists of different steps: Mild medialization of the tibial tubercle in reference to the tubercle–sulcus angle. The tubercle–sulcus angle should be 0° [38] and the TT-TG distance 10–15 mm. The second step consists of shortening and doubling of the medial soft tissue structures (retinaculum, patellofemoral ligament). The last step is the lengthening of the lateral soft tissue structures; tightness is controlled in extension and flexion (in about 60°).

The surgical procedure begins with a parapatellar lateral incision and lateral arthrotomy under consideration of the lengthening of the lateral soft tissue structures. The tibial tubercle is partially detached, moved medially, and temporarily fixed with a Kirschner-wire in the planned position (Fig. 34.21). The tubercle–sulcus angle must be controlled in 90° of knee flexion. When the tubercle–sulcus angle is 0°, then the tibial tubercle is fixed definitively with one or two screws. The lateral soft tissue structures are temporarily adapted in 60° of knee flexion with some sutures. The position of the patella, the lateral displacement, and the patella glide are then controlled. The patella should remain in the trochlea; the displacement and glide of the patella to medial and lateral should be one to two quadrants.[38] If this is present, no doubling of the medial soft tissue structures is necessary. If the patellar glide or lateral patellar displacement are still pathologic (more than two quadrants), then shortening of the medial patellofemoral ligament in 40° of flexion and the medial retinaculum may be necessary.

#### 34.3.1.5 Postoperative Rehabilitation

First therapeutic aim after surgery is healing of the osteotomy, quadriceps muscle activation, and static and dynamic normalization of the patella balancing in the trochlea. This requests partial weight bearing for 4 weeks with a maximum of 15 kg load and 30 kg until the 7th week after surgery. Straight leg raise is prohibited during this period. Full weight bearing is allowed after healing osteotomy has been confirmed by conventional radiographs. Bicycle and swimming exercises can be initiated 4 weeks after surgery. After 4 months, no restriction in activities is advised.

#### 34.3.1.6 Summary

Medialization of the tibial tubercle has one specific indication: increased TT-TG distance in CT scans (>20 mm) with symptomatic patellar (sub-) dislocation.[10] All different underlying pathologies must be respected for the treatment. Overcorrection of the tibial tubercle to medial must be strictly avoided. Wrong indications for medialization of the tibial tubercle may cause medial patellofemoral and/or femorotibial osteoarthritis.

Anteromedially tubercle transfer can be indicated when lateralization of the patella combined with lateral cartilage destruction is found.[28]

## References


1. Albee FH. The bone graft wedge in the treatment of habitual dislocation of the patella. *Med Rec*. 1915;88:257-259.
2. Barnett AJ, Prentice M, Mandalia V, et al. Patellar height measurement in trochlear dysplasia. *Knee Surg Sports Traumatol Arthrosc*. 2009;17:1412-1415.
3. Bereiter H. Die Trochleaplastik bei Trochleadysplasie zur Therapie der rezidivierenden Patellaluxation. In: Wirth CJ, Rudert M, eds. *Das Patellofemoral Schmerzsyndrom*. Darmstadt: Steinkopff; 2000:162-177.
4. Bereiter H, Gautier E. Die Trochleaplastik als chirurgische Therapie der rezidivierenden Patellaluxation bei Trochleadysplasie des Femurs. *Arthroskopie*. 1994;7:281-286.
5. Bernageau J, Goutallier D, Debeyre J, et al. Nouvelle technique d'ecploration de l'articulation fémoro-patellaire. Incindinces axiales quadriceps contracté et décontracté. *Rev Chir Orthop Reparatrice Appar Mot*. 1969;61(suppl 2):286-290.
6. Biedert RM. Is there an indication for lateral release and how I do it. Paper presented at: International Patellofemoral Study Group; 2000; Garmisch-Partenkirchen,Germany.
7. Biedert RM. *Patellofemoral Disorders: Diagnosis and Treatment*. New York: Wiley; 2000.
8. Biedert RM. Measurements of the length of the proximal and distal trochlea and the trochlear depth on sagittal MRI in patients wieht lateral patellar subluxation. Paper presented at: International Patellofemoral Study Group; 2005; Lausanne, Switzerland.
9. Biedert RM. Trochlea dysplasia: indications for trochleoplasty (deepening) and raising/shortening/lengthening of flat/short lateral trochlea. Paper presented at: International Patellofemoral Study Group; 2006; Boston, MA, USA.
10. Biedert RM. Osteotomies. *Orthopade*. 2008;37:872-883.
11. Biedert RM, Albrecht S. The patellotrochlear index: a new index for assessing patellar height. *Knee Surg Sports Traumatol Arthrosc*. 2006;14:707-712.
12. Biedert RM, Bachmann M. Anterior-posterior trochlear measurements of normal and dysplastic trochlea by axial magnetic resonance imaging. *Knee Surg Sports Traumatol Arthrosc*. 2009;17:1225-1230.
13. Biedert RM, Gruhl C. Axial computed tomography of the patellofemoral joint with and without quadriceps contraction. *Arch Orthop Trauma Surg*. 1997;116:77-82.
14. Biedert RM, Netzer P, Gal I, et al. The lateral condyle index: a new index for assessing the length of the lateral articular trochlea. Paper presented at: International Patellofemoral Study Group; 2006; Boston, MA, USA.
15. Blackburne JS, Peel TE. A new method of measuring patellar height. *J Bone Joint Surg*. 1977;59-B:241-242.
16. Bruce WD, Stevens PM. Surgical correction of miserable malalignment syndrome. *J Pediatr Orthop*. 2004;24: 392-396.
17. Carrillon Y, Abidi H, Dejour D, et al. Patellar instability: assessment on MR images by measuring the lateral trochlear inclination-initial experience. *Radiology*. 2000;216: 582-585.
18. Caton J, Deschamps G, Chambat P, et al. Patella infera. Apropos of 128 cases. *Rev Chir Orthop Reparatrice Appar Mot*. 1982;68:317-325.
19. Dejour D, Le Coultre B. Osteotomies in patello-femoral instabilities. *Sports Med Arthrosc*. 2007;15:39-46.
20. Dejour D, Locatelli E. Patellar instability in adults. *Surg Tech Orthop Traumatol*. 2001;55:1-6.
21. Dejour H, Walch G, Neyret P, et al. Dysplasia of the femoral trochlea. *Rev Chir Orthop Reparatrice Appar Mot*. 1990;76:45-54.
22. Dejour H, Walch G, Nove-Josserand L, et al. Factors of patellar instability: an anatomic radiographic study. *Knee Surg Sports Traumatol Arthrosc*. 1994;2:19-26.
23. Dejour H, Walch G, Nove-Josserand L, et al. Factors of patellar instability: an anatomoradigraphic analysis. In: Feagin JA Jr, ed. *The Curcial Ligaments. Diagnosis and Treatment of Ligament Injuries About the Knee*. New York: Churchill Livingstone; 1994:261-367.
24. Delgado ED, Schoenecker PL, Rich MM, et al. Treatment of severe torsional malalignment syndrome. *J Pediatr Orthop*. 1996;16:484-488.
25. Diks MJF, Wymenga AB, Anderson PG. Patients with lateral tracking patella have better pain relief following CT-guided tuberosity transfer than patients with unstable patella. *Knee Surg Sports Traumatol Arthrosc*. 2003;11:384-388.
26. Donell ST, Joseph G, Hing CB, et al. Modified Dejour trochleoplasty for severe dysplasia: operative technique and early clinical results. *Knee*. 2006;13:266-273.
27. Feinstein WK, Noble PC, Kamaric E, et al. Anatomic alignment of the patellar groove. *Clin Orthop Relat Res*. 1996;331:64-73.
28. Fulkerson JP, Becker GJ, Meaney JA, et al. Anteromedial tibial tubercle transfer without bone graft. *Am J Sports Med*. 1990;18:490-496.

29. Goodfellow J, Hungerford DS, Zindel M. Patello-femoral joint mechanics and pathology. 1. Functional anatomy of the patello-femoral joint. *J Bone Joint Surg*. 1976;58-B:287-290.
30. Grelsamer RP, Proctor CS, Bazos AN. Evaluation of patellar shape in the sagittal plane. A clinical analysis. *Am J Sports Med*. 1994;22:61-66.
31. Grelsamer RP, Tedder JL. The lateral trochlear sign. Femoral trochlear dysplasia as seen on a lateral view roentgenograph. *Clin Orthop Relat Res*. 1992;281:159-162.
32. Heegaard J, Leyvraz PF, Curnier A, et al. The biomechanics of the human patella during passive knee flexion. *J Biomech*. 1995;28:1265-1279.
33. Heegaard J, Leyvraz PF, Van Kampen A, et al. Influence of soft structures on patellar three-dimensional tracking. *Clin Orthop Relat Res*. 1994;299:235-243.
34. Hille E, Schulitz KP, Henrichs C, et al. Pressure and contract-surface measurements within the femoropatellar joint and their variations following lateral release. *Arch Orthop Trauma Surg*. 1985;104:275-282.
35. Hoppenfeld S, DeBoer P. *Surgical Exposures in Orthopaedics: The Anatomic Approach*. Philadelphia: Lippincott Williams & Wilkins; 2003.
36. Insall J, Salvati E. Patella position in the normal knee joint. *Radiology*. 1971;101:101-104.
37. James SL, Bates BT, Osternig LR. Injuries to runners. *Am J Sports Med*. 1978;6:40-50.
38. Kolowich PA, Paulos LE, Rosenberg TD, et al. Lateral release of the patella: indications and contraindications. *Am J Sports Med*. 1990;18:359-365.
39. Lee TQ, Anzel SH, Bennett KA, et al. The influence of fixed rotational deformities of the femur on the patellofemoral contact pressures in human cadaver knees. *Clin Orthop Relat Res*. 1994;302:69-74.
40. Lustig S, Servien E, Aït Si Selmi T, et al. Factors affecting reliability of TT-TG measurements before and after medialization: a CT scan study. *Rev Chir Orthop Reparatrice Appar Mot*. 2007;92:429-436.
41. Malaghem J, Maldague B. Depth insufficiency of the proximal trochlear groove on lateral radiographs of the knee: relation to patellar dislocation. *Radiology*. 1989;170:507-510.
42. Masse Y. Trochleoplasty. Restoration of the intercondylar groove in subluxations and dislocations of the patella. *Rev Chir Orthop Reparatrice Appar Mot*. 1978;64:3-17.
43. Müller W, Wirz D. Anatomie, Biomechanik und Dynamik des Patellofemoralgelenks. In: Wirth CJ, Rudert M, eds. *Das Patellofemorale Schmerzsyndrom*. Darmstadt: Steinkopff; 2000:3-19.
44. Pagenstert GI, Bachmann M. Klinische Untersuchung bei patellofemoralen Problemen. *Orthopade*. 2008;37: 890-903.
45. Percy EC, Strother RT. Patellalgia. *Physician Sportsmed*. 1985;13:43-59.
46. Schoettle PB, Zanetti M, Seifert B, Pfirrmann CW, Fucentese SF, Romero J. The tibial tuberosity-trochlear groove distance: a comparative study between CT and MRI scanning. *Knee*. 2006;13(1):26-31.
47. Schoettle PB, Zanetti M, Seifert B, et al. The tibial tuberosity-trochlear groove distance; a comparative study between CT and MRI scanning. *Knee*. 2006;13:26-31.
48. Scuderi GR. Surgical treatment for patellar instability. *Orthop Clin North Am*. 1992;23:619-630.
49. Seil R, Muller B, Georg T, et al. Reliability and interobserver variability in radiological patellar height ratios. *Knee Surg Sports Traumatol Arthrosc*. 2000;8:231-236.
50. Servien E, Neyret P, Si Selmi TA, et al. Radiographs. In: Biedert RM, ed. *Patellofemoral Disorders: Diagnosis and Treatment*. New York: Wiley; 2004:87-100.
51. Tecklenburg K, Dejour D, Hoser C, et al. Bony and cartilaginous anatomy of the patellofemoral joint. *Knee Surg Sports Traumatol Arthrosc*. 2006;14:235-240.
52. van Huyssteen AL, Hendrix MR, Barnett AJ, et al. Cartilage-bone mismatch in the dysplastic trochlea. An MRI study. *J Bone Joint Surg*. 2006;88-B:688-691.
53. van Kampen A, Huiskes R. The three-dimensional tracking pattern of the human patella. *J Orthop Res*. 1990;8: 372-382.
54. Verdonk R, Jansegers E, Stuyts B. Trochleoplasty in dysplastic knee trochlea. *Knee Surg Sports Traumatol Arthrosc*. 2005;13:529-533.
55. Von Knoch E, Böhm T, Bürgi ML, et al. Trochleaplasty for recurrent patellar dislocation in association with trochlear dysplasia. *J Bone Joint Surg Br*. 2006;88-B:1331-1335.
56. Wagenaar F, Koeter S, Anderson P, et al. Conventional radiography cannot replace CT scanning in detecting tibial tubercle lateralisation. *Knee*. 2007;14:51-54.

# Sulcus Deepening Trochleoplasty

35

David Dejour and Paulo Renato F. Saggin

## 35.1 Introduction

Trochlear dysplasia is defined as abnormal shape of the trochlea. It can be shallow, flat, or convex (Fig. 35.1). This anatomic status fails to provide adequate constraint to the normal patellar tracking. Trochlear dysplasia is found in 96% of the population with objective patellar dislocation (at least one true dislocation).[8] This clearly demonstrates its importance in the genesis of the instability. Trochleoplasty is the surgical procedure used to correct trochlear dysplasia. Sulcus deepening trochleoplasty is one of the techniques. It was described by Masse in 1978.[12] Later, Henri Dejour has modified and standardized the procedure.[7]

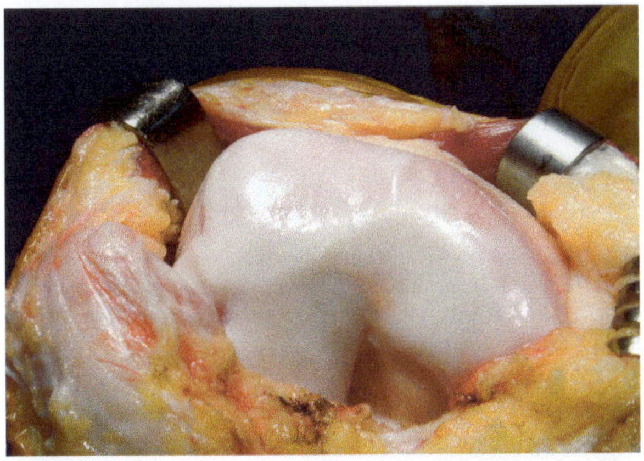

**Fig. 35.1** High-grade trochlear dysplasia (anterior view of a right knee). There is no sulcus, and in the lateral aspect (left) a big bump can be observed

## 35.2 Radiologic Features and Classification

X-ray lateral projections of normal trochleae (obtained with perfect superimposition of both femoral condyles) will typically show the contour of the facets, and posterior to them, the line representing the deepest points of the groove.[10,11] The line representing the bottom of the groove is continuous with the intercondylar notch line, and extends anteriorly and proximally. It may end posteriorly to the condyles line (type A) or join the medial condyle line in the superior part of the trochlea (type B).[7]

Trochlear dysplasia, on lateral projections, is defined by the crossing sign, where the radiographic line of the trochlear sulcus crosses (or reaches) the projection of the anterior part of the femoral condyles or trochlear facets. The crossing point represents the exact location where the groove reaches the same height of the femoral condyles, meaning that the trochlea becomes flat in this exact location. The position of the trochlear groove is abnormally prominent in relation to the anterior femoral cortex. While in normal knees it is usually at a mean distance of 0.8 mm posterior to a line tangent to the anterior femoral cortex, in knees with dysplastic trochlea its mean position is 3.2 mm forward this same line[8] (Fig. 35.2).

Two other features are typical of dysplastic trochleae on lateral views: the supratrochlear spur and the double contour sign. The supratrochlear spur can be clearly identified during the surgical exposure, located in the superolateral aspect of the trochlea. It corresponds to an attempt of containing the lateral displacement of the patella. The double contour represents the subchondral bone of the medial hypoplastic facet, seen

P.R.F. Saggin (✉)
Instituto de Ortopedia e Traumatologia (I.O.T.),
Passo Fundo, RS, Brazil
e-mail: paulosaggin@yahoo.com.br

V. Sanchis-Alfonso (ed.), *Anterior Knee Pain and Patellar Instability*,
DOI: 10.1007/978-0-85729-507-1_35, © Springer-Verlag London Limited 2011

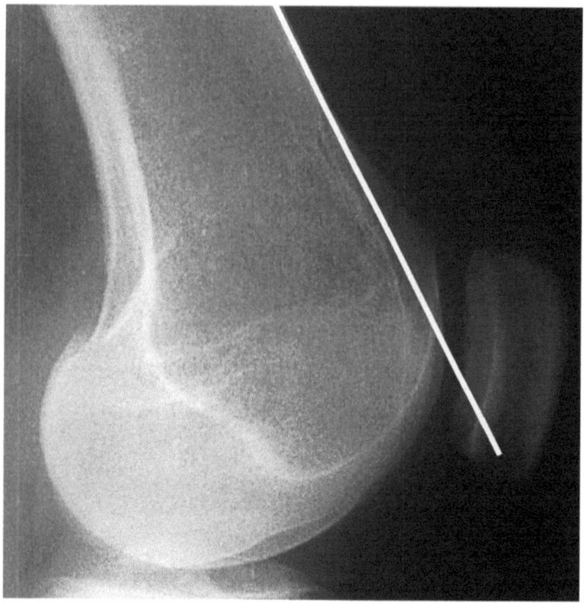

**Fig. 35.2** The trochlear bump is calculated as the amount of trochlea which is in front of a line parallel to the anterior femoral cortex. Alternatively, the sulcus floor position can also be calculated from this line

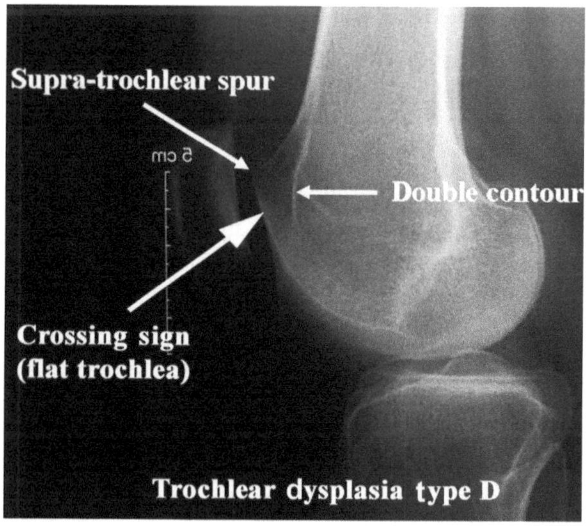


**Fig. 35.3** To analyze the trochlear dysplasia a true profile is needed with a perfect superimposition of the posterior femoral condyles. The three trochlear dysplasia signs are: (1) the crossing sign; (2) the supratrochlear spur; and (3) the double-contour which goes below the crossing sign

posterior to the lateral one on this projection (Fig. 35.3). Based on these signs, trochlear dysplasia may be classified in four types (Fig. 35.4)[6,16]:

- Type A: presence of crossing sign on the lateral true view. The trochlea is shallower than normal, but still symmetric and concave.
- Type B: crossing sign and trochlear spur. The trochlea is flat or convex in axial images.
- Type C: there is the presence of the crossing sign and the double-contour sign on the lateral view, representing the densification of the subchondral bone of the medial hypoplastic facet. There is no spur, and in axial views, the lateral facet is convex and the medial hypoplastic.
- Type D: combines all the mentioned signs: crossing sign, supratrochlear spur, and double-contour sign. In axial view, there is clear asymmetry of the facets height, also referred to as a cliff pattern.

Axial views obtained at 45° (Merchant) will allow the measurement of the sulcus angle.[13] From the point of the bottom of the groove, two lines are drawn connecting it with the most superior point of each facet. The mean normal value defined by Merchant was 138° (SD ± 6), and angles greater than 150° are considered abnormal. Abnormal (dysplastic) trochleae will show higher angles, and at times, no measurement can be made, since there is no sulcus. Alternatively, 30° views will provide those measurements with better trochlear shape assessment.[5] The subjective impression of the trochlear shape is very important, and should be taken in no more than 45° of knee flexion. Greater flexion angles show the lower part of the trochlea, where it becomes deeper, and the examiner can miss the trochlear dysplasia.

The computerized tomography scan will help the x-ray analysis by giving a complete analysis of the trochlea, from the top to the lower part. Tridimensional reconstruction can also be obtained for global shape assessment. Magnetic resonance imaging is another modality in which dysplasia is well documented and the cartilaginous shape of the sulcus can be evaluated.

## 35.3 Function and Biomechanics

To understand the principles of modifying trochlear shape, its function must be well understood. The lateral facet of the trochlea is oriented obliquely in both sagittal and coronal planes. It deviates anteriorly and laterally from the bottom of the groove. The articulating opposed lateral patellar surface follows this orientation. The

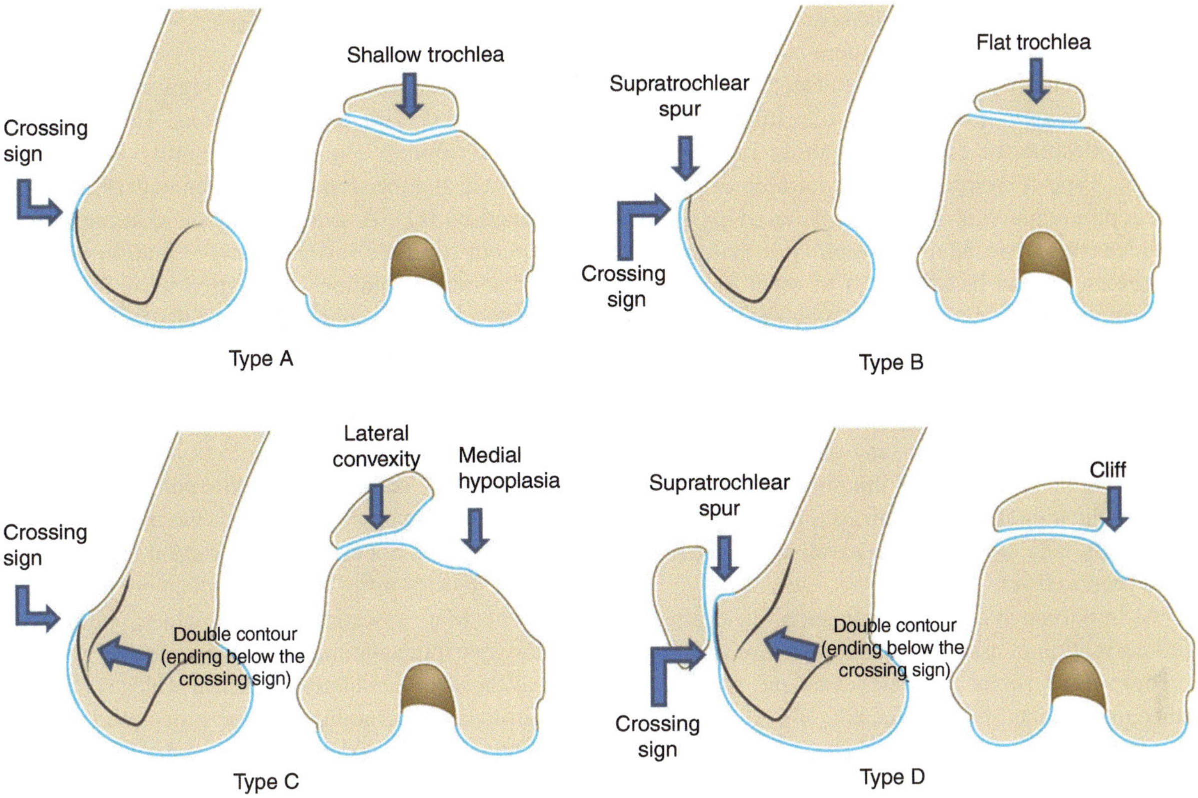


**Fig. 35.4** Trochlear dysplasia classification according to David Dejour

patella rests in front of the femoral cortex in total extension, but engages the trochlea in early flexion. A posteriorly directed force, the patellofemoral reaction force, pushes the patella against the trochlea, and as a result of the articulating surfaces orientation, a medial vector is created, directing patellar tracking.[2] The mediolateral tracking of the patella has been shown as highly erratic in cases of trochlear dysplasia.[3]

From this biomechanical explanation, one conclusion is obvious: the trochlea guides patellar tracking. Not only patellar subluxation or lateral displacement is dependent on trochlear shape, but also patellar tilt. There is a high statistical correlation between patellar tilt and the type of trochlear dysplasia.[16] The more severe the dysplasia, the higher the patellar tilt.

Other feature, not included in trochlear function, but derived from the same principle is that patellofemoral reaction force depends on the trochlear prominence. The bigger the trochlear prominence, the greater the compressive reaction force, thus creating an "antimaquet" effect. Inversely, by diminishing the protrusion, the reaction force is also expected to be diminished.

## 35.4 Goals

Deepening trochleoplasty is proposed to correct trochlear dysplasia, creating a new and more anatomic sulcus and restoring patellar stability. It also corrects the excessive trochlear prominence, thus decreasing the patellofemoral reaction force.

## 35.5 Indications

Trochleoplasty indications are precise: high-grade trochlear dysplasia with patellar instability and/or abnormal patellar tracking, in the absence of established osteoarthritis. Open growth plates are a contraindication to this type of trochleoplasty. The type of dysplasia should be observed when indicating the procedure, since not all procedures fit all deformities. Types B and D are the most suitable to sulcus deepening trochleoplasty.

Patients with type C dysplasia are not good candidates to the procedure, since there is no prominence to be corrected. They can be submitted to an alternative procedure (lateral facet elevating trochleoplasty), despite the controversy about its long-term results. Type A dysplasia is not suitable to any trochlear procedure. It is also not considered high-grade trochlear dysplasia. Major instability or maltracking, if present, should be attributed to other anatomical abnormalities (excessive tibial tubercle – trochlear groove distance, excessive patellar tilt, or patella alta).

The degree of instability should also be taken into account. Trochleoplasty, as any other surgical procedure, is liable to failure, and this should be considered when indicating the procedure to a patient with mild symptoms, and when no conservative treatment has been proposed yet.

As important as a precise indication, the evaluation and correction of associated abnormalities have to be accomplished (tibial tubercle–trochlear groove distance, patella alta, and patellar tilt). TT-TG correction is not always necessary as the trochleoplasty procedure lateralizes the groove, thus diminishing the TT-TG distance. The sulcus deepening trochleoplasty should be understood as part of the *menu à la carte* (specific procedures for each of the main factors in patellar instability). We routinely associate a soft tissue procedure to the trochleoplasty. Formerly, a VMO plasty was added. Since 2003 medial patellofemoral ligament (MPFL) reconstruction is the procedure of choice.

## 35.6 Surgical Technique

The procedure is performed under regional anesthesia, complemented with patient sedation. The patient is positioned supine. The entire extremity is prepared and draped, and incision is performed with the extremity flexed by 90°. A straight midline skin incision is carried out from the superior patellar margin until the tibiofemoral articulation. The extremity is then positioned in extension and a medial full thickness skin flap is developed. The arthrotomy is performed through a midvastus adapted approach: medial retinaculum sharp dissection starting over the 1–2 cm medial border of the patella, and blunt dissection of VMO fibers starting distally, at the superomedial pole of the patella, extending approximately 4 cm into the muscle belly.

The patella is not everted but a careful inspection of chondral injuries using ICRS classification and proper treatment (flap resection, microfracture, autologous chondrocyte implantation) is done if requested, and then the patella is retracted laterally. The trochlea is exposed and peritrochlear synovium and periosteum are incised along their osteochondral junction, and reflected from the field using a periosteal elevator (Fig. 35.5). The anterior femoral cortex should be visible to orientate the amount of deepening. Changing the degree of flexion-extension of the knee allows a better view of the complete operatory field and avoids extending the incision.

Once the trochlea is fully exposed, the new one is planned and drawn with a sterile pen. The new trochlear groove is drawn using as starting point the intercondylar notch. From there, a straight line representing it is

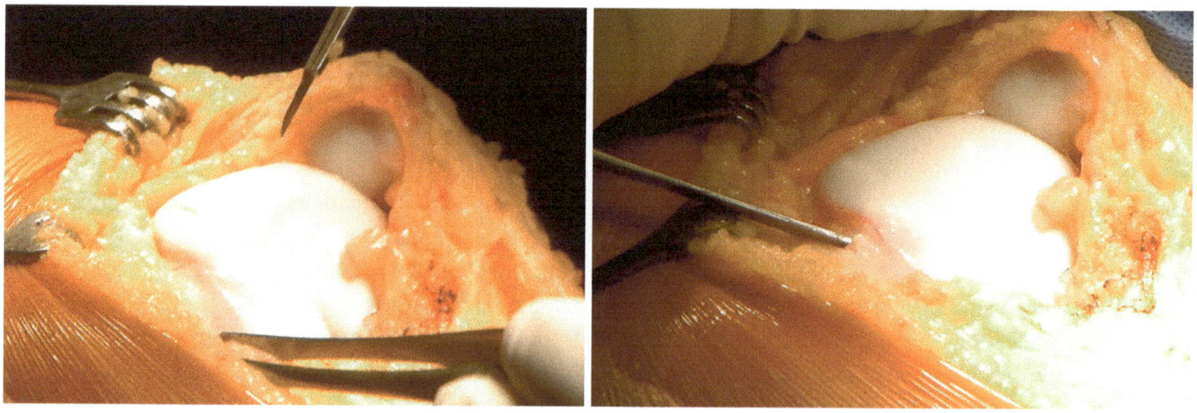

**Fig. 35.5** Surgical exposure. The periosteum is incised along the osteochondral edge and reflected away from the trochlear margin. The anterior femoral cortex should be visible to guide the bone resection

directed proximally and 3–6° laterally. The superior limit is the osteochondral edge. Two divergent lines are also drawn, starting at the notch and going proximally through the condylotrochlear grooves, representing the lateral and the medial facet limits. They should not enter the tibiofemoral articulation (Fig. 35.6).

The next step is accessing the under surface of the femoral trochlea. For this purpose, a thin strip of cortical bone is removed all around the trochlea. The width of the strip is equal to the prominence of the trochlea from the anterior femoral cortex, i.e., the bump formed. A sharp osteotome is used and gently tapped. A rongeur is used next, to remove the bone.

Subsequently, cancellous bone must be removed from the under surface of the trochlea. A drill with a depth guide set at 5 mm is used to ensure uniform thickness of the osteochondral flap, thus maintaining an adequate amount of bone attached to the cartilage. The guide also avoids injuring the cartilage or getting too close to it; otherwise thermal injury could be produced. The shell produced must be sufficiently compliant to allow modeling without being fractured. Cancellous bone removal is extended until the notch. More bone is removed from the central portion where the new trochlear groove will rest.

Light pressure should be able to model the flap to the underlying cancellous bone bed in the distal femur. The groove, and sometimes the lateral facet external margin, should be cut to allow further modeling, which is done by gently tapping over a scalpel (Fig. 35.7).

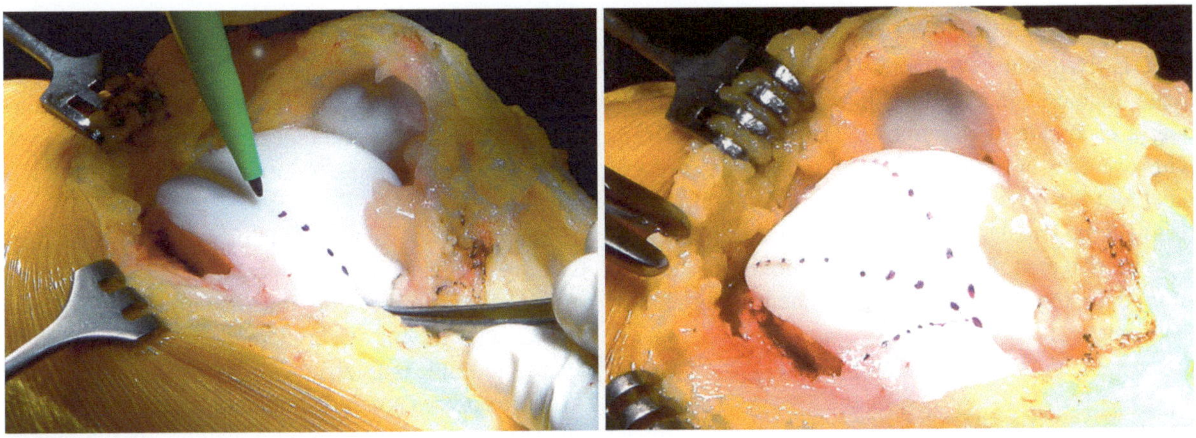

**Fig. 35.6** After the surgical exposure, the new trochlea is drawn. From the intercondylar notch, the bottom of the sulcus and the facets are planned

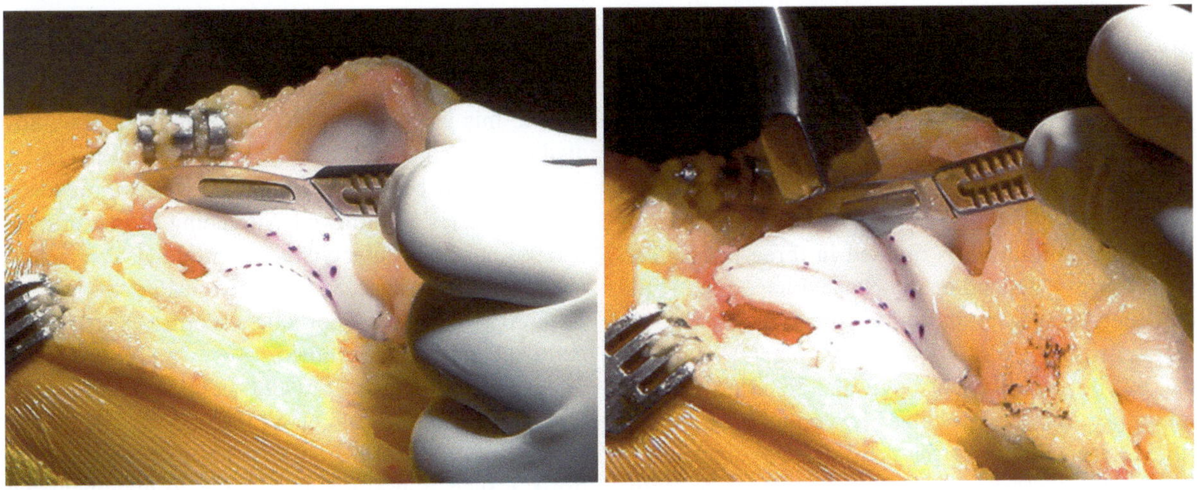

**Fig. 35.7** In order to allow further modeling to the underlying bone bed, the osteochondral flaps may be cut in the sulcus and facets lines

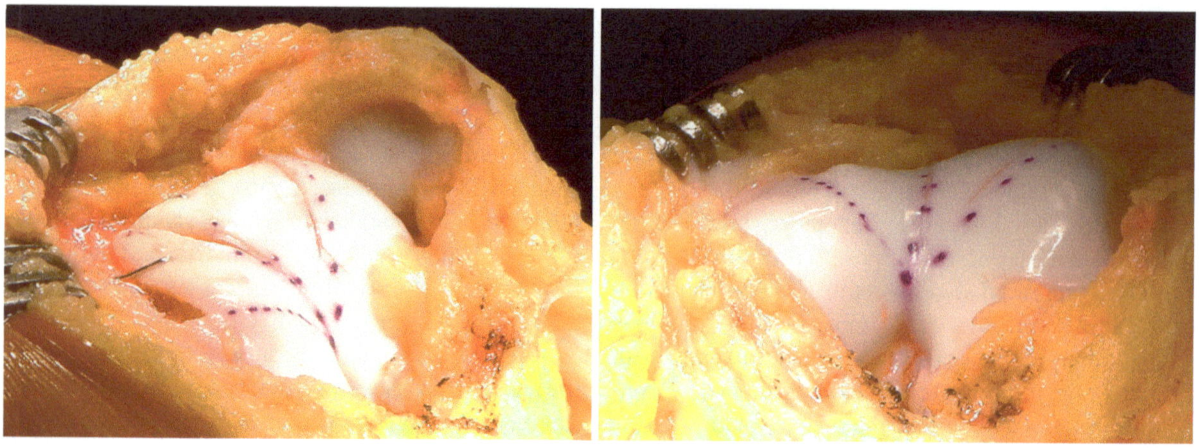

**Fig. 35.8** Lateral and anterior views of dysplastic trochlea after trochleoplasty. Notice that the sulcus and facets relationship resembles a "normal trochlea"

If the correction obtained is satisfactory, the new trochlea is fixed with two staples (K-Wires of one millimeter diameter modeled upon the trochlear shape), one in each side of the groove. The staples are fixed with one arm in the cartilaginous upper part of each facet and the other arm in the anterior femoral cortex (Fig. 35.8). Patellar tracking is tested and measures may be obtained. Periosteum and synovial tissue are sutured to the osteochondral edge and anchored to the staples.

## 35.7 Postoperative Care

Trochleoplasty does not need weight protection or range of motion limitation. Movement like CPM (continuous passive motion) may also improve cartilage healing. Quadriceps wasting is another negative outcome of immobilization. The main principles guiding trochleoplasty rehabilitation are presented here, but the associated procedures performed have to be taken into account, and rehabilitation has to fit them too.

The rehabilitation is divided in three phases and specific goals depend on the phase. Phase 1 starts the day after the surgery and ends at the 45th day. Passive and active range of motion is encouraged to improve the nutrition of the cartilage and to allow further modeling of the trochlea by patellar tracking. Immediate weight bearing is allowed (with crutches and an extension brace for 4 weeks). Walking without the brace is allowed generally after 1 month depending on the quadriceps recovery. Range of motion is gradually regained (avoiding forced or painful postures). Dynamic quadriceps strengthening with weights on the feet or tibial tubercle is prohibited; only isometric contraction and stimulation are allowed.

Phase 2 goes from the 46th day until the 90th day. Cycling is possible with weak resistance initially. Active ascension of the patella can be performed seated, with the leg stretched and the knee unlocked, by static and isometric quadriceps contractions. Active exercises are added but dynamic and isometric quadriceps strengthening with weights on the feet or tibial tubercle is still forbidden. The anterior and posterior muscular chains are stretched. Weight-bearing proprioception exercises are started when full extension is complete, first in bipodal stance and later in monopodal stance when there is no pain.

Phase 3 is passed from the fourth until the sixth month: this is the sports phase. Running can be initiated on a straight line. Closed kinetic chain muscular reinforcement between 0° and 60° with minor loads but long series are allowed. Stretching of the anterior and posterior muscular chains is continued. The patient is encouraged to proceed with the rehabilitation on his own. After 6 months sports on a recreational or competitive level can be resumed.

Six weeks postoperatively control radiographs, including AP and lateral views (Fig. 35.9) and an axial view in 30° of flexion, are taken. After 6 months a control CT scan is performed in order to document the obtained correction (Fig. 35.10).

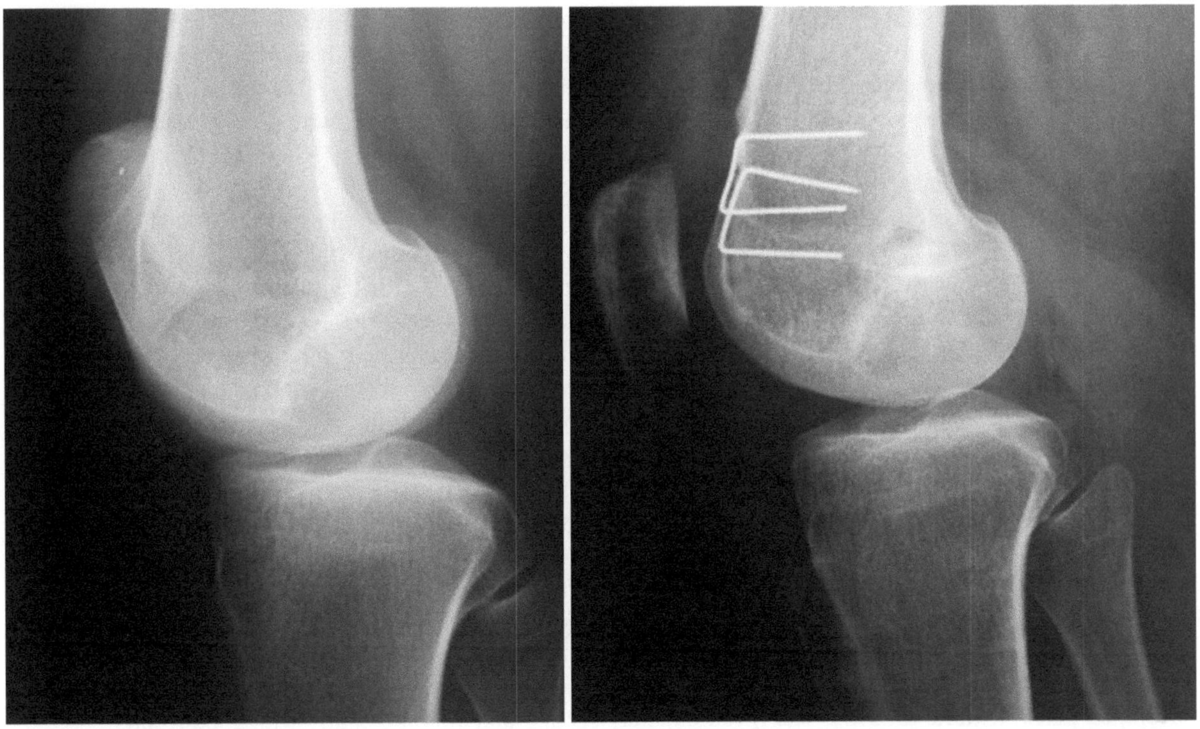

**Fig. 35.9** Pre- and postoperative lateral x-rays showing the resection of the supratrochlear bump and trochlear prominence correction. Additionally, patellar tilt is clearly improved

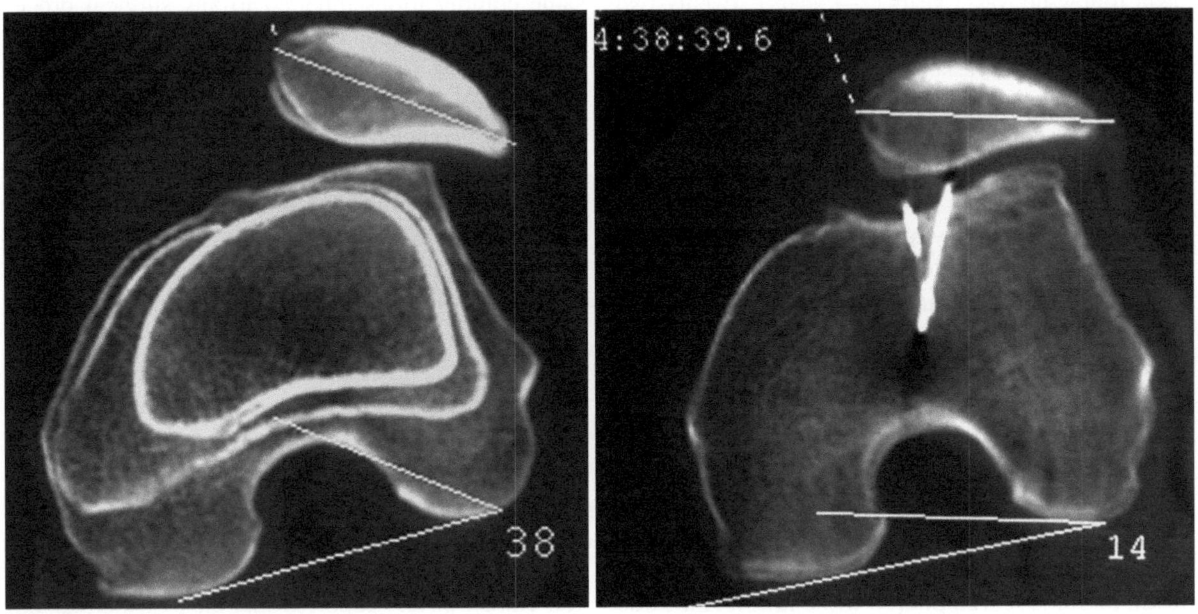


**Fig. 35.10** CT scan axial views before and after trochleoplasty. The trochlear sulcus is restored and patellar tilt is corrected. Patellar subluxation is also improved

## 35.8 Results

Two series reviewing deepening trochleoplasty were published in the *10èmes Journées Lyonnaises de Chirurgie du Genou* in 2002:

The first group included 18 patients, who failed patellar surgery for instability. The mean age at surgery was 24 years. There were no patients lost to follow-up. The mean follow-up was 6 years (2–8 years). The new surgery was six times indicated for pain and 12 times for recurrence of instability. The average number of surgeries before the trochleoplasty was two. The deepening trochleoplasty was associated to a tibial tubercle medialization in eight patients, in six to a tibial tubercle distalization, and all to a VMO plasty. All patients were reviewed clinically with the IKDC form and radiographically. Sixty five percent were satisfied or very satisfied. The knee stability was rated 13 times A and five times B. Twenty eight percent of the patients had residual pain, and this was correlated to the cartilage status at surgery. Two patients developed patellofemoral arthritis. The mean patellar tilt was 35° (18–48°) in the preoperative setting, and improved to 21°(11–28°) with the quadriceps relaxed and 24° (16–32°) with the quadriceps contracted after the surgery.

In the second group there were 44 patients. They had no antecedents of patellofemoral surgery. The mean follow-up was 7 years (2–9 years). Twenty-two tibial tubercle medializations, 26 distalizations, and 32 VMO plasties were associated at the time of surgery. These patients were also reviewed clinically with the IKDC form and radiographically. Eighty five percent were satisfied or very satisfied. The knee stability was rated 31 times A and 13 times B. Five percent had residual pain, but this was not correlated to the cartilage status at surgery. No patellofemoral arthritis was noted. The mean patellar tilt preoperatively was 33° (24–52°), and improved postoperatively to 18° (9°–30°) with the quadriceps relaxed and 22° (14–34°) with the quadriceps contracted.

Verdonk et al.[17] described 13 procedures (deepening trochleoplasty) with a mean follow-up of 18 months. Patients were assessed using the Larsen–Lauridsen score considering pain, stiffness, patellar crepitus, flexion, and loss of function. Seven patients scored poorly, three fairly, and three well. On a subjective scoring system, however, six patients rated the result as very good, four as good, and one as satisfactory. Only two patients found the result inadequate and would never undergo the procedure again. Thus, 77% were satisfied with the procedure.

Donnel et al.[9] described 15 patients (17 knees) submitted to deepening trochleoplasty with a mean follow-up of 3 years. Trochleoplasty was indicated if there was a boss greater than 6 mm, and associated procedures were performed as required. Of the 17 knees, 9 had undergone previous surgery for patellar instability. The boss height was reduced, postoperatively, from an average of 7.5 to 0.7 mm. Tracking became normal in 11 knees and 6 had a slight J-sign. Seven knees had mild residual apprehension. Seven patients were very satisfied, six were satisfied, and two were disappointed. The Kujala score improved from an average of 48 to 75 out of 100.

A different procedure (Bereiter's trochleoplasty[4]) has also been documented in two series by von Knoch et al.[18] and Schottle et al.[14] with good results.

## 35.9 Complications

Patients submitted to trochleoplasty are at risk for the same complications inherent to any surgical procedure – infection, deep venous thrombosis, etc. Specific complications include trochlear necrosis, incongruence with the patella, hypo- or hypercorrection, and cartilage damage. Schottle performed biopsies in three patients after trochleoplasty, showing cartilage cell viability and flap healing. He concluded that the risk of cartilage damage is low.[15]

Incongruence with the patella is another concern. Studies with longer follow-ups are needed before any assumptions can be made about its consequences. Also, arthritis development is multifactorial, and all patients operated on for patellofemoral instability seem more prone to degeneration than those treated conservatively.

Arthrofibrosis incidence varies between series, but is always a possibility in patellofemoral surgery. Verdonk et al.[17] reported 5 cases in 13 patients, while von Knoch et al.[18] reported that all patients had full range of motion in the final visit. The number of previous or associated procedures is variable, and this can interfere with data interpretation.

Recurrence of instability is very rare after such procedure, and is more likely to result from missed associated abnormalities. The procedure results for pain are not consistent, and although it seems to improve it, some patients may complain of worsening.

## 35.10 Alternative Procedures

### 35.10.1 *Lateral Facet Elevating Trochleoplasty*

This procedure was pioneered by Albee in 1915.[1] It consists of an oblique osteotomy under the lateral facet, where a corticocancellous bone wedge is interposed, with the apex medial and the base lateral. The osteotomy advances until the place of the trochlear groove, but does not disrupt it, producing a hinge in its medial aspect. The result is that it elevates the more lateral aspect of the trochlear lateral facet, and also increases its obliquity, thus increasing the containment force acting on the patella. At least 5 mm of subchondral bone should be maintained to avoid trochlear necrosis.

It is effective for patellar containment, but at the same time it increases the patellofemoral reaction force when it increases the trochlear protuberance. Pain and arthritis may result from this.

### 35.10.2 *Bereiter Trochleoplasty*

This technique was described by Bereiter and Gautier in 1994.[4] In this method, a lateral parapatellar approach is performed, the trochlea exposed, and the synovium dissected away from it. Then, a thin osteochondral flake with 2 mm of subchondral bone is elevated from the trochlea extending until the intercondylar notch. The distal femoral subchondral bone is deepened and refashioned with osteotomes and a high-speed burr. Next, the osteochondral flap is seated in the refashioned bed, and fixed with 3 mm wide vicryl bands, passing through the center of the groove and exiting in the lateral femoral condyle. The periosteum is reattached to the edge of the cartilage and closure of the wound is performed.

## 35.11 Conclusion

Deepening trochleoplasty is a very rare procedure in the objective patellar dislocation group. It concerns only patients with high-grade trochlear dysplasia types B or D and abnormal patellar tracking. It is part of the "menu à la carte" which leads to the correction of the anatomical abnormalities, one by one. The technical procedure is highly demanding and prone to complications. It is, however, very effective in providing stability.

## References


1. Albee F. Bone graft wedge in the treatment of habitual dislocation of the patella. *Med Rec*. 1915;88:257-259.
2. Amis AA. Current concepts on anatomy and biomechanics of patellar stability. *Sports Med Arthrosc*. 2007;15:48-56.
3. Amis AA, Oguz C, Bull AM, et al. The effect of trochleoplasty on patellar stability and kinematics: a biomechanical study in vitro. *J Bone Joint Surg*. 2008;90-B:864-869.
4. Bereiter H, Gautier E. Die trochleaplastik als chirurgische therapie der rezidivierenden patellaluxation bei trochleadysplasie des femurs. *Arthroskopie*. 1994;7:281-286.
5. Davies AP, Bayer J, Owen-Johnson S, et al. The optimum knee flexion angle for skyline radiography is thirty degrees. *Clin Orthop Relat Res*. 2004;423:166-171.
6. Dejour D, Le Coultre B. Osteotomies in patello-femoral instabilities. *Sports Med Arthrosc*. 2007;15:39-46.
7. Dejour H, Walch G, Neyret P, et al. Dysplasia of the femoral trochlea. *Rev Chir Orthop Reparatrice Appar Mot*. 1990; 76:45-54.
8. Dejour H, Walch G, Nove-Josserand L, et al. Factors of patellar instability: an anatomic radiographic study. *Knee Surg Sports Traumatol Arthrosc*. 1994;2:19-26.
9. Donell ST, Joseph G, Hing CB, et al. Modified Dejour trochleoplasty for severe dysplasia: operative technique and early clinical results. *Knee*. 2006;13:266-273.
10. Maldague B, Malghem J. Significance of the radiograph of the knee profile in the detection of patellar instability. Preliminary report. *Rev Chir Orthop Reparatrice Appar Mot*. 1985;71(suppl 2):5-13.

11. Malghem J, Maldague B. Depth insufficiency of the proximal trochlear groove on lateral radiographs of the knee: relation to patellar dislocation. *Radiology*. 1989;170:507-510.
12. Masse Y. Trochleoplasty. Restoration of the intercondylar groove in subluxations and dislocations of the patella. *Rev Chir Orthop Reparatrice Appar Mot*. 1978;64:3-17.
13. Merchant AC, Mercer RL, Jacobsen RH, et al. Roentgenographic analysis of patellofemoral congruence. *J Bone Joint Surg*. 1974;56-A:1391-1396.
14. Schottle PB, Fucentese SF, Pfirrmann C, et al. Trochleaplasty for patellar instability due to trochlear dysplasia: a minimum 2-year clinical and radiological follow-up of 19 knees. *Acta Orthop*. 2005;76:693-698.
15. Schottle PB, Schell H, Duda G, et al. Cartilage viability after trochleoplasty. *Knee Surg Sports Traumatol Arthrosc*. 2007;15:161-167.
16. Tavernier T, Dejour D. Knee imaging: what is the best modality. *J Radiol*. 2001;82:387-405; 407-408.
17. Verdonk R, Jansegers E, Stuyts B. Trochleoplasty in dysplastic knee trochlea. *Knee Surg Sports Traumatol Arthrosc*. 2005;13:529-533.
18. von Knoch F, Bohm T, Burgi ML, et al. Trochleaplasty for recurrent patellar dislocation in association with trochlear dysplasia. A 4 to 14-year follow-up study. *J Bone Joint Surg*. 2006;88-B:1331-1335.

# Rotational Tibial Osteotomy

# 36

Robert A. Teitge and Roger Torga-Spak

## 36.1 Background

An abnormal increase in external tibial torsion was one of the components of the "Miserable Malalignment" syndrome described by Stan James in 1979.[10] It is becoming recognized that these various miserable malalignment components: increased femoral anteversion, squinting patella, genu varum, patella alta, increased Q-angle, external tibial rotation, tibia varum and compensatory pronation of the foot, described by James may exist independent of one another and they may independently contribute to anterior knee pain and to patellar instability.

The geometry of the lower extremity skeleton largely determines the direction of load application at the patellofemoral (PF) joint with the amount of load depending on the body mass, the length of the lever arms, the surface area of the PF joint and the velocity of the moving system and the force of muscles which provide acceleration and deceleration. Deviations from normal horizontal plane limb alignment may result in the knee joint flexion–extension axis which advances obliquely as the body moves forward. Anatomic deviations from normal include femoral anteversion or retroversion, excess internal or external tibial torsion, genu valgum or varus, hyperpronation, and Achilles contracture.

If the knee joint axis is twisted out of its normal horizontal plane alignment while the quadriceps is contracting a side-directed force is created which acts on the patella attempting to displace it causing an increased strain on the PF ligaments and retinaculum and an imbalanced direction of force on the PF articular surface.

If these side-directed vectors exceed biological tolerance, for example, an inward pointing of the knee increases the lateral direction of pull of the quadriceps, so the pull on the medial patellofemoral ligament (and also medial retinaculum and medial meniscopatellar ligament) is increased and the direction of pressure on the patella is altered creating an increase on the lateral facet and a decrease on the medial facet (Fig. 36.1), either instability or arthrosis may result. The radiographic appearance of subchondral density under the patellar facets is a useful clue to the mechanical environment (Fig. 36.2). In the absence of overt tissue failure, pain may be the only symptomatic manifestation of this increased side-directed vector.

With normal gait the knee joint axis lies perpendicular to the direction of forward motion with a small (<10°) turning inward and outward.[12] The foot

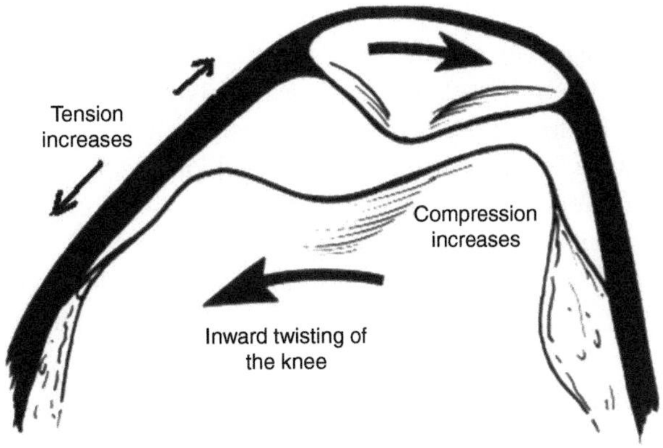


**Fig. 36.1** When the knee joint is twisted medially and the body is moving forward, there is an increase in tension on the medial PF ligaments, while the lateral PF joint is compressed

R. Torga-Spak (✉)
Faculty of Orthopaedics and Traumatology, Department of Surgery, Instituto Universitario CEMIC, Buenos Aires, Argentina
e-mail: rtorgaspak@gmail.com

V. Sanchis-Alfonso (ed.), *Anterior Knee Pain and Patellar Instability*,
DOI: 10.1007/978-0-85729-507-1_36, © Springer-Verlag London Limited 2011

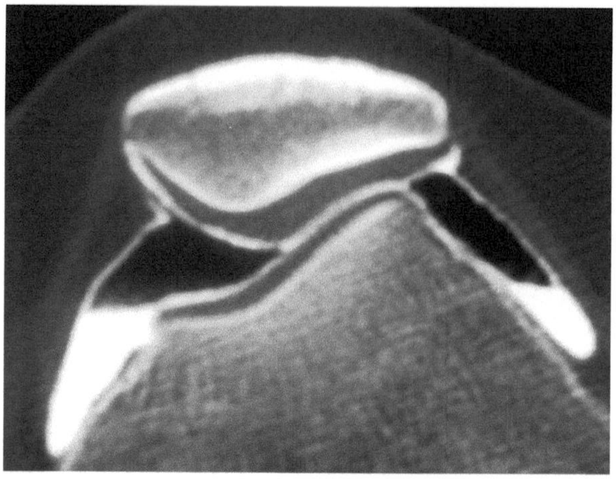

**Fig. 36.2** Increased sclerosis in the lateral patellar facet subchondral bone is indicative of a localized chronic increase in pressure. This double contrast CT arthrogram demonstrates intact articular cartilage on both the patella and the trochlea with an increased compression of cartilage at the lateral facet

also tends to move in a fairly constant direction (foot progression angle).[17] The foot progression angle (FPA) is generally defined as the angle between the long axis of the foot and the direction of body progression and averages between 10° and 15°.[13,17] It has been shown that the FPA remains similar despite differences in the torsion of the tibia or femur.[17] It is likely that this is because proper ankle dorsiflexion cannot occur during gait if the ankle joint axis is not aligned with the direction of forward movement or because this presents the most stable position of the foot on the ground. Hip rotation must vary if there are changes in the torsion of the long bones and the FPA stays constant. Alterations in both femoral and tibial torsion changes the effective lever arm of the hip stabilizers[1] and may account for the frequency of soft tissue complaints around the hip and pelvis as well as the increased pelvic tilt and lumbar lordosis seen in these patients. Examples of the change in the position of the hip and knee with a constant foot progression angle and changes in tibial torsion are seen in Fig. 36.3.

Figure 36.3 drawings show a constant foot progression angle of 13° (Seber average FPA) for a normal male torsional alignment, a normal female torsional alignment, and a female with 30° excess external tibial torsion. One can study the variations in knee joint axis progression with these common tibial torsion patterns. Yoshioka[22-24] has found identical femoral anteversion in both males and females, equal genu valgus in both males and females, but an increase in external tibial torsion and an increase in foot external rotation in females over males. This increase in external foot rotation may account for the apparent increased genu valgus in females, for the increased incidence of PF symptoms in females and even for the increased incidence of ACL tears in females.

## 36.2 Tibial Torsion Measurements

To measure limb alignment in the horizontal (Transverse) plane a CT rotational study is obtained. This is a CT scan which overlaps cuts from the femoral head, base of the femoral neck or lesser trochanter, the distal femur, the proximal tibia, the tibial tuberosity, and the ankle joint (see Chap. 14). These cuts allow lines to be drawn representing the axes of the proximal and distal tibia and proximal and distal femur to define the long bone torsion. Additionally trochlear dysplasia, patellar tilt, patellar shift, the density of the subchondral trabeculae, knee torsion, and the tibial tuberosity–trochlear groove offset (TT-TG), may be recognized.

The measurement of tibial torsion by CT has not been standardized. Jakob et al.[9] described a common sense method superimposing cuts across the proximal tibia and distal ankle joint. We have attempted to use the anatomic measurements of the tibia described by Yoshioka et al.[24] as a basis for measuring the proximal tibial reference line (Fig. 36.4). Blinded repeat measurements made by our orthopedic radiologist have produced a measurement variation of less than 1° indicating that reproducible measurements are possible. Le Damany[11] has reported 23.7° to be normal tibial torsion. Seber et al.[17] calculated external tibial torsion to be 30° (range: 16–50°) in a group of 50 "normal" (asymptomatic) men, but their measurement technique was unique in selecting the location for drawing the proximal tibial reference line. Eckhoff et al.[6] noted variations between 15° and 30°. Turner[20] found 19° (SD, 4.8°) in a control group and 24.5° (SD, 6.3°) in a group with unstable patella. The CT measurements of Sayli et al.[16] averaged 30–35°. Tamari et al.[19] have recently demonstrated a lack of reliability between currently used measurement methods and this is a major stumbling block in answering the question of how much of an influence does altered tibial torsion

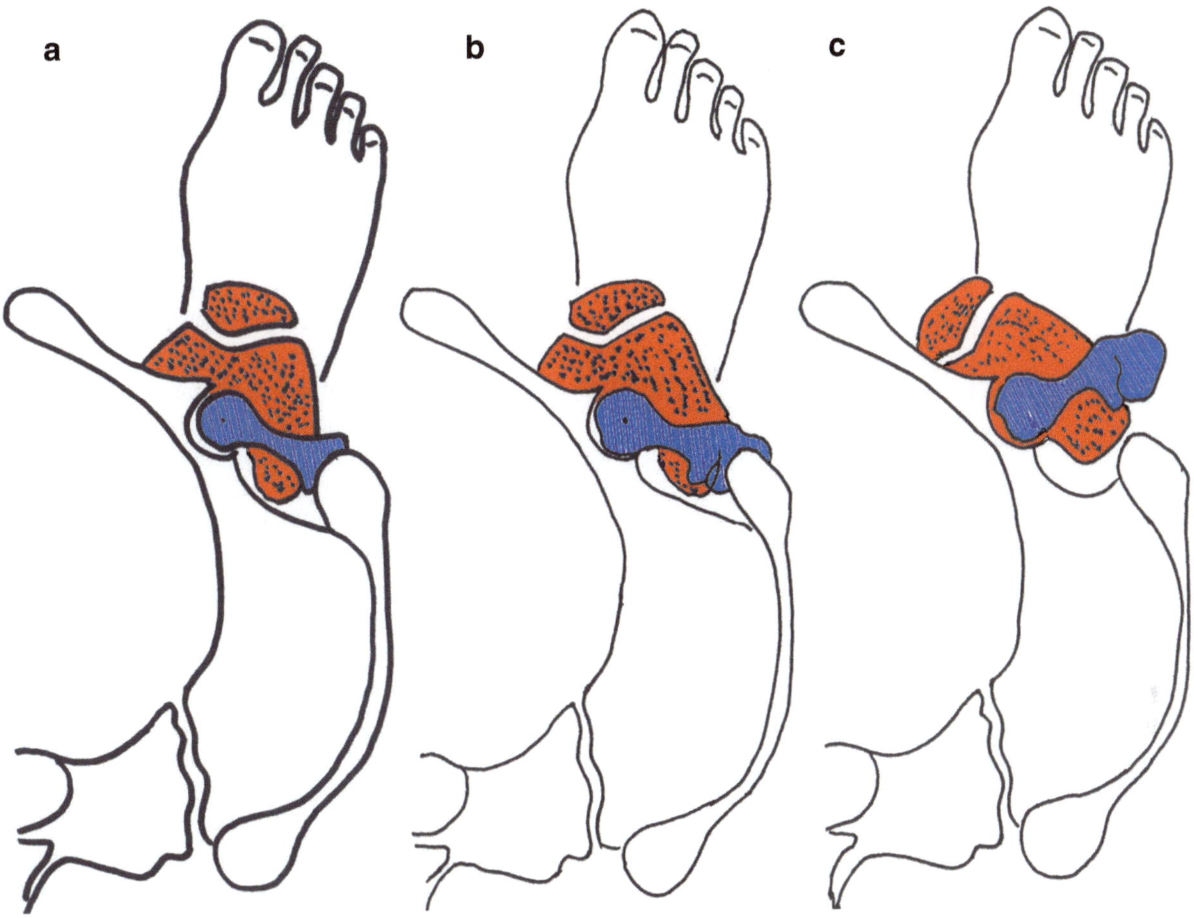


**Fig. 36.3** (**a**) Normal male with femoral anteversion of 13° and external tibial torsion of 21°. Note that with a foot progression angle of 13°, the knee joint faces slightly outward. (**b**) Normal female: 13° femoral anteversion, 27° tibial torsion (external). Note that knee joint is pointing slightly inward, and the greater trochanter slightly more anterior than the normal male. (**c**) Female with 30° increase in tibial torsion. To keep the foot progression angle normal the knee joint axis points inward nearly 30° causing increased strain on the medial knee and increased lateral PF pressures. The hip appears markedly internally rotated with the greater trochanter pointing somewhat anteriorly

play in PF instability and when osteotomy may be useful. In addition to the above method taken after Yoshioka's anatomic measurements, we also use the femoral epicondylar axis as the proximal reference for tibial torsion because we are interested in the relationship of the knee joint axis to the ankle joint axis. The error of twisting across the knee joint while obtaining the CT must be avoided to use this reference. Cobb et al.[3] pointed out "there has been no universally accepted tibial frame of reference" and proposed a new method to locate more accurately the horizontal plane axis at the proximal tibia. They used CT cuts taken at the top of the tibia and placed concentric circles over the medial and over the lateral tibial plateau such that the center of the circles could be connected to create an axis. Yoshioka's anatomical study[22] reported a lateral torsion of 21° in males and 27° in females, a significant difference and the only femoral or tibial difference he noted between males and females. If this observation is confirmed, it is of major importance as it may explain the widely quoted difference between men and women in the frequency of PF disorders. It may also explain the reported increased incidence of ACL tears in women.

The goal of tibial rotational osteotomy is to realign the knee joint axis with the ankle joint axis in the transverse plane leaving the trochlear–tubercle relationship normal. To reestablish the normal tibial torsion it

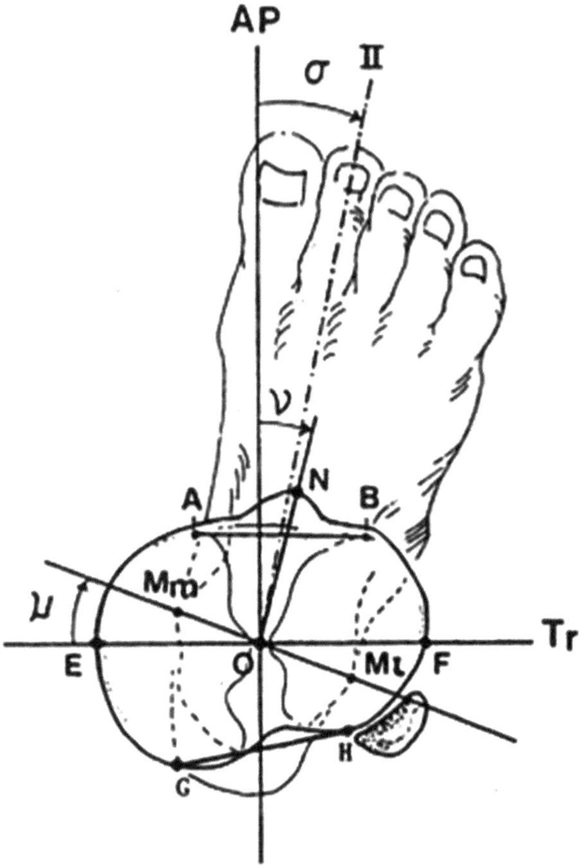


**Fig. 36.4** The measure of tibial torsion is the angle μ measuring the angle between the transverse axis of the proximal tibia ($T_r$) and the ankle joint axis $M_m$-$M_L$ (From Yoshioka et al.[24])

probably makes little difference at what level between the tuberosity and the ankle joint the osteotomy is performed. The Q-angle and TT-TG (tibial tubercle–trochlear groove distance) are important biomechanical arrangements which should not be changed. Rotational osteotomy of the tibia should therefore be performed below the level of the tibial tuberosity. Huberti and Hayes[8] showed that increasing the Q-angle by 10° increased PF contact pressure by 45% and decreasing the Q-angle by 10° increased the PF pressure by 53%. Van Kampen and Huskies[21] has determined during biomechanical studies that altering tibial rotation had a greater influence on PF tracking and pressure than either anterior tuberosity elevation or lateral retinacular release. These observations suggest that any alteration of the normal trochlea–tibial tuberosity relationship may have unrecognized biomechanical consequences. If the tibial tuberosity is located in an abnormally lateral position relative to the horizontal axis of the proximal tibia then a rotational osteotomy above the tibial tuberosity may be considered. However, if the knee joint axis advances sideways to the direction of forward motion of the body, this axial obliquity will not be changed by moving the tibial tubercle. If a 10° decrease in Q-angle from normal increased PF pressure by 53%,[8] then a 20° internal rotation of the tubercle as a consequence of 20° internal rotational tibial osteotomy at a level proximal to the tibial tuberosity to correct a 20° increase in external tibial torsion could be disastrous.

While the goal of operative treatment is to normalize the biomechanics through restitution of normal anatomy, the morbidity of surgery may dictate otherwise. When multiple anatomic abnormalities exist, it is not known which may be more important. If a patient has recurrent patellar lateral subluxation, articular cartilage damage, trochlear dysplasia, patella alta, an Achilles contracture, a femoral anteversion of 45°, an external tibial torsion of 45°, and a genu valgum of 10° is it best to perform a varus, external rotational femoral osteotomy, a distalization of the tibial tuberosity, a reconstruction of the medial patellofemoral ligament, a trochlear osteotomy, an internal rotation osteotomy of the tibia, and an Achilles lengthening? These abnormal findings are often quite subtle but combinations are surprisingly common. The surgical approach to correct all abnormalities may be quite logical from the biomechanical view but excessive from the surgical morbidity view. A biomechanical solution with osteotomy may mean that the ligament reconstruction is not necessary as the displacing forces are reduced and cartilage restoration is not necessary because the compressive forces are reduced and changed in direction. As yet no biomechanical studies indicate which surgery alters biomechanics the most.

Our experience suggests that for most cases with torsion of the femur or tibia exceeding 30° from normal surgery is indicated. For those with torsion exceeding 20° from normal, surgery is thought to be beneficial but for cases with abnormality less than 20° the accuracy of surgery or the morbidity may not justify the smaller biomechanical changes. Turner's data however found 19° average external torsion in a control group and 24.5° in a patellar instability group and Takai found 9° average femoral anteversion in a control group and 23° average in a PF arthrosis group, so it is possible that very small limb torsional differences are significant.

## 36.3 Surgical Technique

Our personal experience is most with osteotomy of the proximal tibia below the tubercle. I have seen slower union with rotational osteotomy in the mid diaphysis fixed with an intramedullary nail and the control of alignment in the coronal and sagittal plane can be more difficult when there is an abrupt change in the patients' intramedullary canal. For fixation of a proximal tibial osteotomy (below the level of the tuberosity) I have seen more rapid union using the angled blade plate for compression of the osteotomy surfaces. However, the geometry of the proximal tibia makes the blade insertion always a problem because rotational correction requires the side plate must lie along the flat surface of the tibia; thus the angle at which the blade is inserted into the proximal fragment will determine rotational correction. The precise direction for blade insertion is not easily referenced off the relatively flat surface of the tibia. Control of varus–valgus is also difficult after blade insertion when tension is applied to the plate with the articular tension device as the tension is applied eccentric to the central axis of the tibia and therefore pulls the distal fragment toward the tensioned side. My experience with locking plates is that healing is much slower than with rigid compression. The locking plates allow greater ease of rotational control but a distortion of varus valgus correction still can occur if compression is applied to the osteotomy. Tensioning of a locked plate which is fixed first to the proximal fragment may also result in the distal plate sitting well off the bone producing an unsatisfactory prominence which can tent the anterior compartment muscle laterally or the sparse subcutaneous tissue if the plate is placed medially. Locking plates without high compression of the osteotomy fragments definitely result in delayed union time and more postoperative discomfort. Comparing laterally placed compression plates with medially placed locking plates in the same patient, patients have preferred the lateral plate location. Comparing laterally placed compression blade plates with medially placed compression blade plates, patients have also preferred the lateral location.

To monitor the rotational correction we still place two 2.5 mm K-wires from anterior to posterior in the tibia one proximal and one distal to the anticipated level of osteotomy. These may be parallel or they may subtend the desired angle of correction in the transverse plane but an attempt is made to place them parallel in the sagittal plane. If they are parallel then the angle between the two after manipulation of the osteotomy fragments indicates the angular change in torsion. If they have been placed at an angle to each other which equals the desired correction then the pins are brought parallel to indicate the desired correction. It is important to have these as reference points before the osteotomy is cut. Comparison of the pin alignment in the sagittal plane will indicate whether a change in flexion or extension has occurred. To estimate any change in varus or valgus, radiographic control using an alignment rod extended from the center of the hip joint to the center of the talus is used. However, it must be noted that small changes in inward or outward rotation of the limb will change the apparent varus–valgus measurement. Currently this author uses a navigation system (Praxim) which indicates the changed alignment in all three planes (transverse, coronal, and sagittal) (Fig. 36.5). It is

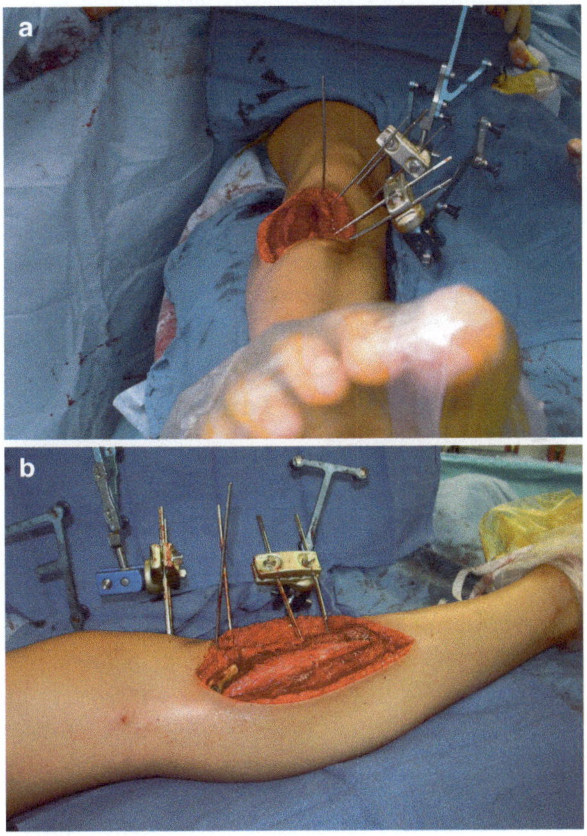

**Fig. 36.5** Internal rotational osteotomy of the tibia for correction of 30° excess external tibial torsion. (**a**) Note that K-wires which were set parallel and located above and below the osteotomy are now separated by the 30° internal rotation of the distal fragment. (**b**)Navigation reflectors (trackers) are attached to the distal fragment below the osteotomy, the proximal fragment above the osteotomy and the femur

impressive that small changes in all three planes are usually present and the manipulation of the fragments to a realignment which is precise in all three planes is difficult to obtain and difficult to hold while fixation is applied. In the author's experience the precision and confidence is greatly improved using navigation but the time and effort to obtain the correction is also increased. If a blade plate is used and the blade is inserted at the correct angle the osteotomy fixation is easier to obtain but it is more difficult to change if an error has been made in blade insertion

## 36.4 Post-op Rehabilitation

Aftercare is essentially that of any well-fixed fracture. After osteotomy I drain the wounds, begin continuous passive motion and foot compression pumps in the recovery room, use no external immobilization, and encourage full range of knee motion. I recommend crutches with approximately 20 kg weight bearing. At times if the patient is anxious I will allow a knee immobilizer temporarily for comfort or confidence to encourage ambulation. Usually weight bearing can be increased by 4 weeks, so full weight bearing can be achieved in 6 weeks. Resistive exercises are delayed until the bone shows evidence of healing.

## 36.5 Results of Tibial Torsional Realignment

Ficat and Hungerford[7] reported one case of recurrent patellar subluxation which responded to osteotomy of both the femur and tibia. Cooke et al.[4] operated on nine knees in seven patients with inwardly pointing knees and patellofemoral complaints. The authors found this group of patients to have a combined abnormal varus and external torsion of the tibia. The operation performed was derotation valgus Maquet osteotomy with associated lateral release. After a 3-year follow-up period the outcome assessments were excellent for all the cases. Meister and James[14] reported on eight knees in seven patients with severe rotational malalignment of the lower extremities associated with debilitating anterior knee pain. The rotational deformity consisted of mild femoral anteversion, severe external tibial torsion, and mild tibia vara and pes planovalgus. Internal rotation tibial osteotomy was performed proximal to the tibial tubercle with an average correction of 19.7°. At 10 years average follow-up all but one patient obtained a subjective good or excellent result while functionally all had a good or excellent result. Server et al.[18] performed 35 tibial rotational osteotomies in 25 patients with increased lateral tibial torsion and with symptoms suggesting patellofemoral subluxation. At 4.3 years follow-up the results were good or excellent in 88.5% of the patients and all the patients except two were not satisfied with the procedure. Delgado et al.[5] treated operatively nine patients with 13 affected extremities with patellofemoral pathology related to torsional malalignment. The procedures performed were femoral external rotation osteotomy, tibial internal rotation osteotomy, or both. No additional soft tissue procedure that would alter patellar tracking was carried out. At 2.6 years average follow-up all the patients had an improvement in gait pattern, extremity appearance, and a marked decrease in knee pain. Bruce and Stevens[2] reviewed the results of correction of miserable malalignment syndrome in 14 patients with 27 limbs. The patients presented significant patellofemoral pain in association with increased femoral anteversion and tibia external rotation. Ipsilateral femoral external rotational osteotomy and tibia internal rotation osteotomy were performed in all the cases. At an average 5.2 years follow-up, all of the patients reported full satisfaction with their surgery and outcomes. Paulos et al.[15] has recently found that the clinical outcome of patients treated with rotational tibial osteotomy are better than a control group treated with anteriormedial tubercle transfer.

Each patient presents with different problems and different structural failures thus outcome measures fail to reveal the complete patient profile. Pain in the absence of instability or chondral disease is the most common early presentation. The only objective measurements may be that of abnormal limb torsion. Patients after surgery have reported returning to painless cross country running after not being able to walk to university classes before correction, the loss of bunions, the loss of radiating pain down the lateral side of the limb from pelvis to lateral ankle after 40 years without relief, the loss of retropatellar crepitation on stairs, the first ability to ride a bicycle without pain and to ski without pain. Exercise which constrains the pelvis and feet such as bicycle, classic cross country skiing, or elliptical machines are a particular problem for these patients as there is no escape for the inward pointing knee. Strong hip abduction is a benefit for patients with femoral anteversion as it may allow the patient to be active with a knee which points forward thus relieving knee pain, but as the hip abductor is working at a mechanical disadvantage it will often fatigue and the knee joint must point medially to gain mechanical leverage at the hip. This inward limb rotation forces an increased pronation at the foot such that medial arch strain, posterior tibial tendon strain and bunions are more common. This chronic foot pronation may allow an increase in equinus ankle contracture which then accentuates internal limb rotation. Excess external tibial torsion with normal femoral torsion presents a different problem. The knee points inward because this is necessary for proper ankle dorsiflexion during gait. The medial knee pain is common as the quadriceps increases the lateral vector on the patella when the foot is pointing forward. The hip abductors however are working at near normal mechanical advantage, so pelvic strengthening is less likely to be useful.

## 36.6 Conclusions

1. Miserable malalignment as described by James exists and must be recognized in the patient with PF pain, instability, or arthrosis.
2. Torsional limb malalignment may present with only pain or may coexist with patellar instability and/or patellar chondrosis and it may be a biomechanical contributor to the etiology of both instability and arthrosis, but all three conditions (alignment, instability, and cartilage injury) must be evaluated independently.
3. Restoration of normal limb alignment in all three planes is thought to restore the normal direction of the force vectors which cross the knee joint.
4. The transverse (horizontal) plane is frequently overlooked and is best evaluated with a CT scan which allows the axis of the hip, knee, and ankle to be measured relative to each other.
5. Realignment of the femur and tibia by rotational osteotomy may not only be appropriate but necessary. It is the only reasonable surgical treatment for PF symptoms which are due to horizontal skeletal malalignment.
6. Surgery for instability or for cartilage restoration is more likely to fail in the mechanical environment of persistent lower limb maltorsion.
7. Surgical morbidity must not be underestimated.

## References


1. Arnold AS, Komattu AV, Delp SL. Internal rotation gait: a compensatory mechanism to restore abduction capacity decreased by bone deformity. *Dev Med Child Neurol.* 1997;39:40-44.
2. Bruce WD, Stevens PM. Surgical correction of miserable malalignment syndrome. *J Pediatr Orthop.* 2004;24:392-396.
3. Cobb JP, Dixon H, Dandachli W, et al. The anatomical tibial axis: reliable rotational orientation in knee replacement. *J Bone Joint Surg.* 2008;90-B:1032-1038.
4. Cooke TD, Price N, Fisher B, et al. The inwardly pointing knee. An unrecognized problem of external rotational malalignment. *Clin Orthop Relat Res.* 1990;260:56-60.
5. Delgado ED, Schoenecker PL, Rich MM, et al. Treatment of severe torsional malalignment syndrome. *J Pediatr Orthop.* 1996;16:484-488.
6. Eckhoff DG, Brown AW, Kilcoyne RF, et al. Knee version associated with anterior knee pain. *Clin Orthop Relat Res.* 1997;339:152-155.
7. Ficat RP, Hungerford DS. *Disorders of the Patello-femoral Joint.* Baltimore: Williams & Wilkins; 1977:103.
8. Huberti HH, Hayes WC. Patellofemoral contact pressures. The influence of q-angle and tendofemoral contact. *J Bone Joint Surg.* 1984;66-A:715-724.
9. Jakob RP, Haertel M, Stussi E. Tibial torsion calculated by computerized tomography and compared to other methods of measurement. *J Bone Joint Surg.* 1980;62-B:238-242.
10. James SL. Chondromalacia of the patella in the adolescent. In: Kennedy JC, ed. *The Injured Adolescent Knee.* Baltimore: Williams & Wilkins Co; 1979.
11. Le Damany P. La torsion du tibia, normale, pathologique, expérimentale. *J Anat Physiol.* 1909;45:598-615 (cited by Jakob).
12. Levens AS, Berkeley CE, Inman VT, et al. Transverse rotation of the segments of the lower extremity in locomotion. *J Bone Joint Surg.* 1948;30-A:859-872.
13. Lösel S, Burgess-Milliron MJ, Micheli LJ, et al. A simplified technique for determining foot progression angle in chil-dren 4 to 16 years of age. *J Pediatr Orthop.* 1996;16:570-574.
14. Meister K, James SL. Proximal tibial derotation osteotomy for anterior knee pain in the miserably malaligned extremity. *Am J Orthop.* 1995;24:149-155.
15. Paulos L, Swanson SC, Stoddard GW, et al. Surgical correction of limb malalignment for instability of the patella: a comparison of 2 techniques. *Am J Sports Med.* 2009; 37:1288.
16. Sayli U, Bolukbasi S, Atik OS, et al. Determination of tibial torsion by computed tomography. *J Foot Ankle Surg.* 1994; 33:144-147.
17. Seber S, Hazer B, Kose N, et al. Rotational profile of the lower extremity and foot progression angle: computerized tomographic examination of 50 male adults. *Arch Orthop Trauma Surg.* 2000;120:255-258.

18. Server F, Miralles RC, Garcia E, et al. Medial rotational tibial osteotomy for patellar instability secondary to lateral tibial torsion. *Int Orthop*. 1996;20:153-158.
19. Tamari K, Tinley P, Briffa K, et al. Validity and reliability of existing and modified clinical methods of measuring femoral and tibiofibular torsion in healthy subjects: use of different reference axes may improve reliability. *Clin Anat*. 2005;18:46-55.
20. Turner MS. The association between tibial torsion and knee joint pathology. *Clin Orthop Relat Res*. 1994;302:47-51.
21. Van Kampen A, Huskies R. The three-dimensional tracking pattern of the human patella. *J Orthop Res*. 1990;8: 372-382.
22. Yoshioka Y, Cooke TDV. Femoral anteversion: assessment based on function axes. *J Orthop Res*. 1987;5:86-91.
23. Yoshioka Y, Siu D, Cooke TDV. The anatomy and functional axes of the femur. *J Bone Joint Surg*. 1987;69-A:873-880.
24. Yoshioka Y, Siu DW, Scudamore RA, et al. Tibial anatomy and functional axes. *J Orthop Res*. 1989;7:132-137.

# Rotational Femoral Osteotomy

# 37

Robert A. Teitge and Roger Torga-Spak

## 37.1 Introduction

Skeletal alignment in all three planes has a great influence on patellar tracking and loading. The source of patellofemoral loading is extraarticular; this is the reason that operations limited to the knee joint frequently fail if this is not recognized. The treatment of skeletal malalignment requires the correct bony operation. If there is genu valgum because of a short lateral femoral condyle, a femoral varus osteotomy is indicated. If the genu valgum is the result of a valgus bow to the tibia then a varus osteotomy of the tibia near the deformity is indicated. Genu varum with medial trochlear degeneration should be treated with tibial valgus osteotomy. Inward pointing knees with secondary lateral subluxation should be treated with external rotation femoral osteotomy if it is caused by increased femoral anteversion; internal rotation tibial osteotomy if it is caused by increased external tibial torsion. Combined deformities are not uncommon and the type of osteotomy and location depends on the deformity.

## 37.2 Surgical Technique

The technique we use is the standard Arbeitsgemainshaft für Osteosynthesefragen (AO) technique for a hip osteotomy using a fixed angled blade plate.[1] An early series of osteotomies was performed with a locked intramedullary nail, which revealed a wider range of correction accuracy, a greater incidence of delayed union, more blood loss (probably because of reaming the intramedullary canal), and more pain (probably because of greater relative instability) than patients fixed with an angled blade plate.

The intertrochanteric region is selected over a supracondylar osteotomy to reduce scarring of the quadriceps near the knee joint and to allow a longer bone length for the thigh muscles to adjust to a new direction. In fact, it is unknown if there is any difference in outcome wherever the osteotomy level is selected. If a patient has an associated genu valgum or varus, then the tibiofemoral angle abnormality needs to be corrected near the knee joint, and the supracondylar femur is selected for combined rotational and angular correction.

For an intertrochanteric osteotomy, the standard lateral approach to the hip is used, but the fascia is opened more anteriorly than normal as this seems to reduce the incidence of late trochanteric pain and fascia dehiscence over the plate. The osteotomy is arbitrarily placed at the upper level of the lesser trochanter. A 95° condylar blade plate is generally used because this allows a fairly low profile of the implant when compared with other types of blade plates. The flat surface of the blade increases surface contact area, providing greater stability when the plate is placed under tension. After exposure of the proximal lateral femur, the condylar plate guide which is a mirror image of the plate is placed along the lateral femur until it has a smooth match or fit as seen with the image intensifier and when the line extended along the top of the guide is within the neck, extending into the lower half of the femoral head. The top of the guide indicates the location for insertion of the U-shaped seating chisel. The seating chisel is driven into the neck, and its insertion is followed with the image intensifier in both the anteroposterior (AP) and lateral planes. It is also necessary to hold the seating

R. Torga-Spak (✉)
Faculty of Orthopaedics and Traumatology, Department of Surgery, Instituto Universitario CEMIC, Buenos Aires, Argentina
e-mail: rogerts@traumatologiapenta.com.ar

V. Sanchis-Alfonso (ed.), *Anterior Knee Pain and Patellar Instability*,
DOI: 10.1007/978-0-85729-507-1_37, © Springer-Verlag London Limited 2011

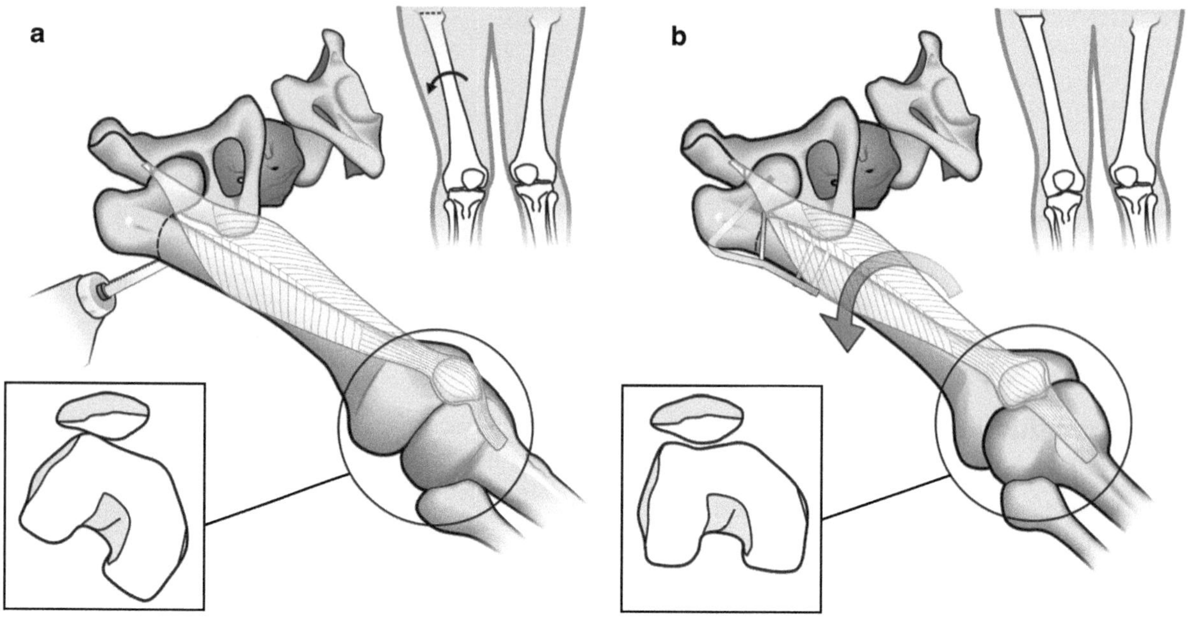


**Fig. 37.1** (**a**) The transverse osteotomy is performed at the level of the top of the lesser trochanter. (**b**) The distal fragment is rotated externally until the desired rotation is obtained

chisel with the slotted hammer so that the side plate will be aligned with the lateral shaft of the femur distally. When the seating chisel has been fully seated, the blade length is noted, and the seating chisel is removed. A 2-mm K-wire is inserted into the seating chisel track to mark the site for later blade insertion. K-wires of 2.5 mm diameter to be used as references are placed parallel one above and one below the level of the proposed osteotomy. The transverse osteotomy is performed at the level of the top of the lesser trochanter (Fig. 37.1). The distal fragment is rotated externally (in the case of excessive femoral anteversion) until the desired rotation is indicated by the desired angular separation of the K-wire. The articulated tension device is screwed onto the femoral shaft distally in line with the distal fragment, and compression of the osteotomy is achieved when tension is applied to the distal end of the plate. We normally strive for 150-kp compression as indicated by the color coding on the Synthes (Paoli, PA) device. The compression can be held by one screw but two are placed in the distal end of the plate, and a third screw is usually placed through the plate and oblique across the osteotomy to hold the blade from backing out of the proximal fragment, to provide additional interfragmentary compression, and to improve rotational control (Fig. 37.1).

## 37.3 Results of Femoral Torsional Realignment: Clinical Data

From 1989 to 2005, 72 knees in 53 patients with excessive femoral anteversion and patellofemoral dysfunction were treated with intertrochanteric femoral osteotomy. All patients were evaluated preoperatively and postoperatively with Kujala, Lysholm, and Tegner scores at a minimum of 24 months.

Follow-up was available in 66 of 72 (92%) knees at a mean of 9.7 (2–17) years. Kujala scores improved from 53 to 86 ($P<0.01$). Lysholm scores improved from 49 to 89 ($P<0.01$). Tegner activity scores improved from 2.2 to 4 ($P < 0.01$). Patients reported an average improvement in symptoms of 91%. Fifty-five percent said surgery relieved their symptoms 100%. No patients reported no improvement or worsening of symptoms as a result of the surgery. All but three patients would have surgery again.

## Reference

1. Müller ME, Allgower M, Schneider R, Willenegger H. *Manual of Internal Fixation: Techniques Recommended by the AO-ASIF Group*. Berlin: Springer; 1977.

# Patella Infera and Patella Alta

# 38

Paulo Renato F. Saggin and David Dejour

## 38.1 Patella Infera

Patella infera represents the low position of the patella in relation to the femur and the tibia. Two terminologies are used to qualify this low position of the patella: "patella baja" or "patella infera." As the Latin form is the common way to describe the high position of the patella (patella alta), it is coherent to define patella infera as the appropriate term. Evocated for the first time by A. Trillat, patella infera was described by J. Caton and G. Deschamps in 1982.[2]

Its real importance lies in the biomechanical abnormality caused by the inferior situation of the patella in relation to the knee. While normal patellae are not engaged in the trochlea in extension, in cases of patella infera the patella is always in contact with the trochlea. It is most of the time a complication of a traumatic event or a previous surgery on the knee. Rarely, it is a constitutional position of the patella and is not pathological.

### *38.1.1 Etiology*

Patella infera can be divided into two mechanicals and one inflammatory etiology.

P.R.F. Saggin (✉)
Instituto de Ortopedia e Traumatologia (I.O.T.),
Passo Fundo, RS, Brazil
e-mail: paulosaggin@yahoo.com.br

#### 38.1.1.1 Mechanical

The Muscular origin is secondary to a quadriceps insufficiency, like in poliomyelitis, femoral nerve palsy or an extensor mechanism rupture or malformation.

Iatrogenic etiology concerns previous tibial tubercle osteotomy and excessive distal transfer, or failed surgeries performed for various purposes.

#### 38.1.1.2 Inflammatory

This etiology is found isolated, or combined to the mechanical causes. There is global retraction of the medial and lateral retinacula, and the patellar tendon retraction will occur in a second step. This explains why the patella has no medio-lateral mobility, and why there is greater stiffness if compared to the mechanical etiologies.

### *38.1.2 Clinical Presentation*

#### 38.1.2.1 History

In almost all cases, patella infera is acquired after a history of quadriceps rupture or patellar fracture, femur fracture, tibia fracture, or after any surgery for patellar painful syndrome, patellar instability, or even an inespecific surgery of the knee.

It is important for the clinician to know how the postoperative care has been managed after those surgeries; a high number of reflex sympathetic dystrophy is found in this population. The delay between pain and surgery, the efficacy of pain management, the type of immobilization, and the delay to recovery quadriceps contraction after the surgery are noted.

V. Sanchis-Alfonso (ed.), *Anterior Knee Pain and Patellar Instability*,
DOI: 10.1007/978-0-85729-507-1_38, © Springer-Verlag London Limited 2011

#### 38.1.2.2 Functional Signs

The patient describes pain below the patella as a bar, or around the patella. The pain is described as a burning sensation, usually permanent and increased by activities. The patient usually says that his knee is "clamped in a vise." The pain can also have an inflammatory pattern, with night pain. Sometimes the pain resembles patellar painful syndrome, with pain in ascending or descending stairs, locking episodes, or reflex instability while walking. Patients frequently have a reduced walking perimeter.

#### 38.1.2.3 Clinical Signs

When the patient is lying supine on the exam table with the knee flexed, if the patellar index is below 0.6, the knee will have the aspect of a "postpatellectomy knee." The shape of the patella disappears because the patella is entrapped into the notch. Flexion is limited in active or passive motion; rarely there is lack of extension.

The most typical sign is that the patient is not able to maintain monopodal weight bearing with the knee flexed between 30° and 60°, because of the permanent hyperpressure on the cartilage. This probably explains why the walking perimeter is limited by pain.

Patellar mobility is restricted in any direction. It is important to check the quadriceps efficiency and activation because they will be important for prognosis and treatment. It is also very important to make a careful analysis of other potential sources of pain, such as superficial skin pain and neuropathic pain. Psychological analysis of the patient must be taken into account. The patients' expectation is a major factor to be considered.

### 38.1.3 X-Ray Analysis

The standard X-Ray protocol will be able to confirm the diagnosis and most of the time will determine the etiology of the patella infera.

The bone quality has to be analyzed in order to discover pathologic osteoporosis (observed in RSD), or sequellae of patella, femur, or tibia fractures. The AP view still allows the diagnosis of associated femorotibial pathology.

Patella infera is diagnosed on the lateral view. The patellar height must be measured using an identified index. The main indexes used in the literature are:

- The Caton–Deschamps index[3]: is the ratio between the distance from the lower edge of the patellar articular surface to the anterosuperior angle of the tibia outline (AT), and the length of the articular surface of the patella (AP). A ratio (AT/AP) of 0.6 and smaller determines patella infera, and a ratio greater than 1.2 indicates patella alta (Fig. 38.1).
- The Insall–Salvati index[6]: is the ratio between the length of the patellar tendon (LT) and the longest sagittal diameter of the patella (LP). Insall determined that this ratio (LT/LP) is normally 1. A ratio smaller than 0.8 indicates a patella infera and greater than 1.2 patella alta (Fig. 38.2).
- The Blackburne–Peel index[1]: is the ratio between the length of the perpendicular line drawn from the tangent to the tibial plateau until the inferior part of the articular surface of the patella (A) and the length of the articular surface of the patella (B). The normal

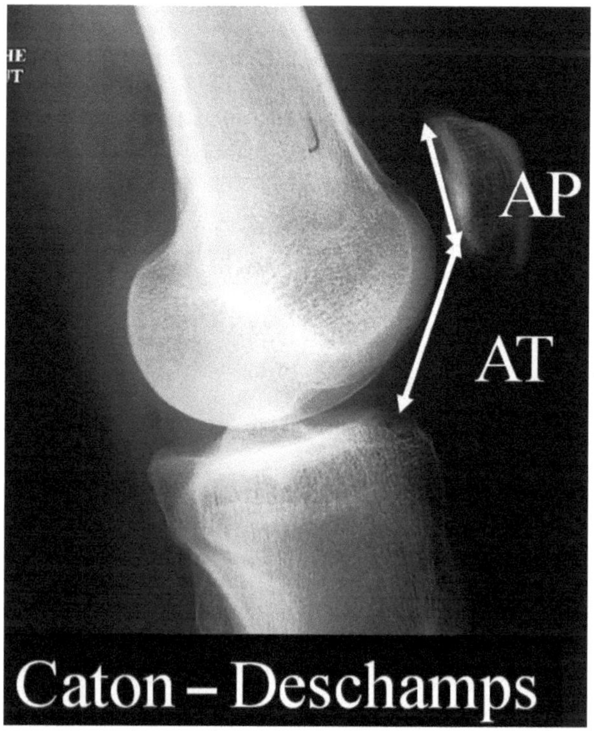


**Fig. 38.1** The Caton–Deschamps index (AT/AP) is the ratio between the distance from the lower edge of the patella's articular surface to the anterosuperior angle of the tibia outline (*AT*), and the length of the articular surface of the patella (*AP*)

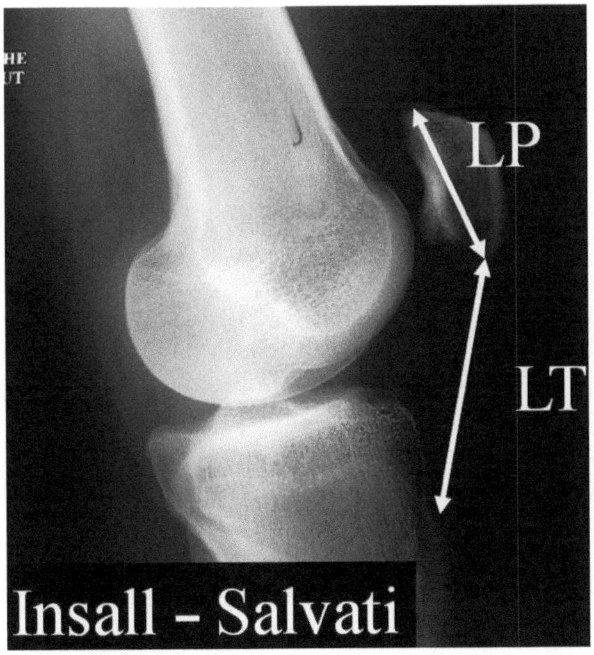


**Fig. 38.2** The Insall–Salvati index (LT/LP) is the ratio between the length of the patellar tendon (*LT*) and the longest sagittal diameter of the patella (*LP*)

ratio (A/B) was defined as 0.8. In patella infera it is smaller than 0.5, in patella alta greater than 1.0 (Fig. 38.3).

The axial view at 30° of flexion gives a good complementary analysis. It shows a typical aspect of the patella infera called the "sunset aspect." As the patella is entrapped into the notch, the joint line disappears, and it can give a false diagnosis of global joint line narrowing, like in arthritis (Fig. 38.4).

### 38.1.4 MRI

This exam is indicated in the preoperative planning. It will show clearly the insertion of the patellar tendon, the exact tendon length, and on the axial slices the patellofemoral cartilage can be analyzed.

### 38.1.5 Bone Scan

This exam is part of the pre-op checking. It shows if there is RSD and if this one is still active, thus delaying the surgical treatment.

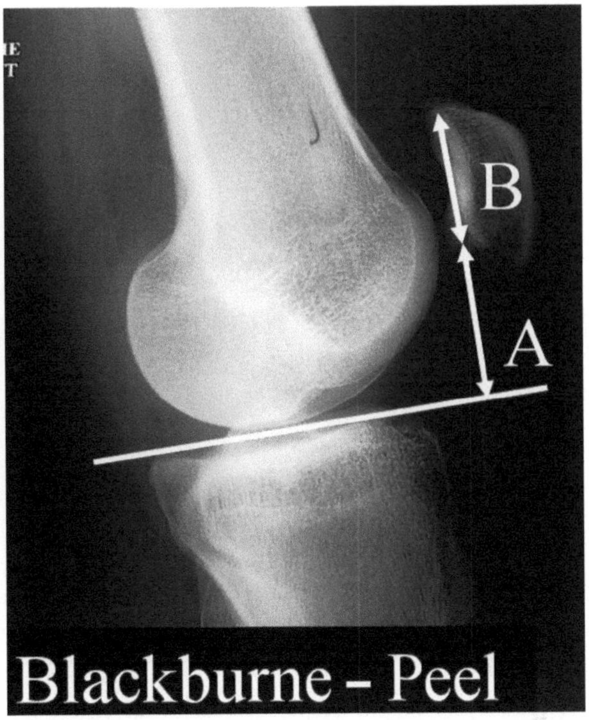


**Fig. 38.3** The Blackburne–Peel index (A/B) is the ratio between the length of the perpendicular line drawn from the tangent to the tibial plateau until the inferior part of the articular surface of the patella (*A*) and the length of the articular surface of the patella (*B*)

### 38.1.6 Treatment

Nonoperative treatment is the first step. It may be tried, but it cannot change the patellar height. The slow and gentle rehabilitation consists of passive patellar mobilization, quadriceps stimulation, passive and active motion and stretching exercises. The aquatic activities such as walking or swimming, and cycling are allowed to decrease pain and the inflammatory syndrome. Nonoperative management lasts for 3–6 months after the first visit.

#### 38.1.6.1 The Operative Treatment

The technique will differ according to the etiology. When the problem's origin is in the tibial tubercle, a proximal transfer will correct it. When the origin is in the soft tissues, and especially when the patellar tendon is retracted, the procedure of choice is patellar tendon lengthening. In cases of inflammatory origin,

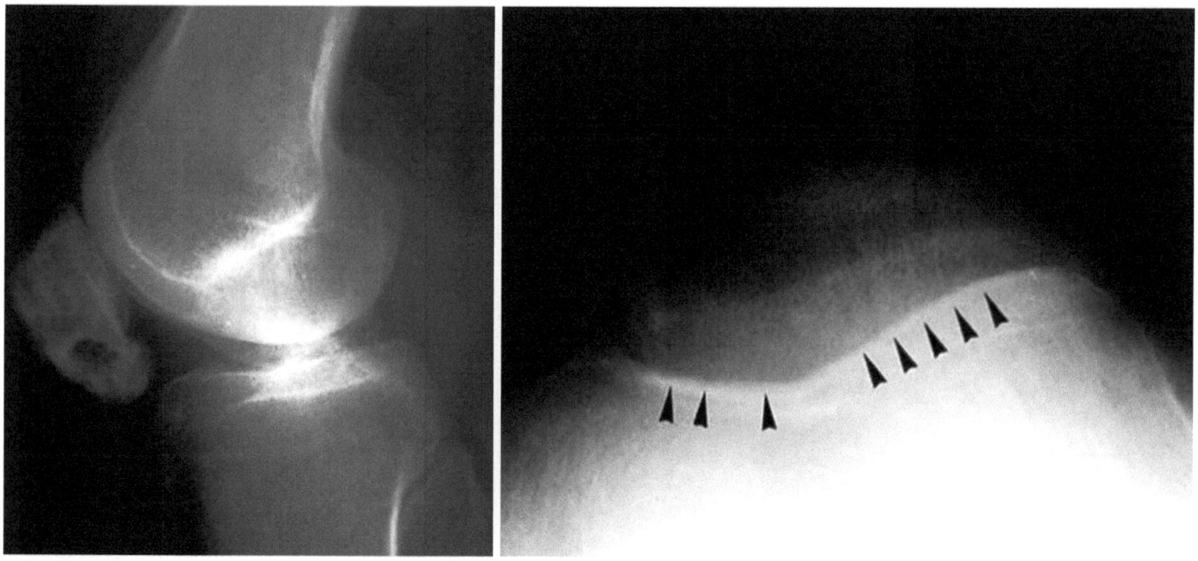

**Fig. 38.4** Patella infera. On the lateral view, the distance from the lower edge of the patella's articular surface to the anterosuperior angle of the tibia outline is almost zero. On the axial view, the "sunset pattern" is shown as the articular space cannot be seen

an arthrolysis should be performed. In all cases, the medial and lateral retinacula must be released and/or lengthened; the fat pad must be removed. The postoperative goal is to reach a patellar index equal to 1 according to the Caton–Deschamps index.

#### 38.1.6.2 Proximal Transfer of the Tibial Tubercle[2]

After an anteromedial approach, dissection of the patellar tendon and section of the peripatellar retinacular tissue are performed. An arthrotomy allowing arthrolysis of the knee and verification of the intra-articular space (this may also be done under arthroscopy) is then carried out. The tibial tubercle, after section of the medial and lateral retinaculae, is detached with a hammered chisel and is transferred upward according to the preoperative planning, generally between 1 and 2 cm. It is fixed with two bicortical screws perpendicular to the tibial shaft. The distal screw maintains the height of the patella, while the second more proximal screw allows correction of the lateral position of the patellar tendon, depending on the preoperative TT-TG measurement. The medial retinaculum is then lengthened and the lateral is left open or lengthened. One should take care that the patellar tendon is not folded when suturing the medial retinaculum.

Postoperative care includes a brace in full extension. Full weight bearing is allowed immediately. Range of motion (ROM) exercises are started on the first postoperative day; in order to avoid excessive stress on the fixation of the tibial tubercle, flexion is limited to 100°. After 45 days, the splint is removed, full flexion is allowed, and closed kinetic chain exercises between 0° and 60° permit muscle strengthening. Return to sports activities is allowed at 6 months.

#### 38.1.6.3 The Patellar Tendon Lengthening[4]

The procedure starts by an anteromedial approach from the superior part of the patellar tendon until the medial edge of the tibial tubercle, followed by extensive dissection of the patellar tendon's medial and lateral aspects. It is often necessary to free the inferior and posterior aspect of the tendon and to perform an arthrolysis of the medial and lateral gutters. The arthrotomy allows to check the status of the patellar cartilage and to cut the fibrous adhesions of the suprapatellar pouch. Patellar tendon lengthening is then carried out by dividing it through the middle over its whole length (Z-plasty). The lateral part remains anchored to the tibia while the medial part remains anchored on the medial aspect of the patella. The patella should rise naturally, and the tendon's stumps slide over each other.

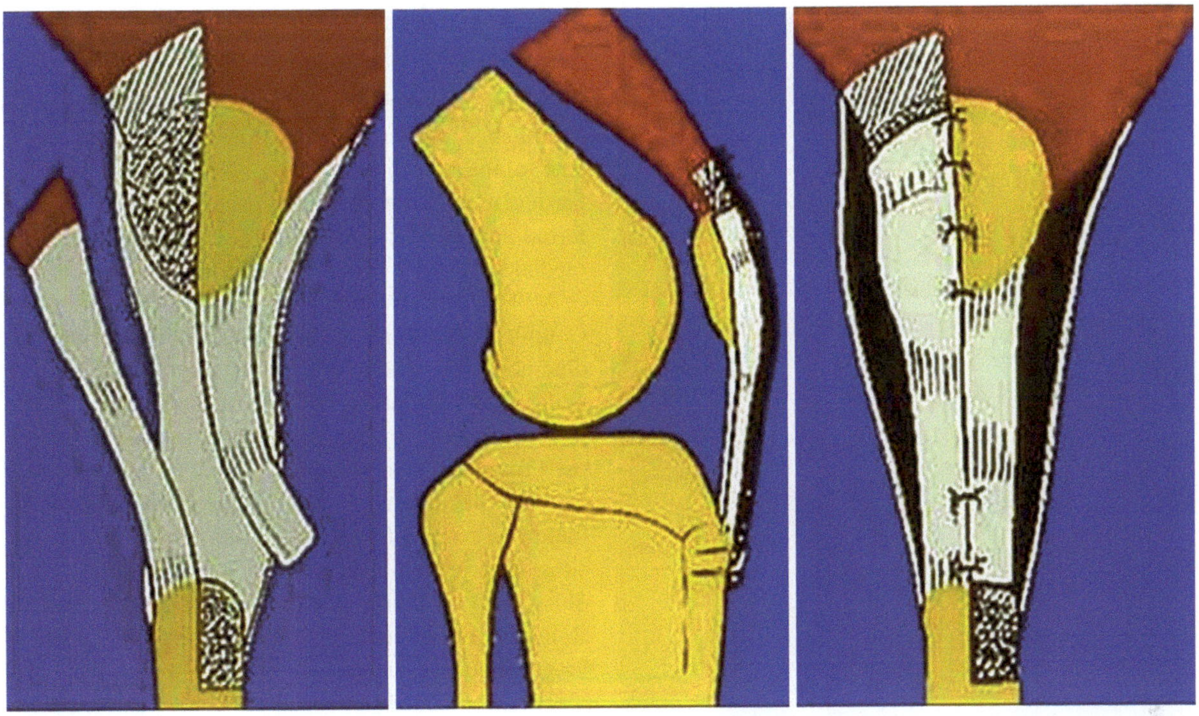

**Fig. 38.5** Patellar tendon Lengthening (DeJour).The three steps: (1) Z plasty of the patellar tendon; (2) perioperative x-ray evaluation of the patellar height; (3) fixation with stitches protected with a metallic wire for 6 months

A perioperative lateral X-ray is taken at 30° flexion to check and measure the patellar height. If the lengthening is correct the patellar tendon edges are then sutured. This suture has to be protected by an absorbable PDS band, a semitendinous tendon, or a metallic wire. The best and the most secure option is to use a metallic wire which goes from the mid part of the patella to the tibial tubercle. This maintains the right length, protects the tendon, and allows more aggressive rehabilitation. The metallic wire has to be removed at 6 months post-op. The lateral retinaculum is left completely open or lengthened and the medial retinaculum is closed after a lengthening plasty (Fig. 38.5).

Postoperative care includes a brace in extension. Full weight bearing is allowed immediately. Range of motion (ROM) exercises are started on the first postoperative day, but flexion is limited to 100º. During the period of rest, the patient should keep knee flexion at 20° to maintain some tension on the patellar tendon. After 45 days, the splint is removed, and full flexion is allowed. Return to sports is permitted at 6 months.

## 38.2 Patella Alta

Patella alta is one of the four anatomical factors leading to patellar instability (the others are trochlear dysplasia, excessive TT-TG, and patellar tilt). The patella engages the femoral trochlea late in flexion, which predisposes to instability (Fig. 38.6). As in patella infera, the diagnosis is established on the lateral view, where appropriate measurements are performed.

Patella alta correction is performed through distal transfer of the tibial tubercle. Associated abnormalities should be corrected simultaneously to achieve patellar stability.

Tibial tubercle transfers are commonly performed to realign the extensor mechanism (medializations). The first description of a tibial tubercle transfer was done by Roux in 1888 and then further modified by other authors like Emslie and Trillat,[10] Maquet,[7] and Fulkerson.[5] The procedure involves displacing the insertion of the patellar tendon through an osteotomy of its insertion.

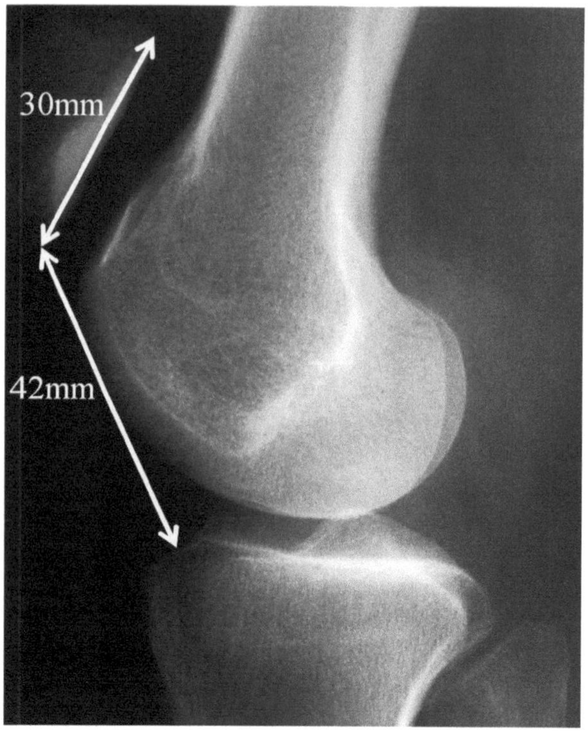


**Fig. 38.6** Patella alta. The Caton–Deschamps index is 1.4

### 38.2.1 Surgical Technique

In the earlier descriptions of tibial tubercle transfers, a lateral incision was used. Following the advances of patellofemoral surgery, and of knee arthroplasty in particular, an anteromedial incision is now the preferred approach. This allows also the association of a medial soft tissue procedure like VMO advancement or MPFL reconstruction with no additional incisions. Complete exposure of the tibial tubercle must be obtained, regardless of the type of transfer that is being undertaken. The proximal limit of the insertion of the patellar tendon is identified, and the outline of the osteotomy is traced with a scalpel in the periosteum.

The tibial tubercle is detached completely, and will, therefore, require fixation with two screws. The screw sites are prepared prior to the actual osteotomy, 2 cm apart. An oscillating saw or an osteotome is used to fashion a bone block with at least 6 cm. The block length should be increased by the amount of distal displacement planned.

In order to decrease the risk of nonunion, the cut must be made sufficiently deep in cancellous bone.

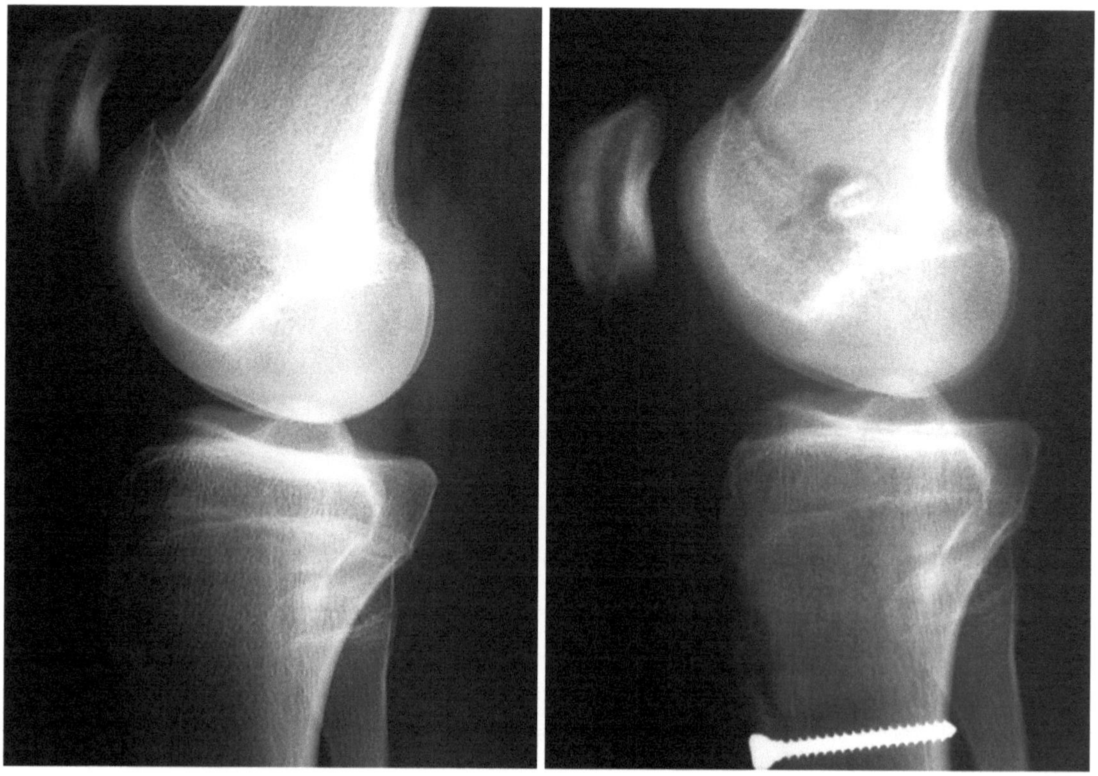

**Fig. 38.7** Pre and postoperative lateral views of patella alta. After the distal tibial tubercle transfer, the patellar height is corrected (1.5 preoperatively to 1 postoperatively)

The proximal portion of the tibial tubercle is pried off, and grasped with bone-holding forceps while the distal portion is being cut to the required length. The distal portion is tapered and trimmed to fit flush into its bone bed. It must not stand proud, since any prominence would interfere with kneeling. The block is held in its distalized position, and fixation is started at the lower screw site. The screws are inserted perpendicular to the anterior border of the tibia to avoid proximal displacement during lagging, with loss of correction. Bicortical fixation is required for proper lagging of the tibial tubercle.

Tibial tubercle distal transfer induces a medialization of 3–4 mm because of tibial torsion, and this phenomenon should be considered if simultaneous medialization is being performed, as it can contribute to "overmedialization."[9] Additional medialization may be achieved after the first screw has been inserted but not tightened. Once the desired amount of medialization has been obtained, the second screw is inserted (Figs. 38.7 and 38.8).

### 38.2.2 Patellar Tendon Tenodesis

This is an adjuvant procedure to distal tibial tubercle transfer surgeries described by Neyret et al.[8] It is indicated when the patient has a patellar tendon length superior to 52 mm, which represents a too long tendon. This measure can be found by radiographic examination, but it is far more reliable when MRI is employed. After the tibial tubercle osteotomy for distalization, as described above, two anchors with sutures are fixed at both sides of patellar tendon, about 29 mm distal to the tibial plateau level, at the normal tendon insertion. The sutures are tied, attaching the patellar tendon to the underlying bone and thus reducing patellar tendon's length, what can be accessed postsurgically with MRI.

Postoperative care is common to all tibial tubercle osteotomies. The patient wears a straight-leg splint and full weight-bearing is allowed. Range of motion (ROM) exercises is started on the first postoperative day; in order to avoid excessive stress on the fixation

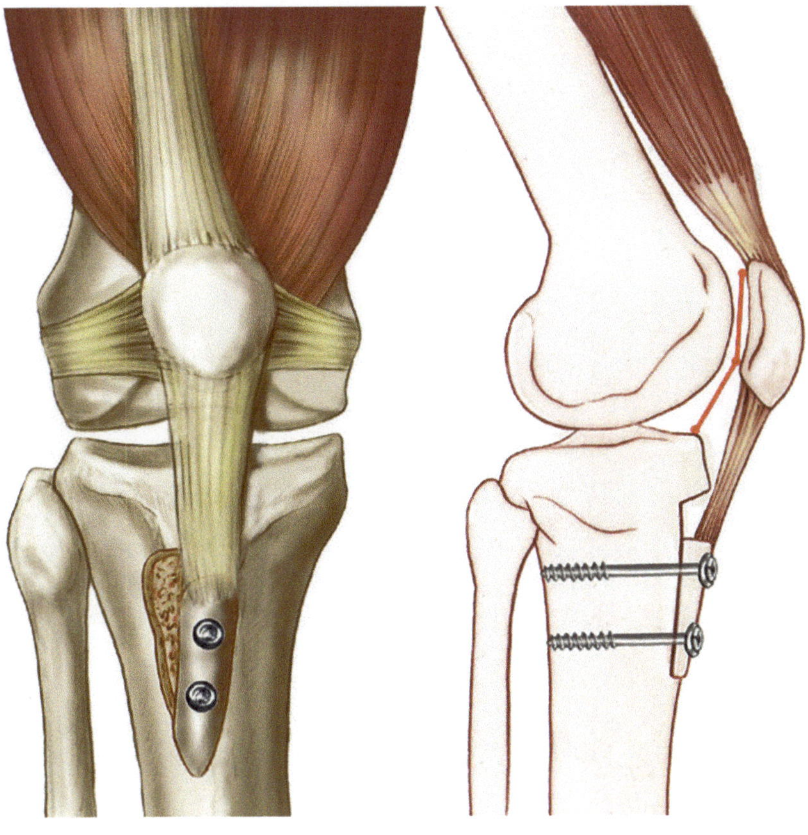

**Fig. 38.8** Medial and distal tibial tubercle transfer. Two screws are used. This procedure is used to correct increased TT-TG distance and patella alta. Caution should be taken to not overmedialize the tubercle, since the distalization procedure alone induces automatic medialization. Screws must be perpendicular to the tibial shaft to allow good compression and avoid proximal displacement during lagging

of the tibial tubercle, flexion is limited to 100°. After 45 days, the splint is removed, and full flexion is allowed. Return to sports activities is permitted 6 months postoperatively.

## References


1. Blackburne JS, Peel TE. A new method of measuring patellar height. *J Bone Joint Surg*. 1977;59-B:241-242.
2. Caton J, Deschamps G, Chambat P, et al. Patella infera. Apropos of 128 cases. *Rev Chir Orthop Reparatrice Appar Mot*. 1982;68:317-325.
3. Caton J. Method of measuring the height of the patella. *Acta Orthop Belg*. 1989;55:385-386.
4. Dejour D, Levigne C, Dejour H. Postoperative low patella. Treatment by lengthening of the patellar tendon. *Rev Chir Orthop Reparatrice Appar Mot*. 1995;81:286-295.
5. Fulkerson JP. Anteromedialization of the tibial tuberosity for patellofemoral malalignment. *Clin Orthop Relat Res*. 1983; 177:176-181.
6. Insall J. Patella position in the normal knee joint. *Radiology*. 1971;101:101-104.
7. Maquet P. Advancement of the tibial tuberosity. *Clin Orthop Relat Res*. 1976;115:225-230.
8. Neyret P, Robinson AH, Le Coultre B, et al. Patellar tendon length – the factor in patellar instability? *Knee*. 2002; 9:3-6.
9. Servien E, Ait Si Selmi T, Neyret P. *Le Genou du Sportif*. Montpellier: Sauramps Medical; 2002.
10. Trillat A, Dejour H, Couette A. Diagnosis and treatment of recurrent dislocations of the patella. *Rev Chir Orthop Reparatrice Appar Mot*. 1964;50:813-824.

# 39 Combined Tibial Tubercle Realignment and MPFL Reconstruction

Joan C. Monllau, Xavier Pelfort, Pablo Gelber, and Marc Tey

## 39.1 Introduction

The etiology of the patellar instability involves multiple factors and it can often be successfully managed with conservative treatment. This is particularly so in cases of primary dislocation. If there is no clinical improvement with nonoperative management, surgery may be considered especially in cases of recurrent patellar dislocation. In these patients, a complete physical examination and some imaging studies are mandatory. With regards physical examination, some risk factors such as Q angle increase, *vastus medialis obliquus* insufficiency, joint laxity, previous surgery, malalignment, or torsion deformities are special concerns that need to be ruled out.[11]

The medial patellofemoral ligament (MPFL) is an extracapsular fascial band that lies within the second of three layers on the medial side of the knee. It has been shown that after a patellar dislocation, a tear to the MPFL occurs in 94% of the patients.[12] For this reason, meticulous assessment of the MPFL is crucial. With the knee at 20–30° of flexion, the examiner tries to subluxate the patella laterally. MPFL deficiency is suspected if the patient is apprehensive during this maneuvre. Furthermore, a specific imaging protocol which includes: conventional radiographs to evaluate patellar height, morphology and osteochondral fractures of the patella, computed tomography scan to assess patellar tilt, TT-TG measurement, and femoral as well as tibial torsion must be done. Magnetic resonance images, to particularly evaluate the MPFL and patellar chondral injuries, should also be performed in all cases of patellar instability.

## 39.2 Indications and Contraindications

Due to the broad spectrum of etiologies and allied conditions, the surgical treatment of patellar instability should be individualized. Patients with a history of recurrent patellar dislocation, disruption of the MPFL on the MRI, a positive test for MPFL insufficiency on physical examination, and an increased TT-TG distance more than 20 mm are the optimal indications for performing a distal realignment combined with a MPFL reconstruction. As do some others,[13] the authors do not consider trochlear dysplasia, lateral femoral condyle dysplasia, or *patella alta* as contraindications for this procedure.

## 39.3 Surgical Technique

The patient is placed in the supine position on the operating table. A high lateral post is used to stabilize the lower extremity. The injured knee is flexed approximately at 90° and maintained with a foot bump. A well-padded tourniquet tied on the proximal operative thigh is recommended.

J.C. Monllau (✉)
Department of Orthopaedic Surgery and Traumatology, Hospital de la Santa Creu i Sant Pau, Universitat Autònoma de Barcelona, Barcelona, Spain

Arthroscopy Unit, ICATME, Institut Universitari Dexeus, Universitat Autònoma de Barcelona, Barcelona, Spain
e-mail: jmonllau@santpau.cat

V. Sanchis-Alfonso (ed.), *Anterior Knee Pain and Patellar Instability*,
DOI: 10.1007/978-0-85729-507-1_39, © Springer-Verlag London Limited 2011

### 39.3.1 Distal Tibial Tubercle Realignment

An anterior longitudinal incision is made from the distal part of the patellar tendon and extending distally around 10 cm following the anterior ridge of the tibia. The patellar tendon is identified and then a subcutaneous lateral patellar retinacular release is performed. Afterward, the patellar tendon tibial attachment as well as the tibial tuberosity (TT) is exposed. For an adequate TT osteotomy, a distal dissection of from 6 to 7 cm is prepared. Two Kirschner wires are drilled to guide the bone cut at the upper and lower part of the TT. Similarly to the osteotomy described by Fulkerson,[2,3] the superior wire is drilled in a 45° oblique direction, with reference to the anteroposterior axis of the tibia, aiming toward the posterolateral tibial corner. This obliquity in the proximal part of the osteotomy is responsible for the anteriorization of the TT at the time it slides medially. On the distal half of the osteotomy, the second wire is drilled in a more perpendicular direction (70° to 80° with respect to anteroposterior axis of the tibia). In this way, the bone cut will get thinner downward as it goes distally. Consequently, the distal part of the osteotomized TT will be more medially than anteriorly moved. Excessive anterior prominence of the TT at the distal part after surgery should be avoided. Subsequently, two 4.5 mm holes are predrilled on the anterior cortex of the TT for later lag-screw compression fixation of the osteotomized bone. Afterward, the TT osteotomy is performed with the help of an oscillating saw and osteotomes. This is when the patellar height can be modified if needed by moving and fixing the osteotomized TT either more distally or proximally on the sagittal plane. After placing the TT in the desired final position, fixation is performed by drilling the second tibial cortex with a 3.5 mm drill and using two cortical 4.5 mm lag compression screws. Once distal realignment is completed, MPFL reconstruction can proceed.

### 39.3.2 MPFL Reconstruction

MPFL reconstruction is necessary in unstable patella since delayed primary repair of the MPFL after primary patella dislocation does not reduce the risk of redislocation.[1] The achievement of correct ligament tension in the MPFL reconstruction is extremely important. Therefore, overtightening of the graft is to be avoided. If the MPFL reconstruction is done first, the performance of the ligament after a distal realignment can be easily modified. Thus, it must always be the last step in the procedure.

To reconstruct the MPFL, the authors' preferred graft is the ipsilateral *gracilis tendon* (GT), as it is long and strong enough to duplicate the MPFL function.[4,6] Additional advantages are little harvest-site morbidity, minor alterations of hamstrings' function as well as the easy passage through the patellar bone drill holes. The GT can be easily seen by dissecting the *pes anserinus* bursa and opening the *sartorius* fascia on its upper half. The GT is then exposed and released with a tendon stripper. A whipstitch suture is performed on each end of the tendon with No. 0 high-resistance nonabsorbable sutures. The tendon is sized by using a set of regular anterior cruciate ligament tunnel sizers, and it is then stored within a moist swab. Later, a 2 cm vertical skin incision is made over the superior medial border of the patella to expose its proximal one third. This area corresponds to the MPFL anatomical origin. According to the GT size, usually 3–4 mm, two convergent drill holes of approximately 10 mm in depth are created leaving a bone bridge of 7–10 mm. Therefore, a V-shaped tunnel is obtained so that the graft forms a loop through the patella. This tunnel is further enlarged and smoothed with the help of a curved mosquito clamp to make posterior tendon passage easier. After this, a suture passer or a lasso loop is used to leave a suture in place. This suture will later be used to pull the graft through the patellar tunnel.

Thereon, another 2–3 cm vertical skin approach is made near the medial femoral epicondyle, where the MPFL has its femoral attachment. The femoral attachment of the MPFL has been localized at a point 10 mm distal to the *adductor tubercle* and posterosuperior to the medial epicondyle.[10] It has fibres spreading proximally toward the *adductor tubercle* and distally toward the superficial medial collateral ligament.[7] Therefore, an area between the medial epicondyle and *adductor tubercle* is considered optimal for reconstruction.[14] In the authors' technique, the hiatus of the *adductor magnus* tendon is instead used as a post for the graft. The use of the *adductor's magnus* as a post for MPFL medial attachment is obviously a variation of the anatomical insertion point of this ligament. However, this position has recently been demonstrated to have quasi-isometric behaviur[9] that does not cause significant changes to the patellofemoral contact pressures with respect to an anatomical reconstruction.[5]

After dissecting the tendon of the *adductor magnus*, another provisional loop suture is made around it as a passer for the graft. Then, a subfascial dissection between both the epicondylar and parapatellar incisions is done with the help of a curved blunt forceps in order to make the pathway for the new ligament.[16] At this point, the graft is first passed through the patella leaving an asymmetrical length at both ends. Next, a loop around the *adductor magnus* tendon with the longer limb of the graft is used to again pass it back through the same subfascial via to the patellar attachment. The knee is cycled several times through full range of motion while keeping the graft under tension. In this way, the graft is prestretched and finally it is sutured at 30° of flexion with some No. 0 high-resistance nonabsorbable sutures so that the patella tilt can be manually lateralized 10 mm. It is important not to over constrain the final construct, which would create a patellar chondral overload in flexion[8] or an extensor lag if it is too tight in extension.[15] Additionally, if the graft is long enough, the remaining tendon can be fixed onto the anterior part of the patella by subperiosteally dissecting the extensor mechanism at this level. It is done in order to avoid a larger bone tunnel thus diminishing the risk of joint penetration or patellar fracture. The wounds are closed in the usual way and once the procedure has finished, the patient is left in a brace locked in full extension.

Further advantages of this procedure are that the MPFL reconstruction turns into a simple soft tissue procedure in which the femoral physeal line is not violated as no tunnel is drilled and no hardware is used to fix the graft to the bone. For this reason, the same technique can also be used in skeletally immature patients, since drilling holes through the physis at the femoral epicondyle is no longer necessary.

## 39.4 Postoperative Management

For the first 2 weeks, patients' knees are maintained in full extension with a knee brace. Full weight bearing with crutches is allowed from the beginning as tolerated. Thereafter, the brace is discontinued. At week 6, knee flexion at 90° is the target. After week 6, free low-demand activities are allowed. Sport-specific drills may be started and gradually progressed after 3 months. Full activity and a return to contact sports may begin 6 months after surgery.

## 39.5 Summary

This chapter describes a combined distal extensor realignment as well as MPFL reconstruction procedure using a hamstring tendon for chronic patellar instability. Although several predisposing factors are involved in lateral patellar dislocation, the authors believe that the MPFL plays a crucial role as a primary restraint among the medial patellar stabilizers. In this chapter, the detailed surgical technique and the rationale for its reconstruction are presented.

## References

1. Christiansen S, Jakobsen B, Lund B, et al. Repair of the medial patellofemoral ligament in primary dislocation of the patella: a prospective randomized study. *Arthroscopy*. 2008;24:881-887.
2. Fulkerson JP. Anteromedialization of the tibial tuberosity for patellofemoral malalignment. *Clin Orthop Relat Res*. 1983;177:176-181.
3. Fulkerson JP, Becker GJ, Meaney JA, et al. Anteromedial tibial tubercle transfer without bone graft. *Am J Sports Med*. 1990;18:490-496.
4. Hamner DL, Brown CH Jr, Steiner ME, et al. Hamstring tendon grafts for reconstruction of the ACL: biomechanical evaluation of the use of multiple strands and tensioning techniques. *J Bone Joint Surg*. 1999;81-A:549-557.
5. Melegari T, Parks B, Matthews L. Patellofemoral contact area and pressure after medial patellofemoral ligament reconstruction. *Am J Sports Med*. 2008;36:747-752.
6. Mountney J, Senavongse W, Amis A, et al. Tensile strength of the medial patellofemoral ligament before and after repair or reconstruction. *J Bone Joint Surg*. 2005;87-B:36-40.
7. Nomura E, Inoue M, Osada N. Anatomical analysis of the medial patellofemoral ligament of the knee, especially the femoral attachment. *Knee Surg Sports Traumatol Arthrosc*. 2005;13:510-515.
8. Ostermeier S, Holst M, Bohnsack M, et al. In vitro kinematics following reconstruction of the medial patellofemoral ligament. *Knee Surg Sports Traumatol Arthrosc*. 2007;15: 276-285.
9. Panagopoulos A, van Niekerk L, Triantafillopoulos IK. MPFL reconstruction for recurrent patella dislocation: a new surgical technique and review of the literature. *Int J Sports Med*. 2008;29:359-365.

10. Phillippot R, Chouteau J, Wegrzyn J, et al. Medial patellofemoral ligament anatomy: implications for its surgical reconstruction. *Knee Surg Sports Traumatol Arthrosc*. 2009;17:475-479.
11. Redziniak D, Diduch D, Mihalko W, et al. Patellar instability. *J Bone Joint Surg*. 2009;91-A:2264-2275.
12. Sallay PI, Poggi J, Speer KP, et al. Acute dislocation of the patella; a correlative pathoanatomic study. *Am J Sports Med*. 1996;24:52-60.
13. Schöttle P, Fucentese S, Romero J. Clinical and radiological outcome of medial patellofemoral ligament reconstruction with a semitendinosus autograft for patella instability. *Knee Surg Sports Traumatol Arthrosc*. 2005;13:516-521.
14. Smirk C, Morris H. The anatomy and reconstruction of the patellofemoral ligament. *Knee*. 2003;10:221-227.
15. Thaunat M, Erasmus P. Management of overtight medial patellofemoral ligament reconstruction. *Knee Surg Sports Traumatol Arthrosc*. 2009;17:480-483.
16. Warren L, Marshall J. The supporting and layers on the medial side of the knee. *J Bone Joint Surg*. 1979;61-A: 56-62.

# Anteromedial Tibial Tubercle Osteotomy (Fulkerson Osteotomy)

40

Jack Farr, Brian J. Cole, James Kercher, Lachlan Batty, and Sarvottam Bajaj

## 40.1 Introduction

The tibial tubercle (interchangeable with tuberosity) is the most distal anchor of the extensor mechanism and can serve as a tool in altering patellofemoral (PF) mechanics. Known collectively as distal realignment procedures, osteotomies of the tibial tubercle are a useful method to treat a variety of PF conditions by allowing coronal, axial, and sagittal plane adjustments of the patellofemoral articulation which redistribute patellar contact pressures (force and contact area) and potentially improve tracking. Numerous tibial tubercle osteotomies have been described in the literature to treat PF pain, chondrosis, and instability. The most notable include medialization, initially described by Roux and later popularized by Elmslie and Trillat, for the treatment of PF instability[30] and anteriorization of the tibial tubercle described by Maquet[18] performed to treat PF pain associated with arthritis. Each of these procedures takes advantage of important technical alterations in patellar kinematics. Anteriorization of the tubercle elevates the distal extensor mechanism and serves to shift patellar contact forces proximally, while medialization results in a decrease of the lateral force vector.

In an effort to avoid complications associated with the Maquet procedure, Fulkerson[11] designed a tubercle osteotomy known as the anteromedialization (AMZ) technique to address PF pain in conjunction with patellar maltracking. The oblique nature of the Fulkerson osteotomy allows for simultaneous anteriorization and medialization of the tibial tubercle. By varying the angle of the osteotomy, the tubercle can be biased to a more anterior or more medial position. Since his initial description, the indications for this procedure have evolved significantly and continue to be refined. This has been primarily driven by the evolution and outcomes of patellofemoral resurfacing procedures as well as improved objective measures of patellar alignment, contact area, and forces.

The tibial tuberosity to trochlear groove (TT–TG) distance, popularized by Dejour et al.[8] Serves as an objective measure of tuberosity position, has helped quantify abnormal tuberosity position and enhanced appropriate candidate identification for all tuberosity osteotomies including the AMZ. This becomes important because patellar contact pressures are very sensitive to distal realignment.[1,17,25] In addition, combining AMZ with PF cartilage restorative procedures such as autologous chondrocyte implantation and osteoarticular grafting procedures within the PF compartment have demonstrated superior results to either procedure performed independently.[10,14,19,21,28]

## 40.2 Indications

When discussing the indications for AMZ it is important to note that as with most patellofemoral surgeries, it should only be performed after the patient has tried and failed nonoperative measures that include a comprehensive "core to the floor"[9] program of rehabilitation, bracing, and orthotics. Indications for AMZ are primarily based upon mechanical and chondral pathologies specific to each individual knee. Malalignment is a term that has different meanings to

J. Farr (✉)
Voluntary Clinical, Orthopaedic Surgery,
IU School of Medicine, OrthoIndy Knee Care Institute,
Cartilage Restoration Center of Indiana, Indianapolis, IN, USA
e-mail: indyknee@hotmail.com

V. Sanchis-Alfonso (ed.), *Anterior Knee Pain and Patellar Instability*,
DOI: 10.1007/978-0-85729-507-1_40, © Springer-Verlag London Limited 2011

different experts, but for the purposes of this chapter it simply means alignment that is different from the average asymptomatic individual. A comprehensive review by Post et al.[23] demonstrated that the "Q" angle was inadequate to use as a measure of malalignment of the tibial tuberosity. Using the objectively measured TT–TG, asymptomatic patients have distances averaging 13 mm and those with instability symptoms have average measurements of over 15 mm.[27] A panel of patellofemoral experts agreed that TT–TG distances of over 20 mm were definitely abnormal and would be potential candidates for moving the tibial tubercle.[15] Patients with isolated chondrosis of the distal or lateral patella, who have excessive lateral patellar tilt and/or subluxation associated with an increased TT–TG distance and minimal trochlear chondrosis are optimal AMZ candidates based on a retrospective review of AMZ outcomes by Pidoriano.[22] It has been argued that rotational tuberosity abnormalities associated with subjective instability and pain may be sufficiently treated with straight medialization or derotation of the tibial tubercle,[20] although Pritsch et al.[24] found 80% of 66 patients undergoing tubercle transfer for patellar instability and pain associated with maltracking required anteriorization based on intraoperative examination. Second, patients who are undergoing PF cartilage restorative procedures have been shown to benefit from a combined AMZ procedure,[10,14,19,21,28] where optimization of the biomechanical environment and decreased stress across the restored cartilage is required. Additionally, in patients undergoing MPFL repair or reconstruction for recurrent lateral patella instability, AMZ may be indicated only in the setting of a significantly increased TT–TG distance. However, it should be noted that while this theoretically decreases the lateral vector forces on the healing MPFL tissues, there is no randomized study of AMZ plus MPFL surgery versus MPFL surgery alone published as of this writing. A summary of AMZ indications is presented in Table 40.1.

**Table 40.1** Summary of indications for anteromedialization

| Summary of AMZ indications: |
| --- |
| • Lateral or distal patella chondrosis with an increased TT–TG distance, excessive lateral tilt/subluxation, and the absence of trochlea chondrosis.<br>• As an adjunct procedure to patellofemoral cartilage restoration in an effort to improve the contact area and decrease PF forces to optimize the biomechanical environment of the new cartilage implant.<br>• Possibly, in conjunction with MPFL repair or reconstruction in patients with markedly increased TT–TG distance. |

## 40.3 Contraindications

Several contraindications to AMZ exist and potential candidates must be assessed carefully prior to surgery. Anteromedialization is contraindicated in patients with a normal TT–TG distance and in patients who have symptoms not explained by an increased TT–TG distance. The condition of the medial PF articulation should be carefully assessed as medialization will significantly increase contact pressures between the medial patellar facet and trochlea.[25] In addition, AMZ is contraindicated for proximal patella, panpatella, and bipolar chondrosis based upon the outcomes from Pidoriano et al.[22]

Advanced chondrosis of the central trochlea has been associated with suboptimal results and is considered a contraindication to AMZ as an isolated procedure.[5,22] Standard contraindications to any osteotomy must also be considered, which includes smoking, infection, inflammatory arthropathy, marked osteoporosis inhibiting adequate fixation, complex regional pain syndrome, arthrofibrosis, inability to minimally weight-bear, and noncompliant patients. A summary of AMZ contraindications is presented in Table 40.2.

## 40.4 Surgical Technique

Techniques for AMZ have classically been described as an isolated procedure; however, AMZ typically includes lateral retinacular release or lengthening to untether the patella allowing the patellar medialization component, and is not uncommonly performed in conjunction with procedures such as MPFL repair/reconstruction or cartilage restorative procedures. These procedures must be taken into consideration when planning the surgical approach.

**Table 40.2** Summary of contraindications to anteromedialization

| Summary of contraindications to isolated AMZ: |
| --- |
| • Normal TT–TG distance<br>• Medial patellofemoral chondrosis (only if not combined with cartilage restoration procedure)<br>• As an isolated procedure, when not combined with cartilage restoration, to treat proximal pole, panpatella, trochlear, or bipolar chondrosis<br>• General contraindications to osteotomy (i.e., smoking, osteoporosis, inflammatory arthropathy) |

### 40.4.1 Preoperative Assessment and Planning

The desired amount of anteriorization and medialization (based on the objective measurement of the TT–TG distance) must be calculated pre-operatively. These two components are considered separately and then basic trigonometric ratios can be used to determine the desired angle for the osteotomy. Anteriorization between 10 and 15 mm is most commonly recommended as it decreases PF stress loads by approximately 20%[7,8] and results in minimal sagittal rotation of the patella. In regards to the medialization component, the goal of the osteotomy is to normalize the TT–TG distance, which based on literature is within a range of 10–15 mm. By varying the slope and the extent of anteriorization, a variety of medialization distances can be achieved. The required angle can be calculated by the inverse tangent of the desired anterior movement divided by the desired medial movement Table 40.3. For example, a 60° osteotomy with 15 mm of elevation will produce 8.7 mm of medialization, which will normalize most tuberosity positions as it is rare for TT–TG distances of over 25 mm. When more medialization is required, the slope may be decreased; a slope of 45° would move the tubercle 15 mm medially with 15 mm of elevation.

### 40.4.2 Setup and Positioning of the Patient

The patient is positioned in the supine position with a side post and a gel-pad under the ipsilateral hemipelvis. This facilitates an initial arthroscopic evaluation of the knee and limits external rotation of the limb during the osteotomy. All extremities are well padded, a tourniquet is applied, and prophylactic antibiotics are administered. General, spinal, epidural, or regional block anesthesia can be used depending upon patient and surgeon preference. A thorough examination under anesthesia includes assessment of range of motion, patella tracking, and patella displacement. The patient is then prepped and draped in standard fashion.

**Table 40.3** Reference guide for osteotomy slope

| Osteotomy slope (°) | Elevation (mm) | Medialization (mm) |
|---|---|---|
| 60 | 15 | 8.7 |
| 50 | 15 | 12.5 |
| 45 | 15 | 15 |

### 40.4.3 Arthroscopic Evaluation

Initially, arthroscopic evaluation and documentation of patellofemoral chondrosis is performed. The areas of chondrosis are regionally mapped using the ICRS region knee mapping system noting that significant patellar chondrosis may lead to termination of the procedure unless concomitant cartilage restoration has been planned. Certainly other contraindications may be discovered at arthroscopy and would also halt proceeding with AMZ. At this stage, based on clinical tilt or CT/MRI documented patellar tilt, an arthroscopic lateral release may be performed if indicated. When combined with PF cartilage restoration the lateral release or lateral lengthening is performed in an open manner to allow direct access for performing the cartilage restoration procedure. Lateral release should allow neutralization of patella tilt and unrestricted central positioning of the patella relative to the trochlea; however, care must be taken to ensure that medial patella subluxation does not occur. It should be noted that lateral lengthening can maintain control not offered by lateral release.[4]

### 40.4.4 Incision and Exposure

The longitudinal incision runs approximately 8–10 cm distally beginning at the patellar tendon insertion to the tibial tubercle. The incision can be extended proximally to allow adequate exposure if concomitant cartilage restoration is being performed. The patella tendon is identified and released from capsule medially and laterally to allow protection with a retractor and later tubercle elevation. The lateral incision is extended distally along the lateral margin of the tibial tuberosity and tibial crest allowing subperiosteal elevation of the anterior compartment musculature and thereby exposing the lateral wall of the tibia. A custom retractor is positioned at the posterior aspect of the lateral tibia in order to protect the posterior neurovascular structures (deep peroneal nerve and anterior tibial artery) (Fig. 40.1).

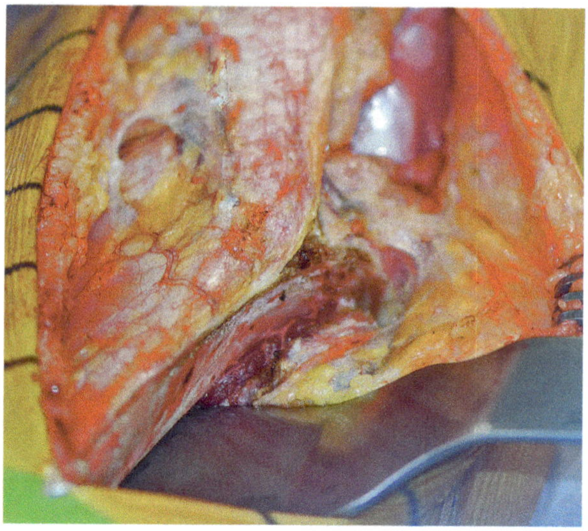

Fig. 40.1 Anterior compartment musculature is elevated from the lateral wall of the tibial with retractor protecting neurovascular structures posteriorly

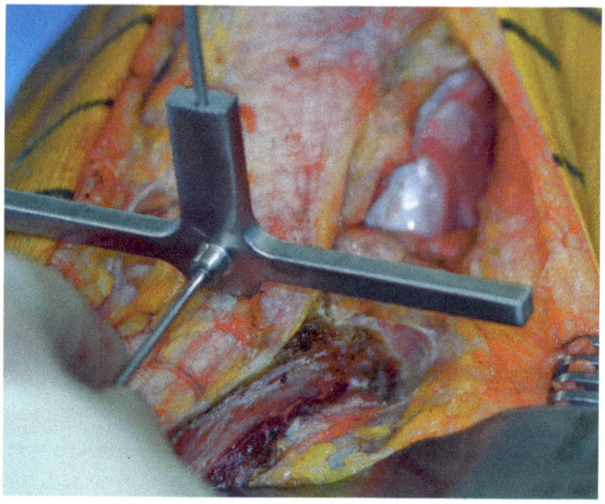

Fig. 40.2 The reference pin guide is orientated so it is perpendicular to the posterior cortex of the tibia

### 40.4.5 Performing the Osteotomy

For the highly experienced surgeon the osteotomy may be performed free-hand. Fulkerson originally used an external fixator pin clamp to direct multiple pins in the osteotomy plane and then complete it with osteotomes.[11] Today, there are two commercially available AMZ osteotomy systems (Tracker, DePuy Mitek, Inc, Raynham, New Jersey and the T3 System, Arthrex, Inc, Naples, Florida). The Tracker system was available first and illustrated detailed surgical techniques using the jig system have been published by both Fulkerson and Farr. The T3 system will be used in this section to illustrate the operative technique; however the approach for each system and steps following fixation of the cutting guide are similar. For the T3 system, an initial reference pin is orientated perpendicular to the posterior cortex of the proximal tibia (Fig. 40.2). The reference pin is inserted through the pin guide into the tibial tuberosity, just distal to the patellar tendon attachment to the tibial tuberosity (Fig. 40.3). Using preoperative calculations for anteriorization and medialization, the desired slope angle guide is assembled with the cutting block and cutting block post. The cutting guide is then placed over the reference pin and the cutting block is positioned immediately medial to the tibial crest beginning directly in line with the medial border of the patella tendon, as it attaches to the tibial tuberosity (Fig. 40.4), and angled laterally to allow a lateral exit of the osteotomy distally. For emphasis, the desired osteotomy forms a triangle shape that tapers distally allowing an exit through the anterior cortex to the lateral wall of the tibia. The desired pedicle length for the osteotomy is approximately 7–10 cm. When correct positioning has been achieved and the entry and exit sites have been confirmed, two break-away pins secure

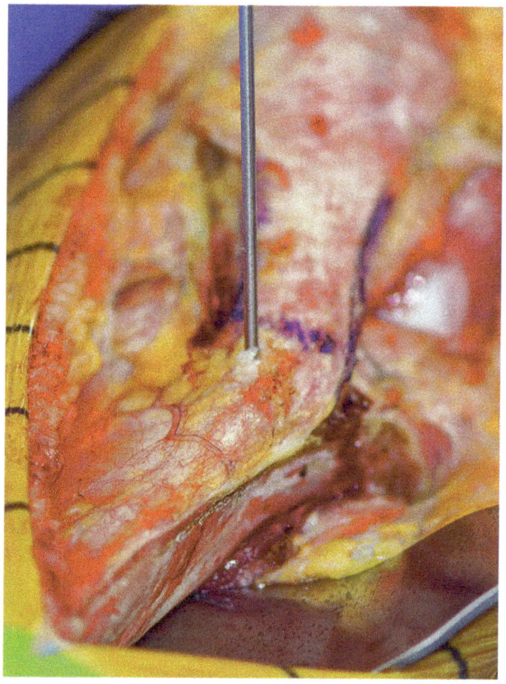

Fig. 40.3 Reference pin is inserted through the guide just distal to Gird's tubercle

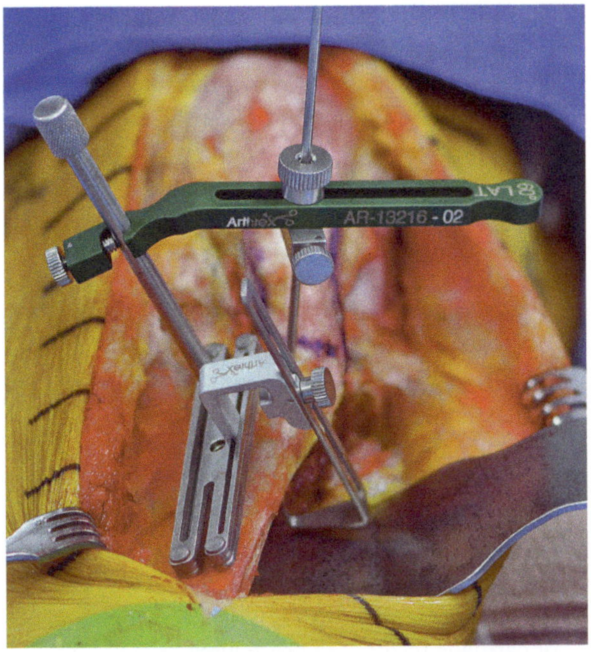


**Fig. 40.4** The cutting guide is placed over the reference pin and the cutting block is positioned medial to the patella tendon

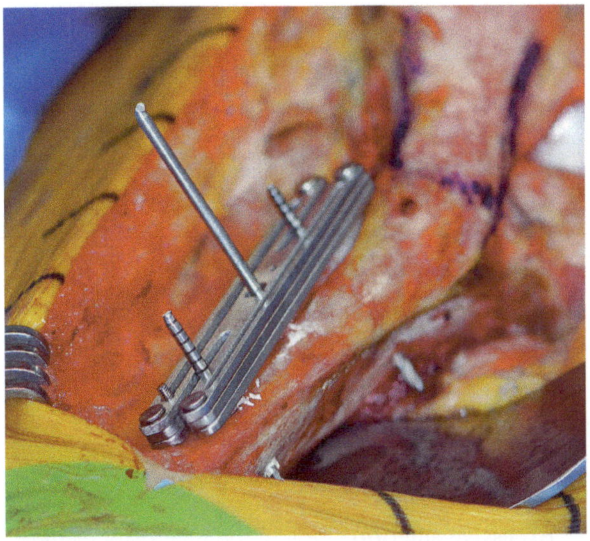

**Fig. 40.5** Break-away pins secure the cutting block after positioning is confirmed

the cutting block in position (Fig. 40.5). With the retractor still protecting neurovascular structures posteriorly, the cut is made with an oscillating saw which is simultaneously cooled with saline (Fig. 40.6). The cutting block is removed and the oscillating saw is directed toward the distal exit of the osteotomy to finish the distal cut. A small osteotome is used to complete the

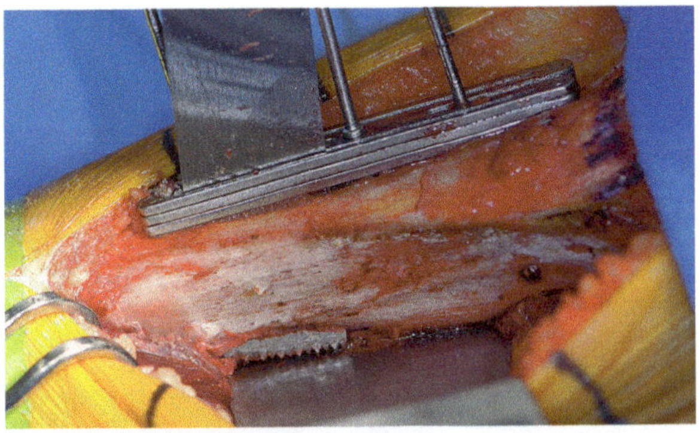

**Fig. 40.6** Oscillating saw cooled with saline creates the initial sloped osteotomy, exiting on the protective retractor

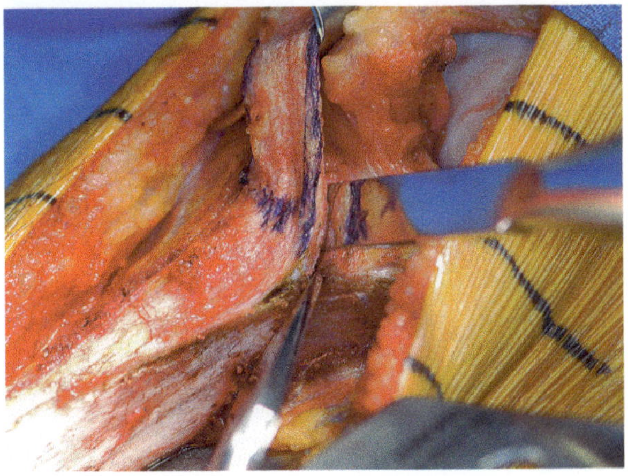

**Fig. 40.7** Proximal cuts are completed with small osteotome

proximal osteotomy, approaching the tibial tuberosity medially and laterally at the level of the patella tendon insertion (Fig. 40.7). The tuberosity is now free.

### 40.4.6 Positioning and Fixation

A ruler is used to measure the required amount of anteriorization and medialization based on preoperative calculations and the pedicle position is adjusted along the osteotomy slope. If required, the pedicles can be moved proximally or distally to address any underlying patella alta or infra. A Kirschner wire is used to temporarily secure the pedicle when correct positioning has been achieved. The tuberosity fragment is then drilled using interfragmentary lag technique and secured using two countersunk 4.5 mm cortical screws (Fig. 40.8). The screws are positioned perpendicular to the osteotomy (angled from the anterolateral aspect of the pedicle to

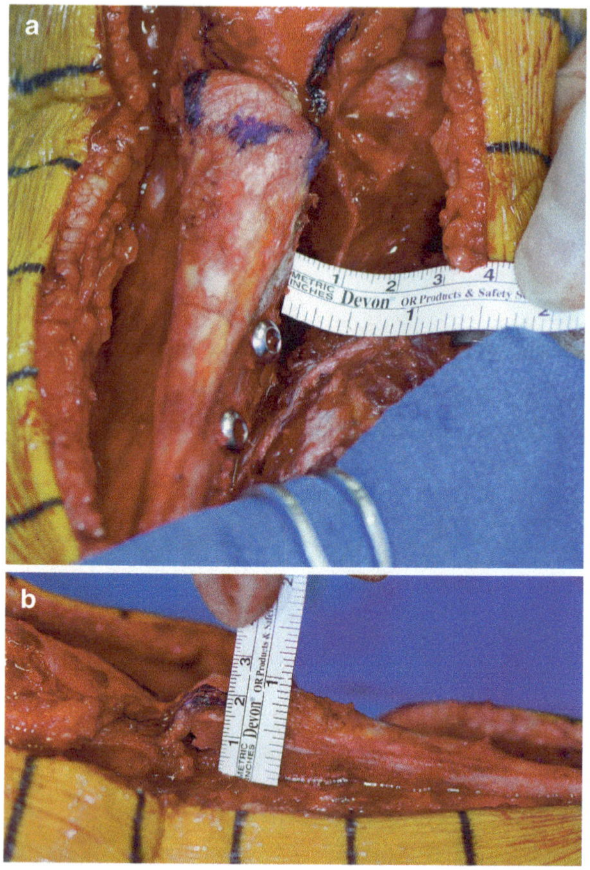


**Fig. 40.8** The distance of medialization (**a**) and anteriorization (**b**) is measured directly and the pedicle is secured with 2–4.5 mm screws

posteromedial tibia) so they are directed away from posterior neurovascular structures. The surgical site is closed in a standard fashion.

## 40.5 Pearls and Pitfalls

### 40.5.1 Pearls

- Preoperative rehabilitation and expectation counseling is extremely important to prepare the patient for surgery and recovery.
- The TT–TG measurement is an objective alternative to the Q-angle, quantifying the concept of tibial tuberosity malalignment.
- The mean TT–TG distance is 13 mm in asymptomatic patients and is considered excessive when above 20 mm.
- The goal is to "normalize" the tibial tubercle position that is keeping within a range of 10–15 mm.
- The required amount of anteriorization and medialization needed for normalization should be considered independently. The required osteotomy angle is determined based upon these values.
- The osteotomy angle is equal to $\tan^{-1}$ of the desired anterior movement ($y$) divided by the desired medial movement ($x$), e.g., Angle = $\tan^{-1}(y/x)$ (For simplicity, see Table 40.3)
- Assessment for patella alta using the Caton–Deschamps ratio (normal range 0.8–1.2) is required to determine if distalization is required.
- Strengthening of proximal core muscles must be a focus of rehabilitation in conjunction with local musculature.
- Anteromedialization can be performed in conjunction with other procedures including lateral release/lateral lengthening, MPFL repair or reconstruction, or cartilage restoration procedures.

### 40.5.2 Pitfalls

- Over medialization of the tibial tubercle can be detrimental secondary to increased medial patellofemoral and tibiofemoral stress.
- Patients should be aware that pain over the screw site is common and they may need removal at a future date.
- Weight bearing too early can lead to a fracture of the proximal tibia if the patient is returned to full weight bearing prior to radiographic healing.[2,12,29]
- The MPFL is recognized as the key restraint to lateral patella dislocation. Isolated tibial tuberosity AMZ is not a substitute for MPFL repair or reconstruction.
- Excessive anteriorization of the tuberosity can lead to skin healing problems and can cause clinically significant sagittal plane rotation of the patella altering contact areas.
- Isolated AMZ performed in the presence of chondrosis will yield poor results when the wear patterns are located in the: proximal patella, panpatella, or trochlea. However, AMZ in conjunction with cartilage restoration procedures in these regions can achieve good results.

## 40.6 Complications

Potential complications include those generally associated with osteotomies of the lower limb. General complications include malunion, nonunion, fracture at the osteotomy site,[12,29] venous-thromboembolism, compartment syndrome, infection, and loss of fixation. Complications specific to AMZ include persistent pain, arthrofibrosis and stiffness, progressive chondral deterioration, symptomatic hardware, complex regional pain syndrome, and intraoperative injury to the neurovascular structures including the popliteal artery and its trifurcation[16] and the deep peroneal nerve.

## 40.7 Postoperative Management

To improve postoperative recovery and prepare for surgery, the patient should undergo a preoperative proximal core and kinetic chain strengthening program (lower back, pelvis, hip thigh, and leg). Postoperatively the patient is treated with standard compression dressings, protective bracing, and cryotherapy, and is monitored for immediate complications. For the first 6 weeks the patient is limited to touch weight bearing with crutches and begins transitioning to full weight bearing after radiographs are noted to be acceptable at 6 weeks. The knee is protected with a hinged knee brace in extension which is unlocked at 2 weeks and discontinued when there is adequate lower extremity control (usually by 8 weeks). Early core proximal strengthening, quadriceps strengthening, and knee range of motion exercises are essential and a close relationship with an experienced physical therapist is key to optimizing the final results. The safe range of motion may need to be modified throughout the rehabilitation process to accommodate for concomitant cartilage restorative procedures.

## 40.8 Conclusions

Multiple case series have reported outcomes of the AMZ procedures (Table 40.4). Despite the heterogeneity in outcome measurements, results demonstrate high percentages of excellent and good results and improvements in objective, subjective, and functional measures. Attention to details related to surgical planning and properly managing patient expectations is most likely to lead to good or excellent results. Newer techniques (i.e., the T3 system) allow the surgeon to objectively determine the inclination of the osteotomy to properly restore patellofemoral mechanics based upon the preoperative planning.

**Table 40.4** Anteromedialization outcomes

| Author, year | Patient number | Mean follow-up (range) | Reported outcomes |
|---|---|---|---|
| Fulkerson[11] | 8 | n/a | Substantial relief of pain and disability for all patients |
| Cameron et al.[6] | 53 | >12 months | 66% Excellent, 16% good, 11% fair, 7% poor |
| Fulkerson et al.[13] | 30 | 35 months (26–50) | 35% Excellent, 54% good or very good, 4% fair, 7% poor |
| Sakai et al.[26] | 21 | 5 years (2–13) | Pain relief in ascending and descending stairs for 20/21 |
| Pidoriano et al.[22] | 37 | 47 months (12–96) | 87% Good to excellent results with lateral or distal lesions, 55% good to excellent results with medial lesions, 20% good to excellent results with proximal or diffuse lesions |
| Bellemans et al.[3] | 29 | 32 months (25–44) | Significant improvements in mean Lysholm (62 preoperative, 92 postoperative, $p<0.001$) and Kujala scores (43 preoperative, 89 postoperative, $p<0.001$) |
| Buuck and Fulkerson[5] | 42 | 8.2 years (4–12) | 86% Good to excellent subjectively, 86% good to excellent on clinical examination |

## References


1. Beck PR, Thomas AL, Farr J, et al. Trochlear contact pressures after anteromedialization of the tibial tubercle. *Am J Sports Med*. 2005;33:1710-1715.
2. Bellemans J, Cauwenberghs F, Brys P, et al. Fracture of the proximal tibia after Fulkerson anteromedial tibial tubercle transfer: a report of four cases. *Am J Sports Med*. 1998; 26:300-302.
3. Bellemans J, Cauwenberghs F, Witvrouw E, et al. Anteromedial tibial tubercle transfer in patients with chronic anterior knee pain and a subluxation-type patellar malalignment. *Am J Sports Med*. 1997;25:375-381.
4. Biedert RM, Friederich NF. Failed lateral retinacular release: clinical outcome. *J Sports Traumatol*. 1994;16:162-173.
5. Buuck D, Fulkerson JP. Anteromedialization of the tibial tubercle: a 4 to 12 year follow up. *Oper Tech Sports Med*. 2000;8:131-137.
6. Cameron HU, Huffer B, Cameron GM. Anteromedial displacement of the tibial tubercle for patellofemoral arthralgia. *Can J Surg*. 1986;29:456-458.
7. Cohen ZA, Henry JH, McCarthy DM, et al. Computer simulations of patellofemoral joint surgery. Patient-specific models for tuberosity transfer. *Am J Sports Med*. 2003;31: 87-98.
8. Dejour H, Walch G, Nove-Josserand L, et al. Factors of patellar instability: an anatomic radiographic study. *Knee Surg Sports Traumatol Arthrosc*. 1994;2:19-26.
9. Deppen R. From the CORE to the floor-interrelationships. In: Donatelli R, Donatelli R, eds. *Sports-Specific Rehabilitation*. Missouri/St. Louis: Elsevier; 2007.
10. Farr J. Autologous chondrocyte implantation improves patellofemoral cartilage treatment outcomes. *Clin Orthop Relat Res*. 2007;463:187-194.
11. Fulkerson JP. Anteromedialization of the tibial tuberosity for patellofemoral malalignment. *Clin Orthop Relat Res*. 1983; 177:176-181.
12. Fulkerson JP. Fracture of the proximal tibia after Fulkerson anteromedial tibial tubercle transfer: a report of four cases. *Am J Sports Med*. 1999;27:265.
13. Fulkerson JP, Becker GJ, Meaney JA, et al. Anteromedial tibial tubercle transfer without bone graft. *Am J Sports Med*. 1990;18:490-496.
14. Henderson IJP, Lavigne P. Periosteal autologous chondrocyte implantation for patellar chondral defect in patients with normal and abnormal patellar tracking. *Knee*. 2006;13: 274-279.
15. International Patellofemoral Study Group-Panel Discussion. Boston, Massachusetts, USA, 2006.
16. Kline AJ, Gonzales J, Beach WR, et al. Vascular risk associated with bicortical tibial drilling during anteromedial tibial tubercle transfer. *Am J Orthop*. 2006;35:30-32.
17. Kuroda R, Kambic H, Valdevit A, et al. Distribution of patellofemoral joint pressures after femoral trochlear osteotomy. *Knee Surg Sports Traumatol Arthrosc*. 2002;10:33-37.
18. Maquet P. Biomechanics of the patello-femoral joint. *Acta Orthop Belg*. 1978;44:41-54.
19. Minas T, Bryant T. The role of autologous chondrocyte implantation in the patellofemoral joint. *Clin Orthop Relat Res*. 2005;436:30-39.
20. Paulos L, Swanson SC, Stoddard GJ, et al. Surgical correction of limb malalignment for instability of the patella: a comparison of 2 techniques. *Am J Sports Med*. 2009;37: 1288-1300.
21. Peterson L, Brittberg M, Kiviranta I, et al. Autologous chondrocyte transplantation. Biomechanics and long-term durability. *Am J Sports Med*. 2002;30:2-12.
22. Pidoriano AJ, Weinstein RN, Buuck DA, et al. Correlation of patellar articular lesions with results from anteromedial tibial tubercle transfer. *Am J Sports Med*. 1997;25:533-537.
23. Post WR, Teitge R, Amis A. Patellofemoral malalignment: looking beyond the viewbox. *Clin Sports Med*. 2002;21: 521-546.
24. Pritsch T, Haim A, Arbel R, et al. Tailored tibial tubercle transfer for patellofemoral malalignment: analysis of clinical outcomes. *Knee Surg Sports Traumatol Arthrosc*. 2007;15:994-1002.
25. Rue JP, Colton A, Zare SM, et al. Trochlear contact pressures after straight anteriorization of the tibial tuberosity. *Am J Sports Med*. 2008;36:1953-1959.
26. Sakai N, Koshino T, Okamoto R. Pain reduction after anteromedial displacement of the tibial tuberosity: 5-year follow-up in 21 knees with patellofomoral arthrosis. *Acta Orthop Scand*. 1996;67:13-15.
27. Schoettle PB, Zanetti M, Seifert B, et al. The tibial tuberosity-trochlear groove distance: a comparative study between CT and MRI scanning. *Knee*. 2006;13:6-31.
28. Steinwachs M, Kreuz PC. Autologous chondrocyte implantation in chondral defects of the knee with a type I/III collagen membrane: a prospective study with a 3-year follow-up. *Arthroscopy*. 2007;23:381-387.
29. Stetson WB, Friedman MJ, Fulkerson JP, et al. Fracture of the proximal tibia with immediate weightbearing after a Fulkerson osteotomy. *Am J Sports Med*. 1997;25: 570-574.
30. Trillat A, Dejour H, Couette H. Diagnostic et traitement des subluxation recidivantes de la rotule. *Rev Chir Orthop Reparatrice Appar Mot*. 1964;50:813-824.

# The Patella Thinning Osteotomy: A New Technique for Patellofemoral Arthritis

**41**

Javier Vaquero and José Antonio Calvo

## 41.1 Introduction

Isolated patellofemoral osteoarthritis (PFOA) is a relatively common and disabling disease. While its radiological incidence is as high as 24% in women and 11% in men aged over 55, it becomes symptomatic in 8% of the women and 2% of the men in this age group.[14] In severe cases, the choice of treatment is difficult, particularly in patients who have not reached their sixth decade, and these patients are still then faced with mutilating patellectomy, patellofemoral arthroplasty, or total knee arthroplasty.[5,11,12,18,20]

Osteotomy of the patella, though not a recent innovation,[10,15] has been long neglected in the treatment of PFOA.[4,8,19] The earliest osteotomies performed in the sagittal plane were intended to improve congruence[10] or reduce the increased intraosseous pressure of the arthritic patella.[15] In the coronal plane, the aim was to improve the alignment of the extensor mechanism by the displacement between the fragments.[6,16] A new technique of coronal thinning osteotomy that, in addition, reduces the patellofemoral pressures as shown experimentally by direct measurement in cadavers[21] can achieve good clinical and radiological results in selected younger patients with isolated PFOA for an extended period of time.

J. Vaquero (✉)
Department of Orthopaedic Surgery,
Universidad Complutense de Madrid,
Hospital General Universitario Gregorio Marañon,
Madrid, Spain
e-mail: vaquerocot@aeartroscopia.com

## 41.2 Indications

The principal indication for this technique is severe symptomatic PFOA, in which alternative treatments probably include patellectomy, patellofemoral arthroplasty, or even total knee arthroplasty. Thinning osteotomy is a less aggressive alternative procedure, principally in patients younger than 60 years.

Wiberg's types 1 or 2 are preferable to obtain a uniform decompressive effect in both facets of the patella after thinning.

It is possible to associate other surgical procedures to treat PFOA (microfractures), and there are no technical problems to correct moderate malalignment of the extensor mechanism or the patellar instability with additional procedures in the same operation.

## 41.3 Contraindications

- Sinovitis or rheumatoid disease of the knee.
- Malalignment of the limb (varus or valgus) greater than 5°.
- Radiological signs of tibiofemoral osteoarthritis.
- Excessive wear of the patella and thickness (less than 20 mm) can be risk factors for fracture after thinning osteotomy (the mean thickness of the arthritic patella is 23.6 mm[13] and a 5 mm thinning does not compromise the patella).

## 41.4 Surgical Technique

The operation is performed under regional anesthesia through a short 10 cm longitudinal incision over the patella and a lateral arthrotomy. Once the lateral

V. Sanchis-Alfonso (ed.), *Anterior Knee Pain and Patellar Instability*,
DOI: 10.1007/978-0-85729-507-1_41, © Springer-Verlag London Limited 2011

retinaculum has been released, the patella is upturned and the osteophytes of the lateral rim are removed with an oscillating saw. We use a patellar clamp to hold firmly the patella. Although a double saw was used to remove a 5 mm thick bone fragment in the experimental study[21] and in the first cases, we are now using a 5 mm side cutting high-speed burr (United American Medical, McMinnville, IN) to remove this thickness of the central patellar bone (Fig. 41.1). With this instrument, which does not influence the final thinning, the technique is now simpler and quicker. We start at the lateral margin by making a through with the burr and we progress with oscillating movements from lateral to medial, maintaining a plane strictly parallel to the anterior cortical of the patella (Fig. 41.2a). Once the osteotomy has been completed, we tight the clamp and collapse the central part of the patella (Fig. 41.2b). We flex the knee a few times to improve the alignment of the extensor mechanism and both fragments are fixed with 3 or 4 divergent biodegradable pins (Orthosorb$^{R}$, Ethicon, Massachusetts) to eliminate postoperative rigid immobilization (Fig. 41.2c). After the apposition of the two fragments, the patella is thinner but always preserves the soft tissues attachment at the proximal and distal poles, and a congruent joint surface (Fig. 41.2d). The apposition of two broad cancellous bone surfaces subjected to compressive forces must favor consolidation. Minimal fixation with 3–4 polydioxanone pins is intended to prevent shearing forces and allow earlier mobilization. The skin is closed with a drain left in place.

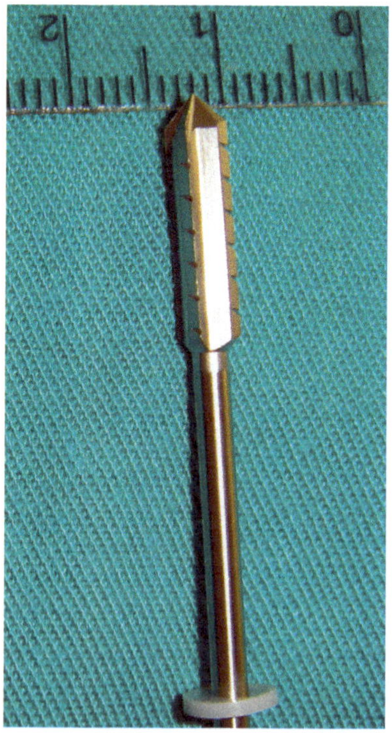

**Fig. 41.1** A 5 mm side cutting high-speed burr used to remove the central patellar bone

## 41.5 Postoperative Management

A brace in extension is worn, which the patient can remove to perform assisted exercises for the first postoperative month. Full weight bearing in extension is allowed. The rehabilitation program was continued for two more weeks to obtain full range of motion. Return to activities occurs at approximately 2 months, once the consolidation is completed.

## 41.6 Pearls and Pitfalls

The burr must be sharp and we recommend a single use. To prevent an oblique cut, we start directing the burr in an AP direction making a pilot hole from lateral to medial in the patella taking care to be strictly parallel to the anterior face of the bone and controlling the exit in the medial margin of the patella (Fig. 41.3). This perforation defines the plane of the osteotomy.

The greatest technical difficulty lays in the need to remove the central portion while causing minimal damage to the soft tissues and the peripatellar vessels. It is extremely important not to free completely the articular fragment to prevent osteonecrosis.

Irrigation is important to reduce thermal damage to bone, but we recommend to keep bone paste as an autologous bone graft.

In case of small or thin patella, we can use a 3.5 mm burr in order to save bone stock.

## 41.7 Clinical Results

From 1991 to 2008, this technique was performed on 31 patients (35 cases) with isolated and painful PFOA with the approval of the local Ethics Committee. We excluded cases with malalignment of the extensor mechanism (Q angle >20° or TT-TG distance over 20 mm) to evaluate

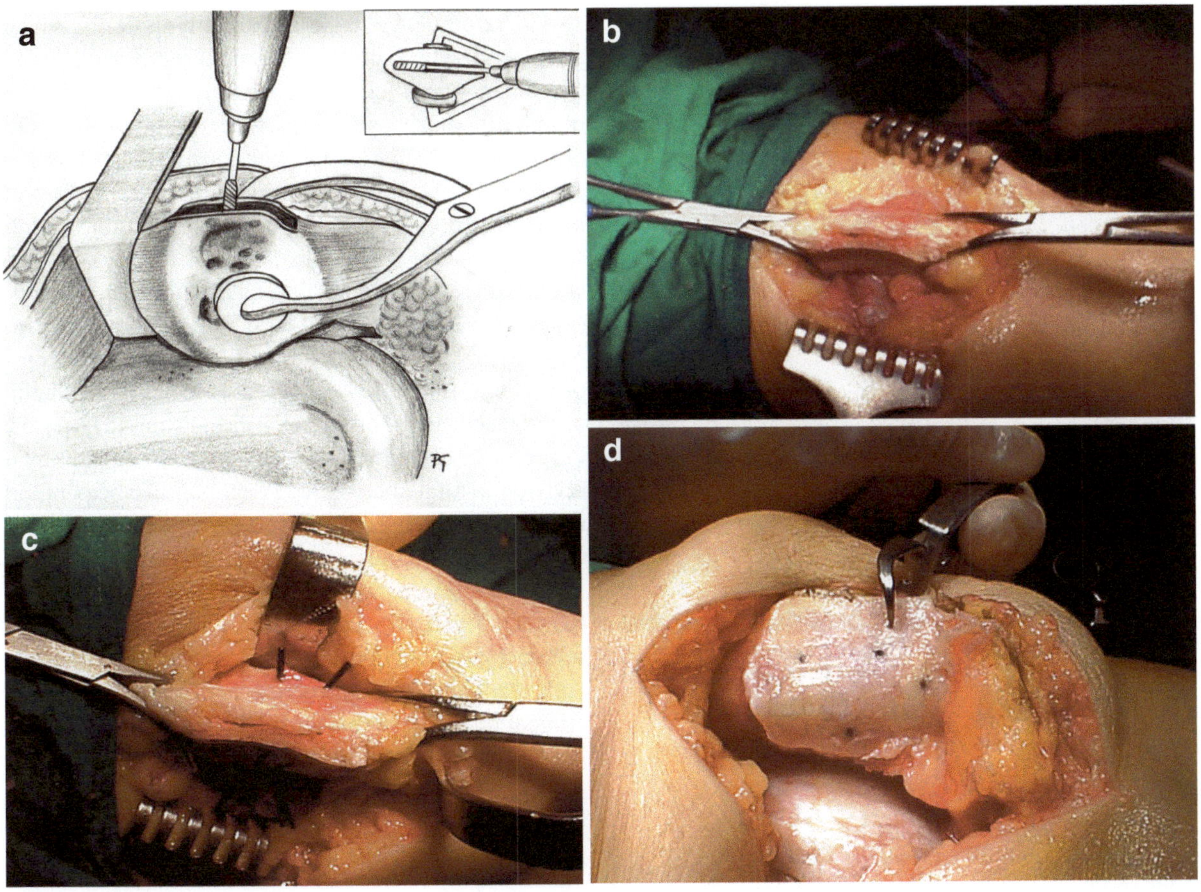


**Fig. 41.2** (**a**) Patella thinning osteotomy: making the through in the lateral rim of the patella. Drawing of the technique that shows the direction of the burr strictly parallel to the anterior face of the patella. (**b**) Patella thinning osteotomy: collapse of the central portion obtaining a thinner patella. (**c**) Patella thinning osteotomy: fixation of fragments with biodegradable pins. Note the osteotomy line. (**d**) Patella thinning osteotomy: final result with a congruent joint surface and preservation of the soft tissues attachments in the proximal and distal poles of the articular fragment (Reproducted and adapted with permission and copyright of the British Editorial Society of Bone and Joint Surgery from Vaquero et al.[22])

the thinning osteotomy without associated surgical techniques, which could influence the results. The results of all the 35 cases followed for 9.1 years (4–18 years) are reported.[22] This group included 7 men (a bilateral case) and 24 women (3 bilateral cases) with a mean age of 61.5 years (44–77 years). All the 31 patients have a follow-up of greater than 4 years and 40% of the cases greater than 10 years. We only lost one patient to follow-up after 5 years. The patients were examined by an independent surgeon who was not involved in the surgery; he explored them clinically and evaluated the radiographs.

All patients reached complete extension and a degree of flexion similar to the contralateral side at the latest follow-up. All the items of the Knee Society Score (KSS) improved, with a significant statistical analysis ($p < 0.05$) during the follow-up. The mean score increased from 131.06 points (76–180) prior to surgery to 166.9 points (110–200) at 5 years of follow-up and 162.21 points (131–200) at 10 years (Table 41.1). The Feller's Patellar Score[7] was used to evaluate the patellofemoral joint. All the items improved and it was particularly marked in pain evaluation. In contrast to KSS score, the gain was maintained over the time. The mean score increased from 14.23 points (7–21) prior to surgery to 24.65 points (12–30) with a follow-up of 5 years and 24.79 points (19–30) with a follow-up of 10 years (Table 41.2).

The subjective assessment of the patients was particularly satisfactory, as all the patients but one said that they felt better after the osteotomy. The SF-36 Health Survey Questionnaire improved principally in Physical Health scores.

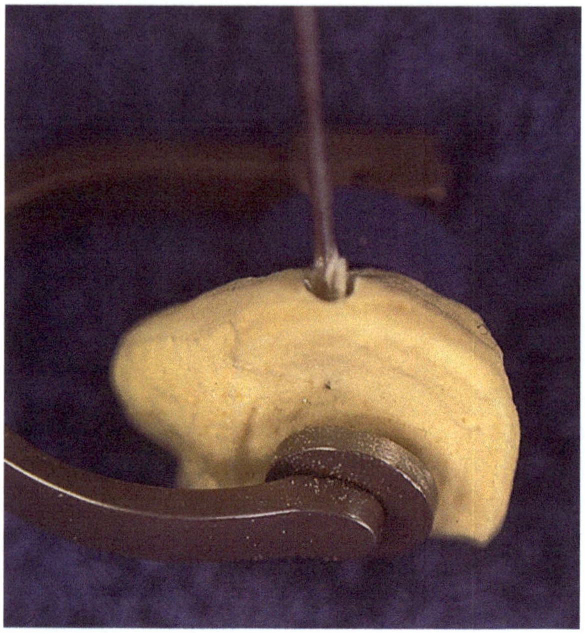

**Fig. 41.3** Pilot hole in saw-bone that determines the correct plane for the osteotomy

The congruence angle and the tilt angle improved postoperatively and the differences were statistically significant ($p < 0.05$) during the follow-up. The degree of patellofemoral osteoarthritis according to Ahlback[2] did not progress after surgery during the follow-up period (Fig. 41.4 a, b). However, the X-rays showed minor radiological femorotibial degeneration in 65% of the cases at a mean follow-up of 4.83 years (1–15). Only four cases have undergone an additional surgery (total knee arthroplasty) at least 5 years postoperative, without any technical complications. A patellar component was implanted in two cases leaving the patella unresurfaced in the other two arthroplasties (Fig. 41.5). Progressive tibiofemoral osteoarthritis necessitating a revision to total knee replacement has also been noted in 12% of the patients following patellofemoral replacement at a mean time of 55 months.[17]

In conclusion, we obtained 80% good results between 4 and 15 years. Barbera and Martinez[3] presented a study using the same technique in 36 patients with a mean age of 55 years and obtained similar clinical results at a shorter follow-up (15 months).

**Table 41.1** Preoperative score and follow-up values of Knee Society Score (KSS)

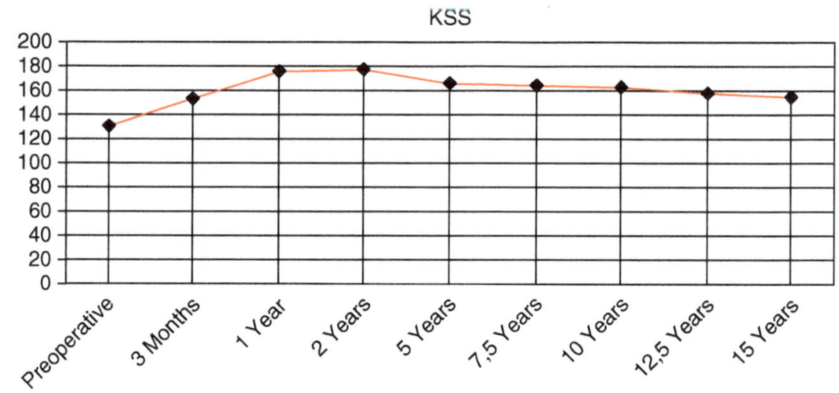


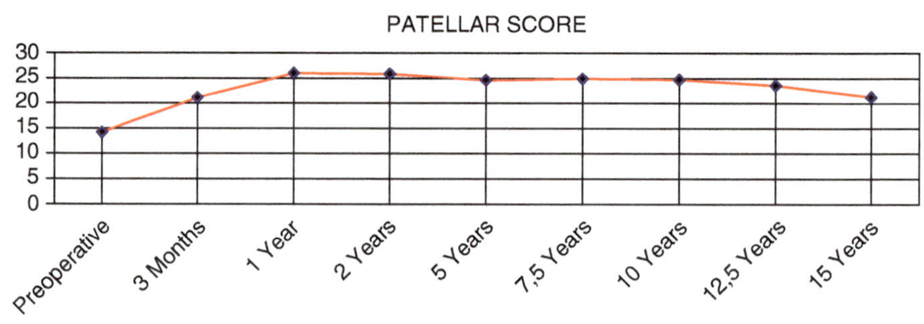


**Table 41.2** Preoperative score and follow-up values of Patellar Score

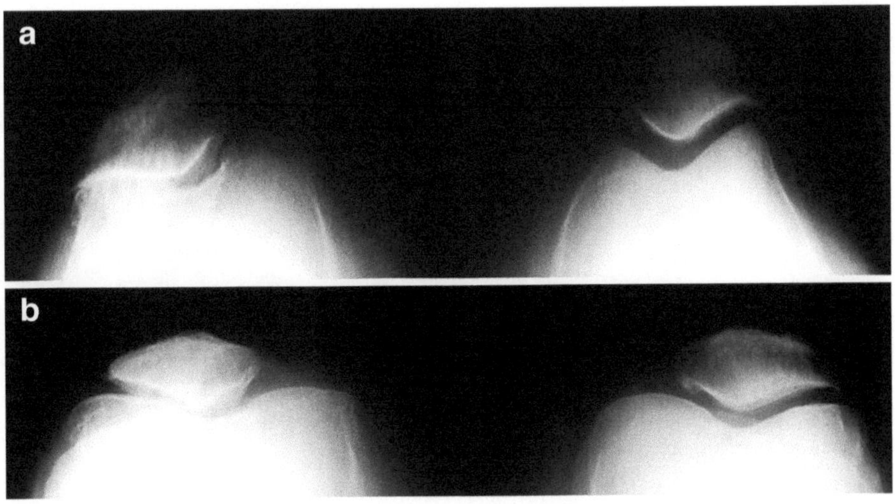


**Fig. 41.4** Skyline view preoperative (**a**) and 5 years (**b**) after a thinning osteotomy on the right side. Note the preservation of the joint line over time

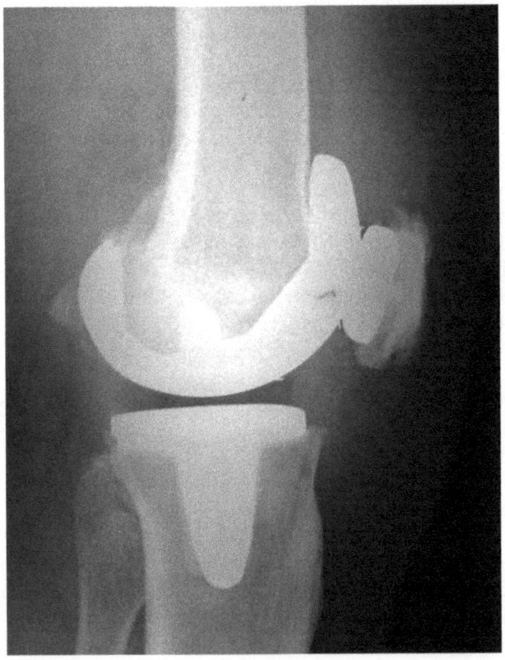

**Fig. 41.5** Total knee arthroplasty implanted without technical complications due to femorotibial osteoarthritis progression 5 years after a patella thinning osteotomy. Lateral view (Reproducted and adapted with permission and copyright of the British Editorial Society of Bone and Joint Surgery from Vaquero et al.[22])

## 41.8 Complications

We only had a major complication in a patient who developed an avascular necrosis of the articular fragment due to a technical error. The osteotomy was oblique and too close to the articular surface, performing a true facetectomy, and the necrotic fragment had to be removed arthroscopically (Fig. 41.6). Only this patient was unsatisfied after surgery. Due to the progression of femorotibial symptoms, it was necessary to perform a total knee arthroplasty with a satisfactory follow-up of 7 years actually.

## 41.9 Conclusion

The improvement following patellar thinning osteotomy is probably due to different factors: reduction in the patellofemoral pressures,[21] decrease of intraosseous pressure,[6,10] lateral retinacular release,[1,9] and the displacement between the fragments during flexion movements prior to the fixation which allows better tracking of the patella.[6] In our experience this new technique gives good results and does not burn any bridges with regard to future total knee replacement.

Patella thinning osteotomy is a conservative technique with good clinical and radiological results in our patients at a mean of 9 years, and a new option for the treatment of isolated patellofemoral osteoarthritis. This osteotomy is a less aggressive alternative for dealing with a difficult clinical problem.

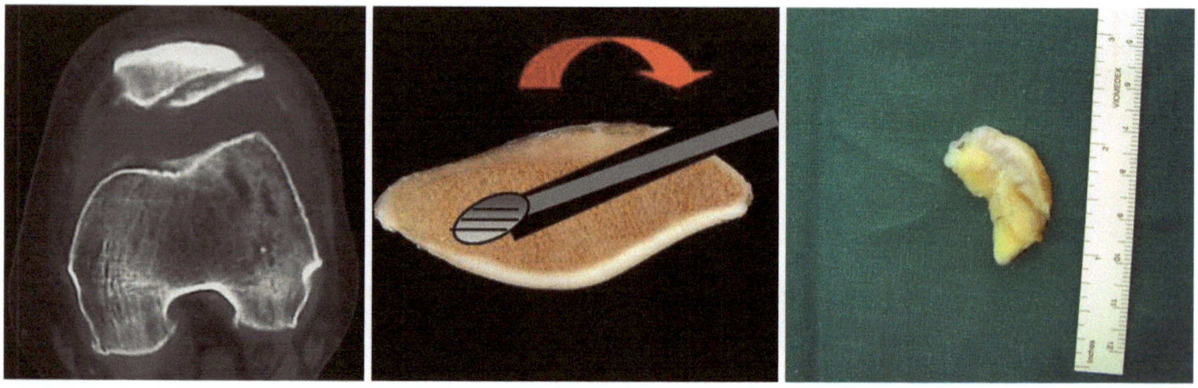

**Fig. 41.6** Skyline view and drawing that shows an oblique osteotomy too close to the articular surface. The necrotic fragment had to be removed arthroscopically 1 year later

## References


1. Aderinto J, Cobb AJ. Lateral release for patellofemoral arthritis. *Arthroscopy*. 2002;18:399-403.
2. Alhbäck S. Osteoarthrosis of the knee. A radiographic investigation. *Acta Radiol Diagn*. 1968;277:7-72.
3. Barberá Castillo ED, Martínez Islas L. Osteotomía de adelgazamiento de patela en artrosis patelofemoral. Resultados funcionales y radiográficos. *Acta Ortop Mex*. 2003;17:273-280.
4. Becker R, Röpke M. Surgical treatment of isolated patellofemoral osteoarthritis. *Clin Orthop Relat Res*. 2008;466: 443-449.
5. Dalury DF. Total knee replacement for patellofemoral disease. *J Knee Surg*. 2005;18:274-277.
6. Deliss L. Coronal plane osteotomy. Preliminary report of its use in chondromalacia patellae. *Proc R Soc Med*. 1977;70: 257-259.
7. Feller JA, Bartlett RJ, Lang DM. Patellar resurfacing versus retention in total knee arthroplasty. *J Bone Joint Surg Br*. 1996;78:226-228.
8. Fulkerson JP. Alternatives to patellofemoral arthroplasty. *Clin Orthop Relat Res*. 2005;436:76-80.
9. Fulkerson JP, Tennant R, Jaivin JS, et al. Histologic evidence of retinacular nerve injury associated with patellofemoral malalignment. *Clin Orthop Relat Res*. 1985;197: 196-205.
10. Hejgaard N, Arnoldi CC. Osteotomy of the patella in the patellofemoral pain syndrome. The significance of increased intraosseus pressure during sustained knee flexion. *Int Orthop*. 1984;8:189-194.
11. Kooijman HJ, Driessen AP, Van Horn JR. Long-term results of patellofemoral arthrosplasty: a report of 56 arthroplasties with 17 years follow up. *J Bone Joint Surg Br*. 2003;85:836-840.
12. Leadbetter WB, Ragland PS, Mont MA. The appropriate use of patellofemoral arthroplasty: an analysis of reported indications, contraindications, and failures. *Clin Orthop Relat Res*. 2005;436:91-99.
13. Lie DT, Gloria N, Amis AA, et al. Patellar resection during total knee arthroplasty: effect on bone strain and fracture risk. *Knee Surg Sports Traumatol Arthrosc*. 2005;13: 203-208.
14. McAlindon TO, Snow S, Coopper C, et al. Radiographic patterns of osteoarthritis of the knee joint in the community: the importance of the patellofemoral joint. *Ann Rheum Dis*. 1992;51:844-849.
15. Morscher E. Osteotomy of the patella in chondromalacia. *Arch Ortop Trauma Surg*. 1978;92:139-147.
16. Nerubay J, Katnelson A. Osteotomy of the patella. *Clin Orthop Relat Res*. 1986;207:103-107.
17. Nicol SG, Loveridge JM, Weale AE, et al. Arthritis progression after patellofemoral joint replacement. *Knee*. 2006;13: 290-295.
18. Parvizi J, Stuart MJ, Pagnano MW, et al. Total knee arthroplasty in patients with isolated patellofemoral arthritis. *Clin Orthop Relat Res*. 2001;392:147-152.
19. Saleh KJ, Arendt EA, Eldridge J, et al. Symposium. Operative treatment of patellofemoral arthritis. *J Bone Joint Surg Am*. 2005;87:659-671.
20. Sisto DJ, Sarin VK. Custom patellofemoral arthroplasty of the knee. *J Bone Joint Surg Am*. 2006;88:1475-1480.
21. Vaquero J, Arriaza R. The patella thinning osteotomy. An experimental study of a new technique for reducing patellofemoral pressure. *Int Orthop*. 1992;16:372-376.
22. Vaquero J, Calvo JA, Chana F, Perez-Mañanes R. The patellar thinning ostotomy in patellofemoral arthritis:four to 18 years follow-up. *J Bone Joint Surg Br*. 2010;92-B:1385-91.

# 42 Cartilage Restoration in the Patellofemoral Joint

Jack Farr, Brian J. Cole, Michael J. Salata, Marco Collarile, and Sarvottam Bajaj

## 42.1 Introduction

The appropriate treatment of patients with anterior knee pain starts with a thorough clinical history and a carefully conducted physical examination. A thorough assessment of the chondral defects and concomitant patho-mechanical factors is critical to the success of any restorative procedure. Co-morbidities such as patella alta, trochlear dysplasia, increased lateral position of the tibial tubercle relative to the femoral sulcus, and secondary soft tissue problems, such as a hypoplastic vastus medialis muscle or a contracted lateral retinaculum must be clearly defined. The standard treatment algorithms used for tibial or femoral chondral lesions cannot be directly extrapolated to the patellofemoral articulation. As an example, Brittberg and Peterson et al. reported successful outcomes for the tibiofemoral joint with autologous cultured chondrocyte transplantation (ACT); however, the same technique reported suboptimal outcomes in the patellofemoral joint as concomitant pathology such as malalignment was not addressed.[1] Peterson et al. next added treatment of the comorbidities to patellofemoral (PF) ACT and reported markedly improved outcomes.[7]

Chondral defects in the patellofemoral joint have varied etiologies. For example, the chondrosis may be genetically related, as with focal or diffuse degeneration secondary to trauma (direct impact or a result of patellofemoral instability) or secondary to repetitive microtrauma (e.g., excessive loads such as in jumping sports), or related to the cumulative microtrauma of biomechanical abnormalities (e.g., chronic patellar subluxation). High-grade (grades III and IV) focal chondral defects (Table 42.1) are reported to occur between 11% to 20% in patients undergoing knee arthroscopy. Of these defects, 11–23% involved the patella and 6–15% involved the trochlea.[1,10,20] Not all of these lesions were symptomatic. In fact, some patients are asymptomatic even at very high functional levels. Kaplan et al. performed MRIs on asymptomatic NBA basketball players and found articular cartilage lesions in 47% of these players, with 50% of these lesions classified as high grade (III or IV). The patella was affected in 35%, and the trochlea in 25% of these players who were asymptomatic.[23] Similarly, Walczak et al. found abnormal cartilage signal on MRI in 57% of asymptomatic NBA players with a 7% incidence of focal defects.[42]

Just as with other PF problems, symptoms and pathology have incomplete correlations. It is not entirely clear why some patients with PF chondral lesions present with pain while others can perform at a high level. Ficat and Hungeford proposed that the elevated intraosseous pressures seen in the face of an articular cartilage lesion could be the source of pain and today with MRI, it is not uncommon to see areas of bone overload associated with chondral lesions as evidenced by "bone bruises."[31] As noted, the articular cartilage is aneural, so pain other than bone may emanate from the soft tissues, including the joint capsule, ligaments, tendons, and synovium. In addition to mechanical factors, pain may be initiated in part by irritation from chondral debris, which activates an inflammatory and nociceptive response. As the true pain generator is often not well defined,

J. Farr (✉)
Voluntary Clinical, Orthopaedic Surgery,
IU School of Medicine, OrthoIndy Knee Care Institute,
Cartilage Restoration Center of Indiana, Indianapolis, IN, USA
e-mail: indyknee@hotmail.com

V. Sanchis-Alfonso (ed.), *Anterior Knee Pain and Patellar Instability*,
DOI: 10.1007/978-0-85729-507-1_42, © Springer-Verlag London Limited 2011

**Table 42.1** Summary of modified outerbridge and ICRS chondral grading scales

| Grade | Modified outerbridge | ICRS |
|---|---|---|
| Grade 0 | Normal | Normal |
| Grade 1 | Softening | A: Near normal<br>B: Soft intact or superficial open lesion |
| Grade 2 | Open fissures, fibrillation to 50% depth | Abnormal lesion to<50%cartilage depth |
| Grade 3 | Open fissure fibrillation to palpable bone (>50% depth) | Severely abnormal<br>A: >50% cartilage depth<br>B: Down to calcified layer<br>C: To but not through bone |
| Grade 4 | Exposed bone | Severely abnormal full-thickness cartilage loss and bone loss |
| Notes | | Add size and site of lesion |

it is crucial to thoroughly evaluate all potential sources of discomfort before attributing symptoms to a chondral defect. This chapter presents the systematic approach to decision-making process for, and surgical treatment of, chondral defects of the PF compartment.

## 42.2 History

A careful clinical history is the first step necessary to make an accurate diagnosis. Patients may report a history of either an insidious onset of symptoms or acute onset after trauma. In addition, it is not uncommon for the mechanism of the PF chondral pathology to be unknown. In general, patients with patellofemoral pathology can be divided in two main groups: anterior knee pain and patellar instability. It is critical to determine which of the patient's symptoms are most prominent: pain or instability, noting that these are not mutually exclusive. The approach of these two subsets is somewhat different and need to be fully explored the patient's main complaint is presented. The character of the anterior knee pain is important to elicit from the patient. Pain from the anterior soft tissues is often described as acute, episodic, and/or localized/poorly localized. Document what activities and positions aggravated the pain. The patient can often perform maneuvers in the office to reproduce pain. Pain due to a chondral etiology mediates through the same tissues that cause pain for other PF pathologies. It is often poorly localized and may be exacerbated by prolonged sitting ("movie theatre sign"). Severe, unrelenting pain that is out of proportion to the patient's exam could be suggestive of a more possible complex regional pain syndrome.

Any history of knee trauma is important. Direct impact injury such as a slip, fall, or "dashboard" type injury may result in anterior knee pain and may damage the patellar or trochlear cartilage even without bone injury. Patellar dislocations may cause damage to the distal medial patellar cartilage and/or lateral femoral condyle. An indirect mechanism is seen with posterior cruciate ligament (PCL) injury. With the posterior displacement of the tibia, PF compartment joint reactive forces are increased.[13] Over time this patellofemoral overload may lead to chondral changes and symptoms of anterior knee pain.

When evaluating the patient with a chief complaint of instability, it is important to determine the amount of energy associated with the first dislocation episode. If the initial episode was a very low energy episode, it should trigger the physician to carefully evaluate for predisposing factors such as generalized ligamentous laxity, patellar alta, trochlear dysplasia, or malalignment. For higher energy dislocations, there is increased risk of chondral pathology with a lower likelihood of significant predisposing anatomic factors. The frequency of and most recent dislocation episode should be recorded, as well as the degree of pain and effusion between instability episodes. Interval pain and effusion symptoms may suggest chondral damage from the recurrent dislocations. In the patient with frequent dislocations, not only is there patholaxity of the soft tissue restraints, there may be significant PF dysplasia and patellar alta that will necessitate a more comprehensive reconstructive procedure. It is important to determine whether the patient is having true dislocation episodes or if they are experiencing subluxations or another phenomenon such as "giving way."[13] This may, indeed, represent patellar instability, but can also be related to a pain reflex causing quadriceps inhibition, secondary to ligament deficiency (e.g., ACL deficiency) or intra-articular effusion that inhibits full quadriceps activation.[37] Patients often report crepitus. This has poor correlation with chondral pathology and may be a result of many factors such as: chondrosis, synovial impingement, or scar tissue. Some patients will also complain of mechanical symptoms of locking or catching. In contrast to the symptoms caused by meniscal pathology, mechanical symptoms from the patellofemoral joint usually occur during activity which loads the patellofemoral compartment such as walking down stairs.

Any previous surgical interventions should be documented. It is ideal if the operative reports and the intraoperative arthroscopy images are obtained and reviewed. The date of the procedure is also very important. If it has been a prolonged period since arthroscopic evaluation, a repeat arthroscopy may be warranted to confirm the diagnosis and to define the lesions by location, region, and grade.

## 42.3 Physical Examination

A focused and detailed physical examination is just as important as the clinical history. The examination entails evaluation of the entire kinetic chain from the foot (pronation vs. cavus) to the tibia (external torsion) to the knee and PF specific exams of the hip. Increased internal rotation increases the suspicion of excessive hip anteversion to the core proximal musculature which will also include the low back and pelvis. Evaluation of muscle weakness of the hip abductors, hip extensors, and pelvic stabilizers is essential. Weakness of these muscles is evaluated by asking the patient to do a single-leg stance on the affected limb which results in a pelvic drop on the contralateral side. Inspection for any deformity or surgical scars should be the first step in the exam. An evaluation of gait should also be performed to assess for any incongruity or abnormality. Both legs should be examined to evaluate for symmetry. The location of the patient's pain should be identified if possible and contributing structures should be carefully assessed. An evaluation for patellar instability should be performed on all patients presenting with symptoms localized to the anterior knee.

Special tests for the PF compartment have been described. Retinacular tightness can be evaluated with the patellar glide and tilt tests. With the knee flexed to 30° the patella is displaced medially. If there is limited medial movement associated with lateral PF facet pain, this is pathognomic of excessive lateral tightness.[13] Lateral retinacular tightness is common in patients with anterior knee pain and is the hallmark of the excessive lateral pressure syndrome described by Ficat.[12] Fulkerson reported tenderness over the lateral retinaculum in 90% of the patients in his series of anterior knee pain.[14] The patellar grind test is an axial compression of the patella on the trochlea and is often positive in the setting of a chondral defect. This test is performed in various angles of flexion in order to establish the location of the chondral defect. As the contact area moves from proximal to distal with knee motion, pain near extension is indicative of a chondral defect in the distal part of patella or trochlea; if the pain is elicited at 90° of flexion, the chondral defect is localized to the proximal aspect of patella or trochlea. The sustained knee flexion test is performed by having the patient flex the knee against resistance for 45 s and then having them extend the knee after a period of 15–30 s.[19] The test is considered positive if pain is reported during the extension period. Patellar and quadriceps tendinosis can present as anterior knee pain, so it is important to palpate the proximal and distal poles of the patella. Hoffa's fat pad should be considered as a source of pain especially in the patient who has undergone a previous arthroscopy.[17]

A patient presenting with instability will usually experience a lateral subluxation or dislocation. The patellar glide test is used to assess the medial and lateral displacement of the patella. It is positive if the patella can be significantly displaced in three or more quadrants.[13] Fairbank's patellar apprehension test, when positive, suggests that instability is a significant problem for the patient. The test is positive when the patient has a defensive contracture of quadriceps during lateral patellar displacement at 20°–30° of flexion. Medial instability is often a consequence of an unnecessary or excessive realignment surgery or lateral release. This can be evaluated by Fulkerson's relocation test.[15] This test is performed by holding the patella in a medial direction with the knee extended. The knee is then flexed while the patella is simultaneously released. This causes the patella to relocate into the trochlea. In patients with medial subluxation this test reproduces the patient's symptom. Patellar tracking can be assessed with the "J" sign. The patient extends the knee from 90° of flexion and the patella moves in a proximal and lateral direction that is similar to an inverted "J." This may be an observation in a patient presenting with PF malalignment or in otherwise normal knees. Likewise, a patella that is always lateral may have linear tracking even though there is malalignment.

Tightness of the quadriceps, hamstring, gastrocnemius muscles, and iliotibial band may contribute to anterior knee pain and should be evaluated. Quadriceps tightness is suggested by: (1) a different degree of flexion of one knee (best documented prone) compared to the other, (2) feeling of tightness in the anterior aspect of the thigh, and (3) elevation of the pelvis due to flexion of the hip.[43] Evaluation of iliotibial band tightness is done using Ober's test. To perform this test the patient lies on the nonpainful side and the examiner flexes the affected knee and hip to 90°. The examiner then abducts and extends the affected thigh, which places the iliotibial band on maximal stretch. Palpation of the iliotibial band just proximal to the lateral femoral condyle during maximal stretch will cause severe pain in patients with excessive iliotibial band tightness. To test pelvic tilt, the Thomas test is performed with full hip flexion while observing pelvic movement.

## 42.4 Imaging

Plain radiographs are a standard part of the diagnostic workup for cartilage-related patellofemoral pain. A standard series includes a standing AP view, 45° (PA "Rosenberg, Shuss or skier view"), a true lateral view, and a low flexion angle axial view (Merchant). The AP view supplemented with a hip to ankle alignment film is used to evaluate the extent of varus or valgus alignment and joint space narrowing. The lateral view is useful for documenting trochlear dysplasia, patellar height (alta or infera), and patellar tilt. Currently, the methods of Caton–Deschamps or Blackburn–Peel are favored over Insall–Salvati. The ratio compares the length of the articular surface of patella and the distance from the most anterior point of articular tibial surface to the most distal point of articular patella surface. Normal ratios are between 0.8 and 1.2. An index greater than 1.3 represents patella alta, and an index less than 0.6 represents patella infera. Dejour et al. have shown that the true lateral radiograph provides more information to assess trochlear dysplasia and patellar tilt than the Merchant view.[2,4,11,17,26] The axial radiograph (Merchant view) is best used to determine information regarding the sulcus angle, joint space narrowing, subchondral sclerosis, and shape of the patella.

CT scan is a useful imaging modality when a tibial tuberosity osteotomy is being considered. The TT–TG (tibial tubercle to trochlear groove) distance can be measured and can guide the surgeon in decision making about the need for an osteotomy. A TT–TG distance of <15 mm is considered normal; values >20 mm are "excessive" and represent malalignment that may be treated with an osteotomy.[4,40] Schutzer et al. identified three patterns of malalignment using CT imaging: type 1 (patellar subluxation without tilt), type 2 (patellar subluxation with tilt), and type 3 (patellar tilt without subluxation).[35] For cartilage specific considerations, a CT arthrogram will allow detailed assessment of lesion position and dimensions. As malposition of the patella relative to the trochlea is often associated with cartilage lesions, additional information may, at times, be obtained from multiple flexion angles (midwaist patellar slices or midwaist patellar cuts comparing quad-active and quad-relaxed views).[34]

Magnetic resonance imaging (MRI) remains essential for the evaluation of osteochondral lesions; in particular the sagittal and coronal image series are useful in evaluating the patellofemoral articulation. MRI has received increased attention due to newly developed high-resolution imaging protocols with the option of enhancement by intravenous gadolinium. This results in sensitivity and specificity approaching 90% for MRI protocols using a 1.5 T magnet with appropriate orthogonal sequences.[32,33,35,44] MRI also allows assessment of bone overload as evidenced with bone edema (bone bruise).

Bone scans are rarely used in standard cases, but can delineate sites of bone overload or in atypical presentations can be an aid in diagnosing complex regional pain syndrome.

## 42.5 Basic Science

The lack of vascular, neural, and lymphatic access to articular cartilage creates an environment of limited repair. Injuries that penetrate the subchondral bone initiate a vascular proliferative response resulting in a combination of normal hyaline cartilage (primarily type II collagen) and a structurally inferior fibrocartilage (primarily type I collagen). Each zone of normal hyaline cartilage has a characteristic composition of chondrocytes, collagen, aggrecan, and fluid dynamics that relate directly to that zone's function. Hyaline cartilage consists of 4 zones with the most superficial zone containing the "lamina splendens" (packed collagen fibers) and a cellular layer of flattened chondrocytes. The preservation of this layer is very important for the deeper layers as it limits passage of large molecules between the synovial fluid and cartilage. The intermediate zone is composed of spherical chondrocytes, proteoglycans, and obliquely oriented collagen fibers. The deep zone is a combination of collagen fibers and chondrocytes oriented perpendicular to the articular surface which allows them to optimally resist compressive loads. The deepest level is the calcified cartilage layer which is separated from the deep zone by the tidemark. There are many classification systems used to describe chondral lesions. We have summarized the most commonly used and present them in Table 42.1.

## 42.6 Patellofemoral Chondrosis Subsets

The cartilage in the patellofemoral articulation is the thickest articular cartilage in the body to accommodate the high loads that are seen in this joint. The variability of bony morphology of this articulation can be a challenge for surgical treatment of the patellofemoral joint. It is useful to categorize patients with PF chondral disease into two categories: those patients with PF chondrosis and associated tibiofemoral chondrosis and those with isolated PF chondrosis. Patients with associated tibiofemoral chondrosis are common. As multiple compartments are affected the outcomes in this patient group are less optimal than in the isolated condition. In order to maximize the outcomes in this patient group the concomitant lesions should be addressed at the same time as the primary procedure. Although, some consideration is given to treating only the most symptomatic lesions as occasionally lesions may be incidental and not clinically relevant. Isolated patellofemoral chondrosis can be divided by etiology into different categories: traumatic, dysplastic, and focal osteochondral defects. The traumatic lesions are subdivided by mechanism into those due to macrotrauma (such as a patellar dislocation or direct blow) and those due to microtrauma (which includes repetitive overuse injuries). Microtraumatic lesions can present with linear fissures of the patella, traumatic delamination, or osteochondral fractures, depending on the degree of knee flexion at the time of the injury. Lesions due to dysplastic conditions result from increased contact pressure. Chondral pathology due to dysplasia can be difficult to treat because of the patellofemoral morphology. These lesions have been treated with soft tissue procedures and TTOs with variable results. Focal osteochondral defects not caused by trauma may be a result of avascular necrosis or osteochondritis dessicans. Lesions secondary to this type of pathology are rare in the patellofemoral joint. Treatment of these lesions requires the surgeon to correct both the underlying bony pathology as well as the chondral defect.

## 42.7 Treatment and Indications/Contraindications

### 42.7.1 *Arthroscopic Chondral Debridement*

Chondroplasty is indicated in low demand patients who have failed nonoperative treatment with therapy, NSAIDs, and injections or as a staging procedure in patients who may undergo a definitive cartilage restorative procedure. Though not a definitive time period, a trial of nonoperative management for 8–26 weeks is reasonable. This procedure is optimal for those patients with mechanical symptoms without widespread degenerative changes. It may be the first line of treatment in younger patients with chondral defects and can be coupled with procedures such as biopsy for ACI for future interventions or planning a definitive major restoration. Goals of this procedure are to stabilize loose chondral flaps and decrease synovial inflammation from recurrent sloughing of articular debris. Chondral debridement is of questionable value in the truly degenerative knee as several studies have failed to show efficacy over nonoperative treatment.[30]

### 42.7.2 Microfracture (Marrow Stimulation)

Microfracture is indicated in younger patients with full-thickness, well-contained, small lesions. It is ideally suited for unipolar disease. Though some authors have reported good outcomes with larger PF lesions, other authors report poor results of marrow stimulation for all patellar lesions.[25,38] Most reports suggest treatment for lesions under 4 $cm^2$[7,24,29] Perhaps the most important aspect of this surgery is the adherence to the postoperative rehabilitation. This procedure is attractive because it is easy to perform and does not require any additional implants.

Marrow stimulation is contraindicated when there is uncorrected malalignment, global, diffuse degenerative change, or an unwillingness or inability to comply with postoperative rehabilitation demands. A relative contraindication is age >40 years based on the Kreuz outcomes.[25]

### 42.7.3 Osteochondral Autograft Transplantation

Osteochondral autograft transplantation is indicated for a patellofemoral lesion of less than 2.5 $cm^2$ when the lesion is contained. It is contraindicated in uncontained lesions, bipolar lesions, or when there is uncorrected malalignment.

### 42.7.4 Autologous Chondrocyte Implantation/Transplantation

ACI is indicated in symptomatic, full-thickness defects of the patellofemoral articulation and in the United States it is a second-line treatment. Larger lesions and bipolar disease can be treated successfully with this technique. This is a treatment option for larger lesions and those lesions that have previously failed other techniques (unless extensive bone loss is present) noting that it is unclear which prior procedures may portend a less optimal result.[28] Results appear to be better with unipolar disease, but focal bipolar disease can be successfully treated. The published series of ACI at the PF compartment often includes significant number of concomitant tibial tuberosity osteotomies; however the technique and discussion of this technique are addressed in a separate chapter in this text (Chap. 40). Relative contraindications to ACI exist when there is subchondral bone collapse or bone loss, uncorrectable malalignment, untreated ligamentous instability, advanced age (>55 years), widespread osteoarthritis, and BMI >30.

### 42.7.5 Osteochondral Allograft Transplantation

Osteochondral allograft transplantation is indicated for patients with symptomatic, large (>3 $cm^2$), full-thickness osteochondral or full-thickness chondral lesions. It is often used for second-line treatment of unstable and irreparable osteochondritis dessicans lesions, failed osteochondral autograft transfers, failed ACI, or in the setting of subchondral bone collapse. The pathology should be monopolar as bipolar lesion treatment has a much lower success rate. Patients with advanced or diffuse degenerative changes involving one or both of the tibiofemoral compartments are contraindicated for this procedure and are better served by knee arthroplasty.

*Authors preference:* For pure chondral pathology, ACI is performed concomitantly with straight anterization if the TT–TG is normal or anteromedialization when the TT–TG is excessive. Isolated bipolar disease of the PF joint in very young and severely symptomatic patients who fail ACI may be treated with fresh OC grafting of both the patella and trochlea given the limited alternatives other than PF resurfacing or total knee arthroplasty. Failed ACI of the PF joint can be treated with revision osteochondral allografting.

## 42.8 Surgical Technique

Prior to any major surgical restoration effort it is important to have a recent and accurate intra-articular evaluation of the patient's anatomy and chondral defect. If recent, high-quality arthroscopic images or video are unavailable, a diagnostic "staging" arthroscopy should be performed at a date prior to the restoration. When ACI is indicated, a biopsy would be harvested at this surgery.

## 42.8.1 *Microfracture*

### 42.8.1.1 Lesion Preparation

Standard arthroscopic evaluation is carried out and the lesion is identified. All other intra-articular pathology should be addressed prior to performing the microfracture. The lesion is debrided with a curette and mechanical shaver to expose the subchondral bone. It is imperative to create a stable "well shouldered" lesion in order to maximize the success of this procedure. A ring curette can be helpful in the patellofemoral joint for this purpose. When preparing a lesion on the undersurface of the patella, it is often helpful to have an assistant provide counter-pressure and stabilize the patella to aid in preparation of the lesion or perform a miniarthrotomy to allow unencumbered access. It is also important to remove the calcified cartilage layer in order to fully prepare the lesion.

### 42.8.1.2 Microfracture

Once the lesion is prepared, a microfracture awl is selected that will allow for perpendicular creation of the holes. The goal is to place the holes 3–4 mm apart and to a depth of 2–4 mm or just until fat globules are seen coming from the underlying marrow (Fig. 42.1). It is often helpful to begin the microfracture at the periphery of the lesion and work from outside in to maximize the amount of holes that can be created. Once the holes have been created the arthroscopy fluid pressure is turned down or off to ensure that blood flows from the created microfracture sites. The arthroscope is withdrawn and the wounds are closed in a standard fashion. A recent basic science study suggests the older form of marrow stimulation, drilling, may have theoretical advantages.[9]

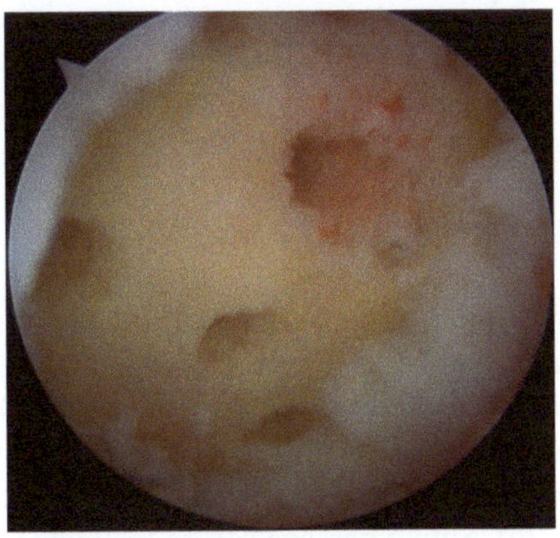

**Fig. 42.1** Marrow stimulation of trochlea

## 42.8.2 *Osteochondral Autograft*

### 42.8.2.1 Exposure

The patient is positioned supine on an operating table. The exposure for this procedure is similar to both ACI and osteochondral allografting utilizing a midline utility approach and either a medial or lateral arthrotomy.

### 42.8.2.2 Recipient Site Preparation

The lesion is sized with commercially available instrumentation and an appropriately sized reamer is selected. The diameter of the reamer should correspond to the diameter of the grafts that are harvested and each recipient hole should be separated by 1–2 mm. Additionally, it is often helpful to allow for an additional 1–2 mm of depth to aid in graft implantation. The holes can be further dilated to facilitate implantation if desired.

### 42.8.2.3 Graft Harvest

There are three major donor sites available for harvest of autogenous tissue: the lateral femoral condyle above the sulcus terminalis, the superolateral aspect of the intercondylar notch (if uninvolved), or the peripheral aspect of the medial femoral condyle. If the medial condylar donor site is to be used a medial arthrotomy will assist in the harvest. Ideally the largest size plug possible (1 $cm^2$) is harvested. In the case of larger lesions multiple plugs can be harvested. Most commercially available systems have a T-handle device that is used to gather the donor tissue. This device should be placed perpendicular to the articular surface for harvesting. The device is impacted to roughly 15 mm and the plug is then rotated free from the surrounding tissue. The depth of the graft is measured and used as a guide for creation of the recipient hole.

#### 42.8.2.4 Graft Implantation

The graft remains in the delivery tube and is then placed perpendicular to the recipient site and held in place firmly. It is imperative to limit the number of mallet strikes and the force of each strike when impacting the graft with the plunger as excessive force may lead to chondrocyte death. With the graft in place, the tube is removed and gentle impaction is used to seat the graft flush with the surrounding articular surface. For larger defects it is beneficial to prepare each graft and recipient site separately until the defect is filled completely.

### *42.8.3 Autologous Chondrocyte Implantation (ACI)*

PF ACI is often performed in conjunction with a tibial tuberosity osteotomy. The technique for AMZ is discussed in detail in other chapters and this section focuses on ACI. In the United States currently matrix autologous chondrocyte implantation (MACI) or other scaffold techniques are not approved for clinical use by the FDA. The current method utilized in the US involves an open procedure with use of a periosteal patch or off label usage of a collagen patch.[8,16]

#### 42.8.3.1 Exposure

A midline incision is utilized in all cases. If the patient has a previous anterior knee incision, all attempts are made to incorporate this in the skin incision. As previously discussed this procedure is often performed in conjunction with a tibial tubercle osteotomy and if this is planned, the incision should extend from the proximal pole of the patella to 8 cm distal to the tibial tubercle. If an ACI is performed in isolation, the incision can end at the level of the tibial tubercle. Sharp dissection is carried out through the skin and subcutaneous tissue and full-thickness flaps are created. A lateral arthrotomy allows adequate exposure and may have less morbidity as it spares the vastus medialis. The arthrotomy extends from the level of the vastus lateralis to the anterior capsule, being careful to avoid injury to the anterior lateral meniscus. It is helpful to release the fat pad and to dissect the anterior horn of the meniscus from the capsule as this can increase the exposure of the trochlea. Variable amounts of knee flexion are utilized to maximize the view of the trochlea. The patella is subluxated and or everted medially to expose the trochlea.

#### 42.8.3.2 Recipient Site Preparation

A fresh #15 blade is then used to create vertical walls at the periphery of the chondral lesion. A ring curette is then used to debride the chondral defect and remove all abnormal cartilage, fibrocartilage with preservation of the calcified cartilage layer. It is important to create a "well shouldered" recipient site at this point of the procedure (Fig. 42.2a). Great care should be taken not to gouge the underlying subchondral bone so as to avoid bleeding. Once the lesion is prepared, a template is pressed into the defect and is sized to cover the defect. At this point the tourniquet is deflated and care is taken to achieve homeostasis. Often, especially in the case of revision for a failed microfracture, bleeding is encountered. It is imperative to obtain meticulous hemostasis as bleeding in the recipient site may theoretically lead to reduced production of hyaline-like cartilage. The use of thrombin soaked gel-foam and small neuro paddies can assist in this step. If the bleeding is difficult to control a small amount of fibrin glue can be applied to the base of the recipient site and pressure can be applied for 3–5 min. It is important to ensure that there is adequate surrounding cartilage available to pass suture through in order to provide secure fixation of the patch.

#### 42.8.3.3 Patch Preparation and Fixation

The patch is cut to match the template of the defect. Classically, the patch is sutured by passing interrupted 6-0 Vicryl sutures from the patch through the surrounding cartilage to achieve a water tight seal and the ACI cell suspension is injected deep to the patch (Fig. 42.2b). Suture passage can be facilitated by running the Vicryl through mineral oil prior to sewing.

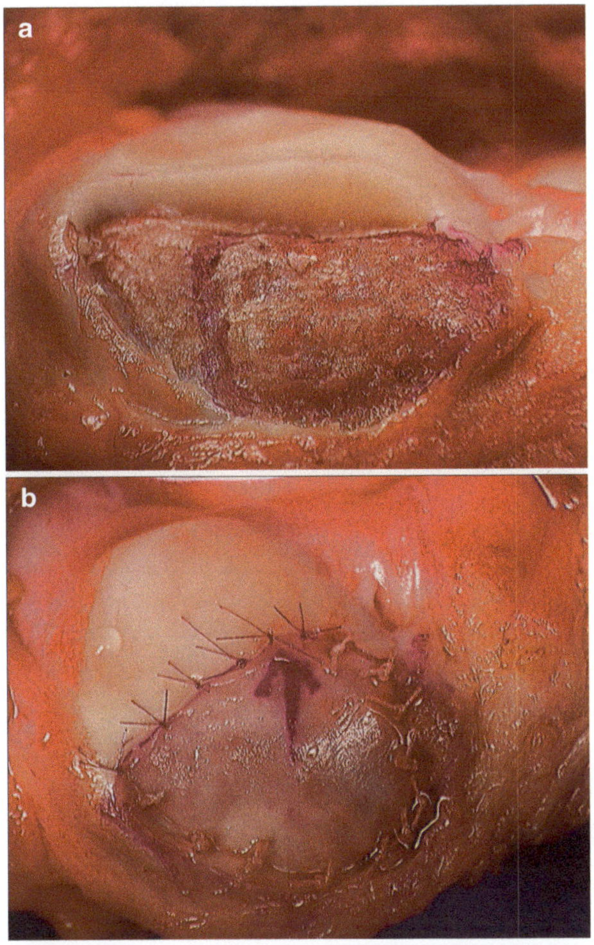


**Fig. 42.2** (**a**) The defect is cleared without penetrating the subchondral bone. Walls are vertical. (**b**) The periosteal patch or collagen patch is secured with suture and sealed with fibrin glue. The suspension of cultured chondrocytes is injected deep to the patch

The knots should be tied on the patch side, near the interface of the patch and surrounding cartilage. Occasionally if there is an area that is uncontained, suture anchors can be placed to provide additional fixation. Alternatively, the cells may be seeded on a collagen patch.[39] Ten minutes after seeding, the patch is sewn into place in the same manner as with the classical use of periosteum. A small area may be left open to allow for injection of the additional chondrocyte suspension.

#### 42.8.3.4 Sealing the Patch

Once sutured into place, fibrin glue is used to complete the seal. Care should be taken to use the minimal amount of glue necessary to ensure an adequate seal. If cells are not seeded, the seal can then be tested with saline.

### 42.8.4 Osteochondral Allografting

#### 42.8.4.1 Preparation of Recipient Site

There are several commercially available systems that can be used to size and prepare both the recipient site and the donor plug. Once the site has been sized a guidepin is placed and a cannulated reamer is used to create a socket with a depth of 6–8 mm. The sidewalls are then trimmed sharply with a fresh #15 blade and the site is irrigated and dried. Once this is complete the depth of the cylindrical socket is measured at the 12, 3, 6, and 9 o'clock positions and this is recorded. Alternatively for a full-area lesion of the patella and/or trochlea, shells may be created free hand.

#### 42.8.4.2 Preparation of the Donor Plug

The ideal donor site is then identified from the fresh osteochondral allograft donor tissue. Though difficult, the goal is to match the native radius of curvature with that of the donor tissue. Once identified the donor is marked with a sizing tube. The donor tissue is fixed in a commercially available jig and a donor-harvesting device is used to core out the donor plug. The graft is then extracted and the measurements made previously of the recipient socket are applied to the donor plug to ensure accurate depth matching.

#### 42.8.4.3 Graft Insertion/Fixation

The recipient site is then dilated an additional 0.5 mm with a commercially available dilation device. The graft is then press-fit into the recipient site with the least amount of force necessary because excessive force has been shown to lead to chondrocyte injury and death. Occasionally an oversized tamp may be required to complete the seating of the graft. For the freehand shell technique, the host bone is cut in the same manner as for a patellofemoral arthroplasty and the shells are shaped to have minimal bone (usually composite thickness of 5–8 mm) with the goal to establish a normal composite thickness (Fig. 42.3a–c). Headless, variable pitch, bioabsorbable screws may be used to fix the shell allografts or to augment the fixation of allograft plugs.

## 42.9 Postoperative Management

Note that if concomitant tibial tuberosity surgery is performed, the weight-bearing recommendations of that procedure take precedence (see Chap. 40).

### 42.9.1 *Microfracture-Trochlear/Patellar Defect*

All patients use continuous passive motion (CPM) from the day of the surgery for a period of 4–6 weeks, 6–8 h per day. Patients with patellar and trochlear groove lesions should be placed immediately in a hinged brace with a 30°–45° flexion stop for at least 8 weeks. Weight bearing in extension as tolerated is allowed immediately postoperatively. After the period of protected flexion, patients begin active range of motion exercises and progress to full flexion. No cutting, twisting, or jumping sports are allowed until at least 6 months after surgery.

### 42.9.2 *Osteochondral Autograft Transplantation*

The postoperative management for this procedure is similar to that of both ACI and osteochondral allografting.

### 42.9.3 *Autologous Chondrocyte Implantation of the Patellofemoral Joint*

The operative extremity is placed into a hinged knee brace locked in full extension postoperatively. Continuous passive motion is initiated on the first postoperative day (0–30°; 1 cycle/min) in 2-h increments for 6–8 h per day. Range of motion is advanced by 15° each week with the use of the continuous passive motion machine and simultaneous unlocking of the brace. The objective is to obtain 90° of flexion by weeks 6–8, but not generally sooner than 4 weeks.

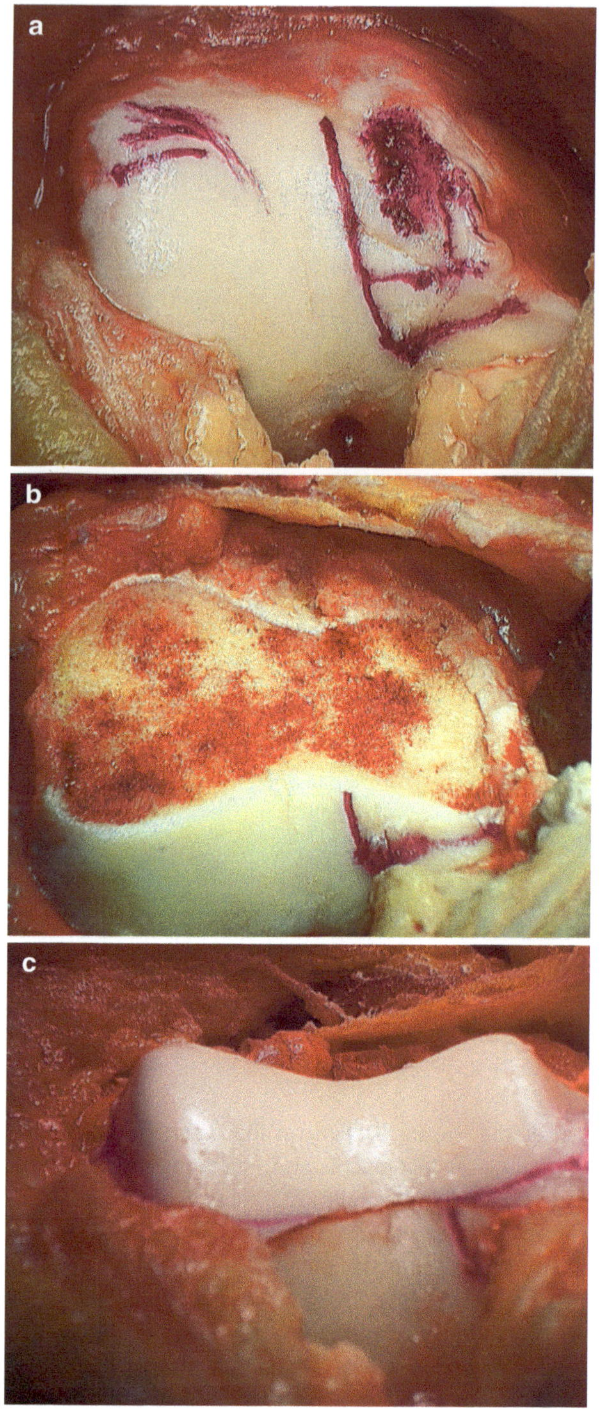


**Fig. 42.3** The area of chondrosis is identified (**a**). The bony cuts are made with a cooled oscillating saw (**b**). The donor graft is shaped to fit the defect and secured (**c**)

Return to full activity is not permitted until 8 months postoperatively to protect the lesion until the cartilage has sufficiently matured.

### 42.9.4 Osteochondral Allograft and Autograft Transplantation

Postoperatively, if the procedure is performed appropriately with a well-contained defect, early weight bearing and motion are encouraged. After a multiple-plug technique, full range of motion and protected weight bearing are advised for the first 4 weeks. At 4 weeks, full weight bearing is allowed. Sporting activities are not recommended until 4–6 months postoperatively.

## 42.10 Outcomes

A detailed description of the studies evaluating outcomes from the various procedures is included in Table 42.2. Below is a summary of these findings.

### 42.10.1 Microfracture

Marrow stimulation techniques result in a repair tissue with inferior wear characteristics. Some authors have reported good results in the treatment of smaller defects (2–3 $cm^2$). However larger lesions and high-demand patients were better treated with autologous chondrocyte implantation or osteochondral grafting.

### 42.10.2 Autologous Chondrocyte Implantation

Recent results of autologous chondrocyte implantation in the patellofemoral joint have been encouraging with good and excellent results even in patients with large defects (average 10 $cm^2$) who had previously undergone an average of three surgeries. It appears that concomitant realignment procedures are an important adjunct in obtaining these favorable results.

### 42.10.3 Osteochondral Grafting: Autograft Transplantation

Transfer of autologous osteochondral plugs is limited by the donor area and donor site morbidity. Based on such limitations, this technique is employed for only small-sized defects. Published studies have reported varying outcomes, suggesting that this technique be suitable for the relatively rare patient who presents with a small isolated chondral defect.

**Table 42.2** Summary of various authors' outcomes of specified patellofemoral surgical techniques

| Procedure | Authors | Reported outcomes |
|---|---|---|
| Microfracture | Blevins et al.[5]<br>Kreuz et al.[25]<br>Steadman et al.[38] | Good results with microfracture in lesions 2–3 $cm^2$ |
| | Miller et al.[27] | Lysholm score 53.8–83, Tegner score 2.9 → 4.5 |
| | Mithoefer et al.[29]<br>Steadman et al.[38]<br>Kreuz et al.[25] | Good midterm outcomes in approximately 80% of patients |
| ACI(PF) | Minas et al.[28]<br>Bentley et al.[3]<br>Bitteberg et al.[6] | Good and excellent results in up to 85% |
| | Yates[45] | No good results without corrective osteotomy 78% good/excellent |
| OA grafting | Hangody et al.[18]<br>Bentley et al.[3] | Good results 80% of patients<br>Others have shown failure rates that approached 100% when used for patellar defects |
| | Jakob et al.[21] | 86% good/excellent |
| Allograft transplantation | Jamali et al.[22]<br>Torga et al.[41] | Graft survival in 60–70% of patients with follow-up of up to 10 years |
| | Shasha et al.[36] | Kaplan–Meier Survival Rate: 5 years – 95%, 10 years – 80%, 15 years – 65%, 20 years – 46% |

### 42.10.4 Osteochondral Grafting: Allograft Transplantation

This type of reconstruction appears to be better suited for the treatment of trochlear defects, though some authors have reported good outcomes with allograft reconstruction of the patella and even bipolar lesions.

## 42.11 Conclusion

Management of patients with a PF joint that presents with pain and dysfunction associated with chondral pathology remains a difficult clinical problem. Attention to the entire PF system including issues pertaining to alignment is paramount in achieving a successful outcome. Similar to the tibiofemoral joint, all comorbidities must be addressed. Multiple options exist to manage the chondral pathology and are chosen based upon defect size and location. Outcomes support good and excellent results similar to that seen with the management of the tibiofemoral joint.

## References


1. Aroen A, Loken S, Heir S, et al. Articular cartilage lesions in 993 consecutive knee arthroscopies. *Am J Sports Med.* 2004;32:211-215.
2. Beaconsfield T, Pintore E, Maffulli N, et al. Radiological measurements in patellofemoral disorders. A review. *Clin Orthop Relat Res.* 1994;308:18-28.
3. Bentley G, Biant LC, Carrington RW, et al. A prospective, randomised comparison of autologous chondrocyte implantation verses mosaicplasty for osteochondral defects in the knee. *J Bone Joint Surg Br.* 2003;85:223-230.
4. Biedert RM. *Patellofemoral Disorders. Diagnosis and Treatment.* West Sussex: Wiley; 2004.
5. Blevins FT, Steadman JR, Rodrigo JJ, et al. Treatment of articular cartilage defects in athletes: an analysis of functional outcome and lesion appearance. *Orthopedics.* 1998;21:761-767.
6. Brittberg M, Lindahl A, Nilsson A, et al. Treatment of deep cartilage defects in the knee with autologous chondrocyte transplantation. *N Engl J Med.* 1994;331:889-895.
7. Brittberg M, Peterson L, Sjiogren-Jansson E, et al. Articular cartilage engineering with autologous chondrocyte transplantation. *J Bone Joint Surg Am.* 2003;85:109-115.
8. Brittberg M, Tallheden T, Sjogren-Sansson B, et al. Autologous chondrocyte used for articular cartilage repair: an update. *Clin Orthop Relat Res.* 2001;391:337-348.
9. Chen H, Sun J, Hoemann CD, et al. Subchondral structure and repair responses following bone marrow stimulation by drilling versus microfracture in rabbit trochleas. ICRS; 2009; Miami.
10. Curl WW, Krome J, Gordon ES, et al. Cartilage injuries: a review of 31,516 knee arthroscopies. *Arthroscopy.* 1997;13:456-460.
11. Dejour H, Walch G, Nove-Josserand L, et al. Factors of patellar instability: an anatomic radiographic study. *Knee Surg Sports Traumatol Arthrosc.* 1994;2:19-26.
12. Ficat P, Ficat C, Bailleux A. External hypertension syndrome of the patella. Its significance recognition arthrosis. *Rev Chir Orthop Reparatrice Appar Mot.* 1975;61:39-59.
13. Ficat P, Hungerford D. *Disorder of the Patellofemoral Joint.* Baltimore: Williams & Wilkins; 1977.
14. Fulkerson JP. The etiology of patellofemoral pain in young, active patients: a prospective study. *Clin Orthop Relat Res.* 1983;179:129-133.
15. Fulkerson JP. A clinical test for medial patella tracking. *Tech Orthop.* 1997;12:165-169.
16. Gomoll AH, Probst C, Farr J, et al. Use of type I/III bilayer collagen membrane decreases reoperation rates for symptomatic hypertrophy after autologous chondrocyte implantation. *Am J Sports Med.* 2009;35:20S-23S.
17. Grelsamer RP, McConnell J. *The Patella. A Team Approach.* Gaithersburg: Aspen Publication; 1998.
18. Hangody L, Rathonyi GK, Duska Z, et al. Autologous osteochondral mosaicplasty. Surgical technique. *J Bone Joint Surg Am.* 2004;86:65-72.
19. Hejgaard N, Arnoldi CC. Osteotomy of the patella in the patellofemoral pain syndrome. The significance increased intraosseous pressure during sustained knee flexion. *Int Orthop.* 1987;8:89-94.
20. Hjelle K, Solheim E, Strand T, et al. Articular cartilage defects in 1,000 knee arthroscopies. *Arthroscopy.* 2002;18:730-734.
21. Jakob RP, Franz T, Gautier E, et al. Autologous osteochondral grafting in the knee: indication, results and reflections. *Clin Orthop Relat Res.* 2002;401:170-184.
22. Jamali AA, Emmerson BC, Chung C, et al. Fresh osteochondral allografts. *Clin Orthop Relat Res.* 2005;437:176-185.
23. Kaplan LD, Schurhoff MR, Selesnick H, et al. Magnetic resonance imaging of the knee in asymptomatic professional basketball players. *Arthroscopy.* 2005;21:557-561.
24. Knutsen G, Engerbretsen L, Ludvigsen TC, et al. Autologous chondrocyte implantation compared with microfracture in the knee. A randomized trial. *J Bone Joint Surg Am.* 2004; 86:455-464.
25. Kreuz PC, Steinwachs MR, Erggelet C, et al. Results after microfracture of full-thickness chondral defects in different compartments in the knee. *Osteoarthritis Cartilage.* 2006;14(11):1119-1125.
26. Merchant AC. Radiography of the patellofemoral joint. *Oper Tech Sports Med.* 1999;7:59-64.
27. Miller BS, Steadman JR, Briggs KK, et al. Patient satisfaction and outcome after microfracture of the degenerative knee. *J Knee Surg.* 2004;17:13-17.
28. Minas T, Bryant T. The role of autologous chondrocyte implantation in the patellofemoral joint. *Clin Orthop Relat Res.* 2005;436:30-39.

29. Mithoefer K, Williams RJ III, Warren RF, et al. The microfracture technique for the treatment of articular cartilage lesions in the knee. A prospective cohort study. *J Bone Joint Surg Am*. 2005;87:1911-1920.
30. Moseley B, O'Malley K, Petersen N, et al. A controlled trial of arthroscopic surgery for osteoarthritis of the knee. *N Engl J Med*. 2002;347:81-88.
31. Post WR. History and physical examination. In: Fulkerson JP, ed. *Disorders of the Patellofemoral Joint*. 4th ed. Philadelphia: Lippincott Williams & Wilkins; 2004.
32. Potter HG, Foo LF. Magnetic resonance imaging of articular cartilage: trauma, degeneration, and repair. *Am J Sports Med*. 2006;34:661-667.
33. Recht MP, Goodwin DW, Winalsky CS, White LM. MRI of articular cartilage: revisiting current status and future directions. A journal review. *Am J Roentegenol*. 2005;185:899-914.
34. Schepsis AA, Fitzgerald M, Nicoletta R. Revision surgery for exertional compartment syndrome of the lower leg: technique, findings and results. *Am J Sports Med*. 2005;33:1040-1047.
35. Schutzer SF, Ramsby GR, Fulkerson JP. Computed tomographic classification of patellofemoral pain patients. *Orthop Clin North Am*. 1986;17:235-248.
36. Shasha N, Krywulak S, Backstein D, et al. Long-term follow-up of fresh tibial osteochondral allografts for failed tibial plateau fracture. *J Bone Joint Surg Am*. 2003;85:33-39.
37. Spencer JD, Hayes KC, Alexander IJ. Knee joint effusion and quadriceps inhibition in man. *Arch Phys Med Rehabil*. 1984;65:171-177.
38. Steadman JR, Briggs KK, Rodrigo JJ, et al. Outcomes of microfracture for traumatic chondral defects of the knee: average 11-year follow-up. *Arthroscopy*. 2003;19:477-484.
39. Steinwachs M. New technique for cell-seeded collagen-matrix-supported autologous chondrocyte transplantation. *Arthroscopy*. 2009;25:208-211.
40. Teitge RA. Plain patellofemoral radiographs. *Oper Tech Sports Med*. 2001;9:134-151.
41. Torga Spak R, Teitge RA. Fresh osteochondral allografts for patellofemoral arthritis: long-term followup. *Clin Orthop Relat Res*. 2006;444:193-200.
42. Walczak BE, McCulloch PC, Kang RW, et al. Abnormal finding on magnetic resonance imaging in asymptomatic NBA players. *J Knee Surg*. 2008;21:27-33.
43. Walsh WM. Patellofemoral joint. In: DeLee JC, Drez D, eds. *Orthopaedic Sports Medicine. Principles and Practice*. Philadelphia: W.B. Saunders Company; 1994.
44. Winalski CS, Gupta KB. Magnetic resonance imaging of focal articular cartilage lesions. *Top Magn Reson Imaging*. 2003;14:131-144.
45. Yates JW. The effectiveness of autologous chondrocyte implantation for treatment of full-thickness articular cartilage lesions in workers' compensation patients. *Orthopedics*. 2003;26:295-301.

# Autologous Osteochondral Mosaicplasty

# 43

László Hangody and Eszter Baló

## 43.1 Introduction

"Modern resurfacing techniques" try to produce a hyaline or hyaline-like surface in the region of a localized, full-thickness cartilage defect. Autologous osteochondral mosaic transplantation technique is one of the recently evolved methods to create hyaline or hyaline-like repair tissue in the pathologic area. During this procedure small-sized osteochondral plugs covered with healthy hyaline cap from the patellofemoral periphery are transplanted to the defect of the weight-bearing area mainly on femoral condyles but tibial, patellar, trochlear, or other articular surfaces too. It is verified by Hangody and colleagues[9] in German Shepherd dog and Bodó and colleagues[2] in horse mosaicplasty trials and in their clinical data and by several independent author's experimental and clinical studies that the transplanted hyaline cartilage could survive the procedure, composite cartilage layer forms from transplanted hyaline cartilage, fibrocartilage ingrown from the bony base of the defect, and deep matrix integration of the transplanted cartilage is seen to the surrounding tissue at the recipient site. Combinations of different graft sizes allow an 80–100% filling rate and a congruent surface.

The donor sites are filled to the surface with cancellous bone during the first 4 postoperative weeks similar to that prevailing after Pridie drilling. Its surface will be covered by early regenerative tissue at 6 weeks and final coverage will be finished by a central fibrocartilage cap and peripheral hyaline cartilage at 8–10th weeks. This partially nonhyaline coverage of the donor holes separated by host articular cartilage appears to be adequate surface for the biomechanical requirements of the less weight-bearing area.[5,9,11]

Osteochondral autograft transfer was originally introduced by Wilson and colleagues[16] in 1952 and Pap and Krompecher[15] in 1960. These early publications described the use of a single autologous osteochondral block, with successful survival of transplanted hyaline cartilage at a follow-up ranging from 6 months to 10 years. Campanacci and colleagues,[3] Fabbricciani and colleagues,[4] Outerbridge and colleagues,[14] and Yamashita and colleagues[17] have also transplanted single block osteochondral autografts with good medium and long-term outcome. But its clinical use was limited by congruency problems and donor-site availability.

Matsusue and colleagues[13] in 1993 also reported good results 3 years after arthroscopic transplantation of multiple osteochondral fragments, harvested from the same knee, for the treatment of a chondral lesion in a patient with ACL deficiency. Outerbridge[14] published in 1995 the results of transplantation of osteochondral fragments of the patella to the femoral condyle, with relief of symptoms and survival of hyaline cartilage up to 9 years. Together, these reports suggested that osteochondral autografts could provide a durable repair of articular cartilage lesions. However, technical difficulties, limited donor-site availability, and lack of proper instrumentation hampered clinical application.

To eliminate the donor site and congruency problems transplantation of multiple small-sized grafts could provide advantages comparing to one block transfer. The use of multiple small-sized cylindrical grafts allows more tissue to be transplanted while maintaining the integrity of the donor site, and the use

L. Hangody (✉)
Department of Orthopaedics, Uzsoki Hospital,
Budapest, Hungary
e-mail: hangody@t-online.hu

V. Sanchis-Alfonso (ed.), *Anterior Knee Pain and Patellar Instability*,
DOI: 10.1007/978-0-85729-507-1_43, © Springer-Verlag London Limited 2011

of grafts in a mosaic-like implanting fashion would allow progressive contouring by fibrous tissue of the new surface.

The autologous osteochondral mosaicplasty was developed in Hungary in 1991. Conceptually, the technique specifically addressed problems of congruency at the recipient site by the implantation of small-sized grafts sequentially arrayed in a mosaic-like pattern.[7] Inherent to the technique design has been the procurement of these small grafts from less weight-bearing surfaces, thus reducing the potential of donor-site morbidity.[5-11] Following several series of animal trials, cadaver research, and the development of special instrumentation, this technique was introduced into clinical practice in 1992. Matsusue and colleagues[12] and later Bobic[1] developed similar techniques for transplantation of multiple cylindrical osteochondral grafts.

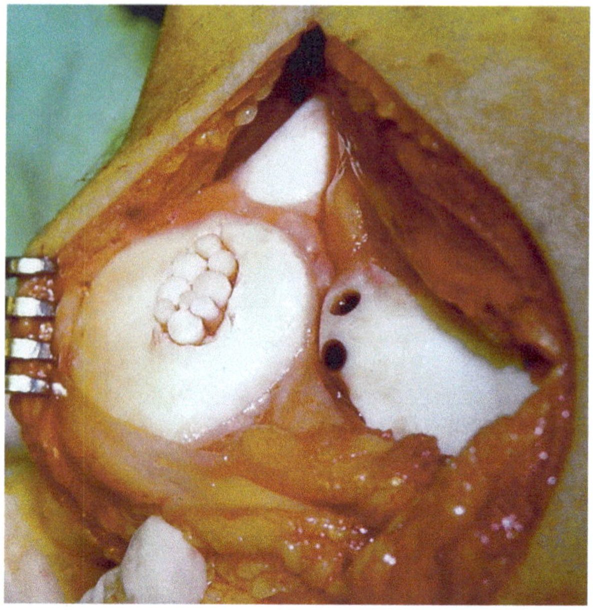

**Fig. 43.2** Open mosaicplasty on the patella – filling by nine grafts of different size

## 43.2 Indications

Basically autologous osteochondral mosaicplasty was developed to treat relatively small and medium-sized (1–4 cm$^2$) focal chondral and osteochondral defects of the weight-bearing surfaces of the femoral condyles and the patellofemoral joint. Small-sized, single focal lesions of femoral condyles represent the best indication for mosaicplasty procedures, but tibial, patellar, and trochlear defects can also be treated by osteochondral grafting (Figs. 43.1–43.4). Multiple defects,

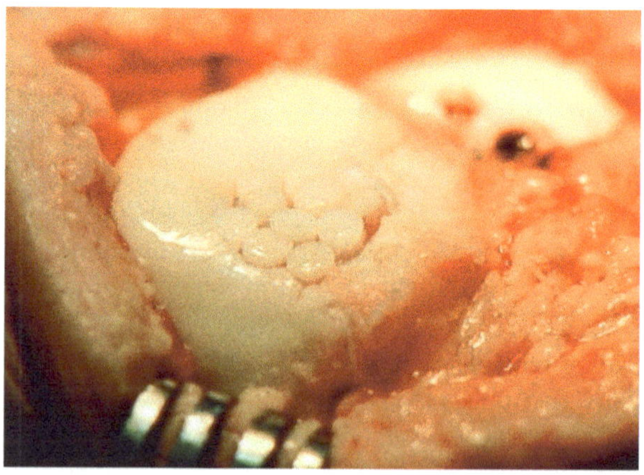

**Fig. 43.1** Open mosaicplasty on the patella – filling by ten grafts of same size

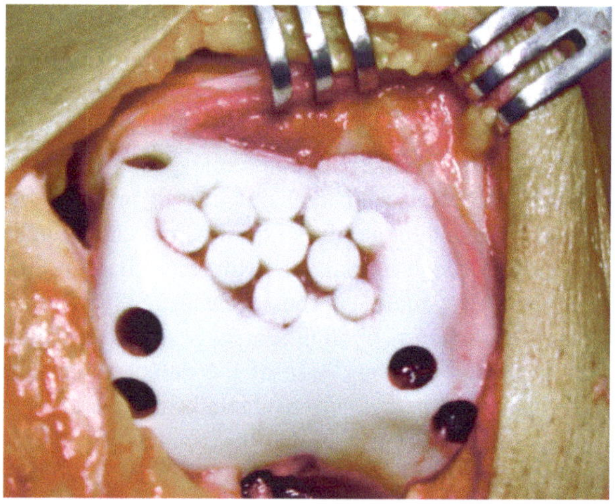

**Fig. 43.3** Open mosaicplasty on the trochlea – graft harvest from the periphery and filling of a central defect

especially kissing lesions may have less promising clinical outcome (Fig. 43.5). Outside the knee talar defects are the most frequent indications, but in exceptional cases capitulum humeri and femoral head lesions can also be treated by mosaicplasty. Donor-site availability and other technical considerations have limited the optimal extent of defect coverage to 1–4 cm$^2$. Usually, both patellofemoral peripheries allow graft

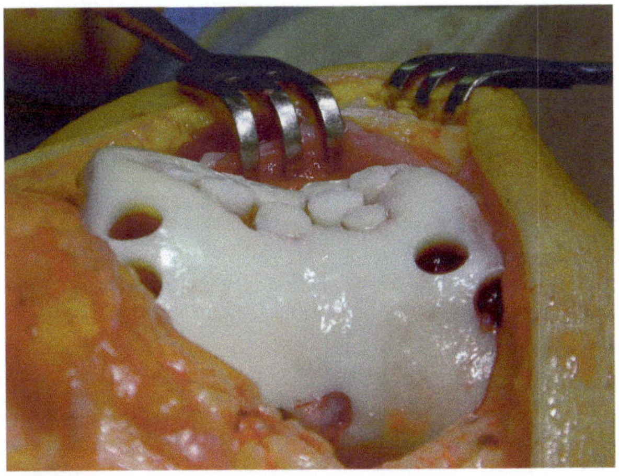

**Fig. 43.4** Open mosaicplasty on the trochlea – perfect congruency according to axial view

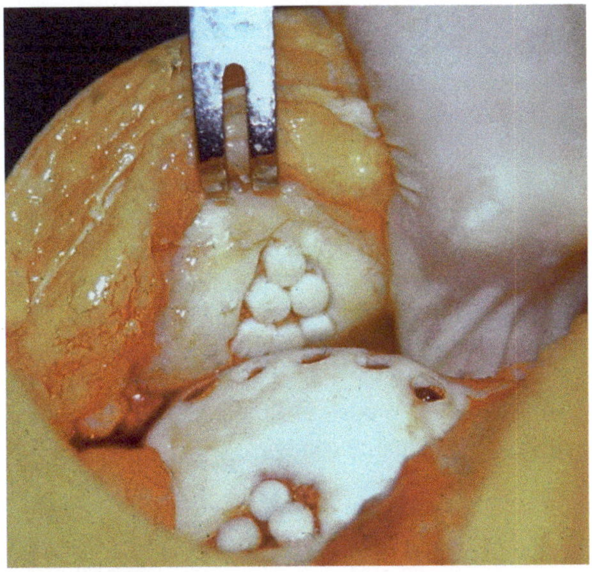

**Fig. 43.5** Mosaicplasty for kissing lesions of patellofemoral joint – exceptional indication

harvest for 3–4 $cm^2$ defects. Defects up to 8–9 $cm^2$ can be covered with mosaicplasty as a salvage procedure, but such extension of the indication can result in a higher rate of donor-site morbidity. Age may be associated with decreased repair capacity and may be a limiting factor. Fifty years of age is the recommended upper age limit for this procedure, which reflects the clinical experiences with single-block osteochondral transfer.

However, localized full-thickness defects of weight-bearing surfaces have usually biomechanical background. Therefore resurfacing is only one element of treatment for full-thickness chondral and osteochondral defects. In every case, it is necessary to treat any accompanying joint abnormalities. Otherwise, early wear of transplanted cartilage or even further degeneration may develop.

Accordingly, treatment for instability, malalignment, meniscal deficiency, patellofemoral shape anomalies or maltraction problems as well as traumatic damages must be incorporated in the operative and postoperative rehabilitation algorithms (if this is possible) in the same step.

## 43.3 Contraindications

Any disadvantageous condition hindering the survival of the transplanted hyaline cartilage on the recipient site can be a contraindication, such as the following:

- Generalized arthritis, rheumatoid and/or degenerative in type
- Infectious or tumor defects

In such cases biochemical alterations in the involved joint's milieu represent poor conditions for graft survival. According to regular indications of the mosaicplasty procedure, osteoarthritis is a contraindication, but in certain motivated patient groups for small-sized focal defects mosaicplasty can be considered as salvage intervention.

- Lack of appropriate donor area
- Age more than 50–55 years
- Osteochondral defects deeper than 10 mm.

## 43.4 Surgical Technique Step by Step

Preoperative preparations should include one-shot antibiotic prophylaxis. General or regional anesthesia with tourniquet control is recommended. The patient is positioned supine with the knee capable of 120° flexion. The contralateral extremity is placed in a stirrup. Standard arthroscopic instrumentation and MosaicPlasty Complete System (Smith & Nephew, Inc., Endoscopy Division, Andover, Massachusetts) is required. Beside these reusable instruments disposable chisels, drillbits, and tamps are also available to provide ideal conditions for precise graft harvest and tunnel preparation. (Dispoposplasty System – Smith & Nephew, Inc., Endoscopy Division, Andover, Massachusetts). A fluid management system may support the procedure.

### 43.4.1 Operative Technique

Choosing an approach for the mosaicplasty – arthroscopic or miniarthrotomy – depends on the type, size, and exact location of the defect determined during arthroscopy. As placing the grafts perpendicular to the surface is paramount to the success of the operation, the first task is to determine whether an arthroscopic or open procedure is required. Although certain trochlear defects can be resurfaced arthroscopically, patellotrochlear and tibial lesions always require an open procedure (Figs. 43.6 and 43.7). Most of the femoral condylar defects can be managed arthroscopically. As for most of these lesions, central anterior medial and central anterior lateral portals will allow correct perpendicular access.

An open procedure may be chosen in the learning curve or when an arthroscopic approach is not practical due to size or location of the lesion. Arthroscopic or open mosaicplasties have the same steps and technique.

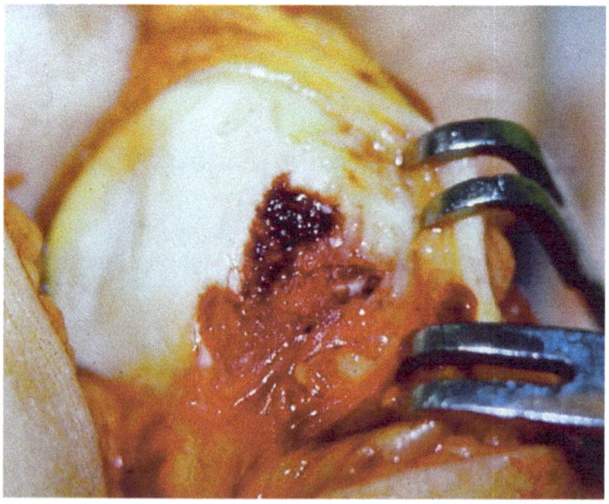

**Fig. 43.6** Fresh traumatic osteochondral lesion of the patella

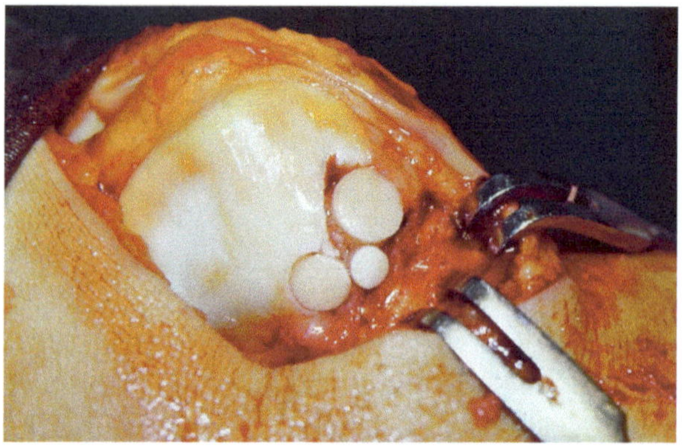

**Fig. 43.7** Filling of the previous defect by three grafts

### 43.4.2 Arthroscopic Mosaicplasty

#### 43.4.2.1 Portal Selection

Perpendicular access to the lesion is critical to proper insertion of the grafts, so careful preparation of working portals has an important role. A 1.2 mm K-wire or 18-gauge spinal needle can be used initially to locate the portal sites. It should be noted that these portals tend to be more central than standard portals due to the inward curve of the condyles. For osteochondritis dissecans lesion on the medial femoral condyle the approach may be necessary from the lateral side. Sometimes standard lateral portal is too oblique; therefore the central patellar tendon portal is used giving good access to the inner positions of both the medial and the lateral femoral condyles.

#### 43.4.2.2 Defect Preparation

Sharp curette and/or proper shaver blades are useful to bring the edges of the defect back to good hyaline cartilage at a right angle. The bony base of the defect should be prepared by an arthroscopic burr (Abrader, Acromionizer) or half-round rasp to eliminate the subchondral sequester layer or refresh subchondral bone. Abrasion arthroplasty of the defect site promotes fibrocartilage grouting from the bony base. Tapping the cutting edge of the guide into the bony base and removal of it can mark the defect site, therefore use the drill guide to determine the number and size (2.7, 3.5, 4.5, 6.5, and 8.5 mm in diameter) of grafts needed. Filling of the defect by same-sized contacting rings allows a filling rate of about 70–80%, but use of additional sizes to cover the dead spaces and cutting the grafts into each other can improve the coverage by up to 90–100%. Finally, measure the depth of the defect with the laser marks of the dilator.

#### 43.4.2.3 Graft Harvest

According to several biomechanical studies all chondral surfaces of the femoral condyles are subjected for loading. However peripheral areas of patellofemoral joint are less weight-bearing surfaces. The medial femoral condyle periphery of the patellofemoral joint above the line of the notch is the most preferred harvest site. The lateral femoral condyle above the sulcus terminalis and, in exceptional cases, the notch area can serve as additional donor areas. In case of arthroscopic mosaicplasty the medial patellofemoral periphery has easier access than the lateral one as fluid distension can promote lateral positioning of the patella and may provide easier perpendicular positioning for the harvesting chisel. Grafts harvested from the notch area are less favorable features, as they have concave cartilage caps and less elastic underlying bone. According to recent publications the proximal tibiofibular articulation may also serve as exceptional donor site.

For graft harvest from the patellofemoral peripheries the best view can be obtained by introducing the scope through the standard contralateral portal. Extend the knee and use the standard ipsilateral portal to check the perpendicular access to the donor site. Extended position should provide perpendicular access to the most superior donor hole. Gradual flexion allows the harvest of additional grafts from the lower portions of the patellofemoral periphery. If the standard portals do not allow a perpendicular approach, use a spinal needle or a K-wire to determine the location of additional harvesting portals.

Once the necessary portal has been determined, introduce the proper-sized tube chisel filled with the appropriate harvesting tamp. This way of harvester introduction may help to eliminate fluid leakage and avoid chondral injuries caused by the sharp cutting edge of the harvester. Once the donor site has been clearly identified, the chisel is located perpendicular to the articular surface. The harvesting tamp is then removed and the harvester should be driven by a hammer to the appropriate depth. The minimal length of the graft should be at least two times its diameter, but, as a rule, take 15 mm long grafts to resurface chondral lesions and 25 mm long plugs for osteochondral defects. It is important to hold the chisel firmly to avoid its shifting at the cartilage–bone interface, producing a crooked graft. Step by step flexion of the knee helps to reach lower harvest sites. The lower limit is the level of the top of the intercondylar notch (sulcus terminalis). Insert the appropriate harvesting tamp into the cross-hole in the tubular chisel and use it as a lever. The chisel should be toggled, not rotated, causing the graft to break free at the chisel tip. Eject the grafts from the chisel by sliding the appropriately sized chisel guard over the cutting end. Use the harvesting tamps to push out the graft onto gauze in a saline-wetted basin. The donor-site holes will eventually be filled up with initial repair tissue by bleeding-mediated mesenchymal stem cell invasion in a few hours. Proper rehabilitation may support a transformation of the primary repair tissue into cancellous bone and fibrocartilage as final coverage (Fig. 43.8).

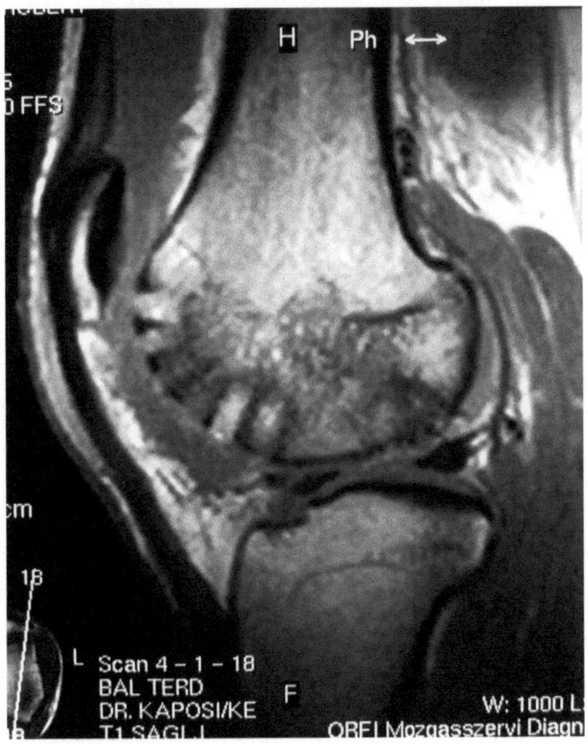


**Fig. 43.8** Magnetic resonance image of mosaicplasty donor sites – minimum 3 mm should be kept between two donor tunnels

During the learning curve, the grafts can also be obtained through a miniarthrotomy (1.5–2.0 cm). Proper site of this approach can be determined by a spinal needle under arthroscopic control.

#### 43.4.2.4 Implantation of the Grafts: "Drill-Dilate-Deliver"

Drill

Flex the knee to reach the recipient site. Fluid management system may promote proper distension and good visualization. Use the dilator as an obturator and introduce again the drill guide. Place these tools to the defected surface and adjust them perpendicularly to the defect site. By rotating the arthroscope, the drill guide and the perpendicularity of the laser mark can be seen from different angles, ensuring proper orientation. Tap the cutting edge of the guide into the subchondral bone. Insert the appropriately sized drill bit and drill to the desired depth. Generally, a recipient hole a few millimeters deeper than the length of the graft is desirable to minimize high intraosseal pressure and avoid prominent graft positioning. Reduce the inflow to minimize leakage. Finally, remove the drill bit and use irrigation to eliminate bone debris.

Dilate

Insert again the conical-shaped dilator into the drill guide. Tap it to the desired depth, depending on the actual stiffness and elasticity of the recipient bone. Stiff bone needs more dilation than normal or soft bone. Hold the drill guide firmly and remove the dilator from the hole.

Deliver

Use the specially designed delivery tamp for graft insertion. First adjust it by turning the handle to initially allow the graft to sit slightly higher than the depth of the defect. Inflow should be stopped to eliminate the graft being forced out of the tube by fluid flow. Deliver the graft under direct visualization into the recipient hole through the drill guide with the delivery tamp. Insert the graft deeper by turning the delivery tamp handle counterclockwise. The graft should be flush to the original articular surface. Remove the drill guide to inspect the graft. If the graft is protruded, reinsert the drill guide and tap the graft down gently with the dilator of the appropriate size. Insert subsequent grafts in a similar manner by placing the drill guide immediately adjacent to the previously placed grafts. The best way is to start with the most posterior graft and implant further grafts in less flexed positions. Such step-by-step graft implantation has several advantages. Dilation of the actual recipient hole allows an easy graft insertion (low insertion force on the hyaline cap), but dilation of the next hole affects surrounding bone to the previously implanted grafts, which can result in a very safe press fit fixation.

Finally, when all of the holes are filled by the grafts, move the knee throughout its range of motion, provoking varus or valgus stress also, depending on the site of the resurfaced area. Introduce suction drainage and close the portals. Use an elastic bandage to fix the appropriate dressing.

The aim of this procedure is to create a composite cartilage surface at the site of the defect. This composite cartilage layer consists, on an average, of 70–80% transplanted hyaline cartilage, and 20–30% integrated fibrocartilage. Mathematically, the use of same-sized contacting rings results in a theoretical 78.5% filling. But, filling the dead spaces with smaller sizes can improve the coverage of the defect. The special design of the instrumentation can accommodate a 100% filling rate but, naturally, such transplantation requires more graft harvesting. Long-term experience has taught that an 80% filling rate correlates with a good clinical outcome. Fibrocartilage results from the natural healing process of the refreshened bony base of the defect. According to experimental data this fibrocartilage fills the space between the transplanted grafts and also eliminates the minimal incongruities of the surface.[9]

### 43.4.3 Open Mosaicplasty

If an arthroscopic approach is impractical, it may be necessary to create a medial or lateral anterior sagittal incision or an oblique incision to perform a miniarthrotomy mosaicplasty. Best position of these approaches can be determined through arthroscopy. At extended knee position a small parapatellar miniarthrotomy provides comfortable approach to reach the donor site, while flexed knee position allows to implant the grafts into the recipient site. Patellotrochlear and tibial implantations may require an extended anteromedial approach. Further steps and technique of the implantation are identical with the arthroscopic procedure.

## 43.5 Postoperative Management

Postoperatively cryotherapy and elastic bandage may help to lessen extreme bleeding from donor tunnels. The drain should be removed at 24 h. Appropriate pain and cool therapy as well as nonsteroidal anti-inflammatory drugs can reduce the complaints of the patient. Postoperative thrombosis prophylaxis is also recommended.

### 43.5.1 Rehabilitation Protocol

Autologous osteochondral mosaicplasty permits immediate full range of motion (ROM), but requires 2 weeks nonweight bearing and further 2–3 weeks partial weight-bearing (30–40 kg) period after the operation. The initial nonweight-bearing phase is recommended to prevent graft subsidence during osseous integration. This period may be supported by controlled passive motion (CPM) to promote cartilage metabolism and moderate soft-tissue oedema around the joint. CPM (6 h per day) in the first 7–10 days is also useful to contour the shape of the initial repair tissue at donor sites and between the grafts. Partial weight bearing supports fibrocartilage repair around implanted cylindrical plugs, further enhancing secure graft incorporation. Normal daily activity can be achieved in 8–10 weeks. High-demand sporting activity should be delayed till after 5–6 months. This protocol can be modified easily in accordance with established guidelines for concurrent ACL reconstruction, high tibial osteotomy, meniscus reinsertion, meniscus resection, and other concomitant procedures (Table 43.1).

## 43.6 Pearls and Pitfalls

The most common problems of this challenging procedure are technical: perpendicular harvest and implantation of the grafts are crucial for success. Oblique harvest and/or insertion may result in surface step-offs. Careful visualization from various angles can detect such issues.

Another frequent mistake is to implant a graft deeper than the desired level. Appropriate use of the delivery tamp can help avoid overinsertion. If the graft has been inserted too deep, the following steps are recommended. Insert the drill guide next to the previously implanted graft. Drill the appropriate recipient hole. Remove the guide and use the arthroscopic probe to lift the previously implanted graft to the proper level. The recipient hole adjacent to the implanted graft should provide enough room for such manipulation. As soon as the expected graft level has been achieved, continue the recommended protocol for the rest of the insertions.

Dilation of the adjacent tunnel will provide perfect press fit fixation of the previously implanted graft.

## 43.7 Clinical Results

Between February 6, 1992 and August 31, 2006 1,097 mosaicplasties were done at the author's institution: 789 implantations on the femoral condyles, 147 in the patellofemoral joint, 31 on the tibia condyles, 98 on talar domes, 8 on the capitulum humeri, 3 on humeral heads, and 11 on femoral heads. Two-thirds of the patients were operated because of a localized Grade III or Grade IV cartilage lesion whereas about one-third underwent surgery because of osteochondral defects. In 81% of the patients, concomitant surgical interventions also have been done, which had an influence on the clinical results of the mosaicplasty procedures. The majority of these concomitant procedures were anterior cruciate ligament reconstructions, realignment osteotomies, meniscus surgery, and patellofemoral realignment procedures.

Results of these resurfacing procedures were evaluated at regular intervals by standardized clinical scores, radiographs, and, in selected cases, by magnetic resonance imaging (MRI), and in certain cases second-look arthroscopy, histological evaluation of biopsy materials, and cartilage stiffness measurement. Femoral, tibial, and patellar implantations were evaluated by the modified Hospital for Special Surgery (HSS), modified Cincinnati, Lysholm and International Cartilage Repair Society (ICRS) scoring systems, while possible

**Table 43.1** Mosaicplasty rehabilitation protocol

| | |
|---|---|
| NO IMMOBILIZATION![a] | |
| *Ambulation*[b] | |
| Two-crutch ambulation, nonweight bearing | Immediate |
| Two-crutch ambulation, partial loading (30–40 kg) | 2–4 weeks |
| Discontinue crutches, full weight bearing | 4–5 weeks |
| Functional exercises | |
| Form walking, gait evaluation | 4–5 weeks |
| Step-up | 4–5 weeks |
| Step-down | 5–6 weeks |
| *Range of motion* | |
| EARLY RANGE OF MOTION ENCOURAGED | |
| CPM for 2–4 $cm^2$ lesions (in painless range) | Immediate (first week) |
| Full extension, flexion as tolerated | Immediate |
| Stationary bicycle | 3 weeks |
| Strength return | |
| **Quadriceps** | |
| *Open chain exercises, leg raises* | *Immediate* |
| *Concentric contraction to full extension* | *1 week (or earlier if tolerated)* |
| Concentric contraction against resistance | 2 weeks |
| Isometric exercises in different angles | Immediate |
| Eccentric exercises against resistance | 3–4 weeks |
| **Hamstrings** | |
| Isometric exercises in different angles | Immediate |
| Concentric and eccentric strengthening | 1–2 weeks |
| Against resistance | 3–4 weeks |
| **Closed chain exercises**[c] | |
| Pushing a soft rubber ball with foot | Immediate |
| Closed chain exercises with half weight bearing | 2–3 weeks |
| With full weight bearing | 5–6 weeks |
| Stationary bicycle with resistance | 2–4 weeks (If 90° knee flexion achieved) |
| Stairmaster | 6–8 weeks |
| Proprioception return | |
| Balance exercises standing on both feet | 5–6 weeks |
| Standing on one foot (hard ground) | 6–8 weeks |
| Standing on one foot (trampoline or aerostep) | 8–10 weeks |
| Return to activity | |
| Jogging | 10 weeks |
| Straight-line running | 3 months |
| Directional changes | 4–5 months |
| Sport specific adaptations | 5 months |
| Shear forces | 5 months[d] |
| Sport activity | 5–6 months[e] |

(continued)

**Table 43.1** (continued)

| | |
|---|---|
| **Special viewpoints:** | |
| *Weight bearing at different defects of knee:* | |
| FEMUR or TIBIA CONDYLE, chondral defect, $d < 15$ mm | |
| Partial weight bearing | 1 week<br>1–3 weeks |
| FEMUR or TIBIA CONDYLE, chondral defect, $d \geq 15$ mm | |
| Nonweight bearing<br>Partial weight bearing | 2 weeks<br>2–4 weeks |
| Femur or tibia condyle, osteochondral defect | |
| Nonweight bearing<br>Partial weight bearing | 3 weeks<br>3–5 weeks |
| PATELLAR defect, $d < 15$ mm | |
| Partial weight bearing | 2 weeks |
| PATELLAR defect, $d \geq 15$ mm | |
| Partial weight bearing | 3 weeks |
| *Quadriceps strengthening and patellar mobilization – differences at patellar defects:* | |
| Vastus medialis strengthening! | |
| Isometric exercises in extension | Immediate |
| Patellar mobilization | Immediate! |
| Isometric exercises in different angles | 1 week |
| Open chain exercises | 2 weeks |
| Against resistance | 3–4 weeks |
| Eccentric exercises against resistance | 4–5 weeks |
| Closed chain exercises | 2–3 weeks |
| *Retinaculum patellae reconstruction combined with mosaicplasty:* | |
| 2–4 weeks nonweight bearing (up to the mosaicplasty)<br>Two more weeks partial weight bearing<br>0–45° ROM for 4 weeks | |

[a]The main point of the rehabilitation is to ensure the early motion of treated joint to promote appropriate nutrition of transplanted cartilage. Cool therapy can be used during the first week to avoid postoperative bleeding and decrease post-op pain. In a case of a concomitant procedure requiring external fixation of the affected joint (e.g., meniscus reinsertion), limitation of ROM for a short period by bracing can be allowed

[b]Extent, type (chondral or osteochondral), and location of the defect may modify weight bearing (see previous page)

[c]Partial loading promotes to transform connecting tissue (between transplanted plugs) into fibrocartilage, so these exercises are mainly important, extremely in the half-weight bearing period. On the other hand, with some closed chain exercises (e.g., cycling) it is possible to ensure cyclic loading that makes the fluid and nutrition transport much more efficient between synovial fluid and hyaline cartilage

[d]Approximately 4–5 months are needed to form a composite hyaline-like surface on transplanted area, which tolerates shear forces

[e]Depending on depth and extent of the defect, if strength, power, endurance, balance, and flexibility are not satisfying, sport activity is allowed only later

donor-site disturbances were evaluated by the Bandi scoring system. Patients with talar lesions were subjected to the Hannover ankle evaluations and for possible donor-site morbidity – for the Bandi scoring system. During the above-mentioned period, 98 second-look arthroscopies were done to check the quality of the resurfaced area and to check the morphologic features of the donor sites. These second-look arthroscopies were performed in 31 patients (2 months to 11 years) because of persistent or recurrent pain, swelling, or postoperative intraarticular bleeding; in 26 patients (1–9 years) because of a second trauma. In 41 patients second-look arthroscopies were indicated at 4–7 months postoperatively to evaluate the quality of the resurfaced area and to determine the earliest date to return to the professional sports activity. In a limited series – 25 patients – cartilage stiffness measurements were performed by an arthroscopic indentometric device. During these evaluations a computerized indentometric device performed cartilage stiffness measurements at 10 N pressure.

Analysis of clinical scores has shown good to excellent results in 92% of patients with femoral condylar implantations, in 87% of tibial resurfacements, in 74% of patellar and/or trochlear mosaicplasties, and in 93% of talar procedures. Moderate and severe donor-site disturbances were present in 3% of patients according to Bandi score (evaluations were done in a 1–10 years interval). Good gliding surfaces, histologically proven survival of the transplanted hyaline cartilage, and acceptable fibrocartilage covering of the donor sites were found in 81 of the 98 control arthroscopies (Figs. 43.9–43.11). Slight or severe degenerative changes were seen at the recipient and/or donor sites in 17 cases (6 chondral lesions and 11 osteochondritis dissecans). Twenty-five patients were tested by the Artscan 1,000 device (Artscan Oy, Helsinki, Finland) during control arthroscopy, as well. Stiffness of the resurfaced area in 80% of the cases was measured similar to the surrounding, healthy hyaline cartilage.

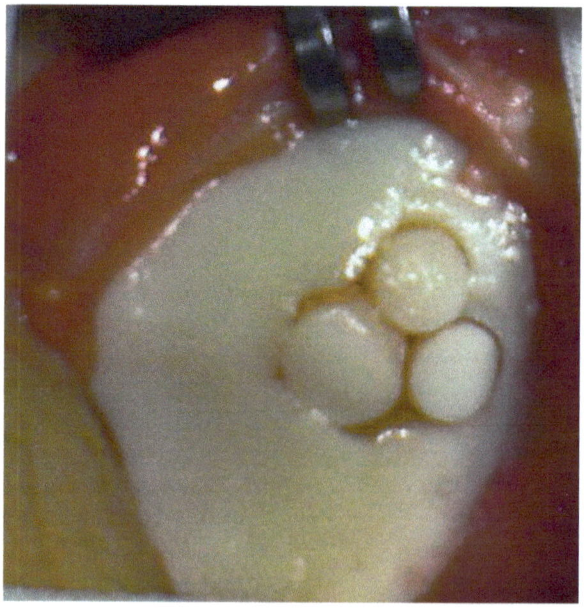

**Fig. 43.9** Mosaicplasty by three grafts in the centre of the patella

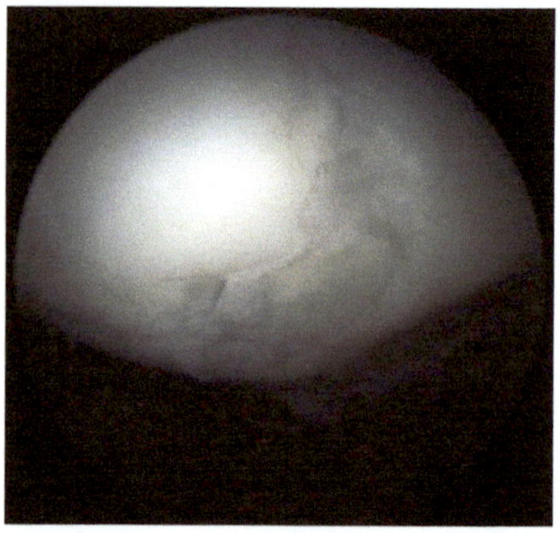

**Fig. 43.10** Two-year-old control arthroscopy of the previous implantation – congruent hyaline-like coverage of the defect

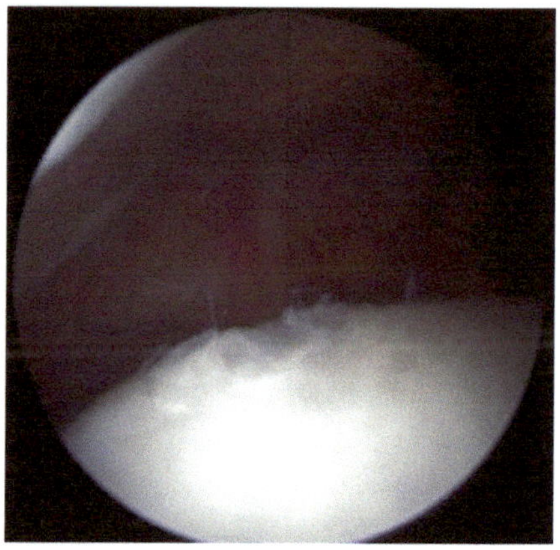

**Fig. 43.11** Two-year-old control arthroscopy of a mosaicplasty donor site – congruent fibrocartilage coverage of the donor tunnel

Postoperative complications are as follows: four deep infections and 56 painful hemarthrosis. Arthroscopic or open debridement solved all deep infections and 12 cases of hemorrhages also required arthroscopic or open debridement. Rest of patients with hemarthrosis were treated by aspiration and cryotherapy. Four patients had minor thromboembolic complications.

As at any other type of cartilage repair, mosaicplasties of the patellofemoral joint have less advantageous clinical outcome than femoral or talar applications. However it would be important to solve this frequent problem, because small-sized cartilage defects in patellofemoral joint can often lead to further degeneration and early osteoarthritis.

Since full-thickness cartilage damages of the patellotrochlear junction can involve associated problems – not infrequently – traumatic or biomechanical in origin; recognition and treatment of these abnormalities are essential simultaneously with resurfacing procedure if possible to ensure a favorable and enduring outcome. Congenital shape anomalies of the patellotrochlear surfaces, alignment problems of the quadriceps traction, patellar subluxation or dislocation, patellofemoral hyperpression as well as posttraumatic disorders represent the most common background of symptomatic deep cartilage lesions of the patellofemoral junction. Effective treatment of full-thickness defects on the patellotrochlear surfaces requires careful patient selection, a comprehensive operative plan, and a well-organized treatment course. There are a lot of different surgical procedures to improve these biomechanical deficiencies, but none of them provide similar long-lasting good outcome than femoral or tibial procedures. Shape anomalies of the patellar or trochlear surfaces represent one of the most difficult problems of the patellotrochlear junction. Osteotomies on the patella and especially on the femoral trochlea are rare and less popular techniques to make a positive influence on the congruency conditions. Soft tissue or bony corrections of traction malalignment and hyperpression are more frequent and have more positive effect to protect the patellofemoral cartilage in selected cases. Since structure of the bone of the patella provides less favorable surroundings than femoral condyles, transplanted osteochondral plugs have less chance to survive in patella.

In spite of these disadvantageous experiences a well-considered therapeutical strategy can promote an acceptable clinical outcome.

## 43.8 Complications

Septic or thromboembolic complications may negatively impact the clinical outcome. Attention to aseptic technique, antibiotic prophylaxis, and antithrombotic prophylaxis can decrease the chance of these complications.

Concerns regarding donor-site morbidity remain an integral part of the current study. A recent biomechanical study demonstrated relatively high loading forces in the donor area but stated that to date there has been no evidence that graft harvest would result in further degenerative changes. With 17 years of follow-up in our population, in case of proper indication long-term donor-site morbidity does not occur frequently. Patellofemoral complaints, such as pain or swelling after strenuous physical activity, follow the mosaicplasty procedure in fewer than 3% of cases. However, extensive graft harvest or graft harvest in spite of already existing patellofemoral degeneration can result in higher donor-site morbidity rate.

The patients with talar, capitellar, femoral, and humeral head lesions who had knee surgery only for procurement of the osteochondral plugs served as the donor-site controls. Those patients, with a rare exception, had no long-term symptoms in the knee. The symptoms in the knee resolved within 6 weeks in 95% of patients with a talar lesion and were completely resolved at 1 year in 98% of them. We think that full recovery of the donor site is due to the peripheral position chosen for the donor area and the small size and proper spacing of the individual grafts. These elements allow the joint to reconstitute structurally and to accept the relatively low loads in these parts of the knee.

However, excessive postoperative bleeding from donor tunnels occurred in 8%. Precise postoperative drainage, cooling therapy, and elastic bandages can diminish the chance of this complication.

## 43.9 Summary

Nowadays one of the most frequently used methods to treat focal full-thickness chondral or osteochondral defects on the weight-bearing area is autologous osteochondral mosaicplasty. The main point of this method is to harvest small, different-sized osteochondral grafts from the less weight-bearing area of the knee and to transplant them to the defect of the weight-bearing surface. Later gaps between transplanted plugs are filled with fibrocartilage. The new composite cartilage surface consists of about 80–90% transplanted hyaline cartilage and 10–20% regenerative fibrocartilage with same biomechanical characteristics that the healthy hyaline surface has. This chapter reports about indications and contraindications of mosaicplasty particularly among patellofemoral diseases. Surgical procedure step by step and postoperative management are also detailed. Complications and their treatments are described. The author's clinical experiences with mosaicplasty are also summarized during 17 years follow-up.

Some pearls and pitfalls are also presented that the author met in his clinical practice using mosaicplasty.

## References


1. Bobic V. Arthroscopic osteochondral autogenous graft transplantation in anterior cruciate ligament reconstruction: a preliminary clinical study. *Knee Surg Sports Traumatol Arthrosc*. 1996;3:262-264.
2. Bodó G, Hangody L, Zs S, et al. Arthroscopic autologous osteochondral mosaicplasty for the treatment of subchondral cystic lesion in the medial femoral condyle in a horse. *Acta Vet Hung*. 2000;48:343-354.
3. Campanacci M, Cervellati C, Dontiti U. Autogenous patella as replacement for a resected femoral or tibial condyle. A report of 19 cases. *J Bone Joint Surg*. 1985;67-B:557-563.
4. Fabbricciani C, Schiavone PA, Delcogliano A, et al. Osteochondral autograft in the treatment of osteochondritis dissecans of the knee. AOSSM Annual Meeting; 1991; Orlando, FL.
5. Hangody L. The biology of cartilage repair. In European instructional course lectures. *Br Ed Soc Bone Joint Surg*. 1999; 4:112–118.
6. Hangody L, Kárpáti Z. A new surgical treatment of localized cartilaginous defects of the knee. *Hung J Orthop Trauma*. 1994;37:237-243.
7. Hangody L, Kish G, Kárpáti Z. Osteochondral plugs: autogenous osteochondral mosaicplasty for the treatment of focal chondral and osteochondral articular defects. *Oper Tech Orthop*. 1997;7:312-322.
8. Hangody L, Kish G, Kárpáti Z, et al. Arthroscopic autogenous osteochondral mosaicplasty for the treatment of femoral condylar articular defects. *Knee Surg Sports Traumatol Arthrosc*. 1997;5:262-270.
9. Hangody L, Kish G, Kárpáti Z, et al. Autogenous osteochondral graft technique for replacing knee cartilage defects in dogs. *Orthop Int*. 1997;5:175-181.
10. Hangody L, Kish G, Kárpáti Z, et al. Treatment of osteochondritis dissecans of the talus: the use of the mosaicplasty technique - preliminary report. *Foot Ankle Int*. 1997;18:628-634.
11. Kish G, Módis L, Hangody L. Osteochondral mosaicplasty for the treatment of focal chondral and osteochondral lesions of the knee and talus in the athlete. *Clin Sports Med*. 1999;18:45-66.
12. Matsusue Y, Kotake T, Nakagawa Y, et al. Arthroscopic osteochondral autograft transplantation for chondral lesion of the tibial plateau of the knee. *Arthroscopy*. 2001;17(6): 653-659.
13. Matsusue Y, Yamamuro T, Hama H. Arthroscopic multiple osteochondral transplantation to the chondral defect in the knee associated with anterior cruciate ligament disruption-case report. *Arthroscopy*. 1993;9:318-321.
14. Outerbridge HK, Outerbridge AR, Outerbridge RE. The use of a lateral patellar autogenous graft for the repair of a large osteochondral defect in the knee. *J Bone Joint Surg*. 1995;77-A:65-72.
15. Pap K, Krompecher I. Arthroplasty of the knee – Experimental and clinical experiences. *J Bone Joint Surg*. 1961;43-A: 523-537.
16. Wilson WJ, Jacobs JE. Patellar graft for severely depressed comminuted fractures of the lateral tibial condyle. *J Bone Joint Surg*. 1952;34-A:436-442.
17. Yamashita F, Sakakida K, Suzu F, et al. The transplantation of an autogenic osteochondral fragment for osteochondritis dissecans of the knee. *Clin Orthop*. 1985;210:43-50.

# Patellofemoral Allografts

# 44

Robert A. Teitge and Roger Torga-Spak

## 44.1 Introduction

If the articular cartilage has been lost and osteoarthritis develops, two alternatives are available: (1) restoration of the normal extra-articular anatomy and stability, and (2) replacement of the articular cartilage. Options for articular cartilage replacement are biologic or prosthetic.

Osteochondral allografts have a long clinical history and have demonstrated >75% clinical success in the treatment of knee joint defects.[1-4] The procedure consists of transplanting a shell of subchondral bone and mature articular cartilage into the damaged area of the joint. The transplant can be either unipolar (only one surface is transplanted) or bipolar (if two reciprocal articulating surfaces are transplanted) (Fig. 44.1). Chondrocyte viability is vital to the success of cartilage transplantation. Because chondrocyte survival is diminished after freezing, and as time elapses, fresh allografts improve the prospects of preserving chondrocyte viability.[8-12] Rejection is less of a concern for articular cartilage transplantation than for other tissues because the chondrocyte surface cell antigens are isolated from the immunologic cells of the host by the complex high-molecular-weight matrix that surrounds the lacunae.[5-7]

R. Torga-Spak (✉)
Faculty of Orthopaedics and Traumatology, Department of Surgery, Instituto Universitario CEMIC, Buenos Aires, Argentina
e-mail: rtorgaspak@gmail.com

## 44.2 Surgical Technique

The knees should be harvested under sterile conditions in an operating room, cooled in sterile bags in ice water, and transported intact to the operating room where the procedure will be performed. It is recommended that patients receive the allografts within 24 h of donor procurement. In our experience donors and recipients were not HLA or blood-type matched; however size was matched in gross terms (A, large; B, medium; C, small).

A standard median parapatellar approach is used and the patella is inverted. An oscillating saw is used to cut the recipient patella in the coronal plane, creating a flat surface with no articular cartilage. The trochlear osteotomy is performed extending from the proximal articular cartilage bone junction distally to the sulcus terminale. Care must be taken to avoid the anterior femorotibial contact surface. The donor knee is opened and an attempt is made to cut the donor graft so that the cut surface would match the surface created in the recipient's knee. A pressure lavage system is used to remove as much cellular material as possible from the donor bone without injuring the articular cartilage. The grafts are fixed with 3.5-mm lag screws from the anterior surface of the recipient patella and along the margins of the femoral trochlea. No screws are placed through the articular cartilage. If the recipient knee has a previous patellectomy, holes are placed in the cancellous surface of the cut donor patella, which is then sutured into the posterior surface of the quadriceps tendon. After a standard closure, motion is begun immediately with a continuous passive motion machine and weight bearing is allowed as tolerated by pain.

V. Sanchis-Alfonso (ed.), *Anterior Knee Pain and Patellar Instability*,
DOI: 10.1007/978-0-85729-507-1_44, © Springer-Verlag London Limited 2011

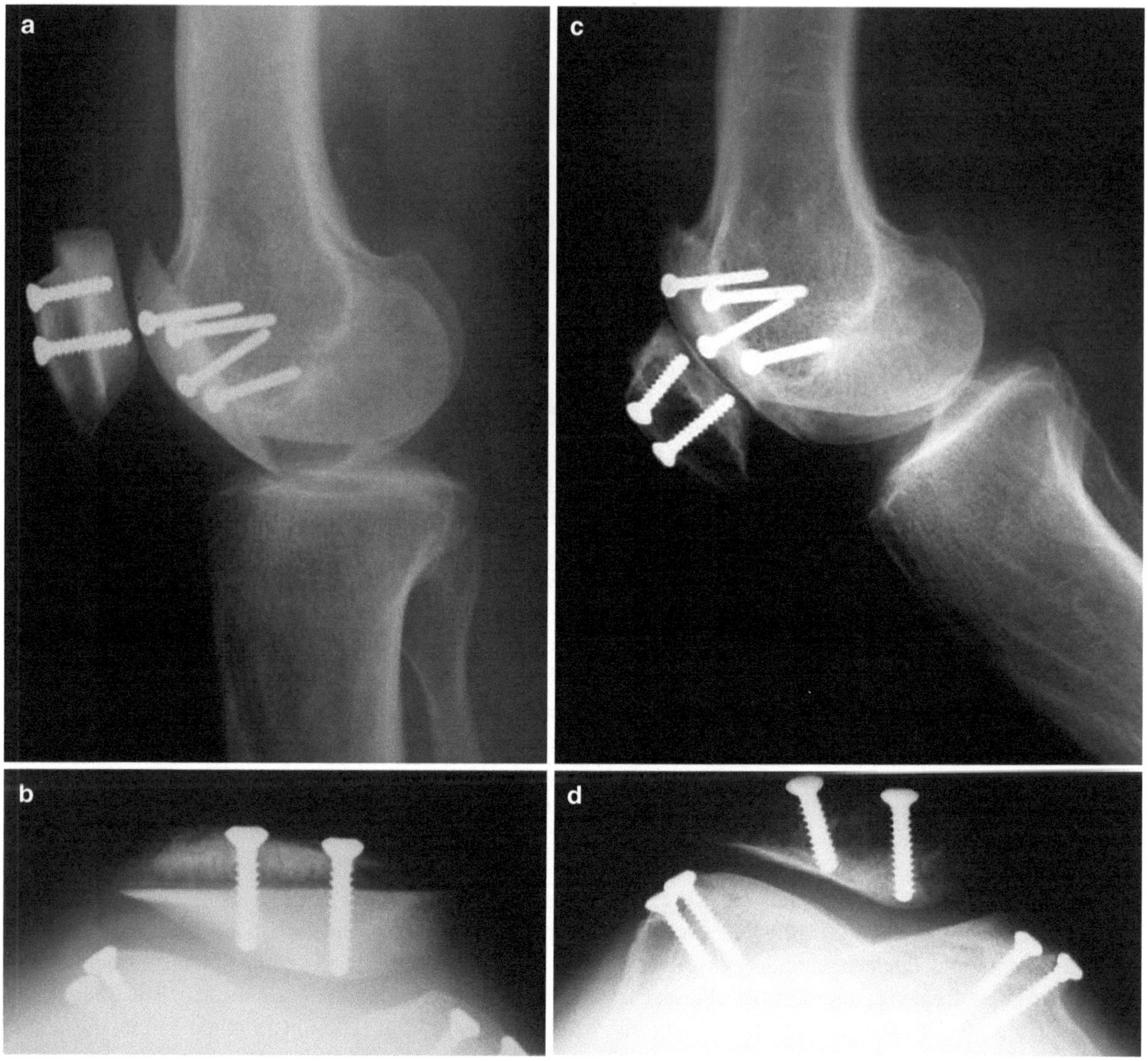


**Fig. 44.1** (**a**) Immediate postoperative lateral view after bipolar transplant. (**b**) Immediate postoperative axial view after bipolar transplant. (**c**) Lateral view after 5 years of bipolar patellofemoral transplant. (**d**) Axial view after 5 years of bipolar patellofemoral transplant

## 44.3 Our Experience

In the past 20 years 11 patients have undergone 14 fresh patellar and trochlear allografts. All of the patients had prior surgeries (average 4.4 surgeries) for patellofemoral arthrosis and chondrosis. The most frequently performed prereplacement procedure in this series was shaving chondroplasty leaving a painful patella with exposed subchondral patellar bone and progressive degenerative changes on the trochlear side. The 11 patients in this series were all severely disabled, including 1 who was in a wheelchair. Most of the patients were referred to our center to be evaluated for total joint replacement. Eight of the 11 patients were believed to have a history of instability, based upon the multiple unsuccessful surgical procedures that had been performed. At an average 10 years follow-up we observed 3 failures and 11 good to excellent results. Overall 9 of 11 patients were very satisfied or satisfied with the procedure and all but 1 of the patients stated that she would have the procedure again.

Isolated patellofemoral joint osteoarthritis is the consequence of trauma, chronic instability, or bony malalignment. The last two factors have to be corrected for biological patellar resurfacing to succeed. If instability and overload due to bony malalignment are not identified and corrected, the allograft will follow the same deterioration as the original articular cartilage. Long bone osteotomies in conjunction or after transplantation were performed in seven cases (four tibial and three femoral osteotomies) in our series.

## 44.4 Complications

All patients developed a low degree of synovitis for as long as 12 months postimplantation in our series. One patient presented a skin rash 2 weeks after allograft that resolved with a course of prednisone. The most common reason for reoperation was symptomatic hardware.

## References


1. Aubin PP, Cheah HK, Davis AM, et al. Long-term followup of fresh femoral osteochondral allografts for posttraumatic knee defects. *Clin Orthop Relat Res*. 2001;391:318-327.
2. Bugbee WD, Convery FR. Osteochondral allograft transplantation. *Clin Sports Med*. 1999;18:67-75.
3. Garrett JC. Fresh osteochondral allografts for treatment of articular defects in osteochondritis dissecans of the lateral femoral condyle in adults. *Clin Orthop Relat Res*. 1994;303:33-37.
4. Gross AE. Repair of cartilage defects in the knee. *J Knee Surg*. 2002;15:167-169.
5. Langer F, Gross AE. Immunogenicity of allograft articular cartilage. *J Bone Joint Surg*. 1974;56:297-304.
6. Langer F, Gross A. The clinical and immunological assessment of frozen bone allografts. *Acta Med Pol*. 1978;19:271-275.
7. Oakeshott RD, Farine I, Pritzker KP, et al. A clinical and histologic analysis of failed fresh osteochondral allografts. *Clin Orthop Relat Res*. 1988;233:283-294.
8. Rodrigo JJ, Thompson E, Travis C. Deep-freezing versus 4 degrees preservation of avascular osteocartilaginous shell allografts in rats. *Clin Orthop Relat Res*. 1987;218:268-275.
9. Shelton WR, Treacy SH, Dukes AD, et al. Use of allografts in knee reconstruction: I. basic science aspects and current status. *J Am Acad Orthop Surg*. 1998;6:165-168.
10. Stevenson S, Dannucci GA, Sharkey NA, et al. The fate of articular cartilage after transplantation of fresh and cryopreserved tissue-antigen-matched and mismatched osteochondral allografts in dogs. *J Bone Joint Surg*. 1989;71:1297-1307.
11. Williams RJ III, Dreese JC, Chen CT. Chondrocyte survival and material properties of hypothermically stored cartilage: an evaluation of tissue used for osteochondral allograft transplantation. *Am J Sports Med*. 2004;32:132-139.
12. Williams SK, Amiel D, Ball ST. Prolonged storage effects on the articular cartilage of fresh human osteochondral allografts. *J Bone Joint Surg*. 2003;85:2111-2120.

# Patellofemoral Arthroplasty: Pearls and Pitfalls

45

Ronald P. Grelsamer and Jason Gould

## 45.1 Introduction

There has been a proliferation of new patellofemoral implants, which reflects an increasing interest in this topic on the part of the orthopedic community. The procedure is a niche procedure reserved for patients with isolated patellofemoral arthritis who are unlikely to develop femorotibial arthritis in their lifetime, and for patients considered too young or too active to receive a total knee replacement. Other options include biological repair, tibial tuberosity transfers, patellectomy (partial or total), and total joint replacement surgery.

## 45.2 History

The practice of resurfacing the patella in the face of patellofemoral arthritis predates the total knee replacement by more than 10 years.[10] McKeever was the first to describe a patellar resurfacing operation when, in 1955 he described fixing a metallic implant to the undersurface of the patella by way of a transverse screw.

In 1975, Aglietti[2] introduced a polyethylene patella. Worrell designed the last of the isolated patellar implants, a cobalt-chrome device that he reported on with short follow-up in 1979[20] and then again in 1986.[21]

R.P. Grelsamer (✉)
Mount Sinai Medical Center, New York, NY, USA
e-mail: ronald.grelsamer@mountsinai.org

In 1979, independent of each other, Lubinus[14] in Europe and Blazina[5] in California introduced the concept of a patellofemoral replacement (PFR), where both the patella and the trochlea would be resurfaced. Despite some confusion in the literature[16] this is a separate and distinct operation from the simple patellar resurfacing of McKeever, Aglietti, or Worrell. The benefits of a patellofemoral replacement relative to a total knee replacement included less surgical dissection, less bone resection, preservation of the femorotibial compartments and cruciates, no blood transfusions, and less expense.

The original descriptions of the procedure did not include strict indications. Technical pitfalls were not completely appreciated, and little emphasis was placed on realignment of the extensor mechanism. Accordingly, reports pertaining to earliest designs were disappointing. This led to refinements of the implant and of the surgical technique in Europe, and to near abandonment of the entire concept in the United States.

The literature of the last 15 years has been much more encouraging, if not outright enthusiastic.[1,3,4,6,8,11,12,15,18,19]

The occasional poor results reported in the above series have one major feature in common: the failure on the surgeon's part to appreciate present or incipient femorotibial arthritis. Patients whose patellofemoral arthritis lacks a clear origin are more likely to develop arthritis in the remainder of their knee. Conversely, patients with well-defined conditions that affect the patellofemoral compartment, such as malalignment, dysplasia, or trauma, do best. When one removes the suboptimally selected patients from the above cohorts, the results of patellofemoral arthroplasty are clearly promising.

V. Sanchis-Alfonso (ed.), *Anterior Knee Pain and Patellar Instability*,
DOI: 10.1007/978-0-85729-507-1_45, © Springer-Verlag London Limited 2011

## 45.3 Indications

The indication for a patellofemoral replacement is pain emanating from an arthritic patellofemoral compartment.[10] It can be challenging to determine if this is the patient's sole source of pain, as a large number of conditions can refer pain to the anterior aspect of the knee. These include overuse, abnormal patellar tilt, plicae, neuromas, tendonitis, synovitis, focal lesions within the patella, as well as referred pain from elsewhere in the knee or distant sites such as the hip or spine. In addition to observable pathology, a patient's pain may lie with abnormal intraosseous pressures, abnormal levels of substance P,[9] or other invisible factors. Our improved ability to image the patellofemoral articulation has not improved our ability to treat patellofemoral pain,[9] and this was well articulated by Insall when he wrote "Curiously, neither the widespread use of arthroscopy nor the advent of new diagnostic tests such as CT scanning and magnetic resonance imaging have cast much light" on the enigma of patellofemoral pain.[10]

A patellar cartilage lesion, for example, is not automatically the source of a patient's pain. Rest pain should arouse suspicion for nerve-related pain, such as a neuroma, reflex sympathetic dystrophy (RSD)/complex regional pain syndrome (CRPS), or a radiculopathy.

A key sign of symptomatic patellofemoral arthritis on the physical examination is tenderness of one patellar facet or the other. The surgeon assesses this by gently curling his fingers under the lateral (or medial) border of the patella (in applying such pressure, the surgeon is simultaneously applying pressure to all the soft tissues between the skin and bone – including the retinaculum and the synovium. The specific source of pain can therefore be debated).

In order to determine whether the arthritis is truly isolated the surgeon must order a complete set of radiographs. These include not just standing anteroposterior radiographs, a true lateral projection, and a Merchant view, but also the standing tunnel view, also known as the Rosenberg view.[17] This view alone will reveal arthritis that is localized to the posterior aspect of a femorotibial compartment. An MRI and an arthroscopy are also useful in evaluating the femorotibial compartments, as is a nuclear bone scan. In fact, the nuclear bone scan is the only imaging modality that assesses the knee's metabolic activity.[9]

Inflammatory arthritis as a cause of patellofemoral arthritis is a major pitfall in patellofemoral replacement surgery, as the patellofemoral compartment can simply be the first compartment affected. Therefore, serum analysis for rheumatoid arthritis is warranted and a workup for Lyme disease can also be considered (this infection is ubiquitous in the United States).

## 45.4 Choice of Implants

Patellofemoral replacements fall into two general design categories differentiated by their approach to the trochlea: resurfacing versus resection.

A resurfacing (inlay) system places a V-shaped or U-shaped metallic piece within the trochlea. This is the classic approach, first espoused by Blazina, by Bechtol, and by Lubinus. In a resection (onlay) system the trochlea and the anterior aspect of the femoral condyles are removed en bloc, as with the anterior cut and trochlear preparation of a total knee replacement.

### *45.4.1 Resurfacing Designs*

(a) Off-the-Shelf. The surgeon sculpts the trochlea to match the off-the-shelf implant. Every trochlea features a different morphology (Fig. 45.1). Patients with trochlear dysplasia require particularly meticulous work. These subjects tend to have flatter trochleas, if not areas of outright convexity. Although patients with trochlear dysplasia are rare in the general population, they form a large percentage of patients undergoing PFR surgery.
The dysplasia of the trochlea can lead to a suboptimal fit of the trochlear component, and one or both flanges may be unsupported by bone. The gaps can be filled with cement.
(b) Custom Trochlea. A computerized tomography (CT) scan is taken of the patient's trochlea. The scan is used to create a three-dimensional model of the distal femur, from which a custom trochlear component is manufactured (Fig. 45.1). This assures an excellent fit without the time expenditure of the trochlear shaping. The side of the trochlear implant facing the patella has a fixed radius of curvature designed to accept a standard, round patellar button (Fig. 45.2).

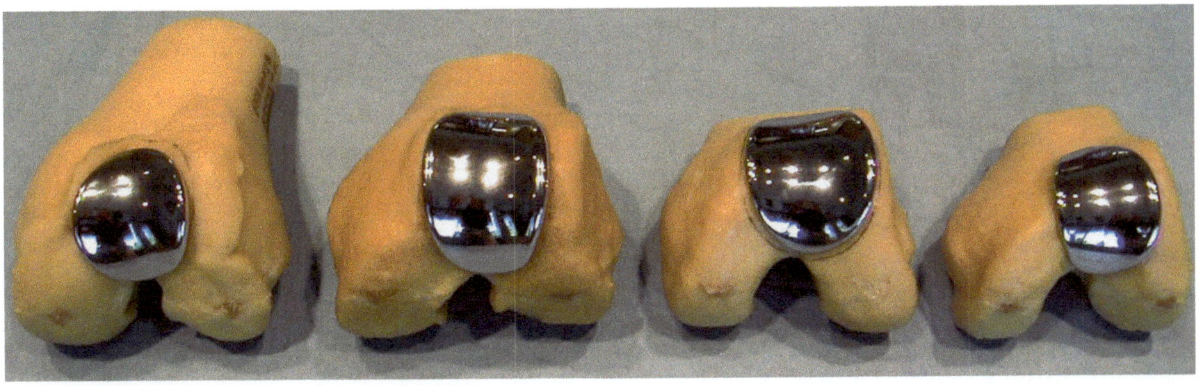

**Fig. 45.1** There exist dramatic variations in trochlear anatomy. This is particularly true in candidates for patellofemoral replacement surgery (Reprinted with permission from Kinamed, California USA)

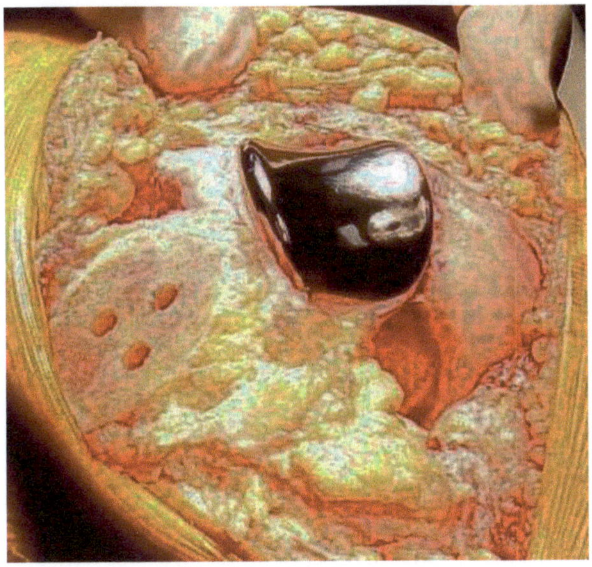

**Fig. 45.2** Custom trochlear component manufactured from a CT scan of the patient's trochlea (Reprinted with permission from Kinamed, California USA)

### 45.4.2 Resection (Onlay) Design

The anterior aspect of the femoral condyles is resected flush with the anterior cortex. The trochlear component has a flat undersurface that rests on this cut surface. The surgeon may not have ready access to the epicondyles, and Whiteside's line may not be of any use with a seriously dysplastic trochlea, leaving some surgeons to resort to a computerized navigation system.[7] The trochlea must be cut or milled. The surgeon chooses among different off-the-shelf sizes.

## 45.5 General Principles

Some technical principles apply to all replacements.

Performing a patellofemoral replacement is not a substitute for a patella realignment. A patella that tends to sublux or dislocate laterally will do so even after the replacement surgery. The surgeon must identify the factors that are causing the patella to track poorly. These can include any combination of a tight lateral retinaculum, a deficient vastus medialis obliquus (VMO), a deficient medial patellofemoral ligament (MPFL), a lateralized tibial tuberosity (increased Q angle), and a dysplastic trochlea.

If the tibial tuberosity is lateralized (trochlear groove–tibial tuberosity distance > approximately 20 mm with the knee extended), the surgeon may choose to medialize it, if the lateral retinaculum is tight, he/she may release it, and if the medial soft tissues are deficient, the surgeon must plicate them. I have not had to reconstruct an MPFL (yet?).

The inferior tip of the trochlear component must not be distal to the trochlea, lest it abut against the tibial spines and become a source of pain. This pitfall is easy to avoid when the trochlea has a normal shape, but harder to avoid when the trochlea is distorted and includes an inferior osteophyte. This inferior osteophyte closes down the femoral notch, leaving just a small opening through which the cruciates can just be visualized. With the use of gouges, osteotomes, and/or rongeurs, the osteophyte must be removed until the notch has a normal appearance. Then, and only then, can the inferior limit of the trochlea be determined, and it is against this lower portion of the trochlea that the inferior portion of the trochlear implant must rest.

The inferior tip of the trochlear implant must not be proud relative to the surrounding cartilage.

If the proximal edge of the trochlear component lies proximal to the native trochlea it should rest directly on the anterior cortex of the distal femur to avoid catching in the early degrees of flexion. This is particularly important if the entire patella lies proximal to the trochlea in full extension.

## 45.6 Summary

Patellofemoral Replacement surgery, popular in Europe for the last 25 years, is gaining popularity in the United States.[10,13] This is reflected in the proliferation of patellofemoral implants.

Nevertheless, it remains a niche procedure that is best indicated for patients who are unlikely to develop arthritis in their femorotibial compartments. The least satisfying results have been obtained in patients whose arthritis is of unknown etiology and who are young enough to develop femorotibial arthritis.

On the other hand, the procedure requires far less surgical dissection than a standard total knee replacement and leads to far less blood loss. It can appeal to patients who would otherwise refuse knee replacement surgery.

The key technical points are: not placing the trochlear component too far distally, not leaving either the proximal or distal portion of the trochlea proud, and not leaving the patella unstable.

## References


1. Ackroyd CE, Newman JH, Evans R, et al. The Avon patellofemoral arthroplasty: five-year survivorship and functional results. *J Bone Joint Surg Br*. 2007;89:310-315.
2. Aglietti P, Insall JN, Walker PS, et al. A new patella prosthesis. Design and application. *Clin Orthop Relat Res*. 1975;107:175-187.
3. Argenson JN, Guillaume JM, Aubaniac JM. Is there a place for patellofemoral arthroplasty? *Clin Orthop Relat Res*. 1995;321:162-167.
4. Arnbjornsson A, Ryd L. The use of isolated patellar prostheses in Sweden 1977-1986. *Int Orthop*. 1998;22:141-144.
5. Blazina M, Fox J, Del Pizzo W, et al. Patellofemoral replacement. *Clin Orthop Relat Res*. 1979;144:98-102.
6. Cartier P, Sanouiller JL, Grelsamer R. Patellofemoral arthroplasty. 2-12-year follow-up study. *J Arthroplasty*. 1990; 5:49-55.
7. Cossey AJ, Spriggins AJ. Computer-assisted patellofemoral arthroplasty: a mechanism for optimizing rotation. *J Arthroplasty*. 2006;21:420-427.
8. De Cloedt P, Legaye J, Lokietek W. Femoro-patellar prosthesis. A retrospective study of 45 consecutive cases with a follow-up of 3-12 years. *Acta Orthop Belg*. 1999;65:170-175.
9. Dye SF. The pathophysiology of patellofemoral pain: a tissue homeostasis perspective. *Clin Orthop Relat Res*. 2005;436:100-110.
10. Grelsamer RP, Stein DA. Patellofemoral arthritis. *J Bone Joint Surg Am*. 2006;88:1849-1860.
11. Kooijman HJ, Driessen AP, van Horn JR. Long-term results of patellofemoral arthroplasty. A report of 56 arthroplasties with 17 years of follow-up. *J Bone Joint Surg Br*. 2003; 85:836-840.
12. Krajca-Radcliffe JB, Coker TP. Patellofemoral arthroplasty. A 2- to 18-year followup study. *Clin Orthop Relat Res*. 1996;330:143-151.
13. Lonner JH. Patellofemoral arthroplasty. *J Am Acad Orthop Surg*. 2007;15:495-506.
14. Lubinus H. Patella glide bearing total replacement. *Orthopedics*. 1979;2:119-127.
15. Mertl P, Van FT, Bonhomme P, et al. Femoropatellar osteoarthritis treated by prosthesis. Retrospective study of 50 implants. *Rev Chir Orthop Reparatrice Appar Mot*. 1997; 83:712-718.
16. Mont M, Haas S, Mullick T, et al. Total knee arthroplasty for patellofemoral arthritis. *J Bone Joint Surg Am*. 2002;84:-1977-1981.
17. Rosenberg TD, Paulos LE, Parker RD, et al. The forty-five-degree posteroanterior flexion weight-bearing radiograph of the knee. *J Bone Joint Surg Am*. 1988;70:1479-1483.
18. Sisto DJ, Sarin VK. Custom patellofemoral arthroplasty of the knee. *J Bone Joint Surg Am*. 2006;88:1475-1480.
19. Smith AM, Peckett WR, Butler-Manuel PA, et al. Treatment of patello-femoral arthritis using the Lubinus patello-femoral arthroplasty: a retrospective review. *Knee*. 2002;9:27-30.
20. Worrell RV. Prosthetic resurfacing of the patella. *Clin Orthop Relat Res*. 1979;144:91-97.
21. Worrell RV. Resurfacing of the patella in young patients. *Orthop Clin North Am*. 1986;17:303-309.

# The Patellofemoral Arthroplasty: The Great Solution, the Great Problem

46

Vicente Sanchis-Alfonso

## 46.1 Introduction

Unfortunately, many orthopedic surgeons believe that the definite solution for eliminating anterior knee pain in a young patient with multiple operations is the patellofemoral prosthesis ("The Great Solution"). But, they fail to ask themselves the most important question; what is causing the pain? When a patellofemoral prosthesis is implanted in these young patients without finding out the cause of the pain, a more serious problem could be created with a worse solution ("The Great Problem"). The cases we present spotlight this abuse.

## 46.2 Case # 1

A 29-year-old woman whose left knee was operated on seven times by four different surgeons, beginning at the age of 20 (arthroscopic shaving, patella osteotomy, tibial tubercle anteromedialization with lateral patellar retinaculum release, and finally a patellofemoral arthroplasty, with primary repair and augmentation of a chronic patellar tendon rupture). Her initial diagnosis was chondromalacia patellae, and her clinical results were worse after each surgery. She comes to my office for an opinion about the possibility of eliminating her anterior knee pain and instability (seventh opinion). She has severe and constant left anterior knee pain even during rest (eight in the visual analog pain scale), she also has evident instability during activities of daily living, she goes up and down stairs one step at a time, she is very limited in her activities of daily living, she even has difficulties getting up from a chair without using the armrest (preoperative Lysholm 26, preoperative IKDC 25, preoperative Tegner activity scale of level 1). She used to work as a hairdresser but no longer can because she is unable to stand up for long periods of time. She only tolerates activities where she can sit.

The patient is 1.68 m tall and weighs 69 kg. The physical examination shows a central anterior scar. An evident chronic patellar tendon rupture is seen, with a very high riding patella (Fig. 46.1). The patient told us that her surgeon explained that this had happened during a knee manipulation by the physical therapist after the anteromedialization surgery, although it could also be due to a devascularization caused by the surgical procedure[8] (unfortunately some orthopedic surgeons always

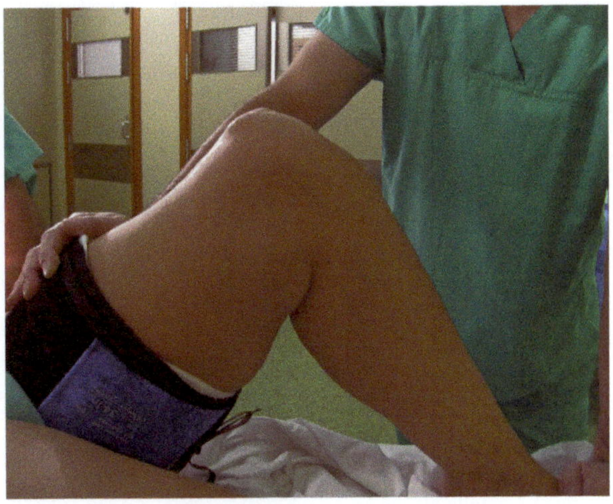

**Fig. 46.1** Physical examination shows a patella alta

V. Sanchis-Alfonso
International Patellofemoral Study Group,
International ACL Study Group,
Hospital 9 de Octubre, Hospital Arnau de Vilanova,
School of Medicine, Catholic University of Valencia,
Valencia, Spain
e-mail: vicente.sanchis.alfonso@gmail.com

V. Sanchis-Alfonso (ed.), *Anterior Knee Pain and Patellar Instability*,
DOI: 10.1007/978-0-85729-507-1_46, © Springer-Verlag London Limited 2011

blame their failures and problems on somebody else). The knee's range of motion is normal, emphasizing that the knee extension is complete. She has mild joint effusion, her limb has normal knee alignment (physiological valgus). Neurological and vascular exam is normal. Blood test shows a sedimentation rate of 10 and a C-reactive protein of seven.

The radiographic study showed a patella alta and a patellofemoral prosthesis in an apparent good condition (Fig. 46.2). An MRI cannot be performed because the prosthesis caused a lot of artifacts. A CT scan showed a correct rotational alignment of the femoral shield. A bone scan with Tc 99m was performed, showing a higher uptake in both internal and external femoral condyles in the loading area (Fig. 46.3). However, the Gallium bone scan was negative.

The kinetic and kinematic study during stair descent test that we routinely perform in the Instituto de Biomecánica de Valencia (IBV) in all our extensor mechanism revision surgeries revealed the following defense mechanisms in our patient: reduction of the extensor moment and reduction of the ground reaction force; we also found an increase in the abductor moment, hence a tibiofemoral overload (Fig. 46.4). The extensor moment reduction entails the suppression of one of the impact absorption mechanism of the knee. This is clearly going to favor the development of a tibiofemoral osteoarthritis.

All the possible therapeutic options with their pros and cons are discussed with the patient, who by the way is very cooperative and psychologically stable. Option 1, do nothing. Option 2, complete extensor mechanism allograft (quadriceps tendon–patella–patellar tendon–proximal tibia insertion) with a possible revision of the femoral shield, or conversion into a total knee arthroplasty. And option 3, complete extensor mechanism allograft plus femoral trochlea allograft (complete bipolar extensor mechanism allograft). The patient chooses option 3. Following medical clinical practice ethical principles[4] the patient is aware that in the medical literature, as far as we know, there are no published cases of such young recipients of a complete extensor mechanism allograft (they are all over 57 years old), which concerns us because the level of demand on the extensor mechanism of a young patient is higher than that of an older patient. Nevertheless it seems that this technique is nowadays quite well standardized.[2]

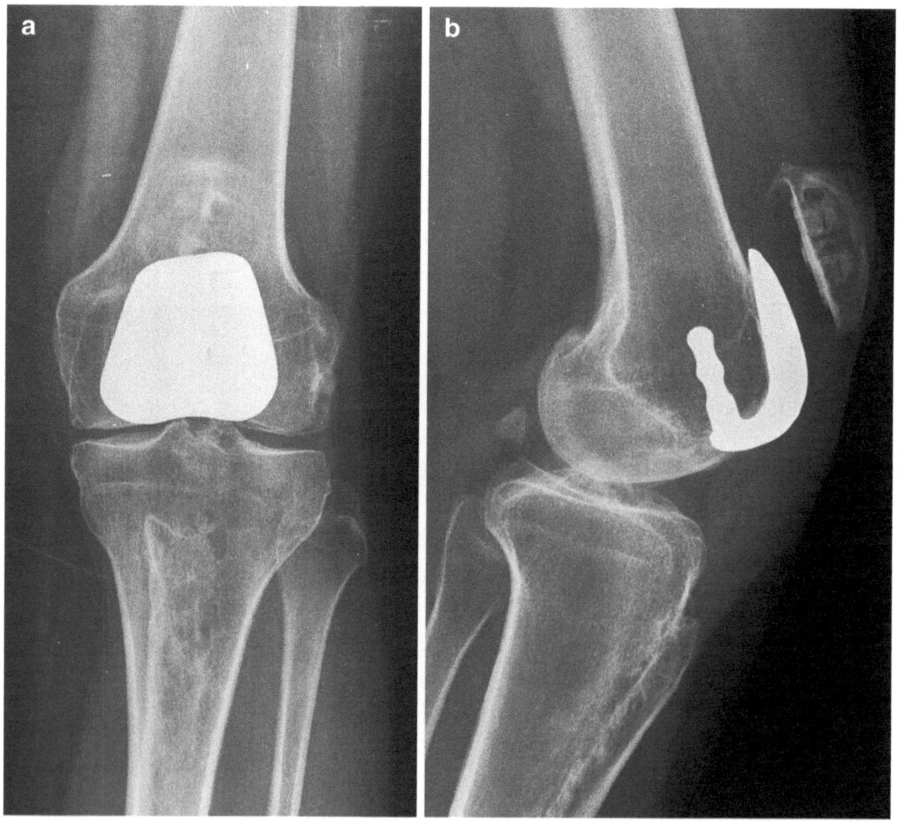


**Fig. 46.2** Anteroposterior (**a**) and lateral (**b**) radiographs of the left knee showing a patella alta and a patellofemoral arthroplasty

Another fact that is unique to this case is the simultaneous transplantation of the femoral trochlea. However, bipolar transplants of trochlea and patella have in fact been described in young people with a high percentage of good results.[10,20] The risks involved in this type of surgery (ruptures, graft attenuation, infection, skin problems) that could require an arthrodesis are discussed in detail with the patient. Finally we insist once again on the fact that it is an unusual procedure, but the patient is determined to undergo this radical knee reconstruction and she therefore signs the written informed consent document.

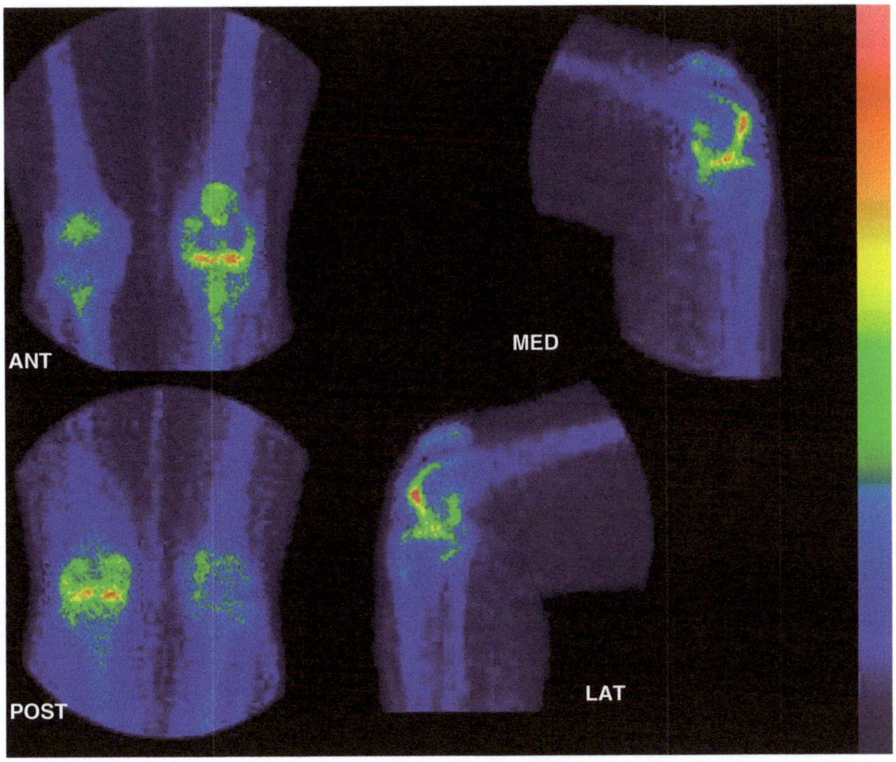


**Fig. 46.3** Standard technetium 99 methylene diphosphonate bone scan showing increased osseous metabolic activity in femoral condyles

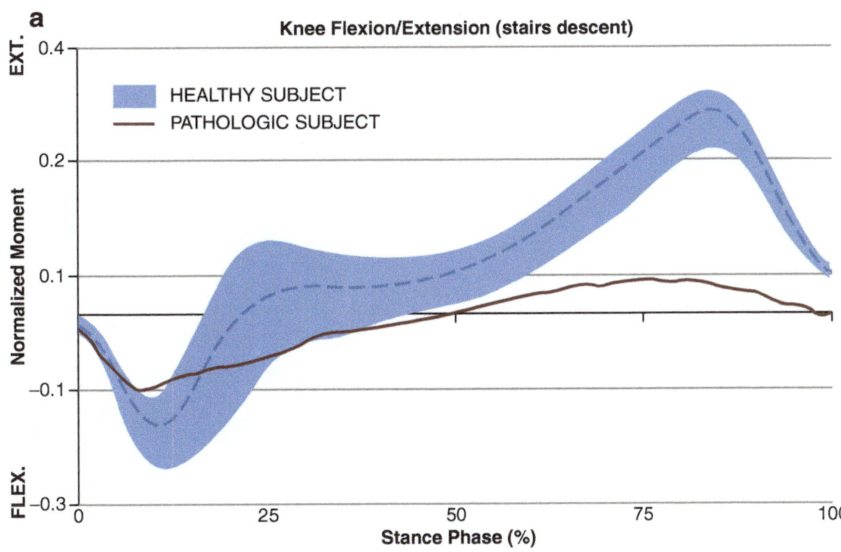


**Fig. 46.4** (**a**) Knee flexion–extension moment during stair descending test. (**b**) Vertical ground reaction force during stair descending test. (**c**) Knee abduction moment during stair descending test

**Fig. 46.4** (continued)

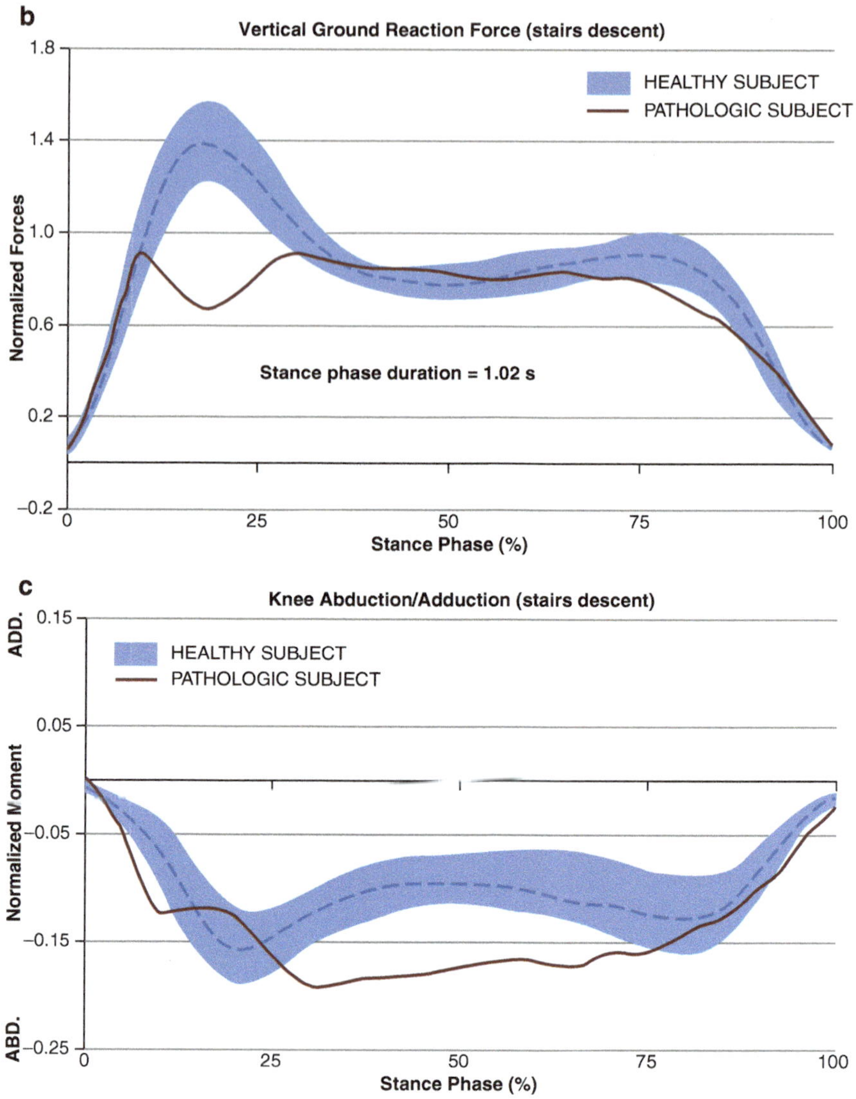


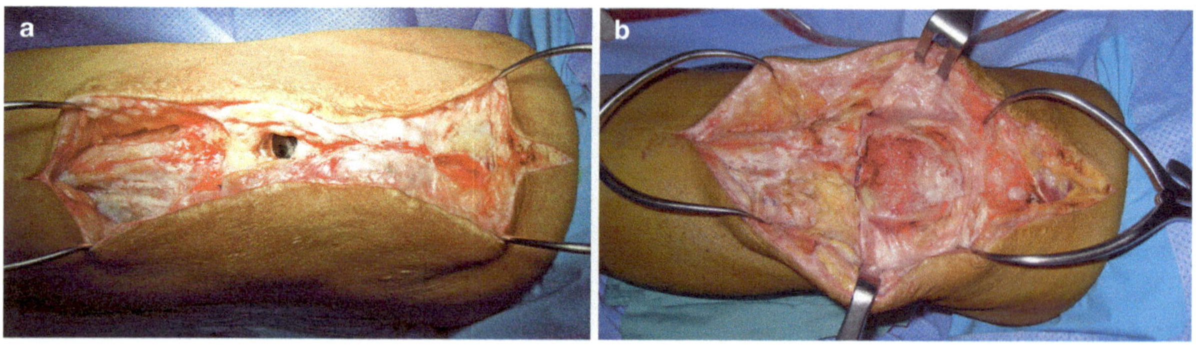


**Fig. 46.5** (**a**) Intraoperative photograph showing a complete absence of the patellar tendon. (**b**) Femoral trochlea after removing the femoral shield of the patellofemoral prosthesis

During surgery we found a complete absence of the patellar tendon and a clear loosening of the femoral shield of the patellofemoral prosthesis (Fig. 46.5). We also found initial ill-defined degenerative changes in the loading area of both femoral condyles. The synovial fluid was sent for culture, and the results came back negative. We performed a reconstruction of the extensor mechanism with a nonradiated cryopreserved allograft of quadriceps tendon–patella–patellar tendon–proximal tibia insertion following the technique described by Burnett et al.[2] (Fig. 46.6) associated with a femoral trochlea allograft for which we used a cryopreserved distal left femur from a young donor without degenerative changes or a trochlear dysplasia (Fig. 46.7). Before implanting the allograft we performed a culture of both (distal femur and complete extensor mechanism), right after we took them out of the plastic bags they came in, and the results came back negative. The quadricipital end of the allograft was sutured with tension to the recipient's quadricipital tendon with the knee in full extension (Fig. 46.6b). Knee flexion is not evaluated during surgery. We follow the postoperative and physical therapy protocol designed by Burnett et al.[2] The patient receives oral antibiotic infection prophylaxis with one capsule of Tavanic every 12 h and one capsule of Zyvoxid every 12 h for 1 month after surgery.

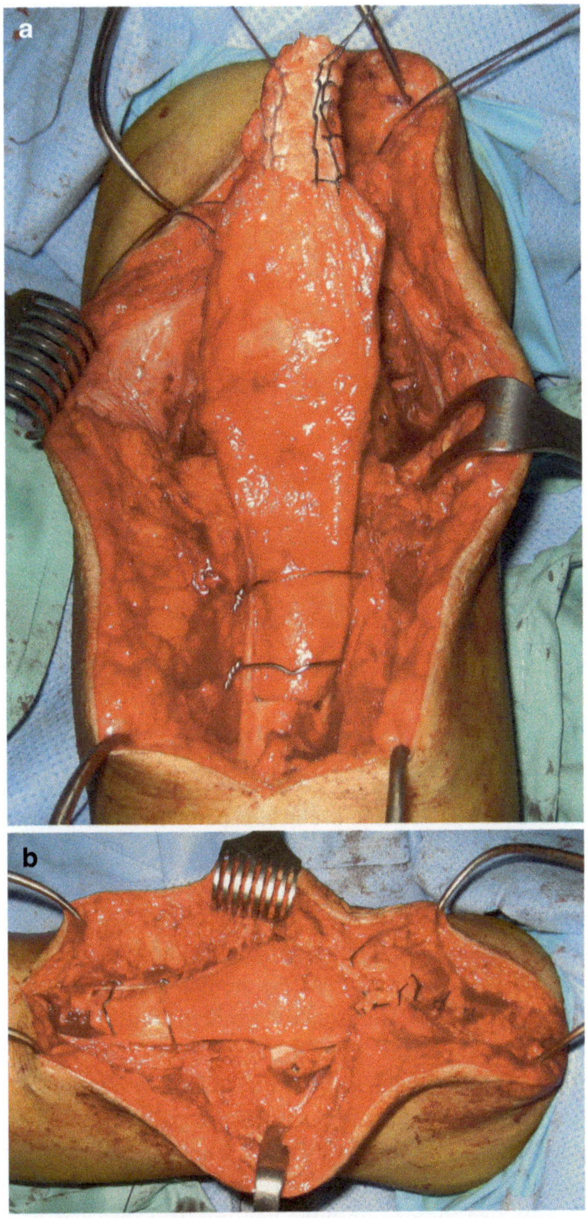

**Fig. 46.6** (**a**) Intraoperative photograph of the allograft extensor mechanism in situ. Fixation of the tibial allograft with stainless steel wires. Two sutures placed in the allograft quadriceps allow the allograft to be tensioned proximally. (**b**) Good coverage of the allograft with autologous soft tissue

### 46.2.1 Comments About Case # 1

The patellofemoral joint is the joint most frequently operated on without any clear pathophysiogical basis. This often happens under the guise of the broad diagnosis of "chondromalacia patellae," a generalization that has been used since the beginning of the twentieth century with no etiologic, diagnostic, therapeutic, and certainly no prognostic implications.

We are dealing with a patellar tendon chronic rupture in a young patient with a patellofemoral arthroplasty with aseptic loosening of the femoral component. We say the loosening was aseptic because the preoperative blood test (SR and CRP) and the Gallium bone scan were normal. Also, during surgery the synovial fluid culture was negative.

A GREAT PROBLEM: Patellar Tendon Chronic Rupture/Complete Extensor Mechanism Allograft: A GOOD SOLUTION?

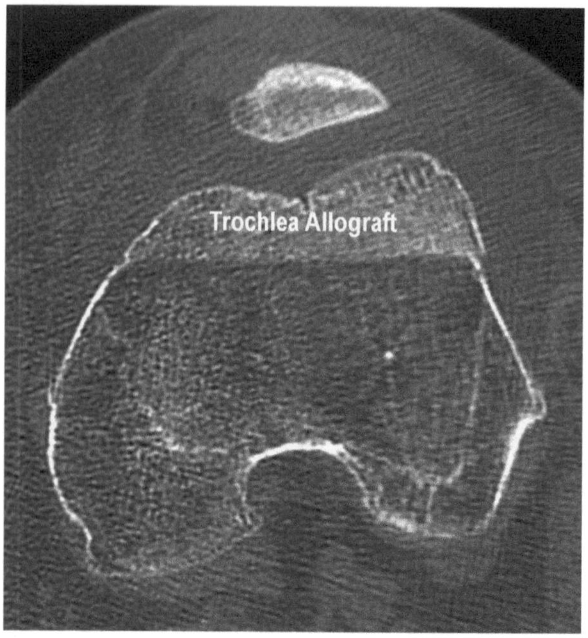


**Fig. 46.7** Postoperative CT at 3 months follow-up. Femoral trochlea allograft without degenerative changes or a trochlear dysplasia (FTA)

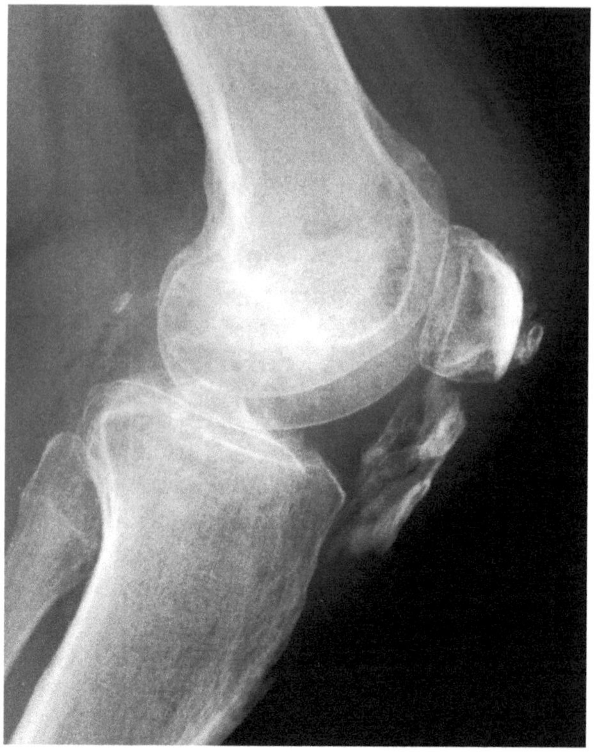

**Fig. 46.8** Extensive posttraumatic ossification of the patellar tendon

When confronting a chronic patellar tendon rupture we have different options. We opted for a complete extensor mechanism allograft because the rupture was very chronic and we could not foresee how retracted the quadriceps muscle and quadriceps tendon would be and besides, the patella had a polyethylene button. The greatest problem with this type of transplant is the healing between the donor's and the recipient's quadriceps tendon. Some authors have gotten around this problem by using a graft of "patella–patellar tendon–tibial tubercle",[13] creating a crest in the graft's patella and a groove in the recipient patella to give rise to bone on bone healing. But this was not an option in our case because of the patellar bone deficit (previous osteotomy to implant the patellar prosthetic button) ("A Great Problem"). However, the healing problem between the donor and recipient quadriceps tendon could also be related to the age of the complete extensor mechanism transplant cases published (over 57 years old). In our case the patient was young and we achieved good coverage of the allograft with autologous soft tissue (Fig. 46.6b) that will most likely be a source of revascularization and cell repopulation of the allograft, like in the ACL allografts.[18]

A complete extensor mechanism allograft would be indicated for a chronic nonreparable patellar or quadriceps tendon rupture or when a primary suture has failed (as in the case we present), nonreparable comminuted patella fractures, severe heterotopic ossification of the extensor mechanism[15] (Fig. 46.8), severe patella infera with arthrofibrosis of the extensor mechanism, patellar tumors with extension to the extensor mechanism, and when converting a knee arthrodesis into a total knee arthroplasty.[2,14] It would be contraindicated in patients with an infection, patients that cannot participate in the postoperative physical therapy, or when a primary repair with or without autologous tissue augmentation is possible.

It is interesting to highlight some of the aspects of the surgical technique of our case. It is recommended that the allograft has 5 cm of quadriceps tendon so that it can be fully covered by the recipient's own quadriceps tendon and sutured with nonabsorbable material.[2] The allograft must be placed with tension and the knee in full extension; we do not evaluate knee flexion after suturing the tendon.[2,3,17] This does not pose a problem in recuperating flexion.[2] Placing the graft without tension is dooming it to failure.[5,6] Finally it is important to achieve good allograft coverage with the recipient's tissue that could act as a source of cell repopulation and thusly reducing the risk of infection.[2]

A GREAT PROBLEM: Loosening of the Femoral Component/A Trochler Allograft: A GOOD SOLUTION?

With the loosening of the femoral component we had two options. Either to implant a new femoral shield or to do a trochlear allograft. When doing an allograft that includes the patella, resurfacing (patellar button) is not recommended because it could weaken the graft and also because allogenic tissue has no sensitivity. In fact, a high percentage of patellar complications with resurfacing have been presented.[5,6] Since we are dealing with a young patient in whom a partial or total arthroplasty is a relative contraindication, and a patellar button with a complete extensor mechanism allograft is not recommended, we chose the second option: a femoral trochlea allograft. Moreover, this type of surgery does not preclude a total knee replacement, and moreover a functioning extensor mechanism is necessary to perform a total knee arthroplasty. This is another aspect in favor of doing a complete extensor mechanism allograft. We are perfectly aware of the problems related to the use of cryopreserved osteoarticular allografts, but due to the great difficulties we have in our area to access fresh allografts we opted for this solution ("Another Problem"). Good results have been achieved with the use of massive fresh-frozen allografts as subtitutes for irreparable tibial plateau destruction following fractures in young patients (JC Monllau, MD personal communication). Despite the degenerative changes in both femoral condyles we decided to leave them alone, since doing a total knee arthroplasty would be a relative contraindication because of the patient's age. Also, restoring the extensor mechanism allows the quadriceps to act as a load absorption system, relieving an overloaded tibiofemoral joint. With this, possibly, we will delay the development of the tibiofemoral osteoarthritis and therefore delay the need for a total knee arthroplasty.

It is interesting to highlight some of the aspects of the surgical technique of our case. When performing a trochlear allograft we must chose a distal femur on the same side, in our case it was the left side, without femoral dysplasia. It has been said that the trochlear prominence increases the patellofemoral compression force which contributes to patellofemoral osteoarthritis (antiMaquet effect). Since in our case the trochlea was slightly prominent we maintained the distal Maquet effect achieved by the previous tibial tubercle anteromedialization surgery, when placing the allograft (tibial bone chip), to compensate for our slightly prominent trochlea and thus reducing patellofemoral overload. This way we also avoid proximal migration of the allograft.

## 46.3 Case # 2

A 34-year-old woman whose left knee was operated on three times (arthroscopic shaving with lateral retinacular release and Pridie drilling, proximal and distal realignment, and finally a patellofemoral arthroplasty) comes to my office for an opinion about the possibility of eliminating her severe chronic knee pain, effusion, and instability. Her initial diagnosis, before the first operation, was "chondromalacia patellae". The pain and impairment got worse and worse with each surgical procedure (pain according to the visual analog pain scale: 6 before the first operation, 7 after the first operation, 9 after the second operation, and 10 after the patellofemoral arthroplasty; impairment according to the Lysholm score: 43 before the first operation, 29 after the first operation, 17 after the second operation, and 19 after the patellofemoral arthroplasty). After the third operation the pain is constant, even during rest. She also has evident instability during activities of daily living. She uses two crutches. She goes up and down stairs one step at a time. She is very limited in her activities of daily living.

Physical examination revealed anterior and posterior knee pain, joint effusion, a positive apprehension sign upon pressing the patella medially, and a positive Fulkerson's relocation test.

Conventional radiography, including sky-line views, revealed no abnormalities. Stress axial radiography revealed a medial patellar instability (Fig. 46.9).

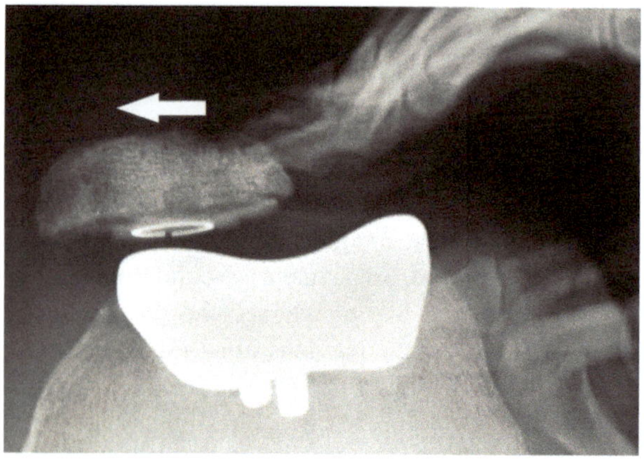

**Fig. 46.9** Axial stress radiograph of the left knee showing an iatrogenic medial subluxation of the patella

The kinetic and kinematic study during stair descent test revealed: reduction of the knee joint flexion angle during stair descent (Fig. 46.10), reduction of the extensor moment and reduction of the ground reaction force (Fig. 46.11).

### 46.3.1 Comments About Case # 2

The excessive high number of surgical procedures performed in some cases in patients with anterior knee pain reflects the inaccurate existing therapeutic concepts in resolving this problem surgically. Unfortunately, in some cases the treatment performed is not

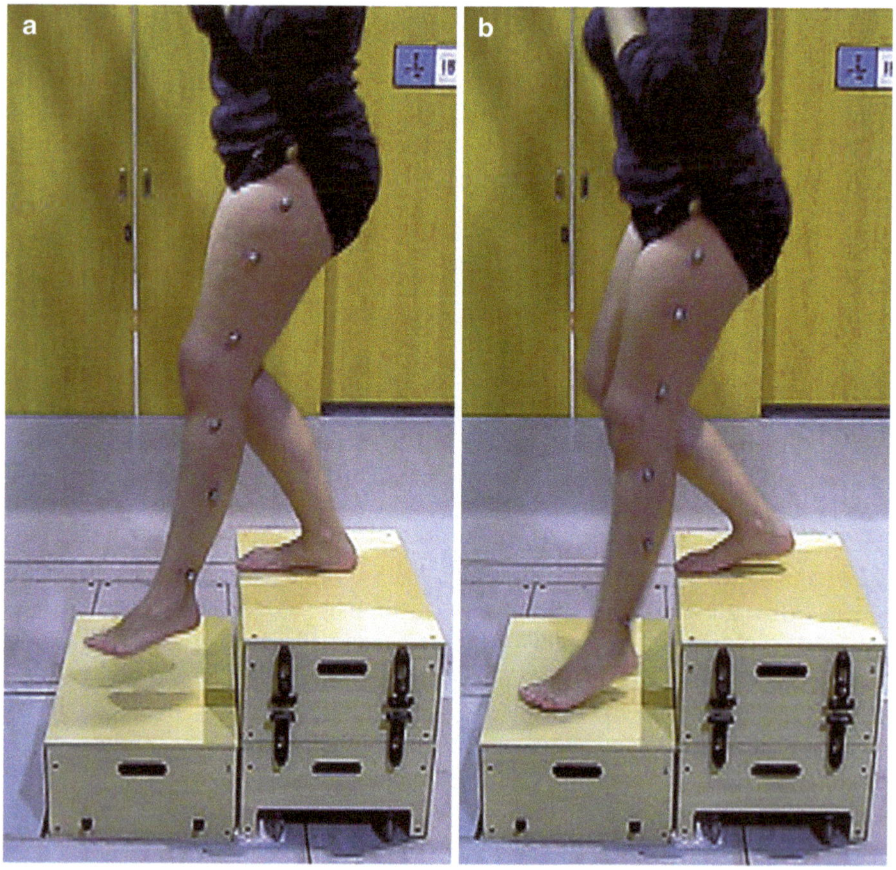


**Fig. 46.10** Knee joint angle during stair descent (Knee extension pattern). One factor that could contribute to the knee extensor moment reduction is the decrease of knee flexion angle during the stance phase of stair ambulation. It would be a strategy to reduce the extensor moment and therefore pain during stair descent. We speculate that the knee extension pattern during stair descent is a strategy to avoid instability and therefore pain. Due to this knee extension pattern, the posterior muscles work in a chronic manner in an elongated eccentric condition; this situation could be responsible for the posterior knee pain in our patient

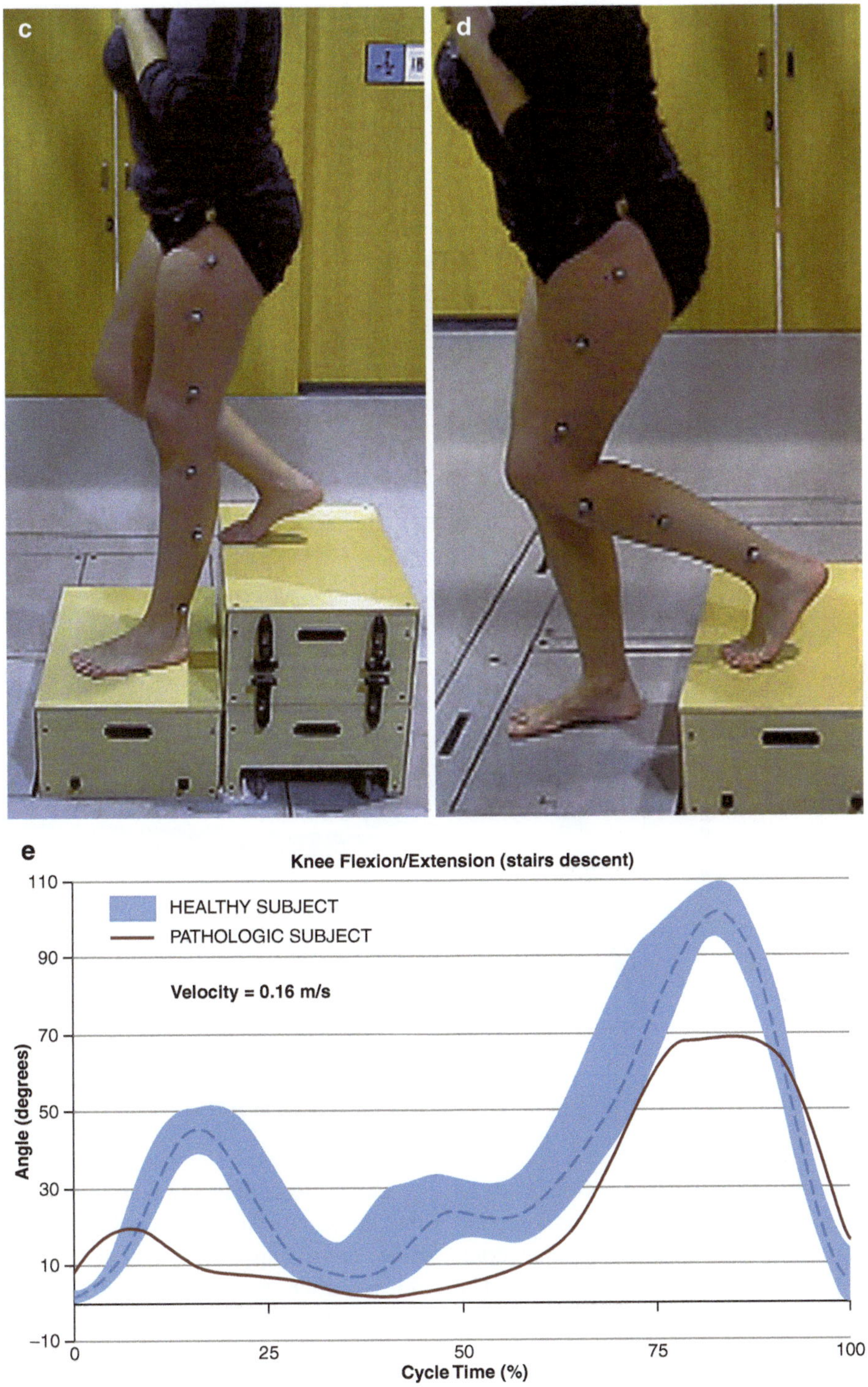


**Fig. 46.10** (continued)

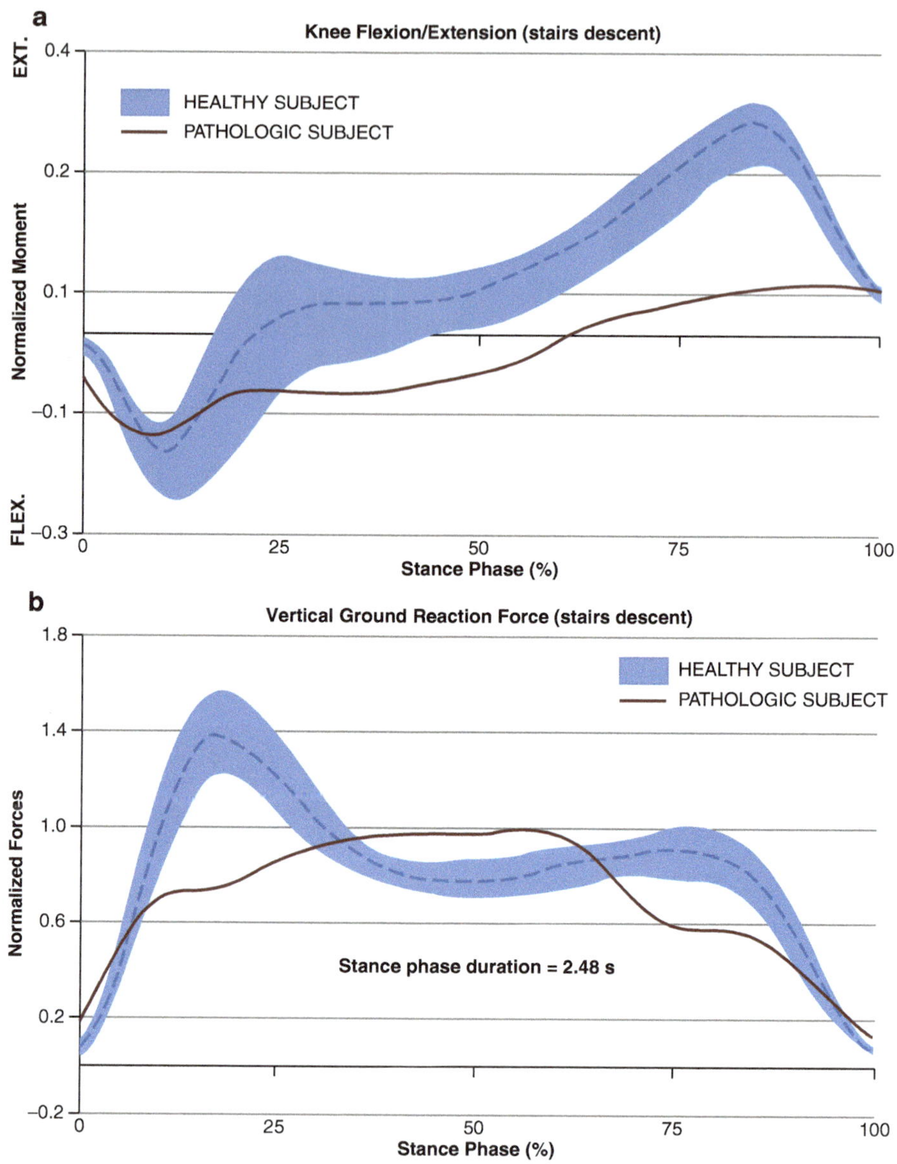


**Fig. 46.11** (**a**) Flexion–extension knee moments during stair descent. (**b**) Ground force reactions during stair descent

the result of a clear diagnosis and/or a correct analysis of the underlying pathology. This explains the catastrophic long-term outcomes and the chronic complaints of some patients with anterior knee pain. The major problem in our series of multioperated patients is medial patellar subluxation with instability.

> The hallmark of medial patellar instability is the patient that experiences pain and dysfunction out of proportion to what they were experiencing before their surgery for patellar realignment.

Our patient, after the patellofermoral arthroplasty, had the same symptoms she had after her first procedure, consisting of an "innocent" lateral retinacular release, after an "absurd diagnosis" of "chondromalacia patellae", only worse. The apprehension test and the Fulkerson relocation test performed after her third operation, according to the patient, caused the same type of pain she had after her initial lateral retinacular release, and that led her to a combined proximal (Insall) and distal (Emslie-Trillat) realignment surgery and then to a patellofemoral prosthesis, neither of which solved her pain. At no time was this patient examined physically or radiographically to rule out an iatrogenic medial patellar instability after her lateral retinacular release. It is therefore necessary to emphasize over and over again, the importance the physical examination has on the origin of the anterior knee pain in order to therefore plan a rational treatment. Moreover, we must remember again that the most frequent problem in multioperated patients is iatrogenic medial patellar instability.

THE PROBLEM: A Patellofemoral Arthroplasty Cannot Stabilize a Highly Imbalance Patellofemoral Joint/THE SOLUTION: Reconstruction of the Lateral Patellofemoral Ligament

Patellofemoral joint replacement is a salvage procedure indicated only when the surgeon proves that the source of pain is from patellofemoral arthrosis or chondropathy. It is not a substitute for a patella realignment. A patella that tends to dislocate medially, as in our case, will do so even after the replacement surgery. The surgeon must identify the factors that are causing the patella to track poorly (in our case an insufficiency of the lateral patellofemoral ligament, LPFL) and treat it. Anterior knee pain and dysfunction from patellar instability, resulting from soft tissue imbalance were the main cause of failure with patellofemoral joint replacement but they are much less common now.[12] The patellofemoral arthroplasty cannot be expected to stabilize a highly imbalanced patellofemoral articulation. The objective of treatment must be recentering of the patella in the trochlea by reconstruction of the LPFL or the medial patellofemoral ligament, in our case the LPFL. This case emphasizes once again the importance of overloading the retinacular structures in the genesis of anterior knee pain.

I cannot emphasize enough the importance of the lateral retinaculum: lengthening of the lateral retinaculum

The lateral patellar retinaculum is an important anatomic structure, which interplays with the intraarticular components and the dynamic structures to ensure patellofemoral stability.[7,8,16,19] Hughston and Deese[9] reported the increased possibility of medial subluxation in 50% of patients treated with lateral retinacular release. Biedert found in 78% of his patients disabling medial subluxation of the patella with a severe imbalance of the patellofemoral gliding mechanism following lateral retinacular release.[1] Our case serves as a warning for the generalized use of lateral retinacular release. Therefore, we believe that it would be interesting to consider the lengthening of the lateral retinaculum described by Roland Biedert[1] as an alternative to lateral retinacular release. The lateral retinaculum consists of a superficial oblique and deep transverse part (Fig. 46.12a). Lengthening is started by incising longitudinally the superficial oblique retinaculum about 5 mm from its attachment to the lateral border of the patella, down to the ligamentum patellae. Then it is separated from the deep transverse retinaculum by preparing with a knife in the dorsal direction (Fig. 46.12b). As much dorsal as possible, then the deep transverse ligament is incised also longitudinally and the synovial layer opened (Fig. 46.12c). This releases the increased tension of the lateral structures. The two parts of the lateral retinaculum are sutured together in 90° of knee flexion (Fig. 46.12d). This makes it impossible that the retinaculum is too tight. The mobility of the patella should be 1–2 quadrants to the medial and the lateral side in full extension, guaranteeing a normal balance of the patella in the trochlea.

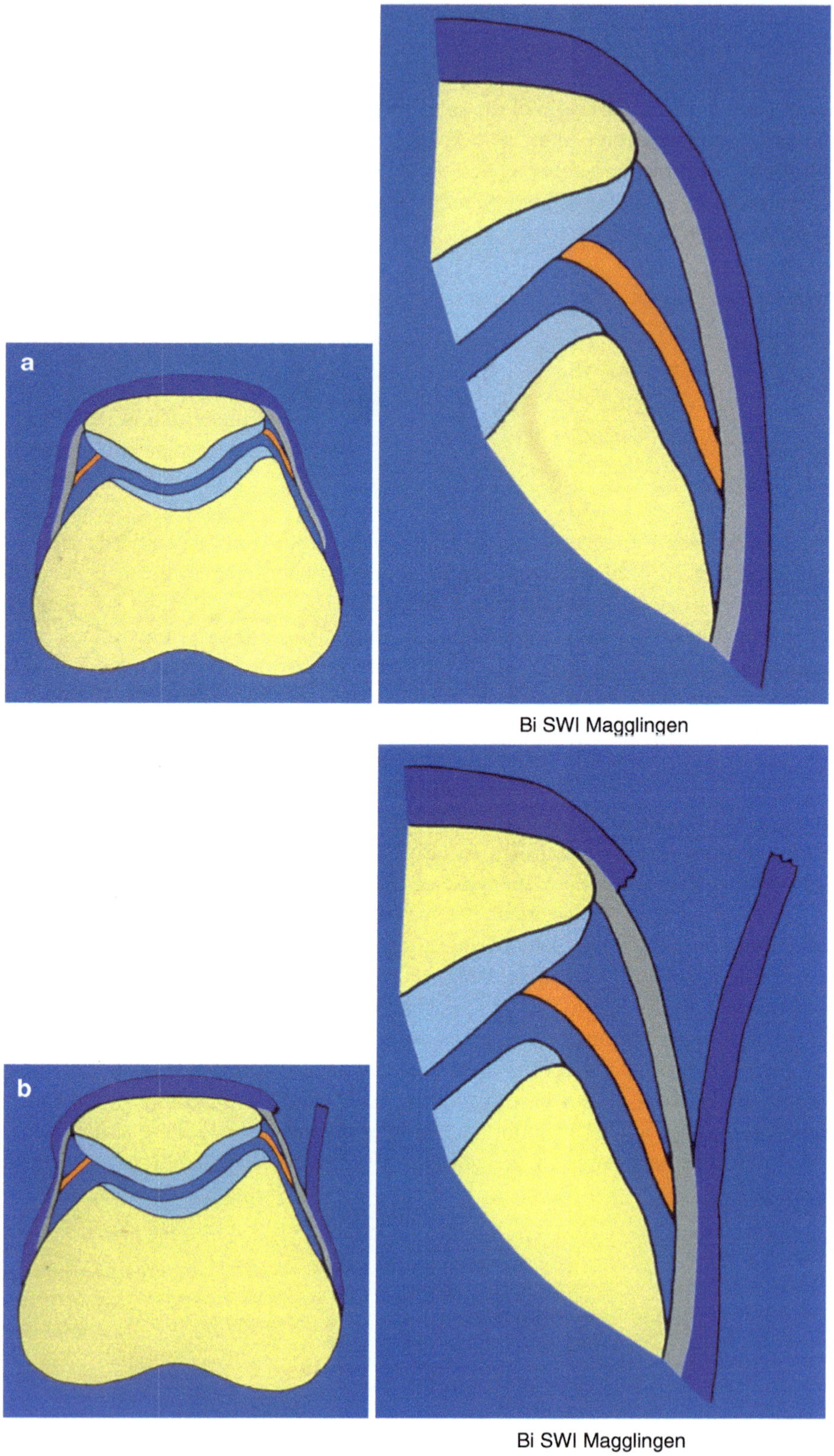


**Fig. 46.12** Schematic diagram showing the lengthening of the lateral retinaculum (Technical note according to Roland M. Biedert)

**Fig. 46.12** (continued)

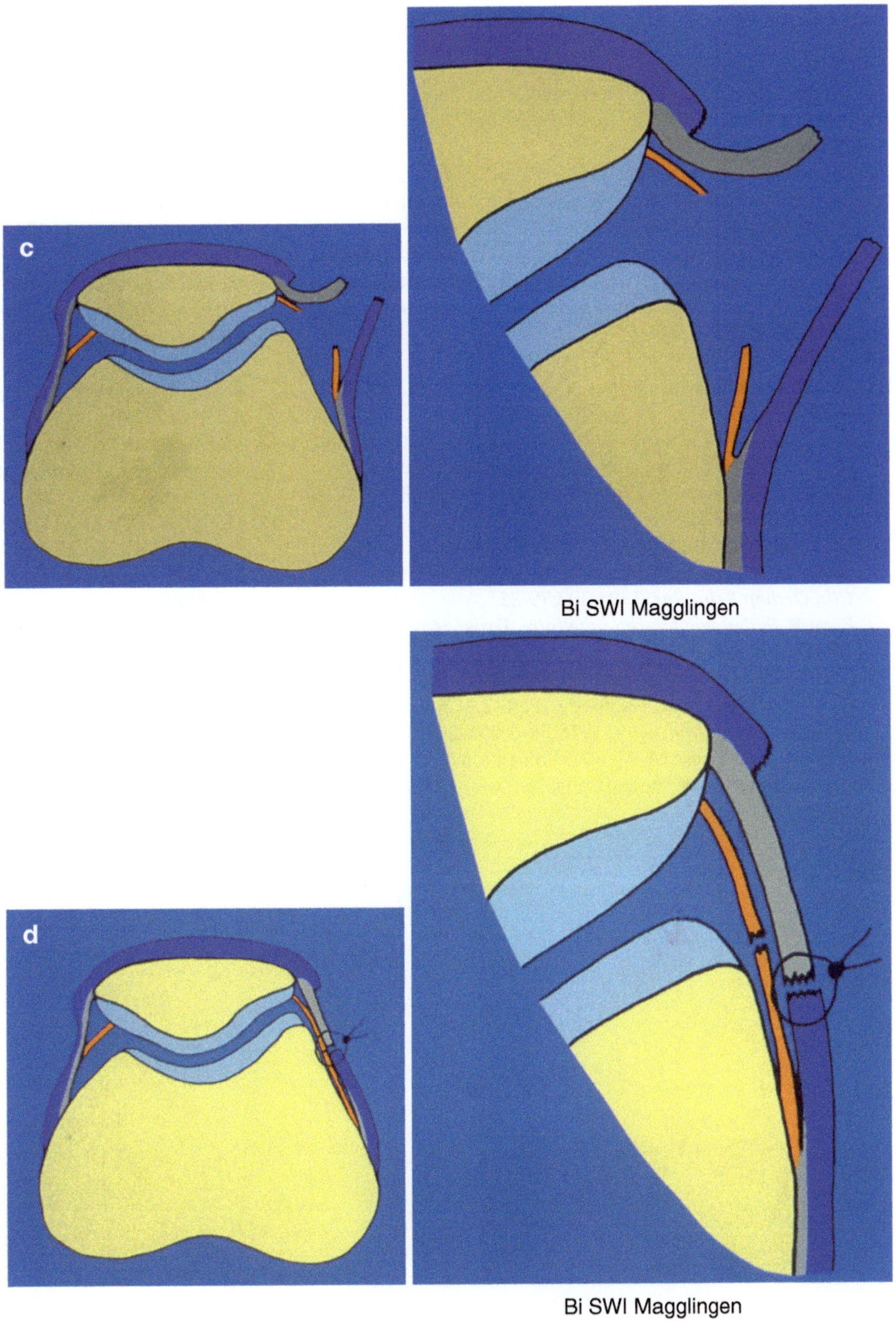

## References


1. Biedert RM. Complicated case studies. In: Sanchis-Alfonso V, ed. *Anterior Knee Pain and Patellar Instability*. Springer: London; 2006.
2. Burnett RSJ, Berger RA, Della Valle CJ, et al. Extensor mechanism allograft reconstruction after total knee arthroplasty. *J Bone Joint Surg*. 2005;87-A:175-194.
3. Burnett RSJ, Berger RA, Paprosky WG, et al. Extensor mechanism allograft reconstruction after total knee arthroplasty. A comparison of two techniques. *J Bone Joint Surg*. 2004;86-A:2694-2699.
4. Capozzi JD, Rhodes R, Chen D. Ethics in practice. Discussing treatment options. *J Bone Joint Surg*. 2009;91-A:740-742.
5. Emerson RH Jr, Head WC, Malinin TI. Reconstruction of patellar tendon rupture after total knee arthroplasty with an extensor mechanism allograft. *Clin Orthop Relat Res*. 1990;260:154-161.
6. Emerson RH Jr, Head WC, Malinin TI. Extensor mechanism reconstruction with an allograft after total knee arthroplasty. *Clin Orthop Relat Res*. 1994;303:79-85.
7. Ficat P. *Pathologie fémoro-patellaire*. Paris: Masson & Cie; 1970.
8. Goodfellow JW, Hungerford DS, Woods C. Patellofemoral joint mechanics and pathology. Part 2. Chondromalacia patellae. *J Bone Joint Surg*. 1976;58-B:291-299.
9. Hughston JC, Deese M. Medial subluxation of the patella as a complication of lateral release. *Am J Sports Med*. 1988;16:383-388.
10. Jamali AA, Emmerson BC, Chung C, et al. Fresh osteochondral allografts: results in the patellofemoral joint. *Clin Orthop Relat Res*. 2005;437:176-185.
11. Leopold SS, Greidanus N, Paprosky WG, et al. High rate of failure of allograft reconstruction of the extensor mechanism after total knee arthroplasty. *J Bone Joint Surg*. 1999;81-A:1574-1579.
12. Lonner JH. Patellofemoral arthroplasty. In: Lotke PA, Lonner JH, eds. *Knee Arthroplasty*. Philadelphia: Lippincott Williams & Wilkins; 2009.
13. Malhotra R, Garg B, Logani V, et al. Management of extensor mechanism deficit as a consequence of patellar tendon loss in total knee arthroplasty. *J Arthroplasty*. 2008;23:1146-1151.
14. Malhotra R, Sharma L, Kumar V, et al. Giant cell tumor of the patella and its management using a patella, patellar tendon, and tibial tubercle allograft. *Knee Surg Sports Traumatol Arthrosc*. 2010;18(2):167-169.
15. Matsumoto H, Kawakabo M, Otani T, et al. Extensive post-traumatic ossification of the patellar tendon. *J Bone Joint Surg*. 1999;81-B:34-36.
16. Müller W. *Das Knie*. Heidelberg: Springer; 1982.
17. Nazarian DG, Booth RE Jr. Extensor mechanism allografts in total knee arthroplasty. *Clin Orthop Relat Res*. 1999;367:123-129.
18. Sanchis-Alfonso V, Monteagudo-Castro C, Roselló-Sastre E, et al. Value of the Hoffa fat pad in recellularization of allografts used to replace the ACL. *Orthop Int*. 1996;4:281-290.
19. Terry GC. The anatomy of the extensor mechanism. *Clin Sports Med*. 1989;8:163-177.
20. Torga-Spak R, Teitge RA. Fresh osteochondral allografts for patellofemoral arthritis: long-term follow-up. *Clin Orthop Relat Res*. 2006;444:193-200.

# Part V

# Personal Reflections on Anterior Knee Pain and Patellar Instability

# A Philosophy of the Patellofemoral Joint: A Logical Clinical Approach

47

Alan C. Merchant

*Philosophy: The study of the general principles of a particular subject, phenomenon, or field of inquiry.*

*Oxford English Dictionary, Oxford University Press*

## 47.1 Introduction

During orthopedic residency (1959–1962), our chairman and professor, Dr. Carroll Larson, taught us how to evaluate and treat enigmatic conditions that had no clear-cut methods to make the diagnosis and no established treatment plan. The key was to develop a theory or pathomechanical/pathophysiologic concept of the disease process that could best explain the patient's symptoms and thus guide the treatment. This theory should fit current information known about the disease or condition and be able to be modified by future research studies. His example at that time was low back pain and degenerative disc disease of the lumbar spine. His indications for low back surgery were surprisingly simple: (1) Increasing neurologic deficit or (2) intractable pain. A short time in clinical practice taught us that the second indication was not so simple after all. One person's discomfort is another person's intractable pain, another challenge when learning the "Art of Medicine."

At that time, there were only two diagnoses applied to the patellofemoral joint, either "chondromalacia patellae" or recurrent dislocation (subluxation) of the patella. If surgery became necessary for "chondromalacia," the surgeon used a scalpel for open patellar shaving. If the lesion was to subchondral bone, multiple drill holes were performed. The Hauser procedure was the standard operation to treat recurrent dislocation of the patella.[14] Unfortunately, in my early days of practice, it was not rare to see a patient for "giving way" of the knee that had *not* been cured by a prior open meniscectomy.

When I became fascinated with patellofemoral disorders in 1970, two things became apparent. (1) There was a need for a more simple, accurate, and reproducible method to radiograph and evaluate the patellofemoral joint. (2) We lacked a concept or pathomechanical theory of the patellofemoral joint to explain the cause of each patient's symptoms. Development of accurate and reproducible radiographs of the patellofemoral joint in axial projection solved the first of these two problems.[26] This led to a pathomechanical/pathophysiologic theory about patellofemoral disorders, and then logically to a clinical etiology-based classification.[22] I have used the term "patellofemoral dysplasia" to describe this pathomechanical and pathophysiologic theory for a large group of patellofemoral disorders that are unrelated to trauma in a normal knee. Subdividing this very large group based upon increasing severity created more manageable diagnostic categories: lateral patellar compression syndrome, chronic patellar subluxation, recurrent patellar dislocation, and chronic patellar dislocation. Once the etiology is known, treating the cause or causes of a problem leads to a logical treatment plan.

A.C. Merchant
Department of Orthopedic Surgery,
Stanford University School of Medicine,
Stanford, CA, USA

Department of Orthopedic Surgery, El Camino Hospital,
Mountain View, CA, USA
e-mail: kneemd@sbcglobal.net

V. Sanchis-Alfonso (ed.), *Anterior Knee Pain and Patellar Instability*,
DOI: 10.1007/978-0-85729-507-1_47, © Springer-Verlag London Limited 2011

## 47.2 Patellofemoral Dysplasia

Patellofemoral dysplasia can be defined as: *a cluster of physical abnormalities, varying from mild to severe, that affect the normal function of the patellofemoral joint*. The severity and combination of these abnormalities in any given patient will dictate that patient's symptoms. Therefore, whether the patient has somewhat mild abnormalities and suffers from intermittent and activity-related anterior knee pain or has severe deficits and demonstrates frequent recurrent dislocation of the patella, the clinician must search for each one of these abnormal factors, assess its severity, and develop a treatment plan to correct these factors for each individual patient. There is no "best" treatment plan or operation for either the symptom of anterior knee pain or the diagnosis of recurrent dislocation of the patella.

Patellofemoral dysplasia should be considered a continuum of these multiple abnormalities ranging from mild to severe. When or how each patient will become symptomatic is determined by a second and very important factor, his or her activity level. This activity level can be continuously variable from sedentary to strenuous competitive sports. These two continua, the factors of patellofemoral dysplasia and each individual's activity level, have an inverse relationship to one another and determine when each individual patient will cross the threshold from asymptomatic to symptomatic (Fig. 47.1). This concept, published in 1991,[23] was given validity when Dye published his paper on the pathophysiology of patellofemoral pain describing the envelope of function 5 years later.[11]

If the theory of patellofemoral dysplasia is valid, an examination of each of these abnormalities affecting the normal function of the patellofemoral joint should be able to demonstrate how each one acting alone or in combination can cause the major symptoms of patellofemoral disorders: pain and instability. Each abnormality should be measured in the most accurate manner possible in order to assess its presence as well as its severity. In order to discuss each physical abnormality, they will be listed here, not in the order of importance, but rather in the order in which the clinician will encounter them during the initial evaluation of a patient. Of these six abnormal factors, four are best discovered by physical examination and two by radiography. Computed tomography (CT) and magnetic resonance imaging (MRI) are rarely necessary.

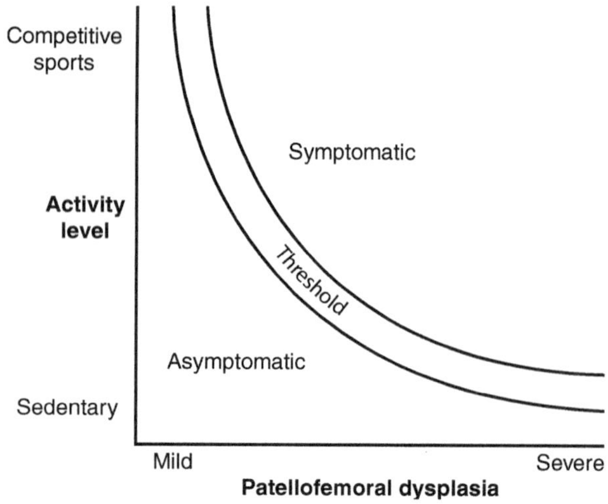


**Fig. 47.1** This diagram shows the inverse relationship between severity of patellofemoral dysplasia and activity level, which determines when any given patient will cross the symptomatic threshold (From reference Merchant[23], with permission)

### 47.2.1 *Vastus Medialis Obliquus Deficiency*

Normally, the vastus medialis obliquus (VMO) inserts into the upper third to one half of the medial edge of the patella. When deficient, it will insert higher into the medial edge of the quadriceps tendon, or will be absent, leaving a characteristic hollow on the medial aspect of the knee with the quadriceps contracted to hold the knee at 30° flexion with the foot unsupported (Fig. 47.2). Studies using both ultrasonography and CT have demonstrated a significant degree of correlation between VMO abnormalities and anterior knee pain.[16,19] However, there is no simple clinical method to measure VMO deficiency, but by observing every knee, the clinician will soon be able to assess VMO deficiencies and grade them as mild, moderate, or severe. By weakening the medial vector, a deficient VMO will increase the lateral vector of the quadriceps and thus increase the "dynamic" Q angle originally described by Brattstrom.[6]

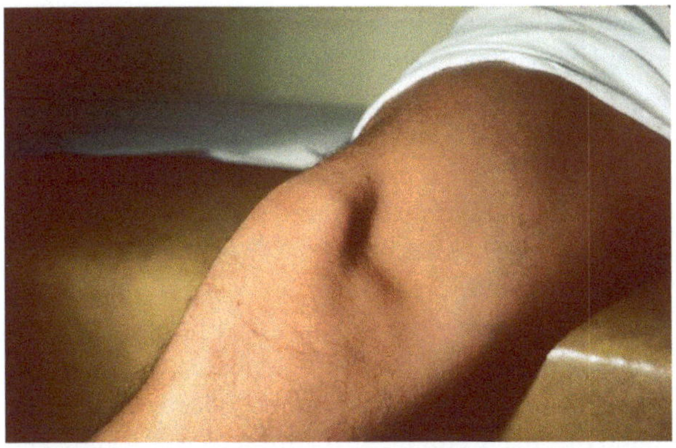

**Fig. 47.2** With the quadriceps contracted holding the knee at 30° flexion and with the foot unsupported, a deficient vastus medialis obliquus will leave a characteristic hollow on the medial aspect of the knee

### 47.2.2 Lax Medial Patellofemoral Ligament

Laxity of the medial patellofemoral ligament (MPFL) is best examined by the lateral glide test with the knee supported at 30° flexion and the quadriceps relaxed. By mentally dividing the patella into vertical quadrants and pushing the patella laterally, the normal patella will move about one quadrant or one fingerbreadth. Severe MPFL laxity will frequently elicit an apprehension response from the patient. Significant laxity usually means that the MPFL has been torn and remains elongated from a previous dislocation leaving the patella vulnerable to repeated dislocations. However, the clinician should be alert to the possibility of the patient with hyperelastosis and hypermobile patellas.

### 47.2.3 Tight Lateral Retinaculum

Examination for a tight lateral retinaculum (LR) is done by the medial glide test, again with the knee supported at 30° flexion and the quadriceps relaxed. The normal medial glide of the patella is approximately one fingerbreadth. Some clinicians prefer to assess the LR by the lateral tilt-up test. Again by testing every patient that requires a knee examination, the clinician will soon learn to grade the LR tightness as normal, mild, moderate, or severe.

### 47.2.4 Increased Quadriceps (Q) Angle

The Q angle is one of the most important factors affecting the normal function of the patellofemoral joint. Since the nineteenth century multiple operations have been devised and used successfully to move the tibial tubercle and the patellar ligament from lateral to medial thus decreasing the Q angle. Therefore, it is only logical to measure this angle during every knee examination to learn if the Q angle is increased and by what degree. Despite its recognized importance, the Q angle has had a fascinating and somewhat checkered history. It was first described by Brattstrom, who defined the Q angle as the complementary angle of the angle formed by the *resultant line of force of the quadriceps muscle* and a line from the center of the patella to the center of the tibial tubercle.[6] This definition accounts for the actual angular and muscular lateralizing forces acting on the patella. We might call this the "dynamic" Q angle. With no simple clinical method to measure the resultant line of quadriceps force, the line from the anterior superior iliac spine (ASIS) to the center of the patella was chosen as a surrogate by subsequent authors, yet still naming it the Q angle. A more specific term would have been the "anatomic" Q angle. In this discussion we will accept the convention and call this anatomic Q angle the "Q angle," but to avoid confusion we will use the term "dynamic Q angle" when referring to its original quadriceps-line-of-force definition.

A plethora of papers have been written attempting to define the normal Q angle over the last several decades, but there has been no agreement on a standard technique or a proper instrument to use for this measurement. Post reviewed seven different articles that attempted to define the Q angle in the normal population.[30] These different authors reported their results with the subjects supine, sitting, or standing. They measured knees extended at 0° and flexed to 10°, 30°, 45°, or 90°. A few authors reported using a long protractor to reach the ASIS, but the majority failed to report exactly what instrument was used. As one would expect, these average "normal" Q angles from these articles varied widely from 5° to 23° with standard deviations ranging widely from 0.08° to 5° as well. Most reports also failed to test for intraobserver and interobserver reliability. There was one area of nearly universal agreement: women had larger Q angles than men, and this difference was caused by the wider pelvis in women compared with men. After studying the confusing literature about the Q angle, Post came to the conclusion that Q angle measurements had "no direct correlation with the incidence of patellofemoral disorders (that) is well established by scientific criteria." He went on to state "no solid data links specific Q angle measurements to diagnosis or results of treatment." Finally he questioned: "Should the Q angle even be measured?"[30]

A couple of decades ago, I came to the conclusion that, if the Q angle was worth measuring, it should be measured easily, consistently, and accurately. The easiest position for the patient is supine with the knee at 0° and the limb in neutral rotation. With the knee fully extended, the tibial tubercle reaches its maximum external rotation due to the terminal "screw home" mechanism. Because it is the tibial tubercle's relationship to the trochlear groove that we actually wish to measure, the examiner should be certain to position the patella so that it is centered in line with the trochlea, especially in cases of patella alta. If a tight retinaculum prevents the patella from being centered manually, this abnormality should be recorded. For accuracy, I created a protractor with one limb long enough to reach the ASIS. Grelsamer et al. used this protractor to gather data for their seminal paper about the Q angle.[13] ("A similar and simpler protractor can be made by carefully gluing a 22 inch (56 cm) section of a wooden yardstick ["meter-stick" internationally] to a short plastic goniometer.) They reported the most accurate measurement of normal male and female Q angles yet published. The average male Q angle was 13.3° and the average in females was 15.7°. They demonstrated that this small 2.4° difference between men and women disappeared when the measurements were corrected for the difference in average height between men and women. They demonstrated trigonometrically that the Q angle decreases 0.2° for each centimeter of added height. Men and women of similar height have similar Q angles. In addition, they also disproved the common assumption that this difference was due to a wider pelvis in women compared with men. Measuring between the ASISs they found no difference between the average male and female pelvis. It seems that the female pelvis appears wider only when measured at the pelvic brim. They found interobserver reliability to be in substantial agreement, and intraobserver reliability was excellent.

Given the confusion and lack of accuracy in the literature about the Q angle, many surgeons have turned to a special scanning technique using MRI and CT to measure lateralization of the tibial tubercle in reference to the trochlear groove, the TT-TG distance. This technique by necessity enforced a standardization not found in prior studies about the Q angle. All subjects were positioned supine, the knee was fully extended, and patellar position was ignored in favor of the trochlear groove. In a review of radiological measurements of the patellofemoral joint, Beaconsfield et al. found that the average TT-TG distance was 13 mm and the upper limit of normal was 20 mm.[2] With the advent of this standardized and accurate method of assessing lateralization of the tibial tubercle as a substitute for measuring the Q angle, many reports have now confirmed that there *is* a direct correlation between lateralization of the tibial tubercle and the incidence of patellofemoral disorders established by scientific criteria.[17,27-29,33,35]

These findings confirmed my years of clinical experience with measuring the Q angle accurately using a standardized method. Aside from the huge difference in cost, the TT-TG measurement has another major clinical disadvantage. The TT-TG distance cannot be transferred directly to the patient in the operating room. Because these scanning techniques normalize the image to correct for knee size, a TT-TG distance of 20 mm does *not* mean that transferring the tibial tubercle 7 mm medially on that patient at surgery will correct the TT-TG to a normal 13 mm. Whereas, by using an accurate, standardized Q angle measurement, that same technique can be used in surgery with the help of a sterilized metal goniometer and a cautery cord stretched to the ASIS to achieve the accurate angular correction desired.

### 47.2.5 Patella Alta

Assessing the severity of patella alta is important for two reasons. First, it allows the patella to escape the confines of the trochlea earlier during active knee extension, and this leads to an increased risk of patellar subluxation and dislocation. Second, because the contact area of the patellar articular surface is small in early flexion and increases with increasing flexion to accommodate the increased compression force, a high

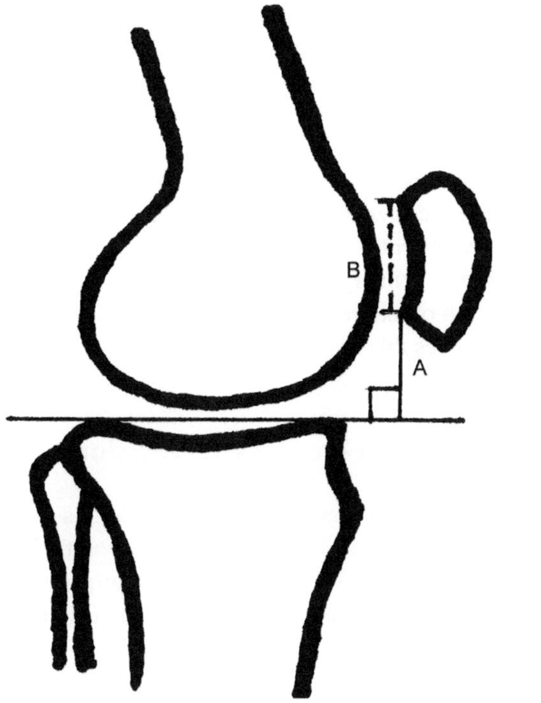


**Fig. 47.3** Blackburn–Peel technique for measuring patellar height ratio. *A* vertical distance above the tibial plateau. *B* patellar articular height. *A/B* patellar height ratio. Normal mean ratio = 1:1. ±0.2

patella will have a contact area that is too small to withstand the increased joint reaction force during increased flexion. This can lead to anterior knee pain and secondary chondromalacia patellae. Berg compared the various radiographic techniques for measuring patellar height ratios and found that the Blackburne–Peel technique (Fig. 47.3) was the most accurate, reliable, and reproducible.[3] The normal ratio is 1:1, ±20%.

### 47.2.6 Trochlear Dysplasia

Trochlear dysplasia, most simply described as a flattening of the trochlear groove, is the most important factor affecting normal patellofemoral function, and yet it remains the most difficult to correct surgically. Senavongse and Amis performed an elegant cadaveric study showing the prime importance of the trochlear groove.[31] They demonstrated that releasing the VMO reduced patellar stability by 30%, cutting the MPFL reduced stability by 49% (but only in full knee extension), but flattening the trochlea decreased patellar

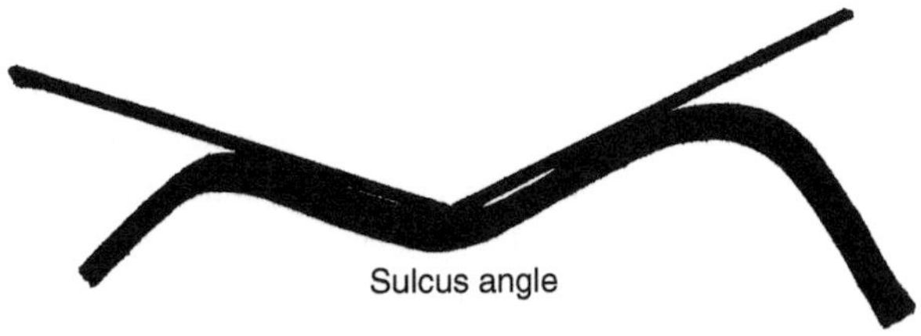


**Fig. 47.4** Sulcus angle measurement from an accurate axial view radiograph with the knee flexed 45°. In 100 normal subjects, the sulcus angle mean = 138°, range = 126–150°

stability by 70%. That is why the most common and successful operations to correct patellar instability rely on changing other factors that guide patellar excursion to compensate for this flattening and take advantage of whatever shallow groove is present.

The simplest method to assess trochlear dysplasia is to measure the sulcus angle on an accurate axial view radiograph taken at 45° knee flexion (Fig. 47.4). In 100 asymptomatic subjects, we found the mean sulcus angle to be 138° and the range was 126–150°.[26] In 25 patients with recurrent dislocation of the patella the mean sulcus angle was 146°, which is within the "normal" range. This demonstrates once again that the etiology of patellofemoral disorders is multifactorial, and while trochlear dysplasia is a very important factor, the other five factors must be considered as well.

Dejour et al. have popularized a technique to assess and classify trochlear dysplasia from a true lateral view of the knee.[9] It has the advantage of showing the trochlea at its proximal extremity. Davies et al. evaluated this technique along with patellar tilt, patellar height, and the sulcus angle in order to identify a rapid and reproducible radiological feature that would indicate the need for further analysis.[7] They found that if the sulcus angle was normal, analysis of the other radiological features was unlikely to reveal additional useful information. In addition, the severity of those other features of dysplasia correlated with an increasing sulcus angle. Therefore, it would seem best in the clinical setting to obtain a true lateral radiograph for further trochlear analysis only if surgery is being planned.

The study of trochlear dysplasia has given us insights into the understanding of and reasons for the unusual frequency of anterior knee pain as a presenting symptom. When Aglietti et al. repeated our axial radiographic measurements of patellofemoral congruence on normal subjects, the averages were nearly identical, but their standard deviation was approximately one half of ours.[1,26] We had assumed that asymptomatic subjects would be "normal," whereas, they also rejected any subject with an abnormal knee examination. Applying their standard deviation to our raw data demonstrated that 20% of an asymptomatic population actually had radiographic abnormalities of the patellofemoral joint. This represents a very large group of people who are at risk for developing pain or instability with increased activity, relatively minor injuries, or just the passage of time.

I have developed a hypothesis to explain this high degree of variability in trochlear morphology and the unusually high frequency of patellofemoral symptoms. This high degree of osseous morphologic variability does not appear anywhere else in the knee. Dye's study on the evolutionary development of the knee demonstrated that the bi-lobed, cam shape of the distal femur could be traced to about 350 million years ago.[10] The patella and its trochlear groove first appeared about 70 million years ago. The earliest skeletal fossils showing indications of an upright, bipedal gait date to only about 4 million years ago. Heiple and Lovejoy[15] and Lovejoy[20] have shown that the trochlear grooves of bipedal hominids are deeper with a more prominent lateral condyle than those of quadruped apes (Fig. 47.5) Efficient bipedal gait requires the knees and feet to move toward the midline of the body, increasing the valgus angle at the knee as well as the dynamic Q angle. A deeper trochlea with a more prominent lateral anterior condyle functions to prevent lateral dislocation of the patella during erect bipedal gait. In addition, Bose et al. have demonstrated that the VMO, which applies a medial vector to the patella, is peculiar to humans.[5] Because the deeper and asymmetric shape of the human trochlea is a recent evolutionary development, it demonstrates a wide variability and an increased incidence of flattening. Furthermore, it has not been corrected by natural selection because the negative effects of this abnormality often appear after the age of primary reproduction and therefore beyond the reach of natural selection. Such circumstantial evidence gives this hypothesis firm support.[21]

## 47.3 Logical Treatment Decisions

"The etiology of patellofemoral disorders is multifactorial" has almost become a mantra for those who study this joint. Why then are we surprised when studying associations we learn that there is no good correlation between one of these multiple factors, the Q angle for example, and anterior knee pain or patellar instability? We should not investigate one factor at a time, but examine these six factors as a group. Here is a *reductio ad absurdum* to illustrate this point. Let us assume a study of anterior knee pain with a cohort of only six patients. Assume that each patient has a different severely abnormal factor listed above. Each factor individually would show a very poor correlation of only 0.17 with anterior knee pain. However, when considered as a group of six abnormal factors, the correlation with anterior knee pain will be perfect at 1.0. If the clinician focuses on these six abnormal factors,

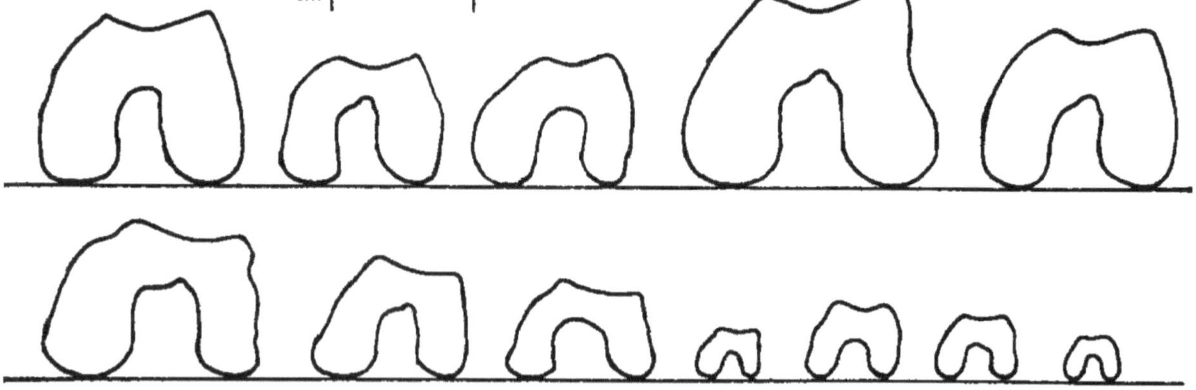


**Fig. 47.5** These drawings are traced outlines from scale photographs of distal femurs arranged (or *reversed*) so that the lateral condyle is to the *right*. Primates with erect bipedal gait are on the top row, and primates with quadripedal gait are shown on the *bottom* (Redrawn from reference Heiple and Lovejoy[15])

the treatment of patellofemoral disorders becomes much easier.

## 47.4 Safe Knee Exercises

The nonoperative treatment of anterior knee pain and instability is not the subject for this chapter; however, there is one modality that deserves emphasis because it has proved so successful in practice during the last four decades. That modality is Progressive Resistive Isometric Quadriceps Exercise. Very few patients understood that term, so I would ask them to do Straight Leg Weight Lifting. This is a rehabilitation exercise, but can be used initially for sports conditioning. Because moving the knee after injury or surgery is painful, we all use straight leg raising exercises as soon as possible, and then add ankle weights to rehabilitate the quadriceps. Adding weights beyond about 7 lb (3.2 kg) will risk straining the hip or low back. For treating athletes with "chondromalacia," DeHaven et al. used a weight bench technique or an assistant with the patient sitting to achieve weight goals of 30 lb (13.6 kg) and above with excellent results.[8] Referral of the patients to different physical therapy departments for this technique was eminently unsuccessful. Lacking our own therapist, I decided to convert this isometric weight lifting with the knee immobile in full extension to a home exercise shown in Fig. 47.6. Demonstrating the exercise, modifying the printed instructions for each patient, and then monitoring progress at decreasing time intervals certainly took more effort, but the results were worth it. The goal for a person of average stature was set at 20 lb (9.1 kg) with adjustments for size, body build, and age. Most patients would start to improve at about 15 lb (6.8 kg) and approximately 90% of patients with anterior knee pain would be well at the 20-lb (9.1 kg) goal.

Straight leg weight lifting as a home exercise has many advantages. With the knee in full extension, the patient is able to load the quadriceps progressively without causing patellofemoral joint pain. It cannot damage the knee when done properly and, therefore, is the safest knee exercise. The patient can exercise daily and can appreciate the progress as weights are added. It actively involves the patients in their own recovery, and if successful, the patient can proceed to sport-specific rehabilitation. If it should fail to give relief, the patient will approach surgery with a strong quadriceps and a complete understanding of the postoperative rehabilitation. Therefore, all patients should do

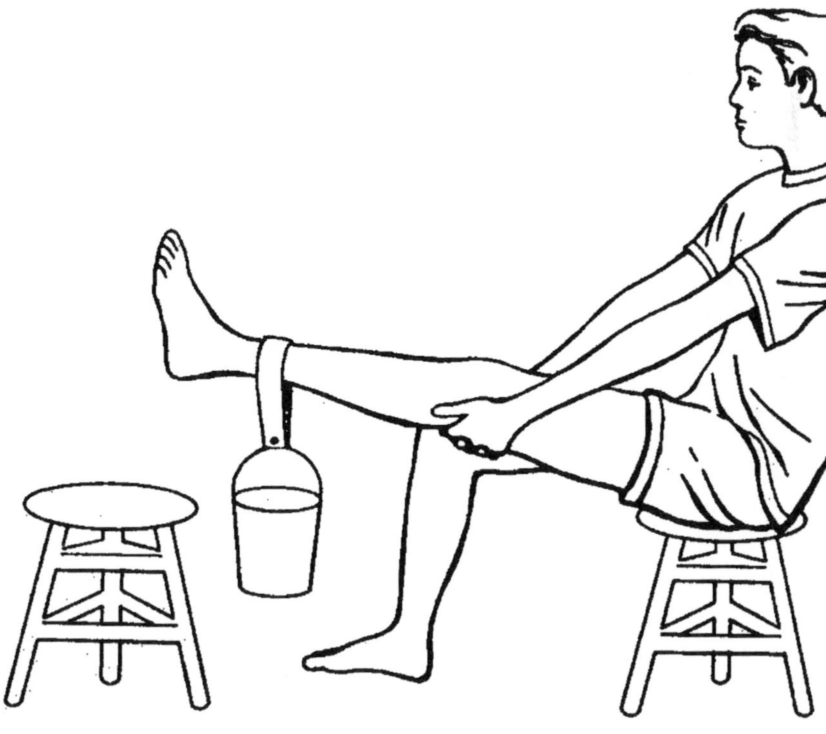

**Fig. 47.6** This drawing depicts safe straight leg weight lifting (or isometric progressive resistive quadriceps) exercises (From reference Merchant[23], with permission)

these exercises even when surgery is planned from the beginning. Each patient understands that the operation only provides half the result, the other half is up to them. It also serves as an excellent preoperative test when treating pain with a paucity of physical findings to determine the level of symptoms and each patient's commitment to his or her recovery. Getting to know the patient, learning about his or her reaction to pain, and discovering the patient's ability and willingness to follow directions are all better to know before surgery rather than after.

## 47.5 Logical Surgical Decisions

Once the surgeon has assessed the six factors and their severity listed above, the choice of surgical corrections becomes logical and individualized. Two of the six are very difficult to correct, a deficient VMO and a shallow trochlea. However, they must be carefully evaluated to determine what surgery can be performed to compensate for these deficiencies.

*The deficient VMO* increases the dynamic Q angle. Therefore, when planning a medial tibial tubercle transfer, just normalizing the Q angle might not be enough in a patient with a shallow trochlea and deficient VMO. A compensatory overcorrection to 7–10° would be better.

*A lax MPFL* almost always means the ligament has been torn from a previous dislocation. When the most popular operation for recurrent dislocation of the patella was medial tibial tubercle transfer, lateral retinacular release, and medial capsular reefing, it became apparent that if the trochlear depth were relatively normal, the surgery would be successful. However, if the trochlea was shallow, the capsular reefing (MPFL repair) usually stretched out in 4 or 5 years allowing further dislocations. We should remain skeptical about reports of isolated MPFL repair for acute patellar dislocations until there is at least a 5-year follow-up for those with very shallow trochleas. Likewise, the results of long-term follow-up of MPFL repair for acute dislocations should be correlated with sulcus depth, because a significant number of acute dislocators with normal trochleas would not have dislocated again without surgery.

*A tight lateral retinaculum* should always be released when performing patellofemoral surgery. This theory of patellofemoral dysplasia, though it was developed years later, explained our earlier success treating both pain and instability using the isolated retinacular release.[25] Overrelease should be avoided by releasing the tight LR approximately 1 cm lateral to the patella and ending the release proximally at the muscular fibers of the vastus lateralis. The one exception is for those rare cases, usually a child, where the entire quadriceps and extensor mechanism is rotated laterally around the distal femur. Open surgery is required to reposition the patella anteriorly and derotate the quadriceps as well. After the lateral retinaculum has been released, the dissection proceeds posteriorly. The entire distal vastus lateralis needs to be lifted anteriorly and dissected off the lateral intermuscular septum to achieve this derotation quadricepsplasty. A secure medial imbrication will maintain the quadriceps and patellar position providing reasonable function until puberty, when definitive tibial tubercle transfer and MPFL autograft reconstruction can be achieved.

*An increased Q angle* almost always needs to be corrected by medial tibial tubercle transfer, one of the safest and most secure techniques available. Remember to check for and release tight lateral retinacular tissues as the tubercle is medialized. The transfer can be done through a short vertical incision that is not prone to stretching and is cosmetically acceptable. By carefully measuring the Q angle in surgery, an overcorrection to a 5° Q angle can be achieved when dealing with a very flat sulcus and the patella tethered by a MPFL reconstruction. If anteriorization is needed in addition, it can be achieved by deeper V-shaped cuts using local bone or bone grafts, thereby avoiding more extensive surgery on the upper tibia with its risk of stress fracture.[24]

*Patella alta* usually needs to be corrected only when it is severe enough to affect the normal function of the patellofemoral joint. Distal tibial tubercle transfer, combined with medial transfer if necessary, can be performed. Careful measurement of preoperative radiographs accounting for magnification is necessary to avoid overcorrecting a patella alta to a patella infera, which is much worse.

*A dysplastic (shallow) trochlea* needs to be carefully considered when planning patellofemoral surgery. In the great majority of cases, compensation for a very shallow trochlea can be achieved by decreasing the Q angle to about 5° using a medial tibial tubercle transfer and increasing the strength of the

MPFL by autograft ligament reconstruction. There are a few cases of trochlear dysplasia in which the groove is flat or almost flat. In these cases, it is very disappointing to learn that what appeared to have been an excellent static realignment at surgery becomes a poor dynamic alignment once the patient is awake and undergoing rehabilitation. To avoid this problem it has been extremely helpful to use selective epidural analgesia so that the patient can be awakened during surgery in order to actively extend the knee. If the patellar excursion is not correct, the repair can be adjusted and the patient awakened again for another test.

For those very rare patients who have a convex instead of a concave trochlea, trochleoplasty is being performed in a few centers. Different techniques are being used and still others are being proposed. At this writing, there are very few studies that report results and almost none with long-term follow-up. For the clinician-surgeon a paraphrase of the sixth stanza of the Hippocratic oath seems appropriate. "I will not *perform trochleoplasty*, even for patients in whom the disease is manifest; I will leave this operation to be performed by practitioners, specialists in this art."

In summary, the surgical treatment of this large and varied group termed patellofemoral dysplasia will depend upon the severity of the symptoms and the physical findings of each patient. The complexity of the surgery will increase in correlation with the severity of these abnormalities. Given a patient who has recurrent dislocation of the patella, an arthroscopic lateral retinacular release will suffice if the Q angle is normal, if the trochlea is only somewhat shallow, if the lateral retinaculum is tight, and if the patient's activity level is not extreme. In a patient who has unrelenting, severe anterior knee pain with a normal trochlea, slightly tight lateral retinaculum, and a severely increased Q angle, an arthroscopic lateral release plus medial tibial tubercle transfer will be necessary. A lateral release alone will fail. As mentioned above, the patient who has recurrent dislocation of the patella with a very flat sulcus will need tibial tubercle transfer decreasing the Q angle below normal as well as reconstruction of the MPFL. In the final analysis, the surgical treatment for the pain and instability of patellofemoral dysplasia can be simplified to: "Find out what's wrong, and fix it."

## 47.6 Patellofemoral Dysplasia and Symptoms

It is self-evident that abnormalities within this cluster of six physical factors that guide the patella can cause instability, but it is less clear how these factors might cause anterior knee pain. Fulkerson has proposed that areas of microscopic neuropathy within the lateral retinaculum cause tenderness and pain when it is under abnormal tension.[12] This is certainly one source of anterior knee pain and tenderness. It is well accepted that abnormal loads on articular cartilage can cause its physical degradation eventually leading to osteoarthrosis and pain. However, that does not explain the cause of pain when articular cartilage is subjected to abnormal stress while it remains intact, given the fact that articular cartilage has no nerves.

A study by Besier et al. may possibly explain how stress on articular cartilage that is aneural might cause anterior knee pain.[4] Working from images of the patellofemoral joint taken of the knee during a semisquat in an open-gantry MRI, they used finite element analysis of the articular cartilage to demonstrate that greater loads were experienced adjacent to the subcondral bone than at the bearing surface, especially near the lateral margins (Fig. 47.7). If these maximum loads occur right next to the subcondral bone, it stands to reason that this stress would be transmitted directly to the adjacent bone, which is well innervated. This study was done with a normal knee and a congruent patellofemoral joint. One can logically assume that a knee with the added force of an increased Q angle (either anatomic, dynamic, or both) or one with an incongruent patellofemoral joint would generate much higher and abnormally focused stress on the articular cartilage and subcondral bone.

The reaction of articular cartilage at the macro level to a given force has a temporal component as well. Various experimental models have shown that when a given force is applied directly, the cartilage will deform, then recover over time when the force has been released. However, if that same force is applied in a cyclical manner over time, the structural integrity of the cartilage will degrade with an appearance similar to osteoarthritis.[18]

Homeostasis of articular cartilage depends, at least in part, on the mechanical loads experienced during the activities of daily living, but there is evidence to show that even before physical breakdown, there are

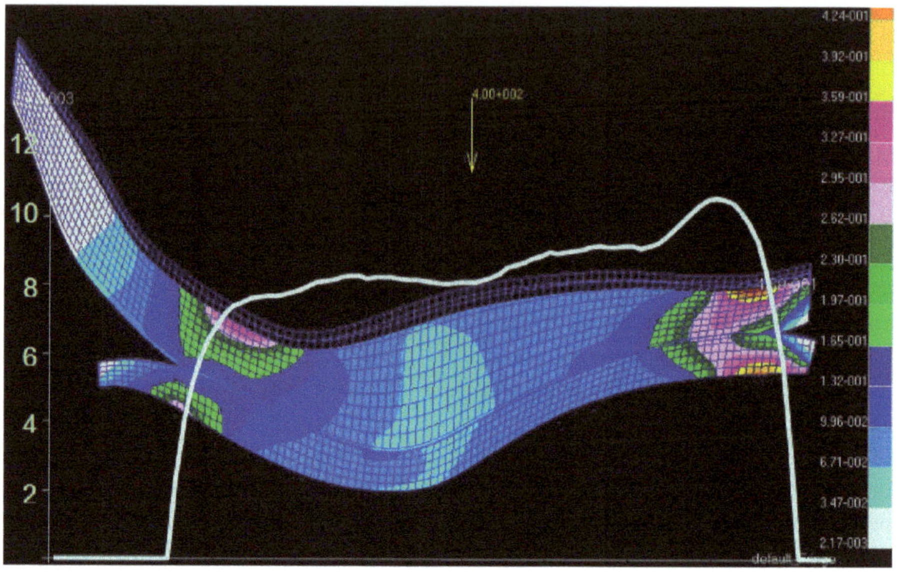


**Fig. 47.7** Finite element analysis showing cartilage stress distributions during a static squat with the knee at 60° of flexion from an MRI image. Note stress concentrations adjacent to the subchondral bone (Image courtesy of Besier et al.[4], Ph.D.)

changes occurring at the cellular level that could account for either pain and progressive degradation or homeostatic restoration and resistance to such damage. Smith et al. studied two different types of mechanical loads on adult human articular chondrocytes in high-density monolayer culture.[32] A summary of their findings is fascinating. When intermittent hydrostatic pressure at physiologic levels was applied to these chondrocytes, they found increased aggrecan and Type II collagen gene expression and induced changes in the cell-associated proteins. Aggrecan, Type II collagen, and cell-associated proteins are important components to maintain the health and induce repair of the extracellular matrix of articular cartilage. When added to cultured chondrocytes, bacterial lipopolysaccharide has an inhibitory effect on matrix protein expression. They found that hydrostatic pressure counteracted this inhibitory effect on the cells. Next, these authors tested the cellular response to a second type of mechanical load, sheer stress, using a rotating cone viscometer. After application of this sheer stress, they demonstrated increased release of the proinflammatory mediator, nitric oxide, decreased aggrecans and Type II collagen expression, and induced molecular changes associated with programmed cell death or apoptosis.

The studies referenced above offer explanations for anterior knee pain in a variety of clinical settings. Repetitive overuse from sports or recreational activities in an anatomically normal knee could be expected to generate sufficient shear stresses to initiate the cascade of cellular changes that lead to loss of tissue homeostasis, anterior knee pain, and synovial inflammation. The same overuse or minor trauma in a knee with even minor abnormalities of one or more of the six anatomic factors discussed above would experience pain and inflammation even earlier than would the normal knee. We are frequently asked to help patients in this situation because the knee has not recovered to a state of homeostasis and health in the time normally expected by the patient. For example, a person with an increased Q angle and a deficient VMO who is asymptomatic at his or her activity level could suffer a patellar contusion from a fall or dashboard injury. Pain from the injury will likely cause the patient to rest the knee with subsequent quadriceps deconditioning. As the pain resolves and the person resumes their usual activities, the weakened quadriceps plus the preexisting anatomic deficiencies may well cause an imbalance of the extensor mechanism, increase the sheer stress, and precipitate pain and inflammation. These are the cases that recover nicely by getting the patient back into his or her "envelope of function," as Dye so aptly puts it,[11] restoring homeostasis, and rehabilitating the quadriceps. In addition, there are those patients who have more severe abnormalities of this cluster of factors. Some will have unrelenting pain with or without cartilage degradation (either secondary chondromalacia or secondary patellofemoral osteoarthritis), and some will have recurrent dislocation of the patella. It is this group of patients that, after a trial of appropriate rehabilitation, will frequently need careful analysis of the six factors of patellofemoral dysplasia and appropriate surgical correction of the ones that can be corrected. Finally, patients with significant patellofemoral arthritis come to us with a history of pain extending back for only a few months. The explanation for this discrepancy lies in the large functional reserve of articular cartilage. Its major functions of reducing friction and cushioning subchondral bone from stress concentration continue almost unaffected until approximately 75% of its normal thickness has worn away.[34]

## 47.7 Summary

The philosophy of the patellofemoral joint presented here, focusing on the six possible abnormal factors affecting the normal function of this enigmatic joint, has addressed the areas of possible confusion in clinical practice. It has provided a framework and logical guidelines for successful diagnosis, treatment, and surgical correction of patellofemoral disorders. In addition, this philosophy has supplied a pathomechanical/pathopysiologic explanation for the primary symptoms of patellofemoral disorders, pain, and instability. While the environment of clinical private practice did not allow testing this theory using the currently fashionable levels of evidence, what better evidence-based medicine could there be than a successful orthopedic practice in one community in one hospital in one location focused on the patellofemoral joint for 35 years?

## References

1. Aglietti P, Insall JH, Cerulli G. Patellar pain and incongruence. I: measurements of incongruence. *Clin Orthop Relat Res*. 1983;122:217-224.
2. Beaconsfield T, Pintore E, Maffulli N, et al. Radiological measurements in patellofemoral disorders. A review. *Clin Orthop Relat Res*. 1994;308:18-28.
3. Berg EE, Mason SL, Lucas MJ. Patellar height ratios: a comparison of four measurement methods. *Am J Sports Med*. 1996;24:218-221.
4. Besier TF, Gold GE, Beaupre GS, et al. A modeling framework to estimate patellofemoral joint cartilage stress in vivo. *Med Sci Sports Exerc*. 2005;37:1924-1930.
5. Bose K, Kanagasuntheram R, Osman MBH. Vastus medialis oblique: an anatomic and physiologic study. *Orthopedics*. 1980;3:880-883.
6. Brattstrom H. Shape of the intercondylar groove normally and in recurrent dislocation of the patella: a clinical and x-ray anatomical investigation. *Acta Orthop Scand*. 1964;68(suppl):1-147.
7. Davies AP, Costa ML, Donnell ST, et al. The sulcus angle and malalignment of the extensor mechanism of the knee. *J Bone Joint Surg Br*. 2000;82:1162-1166.
8. Dehaven KE, Dolan WA, Mayer PJ. Chondromalacia patellae in athletes. *Am J Sports Med*. 1979;7:5-11.
9. Dejour H, Neyret P, Walch G. Factors in patellar instability. In: Aichroth PM, Cannon WD Jr, Patel DV, eds. *Knee Surgery: Current Practice*. London: Martin Dunitz Limited; 1992.
10. Dye SF. An evolutionary perspective of the knee. *J Bone Joint Surg Am*. 1987;69:976-983.
11. Dye SF. The knee as a biologic transmission with an envelope of function: a theory. *Clin Orthop Relat Res*. 1996;325: 10-18.
12. Fulkerson JP, Tennet R, Jaivin JS, et al. Histologic evidence of retinacular nerve injury associated with patellofemoral alignment. *Clin Orthop Relat Res*. 1985;197:196-205.
13. Grelsamer RP, Dubey A, Weinstein CH. Men and women have similar Q angles: a clinical and trigonometric evaluation. *J Bone Joint Surg Br*. 2005;87:1498-1501.
14. Hauser EW. Total tendon transplant for slipping patella. *Surg Gynecol Obstet*. 1938;66:199-203.
15. Heiple KG, Lovejoy CO. The distal femoral anatomy of Australopithecus. *Am J Phys Anthropol*. 1971;35:75-84.
16. Jan MH, Lin DH, Lin JJ, et al. Differences in sonographic characteristics of the vastus medialis obliquus between patients with patellofemoral pain syndrome and healthy adults. *Am J Sports Med*. 2009;37:1743-1749.
17. Jones RB, Bartlett EC, Vainright JR, et al. CT determination of tibial tubercle lateralization in patients presenting with anterior knee pain. *Skeletal Radiol*. 1995; 24:505-509.
18. Kempson GE. Mechanical properties of articular cartilage. In: Freeman MAR, ed. *Adult Articular Cartilage*. 2nd ed. Kent: Pitman Medical Publishing; 1979.
19. Lin YF, Lin JJ, Jan MH, et al. Role of the vastus medialis obliquus in repositioning the patella: a dynamic computed tomography study. *Am J Sports Med*. 2008;36:741-746.
20. Lovejoy CO. The natural history of human gait and posture. Part 3. The knee. *Gait Posture*. 2007;25:325-341.
21. Lovejoy CO. Personal communication. 2009.
22. Merchant AC. Classification of patellofemoral disorders. *Arthroscopy*. 1988;4:235-240.
23. Merchant AC. Patellofemoral disorders: biomechanics, diagnosis, and non-operative treatment. In: McGinty JB, Casperi RB, Jackson RW, Poehling GG, eds. *Operative Arthroscopy*. New York: Raven; 1991.
24. Merchant AC. Patellofemoral joint disorders. In: Chapman MW, ed. *Chapman's Orthopaedic Surgery*. 3rd ed. Philadelphia: Lippincott Williams & Wilkins; 2001.
25. Merchant AC, Mercer RL. Lateral release of the patella: a preliminary report. *Clin Orthop Relat Res*. 1974;103: 40-45.
26. Merchant AC, Mercer RL, Jacobsen RH, et al. Roentgenographic analysis of patellofemoral congruence. *J Bone Joint Surg Am*. 1974;56:1391-1396.
27. Metin-Cubuk S, Sindel M, Karaali K, et al. Tibial tubercle position and patellar height as indicators of malalignment in women with anterior knee pain. *Clin Anat*. 2000;13: 199-203.

28. Miyanishi K, Nagamine R, Murayama S, et al. Tibial tubercle malposition in patellar joint instability: a computed tomography study in full extension and at 30 degree flexion. *Acta Orthop Scand.* 2000;71:286-291.
29. Muneta T, Yamamoto H, Ishibashi T, et al. Computerized tomographic analysis of tibial tubercle position in the painful female patellofemoral joint. *Am J Sports Med.* 1994;22:67-71.
30. Post WR. Clinical evaluation of patients with patellofemoral disorders. *Arthroscopy.* 1999;15:841-851.
31. Senavongse W, Amis AA. The effects of articular, retinacular, or muscular deficiencies on patellofemoral joint stability. *J Bone Joint Surg Br.* 2005;87:577-582.
32. Smith RL, Carter DR, Schurman DJ. Pressure and shear differentially alter human articular chondrocyte metabolism. *Clin Orthop Relat Res.* 2004;427S:S89-S95.
33. Tsujimoto K, Kurosaka M, Yoshiya S, et al. Radiographic and computed tomographic analysis of the position of the tibial tubercle in recurrent dislocation and subluxation of the patella. *Am J Knee Surg.* 2000;13:83-88.
34. Weightman B, Kempson GE. Load carriage. In: Freeman MAR, ed. *Adult Articular Cartilage.* 2nd ed. Kent: Pitman Medical Publishing; 1979.
35. Wittstein JR, Bartlett EC, Easterbrook J, et al. Magnetic resonance imaging evaluation of patellofemoral malalignment. *Arthroscopy.* 2006;22:643-649.

# Epilogue

As this work is published, at the beginning of the twenty first century, a new perspective of the classic orthopedic enigma of the patellofemoral pain problem is becoming increasingly accepted. It is clear that the decades-old paradigm of a pure structural and biomechanical explanation for the genesis of patellofemoral pain is inadequate, and that a new era has begun with biological factors now being given more consideration. A variable mosaic of pathophysiologic events (often due to simple overload) such as patellofemoral synovitis, retinacular neuromas, patellar tendonitis, and painful increased osseous remodeling of the patellofemoral joint – processes when taken together can be characterized by the term "loss of tissue homeostasis" – can be seen as providing new and alternative explanations for the conundrum of anterior knee pain. It clinically matters little what structural factors may be present in a given joint (such as chondromalacia, patellar tilt, or a Q angle above a certain value) if the pain-free condition of tissue homeostasis is achieved and maintained. Despite recent conceptual advances – represented by this newer biological perspective – much remains to be discovered regarding the patellofemoral joint before it can be said to be fully understood.

Better methods of determining dynamic patellofemoral joint reaction forces and kinematics need to be developed utilizing perhaps cine-CT or cine-MRI. Actual in vivo measurements are still required, particularly under real-time loading conditions to calibrate any noninvasive external assessment system that may be devised. Methods of geographically manifesting the homeostasis characteristics of all tissues, including soft tissues, need to be developed perhaps with techniques such as fMRI or CT-PET, which could help objectively evaluate the effectiveness of a variety of current and future nonoperative and operative therapies. I envision a day when this information may be displayed in a dynamic three-dimensional hologram with the structural and tissue homeostasis characteristics of the patellofemoral joint being represented by different colors and intensities.

Before advanced imaging techniques can be properly interpreted, further work on the histopathology associated with the genesis of patellofemoral pain needs to be accomplished, such as that currently being carried out by Sanchis-Alfonso. Simple tools that may be helpful to the clinician in assessing a joint's degree of homeostasis, such as the accurate determination of surface temperature through inexpensive hand-held devices, could be developed and calibrated. New methods of treatment aimed at addressing the pathophysiology of loss of tissue homeostasis, which may seem unorthodox from today's perspective, such as the use of the hormone calcitonin in patients with painful increased osseous metabolic activity manifested by an intensely positive bone scan, may in time prove useful – whereas the ill-considered and indiscriminate use of the lateral retinacular release, may not.

Those of us with a specific interest in the research of the patellofemoral joint also face general problems common to all musculoskeletal systems including discovering the factors that result in the induction, persistence, and eventual resolution of muscle atrophy. Subtle but important neuromuscular mechanisms such as the proprioceptive, spinal, and cerebellar systems that determine to a great degree the adaptive temporal sequencing of motor unit contractions, could be better understood and ultimately controlled for therapeutic benefit.

V. Sanchis-Alfonso (ed.), *Anterior Knee Pain and Patellar Instability*,
DOI: 10.1007/978-0-85729-507-1, © Springer-Verlag London Limited 2011

Other mysteries of the patellofemoral joint remain to be answered including, determining why some patients may indefinitely remain asymptomatic despite obvious radiographically identifiable structural abnormalities such as advanced chondromalacia, substantial malalignment, and even established degenerative arthrosis. When the patellofemoral joint is eventually understood in greater depth, the insights discovered should be generally applicable to other subdisciplines within the field of orthopedic surgery and musculoskeletal medicine as well.

Scott F. Dye M.D.
Associate Clinical Professor of Orthopaedic Surgery
University of California, San Francisco
CA, USA

# Index



V. Sanchis-Alfonso (ed.), *Anterior Knee Pain and Patellar Instability*,
DOI: 10.1007/978-0-85729-507-1, © Springer-Verlag London Limited 2011

FSC
www.fsc.org
MIX
Papier | Fördert
gute Waldnutzung
FSC® C083411

Kolibri 360 GmbH
Ferdinand-Jühlke-Straße 7
99095 Erfurt, Deutschland
produktsicherheit@kolibri360.de